# Hand, Elbow & Shoulder: Core Knowledge in Orthopaedics

# Hand, Elbow & Shoulder: Core Knowledge in Orthopaedics

## Thomas E. Trumble, MD
Professor and Chief
Hand and Upper Extremity Surgery Service
Department of Orthopaedics
University of Washington School of Medicine
Seattle, WA

## Jeffrey E. Budoff, MD
Assistant Professor
Hand and Upper Extremity Institute
Department of Orthopaedic Surgery
Baylor College of Medicine
Houston Veterans Affairs Medical Center
Houston, TX

## Roger Cornwall, MD
Pediatric Hand and Upper Extremity Surgeon
The Children's Hospital of Philadelphia
Assistant Professor of Orthopaedic Surgery
University of Pennsylvania School of Medicine
Philadelphia, PA

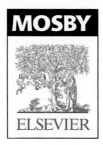

MOSBY

ELSEVIER

# MOSBY
# ELSEVIER

1600 John F. Kennedy Blvd.
Ste 1800
Philadelphia, PA 19103-2899

HAND, ELBOW & SHOULDER: CORE KNOWLEDGE IN ORTHOPAEDICS        ISBN-13: 978-0-323-02769-4
**Copyright © 2006, Mosby, Inc. All rights reserved.**        ISBN-10: 0-323-02769-5

Permissions may be sought directly from Elsevier's Health Sciences Rights Department in Philadelphia, PA, USA: phone: (+1) 215 239 3804, fax: (+1) 215 239 3805, e-mail: healthpermissions@elsevier.com. You may also complete your request on-line via the Elsevier homepage (http://www.elsevier.com), by selecting 'Customer Support' and then 'Obtaining Permissions'.

---

### Notice

Knowledge and best practice in this field are constantly changing. As new research and experience broaden our knowledge, changes in practice, treatment and drug therapy may become necessary or appropriate. Readers are advised to check the most current information provided (i) on procedures featured or (ii) by the manufacturer of each product to be administered, to verify the recommended dose or formula, the method and duration of administration, and contraindications. It is the responsibility of the practitioner, relying on their own experience and knowledge of the patient, to make diagnoses, to determine dosages and the best treatment for each individual patient, and to take all appropriate safety precautions. To the fullest extent of the law, neither the Publisher nor the Editors assume any liability for any injury and/or damage to persons or property arising out or related to any use of the material contained in this book.

---

**Library of Congress Cataloging-in-Publication Data**

Trumble, Thomas.
   Hand, elbow, and shoulder: core knowledge in orthopaedics/Thomas E. Trumble, Jeffrey E. Budoff, Roger Cornwall.
      p. cm.
   ISBN-13: 978-0-323-02769-4        ISBN-10: 0-323-02769-5
   1. Hand–Wounds and injuries. 2. Elbow–Wounds and injuries. 3. Shoulder–Wounds and injuries. 4. Orthopedics. I. Budoff, Jeffrey E. II. Cornwall, Roger. III. Title.
RD776.T78 2006
617.5'7044–dc22                                        2005041524

*Acquisitions Editor:* Kim Murphy
*Developmental Editor:* Anne Snyder
*Project Manager:* David Saltzberg
*Design Direction:* Gene Harris

Printed in China

Last digit is the print number:   9  8  7  6  5  4  3  2

Working together to grow
libraries in developing countries
www.elsevier.com | www.bookaid.org | www.sabre.org

ELSEVIER | BOOK AID International | Sabre Foundation

# Contributors

**BRIAN D. ADAMS, MD**
Professor of Orthopaedic Surgery and Biomedical Engineering, Department of Orthopaedic Surgery and Biomedical Engineering, University of Iowa, Iowa City, IA

**CHRISTOPHER ALLAN, MD**
Assistant Professor, Hand and Microvascular Surgery, Department of Orthopaedics, University of Washington; Attending, Harborview Medical Center, Department of Orthopaedics, Seattle, WA

**MARK E. BARATZ, MD**
Professor of Orthopedics, Drexel University School of Medicine, Philadelphia, PA; Vice Chairman, Department of Orthopaedic Surgery; Director, Division of Hand and Upper Extremities, Allegheny General Hospital, Pittsburgh, PA

**DAVID P. BAREI, MD, FRCSC**
Assistant Professor, Department of Orthopaedics and Sports Medicine, University of Washington, Harborview Medical Center, Seattle, WA

**PHILIP E. BLAZAR, MD**
Assistant Professor, Department of Orthopaedics, Harvard Medical School; Brigham and Women's Hospital, Boston, MA

**JEFFREY E. BUDOFF, MD**
Assistant Professor, Hand and Upper Extremity Institute, Department of Orthopaedic Surgery, Baylor College of Medicine; Houston Veterans Affairs Medical Center, Houston, TX

**DAVID T.W. CHIU, MD**
Professor of Plastic Surgery, New York University; Senior Attending, Director of New York Nerve Center, New York University Medical Center; Institute of Reconstructive Plastic Surgery, New York, NY

**MIHYE CHOI, MD**
Assistant Professor of Surgery, New York University School of Medicine; Attending Physician, New York Medical Center, New York, NY

**LORETTA COADY, MD**
Hand Fellow, SUNY at Buffalo School of Biomedical Science, Buffalo, NY

**MARK S. COHEN, MD**
Professor, Department of Orthopaedic Surgery; Director, Hand and Elbow Section; Director, Orthopaedic Education, Department of Orthopaedic Surgery, Rush University Medical Center, Chicago, IL

**EVAN D. COLLINS, MD**
Department of Orthopaedic Surgery, Baylor College of Medicine, Houston, TX

**ROGER CORNWALL, MD**
Pediatric Hand and Upper Extremity Surgeon, The Children's Hospital of Philadelphia; Assistant Professor of Orthopaedic Surgery, University of Pennsylvania School of Medicine, Philadelphia, PA

**PHANI K. DANTULURI, MD**
Clinical Instructor, Department of Orthopaedic Surgery, Thomas Jefferson University, Jefferson Medical College, Philadelphia, PA

**NICKOLAOS A. DARLIS, MD, PhD**
Fellow, Upper Extremity Surgery, Department of Orthopaedic Surgery, Allegheny General Hospital, Pittsburgh, PA

**LEE DELLON, MD**
Professor, Plastic Surgery and Neurosurgery, Johns Hopkins University, Baltimore, MD; Clinical Professor of Plastic Surgery, Neurosurgery and Anatomy, University of Arizona, Tucson, AZ

**LEIGH S. FRENCH, MSPT**
Medical College of Virginia/Virginia Commonwealth, Physical Therapy; Staff Physical Therapist, Bethesda Hand Rehabilitation, Cincinnati, OH

**PAMELA E. GLENNON, MD**
Hand Surgery Fellow, Department of Orthopaedic Surgery, University of Iowa, Iowa City, IA

**STEVEN H. GOLDBERG, MD**
Chief Resident, Department of Orthopaedic Surgery, Rush University Medical Center, Chicago, IL

**STEPHEN M. HANKINS, MD**
Hand Surgery Fellow, Jefferson Medical College of Thomas Jefferson University, Philadelphia, PA

**EMILY ANNE HATTWICK, MD, MPH**
Attending Hand Surgeon, Department of Orthopedics, Children's Hospital National Medical Center, Washington, DC

**MICHAEL R. HAUSMAN, MD**
Department of Orthopaedics, Mount Sinai School of Medicine, New York, NY

**JAMES P. HIGGINS, MD**
Teaching Faculty, Department of Plastic Surgery, Johns Hopkins University School of Medicine; Attending Hand Surgeon, The Curtis National Hand Center, Department of Orthopaedic Surgery, Union Memorial Hospital, Baltimore, MD

**JOSEPH A. IZZI, JR., MD**
St. Joseph's Health Service of Rhode Island, North Providence, RI; Roger Williams Medical Center, Providence, RI; Former Fellow, The Hospital for Special Surgery, Weill Medical College of Cornell University, New York, NY

**PETER J.L. JEBSON, MD**
Associate Professor, Chief Orthopaedic Hand Service, Department of Orthopaedic Surgery, University of Michigan Medical Center, Ann Arbor, MI

**JOHN A. JIULIANO, MD, MS, BS**
Fellow, Department of Hand and Upper Extremity, Massachussetts General Hospital, Boston, MA; Staff Orthopaedic Surgeon, Washington Hospital Healthcare System, Fremont, CA

**JESSE JUPITER, MD**
Hansjörg Wyss/AD Professor, Harvard Medical School; Director, Orthopaedic Hand Surgery, Massachusetts General Hospital, Boston, MA

**LEONID I. KATOLIK, MD**
Assistant Professor, Department of Orthopaedic Surgery, University of Washington, Seattle, WA

**MICHAEL W. KEITH, MD**
Professor of Orthopedics and Biomedical Engineering, Case Western Reserve University; Chief, Hand Service, Metrohealth Medical Center, Cleveland, OH

**VICTORIA D. KNOLL, MD**
Associated Orthopaedics and Sports Medicine, Plano, TX

**SCOTT H. KOZIN, MD**
Associate Professor, Department of Orthopaedic Surgery, Temple University School of Medicine; Hand and Upper Extremity Surgeon, Shriner's Hospital for Children, Philadelphia, PA

**LISA L. LATTANZA, MD**
Assistant Professor, Chief, Elbow Recontructive Surgery, Department of Orthopaedic Surgery, University of California-San Francisco; Consultant, Shriner's Hospital, Northern California, San Francisco, CA

**MICHAEL E. LEIT, MD, MS**
Clinical Assistant Professor of Orthopaedic Surgery, University of Rochester School of Medicine, Rochester, NY; Assistant Professor of Surgery, Uniformed Services University, Bethesda, MD; Attending, University of Rochester Medical Center, Rochester, NY; Chief Orthopaedic Surgeon, Lakeside Memorial Hospital, Brockport, NY

**JOHN D. LUBAHN, MD**
Chairman, Department of Orthopaedic Surgery, Hamot Medical Center, Erie, PA

**DAVID P. MAGIT, MD**
Clinical Instructor, Department of Orthopaedics and Rehabilitation, Yale University School of Medicine, New Haven, CT

**ANDREW D. MARKIEWITZ, MD, BS**
Assistant Professor, Department of Surgery, Uniformed Services University of the Health Sciences, Bethesda, MD; Volunteer Staff Associate Professor, University of Cincinnati; Hand Surgery Specialists, Inc., Cincinnati, OH

**ALEXANDER D. MIH, MD**
Associate Professor, Department of Orthopaedic Surgery, Indiana University School of Medicine; The Indiana Hand Center, Indianapolis, IN

**STEVEN L. MORAN, MD**
Assistant Professor of Plastic Surgery, Mayo Clinic College of Medicine; Consultant, Department of Orthopedic Surgery and Division of Plastic Surgery, Mayo Clinic, Rochester, MN

**DAVID P. MOSS, MD, BA**
Senior Resident, Department of Orthopaedic Surgery, New York University School of Medicine, Hospital for Joint Diseases, New York, NY

**OWEN J. MOY, MD**
Clinical Professor, Orthopaedic Surgery, State University of New York School of Biomedical Sciences at Buffalo; Director, Hand Fellowship Program, Hand Center of Western New York, Buffalo, NY

**MICHAEL S. MURPHY, MD**
Department of Orthopaedic Surgery, Johns Hopkins University School of Medicine; Attending Hand Surgeon, Department of Orthopaedic Surgery, The Curtis National Hand Center, Union Memorial Hospital, Baltimore, MD

**PETER M. MURRAY, MD**
Associate Professor, Department of Orthopaedic Surgery, Division of Hand and Microvascular Surgery, Mayo Clinic Graduate School of Medicine, Rochester, MN; Consultant, Department of Orthopaedic Surgery, Division of Hand and Microvascular Surgery, Mayo Clinic, Jacksonville, FL

**DOUGLAS MUSGRAVE, MD**
Fellow, Upper Extremity Surgery, Allegheny General Hospital, Pittsburgh, PA

**ARSHAD MUZAFFAR, MD**
Assistant Professor, Department of Plastic Surgery, University of Washington; Attending Physician, Department of Plastic Surgery, Children's Hospital and Regional Medical Center, Seattle, WA

**ROBERT P. NIRSCHL, MD, MS**
Associate Clinical Professor, Department of Orthopaedic Surgery, Georgetown University Medical Center, Washington, DC; Director, Orthopaedic Sports Medicine Fellowship Program, Nirschl Orthopaedic Center for Sports Medicine and Joint Reconstruction, Virginia Hospital Center, Arlington, VA

**MATTHEW J. NOFZIGER, MD**
Orthopaedic Surgeon, Southwestern Vermont Medical Center, Taconic Orthopaedics, Bennington, VT

**SEAN E. NORK, MD**
Associate Professor, Department of Orthopaedics and Sports Medicine, University of Washington, Harborview Medical Center, Seattle, WA

**ANASTASIOS PAPADONIKOLAKIS, MD**
Resident, Department of Orthopaedic Surgery, Wake Forest University School of Medicine, Winston-Salem, NC

**KEITH B. RASKIN, MD**
Clinical Associate Professor of Orthopaedic Surgery, New York University School of Medicine; Former Chief of Hand Surgery, New York University Medical Center, New York, NY

**MARK REKANT, MD**
Philadelphia Hand Center, Philadelphia, PA

**DAVID RING, MD**
Instructor of Orthopaedics, Harvard Medical School; Director of Research, Department of Orthopaedic Surgery, Hand and Upper Extremity Unit, Massachusetts General Hospital, Boston, MA

**DAVID S. RUCH, MD**
Professor, Department of Orthopaedic Surgery, Wake Forest University School of Medicine, Winston-Salem, NC

**IOANNIS SARRIS, MD, PhD**
Fellow, Upper Extremity Surgery, Department of Orthopaedic Surgery, Allegheny General Hospital, Pittsburgh, PA

**JAMES M. SAVUNDRA, MBBS, FRACS**
Consultant Plastic Surgeon, Royal Perth Hospital, Perth, Australia; Consultant Plastic Surgeon, Fremantle Hospital, Fremantle, Australia

**KHEMARIN R. SENG, MD**
Resident, Department of Orthopaedic Surgery, Massachusetts General Hospital, Boston, MA

**ANTHONY M. SESTERO, MD**
Orthopaedic and Hand Surgeon, Northwest Orthopaedic Specialists, P.S., Spokane, WA

**AJAY K. SETH, MD**
Spectrum Orthopedics, Canton, OH

**JOSEPH E. SHEPPARD, MD**
Department of Orthopaedic Surgery, University of Arizona Health Sciences Center, Tucson, AZ

**ALEXANDER Y. SHIN, MD**
Associate Professor of Orthopedic Surgery, Mayo Clinic College of Medicine; Consultant, Department of Orthopedic Surgery, Mayo Clinic, Rochester, MN

**JOSEPH F. SLADE III, MD**
Associate Professor and Director, Hand and Upper Extremity Service, Department of Orthopaedics and Rehabilitation, Yale University School of Medicine, Guilford, CT

**DEAN G. SOTEREANOS, MD**
Professor, Orthopaedic Surgery, Drexel University School of Medicine, Philadelphia, PA; Vice Chairman, Department of Orthopaedic Surgery, Allegheny General Hospital, Pittsburgh, PA

**PETER J. STERN, MD**
Director and Chairman, Norman S. and Elizabeth C.A. Hill Professor of Orthopaedic Surgery, Department of Orthopaedic Surgery, University of Cincinnati College of Medicine; University of Cincinnati, Cincinnati, OH

**DANIEL N. SWITLICK, MD**
Department of Orthopaedic Surgery, University of Arizona Health Sciences Center, Tucson, AZ

**LISA A. TAITSMAN, MD, MPH**
Assistant Professor, Department of Orthopaedics and Sports Medicine, University of Washington; Attending Surgeon, Department of Orthopaedics, Harborview Medical Center, Seattle, WA

**JOHN S. TARAS, MD**
Associate Professor, Drexel University; Chief, Division of Hand Surgery, Thomas Jefferson University Hospital, Philadelphia, PA

**Matthew M. Tomaino, MD, MBA**
Professor of Orthopaedic Surgery, University of Rochester School of Medicine; Chief, Division of Hand and Upper Extremity Surgery, University of Rochester Medical Center, Rochester, NY

**Thomas E. Trumble, MD**
Professor and Chief, Hand and Upper Extremity Surgery Service, Department of Orthopaedics, University of Washington School of Medicine, Seattle, WA

**Christopher J. Veneziano, MD**
Orthopaedic Sports Medicine Fellow, Georgetown University Medical Center, Washington, DC; Orthopaedic Sports Medicine Fellow, Nirschl Orthopaedic Center for Sports Medicine and Joint Reconstruction, Virginia Hospital Center, Arlington, VA

**Peter M. Waters, MD**
Associate Professor, Department of Orthopaedic Surgery, Harvard Medical School; Associate Chief, Department of Orthopaedic Surgery, Children's Hospital; Director, Hand and Upper Extremity Surgery, Children's Hospital, Boston, MA

# Contents

# Preface

The driving force of this text, *Hand, Elbow & Shoulder: Core Knowledge in Orthopaedics,* was to combine the best knowledge about the entire upper extremity, from the fingertips to the shoulder, into a single volume. The editors and authors view the upper extremity as an integrated system that enables the person do everything from throwing a baseball to drawing a picture. My co-editors, Jeff Budoff and Roger Cornwall, were instrumental in forging a clean, cutting-edge text in a well-organized style that provides a ready resource for surgeons preparing for surgery, board examinations, and lectures. We owe a huge debt to our chapter authors who are not only experts on the topic but also exciting innovators in this field. Many surgery texts have whole catalogs of surgical procedures without a single discussion on the biology, whereas research journals contain basic science reports without surgical application. Very few texts merge the core knowledge with the best surgical methods in a well-illustrated text. Our goal has been to bring the best practical material to help attending surgeons, fellows, residents, therapists, and students. We wanted to make a single-volume text that would be portable and functional. We would like to see the text used and abused in operating rooms and clinics. The editors and authors wanted to speak to the working clinicians with a text that would not only benefit their practice but also serve as an educational tool for resident education and board preparation with critical core knowledge. The table of contents is designed to follow the Residency Review Committee requirements for orthopaedic surgery, plastic surgery, and fellowships related to hand, elbow, and shoulder surgery. At the heart of this work, the authors and editors wanted to share their passion for caring for patients and improving the services that are provided. We love the fact that our practice allows us to examine and treat patients in a hands-on way. We hold patients in our hands as we test for stability, sensation, strength, and other necessary abilities. We partner with our patients while designing their rehabilitation programs. We look forward to a bright future in a field that has so much to offer patients—from minimally invasive surgery to joint replacement—with many tremendous innovations. Each text of this nature continues to be a work in progress. We welcome your thoughts on improvements for future editions.

Best Regards,

Thomas E. Trumble, MD
Editor

# Acknowledgments

As the editor of such a fantastic text combining core knowledge with cutting-edge techniques, I would like to recognize my co-editors and authors who burned the late night oil to craft such a beautiful and finely honed educational tool. Our artist, Barney Chiu, worked against impossible deadlines to produce a text that stands out as one of the best illustrated in all of surgery. The editorial staff at Elsevier was remarkable at every stage of publication. For my own part, I remain indebted to:

Wayne O. Southwick, MD, and Richard J. Smith, MD, who taught me that knowledge is the eternal torch that we pass on to the next generation;

Dorothy and Earl Trumble, who taught me that if you mold your gift with compassion it will never be forgotten;

My staff, Lenore Provan and Josette Morton, who often boss me as much as I boss them and who show me that the difference we make as a team produces the best of all possible gifts.

We would also like to acknowledge the editorial assistance of the following individuals, Chad Moloney, PA-C; Magee Saewert, PA-C; Brian Miller, MD; and William Montgomery, MD.

And last but not least, my wife, Maureen, and my daughters, Stacey, Kelley, and Kristin, who have never questioned me when I stayed up through another night to write a book that would help surgeons when the unpredictable happens at the worst possible hour.

We know what it is like to struggle in the middle of the night to save a child's hand or to stabilize the impossible fracture. When you, the surgeon or the therapist, think that no one else feels your frustration or pain, call us and we will try to help any time (1-206-731-3000).

Thomas E. Trumble, MD
trumble@u.washington.edu

# Anatomy and Physical Examination of the Hand

Joseph A. Izzi, Jr.,[*] and Thomas E. Trumble[†]

[*]MD, St. Joseph's Health Service of Rhode Island, North Providence, RI; Roger Williams
Medical Center, Providence, RI; Former Fellow, The Hospital for Special Surgery, Weill
Medical College of Cornell University, New York, NY
[†]MD, Professor and Chief, Hand and Upper Extremity Surgery Service,
Department of Orthopaedics, University of Washington School of Medicine, Seattle, WA

## Introduction

### General Information

- The goal of any type of treatment of the hand is to restore function not only to the affected area but also to the whole upper extremity. Whether obtained for the acutely traumatized hand or the smallest most chronic condition, an accurate and complete history and physical examination are paramount to a successful outcome.
- The history should include information regarding the patient's age, occupation, hand dominance, and recreational activities. Although all of these data are routinely obtained in a standard orthopaedic history and physical examination, there are several important aspects of which the physician should be cognizant. For example, an injury that could be detrimental to something as simple as small finger abduction could severely compromise the capabilities of someone who plays the piano.
- The patient's past medical history is important. A history of diabetes mellitus can cause difficulties in the diagnosis of a compressive neuropathy and/or complicate wound healing in the surgical patient. One also must be aware of conditions in the upper extremity that exist concomitantly with the presenting problem. Does the patient with a hand problem have a prior history of shoulder or elbow problems? Every examination of the hand should begin at the shoulder, especially in patients who had long periods of

disuse or who protected the hand with a sling. The skin, nerves, tendons, muscles, bones, and joints should be thoroughly examined. The size of the muscles is indicative of the amount of use of the hand, and the presence and/or amount of atrophy are indicative of a pathologic processes.

## Nontraumatic Hand Conditions

- A hand with a disability of gradual onset and without any specific traumatic incident often presents a difficult diagnostic problem. In the nontraumatized patient, determine the chief complaint. Is the primary problem pain, stiffness, numbness, snapping, a painless mass, or a combination of these signs? When did the symptoms begin, what makes them better and worse, and have they been progressive? Are there associated problems at night, such as pain or numbness, and do these problems cause the patient to wake up or prevent sleep? Is the patient's function worse in the morning and improve throughout the day, or is there a constant problem? Knowing underlying medical conditions, such as gout, rheumatoid arthritis, or generalized osteoarthritis, can help in making the diagnosis and formulating a treatment strategy. A thorough history may reveal an unusual use of the hand that was a precipitating cause or the history of a degenerative process that reached a point where secondary injury occurred, as in an attritional tendon rupture.

## The Traumatized Hand

- Some fractures and dislocations are readily obvious because of gross deformity and swelling. One of the most common pitfalls in treating hand injuries is overlooking the damage to the soft tissue structures or an additional injury because of an obvious fracture or dislocation. The history in acute injuries should include the time of injury, preliminary treatment by emergency medical technicians or emergency department staff, medications given (especially tetanus and antibiotics if there are open wounds), mechanism of injury (crushing vs. sharp), setting of the injury (i.e., barnyard, kitchen), and whether the injury was work related.

## Physical Examination

- Observation of the resting hand should precede any physical examination. One should observe the attitude of the hand, posture of the digits, color of the skin, presence of atrophy (particularly of the thenar, hypothenar, and first dorsal interosseous regions), calluses, swelling, bruising, vascularity of all the digits, and prior scars. If swelling is present, is the cause trauma, obstruction of blood or lymphatic flow, a trophic condition resulting from injury to the nerves, vasomotor, or self-inflicted? The nails and nail folds should be inspected because they often show signs of undiagnosed systemic diseases, malnutrition, toxicity, and trauma. Additionally, an examination of the unaffected hand is helpful prior to an examination of the affected side. Always look for a second or third coexisting condition that may not be the primary complaint. For example, patients with arthritis of the carpometacarpal joint of the thumb can have coexisting carpal tunnel syndrome and the associated sequelae.

## Embryology and Development

- Although it is beyond the scope of this chapter to go into extensive detail about the embryology and development of the hand, there are several key periods of development to keep in mind. The limb bud generally forms during 4 weeks of gestation. By 33 days of gestation, the hand forms into a paddle without individual digits. Digital separation usually begins at 7 weeks and progresses over the course of week 7. The condensation that will give rise to each of the bones of the hand also occurs at week 7.
- Ossification of the carpal bones begins at the capitate and proceeds in a clockwise direction. Ossification of the capitate usually is present at age 1 year. The hamate is the second carpal bone to ossify at approximately 1 to 2 years, followed by the triquetrum at 3 years, the lunate at 4 to 5 years, the scaphoid at 5 years, the trapezium at 6 years, the trapezoid at 7 years, and the pisiform at 9 years.

## Terminology

- In true anatomic description, the palm is the anterior surface of the hand; however, this descriptive term is seldom used. The hand and digits have a dorsal surface, a palmar or volar surface, and radial and ulnar borders. The palm is subdivided into the thenar, midpalmar, and hypothenar areas. The thenar mass or eminence is the muscular area overlying the palmar surface of the thumb metacarpal. Atrophy of this muscle may be noted in pathologic conditions such as chronic carpal tunnel syndrome. The hypothenar musculature is located overlying the small finger metacarpal. The digits are referred to as the thumb, index finger, long (middle) finger, ring finger, and small finger. Each finger possesses three joints: the metacarpophalangeal (MCP) joint, the proximal interphalangeal (PIP) joint, and the distal interphalangeal (DIP) joint. The MCP joints of the fingers are located at a line drawn from the radial extent of the proximal palmar crease to the ulnar extent of the distal palmar crease. This is important to bear in mind when placing a splint or cast that requires flexion of the MCP joints. The level of the finger webs correlates to the middle third of the proximal phalanges. The thumb has an MCP joint and only one interphalangeal (IP) joint. The carpometacarpal (CMC) or basal joint of the thumb is a unique structure in the hand and is important for thumb mobility.

## Motion

- Active and passive measurements should be taken for each motion of the entire upper extremity, and any discrepancies noted. Pronation and supination of the forearm are measured with the elbow firmly at the side and at a right angle. In pathologic conditions, the amount of forearm rotation should be measured at the forearm because the radiocarpal joint may allow 10 to 20 degrees of motion without forearm rotation. Wrist motion is measured as degrees of dorsiflexion and palmar or volar flexion and radial or ulnar deviation. Ulnar deviation is determined by the angle between the midline of the forearm and the line from the center of the wrist to the third metacarpal. Radial deviation should be measured with the hand in the plane of the forearm because abnormal values can be obtained as the wrist goes into dorsiflexion. Finger motion is measured in degrees of maximal extension and degrees of maximal flexion. Hyperextension is documented as a negative number for calculations of total active motion (TAM) and total passive motion (TPM).
- Motion of the thumb has flexion and extension at the MCP and IP joints but becomes more complex when measuring motion of the CMC joint. Thumb CMC joint motions include palmar and radial abduction, opposition, and retropulsion (Figure 1–1). The thumb should be examined through the full range of circumduction, from

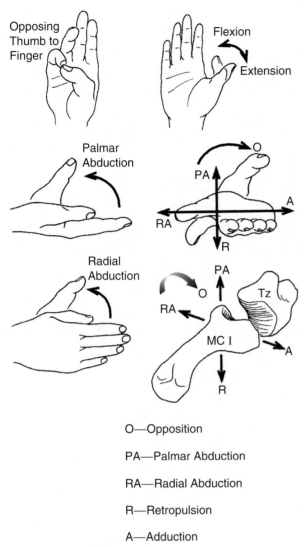

O—Opposition

PA—Palmar Abduction

RA—Radial Abduction

R—Retropulsion

A—Adduction

Figure 1–1:
**The biconcave surfaces of the thumb carpometacarpal joint allow thumb rotation, flexion/extension, and abduction/adduction.** *MCI,* Thumb metacarpal; *Tz,* trapezium. (From Trumble TE, editor: *Principles of hand surgery and therapy.* Philadelphia, 2000, WB Saunders Company.)

the back of the hand to opposition and to touch of the fifth metacarpal head. It also should be fully extended and fully flexed, and it should be able to make the OK sign with the index finger. Abduction of the thumb is measured by the angle between the first and second metacarpals with the thumb spread at right angles to the palm. Opposition is a combination of flexion, adduction, and pronation. Thumb adduction can be measured as the distance between the tip of the thumb and the head of the fifth metacarpal.

- By knowing the normal range of motion of these joints, one can quickly determine what the patient cannot do and where the disability may lie (Table 1–1). Examination of the contralateral limb is particularly important if the patient has hypermobility of the other joints.

| Table 1–1: | Approximate Normal Ranges of Motion |
| --- | --- |

**Elbow Range of Motion**
  Active range of motion
    Flexion: 135+ degrees
    Extension: 0 to −5 degrees
    Supination: 90 degrees
    Pronation: 90 degrees

**Wrist Range of Motion**
  Active range of motion
    Flexion: 80 degrees
    Extension: 70 degrees
    Ulnar deviation: 30 degrees
    Radial deviation: 20 degrees

**Finger Range of Motion**
  Metacarpophalangeal joint flexion and extension
    Flexion: 90 degrees
    Extension: 30–45 degrees
  Proximal interphalangeal joint flexion and extension
    Flexion: 100 degrees
    Extension: 0 degrees
  Distal interphalangeal joint flexion and extension
    Flexion: 90 degrees
    Extension: 20 degrees
  Finger abduction and adduction
    Abduction: 20 degrees
    Adduction: 0 degrees
  Thumb abduction and adduction
    Abduction (palmar abduction): 70 degrees
    Adduction (dorsal adduction): 0 degrees

# Hand and Forearm Anatomy
## Skin

- The skin on the volar aspect of the palm and fingers is tough and thick and possesses no hair follicles (glabrous). It covers a layer of fat with many fibrous septa that hold the skin firmly to the deeper tissues. The septa allow traction when gripping but necessitate a system of creases to prevent the skin from bunching as the hand is closed (Figure 1–2). The skin on the dorsal surface is thin, soft, and pliable, permitting motion of the joints. Because the veins are located dorsally, the dorsum of the hand is a common site for edema, which can limit flexion. The skin on the fingers is fixed to the bone by small ligaments along the radial and ulnar sides of the fingers. The ligaments dorsal to the neurovascular bundles are called *Cleland's ligaments* and those volar to the neurovascular bundles are called *Grayson's ligaments.*

## Nail Bed and Fingertip

- The nail bed complex, also called the *perionychium,* consists of the paronychium and the nail bed itself (Figure 1–3). Proximally the nail fits into a depression called the *nail fold.* The eponychium is the thin membrane that extends onto the dorsum of the nail. Just distal to the eponychium beneath the nail is the lunula, a

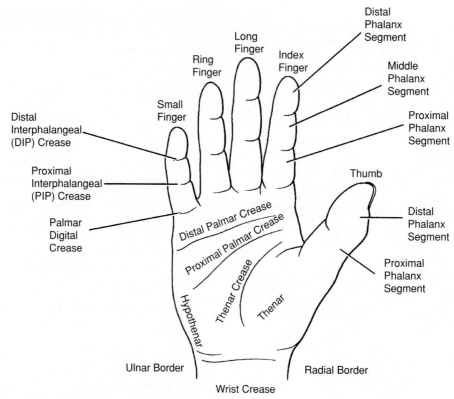

Figure 1–2:

**Surface anatomy of the palm. (From Trumble TE, editor: *Principles of hand surgery and therapy*. Philadelphia, 2000, WB Saunders Company.)**

curved white opacity at the junction of the proximal germinal and distal sterile matrixes on the nail floor. Bacterial infections (paronychia) of the nail most commonly involve the paronychium and can be diagnosed easily on physical examination.

- The fingertip is the area of the digit distal to the insertion of the flexor and extensor tendons on the distal phalanx. The tuft of the distal phalanx is covered by adipose tissue and highly innervated skin tethered to the distal phalanx by numerous fibrosepta. The tuft and the fibrosepta are implicated in infections of the pulp of the distal phalanx called a *felon*.

## Motor Units of the Hand and Wrist

- Motion of the hand and wrist is facilitated through the intrinsic and extrinsic motor units. The tendons and muscles originating proximal to the wrist are extrinsic and those that originate within the hand are intrinsic.

## Osseous Anatomy of the Hand and Wrist

- The radiocarpal joint is an ellipsoid joint composed of the distal radius and its two articular facets for the scaphoid and lunate, respectively. Between the radius and the ulna is the sigmoid notch of the radius, which allows an

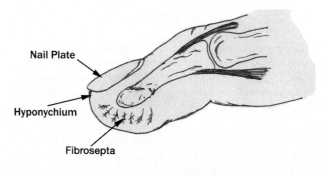

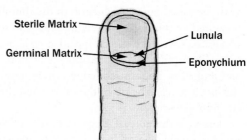

Figure 1–3:

**Dorsal and lateral views of the finger with the anatomy of the nail and nail bed complex. (Courtesy of Jason R. Izzi, D.M.D.)**

articulation with the distal ulna and 270 degrees of rotation. The ulnar styloid is the attachment of the triangular fibrocartilage complex. In the normal intact forearm with neutral ulnar variance and neutral rotation 80% of the forces are transmitted through the distal radius (50% across the scaphoid fossa and 30% across the lunate fossa) and 20% through the distal ulna. These numbers change with wrist and forearm motion and ulnar variance.

## Intercarpal Joints

- The proximal carpal row is composed of the scaphoid, lunate, and triquetrum. The pisiform is a sesamoid bone within the flexor carpi ulnaris (FCU) tendon that articulates with the triquetrum. This articulation can become a source of ulnar-sided wrist pain that is often overlooked. The joints of the proximal row are primarily gliding joints. The scaphoid bone is the link between the proximal and distal rows and is the reason why pathology originating from the scaphoid can cause problems with almost all of the articulations in the wrist. The distal carpal row is made up of the trapezium, trapezoid, capitate, and hamate. With the exception of the trapezium, the bones of the distal carpal row are strongly anchored by their attachments with the metacarpals.

## Metacarpals and Metacarpophalangeal Joints

- The MCP joints are condyloid joints and, unlike the IP joints, allow not only flexion and extension but also abduction and adduction of the proximal phalanx on the metacarpal head. The collateral ligaments of the MCP joints provide stability, where the volar plate prevents hyperextension. All of the volar plates are connected by the strong intermetacarpal ligaments, which help maintain longitudinal and rotational alignment in the case of many metacarpal fractures. Because of the camlike shape of the metacarpal head, the collateral ligaments are lax in extension and taut in flexion. When the MCP joints are included in a cast, they should be flexed to maintain the length of the ligaments, preventing permanent shortening and stiffness.
- Although index and long finger CMC joints are relatively immobile, there is 5 to 10 degrees of flexion at the ring finger CMC joint and 15 to 20 degrees of flexion of the small finger CMC joint. Because of their articulations with the distal hamate facets, the ring and small finger metacarpals rotate toward the middle of the palm with flexion to enhance gripping. However, because of the shape of the articulations with the hamate, subluxations and/or dislocations can occur easily in a fracture situation of the fourth and fifth metacarpal bases.

## Phalanges and Interphalangeal Joints

- The PIP and DIP joints are bicondylar ginglymus (hinge) joints where the collateral ligaments and the volar plate allow only flexion and extension (Figure 1–4).

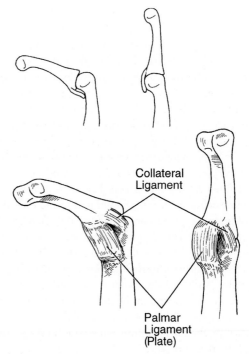

Figure 1–4:
**Anatomy of the palmar plate of the proximal interphalangeal joint. (From Trumble TE, editor: *Principles of hand surgery and therapy*. Philadelphia, 2000, WB Saunders Company.)**

## Metacarpophalangeal and Basal Joints of the Thumb

- The thumb MCP joint is much more complex than the MCP joints of the other digits. Its complexity is compounded by the presence of the sesamoid bones and the thenar musculature. At the ulnar side, a collateral ligament injury can become "complex" if the adductor aponeurosis becomes interposed between the torn ligament and its bony insertion. This forms a "Stener lesion," where the avulsed ligament end cannot heal back to the bone, requiring operative reduction and fixation.
- The basal joint or CMC joint of the thumb is a complex structure, which allows 360 degrees of motion. The thumb metacarpal articulates with the trapezium on biconcave saddle-shaped joints and the trapezium articulates with the scaphoid, trapezoid, and the radial facet of the index finger (see Figure 1–1). This joint is supported by the capsule and the radial, volar, and dorsal CMC ligaments. Perhaps one of the more important ligaments of the basal joint is the volar oblique or "beak" ligament, named for its attachment to the articular margin of the ulnar side of the metacarpal beak. Its origin is the palmar tubercle of the trapezium. The volar oblique ligament is implicated in pathologic conditions of the CMC joint, such as osteoarthritis.

## Ligaments of the Wrist

- The ligaments of the wrist are divided into three groups: the volar radiocarpal, the interosseous, and the dorsal intercapsular, although there is much diversity in the nomenclature of these ligaments. The volar wrist ligaments provide the majority of stability of the radiocarpal joint and maintenance of position of the individual carpal bones.[1] Although there are numerous intercarpal ligaments, the two most important are the scapholunate (SL) interosseous ligament and the lunotriquetral (LT) interosseous ligaments. Tearing of the SL interosseous ligament is implicated in the formation of dorsal intercalated segment instability (DISI), where the SL angle on the lateral radiograph is greater than 60 degrees. Usually, there is also an associated disruption of the volar radiocarpal ligament. Volar intercalated segment instability (VISI) usually results as a disruption of the LT interosseous ligament and the dorsal radiocarpal (DRC) and ulnocapitate (UC) ligaments. In DISI the lunate assumes an extended posture, whereas in VISI the lunate assumes a flexed posture.

- The volar radiocarpal ligaments include the radioscaphocapitate (RSC), long and short radiolunate (LRL and SRL), radioscapholunate (RSL) (ligament of Testut), ulnotriquetral (UT), UC, and ulnolunate (UL) (Figure 1–5). With some exceptions, most of these ligaments can be visualized during wrist arthroscopy. These ligaments are arranged in a double chevron pattern that allows them to adjust the carpal rotation and the ulnar and radial heights of the carpus during ulnar and radial deviation. Between the RSC and LRL ligaments is an area of potential weakness over the capitate-lunate articulation known as the *space of Poirier,* where the capitate can dislocate during a perilunate dislocation.

- The dorsal intercarpal (DIC) and DRC ligaments are important thickenings in the dorsal joint capsule (Figure 1–6). These structures provide important stabilization of the carpal bones. The DRC originates from the dorsal margin of the distal radius, and its radial fibers attach at the lunate and LT interosseous ligament before inserting on the dorsal tubercle of the triquetrum.[2] The DIC originates from the triquetrum and attaches onto the lunate before inserting into the dorsal groove of the scaphoid with extension of the insertion to the trapezium. Because of the importance of these ligaments, some authors recommend a ligament-sparing technique when performing a dorsal capsulotomy.

## Fibroosseous Tunnels of the Wrist

- On the palmar side of the wrist, the carpal tunnel and the Guyon's canal allow the tendons, nerves, and arteries to enter the hand. The bony pillars of the carpal tunnel are made up of the bony ridges of the trapezium and the scaphoid on the radial side and the hook of the hamate and the pisiform on the ulnar side. The roof of the carpal tunnel is the transverse carpal ligament. The contents of the carpal tunnel include the eight extrinsic flexor tendons to the fingers, the flexor pollicis longus (FPL), and the median nerve. The Guyon's canal is located ulnar to the carpal tunnel and contains the ulnar nerve and artery (Figure 1–7). The bony boundaries of the Guyon's canal are the pisiform and the hook of the hamate. The volar carpal ligament forms the roof of Guyon's canal.

## Innervation

- The sensation on the palmar aspect of the hand is provided by the median and ulnar nerves. On the dorsal aspect of the hand, the radial and ulnar nerves provide sensation. The ulnar nerve is the major motor innervation to the intrinsic

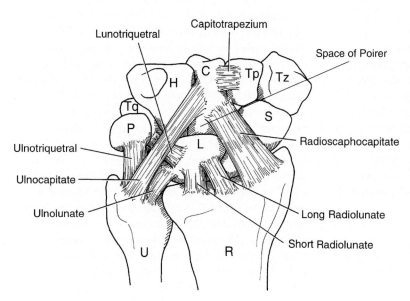

Lunotriquetral
Capitotrapezium
Space of Poirer
Ulnotriquetral
Ulnocapitate
Ulnolunate
Radioscaphocapitate
Long Radiolunate
Short Radiolunate

**Figure 1–5:**
Palmar extraarticular wrist ligaments. *C,* Capitate; *H,* Hamate; *L,* Lunate; *P,* Pisiform; *R,* Radius; *S,* Scaphoid; *Tp,* Trapezoid; *Tz,* Trapezium; *U,* Ulna. (From Trumble TE, editor: *Principles of hand surgery and therapy.* Philadelphia, 2000, WB Saunders Company.)

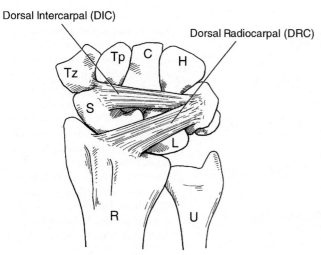

Dorsal Intercarpal (DIC)

Dorsal Radiocarpal (DRC)

Figure 1–6:
**Diagrammatic representation of the extraarticular dorsal wrist ligaments.** *C,* Capitate; *H,* Hamate; *L,* Lunate; *R,* Radius; *S,* Scaphoid; *Tp,* Trapezoid; *Tz,* Trapezium; *U,* Ulna. (From Trumble TE, editor: *Principles of hand surgery and therapy.* Philadelphia, 2000, WB Saunders Company.)

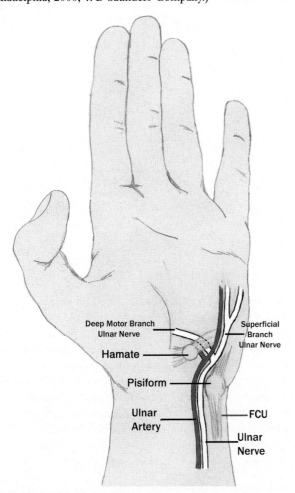

Deep Motor Branch
Ulnar Nerve

Superficial
Branch
Ulnar Nerve

Hamate

Pisiform

Ulnar
Artery

FCU

Ulnar
Nerve

Figure 1–7:
**Schematic representation of the Guyon's canal and its contents.** *FCU,* Flexor carpi ulnaris. (Courtesy of Jason R. Izzi, D.M.D.)

musculature of the hand, except for the muscles supplied by the motor branch of the median nerve.

## Extrinsic Tendons of the Wrist

- On the dorsal aspect of the wrist are six discrete compartments for the extrinsic extensor tendons (Figure 1–8). The compartments prevent bowstringing and provide reliable landmarks for surgical approaches. Additionally, each compartment can have its own unique pathologic process. On the volar aspect of the wrist, the tendons are not arranged as discretely.

### Anatomy of the Extrinsic Extensor Tendons

- Knowledge of the surface anatomy and location of the extensor tendons is crucial for understanding pathologic conditions of the tendons themselves. In addition, the extensor tendon compartments are important intervals for open surgical approaches to the wrist and forearm and for placement of arthroscopy portals.

#### First Dorsal Compartment

- The first dorsal compartment contains the abductor pollicis longus (APL) and the extensor pollicis brevis (EPB) tendons. These tendons represent the radial border of the anatomic snuffbox. As the thumb is brought into radial abduction, the individual tendons can be palpated as they exit distal to the retinaculum. Toward the insertion of these tendons on the thumb metacarpal, the EPB lies on the ulnar side of the APL. The APL can possess two to five separate tendon slips. In up to 60% of the population, there is a separate subcompartment for the EPB or one of the slips of the APL. If all of the compartments are not released during surgery for tenosynovitis, surgical failure may result. Tenosynovitis of the wrist is most commonly seen at the first dorsal compartment and is referred to as *de Quervain's disease.* The provocative maneuver for diagnosis of de Quervain's disease is the Finkelstein test. The Finkelstein test is performed by tucking the patient's thumb inside the closed fingers of a fist (Figure 1–9). The wrist then is brought into ulnar deviation as the forearm is stabilized. Sharp pain in the area of the first dorsal compartment is strong evidence for de Quervain's disease.
- *Pathologic Condition*—de Quervain's disease

#### Second Dorsal Compartment

- The second dorsal compartment is located on the radial side of the Lister's tubercle and contains the extensor carpi radialis longus (ECRL) and the extensor carpi radialis brevis (ECRB). The ECRL inserts on the base of the second metacarpal, and the ECRB inserts on the base of the third metacarpal. To examine the tendons, ask the patient to make a clenched fist. The tendons will be palpable on the radial side of the Lister's tubercle (Figure 1–10). The two tendons are powerful wrist

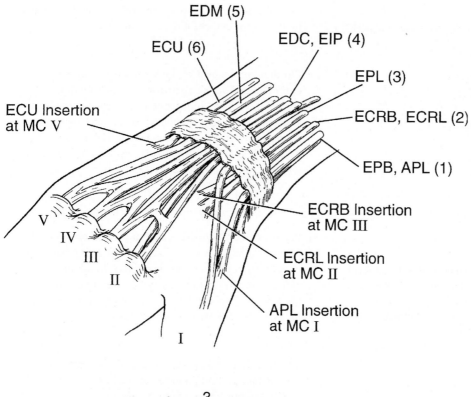

EDM (5)

ECU (6)

EDC, EIP (4)

EPL (3)

ECRB, ECRL (2)

ECU Insertion at MC V

EPB, APL (1)

ECRB Insertion at MC III

ECRL Insertion at MC II

APL Insertion at MC I

V
IV
III
II
I

Figure 1–8:
The six dorsal compartments of the extensor tendons. *APL,* Abductor pollicis longus; *ECRB,* extensor carpi radialis brevis; *ECRL,* extensor carpi radialis longus; *ECU,* extensor carpi ulnaris; *EDC,* extensor digitorum communis; *EDM,* extensor digiti minimi; *EIP,* extensor indicis proprius; *EPB,* extensor pollicis brevis; *EPL,* extensor pollicis longus; *MC,* metacarpal. (From Trumble TE, editor: *Principles of hand surgery and therapy.* Philadelphia, 2000, WB Saunders Company.)

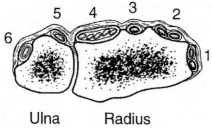

5  4  3  2

6

1

Ulna     Radius

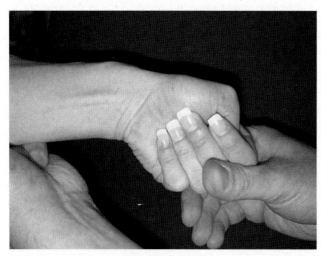

Figure 1–9:
**Clinical photograph of the Finkelstein's test.**

extensors that also cause radial deviation because of their insertions on the radial aspects of the metacarpal bases. However, the ECRB remains the primary location for transfer of a tendon to provide wrist extension because of its more central location causing less radial deviation. Intersection syndrome is tenosynovitis of the second dorsal compartment. Symptoms of intersection syndrome are pain and swelling where the APL and EPB tendons cross the ECRL and the ECRB, approximately 4 cm proximal to the wrist joint.

• *Pathologic Condition*—Intersection syndrome

## Third Dorsal Compartment

• The third dorsal compartment contains the extensor pollicis longus tendon (EPL) (Figure 1–11). The EPL tendon defines the ulnar border of the anatomic snuffbox.

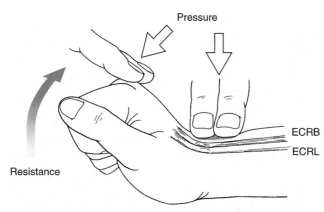

Figure 1–10:
The extensor carpi radialis longus *(ECRL)* and extensor carpi radialis brevis *(ECRB)* extend and radially deviate the wrist. (From Trumble TE, editor: *Principles of hand surgery and therapy.* Philadelphia, 2000, WB Saunders Company.)

At Lister's tubercle, the EPL tendon takes a 45-degree turn before attaching on the base of the distal phalanx of the thumb. Placing the patient's hand flat on a table and then asking the patient to lift only the thumb can allow evaluation of the EPL tendon. Pain and crepitus over the EPL tendon, especially at the Lister's tubercle, can represent impending rupture of the tendon, especially after a fracture of the distal radius. Another cause of attritional rupture of the EPL tendon is rheumatoid arthritis.

- *Pathologic Condition*—Attritional tendon rupture

## Fourth Dorsal Compartment

- The fourth dorsal compartment contains the extensor digitorum communis (EDC) and the extensor indicis proprius (EIP). The EDC inserts on the extensor hoods of all four fingers, and the EIP inserts on the ulnar aspect of the extensor tendon to the index. The ulnar location of the EIP is important for identifying the tendon for transfers. Additionally, the EIP allows full independent extension of the index finger, whereas the EDC provides combined extension of all four fingers (Figure 1–12). The juncturae tendineae are links that

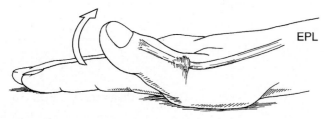

Figure 1–11:
The extensor pollicis longus *(EPL)* tendon extends the interphalangeal joint of the thumb and brings the thumb out of the plane of the palm. (From Trumble TE, editor: *Principles of hand surgery and therapy.* Philadelphia, 2000, WB Saunders Company.)

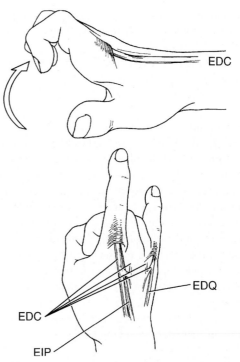

Figure 1–12:
The fourth dorsal compartment consists of the extensor digitorum communis *(EDC)* and the extensor indicis proprius *(EIP).* The fifth compartment contains the extensor digiti minimi. The tendons provide metacarpophalangeal joint extension and extension of the proximal interphalangeal and distal interphalangeal joints in conjunction with the intrinsic muscles. The EIP and extensor digiti minimi provide independent extension of the index and small finger. *EDQ,* Extensor digiti quinti. (From Trumble TE, editor: *Principles of hand surgery and therapy.* Philadelphia, 2000, WB Saunders Company.)

typically occur between the extensor of the middle finger and the index and ring finger. For 80% of the population, the EDC of the small finger consists of only a slip of junctura from the ring finger. The EDC causes MCP joint extension and can be evaluated by asking the patient to extend the fingers. The EIP can be tested by asking the patient to extend the index finger while making a fist. Except in cases of rheumatoid arthritis, primary symptomatic tenosynovitis of the fourth compartment is rare.

- *Pathologic Condition*—Rheumatoid synovitis

## Fifth Dorsal Compartment

- The fifth dorsal compartment contains the extensor digiti minimi (EDM) or extensor digiti quinti (EDQ) tendon and overlies the dorsal radioulnar articulation. The EDQ tendon attaches to the extensor hood on the ulnar side of EDC. The EDQ, similar to the EIP, allows independent extension of the small finger. Because of its location near the radioulnar joint, the tendon can become involved from rheumatoid arthritis of the joint or can rupture because of attritional wear resulting from a dorsally dislocated ulnar head.

- *Pathologic Condition*—Rheumatoid synovitis, attritional rupture

### Sixth Dorsal Compartment

- The sixth dorsal compartment contains the extensor carpi ulnaris (ECU), which lies in a groove between the ulnar styloid process and the ulnar head. With the wrist extended and ulnarly deviated, the ECU tendon can be palpated before its insertion onto the ulnar side of the fifth metacarpal base. A traumatic event can rupture the dorsal carpal ligament, which normally prevents subluxation of the tendon during pronation. Subluxation of the tendon usually is accompanied by pain and an audible snap. Patients with rheumatoid arthritis can similarly have displacement of the tendon or even rupture.
- *Pathologic Condition*—Posttraumatic dislocation, attritional rupture in rheumatoid patients

## Anatomy of the Extrinsic Flexor Tendons

### Wrist Flexor Tendons

- The two major extrinsic flexor tendons of the wrist are the flexor carpi radialis (FCR) and the FCU. To examine the FCR, wrist flexion and radial deviation make the tendon prominent, as it lies radial to the palmaris longus tendon. The FCR (innervated by the median nerve) originates at the medial epicondyle and crosses the scaphoid before inserting distally on the base of the second metacarpal and trapezium. Localized tenosynovitis of the FCR at the wrist level can become severe, necessitating release of the distal extent of the tendon from its sheath. The FCU lies ulnar to the palmaris longus and can be palpated when the wrist is flexed against resistance. The FCU (innervated by the ulnar nerve) also originates from the medial epicondyle and encloses the pisiform at its insertion. Occasionally, the insertion of the FCU can be the site of severe pain when calcific deposits form.
- The palmaris longus tendon bisects the volar aspect of the wrist. The palmaris tendon also originates from the medial epicondyle and inserts distally on the palmar fascia. The palmaris longus is one of the most commonly used tendons for a variety of upper extremity reconstructions. However, it is crucial to examine for the presence of a palmaris longus tendon prior to surgery because this tendon is absent in 7% to 20% of the population. To examine for the presence of a palmaris longus tendon, the patient should flex the wrist and oppose the tips of the thumb and small finger.

### Digital Flexor Tendons

- The flexor digitorum superficialis (FDS) and the flexor digitorum profundus (FDP) are the major extrinsic flexors of the digits, as the fingers themselves do not possess any muscle bellies. The FDS originates from the medial epicondyle and the radial shaft and inserts on the on the palmar middle phalanx to produce flexion of the PIP joint. Proximal to the insertion onto the middle phalanx, the FDS divides into two slips to form Camper's chiasma (Figure 1–13). Anatomically, Camper's chiasma is a long area located over most of the proximal phalanx and is not just a discrete point. The FDP tendon passes between these two slips before attaching on the distal phalanx. As the FDS tendons pass through the carpal tunnel, they are organized in two reproducible layers. The FDSs to the ring and middle fingers are always located palmar to the FDS of the index and small fingers. This anatomic relationship is of particular importance when performing flexor tendon repairs located at this level. A commonly taught way of remembering this relationship is that "34" in reference to the third and fourth digits is greater than "25" corresponding to the second and fifth digits (Figure 1–14). Each muscle of the FDS can function independently. However, absence of the FDS to small finger, seen in up to 30% of the population, prevents isolated flexion of the PIP joint of the small finger. Because the FDP shares a common muscle belly, only the FDS can cause active flexion of the middle, ring, and small fingers while the adjacent digits are held in extension (Figure 1–15).
- The FDP originates from the ulna and inserts on the distal phalanx, promoting flexion of the DIP joint. In contrast to the FDS, the FDP possesses only a single muscle to the long, ring, and small fingers, which prevents independent flexion. The index finger FDP usually has independent function. To test for FDP function, the PIP joint should be held in extension while active flexion of the DIP joint is attempted (Figure 1–16).

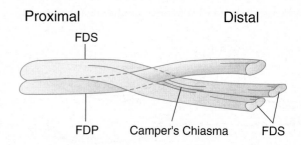

Figure 1–13:
The flexor digitorum profundus *(FDP)* passes through the Camper's chiasma. The vincula provide the blood supply to the flexor tendons. *FDS,* Flexor digitorum superficialis. (From Trumble TE, editor: *Principles of hand surgery and therapy.* Philadelphia, 2000, WB Saunders Company.)

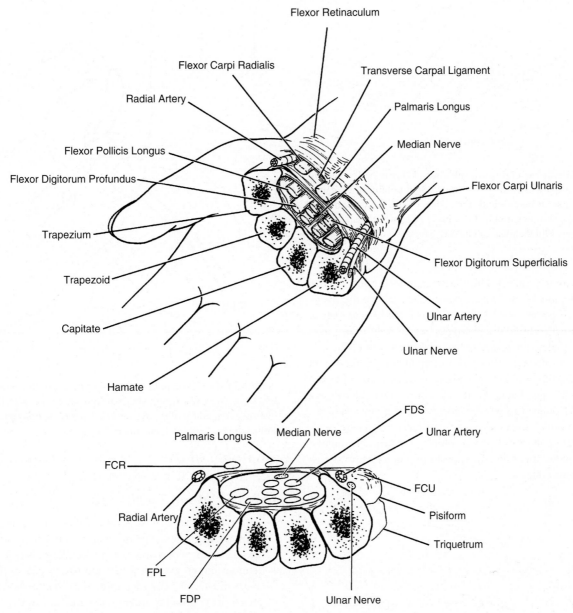

**Figure 1–14:**
The median nerve, all the digital flexor tendons, and the flexor pollicis longus *(FPL)* pass through the carpal tunnel. *FCR,* Flexor carpi radialis; *FCU,* flexor carpi ulnaris; *FDP,* flexor digitorum profundus; *FDS,* flexor digitorum superficialis. (From Trumble TE, editor: *Principles of hand surgery and therapy.* Philadelphia, 2000, WB Saunders Company.)

- The FPL originates from the volar surface of the radius and inserts into the base of the distal phalanx of the thumb, allowing for IP joint flexion (Figure 1–17). Between the FPL and the pronator quadratus at the level of the distal radius is the space of Parona. This is the area where infection can spread from the thumb flexor tendon sheath to the small finger, causing a horseshoe abscess.

## Flexor Tendon Sheath

- At the level of the MCP joints, the digital flexors enter a fibroosseous tunnel also referred to as the *flexor tendon sheath.* The flexor tendon sheath keeps the flexor tendons close to bone, improving the biomechanics of digital flexion and preventing the tendons from bowstringing. The tendon sheath is composed of annular (A) and

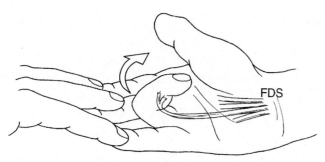

**Figure 1–15:**
Testing the flexor digitorum sublimus *(FDS)* is performed by asking the patient to flex the digits while holding the adjacent digits in extension to block the action of the flexor digitorum profundus. (From Trumble TE, editor: *Principles of hand surgery and therapy*. Philadelphia, 2000, WB Saunders Company.)

cruciate (C) pulleys. There are five annular pulleys: A1 to A5 (Figure 1–18). The two most important of the five annular pulleys are A2 and A4, which are located over the proximal and middles phalanges, respectively. Injury to these pulleys are responsible for bowstringing of the flexor tendons. The A1 pulley is frequently implicated in the pathology of flexor tendon stenosing tenosynovitis or trigger finger. Except in the case of rheumatoid arthritis, the A1 pulley can be released with little biomechanical compromise. In addition to the annular pulleys are three cruciate pulleys: C1 to C3, which are collapsible pulleys that allow finger flexion without impingement of the adjacent pulleys.

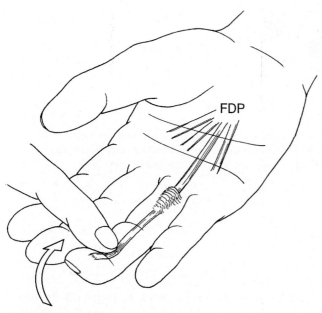

**Figure 1–16:**
Testing of the flexor digitorum profundus *(FDP)* is performed by blocking the proximal interphalangeal joint in full extension. (From Trumble TE, editor: *Principles of hand surgery and therapy*. Philadelphia, 2000, WB Saunders Company.)

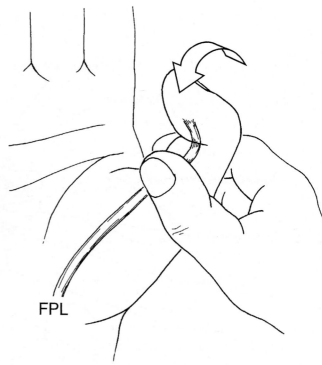

**Figure 1–17:**
Testing of the flexor pollicis longus *(FPL)* is performed by blocking the metacarpophalangeal joint in extension. (From Trumble TE, editor: *Principles of hand surgery and therapy*. Philadelphia, 2000, WB Saunders Company.)

## Anatomy of the Extensor Hood and the Intrinsic Muscles of the Hand

### Extensor Hood Mechanism

- The extensor mechanism of the finger is much more complex than the flexor mechanism. The extensor hood mechanism is where the extrinsic tendons and intrinsic tendons merge to control PIP and MCP motion (Figures 1–19 and 1–20).[3] For each digit, the extensor hood has attachments from the interosseous muscles and a lumbrical muscle. These intrinsic muscles make up the lateral bands, which join distally and insert at the distal phalanx to allow DIP joint extension. Spanning between the two conjoined lateral bands is the triangular ligament, which prevents their volar subluxation. Also stabilizing the lateral bands is the transverse retinacular ligament (located at the level of the PIP joint), which prevents dorsal subluxation. The central slip is the part of the extensor tendon that inserts on the base of the middle phalanx, allowing PIP joint extension.

- Swan-neck deformity is characterized by hyperextension of the PIP joint and flexion of the DIP joint. Common causes of swan-neck deformity include rheumatoid arthritis, mallet finger, laceration of the FDS, and intrinsic contracture. Except in the case of mallet finger (where the terminal extensor tendon is disrupted), the pathophysiology of swan-neck deformity arises from

Figure 1–18:
The flexor tendon sheath is composed of annular pulleys and cruciate pulleys. (From Trumble TE, editor: *Principles of hand surgery and therapy*. Philadelphia, 2000, WB Saunders Company.)

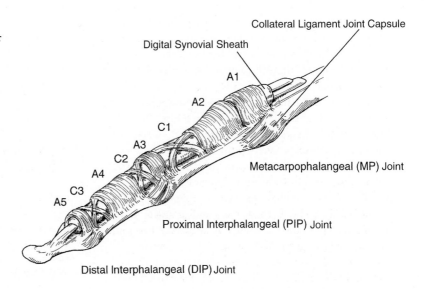

Collateral Ligament Joint Capsule

Digital Synovial Sheath

A1

A2

C1

A3

C2

A4

C3

A5

Metacarpophalangeal (MP) Joint

Proximal Interphalangeal (PIP) Joint

Distal Interphalangeal (DIP) Joint

Transverse Retinacular Ligament

Extensor to Middle Phlanx

Lateral Conjoined Band of Extensor

Oblique Retinacular Ligament (ORL)

Terminal Tendon of Extensor

Transverse Fibers

Oblique Fibers

Sagittal Band

Lateral Tendon of Deep Head of Dorsal Interosseous Muscle

Interosseous Muscle

Flexor Profundus Termination

A5  C3  A4  C2  A3  C1  A2  A1

Flexor Pulleys

Flexor Profundus

Lumbrical Muscle

Flexor Superficialis

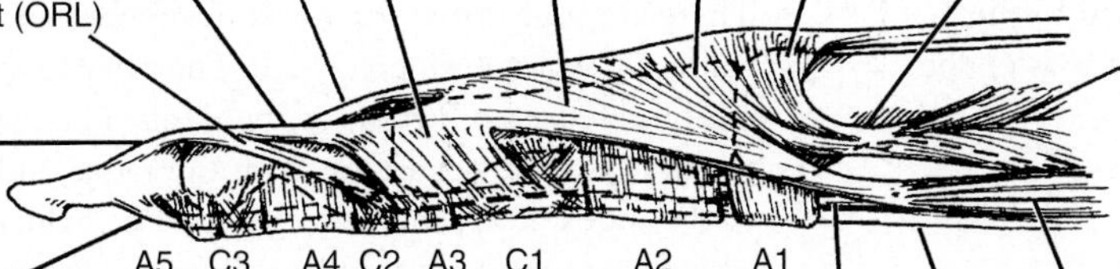

Figure 1–19:
Lateral view of digital extensor tendons and intrinsics. (From Trumble TE, editor: *Principles of hand surgery and therapy*. Philadelphia, 2000, WB Saunders Company.)

Figure 1–20:
Dorsal view of the digital extensor tendon and intrinsics. (From Trumble TE, editor: *Principles of hand surgery and therapy*. Philadelphia, 2000, WB Saunders Company.)

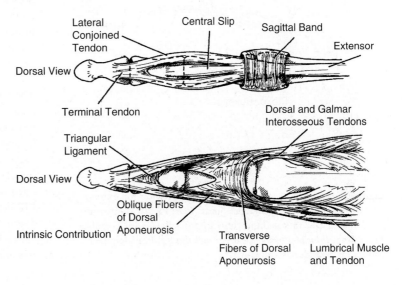

Extrinsic Contribution

Lateral Conjoined Tendon

Central Slip

Sagittal Band

Extensor

Dorsal View

Terminal Tendon

Triangular Ligament

Dorsal View

Intrinsic Contribution

Oblique Fibers of Dorsal Aponeurosis

Dorsal and Galmar Interosseous Tendons

Transverse Fibers of Dorsal Aponeurosis

Lumbrical Muscle and Tendon

stretching of the transverse retinacular ligaments, which allows the lateral bands to sublux dorsal to the axis of the PIP joint. When combined with laxity of the volar plate, hyperextension of the PIP joint and subsequent swan-neck deformity occur.

- Boutonnière deformity is the opposite posture of swan-neck deformity, exhibiting PIP flexion and DIP extension. Rheumatoid arthritis, laceration, or traumatic injury can cause a problem with central slip and subsequent volar subluxation (in contrast to the dorsal subluxation seen in swan-neck deformity) of the lateral bands as a result of incompetence or injury to the triangular ligament. As the lateral bands translate in a palmar direction, they become a flexor at the PIP joint and an extensor at the DIP joint.
- The sagittal band is the most proximal portion of the extensor hood and centralizes the extensor mechanism over the metacarpal head. It is a unique structure in that it encircles the proximal phalanx and attaches to the flexor tendon sheath, which allows extension of the proximal phalanx on the metacarpal head. MCP joint flexion and extension is a complex motion because there are no attachments of either flexor or extensor tendons at the proximal phalanx. Primary extension of the MCP joint is accomplished when the extensor tendon pulls on the sagittal bands, lifting the proximal phalanx from below (Figures 1–21 and 1–22). Located distal to the sagittal band are the transverse and oblique bands of the dorsal hood (see Figure 1–20).

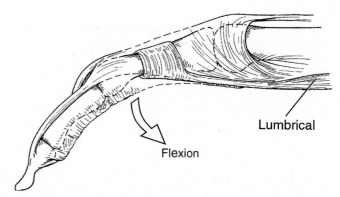

Figure 1–22:
**The transverse band of the extensor mechanism provides for flexion of the metacarpophalangeal joint. (From Trumble TE, editor:** *Principles of hand surgery and therapy.* **Philadelphia, 2000, WB Saunders Company.)**

## Intrinsic Muscles

- The intrinsic muscles assist with MCP joint flexion via their attachments to the extensor mechanism. The lumbrical muscles cross the MCP joint palmar to its axis and dorsal to the axis of the PIP joint before attaching on the middle phalanx. This line of force allows the intrinsic muscles to cause MCP joint flexion and PIP joint extension.
- There are four dorsal interosseous muscles and three palmar interossei (Figure 1–23). The dorsal interossei are responsible for abduction of the digits. The insertions of the dorsal interossei are on both the radial and ulnar sides of the index, long, and ring fingers. The palmar interossei adduct the index, ring, and small fingers. A way to remember the function of the interossei are the words *DAB* and *PAD*, which represent dorsal-abduction and palmar-adduction, respectively.
- The lumbrical muscles originate on each of the FDP tendons and insert on the radial lateral band of the extensor expansion. The lumbrical muscle is the only muscle in the body that originates and inserts on a tendon (Figure 1–24). Another unique attribute of the lumbrical muscle is its ability to relax its own antagonist, the FDP. Innervation of the lumbrical muscles is the ulnar nerve for the ulnar two lumbricals and the median nerve for the radial two lumbricals.
- The intrinsic tightness test is used to examine for contracture of the intrinsic muscles.[4] To perform the intrinsic tightness test, the amount of passive PIP joint flexion is tested with the MCP joints held in extension. Next, the MCP joints are flexed (relaxing the intrinsic muscles) and amount of passive PIP flexion reevaluated. The intrinsic tightness test is positive when there is less passive PIP flexion when the MCP joint is extended (Figure 1–25). Clinically, intrinsic tightness hampers the grasp of large objects, in contrast to extrinsic tightness, which prevents closure of the fist and the grasp of small objects.

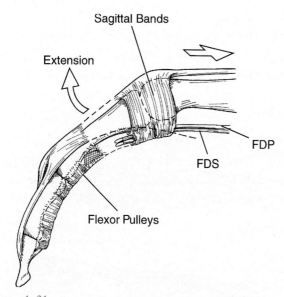

Figure 1–21:
**Sagittal bands of the extensor mechanism provide for extension of the metacarpophalangeal joint.** *FDP,* **Flexor digitorum profundus;** *FDS,* **flexor digitorum superficialis. (From Trumble TE, editor:** *Principles of hand surgery and therapy.* **Philadelphia, 2000, WB Saunders Company.)**

Figure 1–23:
Four dorsal interossei provide abduction and three volar interossei provide adduction of the fingers. (From Trumble TE, editor: *Principles of hand surgery and therapy*. Philadelphia, 2000, WB Saunders Company.)

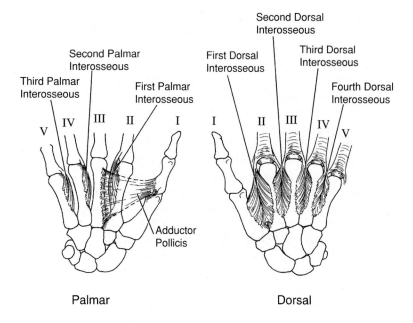

Palmar

Dorsal

## Oblique Retinacular Ligament (of Landsmeer)

- The oblique retinacular ligament (ORL) links the PIP joint and DIP joint extension. Its line of force is analogous to the intrinsic muscles but is applied more distally in the finger. The ORL originates from the periosteum of the proximal phalanx and the A1 and C1 pulleys and inserts on the terminal tendon. With extension of the PIP joint, the ORL, which is palmar at this level, tightens. This tension is transmitted distally, pulling on the terminal tendon as the ORL travels dorsally at the level of the DIP

joint. The ORL becomes contracted in chronic boutonnière deformity. Because of the ORL, Fowler terminal tendon tenotomy can be performed to correct this deformity, with preservation of DIP extension.

## Thenar Muscles

- The muscles of the thenar eminence are the abductor pollicis brevis (APB), flexor pollicis brevis (FPB), opponens pollicis, and adductor pollicis. Muscles located

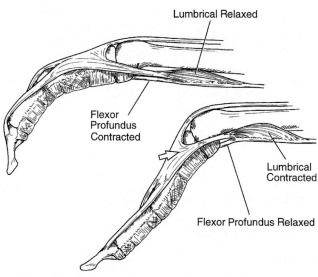

Figure 1–24:
The lumbrical muscles function to flex the metacarpophalangeal joint and extend the proximal interphalangeal joint. (From Trumble TE, editor: *Principles of hand surgery and therapy*. Philadelphia, 2000, WB Saunders Company.)

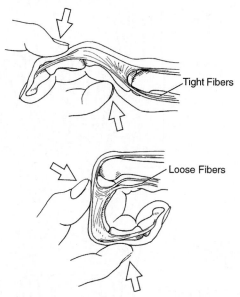

Figure 1–25:
When the intrinsic tightness test is positive, the proximal interphalangeal joint has less passive flexion with metacarpophalangeal extension because the contracted intrinsic muscles are under greater stretch. (From Trumble TE, editor: *Principles of hand surgery and therapy*. Philadelphia, 2000, WB Saunders Company.)

on the radial side of the FPL are innervated by the median nerve; muscles on the ulnar side are innervated by the ulnar nerve (Figure 1–26). The APB (innervated by the median nerve) originates from the transverse carpal ligament and the trapezium and inserts on the radial aspect of the proximal phalanx. Thumb flexion, pronation, and palmar abduction all are caused by action of the APB. The FPB originates from the transverse carpal ligament and trapezium and inserts on the radial sesamoid. There is a dual innervation of the FPB: the median nerve innervates the superficial head and the ulnar nerve innervates the deep head. The APB and FPB obtain opposition and thumb rotation by a combination of action. Located deep to the APB and FPB is the opponens pollicis brevis (OPB). It also arises from the transverse carpal ligament and inserts on the radial aspect of the thumb metacarpal, causing flexion of the thumb metacarpal at the CMC joint. The adductor pollicis (innervated by the ulnar nerve) originates from the third metacarpal and capitate and inserts onto both sesamoids, providing major strength during pinch.

## Hypothenar Muscles

- All of the hypothenar muscles are innervated by the ulnar nerve. These muscles are the abductor digiti quinti (ADQ), flexor digiti quinti (FDQ), and opponens digiti quinti (ODQ). The ADQ originates on the pisiform and inserts on the ulnar aspect of the proximal phalanx of the small finger, providing for abduction of the small finger (see Figure 1–26). The FDQ originates on the hook of the hamate and inserts on the palmar base of the small finger proximal phalanx, causing flexion at the small finger CMC joint. The ODQ is deep to the ADQ and FDQ, originates from the hamate, and inserts on the fifth metacarpal.

# Innervation of the Hand

- Although it is beyond the scope of this chapter to describe the brachial plexus in its entirety, understanding the contributions of the cervical spine to each nerve of the hand is crucial. Sensation and motor innervation in

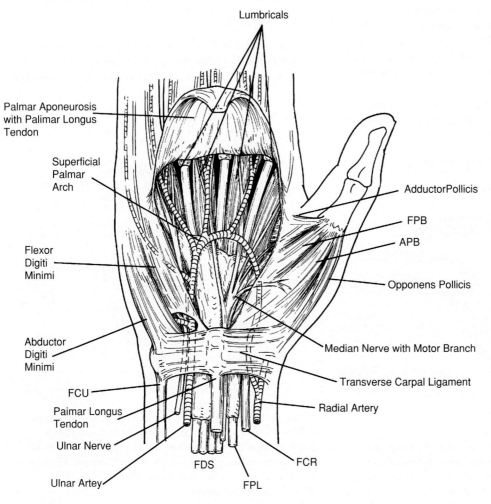

Lumbricals

Palmar Aponeurosis with Palimar Longus Tendon

Superficial Palmar Arch

Flexor Digiti Minimi

Abductor Digiti Minimi

FCU

Paimar Longus Tendon

Ulnar Nerve

Ulnar Artey

FDS

FPL

FCR

Radial Artery

Transverse Carpal Ligament

Median Nerve with Motor Branch

Opponens Pollicis

APB

FPB

AdductorPollicis

Figure 1–26:
The muscles of the thenar eminence include the abductor pollicis brevis *(APB)*, flexor pollicis brevis *(FPB)*, opponens, and adductor pollicis. *FCR,* Flexor carpi radialis; *FCU,* flexor carpi ulnaris; *FDS,* flexor digitorum superficialis; *FPL,* flexor pollicis longus. (From Trumble TE, editor: *Principles of hand surgery and therapy.* Philadelphia, 2000, WB Saunders Company.)

the hand are mediated through the median, radial, and ulnar nerves and their branches. When assessing an injury to one or more of the nerves of the hand, key aspects of the physical examination are indicative of the area of injury (Table 1–2).

## Radial Nerve

- The radial nerve originates from the posterior cord of the brachial plexus (receiving innervation from C5 through T1) and then spirals distally from medial to lateral before emerging between the brachialis and brachioradialis anterior to the lateral epicondyle. Proximal to the elbow the nerve innervates, in order, the anconeus, brachioradialis, and ECRL, before dividing into its posterior interosseous and sensory branch. The radial sensory nerve proceeds distally deep to the brachioradialis until approximately 4 cm proximal to the tip of the radial styloid, where the nerve becomes superficial and passes between the ECRL and the brachioradialis. At this level, the nerve can be injured during placement of an external fixator. As the sensory nerve proceeds distally, it provides for sensation on the dorsum of the thumb and dorsal radial web space (Figures 1–27 and 1–28). At the radial aspect of the wrist, the superficial branch of the radial sensory nerve and the lateral antebrachial cutaneous nerve (the terminal branch of the musculocutaneous nerve) overlap the same sensory territories in 75% of the population. Because of this overlap, treatment of injury or neuroma at this level is fraught with mediocre results.

| Table 1–2: Physical Examination Points Indicative of Nerve Injury[5] |
| --- |
| Sensory Examination |
|   Radial nerve: Dorsal radial hand near the first web space |
|   Median nerve: Pulp of the thumb and index finger |
|   Ulnar nerve: Pulp of the small finger |
| Motor Examination |
|   Median nerve |
|     Intrinsic: Thumb palmar abduction |
|     Extrinsic: All flexor digitorum superficialis tendons |
|     Flexor digitorum profundus to index |
|     Flexor pollicis longus |
|     Flexor carpi radialis |
|   Ulnar nerve |
|     Intrinsic: Hypothenar muscles, first dorsal interosseous (FDIO) |
|     Extrinsic: Flexor digitorum profundus to the small finger |
|     Flexor carpi ulnaris |
|   Radial nerve |
|     Extrinsic: Wrist extension |
|     Finger extension at the metacarpophalangeal joint |
|     Thumb extension |

- After branching from the radial nerve, the posterior interosseous nerve (PIN) dives deep to the fascia of the proximal edge of the supinator (also known as the *arcade of Froshe),* one of the potential sites of compression in radial tunnel syndrome. The PIN innervates the supinator at this level and then all of the extensor muscles of the forearm (see Table 1–3 for the order of innervation).

Figure 1–27:

Sensory patterns of the median ulnar and radial nerves for the palm *(left view)* and dorsum *(right view)* of the hand. (From Trumble TE, editor: *Principles of hand surgery and therapy.* Philadelphia, 2000, WB Saunders Company.)

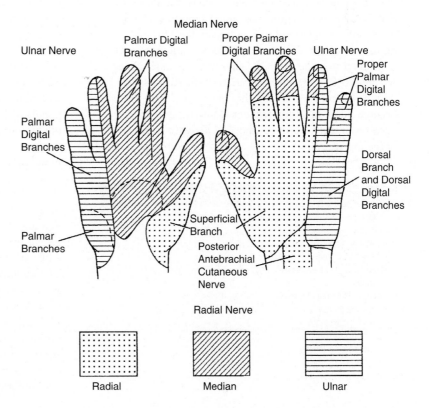

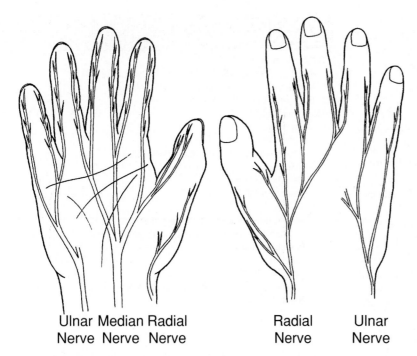

Figure 1–28:
Anatomy of the dorsal sensory nerves of the hand on the palm *(left view)* and dorsum *(right view)*. (From Trumble TE, editor: *Principles of hand surgery and therapy*. Philadelphia, 2000, WB Saunders Company.)

Ulnar   Median   Radial
Nerve   Nerve   Nerve

Radial
Nerve

Ulnar
Nerve

## Median Nerve

- The median nerve originates from both the medial and lateral cords of the brachial plexus (receiving fibers from C6, C7, C8, and T1 and sometimes C5) and travels with the brachial artery before entering the forearm medial to the biceps tendon. The nerve then passes between the two heads of the pronator teres. At the level of the pronator teres, the median nerve gives off its anterior interosseous nerve (AIN) branch, providing innervation to the FDP muscle of the index and middle fingers, the FPL, and pronator quadratus. To test for function of the AIN, ask the patient to make the "OK" sign with the index finger and thumb. Because of the location of the AIN in the deep flexor compartment of the forearm, the AIN can become injured in compartment syndrome and/or fractures of the forearm or elbow. In the volar forearm, all of the forearm flexor muscles are innervated by the

median nerve, except for the FDP to the ring and small fingers and the FCU, which are innervated by the ulnar nerve. The nerve continues distally between the FDS and FDP (innervating the entire FDS). Approximately 5 cm proximal to the wrist flexion crease, the palmar cutaneous branch splits off of the radial side of the nerve and runs between the palmaris longus and the FCR, innervating the skin at the base of the thenar eminence.

- Beneath the transverse carpal ligament, the median nerve enters the hand and gives off its motor branch from the radial side. The motor branch provides innervation to the APB, opponens pollicis, and superficial head of the FPB. There are three variations of the motor branch. The most common (occurring in approximately 50% of the population) is the extraligamentous and recurrent, where the motor branch comes off of the median nerve distal to the transverse carpal ligament before innervating the thenar musculature. In 30% of the population the nerve branches beneath the transverse carpal ligament (subligamentous), and in 20% the nerve is transligamentous, piercing transverse carpal ligament after branching below. To examine the motor branch of the median nerve, ask the patient to oppose the thumb to the small finger while the APB muscle is palpated for contraction.

- The median nerve provides sensation to the palmar aspects of the radial 3½ digits and the dorsum of these digits from the DIP joint to the fingertips (see Figures 1–27 and 1–28). The four sensory nerves begin deep to the superficial palmar arch but become superficial to the arteries in the distal palm. The nerve always lies superficial to the artery within the finger. Innervation of the radial two lumbricals is provided by the common digital nerves.

| Table 1–3:   Radial Nerve Order of Innervation |
|---|
| 1. Triceps |
| 2. Anconeus |
| 3. Brachioradialis |
| 4. Extensor carpi radialis longus |
| 5. Extensor carpi radialis brevis |
| 6. Supinator |
| 7. Extensor digitorum communis |
| 8. Extensor digiti quinti |
| 9. Extensor carpi ulnaris |
| 10. Abductor pollicis longus |
| 11. Extensor pollicis longus |
| 12. Extensor pollicis brevis |
| 13. Extensor indicis proprius |

## Ulnar Nerve

- The ulnar nerve is composed of fibers from the C8 and T1 nerve roots and sometimes a minor contribution from C7. Nearly all of the fibers arise from the lower trunk of the brachial plexus and pass through the medial cord before forming the ulnar nerve. It is important to remember that a large portion of the median nerve and medial antebrachial cutaneous nerve also originate from the medial cord. From the brachial plexus, the ulnar nerve runs along the medial aspect of the arm. At the elbow, the nerve passes in the groove between the medial epicondyle and olecranon process, the cubital tunnel. The ulnar nerve continues distally, enters the forearm between the two heads of the FCU, which it supplies, and then runs between the FCU and the FDP. At this level, the nerve gives off motor branches to the FDP to the ring and small fingers. In the distal third of the forearm, the ulnar nerve gives off the ulnar sensory nerve. Approximately 4 cm proximal to the wrist crease, the ulnar sensory branch exits dorsal to the FCU, providing sensation to the dorsum of the ring and small fingers.
- The ulnar nerve enters the wrist via Guyon's canal. The motor branch of the ulnar nerve innervates the hypothenar muscles (ADQ, FDQ, ODQ) and all of the interossei. The motor branch to the interossei takes an acute turn just distal to the hook of the hamate and usually is visualized during removal of the hook for a fracture (see Figure 1–7). The sensory portion of the ulnar nerve supplies the palmar small finger and the ulnar half of the ring finger (see Figures 1–27 and 1–28). Sensory abnormalities on the dorsum of the hand help distinguish between a lesion of the nerve located proximal versus distal to the branch of the ulnar sensory nerve. Testing for motor function of the ulnar nerve is accomplished through pinch strength. Froment's sign is hyperflexion of the thumb IP joint as a patient with deficient ulnar innervation applies a firm key pinch. When the adductor pollicis is paralyzed, the patient compensates by using the FPL, which causes hyperflexion of the IP joint (Figure 1–29). Other tests of ulnar nerve function include examination of digital abduction to test the interossei.

## Arterial Anatomy

- The arterial anatomy of the hand is one of the greatest areas of variability among patients. There are three main arches for blood supply to the hand: the superficial palmar arch, the deep palmar arch, and the dorsal carpal arch. These three arches are formed by the radial and ulnar arteries and provide a rich collateral circulation to the hand. The main blood supply to the superficial palmar arch is the ulnar artery. This arch is located at Kaplan's cardinal line at the distal extent of the transverse carpal

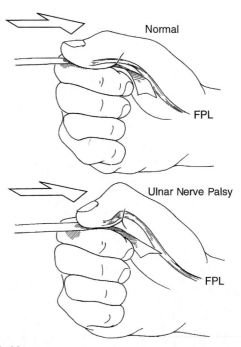

Figure 1–29:

**Positive Froment's sign with thumb interphalangeal joint flexion to compensate for paralysis of adductor pollicis muscle indicates a low ulnar nerve palsy.** *FPL,* **Flexor pollicis longus. (From Trumble TE, editor:** *Principles of hand surgery and therapy.* **Philadelphia, 2000, WB Saunders Company.)**

ligament and is superficial to the median nerve and the long finger flexors. The common digital arteries to the second, third, and fourth web spaces arise from the superficial palmar arch.

- Deep to the median nerve and the long finger flexors is the deep palmar arch. The main blood supply of the deep palmar arch is the radial artery, which also gives a branch to the dorsal carpal arch. The princeps pollicis is a branch of the radial artery just distal to the deep palmar arch. It runs on the palmar aspect of the adductor pollicis before emerging into the subcutaneous tissue at the MCP flexion crease of the thumb. It then branches into the two collateral palmar arteries of the thumb, which run along the flexor sheath, before anastomosing at the fingertip. Other branches, given off while still at the level of the adductor pollicis, include the radialis indicis artery, which supplies the radial digital artery to the index finger, and a branch to the deep palmar arch.
- The dorsal carpal arch is formed by the radial and ulnar dorsal carpal branches. This arch is an important blood supply to the carpal bones, especially the scaphoid. The scaphoid receives its blood supply proximally along the dorsal carpal ridge via the dorsal carpal branch of the radial artery and distally from the volar tuberosity. The dorsal carpal arch extends distally with the dorsodigital arteries, which are important for performing local dorsal hand flaps.

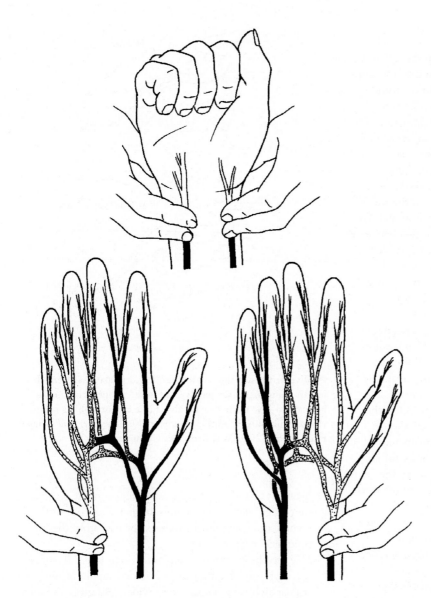

Figure 1–30:
**The Allen test to evaluate patency of the radial and ulnar arteries. (From Trumble TE, editor: *Principles of hand surgery and therapy*. Philadelphia, 2000, WB Saunders Company.)**

- The patency of the palmar arch can be determined by the Allen test (Figure 1–30). To perform the test, the radial and ulnar arteries are occluded with manual pressure while the patient makes a fist several times. Pressure is released from one artery, and capillary refill should be noted in the fingertips within 5 seconds. Failure to provide rapid capillary refill to all the digits after releasing pressure from one of the arteries indicates the patient has a vessel occlusion or an incomplete arch. Similarly, a digital Allen test can be performed at the finger level to assess the digital arteries.

# References

1. Berger RA, Landsmeer JM: The palmar radiocarpal ligaments: a study of adult and fetal human wrist joints. *J Hand Surg Am* 15:847-854, 1990.
   Three palmar radiocarpal ligaments are described: radioscaphocapitate, long radiolunate, and short radiolunate.

2. Viegas SF, Yamaguchi S, Boyd NL, Patterson RM: The dorsal ligaments of the wrist: anatomy, mechanical properties, and function. *J Hand Surg Am* 24:456-468, 1999.
   This study examined the anatomy and mechanical properties of the dorsal radiocarpal and dorsal intercarpal ligaments of the wrist.

3. Smith RJ: Balance and kinematics of the hand under normal and pathologic conditions. *Clin Orthop* 104:92-111, 1974.
   A classic description of the intrinsic mechanism.

4. Zancolli E: In *Structural and dynamic bases of hand surgery*. Philadelphia, 1969, JB Lippincott.
   A detailed discussion, with drawings, of the anatomy and function of the hand.

5. Mackinnon SE, Dellon AL: *Surgery of the peripheral nerve*. New York, 1988, Thieme Medical Publishers.

6. Weaver L, Tencer AF, Trumble TE: Tensions in the palmar ligaments of the wrist. I. The normal wrist. *J Hand Surg Am* 19:464-474, 1994.
   A discussion of the tensions of the palmar radiocarpal ligaments.

7. Hoppenfeld S: Physical examination of the spine and extremities. 1976, Appleton & Lange.
   A classic textbook on the physical examination of the entire musculoskeletal system and the provocative maneuvers for common pathologic conditions.

8. Miller MD, Brinker MR: *Review of orthopaedics,* ed 3, Philadelphia, 2000, WB Saunders.

9. Peimer CA, editors: *Surgery of the hand and upper extremity.* New York, 1996, McGraw-Hill Companies.

10. Green DP, Hotchkiss RN, Pederson WG, editors: *Greens operative hand surgery,* ed 4, New York, 1998, Churchill Livingstone.

11. Trumble TE, editor: *Principles of hand surgery and therapy.* Philadelphia, 2001, WB Saunders.

# Phalangeal Fractures and Dislocations

Joseph F. Slade III* and David P. Magit†

*MD, Associate Professor and Director, Hand and Upper Extremity Service, Department of Orthopaedics and Rehabilitation, Yale University School of Medicine, Guilford, CT
†MD, Clinical Instructor, Department of Orthopaedics and Rehabilitation, Yale University School of Medicine, New Haven, CT

## Introduction

- Although often viewed as trivial injuries, the consequences of maltreated finger injuries can have profound functional consequences. These injuries can prevent full hand function and can limit patients from participating in their chosen vocational and avocational activities. It is not uncommon for stable fractures to be overtreated and unstable fractures to be sometimes neglected. One survey found initial emergency department management was incorrect up to 25% of the time.

- Phalangeal fractures are a common injury that affects all age groups. It is estimated that the annual number of phalangeal fractures treated in emergency rooms in the United States is 341,305 or an incidence per 100,000 of 104.6 for women and 149 for men. The incidence for phalangeal fractures initially treated in an emergency room was highest for individuals aged 0 to 4 years at 207 per 100,000 and decreased for every age group until age over 85 years, when the incidence peaked at 740 per 100,000.[1]

- In a review of hand injuries treated in the emergency room at Yale New Haven Hospital over a 4-month period, fractures represented 11.4% (133/1164) of the injuries distal to the radiocarpal joint. Fractures were second in incidence to lacerations at 61.5% (716/1164). Among these hand fractures, phalangeal fractures represented more than half or 66.5% (95/143) of all the fractures. The distal phalanx was the most frequently injured, representing 31.5% (45/143) of all fractures, with the distal phalanx of the long finger the single most frequently fractured bone representing 10.5% (15/143) of all hand fractures. The fifth metacarpal was the second most fractured bone, representing 9.8% (14/143) of all hand fractures. Fifty-three percent of the phalangeal fractures were on the right side.[2]

## Physical Examination

- The signs of injury usually are obvious: swelling, tenderness, ecchymosis, deformity, and/or skin abrasions. Inspection of the hand reveals a natural attitude and harmony of the digits. The examiner needs to distinguish among fracture, collateral ligament rupture, volar plate rupture, and tendon avulsion. Extension of the wrist results in flexion of the digits, whereas flexion of results in extension. This simple tenodesis test confirms the integrity of the joints, ligaments, and tendons. Each joint is individually examined for congruent gliding through a full arc of motion both actively and passively. Rotational alignment is checked by active flexion of all fingers toward the scaphoid tubercle in the palm of the hand and assessing for digital overlap. If pain prevents active flexion, use of tenodesis with gentle wrist extension can result in digital flexion.

- The joint is stressed to confirm competence of the collateral ligaments. Vascular and neurologic examination are mandatory with any fracture or dislocation. Phalangeal fractures resulting from industrial accidents often are open, requiring review of tetanus immunization and the nature and time of injury.

## Radiologic Examination

- Screening radiographs of the injured hand include three views with the imaging beam centered over the metacarpal phalangeal joint of the long finger: posteroanterior (PA), lateral, and oblique. Focused radiographs are obtained of the injured digit, with PA and lateral views centered on the proximal interphalangeal (PIP) joint. These focus images help detect subtle joint subluxation, dislocations, and fractures. Comparison radiographs of the opposite hand provide a valuable reference to interpret radiographic anomalies. When indicated, stress views can be obtained with the administration of a digital block of lidocaine, performed after documenting the neurologic status of the digit.

## Emergency Room Management

- Closed reduction to align the fracture fragments can be performed via axial traction, followed by reversal of the deformity. For digital fractures, the intrinsics can be relaxed by flexion of the metacarpophalangeal (MCP) joints. The important exception to this use of traction is in simple MCP dislocations, where traction poses the risk of converting a subluxation to a complex dislocation, trapping the volar plate within the joint. Once the reduction is performed, the digit is examined to determine the stability of the reduction.
- A radial or ulnar gutter type splint with the MCP joints flexed as close to 90° as possible will hold the digits aligned while relaxing the intrinsics and preventing collateral ligament contracture. In the case of a stable fracture, "buddy taping" the injured digit to an adjacent uninjured digit may be adequate.
- Postreduction x-ray films should be obtained in two planes. Analysis of sagittal alignment on the lateral view is difficult, and a series of oblique radiographs or computed tomographic scans may be needed to confirm that correct alignment has been achieved. Follow-up with new radiographs 1 week after initial reduction is required to confirm maintenance of alignment. Delay of follow-up beyond 1 week makes salvage of lost reduction more difficult.

## General Principles of Treatment

- The goal of treatment is to restore the normal function of the finger. Restoration of bony anatomy is a basis of returning normal function; however, anatomic reduction should not be obtained at the expense of soft tissue

scarring and loss of motion. Early motion must be achieved through the inherent stability of the fracture, splinting, or adequately secure internal fixation. Unstable fractures of the phalanges tend to angulate in the sagittal plane because of the deforming forces created by the intrinsic and extrinsic tendon system of the hand.

## Management

### Nonoperative

- Closed, nondisplaced, or minimally displaced fractures with acceptable alignment that result from low-energy trauma usually have intact supporting tissues, are stable, and can be treated with protected mobilization. Fractures with rotational or angular malalignment can be treated with closed reduction and splinting in an intrinsic plus position. These unstable injuries must be closely monitored (Box 2–1).

### Operative

- Fractures with articular step-off, open fractures, fractures with significant shortening, and fractures that do not respond to closed reduction are indications for surgical treatment. Surgical placement of internal fixation should be performed with minimal soft tissue disruption so as to limit scarring, but it also must be rigid enough to allow immediate active motion. Surgical intervention carries a risk of iatrogenic stiffness if early mobilization is not instituted (Box 2–2).
- Although the principles of fracture treatment have not changed, improvements in techniques and equipment have created new options for management. Methods of dynamic external fixation have been developed that aid in treating difficult articular fractures. Advances in minimally invasive techniques guided by fluoroscopy and arthroscopy allow the introduction of rigid fixation while preserving the delicate soft tissue envelope of the

---

### Box 2–1

- A radial or ulnar gutter-type splint with the MCP joints flexed as close to 90 degrees as possible holds the digits aligned while relaxing the intrinsics and preventing collateral ligament contracture.

---

### Box 2–2   Indications for Surgical Treatment

- Fractures with articular step-off
- Open fractures
- Fractures with significant shortening
- Fractures that did not respond to closed reduction

phalanges. Rigid miniplates are available for internal fixation of selected fractures. Headless cannulated compression screws buried within bone permit rigid fixation of oblique fractures while permitting early motion without interference from exposed hardware against gliding tendons. Intramedullary fixation with Kirschner wires or new curved blunt nails introduced with an awl allows early motion of shaft fractures.

## Rehabilitation

- Early motion prevents adhesions of the gliding soft tissues of the extensor and flexor tendon systems and contracture of the joint capsules. Immobilization of fingers much beyond 4 weeks leads to long-term stiffness as the result of extensor tendon and joint capsular scarring. Fractures treated with closed reduction and splinting are mobilized after 3 to 4 weeks, once a secure fibrous union has occurred. Even if splinting of one joint is needed, splints should be made small enough to allow early motion of uninjured joints, such as the PIP joint in cases of distal phalanx or distal interphalangeal (DIP) joint fractures.

## Fractures of the Distal Phalanx

### Tuft Fractures

- Fractures of the distal phalanx are the most common hand fracture. Distal tuft fractures most commonly result from a crushing injury and frequently coincide with a nail bed injury. A subungual hematoma involving 50% of the nail often suggests a nail bed laceration and in the past was thought to be an indication for removal of the nail and direct repair of the lacerated nail bed with absorbable suture. However, a study showed that in children with tuft fractures and subungual hematomas of any size, there was no advantage to removal of the nail and repair if the nail bed and nail margins were intact.[3] Trephination of the nail helps relieve pain in these cases. The intact nail often serves as a splint for the fractures. In cases with disrupted nail or nail margins, repair of the underlying nail bed with fine absorbable sutures is indicated. Cases with a disrupted or avulsed nail may also require more prolonged splinting or internal fixation with a Kirschner wire.

### Classification

- Tuft fractures are classified as simple or comminuted.

### Management

#### Nonoperative

- Because of the few deforming forces about the distal phalanx, these fractures usually can be treated in a closed manner with simple splinting, closed reduction and splinting, or closed reduction and percutaneous fixation.

#### Operative

- Irreducible fractures resulting from interposition of the nail fold between the fracture fragments can require open extirpation of the nail fold with reduction and internal fixation of the fracture fragments.[4]

### Rehabilitation

- Most tuft fractures can be protected by 2 to 3 weeks of simple splinting, including the DIP joint but leaving the PIP free. Because of the injury to the fingertip, which is the terminal sensory organ, patients must be warned that they will often have decreased functionality caused by hyperesthesia, cold intolerance, and numbness even 6 months after the injury. Motion of the DIP is started at 2 to 3 weeks with continued protection during active use until pain resolves. A fibrous nonunion can result but can be asymptomatic.[5]

## Shaft Fractures

### Classification

- Fractures of the distal phalangeal shaft may be transverse or longitudinal. Transverse fractures can be characterized as stable or unstable (Figure 2–1).

### Management

#### Nondisplaced Fractures

- Nondisplaced fractures generally have an intact soft tissue envelope that provides stability. Treatment consists of 3 to 4 weeks of splint immobilization including the DIP joint, followed by gentle DIP motion. Displaced fractures result

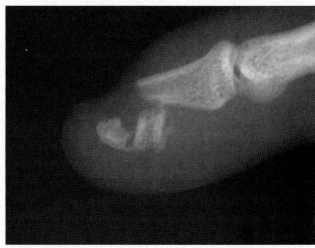

Figure 2–1:
**Unstable transverse shaft fracture of the distal phalanx.**

from higher-energy trauma that causes greater soft tissue compromise.

## Displaced Fractures

- Transverse diaphyseal fractures often are associated with subluxation of the nail plate out of the eponychial fold, with damage to the sterile or germinal matrix. After appropriate irrigation, debridement, antibiotics, and nail bed repair, the bony reduction may require percutaneous K-wire fixation.
- Nonunions of the shaft often can be successfully aided in healing by adequate stabilization with two parallel Kirschner wires placed percutaneously. As the tip of the distal phalanx lies in the dorsal half of the fingertip, the wire should be inserted just a few millimeters palmar to the nail plate.

# Intraarticular Fractures

- Distal articular fractures occur from the dorsal base and include either mallet fractures or pilon-type fractures, or from the volar base, which involves avulsion of the profundus tendon.

## Mallet Fractures of the Base of the Distal Phalanx

### Mechanism of Injury

- The majority of fractures of the base of the distal phalanx are "mallet injuries," occurring because of an axial load with resultant disruption of the terminal extensor mechanism with an attached bone fragment.

### Management

#### Nonoperative

- Mallet injuries with and without a bony fragment can be effectively treated with 6 to 8 weeks of extension splinting of the DIP joint, followed by 1 month of night splinting. Bone fragments retained within the extensor tendon allow greater healing potential. The PIP can be left free, as immobilization of the PIP joint and its resultant stiffness can cause more morbidity than the original injury. Patients are counseled to expect a slight extensor lag (5 degrees) under the best circumstances, with mild loss of total motion. If the extensor lag recurs after splinting, the splinting program is reinstituted for an additional 1 or 2 months. Chronic mallet injuries do well with splinting started as late as 3 months.

#### Operative

- Internal fixation of mallet fingers is recommended in cases of volar subluxation of the distal phalanx or in cases where the dorsal component is greater than $\frac{1}{3}$ of

the joint surface.[6] Because open reduction carries significant risk of complications, percutaneous internal fixation using Kirschner wires for reduction and fixation is the preferred technique. Numerous published series have shown the safety and effectiveness of percutaneous reduction and pinning of mallet injuries. Regardless of the wire configuration used, a congruent reduction of the volar distal phalangeal component with the head of the middle phalanx must be confirmed on the lateral x-ray film.

## Pilon-Type Fractures of the Base of the Distal Phalanx

- Dorsal fracture dislocation can result from an impaction injury of the volar base of the distal phalanx in a manner analogous to the pilon fractures of the PIP. Significant comminution of the articular surfaces may result.

### Management

#### Nonoperative

- Initial treatment is closed reduction, extension block splinting, and closed pinning if needed. Open reduction internal fixation (ORIF) can be difficult, and all attempts at closed treatment should be made.

#### Operative

- Volar plate arthroplasty of the DIP joint for badly comminuted volar fractures or chronic dorsal dislocations remains a good option[7] (for discussion see discussion in PIP section later).

## Flexor Tendon Avulsions

- Flexor digitorum profundus (FDP) tendon avulsions can occur with or without bony avulsions. With avulsion of the FDP tendon, the vinculum or a large bony fragment may prevent retraction of tendon stump. The ring finger is the most commonly injured digit, reported in 75% of all cases.

### Examination

- Although patients often complain of an inability to flex the DIP joint, the clinical examination usually demonstrates normal passive motion. The injury is frequently missed by either the patient or the primary care providers, who misdiagnose the injury as a "sprained" finger.

### Classification[8]

#### Type I

- The vincula are ruptured, and the proximal tendon retracts to the palm. The tendon then is rendered avascular, leading to poor long-term results. These require repair in 7 to 10 days and ideally with 24 to 48 hours.

### Type II

- The tendon is held at the level of the PIP joint, with the vincula remaining intact. These injuries, which are the most common subtype, have better prognosis for treatment because of the preserved blood supply. Delayed repair out to 6 weeks from the time of injury is possible.

### Type III

- These injuries have a large bone fragment that becomes ensnared and prevents retraction beyond the A4 pulley (Figure 2–2). Delayed repair is possible in these cases.

## Management

- For all injury types, anatomic repair of the tendon to its insertion is the goal of treatment. Surgical repair of the tendon avulsion includes the use of a heavy, nonabsorbable pullout suture tied over a button. The button can be placed either dorsally with the sutures brought out transosseously through the nail bed or distally with the sutures brought out just volar to the tip of the distal phalanx. The latter method has a lower incidence of nail growth disruption.
- Fully retracted tendons are difficult to reinsert after the first several weeks, although successful reinsertion with good functional motion has been performed up to 1 month after injury.
- For large bony fragments (type III), ORIF with small screw fixation is possible.

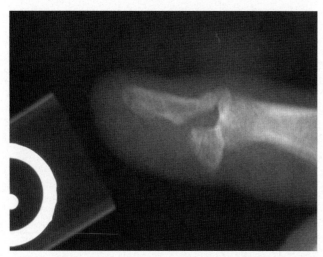

Figure 2–2:
**The flexor digitorum profundus tendon is avulsed with a large bony fragment. The large bony fragment prevents retraction of tendon stump. Classified as a type III injury. (From Leddy JP, Packer JW: Avulsion of the profundus tendon insertion in athletes.** *J Hand Surg [Am]* 2:66-69, 1977.)

# Intraarticular Fractures of the Proximal and Middle Phalanges

## DIP and PIP Joint Dislocations

### DIP Joint Dislocations

#### Management

##### Nonoperative

- Closed injuries can be reduced with longitudinal traction with the distal phalanx held in flexion.
- See Box 2–3

##### Operative

- Because of the thin soft tissue envelope, these injuries often are open in more than 60% of cases.
- Open dislocations are treated with appropriate antibiotics and irrigation and debridement, followed by open reduction.
- Postreduction radiographs must show concentric reduction.
- Irreducible dislocations often result from interposed soft tissue, most commonly from the proximal volar plate or the flexor tendon trapped over the condyle of the middle phalanx. The flexor tendon usually remains attached to the distal phalanx, but this situation must be confirmed after reduction.
- Irreducible volar dislocations often demonstrate splitting of the extensor mechanism, with the extensor tendon interposed within the joint. Pinning of the DIP can help to maintain the reduction and avoid excess pressure on the skin.

#### Rehabilitation

- The DIP joint is splinted in flexion for 2 to 3 weeks, with a protected motion program started after 1 week.
- The rare volar dislocation is reduced and immobilized in a DIP extension splint for 6 to 8 weeks.

### Proximal Interphalangeal Joint Dislocations

#### Dorsal Proximal Interphalangeal Dislocations

- Dorsal dislocations of the PIP joint are the most common joint injuries of the hand.[9]

---

| **Box 2–3    Clinical Anatomy** |
| --- |
| - The DIP joint is a bicondylar "hinge joint" with collateral ligaments, volar plate, and tendon insertions. The joint is stabilized by its articular congruity and by stout capsular ligaments that permit motion in the plane of flexion and extension. |
| - Dislocations of the DIP joint are most often dorsal or lateral. |
| - The mechanism of injury may be hyperextension, hyperflexion, lateral deviation, impaction, or shear. |

- The mechanism of injury is believed to be either hyperextension of the PIP joint or axial loading of the flexed fingertip with hyperextension of the PIP joint and shearing of the volar plate from the base of the middle phalanx.
- The palmar plate fails at its distal attachment with a chip avulsion from the base of the middle phalanx. Pure dislocations often preserve the collateral ligaments.
- See Box 2–4

## Classification

- Eaton and Malerich described and classified injuries to the PIP joint with displacement in the sagittal plane into three types (Table 2–1). Type I injuries are a simple hyperextension injury; type II and III injuries occur from a shear force with dorsal displacement. Type II injuries represent dorsal dislocations with no fracture. Type III injuries represent fracture-dislocations and can be subgrouped based on fracture pattern into IIIA (stable) and IIIB (unstable).[10]

---

### Box 2–4    Clinical Anatomy

- The PIP joint is a hinge joint composed of two condyles with an arc of motion of 110 degrees.
- The condyles are asymmetric and permit 9 degrees of supination through flexion. The proper collateral ligament is the primary stabilizer and inserts on the volar third of the base of the proximal phalanx.
- The accessory collateral ligaments stabilize the volar plate and insert on the lateral margins.
- The volar plate is thick distally and dense only at its lateral insertion. Proximally, the plate is thin and allows for collapse, much like an accordion during flexion.
- Stability is conferred during joint loading by articular congruity.
- The stout capsular ligaments provide a powerful check against angular and torsional forces. PIP dislocations can occur in a dorsal, volar, or lateral direction.

---

## Management

### Nonoperative

- Type I dorsal dislocations can be treated with buddy taping and early motion.
- Reduction of type II dorsal dislocation is accomplished with longitudinal traction under local digital block. After reduction, radiographs of the digit are obtained with imaging beam focused on the PIP joint to confirm that a concentric reduction has been obtained. Assessment of stability follows congruous reduction. Functional stability is tested by actively flexing and extending the joint through a full arc of motion. Stability of the collateral ligaments is also tested with the passive lateral stress test, both in full extension and in 30 degrees of flexion.

### Operative

- Chronic dorsal PIP fracture dislocations result in stiffness and pain of the PIP joint if not treated. Chronic dislocation is treated with open reduction. If unstable or significant joint destruction is present, volar plate arthroplasty is the recommended treatment.

## Rehabilitation

- If stable, active motion with protective extension splinting is initiated. If unstable, the point of dislocation is identified, the joint is flexed 10 degrees farther than the point of dislocation, and an extension block splint is applied. Each week the splint is extended 10 degrees.
- The most common complication is a flexion contracture of the PIP joint resulting from scar contracture of the healing volar plate. This stiffness can be prevented by an early aggressive range of motion program emphasizing full passive extension exercises.

## Dorsal Fracture Dislocations and Pilon Fractures of the Proximal Interphalangeal Joint

- Dorsal fracture dislocations of the PIP joint are Eaton type III injuries. Cadaver studies have shown that an injury sustained by a fully extended PIP joint often

---

### Table 2–1:  Eaton Classification of Dorsal Proximal Interphalangeal Fracture-Dislocations

| I | II | IIIA | IIIB |
|---|---|---|---|
| Hyperextension | Dorsal Dislocation | Stable | Unstable |
| Volar plate avulsion off middle phalanx | Volar plate rupture and split collaterals | Fracture <40% of volar articular surface | Fracture >40% of volar articular surface |
| Buddy taping and early active flexion preventing the last 20° of extension | Extension block splinting or buddy tape | Extension block splinting or open reduction internal fixation | Operative choices |

Adapted from Eaton RG, Littler JW: Joint injuries and their sequelae. *Clin Plast Surg* 3:85-98, 1976.

results in a fracture-dislocation, whereas loading of the joint in moderate flexion results in a pilon fracture. Full extension of the joint causes laxity in the collateral ligaments, which permits dorsal gliding of the middle phalanx and shearing of the volar base and plate. This is similar to the mechanism of dorsal dislocation, but with fracture dislocations there is a shearing off of the volar base of the middle phalanx on the proximal phalanx head and a dorsal dislocation of the middle phalanx as it travels proximally.

- If the PIP joint is partially flexed, the collateral ligaments tighten as they glide over the condyle of the proximal phalanx and firmly seat the base of the middle phalanx on the head of the proximal. This situation can result in a pilon fracture of the base of the middle with displaced volar and dorsal articular fragments and a depressed central articular fragment. The forces acting on the middle phalanx result from both the intrinsic and extrinsic tendon systems.

- With disruption of the connection from the more distal phalangeal shaft to the bony and ligamentous support of the articular surface, the flexor tendon forces draw the fractured shaft of the middle phalanx proximally. With dorsal fracture dislocations of the PIP joint, these deforming forces tend to rotate the distal portion of the middle phalanx palmarly and the proximal end of the middle phalanx dorsally while drawing it proximally. With volar dislocation, the reverse situation exists. Pilon fractures results in a "mushrooming of the base of middle phalanx."

- These deforming forces explain the difficulty in maintaining a concentric reduction of the fracture-dislocation. Any treatment selected must balance the forces acting on the injured joint to maintain a concentric reduction throughout a full range of motion.

### Management

- The goal of treatment of these injuries is a congruous articular surface and full range of motion.[11]

#### Nonoperative

- For dorsal fracture-dislocations involving less than 30% of the articular surface, closed treatment with extension block splinting can yield satisfactory results.

#### Operative

- Complex fractures involving greater than 40% of the articular surface of the base of the middle phalanx are inherently unstable and often require some form of surgical stabilization.

- The options for treatment include skeletal traction, static or dynamic external fixation, dynamic traction with passive motion, dynamic traction with active motion, volar plate arthroplasty, closed reduction and transarticular

Kirschner wire fixation, and ORIF with or without bone graft.

1. Extension Block Splinting
   - This treatment is contraindicated for dorsal fracture dislocations with greater than 40% joint involvement. It requires such extreme flexion to prevent redislocation that flexion contracture is a common complication.

2. Closed Reduction and Kirschner Wire Fixation
   - Newington, Davis, and Barton[12] reported a 16-year follow-up of 10 patients, showing minimal degenerative articular changes with satisfactory long-term clinical results.

3. Open Reduction Internal Fixation
   - ORIF is only feasible in the PIP joint when the fracture fragments are large enough to allow secure fixation. Weiss[13] reported good results using ORIF with volar cerclage wiring. Williams et al.[14] reported 100% bony union and good clinical results after using hemi-hamate autograft secured with miniscrews. ORIF can be associated with complications, including loss of motion, infection, chronic instability, and degenerative arthritis.
   - Pilon fractures of the base of the middle phalanx are best treated by dynamic external fixation with limited percutaneous reduction.[9,15,16] ORIF of pilon fractures is indicated only when single large fracture fragments can be rigidly fixed but is prone to soft tissue problems and joint stiffness. The best results have been reported for dynamic distraction, with improved safety and equivalent clinical and radiographic results compared to open reduction. Skeletal traction provides better range of motion with fewer complications than splinting or ORIF for treatment of PIP pilon fractures. Stern et al.[17] examined three types of treatment of pilon fractures of the PIP joint. These authors and others found that skeletal traction provided results radiographically and clinically superior to ORIF with far fewer complications. Long-term follow-up radiographs showed remodeling of the articular surface of the base of the middle phalanx.

4. External Fixation
   - External fixation and closed reduction through distraction or ligamentotaxis has several biologic advantages over internal fixation, including preservation of blood supply to small articular fragments and as the capacity for early motion of the PIP joint.
   - Fractures that are unstable after open repair of joint surface or joint resurfacing arthroplasty can be splinted with external fixation and permitted early motion.
   - A variety of PIP external fixator devices have been described over the past 60 years. Schenck[18] added

the concept of passive motion to distraction and developed a thermoplastic banjo-type splint based off the forearm, which was attached via rubber bands to transosseous traction pins placed through the middle phalanx. External fixators connected to both the proximal and middle phalanges, such as the PIP compass hinge designed by Kasparyan and Hotchkiss,[19] provided better stability but less traction.

● Combining the benefits of traction, early motion, and more rigid fracture stabilization, Slade et al.[16] developed a dynamic distraction external fixator connecting the middle and distal phalanges. It is made in the operating room of three 0.045-inch Kirschner wires placed in both the proximal and middle phalanges and connected to each other by dental rubber bands. This combination creates simultaneous traction and joint stability[16] (Figure 2–3).

## Technique of Application of Proximal Interphalangeal Dynamic Distraction External Fixation

○ Concentric reduction of the joint must be obtainable prior to frame application.
  ▪ Closed reduction
  ▪ Limited open reduction, if closed not successful
○ The dynamic distraction external fixator is assembled using three 0.045-inch K-wires placed parallel to each other and perpendicular to the lateral axis of the digit.
○ The lateral axis of the finger is a plane where the dorsal forces acting on the skin are perfectly balanced by the palmar forces, resulting in minimal soft tissue gliding, an important feature in pin placement to reduce pin tract infection.
○ Using a mini C-arm fluoroscopy for pin placement, the first K-wire is placed through the rotational center of the head of the proximal phalanx as seen on the lateral fluoroscopic view.
○ The free ends of the wire on both sides are bent at right angles and distally along the long axis of the digit. The ends of the wire are formed into hooks for application of the dental loop rubber bands.
○ A second parallel 0.045-inch K-wire is passed through the distal metaphysis or condyle of the middle phalanx. The free ends of this wire also are bent at a right angle and directed distally. This wire is parallel to the first wire, and its ends also are fashioned into hooks for attachment of the dental loops.
○ The proximal and distal pins are bent into hook forms, with a 2.5-cm distance between the hooks. These two wires bridge the joint and with the dental loop rubber bands become the engine for continuous distraction to maintain concentric joint reduction. Ligamentous traction maintains reduction by transferring the forces of distraction to the surrounding soft tissue of the joint, which hold the fracture alignment.

○ The final K-wire (may be 0.035 inch) is parallel to other two wires and passes through the middiaphysis of the middle phalanx in the midaxial line. Its free ends are cut short and bent around the limbs of the first wire to maintain the alignment of the first wire in the same plane with the digit as it courses through its flexion and extension arc of motion (Figure 2–4). This wire acts as a fulcrum. It reduces the forces required for reduction by providing a block to the translation of the middle phalanx.
○ Dental loop rubber bands are applied between the two hooks in sufficient quantity (usually three for each pair of hooks) to distract the joint and maintain its reduction throughout full range of motion. Joint

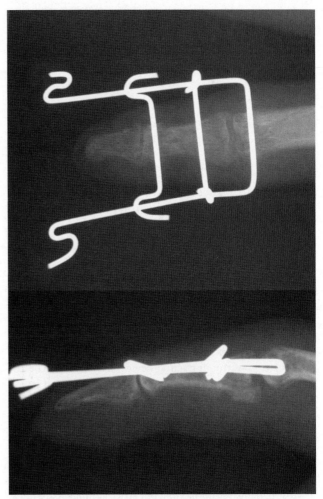

Figure 2–3:
The dynamic distraction external fixator combines the benefits of congruent joint reduction by continuous traction and active early motion. This device is constructed from materials available in the operating room, three 0.045-inch Kirschner wires, and dental rubber bands. (From Slade JF, Baxamusa TH, Wolfe SW: External fixation of proximal interphalangeal joint fracture dislocations. *Atlas Hand Clin* 5:1-29, 2000.)

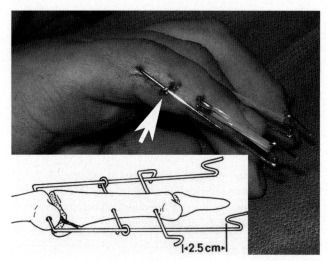

Figure 2–4:
**The key to assembly of the dynamic distraction fixator is the placement of the first K-wire through the rotational center of the head of the proximal phalanx. This is accomplished with fluoroscopic imaging.**

reduction through a complete arc of motion is confirmed with radiographic imaging.

*Postoperative Management*

- Successful restoration of hand function is greatly aided by supervised hand therapy for both active and passive motion at both interphalangeal joints.
- Patients are started on an active and passive motion protocol when swelling has decreased and joint motion has increased, usually within a few days following surgery.
- Weekly radiographs are obtained to confirm joint reduction. If dorsal subluxation is identified, traction is increased by applying more dental loop rubber bands until reduction is achieved.
- This is a powerful distraction device, and care must be taken not to overdistract the joint. This is corrected by decreasing the number of rubber bands used for traction.
- All external fixators are at risk for infection. Daily local wound care to pin tract sites is provided with dilute hydrogen peroxide. If cellulitis is detected, oral antibiotics and rest are applied. If infection cannot be controlled, the offending pin is removed and formal traction is applied.
- Most patients regain flexion, but strict compliance with a supervised hand rehabilitation program is required to regain full active extension of the PIP joint.
- The device is removed when radiographs demonstrate bony union, usually at 6 to 7 weeks. Prior to device removal, lateral radiographs with the rubber bands removed are obtained in full flexion and extension to confirm that concentric joint reduction is maintained out of traction.

Therapy is continued after splint removal for one to two months, to recover motion and strengthen the hand.

5. Volar Plate Arthroplasty

- As originally described by Eaton and Malerich, the volar plate is incised laterally and released from the collateral ligaments, then released from its distal attachments. A trough is created across the middle phalanx near the junction between the intact articular surface and the fracture zone. The volar plate then is advanced into the defect and held in place with sutures or trans-osseus wires that are secured over a dorsal button or on the dorsum of the middle phalanx beneath the extensor mechanism.[10]
- Volar plate arthroplasty has been advocated for treatment of acute unstable and chronic dorsal fracture dislocations.[20,21] Reconstructions performed early have resulted in better results than reconstructions performed late. The most common complication of volar plate arthroplasty is recurrent dislocation, particularly when greater than 50% of the articular surface is involved. Filling any gap that remains behind the advanced volar plate with bone graft can help prevent this complication. Williams et al[14] recommended the use of a osteochondral graft obtained from the hamate. Failure to create a symmetric trough in the base of the proximal phalanx results in an angular deformity of the joint. Dynamic distraction fixation can facilitate early motion without risking redislocation.

### Rehabilitation

- Salter noted the importance of early motion in the recovery of full joint function, and he revolutionized our rehabilitation protocols by emphasizing early passive joint motion for the beneficial effects on both the joint surface cartilage healing and nutrition and on the surrounding soft tissue. Regardless of technique, all restrictions on motion are removed with radiographic signs of healing usually at 5 to 6 weeks. Therapy is continued for 1 to 2 months after splint removal, both to recover motion and to strengthen the hand.

### Complications

- The most common complications of PIP fracture-dislocation treatment are redisplacement, flexion contracture, and DIP joint stiffness. Angular deformity can result in fractures treated by volar plate arthroplasty, whereas pin tract infection is common in external frames.

## Volar Proximal Interphalangeal Dislocations

- Volar PIP dislocations, which are far less common than dorsal dislocations, have been described in two forms. A straight volar dislocation of the PIP joint results in a disruption of the central slip. A volar rotary subluxation represents the rotation of the middle phalanx base around an intact collateral ligament.

### Straight Volar Dislocations

*Management*

- Straight volar dislocations can be treated with closed splinting if reduction can be achieved. If a dorsal bony avulsion is present, internal fixation may be necessary. Global instability is best treated with immediate open repair.

*Rehabilitation*

- Postoperatively, the PIP joint is held in extension for 6 weeks and the DIP joint is started on active and passive motion to allow the central slip injury to heal and prevent the development of a chronic boutonnière deformity.

### Volar Rotatory Subluxation

*Management*

- Volar rotary subluxation results from a compressive force applied to a semiflexed PIP joint. There is a complete disruption of the central tendon or split between the central tendon and the lateral band as the condyle buttonholes through this tear. The collateral ligament fails proximally and the palmar plate fails distally.
- Reduction of the straight volar dislocation is accomplished by longitudinal traction, but reduction of the volar rotary subluxation can be more difficult, as the condyle becomes trapped between the lateral band and the central slip. Reduction can occur by flexion of the MCP and PIP joint. This maneuver relaxes the lateral band, and gentle manipulation of the middle phalanx frees the condyle. Open reduction, however, usually is required because of swelling from failed attempts at reduction.

*Rehabilitation*

- After reduction, assess the continuity of the central tendon. If the central tendon is intact, a short period of immobilization is followed by controlled early motion. If the central slip is disrupted, the tendon should be repaired and the rehabilitation should be dictated by the central slip repair as described in chapter 13.

## Lateral Proximal Interphalangeal Joint Dislocations

- These dislocations result from rupture of one collateral ligament and the volar plate.

- Examination reveals asymmetric joint swelling and tenderness over the collateral ligament. Stability is tested in extension to test the primary (collateral ligaments) and secondary (volar plate) stabilizers. Radiographs show a chip avulsion at ligament origin or an avulsion at the base of the middle phalanx. A complete tear shows greater than 20 degrees of angulation to lateral stress.

### Management

- All partial and most complete tears are treated with 1 to 2 weeks of static splinting, followed by protected motion.
- Surgical indications include interposed soft tissue or a displaced fracture. An irreducible rotatory dislocation results from interposition of the lateral band into the joint. These injuries usually result in stiff joints, not instability. In the rare case of chronic instability, the collateral ligament can be reconstructed.

## Condylar Fractures

- Torsional and valgus impaction injuries to the DIP and PIP joints can result in condylar fractures of the head of the middle or proximal phalanx. These fractures are sometimes missed, being diagnosed as a severe sprain by the patient. Moreover, what is first seen as a nondisplaced condylar fracture may later displace into an angular malunion.
- In addition to the standard PA and lateral views, an oblique x-ray film may be needed to fully visualize the fracture.

### Classification[22]

- Type I: Stable, nondisplaced unicondylar
- Type II: Unstable, unicondylar
- Type III: Bicondylar or comminuted
- Weiss and Hastings[23] modified London's classification for middle phalangeal fractures by subdividing the type I and II unicondylar fractures into four classes determined by the orientation of the fracture line:
  - Class I: Volar oblique
  - Class II: Long sagittal
  - Class III: Dorsal coronal
  - Class IV: Volar coronal

### Management

- Untreated, this intraarticular fracture can lead to significant disability. Open reduction is necessary if percutaneous fixation cannot maintain anatomic reduction. Because of the torsional forces on these fractures, best fixation is achieved with two or more Kirschner wires or screws.

### Nonoperative

- Nondisplaced London type I unicondylar fractures can be treated with splint immobilization for 3 to 4 weeks, with close weekly follow-up to monitor for displacement. However, especially in the proximal phalanx, these fractures carry a high risk of displacement. Patients must be warned of the potential need for surgical treatment of the fracture.

## Operative

Operative management is indicated for the first sign of displacement.

### *London Type II Fractures*

#### *Closed Reduction and Percutaneous Pinning*

- Surgical treatment should first be attempted with percutaneous fixation with two laterally placed wires or small 1.0-mm or 1.2-mm screws. If the fracture pattern allows stability with compression, a single screw may suffice.

#### OPEN REDUCTION INTERNAL FIXATION

- If an anatomic reduction is not achieved percutaneously with pointed bone-holding clamps, open reduction is indicated via a lateral incision or a dorsal incision curved toward the side of the injured condyle. Approach to the head of the middle phalanx is attempted lateral to the terminal extensor tendon. For the PIP joint, the fracture is approached between the central slip and the lateral band to prevent disruption of the central slip. Care is taken to maintain the condylar fragment's collateral ligament attachments, which provide much of the blood supply to the condyle. Loss of the collateral attachment may result in osteonecrosis of the condylar fragment. Under direct vision, the fractured condyle can be reduced and secured to the opposite condyle and diaphyseal shaft with two screws or a screw and an antirotation Kirschner wire.

### *London Type III Bicondylar Fractures*

- These fractures usually are too unstable to allow closed reduction and percutaneous fixation. If the fracture line between the condyles and the shaft is in a short oblique pattern, it may be possible to fix both condyles to the shaft with individual lag screws. However, in the more common transverse fracture pattern, a 90-degree condylar plate usually is required, as collapse may occur with screws alone. Fixation proceeds with lag screw fixation of one condyle to the other, followed by plate fixation of the condyles to the shaft. Occasionally bone grafting at the metaphysis is necessary to prevent undue shortening of the digit in highly comminuted fractures. Careful preoperative planning is required because of this implant's small size and unforgiving tolerances of application. Complications of using the 90-degee condylar plate include infection, joint stiffness, and tendon adhesion.

- Weiss and Hastings class I and II fractures can be well held with multiple screws or Kirschner wires. Class III and IV fractures are difficult because of their multiplanar nature. Class IV fractures have the poorest outcome. Fixation can be achieved with small screws or smooth or threaded wires.

### **Rehabilitation**

- If adequate stability can be achieved with internal fixation, motion should begin after a short period of postoperative immobilization.

# Fractures of the Middle and Proximal Phalanges

## **Extraarticular Shaft Fractures**

### **Classification**

- Closed extraarticular fractures of the proximal and middle phalanges can be transverse, oblique, spiral, or comminuted. Fracture displacement and stability after closed reduction guide the treatment options.

### Nondisplaced Fractures

- Most nondisplaced extraarticular fractures can be treated with buddy taping for 3 to 4 weeks. For spiral fractures or others with potential for instability, splinting can be used for 3 weeks, with close follow-up to monitor for any displacement.

### Displaced Fractures

- Displaced fractures can be unstable, even if reduced, and can be difficult to hold in reduction. Oblique, spiral, or comminuted fractures tend toward instability, whereas transverse fractures in adults or Salter II metaphyseal fractures in children tend to be stable once they are reduced. Fractures at the bases of the phalanges often are unstable because of deforming muscular forces. Transverse fractures of the proximal phalanx are deformed into an apex-palmar direction. The insertions of the interossei into the base of the proximal phalanx flex it down, and the insertion of the central slip into the middle phalanx extends the distal piece. Fractures of the middle phalanx distal to the insertion of the superficialis tendon deform in a similar manner.

- Proximal phalanx fractures can lead to extensor tendon dysfunction often caused by extensor tendon adhesions and bony malunion. Malunion can result from either apex volar angulation or shortening from fracture comminution. In a cadaveric study, Vahey, Wegner, and Hastings[24] found a linear relationship between proximal phalangeal shortening and extensor lag. The authors also found that apex palmar angulations of 16, 27, and 46 degrees correlated with PIP lags of 10, 24, and 66 degrees, respectively.[24]

## Management

### Closed Reduction

- As for all fractures, reduction of phalangeal fractures is achieved by axial traction, accentuation of the deformity to unlock the fracture fragments, and reversal of the deformity. For shaft fractures, relaxing the tension of the intrinsic musculature by flexing the MCP joint aids in closed reduction. Once reduced, rotational alignment is confirmed clinically, the hand is splinted in a functional position with the MCP joint flexed and IP joints extended, and radiographs are obtained.

### Closed Reduction and Percutaneous Fixation

- Displaced fracture fragments may ensnare the surrounding soft tissues, preventing reduction. An irreducible fracture may be result from entrapment of the Grayson or Cleland ligaments or the flexor tendon sheath in the fracture site. Percutaneous fixation is most suitable for fractures with minimal soft tissue disruption that can be reduced in a closed or percutaneous manner.

### Base Fractures

- These fractures tend toward a hyperextension deformity of the distal fragment and can be rigidly fixed either with crossed Kirschner wires through the base or via a transmetacarpal head pin. If a transmetacarpal head pin is used, the MCP joint should be pinned in at least 70 degrees of flexion to prevent contracture of the collateral ligaments in extension. When using bicortical crossed Kirschner wires for transverse fractures, the wires should not cross at the fracture site or rotational stability will be lost. Kuhn et al.[25] reported the results of avulsion fractures of the base of the proximal phalanx associated with collateral ligament instability. They noted good results after 10 patients were treated with ORIF using a volar A1 pulley approach.

### Short Oblique and Transverse Fractures

- A Kirschner wire can be used longitudinally as an intramedullary rod. The wire can be passed down the shaft of the phalanx retrograde entering at the head, or the wire can be passed antegrade through the base or even through the metacarpal head into the phalangeal shaft.[26]

### Long Oblique or Spiral Fractures

- These fractures are prone to rotational malalignment. Once the fracture has been reduced, the reduction can be held by percutaneous bone-holding forceps. Fixation is achieved by compression screws or K-wires placed at right angles to the fracture line (Figure 2–5). Placing

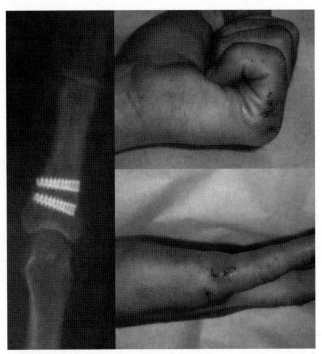

Figure 2–5:

**Long oblique or spiral fractures can be repaired with traditional lag screws. The risk is that screws placed close to the joint will block gliding of the joint capsule, restricting joint motion. Use of headless screws prevents these complications and permits early motion. Shown here are mini-acutrak screws (Beaverton, Oregon) used to repair a long oblique fracture and start early motion.**

the screws from the midaxial position prevents injury to the flexors and extensors. The phalangeal shaft is kidney bean shaped in cross section, so care must be made to avoid tethering the flexor tendon with a screw or pin.

- Studies have challenged the traditional notion that ORIF with screws provides superior fixation to closed reduction and K-wire fixation. In a prospective randomized trial comparing closed reduction and K-wire fixation versus ORIF with screws, no significant difference in the functional recovery rates or in the pain scores for the two groups was noted.[27]

### Rehabilitation

- Early follow-up with radiographs is essential to monitor for loss of reduction. Protected motion can be started at 3 to 4 weeks. As in all techniques, motion should be started as soon as possible and no later than 4 weeks after surgery.

### Open Reduction Internal Fixation

- Open techniques allow the opportunity for anatomic reduction and stable fixation. However, the brittle cortical bone and small fracture fragments require sharp drill bits and appropriate drill guides, avoidance of screw

- Irreducible fractures
- Fractures with segmental bone loss requiring grafting
- Inadequate fixation by percutaneous methods

placement at the tips of spiral fragments, and gentle reduction techniques to prevent worsening of the fracture pattern. Fixation techniques include K-wires, screws, plate fixation techniques, intraosseous wiring, tension band wiring, intramedullary fixation techniques, and external fixation (Figure 2–6). The choice of technique depends upon the fracture pattern and degree of soft tissue injury. The goal is to provide maximal stability with minimal soft tissue injury and minimal prominence of the fixation device, hopefully obviating the need for later removal. Open techniques such as wiring and plating usually are reserved for open fractures with significant tissue injury. Segmental bone loss or comminution requires bone grafting and plate fixation (Box 2–5).

## Approaches

- The midaxial or lateral approach provides exposure with minimal disruption to tendon or neurovascular structures. Through a lateral approach, with elevation at the level of the periosteum, both fracture reduction and rigid fixation can be accomplished without risk of late tendon scarring to hardware. Proximal phalanx fractures can be approached by excision of the ulnar sagittal band. Laterally

based implants, such as the 90-degree condylar plate, do not interfere with the extensor tendons. Cadaveric studies have demonstrated similar biomechanical properties to the more traditional dorsal approach.[28]

- Some believe that the dorsal approach gives better exposure of the proximal and middle phalanges, even though the approach requires incision and repair of the extensor mechanism and risks scarring of the extensor tendon to implants. A straight dorsal midline incision is made carefully to preserve the veins and epitenon, and then the extensor mechanism is longitudinally split down to the level of bone.

## Rehabilitation

- When internal plate fixation is used, immediate protected motion must be started to prevent the development of tendon adhesion and stiffness. Motion should be started as soon as possible and no later than 4 weeks after surgery.

### External Fixation

- External fixation is indicated for management of severe soft tissue injuries. The external fixation device may be a temporizing measure until soft tissue coverage is achieved, or the external fixator may be the definitive fixation device. Small, unilateral fixators are placed midaxially. Mini-open techniques allow pin placement while avoiding neurovascular structures. Depending on the soft tissue state and bone healing, the external fixator is removed in 3 to 6 weeks.

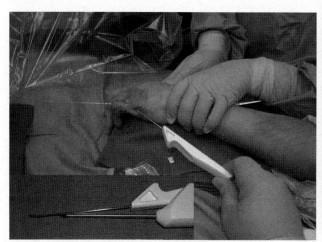
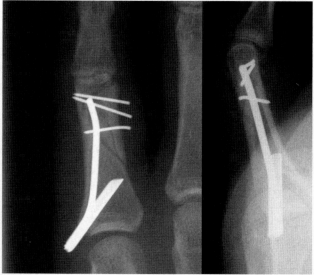

Figure 2–6:

**A,** Percutaneous insertion of a flexible intramedullary rod designed by Orbay. The insert demonstrates the awl and rod assembly. The awl is used to initiate entry into the medullary canal and advancement of the flexible rod. **B,** The rod is inserted in the proximal phalanx and locked at the base.

# Complications

## Loss of Motion

- The most common complication in the treatment of any phalangeal injury is loss of motion. Range of motion exercises within 3 to 4 weeks of injury help prevent long-term loss of motion. Loss of motion may result from intraarticular adhesion formation, capsular and ligamentous contracture, and tendon adhesion formation. Intraarticular stiffness can be prevented by immobilization in the "safe position," with the MCP joints flexed to 90 degrees and the interphalangeal joints extended. Once joint contracture develops, it is treated with aggressive physical therapy. Surgical release of posttraumatic contracted joints has been of some benefit.
- Extraarticular flexor tendon adhesions are a less common but devastating complication of extraarticular fractures. The initial fracture causes an injury to the flexor tendon sheath. Adhesions form between the flexor tendon and the tendon sheath. This situation can be prevented by early mobilization to prevent healing of the tendon to the sheath. Atraumatic technique that minimizes injury to the flexor tendon sheath (i.e., by errant K-wires) also may help prevent flexor tendon adhesions. A patient with flexor tendon adhesions will have full passive flexion and full active extension, with loss of active flexion. If aggressive therapy with blocking exercises does not break the tendons free, open tenolysis followed by early therapy improves motion in most patients.

## Malunion

- Malunion results from loss of closed reduction, failure of internal fixation, and/or inadequate initial reduction. Resultant angular and rotational deformity can result in compromise, often leading to muscle imbalance, grip and pinch weakness, and pain. Rotational deformity also can result in deviation of the digit, often affecting the function of the other digits.[29] Reconstructive osteotomies provide significant benefit to patients with established malunions. Corrective osteotomies have been described both at the malunion site and in situ. Although an osteotomy at the site of the fracture can provide the greatest source of correction of the deformity, it also can result in the formation of adhesions of the surrounding flexor and extensor tendons.[30] Internal fixation with reconstructive in situ osteotomies, including step-cut osteotomies, closing wedge osteotomies, or transverse osteotomies, provide the benefit of restoring alignment and rotation without compromising motion through the creation of soft tissue adhesions.
- Adequate initial evaluation and reduction prevent early treatment gaffes. Vigilant follow-up helps in the detection of failed reduction and internal fixation. Early detection is essential, as revision of internal fixation beyond 3 weeks is extremely difficult.

## Infection

- Infection may result from open fractures (recognized or unrecognized), pin sites, and/or internal fixation devices. Open fractures of the hand generally have a lower infection rate compared to other body sites because of the excellent blood supply to the hand. Nevertheless, finger fractures often result from severe crush injuries, which may yield a large amount of devitalized tissue. Appropriate early debridement and microvascular repair where appropriate helps prevent infection secondary to open fracture. Pin site infections are managed with proper cleansing of the pins and oral antibiotic suppression. In the case of frank osteomyelitis, loose hardware, pyarthrosis, or overlying cellulitis, irrigation and debridement including hardware removal usually are necessary.

## Nonunion

- Symptomatic nonunion of phalangeal fractures is rare, most often resulting from severe comminution and bone loss. Revision internal fixation with intercalary allograft as necessary usually achieves union. Nonunion of distal phalangeal tuft fractures is common and usually asymptomatic. A symptomatic nonunion of a distal phalangeal shaft fracture may result from entrapment of the germinal matrix of the nail bed within the fracture. Distal phalangeal shaft nonunions can be healed with rigid internal fixation with two buried Kirschner wires.

# Conclusion

- Successful treatment of phalangeal fractures and dislocations requires deep respect for the integrity and importance of the soft tissues of the finger and hand. Carefully balancing the need for both rigidity of fixation and early mobilization leads to optimal outcome in treatment of these injuries.

# References

1. Chung KC, Spilson SV: The frequency and epidemiology of hand and forearm fractures in the United States. *J Hand Surg [Am]* 26:908-915, 2001.
   This study thoroughly evaluates the epidemiology of hand and forearm fractures in the United States.

2. Frazier WH, Miller M, Fox RS, et al: Hand injuries: incidence and epidemiology in an emergency service. *JACEP* 7:265-268, 1978.
   This study describes the epidemiology and nature of soft tissue and bony injuries in the hand.

3. Roser SE, Gellman H: Comparison of nail bed repair versus nail trephination for subungual hematomas in children. *J Hand Surg [Am]* 24:1166-1170, 1999.
   Operative and nonoperative treatments were compared in 53 pediatric patients with a subungual hematoma and intact nail and nail folds, with no difference in outcomes seen between the groups.

4. Park CM, Spinner M: Irreducible fractures of the distal phalanx of the hand. *Bull Hosp Joint Dis* 37:24-29, 1976.

5. DaCruz DJ, Slade RJ, Malone W: Fractures of the distal phalanges. *J Hand Surg [Br]* 13:350-352, 1988.
   Study of 110 patients with fractures of the distal phalanx indicates that fewer than one in three patients with such injuries recovered after 6 months.

6. Kronlage SC, Faust D: Open reduction and screw fixation of mallet fractures. *J Hand Surg [Br]* 29:135-138, 2004.
   Twelve patients with mallet fractures treated by open reduction internal fixation with small screws were reviewed.

7. Rettig ME, Dassa G, Raskin KB: Volar plate arthroplasty of the distal interphalangeal joint. *J Hand Surg* 26A:940-944, 2001.
   Volar plate arthroplasty of the distal interphalangeal joint was used to treat 10 patients with impaction of the volar base of the distal phalanx and chronic dorsal subluxation of the distal phalanx at an average of 8 weeks after injury.

8. Leddy JP, Packer JW: Avulsion of the profundus tendon insertion in athletes. *J Hand Surg [Am]* 2:66-69, 1977.

9. Deitch MA, Kiefhaber TR, Comisar BR, Stern PJ: Dorsal fracture dislocations of the proximal interphalangeal joint: surgical complications and long-term results. *J Hand Surg* 24A:914-923, 1999.
   This retrospective study assessed the short-term complications and long-term results of operative treatment of acute unstable dorsal proximal interphalangeal joint dislocations treated by two methods: open reduction internal fixation and volar plate arthroplasty.

10. Eaton RG, Malerich MM: Volar plate arthroplasty of the proximal interphalangeal joint: a review of ten years' experience. *J Hand Surg [Am]* 5:260-268, 1980.

11. Seno N, Hashizume H, Inoue H, Imatani J, Morito Y: Fractures of the base of the middle phalanx of the finger. Classification, management, and long-term results. *JBJS* 79-B:758-763, 1997.
    The authors classified fractures of the base of the middle phalanx into five types and underscored the importance of restoring articular congruency and stability.

12. Newington DP, Davis TR, Barton NJ: The treatment of dorsal fracture-dislocation of the proximal interphalangeal joint by closed reduction and Kirschner wire fixation: a 16-year follow up. *J Hand Surg* 26B:537-540, 2001.
    The authors described ten patients who had sustained eleven unstable dorsal fracture-dislocations of finger proximal interphalangeal joints and who were reviewed at a mean follow-up of 16 years. All were treated acutely by closed reduction and transarticular K-wire fixation of the proximal interphalangeal joint, without any attempt at reduction of the fracture of the base of the middle phalanx, which probably involved 30% to 60% of the articular surface. Seven of ten patients complained of no finger pain pain or stiffness, and none complained of severe pain. There was a mean fixed flexion deformity of 8° at the proximal interphalangeal joint, which had a mean arc of movement of 85°. Although subchondral sclerosis and mild joint space narrowing were observed in some instances, there were no severe degenerative changes. The authors concluded that this technique is a reliable treatment method for these injuries and produces satisfactory long-term results.

13. Weiss AP: Cerclage fixation for fracture dislocation of the proximal interphalangeal joint. *Clin Orthop* 327:21-28, 1996.
    The author describes the technique and results of the volar cerclage wiring technique for PIP fracture dislocations in 12 patients.

14. Williams RM, Kiefhaber TR, Sommerkamp TG, Stern PJ: Treatment of unstable dorsal proximal interphalangeal fracture/dislocations using a hemi-hamate autograft. *J Hand Surg [Am]* 28:856-865, 2003.
    The authors describe the technique and results of hemi-hamate autograft for fracture-dislocations of the PIP joint with fractures involving greater than 50 of the articular surface in 13 patients.

15. Bain GI, Mehta JA, Heptinstall RJ, Bria M: Dynamic external fixation for injuries of the proximal interphalangeal joint. *JBJS* 80B:1014-1019, 1998.
    Operations were carried out to obtain stability, followed by application of a dynamic external fixator in twenty patients with a mean age of 29 years. This provided stability and distraction and allowed controlled passive movement. Most patients (70%) had a chronic lesion, and the mean time from injury to surgery was 215 days (3 to 1953). The final mean range of movement was 12° to 86°. Complications included redislocation and septic arthritis, which affected the outcome, and four pin-track infections and two breakages of the hinge, which did not influence the result. The PIP Compass hinge is a useful adjunct to surgical reconstruction of the injured PIP joint.

16. Slade JF, Baxamusa TH, Wolfe SW: External fixation of proximal interphalangeal joint fracture dislocations. *Atlas Hand Clin* 5:1-29, 2000.
    The use of distraction-external fixation in the treatment of PIP fracture-dislocations is discussed, and the technique of application of the authors' mini K-wire external fixator is described. In a small series of patients treated with this device, the authors report good range of motion without complications.

17. Stern PJ, Roman RJ, Kiefhaber TR, McDonough JJ et al: Pilon fractures of the proximal interphalangeal joint. *J Hand Surg* 16A:844-850, 1991.
    This study reviews three treatment methods in 20 patients, including splint, skeletal traction through the middle phalanx, and open reduction with Kirschner pins, with failure to restore anatomic reduction and normal motion in all patients.

18. Schenck RR: Dynamic traction and early passive movement for fractures of the proximal interphalangeal joint. *J Hand Surg [Am]* 11:850-858, 1986.

19. Kasparyan NG, Hotchkiss RN: Dynamic skeletal fixation in the upper extremity. *Hand Clin* 13:643-663, 1997.
    The authors review the principles and uses of dynamic external fixation in the upper extremity.

20. Durham-Smith G, McCarten GM: Volar plate arthroplasty for closed proximal interphalangeal joint injuries. *J Hand Surg* 17B:422-428, 1992.
    This article describes a current technique of repair for these injuries and its evolution from Eaton's original procedure, with results of 71 cases provided.

21. Dionysian E, Eaton RG: The long-term outcome of volar plate arthroplasty of the proximal interphalangeal joint. *J Hand Surg* 25A:429-437, 2000.
    The authors reported good long-term outcomes in 17 patients following volar plate arthroplasty for a fracture-dislocation of the PIP joint.

22. London PS: Sprains and fractures involving the interphalangeal joints. *Hand* 3:155-158, 1971.

23. Weiss AP, Hastings H: Distal unicondylar fractures of the proximal phalanx. *J Hand Surg* 18A:594-599, 1993.
    The authors review treatment of 38 consecutive patients with distal unicondylar fractures of the proximal phalanx, advocating operative fixation.

24. Vahey JW, Wegner DA, Hastings H: Effect of proximal phalangeal fracture deformity on extensor tendon function. *J Hand Surg* 23A:673-681, 1998.

25. Kuhn KM, Dao KD, Shin AY: Volar A1 pulley approach for fixation of avulsion fractures of the base of the proximal phalanx. *J Hand Surg* 26A:762-771, 2001.
    The authors describe 10 cases of proximal phalanx base avulsion fractures with collateral ligament insufficiency treated with open reduction internal fixation through an A1 pulley approach.

26. Gonzalez MH, Hall RF Jr: Intramedullary fixation of metacarpal and proximal phalangeal fractures of the hand. *Clin Orthop* 327:47-54, 1996.
    The authors describe the use of intramedullary fixation for fixation of fractures of the metacarpal and proximal phalanx.

27. Horton TC, Hatton M, Davis TR: A prospective randomized controlled study of fixation of long oblique and spiral shaft fractures of the proximal phalanx: closed reduction and percutaneous Kirschner wiring versus open reduction and lag screw fixation. *J Hand Surg* 28B:5-9, 2003.
    No significant differences could be found in subjective, radiographic, or functional outcomes between these two types of fixation for unstable phalanx shaft fractures.

28. Ouellette EA, Dennis JJ, Latta LL, et al: The role of soft tissues in plate fixation of proximal phalanx fractures. *Clin Orthop* 418:213-218, 2004.
    The tension band effect of plate fixation and the contribution of soft tissues to that effect were examined biomechanically in human cadaver proximal phalanges, suggesting that laterally placed plates may be as effective as dorsally based plates.

29. van der Lei B, de Jonge J, Robnson PH, Klasen HJ: Correction osteotomies of phalanges and metacarpals for rotational and angular malunion: a long term follow up and a review of the literature. *J Trauma* 35:902-908, 1993.

30. Trumble T, Gilbert M: In situ osteotomy for extra-articular malunion of the proximal phalanx. *J Hand Surg* 23A:821-826, 1998.

# 3

# Fractures and Dislocations Involving the Metacarpal Bone

Andrew D. Markiewitz

MD, BS, Assistant Professor, Department of Surgery, Uniformed Services University of the Health Sciences, Bethesda, MD; Volunteer Staff Associate Professor, University of Cincinnati; Hand Surgery Specialists, Inc., Cincinnati, OH

## Introduction

- Although common, metacarpal fractures produce their share of treatment dilemmas and complications. The border digits, especially the fifth metacarpal, are injured frequently and represent up to 40% of all hand fractures.[1] Callous treatment can result in shortening, rotation, angulation, and tendon imbalances. Treatment should be matched to the stability of the fracture. Recent advances have addressed surgical indications, surgical techniques, and surgical implants.
- Surgery is indicated in fractures with significant malalignment, open fractures, soft tissue injuries (artery, nerve, and tendon), and associated orthopaedic trauma, which necessitate early use of the hand. Damage to the soft tissue envelope further complicates recovery if the damage is underestimated. Despite optimal treatment and rehabilitation, dissatisfying results may occur.
- Typically given less credit than they deserve, metacarpal bones fill an essential role in the hand. They provide the hand space to grasp and to hold objects spanning the distance from the carpus to the phalanges. Loss of function lessens the patient's strength and motion and may lead to disability. This chapter looks at the anatomy, function, injury patterns, and treatment of metacarpal fractures and dislocations of the carpometacarpal (CMC) and metacarpophalangeal (MCP) joints.

## Anatomy

- The metacarpals stretch from their stable articulations with the carpus to their more flexible associations with the proximal phalanges. At their base, they are bound by intricate ligaments to each other and to the carpus.[2] The shafts are roughly triangular tubes bordered by the interossei muscles, which are the primary deforming force for transverse shaft fractures.[1]
- The metacarpal head has a unique "cam" configuration that provides increased stability with flexion (Figure 3–1). The volar portion of the head is wider than the dorsal portion.[3] Thus, the collateral ligaments, which originate from dorsal on the head, tighten with flexion to further stabilize the joint. Abduction and adduction are seen with joint extension but not with flexion. This multiaxial condyloid joint permits an arc of motion from 15 degrees of hyperextension to 110 degrees of flexion,[4] in addition to abduction, adduction, and circumduction.[5] The volar plate in combination with the contiguous intermetacarpal ligament provides volar stability.[5] The dorsal restraints are less developed. Because of its large articular surface, the head has a limited blood supply, which places it at risk for avascular necrosis with injury or excessive dissection. The thumb sacrifices motion for stability at the MCP joint.

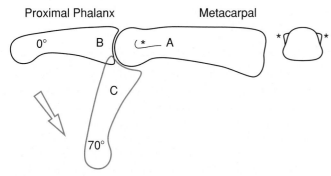

Figure 3–1:
Immobilization should be performed with the metacarpophalangeal joint flexed over 60 degrees to keep the collaterals at length to prevent stiffness. The collaterals are longer with flexion because of the cam effect of the metacarpal head shape.

## Evaluation

- Clinical evaluation combines the patient's history with the physical examination and appropriate studies. In addition to an open wound, alignment remains the key determinant to intervention. Angulation can vary depending on location and the metacarpal involved. Shortening can affect extensor function. Rotation is essentially unacceptable. Thus, the fingers should be examined in extension and flexion. The nails should align well together in extension. As the fingers flex, they should remain aligned and appear to angle toward the scaphoid tuberosity without overlapping. Evaluating the patient's uninjured hand allows appreciation of subtle normal variation. Standard radiographs include posteroanterior (PA), lateral, and oblique radiographs. Injuries to the MCP joint or the metacarpal head are better seen with the Brewerton view, which removes the overlap between the head and base of the proximal phalanx.[6] Seamoids, normally volar to the MCP joint, may be visualized inside the joint. This indicates a trapped volar plate, which can prevent closed reduction in cases of MCP dislocations.[5] Skyline or tangential views can be used if a "fight bite" is suspected[4] (Figure 3–2). Metacarpal base fractures may require computed tomography (CT) to better visualize their relationship to the carpus.

## Surgical Indications

- Most metacarpal fractures remain stable in a cast or a splint. Close follow-up is recommended if immobilization is used for fractures that are relatively nondisplaced but have unstable tendencies. As elucidated by Stern,[7] there are several clear-cut indications for operative intervention: rotational deformity, intraarticular displacement greater than 1 mm, open injuries, segmental bone loss, polytrauma, multiple upper extremity fractures, and associated soft tissue injuries. Shortening and fracture displacement also may warrant consideration. Individual patient factors are included in planning.

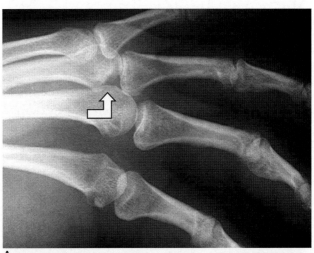

A

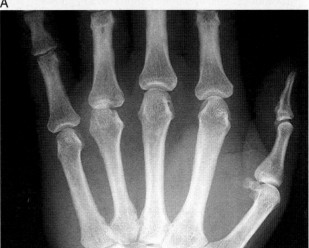

B

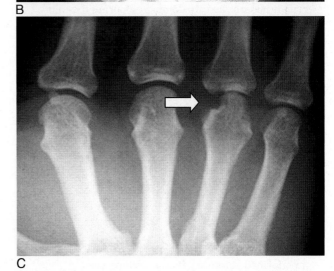

C

Figure 3–2:
Standard radiographs **(A, B)** help in most cases, although specialty films such as the Brewerton view can uncover head deformity from fight bites or boxing injuries **(C)**. The Brewerton view flexes the metacarpophalangeal joint to 65 degrees. The fingers then lie flat on the film with the thumb extended, and the tube angled radially 15 degrees.

# Metacarpal Base

- Fractures of the metacarpal base can be associated with carpal fractures. These injuries can be overlooked because the trauma may be limited as in a clenched fist injury with no discernible metacarpal rotation. Blows to a clenched fist typically produce dorsal injuries to the capitate, the hamate, and the base of the third metacarpal. The volar portion of the metacarpals also may be injured.[8] Because 15% of fourth and fifth metacarpal base fractures are associated with metacarpal neck fractures, cursory evaluation may miss the second injury.[8,9]
- CMC fracture-dislocations are high-energy injuries produced by axial loads combined with shear stresses. Looking at one edge of the spectrum, Garcia-Elias et al.[10] defined these injuries into three groups: axial-ulnar disruptions, axial-radial disruptions (most common), and combined axial-radial-ulnar disruptions. Prognosis is related to the accompanying soft tissue injuries.[10] However, at the lower end of the force spectrum, fracture-dislocations from a longitudinal force may split the arch and lead to its collapse, similar to Lisfranc fracture-dislocations. The flexor carpi ulnaris and extensor carpi ulnaris are deforming forces on the ulnar portion. The metacarpals may also be driven through the carpal bones in a dorsal direction. These fractures shear off the dorsal lip of the CMC joints.[8]
- All of these patterns are difficult to interpret and are frequently missed. However, in the absence of swelling, the clinical examination reveals a flattened arch and a wider hand profile. Although hard to see dorsal fractures on plain radiographs, PA radiographs show overlap of the metacarpals on the carpal bones obscuring the joints (Figure 3–3, A). A lateral radiograph shows dorsal displacement of the metacarpals relative to the carpus (Figure 3–3, B).
- If unable to explain the altered hand appearance on standard radiographs, one should order special plain radiographs (Brewerton view or a 60-degree supinated view [fifth CMC] or a 60-degree pronated view [second CMC]) or a CT scan with 3-dimensional reconstruction (preferred).[10] A 30- to 45-degree pronated PA view helps define the base of the fourth and fifth metacarpal bases. CT scans help define the fragment location and size.[7,11]
- The index, middle, and ring metacarpals are rigidly fixed. Significant force is necessary to fracture and displace these metacarpal bases. Early closed reduction may be possible if performed before significant swelling occurs. Reduction may be impaired by soft tissue interposition, such as muscle, tendon, or capsule. Reduction is essential to prevent late complications of stiffness, loss of flexion, and loss of strength; however, a study showed that 40% of patients with arthrosis at the base of the fifth metacarpal still had acceptable function.[12] Preferably, these fractures are treated with pin fixation or dorsal plates to prevent redisplacement.

## Author's Preferred Treatment

- If the fragments are large, plate and screw reduction may be easily accomplished. Shear fractures of the capitate and hamate may be stabilized with reduction of the carpal bones. Pin fixation may unload the carpus for the first 4 weeks (Figure 3–3, C and D). Small fragments can be reduced and pinned successfully. Malunions limit CMC motion and leave patients with complaints of persistent pain. Reduction of the malunions combined with aggressive therapy may limit patient disability. If symptomatic with joint destruction, fusion is an option.
- Fractures at the base of the thumb and little finger require special consideration. A Bennett fracture involves the base of the first metacarpal (Figure 3–4, A). This is an intraarticular fracture with special anatomic concerns. The thumb metacarpal is deformed by the pull of the extensor pollicis longus tendon, the adductor pollicis tendon, and especially the abductor pollicis longus tendon. Without support from an adjacent metacarpal, the thumb metacarpal may rotate and shorten.
- Rolando and Bennett fractures affect the base of the thumb, and continuity must be restored to prevent early arthritis.[13–16] Closed reduction is difficult and uses traction, pronation, and pressure on the shaft in a volar direction. The volar ulnar portion of the thumb base is the attachment site for the powerful stabilizing anterior oblique ligament. Displacing dorsally and supinating with the effects of the attached tendons, the metacarpal must be reduced to the volar metacarpal fragment. This action improves stability by restoring bony and ligamentous anatomy and minimizes joint incongruity.[6,13] If nondisplaced, cast immobilization is an option. Close monitoring should be used to ensure healing without significant displacement.[14,17] Patients whose articular step-off is greater than 1 mm have more symptoms.[16,18] Larger fragments also should be treated surgically.[14] If displaced, an attempt at closed reduction may be used with pin fixation to prevent redisplacement. Pins should be placed into the second metacarpal base and the trapezium[19] (Figure 3–4, B). Understand that many other fractures, including extraarticular fractures, are lumped into this classification when referred to the specialist (Figure 3–4, C and D).
- Because many Bennett fractures are resistant to closed reduction, treatment often requires open reduction and fixation. The volar (Wagner) approach is performed as follows. The curved approach is made radial to the thenar muscles to expose the shaft and the CMC joint[19]; supination exposes the fragment, and pronation reduces the shaft onto the fragment; fixation techniques depend on fragment size. If screw

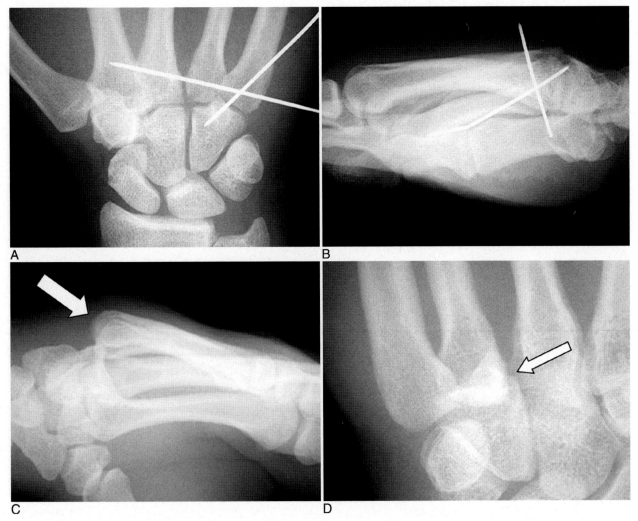

Figure 3–3:
Commonly, injuries to the metacarpal bases include metacarpal fractures, carpal fractures, and dislocations.
**A,** AP view of a fracture-dislocation of the 4–5 carpometacarpal joints. **B,** Lateral view. **C,** Pin fixation, lateral view. **D,** Lateral view.

fixation is rigid, shorter immobilization times may be used, allowing a controlled transition to a splint. If the base is significantly comminuted, traction may be used. Traction can be used against the second metacarpal using K-wires or an external fixation device.

- Rolando fractures are a **Y-** or **T**-shaped intraarticular fracture of the base of the thumb metacarpal. A similar approach to that used for a Bennett fracture can be used with a Rolando fracture. Plate fixation is a better option in Rolando fracture than in Bennett fractures.[20] Comminuted fractures may require traction or external fixation to prevent collapse.

- Similar fractures to a Bennett or Rolando fracture are present in the fifth metacarpal. The flexor carpi ulnaris and extensor carpi ulnaris tendons adduct and shorten the metacarpal.[21] Treatment of these reverse Bennett fractures is similar to that in the thumb.

## Metacarpal Shaft

- Transverse fractures are deformed by the interossei muscles into an apex dorsal position,[22] or they override and shorten. Oblique fractures can rotate and shorten. The index and middle metacarpals accommodate less than 15 degrees of angulation. Typically, the ring and small finger can tolerate up to 40 degrees of angulation resulting from CMC motion at the hamate articulation. The thumb has significant CMC motion; thus, up to 30 degrees of angulation can be tolerated. Age and occupation affect the decision process. Fracture angulation has a theoretical effect on load, tendon excursion, and work to achieve full flexion.[23] Multiple metacarpal fractures, displaced fractures of border metacarpals, and open fractures typically require operative intervention. Reduction is required if excessive angulation or rotation is present. The patient's needs and

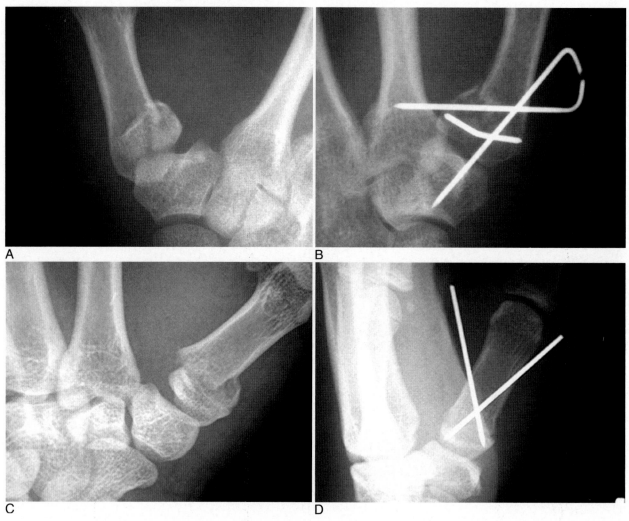

**Figure 3–4:**
Bennett fractures can be treated by closed reduction and percutaneous pin fixation **(A, B)**. A Wagner approach allows exposure if open reduction is necessary. Extraarticular metaphyseal fractures can be treated with plates or K-wires **(C, D)**.

soft tissue damage affect the duration and degree of immobilization.

- Nonoperative treatment uses MCP joint flexion to relax the interossei and uses the collateral ligaments and force on the flexed proximal phalanx to reduce the fracture.[1] Immobilization with at least 60 to 70 degrees of MCP flexion (up to 90 degrees reflects the intrinsic plus position) with the fingers extended limits stiffness. Follow-up radiographs should be obtained weekly for 2 weeks and compared to the original film to prevent loss of reduction. Because tenderness typically resolves between 4 and 6 weeks, the patient can be advanced from cast to splint with buddy straps. Some surgeons discontinue casting between 2 and 3 weeks to limit stiffness.

- With the improvement in surgical implants, management of shaft fractures has become more aggressive. Acceptable shortening has dropped from 1 cm to less than 5 mm. The intermetacarpal ligament may prevent metacarpal shortening more than 6 mm. Extensor lag to this amount

may be accommodated for by MCP hyperextension in the absence of musculotendinous shortening.[24] Minimal rotation may be allowed. However, rotation should not result in finger overlap. Seitz and Froimson[25] noted that 10 degrees of shaft rotation produced 2 cm of fingertip overlap with flexion. Spiral and oblique fractures produce more rotation than do transverse fracture patterns. Familiarity with various surgical implants allows the surgeon to treat each fracture's personality specifically.[25] No one implant is superior for every fracture faced by the practitioner.

- Percutaneous crossed Kirschner pin fixation provides good resistance to torsion in transverse patterns.[26] Adding a longitudinal pin helps improve bending resistance. Perpendicular or transverse pins can be used for index and fifth metacarpal fractures (Figure 3–5, *A*). The MCP joint is flexed to 90 degrees with traction applied. The proximal fragment is secured to the adjacent metacarpal. The distal fragment is reduced to this construct and secured. The final product appears similar to an external fixation device. This fixation to the third or fourth metacarpals can stabilize the border digits. Transverse pins can obviate use of the longitudinal pins through the MCP joint. Closed reduction supplemented with several percutaneous pins can provide stability and limit rotation. One should try to avoid impaling the extensor mechanism. K-wires can be bent and left out of the skin to ease removal; however, they risk infection if left in place too long or in hygiene issues.

- Intramedullary nails, which also avoid the open approach, limit dissection and can allow early motion (Figure 3–5, *B*). Rotational control may be limited, although modifications to the nail are being made. These nails work best in transverse and short oblique fracture patterns.[27] Using fluoroscopy to narrow down the starting point, these nails are started in the metaphyseal flare with an awl. The dorsal skin is loose and can easily be moved proximal and distal. This action allows the incision to be centered. Once started into the medullary canal, the nail is advanced to the fracture site. The fracture is reduced, and the nail is advanced. When the nail is set, the fingers are loaded onto the wrist. The nail is cut and bent. When bent, the nail end lies distal to the entry site if not centered initially. A distal Kirschner pin may be used to supplement fixation and improve rotational control. Immobilization with a splint and buddy straps allows early motion in controlled environments and daily pin care.
- Multiple pre-bent pins can be placed to stack the medullary canal[28] (Figure 3–5, *C*). These pins require a larger drill hole into the metaphyseal area. The smaller pins can be advanced through the metacarpal medullary canal.
- Transverse and short oblique fractures usually are best stabilized by plates (Figure 3–5, *D*), although interosseous

wiring in two perpendicular planes also provides adequate fixation.[29] For long oblique, comminuted, or spiral fracture patterns, low-profile plates or compression screws may provide more stable fixation than screws or pins, allowing early motion. Lag screw fixation uses 2.7-mm screws, with 2.0-mm screws reserved for smaller individuals[1] (Figure 3–5, *E*). Fractures with comminution or poor bone quality do poorly with screws alone.

- Standard dorsal plates remain effective and limit soft tissue dissection compared to lateral plates (Figure 3–5). Titanium plates diminish stress shielding because of lower stiffness.[30,31]
- Bioabsorbable implants have been used more frequently. A biomechanical test indicated stable implant strength and stiffness for up to 8 weeks.[32]

## Author's Preferred Treatment

- A dorsal approach is simply made longitudinally just lateral to the extensor tendon in order to expose the shaft (Figure 3–5). A junctura, if released, should be repaired on closure. The superficial radial nerve and the dorsal branch of the ulnar nerve are at risk radially and ulnarly, respectively. If the fracture is a long oblique, screw fixation works well and is less bulky. Reduction clamps hold the reduction, whereas standard AO technique is used to lag the fragments. Short oblique fractures may benefit from plating with a supplemental lag screw through the plate if possible. Transverse fractures or those with comminution are stabilized with a plate. With stable fixation, splinting and early motion can be used.
- Screws used in a lag fashion provide excellent compression and supplement plate fixation. If the oblique fracture line is twice the bone's diameter, lag screws alone are effective.
- External fixation devices may be useful in the treatment of open fractures with complicated wounds

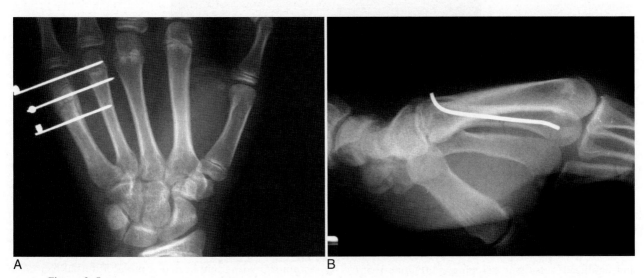

A            B

Figure 3–5:
**Transverse K-wires protect epiphyseal plates (A). Shaft fractures can be managed with various devices, including intramedullary nails (B) or multiple prebent pins (C).**

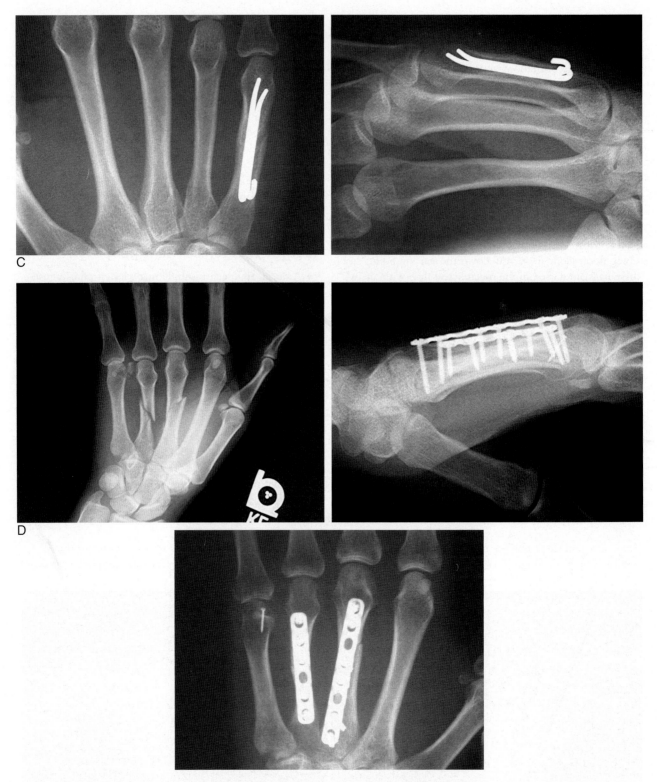

**Figure 3–5, cont'd**
Midshaft transverse and short oblique fragments can be treated with plates, especially if multiple metacarpals are involved (**D**). Long oblique fragments can be reduced with lag screws.

and significant soft tissue stripping[33,34] (Figure 3–5, *F*). New fixators are lower in profile and allow for distraction adjustments in the clinic. External fixation devices are useful, especially in the treatment of open injuries with complicated wounds. External fixation in complex fractures can be effective, with pins placed so as not to interfere with soft tissue management.[34,35] External fixation of unstable fractures has shown 94%

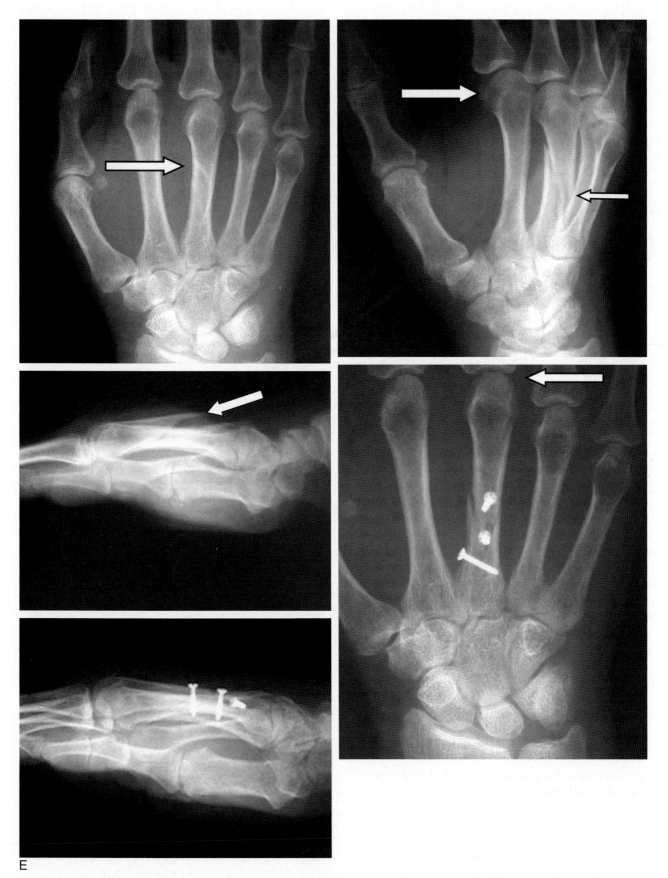

E

Figure 3–5,  cont'd

(E). External fixation is reserved for highly comminuted or open fractures to manage soft tissue issues

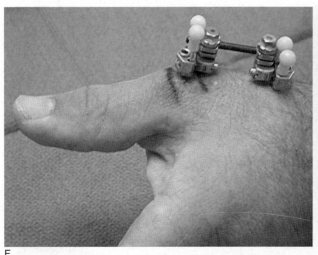
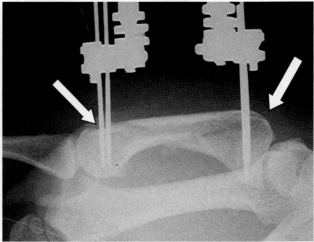

F

Figure 3–5, cont'd
**(F).** The devices can be low profile and rigid enough for early motion.

good or excellent results.[33] Alternatively, Drenth and Klasen[36] recommended transverse pins for open fractures. The pins can be bent dorsally 40 to 60 degrees to prevent interference with motion. Devices may be removed at 6 weeks, depending on healing. Staged procedures can allow the wound to stabilize before definitive bone grafting and internal fixation. Conversion to internal implants is not mandatory but may minimize wound care and ease rehabilitation. External fixation for closed injuries can lead to unnecessary complications.

- Splint use alone for shaft fractures after closed reduction has been shown to be ineffective because of skin breakdown and patient noncompliance.
- Hardware may be removed within 6 months, but a second surgery is required for plates and screws. The procedure also leaves holes that leave the patient at risk for refracture for 6 to 8 weeks. Most hardware is removed for problems with prominence or tendon irritation.

## Metacarpal Neck

- Neck fractures may produce unacceptable prominences in the palm. Although not an issue in most patients, laborers and athletes in racquet or bat sports may have difficulty gripping without discomfort.
- The acceptable degree of angulation is variable and contested in the literature. Up to 30 degrees seems to have no impact in biomechanical studies. However, interobserver and intraobserver variability affect measurement.[36] Although some authors allow up to 70 degrees of angulation,[37,38] angulation of the fifth metacarpal exceeding 30 degrees theoretically leads to decreased finger motion and flexor digiti minimi strength.[37]

Although the fourth and fifth metacarpal necks may tolerate angulation up to 60 degrees, reduction should be considered for angulation greater than 40 degrees. Generally, the second and third metacarpals accept less angulation and should be treated for dorsal angulation exceeding 15 degrees.

- Closed reduction and cast immobilization remain the mainstay of treatment (Figure 3–6). Literature has suggested elastic bandages and splints as options to decrease the need for extended rehabilitation.[38] Plastic splints can reduce the angulation by 50% and is acceptable in stable fracture patterns. Regardless of treatment, functional outcomes at 3 months are similar.
- Fixation should be strongly considered in unstable patterns. Rotation is unacceptable and should be treated

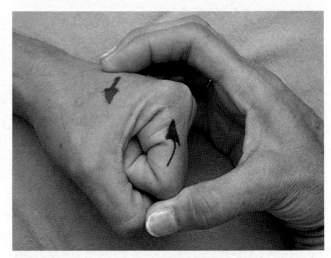

Figure 3–6:
**Reduction technique for metacarpal neck fractures uses pressure up on the flexed proximal phalanx and pressure down on the metacarpal shaft.**

with surgery. Strapping twists the proximal phalanx on its collateral ligaments but does little to change metacarpal alignment.

## Author's Preferred Treatment

- Percutaneous pin techniques are effective in reducing and stabilizing neck fractures.[26] New devices allow for reduction and pinning through one clamp. Used proximal and distal to the fracture line, transverse pins can be supplemented with longitudinal pins. Two pins through the head into the adjacent intact metacarpal head prevent rotation around a single axis. As the fracture callus is undisturbed, infection is reduced and healing progress unaffected.[10] Tendons are avoided, and the hardware is easily removed in the clinic. If buried, a clinic-based procedure is necessary. Fluoroscopy may be required to find the pins.

- The AO/ASIF minicondylar plate allows periarticular fixation from a lateral approach[39] (Figure 3–7, A). This arrangement limits the trauma to the extensor mechanism over the joint. Because this plate is weak in bending, an intact or restored opposite cortex must be achieved. Dorsal plates are prominent under the extensor mechanism and may require early removal (Figure 3–7, B).

# Metacarpal Head Fractures

- Less common, these fractures span a spectrum of injuries. Despite their rarity, attempts have been made to classify them into 10 anatomic groups[40]: collateral ligament injuries; horizontal, oblique, osteochondral, epiphyseal, and vertical fractures; head and neck fractures; comminuted fractures; bone loss; and occult fractures with avascular necrosis.[41] Comminuted head fractures, which represent 31% of the fractures, lose more than 45 degrees of motion.[40]

- Collateral injuries are common, especially in the border digits. A common example is the gamekeeper injury (for discussion, see Chapter 4). Although predominantly a ligament injury, the pattern may include a chip fracture off the metacarpal head. The index finger requires a stable radial collateral ligament because of the demands of pinch. Conversely, the same injury to the little finger produces persistent abduction.[4]

- Instability of the joint upon testing may indicate a need for acute ligamentous repair. Ligamentous injuries span the spectrum of tears in continuity from partial tears to complete tears.[21] Complete tears are unstable without a fixed endpoint. Freeland[22] recommends 2 weeks of immobilization at 30 degrees with gradual increase in motion, even for complete tears.

- If the avulsion fracture is minimally displaced, closed treatment may obviate surgery and may result in a stable joint. Light and Bednar[4] recommend buddy taping and

motion if the fracture is less than 20% of the articular surface.

- Articular injuries to the metacarpal heads may result from direct trauma, such as the common "fight bite." The head is exposed in the fist position, rendering it vulnerable to injury from teeth, walls, and associated hard objects. Although they might not displace, the overriding concern remains the potential for joint contamination. Fight bites must be washed out well. Skin incisions, if made for exposure, may be closed, but the wound should be left open and closed secondarily if large. Antibiotic coverage must be broad and cover *Staphylococcus, Streptococcus,* and anaerobes (e.g., *Eikenella*).

- Articular fragments should be reduced to prevent incongruity. If minimally displaced, close follow-up should verify healing without displacement or avascular necrosis. Early protected motion is the key to preventing motion loss despite accurate reduction. Kirschner wires remain an option for small fragments; however, the newer smaller implants improve stability, allow earlier motion, and prevent pin complications. Reduction can be achieved with wires and exchanged to screws without drilling (i.e., 0.028 wire = 0.7 mm; 0.035 wire = 0.9 mm; 0.045 wire = 1.1 mm; 0.062 wire = 1.6 mm). If necessary based on fracture configuration, screws may need to be buried to avoid impingement along the joint surface (Figure 3–7, C).

- If the fragment is displaced more than 1 mm or involves more than 20% of the articular surface, open reduction and fixation is recommended to prevent ligamentous laxity.[41,42] Firm screw fixation allows early motion and limits stiffness.[4,42] The screw heads should be buried or enter from outside the arc of motion. A Herbert screw can be used if the fracture is intraarticular or small.[4] Bioabsorbable devices may have a role in the treatment of these fractures. Long-term results are better if the joint is accurately reduced; however, this action does not guarantee that all fractures will have an excellent outcome.[3] Comminution, displacement, and soft tissue injury have resulted in a worse prognosis.[3,42]

## Author's Preferred Technique

- A curvilinear incision is made over the MCP joint. The extensor tendon is identified. Leaving a cuff of the extensor mechanism to repair, the surgical incision is carried through the sagittal bands, allowing full exposure of the joint. Although some surgeons prefer exposure through the ulnar sagittal band, one may be served by determining which approach provides better exposure of the fracture for fixation. If the capsule is intact, a transverse incision can be made to alter repair lines. Because the collateral ligaments provide vascular support to the metacarpal head, injury to these structures should be avoided to minimize the risk of avascular necrosis. The

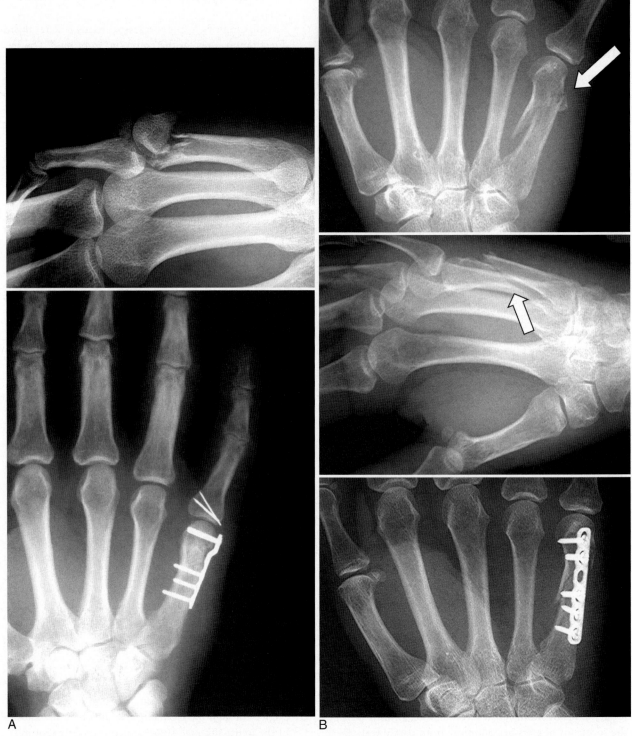

Figure 3–7:
Head and neck fractures can be fixed with pins, screws, or plates. **A,** Condylar plate can be placed on the border metacarpals. (Courtesy TG Sommerkamp.) **B,** If there is enough room distally, a dorsal plate can be adapted.

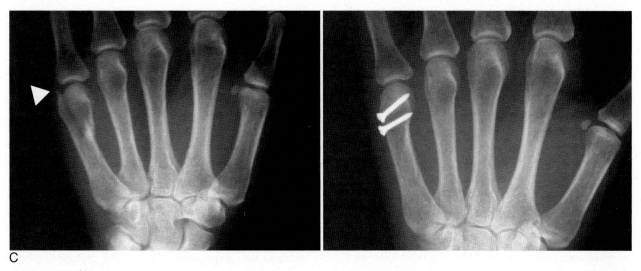

C

Figure 3–7, cont'd
**C,** K-wires can provisionally fix a fragment and then be exchanged with screws. K-wires limit early motion.

joint should be irrigated free of debris, including cartilage fragments that are found floating in the joint, underscoring the shearing nature of these fractures. If too small for fixation, excision of the fragment prevents future locking and pain.[21] Excellent exposure eases reduction of the articular surface. Pins can be used to help with reduction. Wires can be left if the fragments are too small.[41] If the fragments are large enough, the temporary K-wires can be directly exchanged with screws as noted earlier. This exchange allows early motion and circumvents the potential for pin tract infections. Bone graft or substitute may be necessary to fill in behind cartilage if gaps exist when the articular surface is restored. If head and neck fractures coexist, a minicondylar plate may be necessary.[15] Early motion into full flexion must be controlled to allow the extensor mechanism to heal without stretching out.

## Metacarpophalangeal Joint Dislocations

- MCP dislocations are classified as dorsal or volar. Each class can be further typed as reducible (simple) or irreducible (complex). Volar dislocations are relatively rare because of the strong volar restraints; however, with dislocation they usually are irreducible. A host of causes have been described in the few incidents that have occurred.[5] Dorsal dislocations are more common than volar dislocations injuries[43] because of the weak dorsal restraints. The thumb and index are more frequently involved.[5]
- Patients with a dorsal dislocation are unable to move their MCP joints. Slight flexion may be preserved with a volar dislocation. Surface anatomy can be changed with either dislocation pattern. Swelling and pain are present.
- Standard radiographs should be reviewed with an eye to joint preservation and alignment. A change in the joint

space (narrowing) when compared to adjacent MCP joints or the presence of debris in the joint should alert one to the diagnosis.
- Dorsal dislocations are reducible when the phalanx remains in contact with the head and the volar plate remains outside of the joint (Figure 3–8). These dislocations may appear more deforming than volar dislocations, as the joint postures in 60 degrees of extension[21] and the proximal phalanx slides dorsal to the metacarpal head.

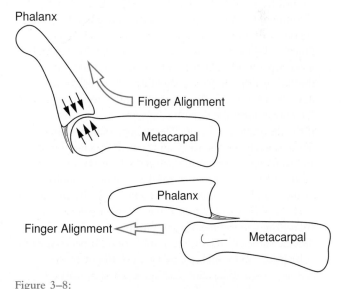

Figure 3–8:
Dislocations of the metacarpophalangeal joint can be simple or complex. If the joint still is opposed, as in a simple dislocation *(top)*, the deformity appears greater, but the volar plate should not become interposed during reduction as long as hyperextension or traction is not performed. Either hyperextension or traction may pull the volar plate dorsally into the joint, decreasing the apparent deformity but converting the dislocation to a complex one, requiring open reduction *(bottom)*.

- The metacarpal head can become trapped in the tendons and ligamentous structures that usually support it. Buttonholing in a volar direction occurs between the natatory ligament, the lumbrical radially, the flexors ulnarly, and the superficial transverse metacarpal ligament proximally.[5] Unfortunately, when approached from the volar side, a neurovascular bundle is found over the metacarpal head.

## Author's Preferred Technique

- Reduction of simple dorsal dislocations uses joint contact as an edge to rotate the phalanx down as the wrist and proximal interphalangeal joints are flexed to relax the extrinsic flexors.[44] The base of the proximal phalanx is pushed along the dorsum of the metacarpal to maintain contact and limit the risk of entrapping the volar plate. Traction is contraindicated because it may convert this reducible simple dislocation into an irreducible complex dislocation by entrapping the volar plate.
- Complex dislocations require open reduction to clear the volar plate from the joint or release the trapped metacarpal head.[44] Complex dislocations are more commonly found with the index and small fingers.[21] As the phalanx slides along the dorsal surface of the head with the dislocation (see Figure 3–8), the volar plate, which now is displaced dorsal to the joint, becomes entrapped. With an entrapped volar plate, the joint space appears widened. These dislocations appear less worrisome than simple dislocations because the fingers are not hyperextended. Glickel, Barron, and Eaton[45] recommend a volar approach extending from the palmar creases to the midaxial line for the index and small fingers. The neurovascular bundle is stretched over the metacarpal head, which pushes it precariously close to the skin waiting to be damaged by a deep cut. The flexor tendon is displaced dorsally and is tense, requiring A1 release for reduction.[44]
- If the dislocation is irreducible, an approach from the dorsal side allows one to avoid the neurovascular bundle and to fix associated head fractures, which can occur in up to 25% of cases.[21,44,45] A similar curvilinear approach or the straight dorsal incision recommended by Becton et al.[46] can be used. Use of a freer or joker can ease the volar plate and the flexor back into place. Anesthesia can provide sufficient relaxation in most cases. If necessary, the volar plate can be split, taking care not to gouge the cartilage. Volar dislocations are approached similarly if they cannot be reduced closed.
- Once reduced, stability should be tested through a range. Testing determines the range of stability, and immobilization should be kept within the range for 2 weeks. After 2 weeks or if the joint is completely stable, the joint should be allowed to flex over the range with extension blocked by at least 10 degrees.[21] The patient is slowly weaned from the splint by 6 weeks,[44] although

protection with straps should be continued during sports activities for remainder of the season.

# Carpometacarpal Joint Dislocations

- These injuries can occur from high-energy trauma, falls, or direct blows. Carpal fractures can occur and should be suspected. Any dislocation leads to tenderness, loss of grip strength,[46] and decreased range of motion. These injuries may be overlooked as the trauma team stabilizes the patient, but a secondary survey should be performed on all trauma patients, looking for non-life–threatening injuries.[46,47]
- Initial radiographs should include PA, oblique (supination or pronation[7]), and lateral views. Forearm rotation with oblique radiographs uncovers the border CMC joints. Disruption in the normal metacarpal cascade, alteration of the CMC joint surfaces, or overlap of bone edges should be suspicious, especially with impaired hand function. Proximal phalangeal fractures can occur frequently with a dislocation.[5] Unfortunately, these injuries can be missed if one is unfamiliar with the views.[47] Therefore, in most cases CT scans remain the standard imaging study for defining the degree of injury. An anatomic and pathomechanical study of the fourth and fifth CMC injuries found common fractures of the dorsal capitate, third metacarpal base, and hamate.[8] Yoshida et al.[9] recommend CT scans because of the complexity of ligament injuries, fractures, and fracture-dislocations.
- The second and third CMC joints form a relatively rigid central unit between the mobile units of the first and the fourth and fifth CMC joints.[43] The second and third metacarpals have tight articulations with each other and their corresponding carpal bones. The third CMC joint involves the capitate, which lies proximal to all the other CMC joints, and forms a "keystone" to the distal transverse arch.[43,48,49] The central units motion produces 1 to 3 degrees of motion compared with 10 to 15 degrees for the fourth CMC joint and 15 to 40 degrees for the fifth CMC joint.[49,50]
- Injuries to the mobile portions (first, fourth, and fifth) are more common than injuries to the central area.[43,44] Because these injuries disrupt the transverse and longitudinal arches,[46] they are more likely to produce unsatisfactory results.[51] The distal edge of the transverse carpal ligament lies volar to the second and third metacarpal bases, placing the median nerve at risk from swelling and injury with volar dislocations of the second and third CMC joints.[52] The deep palmar arch and the ulnar nerve distal to Guyon canal lie volar to the third and fifth CMC joints, respectively.[43] The dorsal branch of the ulnar nerve lies over the dorsum of the fourth and fifth CMC joints and can be easily injured with surgery. This close relationship also exists between branches of

the superficial radial nerve and the first and second CMC joints. Lawlis and Gunther[53] noted that a concomitant ulnar nerve injury produced unsatisfactory results.

- If examined before swelling obscures the surface anatomy, the alignment of the metacarpal bases is distorted by a dorsal dislocation (see Figure 3–3). Although more rare, a volar dislocation is more difficult to identify because of the overlying musculature,[43] except with a volar radial dislocation of the fifth CMC, which, like a hip dislocation, rotates externally and shortens.

- Closed reduction of simple dislocations may be possible if treated early. However, the high energy or shear nature of the injury combined with swelling may prevent stable reduction. Stability should be confirmed before the patient leaves the operating room. Pin fixation is recommended to maintain the reduction[43,50–53] and improve the outcome.[52]

- Close observation during immobilization is necessary to avoid subluxation or redislocation.[43] It has been suggested that the key in multiple metacarpal fractures is reducing the third CMC joint.[43] If possible, a proximal phalanx blocking cast allows early digital motion at the distal and proximal interphalangeal joints. Immobilization and pins are discontinued by 6 weeks. Resistance exercises should be avoided until wrist and digital motion is optimized, although light putty may help break down some adhesions.

- Complex dislocations require an open dorsal approach,[40,44] although the personality of the fracture may alter the approach. CT scans allow definition of the pattern and illuminate the surgical approach to achieve a stable reduction.

- Delay in treatment can lead to chronic pain, weakness, and stiffness. If the delay is more than 3 weeks, open reduction usually is required. If joint destruction has occurred, fusion may be used to relieve pain but limits motion, especially in the border digits. However, posttraumatic arthritis remains a possible outcome despite prompt appropriate treatment secondary to the high degree of force that dislocates the CMC joint. Fusion of the fifth CMC joint should be performed in 20 to 30 degrees of flexion to help with grip and pain relief.[54]

- Dislocation of the thumb CMC joint requires reduction. If reducible and stable, cast immobilization for 6 weeks can be used, followed by splinting and therapy. If unstable after reduction, simple percutaneous pin fixation may be satisfactory for allowing the ligaments to heal. If the dislocation is irreducible, open ligamentous repair or reconstruction improves the chance of a stable joint.[44] If suspected early and treated early, open reduction will not require additional ligament reconstruction. Despite a stable reduction or with a delay in treatment, instability may ensue and require ligamentous reconstruction at a later date. This reconstruction can be done through a modified Wagner approach, clearing the joint of debris and using the flexor carpi radialis tendon as graft.[44]

## Soft Tissue Considerations

- Trauma to the metacarpals may compromise the soft tissue envelope. In the acute event, compartment syndrome may develop and will require release. If a release is necessary, the incisions can be used for standard approaches for shaft fractures. The extensor tendons lie close to the metacarpals. Persistent edema can lead to scarring simply from crush injuries without displaced fractures. The edema can organize and result in disproportionate stiffness refractory to intensive occupational therapy. Sensory nerves track over the wrist. Damage to these nerves, especially the superficial radial nerve and the dorsal branch of the ulnar nerve, may lead to disability from chronic pain and dysesthesias. Skin coverage is limited, and the tissue bed for skin grafting is limited over bone and tendon.

- Skin defects expose bones and tendons, increasing the risk of infection. Wounds must be aggressively washed out and debrided. Use of flaps may be necessary to preserve length or function.[55] Fractures should be fixed at length and grafting performed in an expedient manner to improve the tissue bed.

- The status of the soft tissues remains the main determinant of outcome.[56] To prevent stiffness, early motion remains the mainstay of treatment.

## Splint Use

- With the goal of limiting immobilization, splints have been revisited. Use of splints in managing stable fracture patterns is possible in compliant patients. Splints appear to be better tolerated in patients with metacarpal neck fractures than shaft fractures. Close observation is necessary to manage complications such as loss of reduction and pressure sores. Unfortunately, patients may assume that splint use indicates a lower level of concern regarding their injury.

- Colditz[57] reviewed functional fracture bracing for treatment of metacarpal fractures. Typical bracing requires compression of the surrounding musculature to stabilize the fracture. In the absence of surrounding muscles, the metacarpal brace protects a stable fracture from displacing, allows tendon motion to prevent stiffness and edema, and allows normal healing to continue. Prolonged immobilization can lead to loss of proximal interphalangeal joint extension.[58] Colditz[57] notes that intrinsics prevent bracing from working in most cases, especially multiple metacarpal fractures.

- Advancing a patient to a splint from other means of immobilization in a controlled environment can minimize recovery time and speed the patient's return to work.

## Complications

- As with any fracture, complications may result despite the best surgical decisions and techniques.[57,59] Patients may interpret complications as occurring when their expectations do not match the achieved outcome. Matching their expectations regarding pain, motion, and function to the proposed intervention is key and requires compromise.[22]
- Malunion, rotational deformity, delayed union, and nonunion should be addressed promptly if function is impacted. Bone grafting, reduction, and improved fixation are key elements for a successful outcome. Improved fixation allows earlier motion to prevent stiffness following tenolysis and osteotomy[22,60]; however, stiffness may increase after intervention.
- Intraarticular fractures regardless of anatomic reductions may result in posttraumatic arthritis.[3] Fusion may reduce the pain at the expense of flexibility. The index finger does well with fusion as the stability in pinch is important. Arthroplasty may improve motion but requires stable bone stock. Resurfacing with autogenous bone-cartilage graft has been explored but has been of variable success.[61,62]
- Extensor tendons may adhere to the raw bone surfaces. Prompt fixation allows healing despite early motion.[22] Tenolysis may be necessary and can be performed in conjunction with plate removal. Typically, this release occurs after the bone has healed and extensive therapy has been performed to optimize passive motion. Joint releases may be necessary, although expectations of motion should be realistic. Intrinsic tightness will require release if motion loss is significant.[1] Local anesthesia allows a staged release of tight structures. The outcomes of a second surgery are less than guaranteed.
- Patient factors should be addressed in order to improve healing. The patient's nutritional status should be adequate, and the patient should discontinue smoking.

## Salvage Procedures

- Metacarpal fractures may heal in a malunited position. Prior to salvage, reconstruction can be considered. Reduction of the malunions should be considered. Rotational osteotomies and "cheilectomies" are valid options. A "cheilectomy" removes a bony block around the periphery of the joint,[4] improving motion. If the head is significantly damaged, fusion of the joint, arthroplasty, or a flexible implant may be necessary. However, these options do not come close to the normal function of the MCP joint. Thus, joint preservation remains paramount. Bone stock remaining after injury and the condition of the soft tissues determine the options available. Fusion can be well tolerated at the thumb MCP. The index finger requires stability, so fusion

is recommended[3] but remains less than optimal. It limits flattening of the hand if fused in flexion or limits flexion if fused in extension.[4] Arthroplasty of the central digits leads to more satisfying results and can provide an average of 60 degrees of motion.[63] Autograft replacement from the fourth toe can be used if the metacarpal head is destroyed.[4] Vascularized transfers have been proposed; however, the average motion of 36 degrees seems limited given the risks involved.[64,65] In trauma settings, nonsalvageable portions of adjacent rays can be used.

## Rehabilitation

- The surgeon's job does not stop once the plates and pins have been applied. Intimate involvement in the rehabilitation process optimizes the surgical result by matching the protocol with the surgical stability. If poorly matched, complications may result, requiring further surgery. Although hardware removal by 3 weeks has been described in the literature, a clinical examination reveals when healing has occurred. Clinical healing may precede radiographic healing. Regardless of timing, hardware should be maintained in patients with localized tenderness to prevent reduction loss.
- Early motion protocols and edema control are important for minimizing adhesions and optimizing motion. The therapist monitors and adjusts the patient's progress.
- The rest of the upper extremity should not be neglected during the immobilization phase.
- Fixation rigidity can be checked intraoperatively. If stable, early active and passive motion can be encouraged in a controlled setting.[41] If the construct is less stable, rehabilitation can be delayed up to 3 weeks to allow some healing. Depending on the therapist or patient, motion at the wrist, distal interphalangeal joint, or proximal interphalangeal joint may be allowed to obtain some motion of the extensor mechanism.

## Summary

- Treatment of metacarpal fractures should be matched to their complexity, with an eye to associated injuries. Rehabilitation can be advanced based on fracture or fixation stability. Despite appropriate intervention, patients frequently have complications and should not be routinely assumed to all do well.

## References

1. Diao E, Welborn JH: Extraarticular fractures of the metacarpals. In Berger RA, Weiss A-PC, editors: *Hand surgery,* Philadelphia, 2004, Lippincott Williams & Wilkins.

2. Nakamura K, Patterson RM, Viegas SF: The ligament and skeletal anatomy of the second through fifth carpometacarpal joints and adjacent structures. *J Hand Surg* 26:1016-1029, 2001.

Anatomic study illustrating the complex anatomy of the CMC joints.

3. Margles SW: Intra-articular fractures of the metacarpophalangeal and proximal interphalangeal joints. *Hand Clin* 4:67-74, 1988.

4. Light TR, Bednar MS: Management of intra-articular fractures of the metacarpophalangeal joint. *Hand Clin* 10:303-314, 1994.
   Review of articular fractures that recommends operative treatment and its benefits.

5. Lattanza LL, Choi PD: Intraarticular injuries of the metacarpophalangeal and carpometacarpal joints. In Berger RA, Weiss A-PC, editors: *Hand surgery.* Philadelphia, 2004, Lippincott Williams & Wilkins.

6. Brewerton D: A tangential radiographic projection for demonstrating involvement of metacarpal heads in rheumatoid arthritis. *Br J Radiol* 40:233-234, 1967.

7. Stern PJ: Fractures of the metacarpals and phalanges. In Green DP, Hotchkiss RN, Pederson WC, editors: *Green's operative hand surgery.* New York, 1999, Churchill Livingstone.

8. Cain JE Jr, Shepler TR, Wilson MR: Hamatometacarpal fracture-dislocation: classification and treatment. *J Hand Surg* 12A:762-767, 1987.
   Categorizes fracture-dislocations into three types: dislocation only, dislocation with rim avulsion fracture, and dislocation with coronal split of the hamate.

9. Yoshida R, Shah MA, Patterson RM et al: Anatomy and pathomechanics of ring and small finger carpometacarpal joint injuries. *J Hand Surg* 28A:1035-1043, 2003.

10. Garcia-Elias M, Dobyns JH, Cooney WP III, Linscheid RL: Traumatic axial dislocations of the carpus. *J Hand Surg* 14A:446-457, 1989.
    Comprehensive description of the shear injuries of the hand and carpus. Early treatment is recommended. The outcomes remain guarded and are dependent on soft tissue injuries.

11. Markiewitz AD: Metacarpal fractures. In Trumble TE, editor: *Hand surgery update: hand, elbow, & shoulder*, Rosemont, 2003, American Society for Surgery of the Hand.

12. Bora FW Jr, Didizian NH: The treatment of injuries to the carpometacarpal joint of the small finger. *J Bone Joint Surg* 56A:1459-1463, 1974.

13. Lundeen JM, Shin AY: Clinical results of intraarticular fractures of the base of the fifth metacarpal treated by closed reduction and cast immobilization. *J Hand Surg [Br]* 25:258-261, 2000.

14. Simonian PT, Trumble TE: Traumatic dislocation of the thumb carpometacarpal joint: early ligamentous reconstruction versus closed reduction and pinning. *J Hand Surg* 21:802-806, 1996.
    Stable joints had a decreased risk of instability and improved function; thus, if unstable ligamentous reconstruction is encouraged.

15. Soyer AD: Fractures of the base of the first metacarpal: current treatment options. *JAAOS* 7:403-412, 1999.
    Complete review of assessment and treatment of first metacarpal fractures.

16. Buchler U, McColuum S, Oppikofer C: Use of a mini-condylar plate for metacarpal and phalangeal periarticular injuries. *Clin Orthop* 214:53-58, 1987.
    Comminuted fractures were reduced and held in an anatomic position, with a good result with 9/13. All fractures united.

17. Breen TF, Gelberman RH, Jupiter JB: Intra-articular fractures of the basilar joint of the thumb. *Hand Clin* 4:491-501, 1988.
    Reviews nonoperative and operative treatment for intraarticular fractures.

18. Oosterbos CJ, de Boer HH: Nonoperative treatment of Bennett's fracture: a 13-year follow-up. *J Orthop Trauma* 9:23-27, 1995.

19. Cullen JP, Parentis AM, Churchill VM, Pellegrini VD: Simulated Bennett fracture treated with closed reduction and percutaneous pinning: a biomechanical analysis of residual incongruity of the joint. *J Bone Joint Surg* 79A:413-420, 1997.
    Demonstrated that a step-off less than 2 mm was satisfactory. Recommended reducing the shaft to the volar fragment and trapezium.

20. Trumble TE: Hand fractures. In Trumble TE, editor: *Principles of hand surgery and therapy*, Philadelphia, 2000, WB Saunders.

21. Foster RJ, Hastings HH II: Treatment of Bennett, Rolando, and vertical intraarticular trapezial fractures. *Clin Orthop* 214:121-129, 1987.
    Displaced base fractures develop arthritis quickly. Rolando fractures are best treated with a plate and screws. Trapezial fractures require open reduction internal fixation (ORIF).

22. Freeland AE: Metacarpal fractures. In Freeland AE, editor: *Hand fractures: repair, reconstruction, and rehabilitation.* New York, 2000, Churchill Livingstone.

23. Rosenwasser MP, Quitkin HM: Malunion and other posttraumatic complications in the hand. In Berger RA, Weiss A-PC, editors: *Hand surgery.* Philadelphia, 2004, Lippincott Williams & Wilkins.

24. Birndorf MS, Daley R, Greenwald DP: Metacarpal fracture angulation decreases flexor mechanical efficiency in human hands. *Plast Reconstr Surg* 99:1079-1083, 1997.

25. Seitz WH, Froimson A: Management of malunited fractures of the metacarpal and phalangeal shafts. *Hand Clin* 4:529-536, 1988.

26. Kozin SH, Thoder JJ, Lieberman G: Operative treatment of metacarpal and phalangeal shaft fractures. *JAAOS* 8:111-121, 2000.

27. Klein DM, Belsole RJ: Percutaneous treatment of carpal, metacarpal, and phalangeal injuries. *Clin Orthop* 375:116-125, 2000.
    Technique and indications for percutaneous pin fixation around the hand.

28. Liew KH, Chan BK, Low CO: Metacarpal and proximal phalangeal fractures: fixation with multiple intramedullary Kirschner wires. *J Hand Surg* 25:125-130, 2000.

29. Prevel CD, Eppley BL, Jackson JR et al: Mini and micro plating of phalangeal and metacarpal fractures: a biomechanical study. *J Hand Surg* 20:44-49, 1995.

30. Gonzalez MH, Hall RF Jr: Intramedullary fixation of metacarpal and proximal phalangeal fractures of the hand. *Clin Orthop* 327:47-54, 1996.
    Technique for flexible intramedullary rods and rehabilitation.

31. Fischer KJ, Bastidas JA, Provenzano DA, Tomaino MM: Low-profile versus conventional metacarpal plating systems: a comparison of construct stiffness and strength. *J Hand Surg* 24:928-934, 1999.

32. Lister G: Intraosseous wiring of the digital skeleton. *J Hand Surg* 3:427-435, 1978.
    Classic article on two techniques for osteosynthesis in fractures and fusion.

33. Bozic KJ, Perez LE, Wilson DR et al: Mechanical testing of bioresorbable implants for use in metacarpal fracture fixation. *J Hand Surg* 26:755-761, 2001.

34. Parsons SW, Fitzgerald JA, Shearer JR: External fixation of unstable metacarpal and phalangeal fractures. *J Hand Surg [Br]* 17:151-155, 1992.
    Prospective study of the use of external fixation, with good to excellent results in unstable fracture patterns.

35. Ashmead D IV, Rothkopf DM, Watson RF, Jupiter JB: Treatment of hand injuries by external fixation. *J Hand Surg* 17:956-964, 1992.
    Technique article on treatment of fractures and fusions and rehabilitation using external fixators.

36. Drenth DJ, Klasen H: External fixation for phalangeal and metacarpal fractures. *J Bone Joint Surg [Br]* 80:227-230, 1998.

37. Leung YL, Beredjiklian PK, Monaghan BA, Bozentka DJ: Radiographic assessment of small finger metacarpal neck fractures. *J Hand Surg* 27:443-448, 2002.

38. Ali A, Hamman J, Mass DP: The biomechanical effects of angulated boxer's fractures. *J Hand Surg* 24:835-844, 1999.

39. Kuokkanen HO, Mulari-Keranen SK, Niskanen RO et al: Treatment of subcapital fractures of the fifth metacarpal bone: a prospective randomized comparison between functional treatment and reposition and splinting. *Scand J Plast Reconstr Surg* 33:315-317, 1999.

40. Ouellette EA, Freeland AE: Use of the minicondylar plate in metacarpal and phalangeal fractures. *Clin Orthop* June:38-46, 1996.
    Retrospective review of plate fixation and associated complications.

41. McElfresh EC, Dobyns JH: Intra-articular metacarpal head fractures. *J Hand Surg* 8:383-393, 1983.
    Comprehensive attempt to classify metacarpal head fractures to define management options for each class.

42. Hastings HI, Carroll C IV: Treatment of closed articular fractures of the metacarpophalangeal and proximal interphalangeal joints. *Hand Clin* 4:503-527, 1988.
    Review of articular fractures, which recommends surgical intervention for 2-mm displacement or 20% surface involvement.

43. Shibata T, O'Flanagan SJ, Ip FK, Chow SP: Articular fractures of the digits: a prospective study. *J Hand Surg* 18:225-229, 1993.

44. Jebson PJ, Engber WD, Lange RH: Dislocation and fracture-dislocation of the carpometacarpal joints. *Orthop Rev* February:19-28, 1994.

45. Glickel SZ, Barron OA, Eaton RG: Dislocations and ligament injuries in the digits. In Green DP, Hotchkiss RN, Pederson WC, editors: *Green's operative hand surgery.* New York, 1999, Churchill Livingstone.

46. Becton JL, Christian JD, Goodwin HN, Jackson JG III: A simplified technique for treating the complex dislocation of the index metacarpophalangeal joint. *J Bone Joint Surg* 57A:698-700, 1975.
    Describes the risks and benefits of volar and dorsal approaches to complex metacarpophalangeal dislocations.

47. Smith GR, Yang SS, Weiland AJ: Multiple metacarpal dislocations: a case report and review of treatment. *Am J Orthop* 88:502-506, 1996.

48. Henderson JJ, Arafa MA: Carpometacarpal dislocation: an easily missed diagnosis. *J Bone Joint Surg [Br]* 69:212-214, 1987.

49. Hartwig RH, Louis DS: Multiple carpometacarpal dislocations. *J Bone Joint Surg* 61A:906-908, 1979.

50. Gunther SF: The carpometacarpal joints. *Orthop Clin North Am* 15:259-277, 1984.

51. Weiland AJ, Lister GD, Villarreal-Rios A: Volar fracture-dislocations of the second and third carpometacarpal joints associated with acute carpal tunnel syndrome. *J Trauma* 16:672-675, 1976.

52. Rawles JG: Dislocations and fracture-dislocations at the carpometacarpal joints of the fingers. *Hand Clin* 4:103-112, 1988.
    Description of varous injuries and treatment options.

53. Lawlis JF, Gunther SF: Carpometacarpal dislocations. Long-term follow-up. *J Bone Joint Surg* 73A:52-59, 1991.
    Early reduction and fixation yielded better long-term results. Results were less satisfactory with injuries to the rigid second and third CMC joints.

54. De Beer JD, Maloon S, Anderson P et al: Multiple carpometacarpal dislocations. *J Hand Surg [Br]* 14:105-108, 1989.

55. Clendenin MB, Smith RJ: Fifth metacarpal/hamate arthrodesis for posttraumatic osteoarthritis. *J Hand Surg* 9:374-378, 1984.
    Irregular joints become symptomatic but fare well with fusion.

56. Lee HB, Tark KC, Kang S et al: Reconstruction of composite metacarpal defects using a fibula free flap. *Plast Reconstr Surg* 104:1448-1452, 2000.

57. Colditz JC: Functional fracture bracing. In Hunter JM, Mackin EJ, Callahan AD, editors. *Rehabilitation of the hand: surgery and therapy.* Philadelphia, 1995, Mosby.

58. Duncan RW, Freeland AE, Jabaley ME, Meydrech EF: Open hand fractures: an analysis of the recovery of active motion and of complications. *J Hand Surg* 18:387-394, 1993.

Open metacarpal fractures did better than open phalangeal fractures. Soft tissue damage significantly impacted motion and function.

59. Fusetti C, Meyer H, Borisch N et al: Complications of plate fixation in metacarpal fractures. *J Trauma* 52:535-539, 2002.

60. Page SM, Stern PJ: Complications and range of motion following plate fixation of metacarpal and phalangeal fractures. *J Hand Surg* 23:827-832, 1998.
This review noted a 36% rate of surgical complications, especially in phalangeal fractures.

61. Gollamudi S, Jones WA: Corrective osteotomy of malunited fractures of phalanges and metacarpals. *J Hand Surg [Br]* 25:439-441, 2000.

62. Boulas HJ: Autograft replacement of small joint defects in the hand. *Clin Orthop* 327:63-71, 1996.

63. Seradge H, Kutz JA, Kleinert HE et al: Perichondrial resurfacing arthroplasty in the hand. *J Hand Surg* 9:880-886, 1984.

64. Nagle DG, af Ekenstam FW, Lister GD: Immediate Silastic arthroplasty for non-salvageable intra-articular phalangeal fractures. *Scand J Plast Reconstr Surg* 23:47-50, 1989.

65. Ishida O, Tsai TM: Free vascularized whole joint transfer in children. *Microsurgery* 12:196-206, 1991.

66. Foucher G: Vascularized joint transfers. In Green DP, Hotchkiss RN, editors: *Operative hand surgery.* New York, 1993, Churchill Livingstone.

# CHAPTER 4

# Fractures and Dislocations of the Thumb

John S. Taras[*] and Stephen M. Hankins[†]

[*]MD, Associate Professor, Drexel University; Chief, Division of Hand Surgery, Thomas Jefferson University Hospital, Philadelphia, PA
[†]MD, Hand Surgery Fellow, Jefferson Medical College of Thomas Jefferson University, Philadelphia, PA

## Introduction

- The biomechanical complexity of the hand is particularly exemplified in the function of the thumb.
- The complex kinematics of the thumb result from the precise arrangement of its bony and soft tissue anatomy and its multiple muscle actions.
- The thumb has the unique ability to function in opposition and pinch.
- Injury with subsequent loss of the thumb function impacts hand dexterity more than in any other digit.
- Accurate understanding of the pathomechanics and treatment of injuries to the thumb is essential for successful reconstruction of traumatic injuries.

## Phalangeal Injuries

- Extraarticular fractures of the thumb phalanges are uncommon and usually result from direct trauma.
- These injuries are managed according to fracture pattern and stability.

### Distal Phalanx Fractures

- Distal phalangeal fractures can be classified as longitudinal, transverse, or tuft types.

- Tuft fractures typically are associated with nail matrix injuries, which should be repaired if lacerated.
- Transverse fractures may be unstable because pull of the flexor pollicis longus tendon creates an apex volar deformity. These fractures may require percutaneous pinning if unstable.
- Vertical fractures are rare and require percutaneous reduction with pointed forceps and pinning if displaced.
- Avulsion fractures of the dorsal base of the distal phalanx represent a bony mallet injury. This injury can be treated with extension block splinting for a minimum of 6 to 8 weeks unless there is evidence of volar subluxation, which requires reduction and fixation.
- Avulsion fractures of the volar lip of the distal phalanx usually occur as a result of dorsal interphalangeal (IP) dislocations.
- Intraarticular fractures of the metacarpophalangeal (MCP) and IP joints may be comminuted and require restoration of the articular surface. Open reduction and internal fixation with 2-mm plates can be used to restore length and alignment for severe injuries (Figure 4–1).

### Proximal Phalanx Fractures

- Transverse proximal phalanx fractures angulate apex dorsally because of the surrounding muscle forces.
- Closed reduction usually is stable.

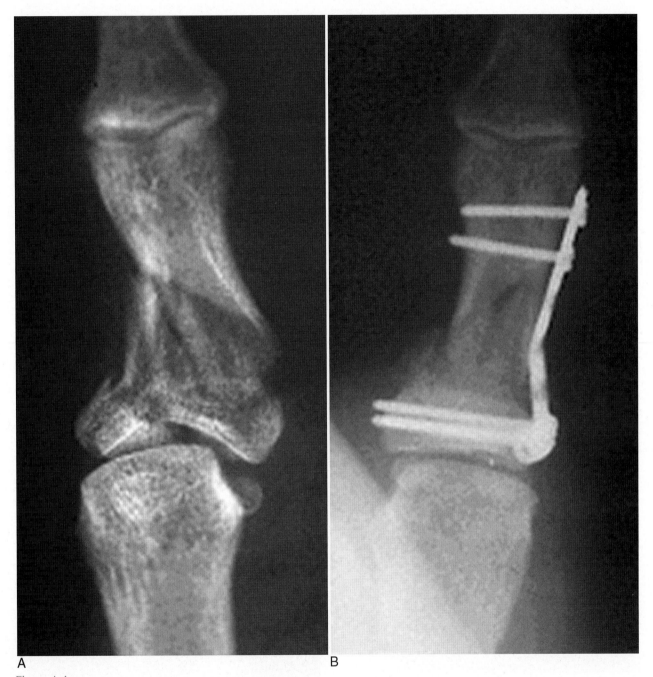

**Figure 4–1:**
A, Comminuted intraarticular proximal phalanx fracture. B, Operative treatment with open reduction and internal fixation and restoration of articular congruity.

- Greater than 20 degrees of angulation may be associated with a significant extensor lag.
- Unstable shaft fractures, including spiral, oblique, and comminuted fracture patterns, can be treated by percutaneous pinning or open reduction and internal fixation.
- Proximal phalanx head and neck fractures should be managed similarly to fractures of the fingers. Metacarpal neck fracture angulation should not exceed 20 degrees.

## Interphalangeal Joint Injuries

- The thumb phalanges and IP joint provide the terminal link in thumb function.
- The thumb IP joint is stabilized by the familiar three-sided box composed of collateral ligaments and volar plate.
- The flexor pollicis longus and extensor pollicis longus are the only tendons that traverse the IP joint of the thumb.
- IP joint dislocations are less common than MCP joint dislocations because of the shorter lever arm of the distal

phalanx and the additional stability provided by the local tendinous insertions.

- Dislocations almost always are dorsal and frequently are associated with skin laceration. Reduction is by longitudinal traction and pressure at the base of the distal phalanx. Joint instability is rare after reduction. The thumb should be immobilized in 20 degrees of flexion for 2 to 3 weeks. Irreducible dislocations have been reported and usually involve proximal volar plate disruption.

## Sesamoid Fractures

- The sesamoid bones almost always are present on the radial and ulnar sides of the MCP joint of the thumb and occur frequently at the thumb IP joint.
- Sesamoid bones are thought to increase leverage and change pull direction of musculotendinous units.
- The mechanism of thumb sesamoid fracture is thought to include hyperextension and direct trauma.
- Diagnosis can be difficult. Oblique radiographic views are needed to ensure fracture visualization (Figure 4–2).
- Usually the injury can be treated with a 4-week period of immobilization with no residual symptoms. Weakness

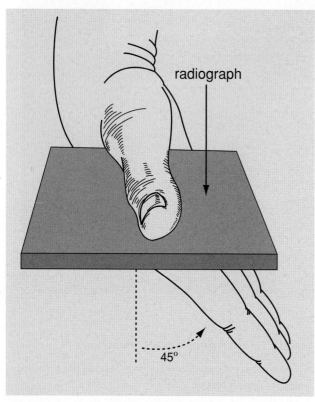

radiograph

45°

Figure 4–2:
**Radiography of the radial sesamoid of the thumb metacar-pophalangeal joint. Abducting the thumb and placing the cas-sette between the thumb and index finger avoids overlap with the hand.** (From Mohler MD, Trumble TE: Disorders of the thumb sesamoids. *Hand Clin* 17:291-301, 2001.)

of the affected thumb may result from widely separated fractures. It may be necessary to operatively reduce these fractures to prevent flexor pollicis brevis weakness.

## Metacarpophalangeal Injuries

### Anatomy and Biomechanics

- The MCP joint of the thumb somewhat resembles those of the fingers.
- The range of flexion is quite variable among individuals, varying anywhere from 30 to 90 degrees. This disparity may be related to the variable shape of the metacarpal head. More spherical heads provide greater range of motion in the flexion-extension arc.
- The joint also allows abduction-adduction and some amount of pronation-supination (Box 4–1).
- The MCP joint has little intrinsic stability because of its bony architecture.
- There is some evidence that limited range of motion predisposes the joint to injury.

### Metacarpophalangeal Dislocations

- The vast majority of MCP dislocations are dorsal, although palmar dislocations have been reported.
- Doral dislocations occur following a hyperextension force in which complete rupture of the volar plate and capsule occurs.
- The collateral ligaments also are injured and sustain at least partial, if not complete, disruption.
- The volar plate rupture usually occurs proximally but may be through or distal to the sesamoids.
- Radiography may assist in making this determination and may be predictive of the reducibility of the injury.
- Volar dislocations reported usually require open reduction.

| Box 4–1 | Thumb Metacarpophalangeal Joint Anatomy |
|---|---|

- Ligamentous stability of the MCP joint is provided by the three-sided box configuration similar to that of the finger proximal interphalangeal (PIP) joints (Figure 4–3).
- The sides of the box consist of the radial and ulnar collateral ligaments.
- The floor of the box is composed of the volar plate but, unlike the PIP joints of the fingers, there is no flexor sheath proximal to the plate.
- Volar support is also provided by the thenar muscles, which insert into the paired sesamoid bones embedded in the distal volar plate.
- The flexor pollicis brevis and adductor pollicis also insert into the adductor and abductor aponeuroses, which provide dynamic lateral stability (Figure 4–4).

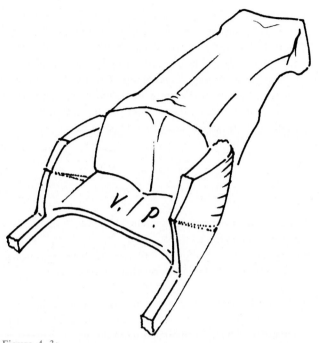

Figure 4–3:
Three-dimensional ligament-box complex consisting of collateral ligaments and volar plate. At least two sides of this box must be disrupted for displacement of the joint to occur. (From Green DP, Hotchkiss RN, Pederson WC: *Green's operative hand surgery,* ed 3. New York, 1999, Churchill Livingstone.)

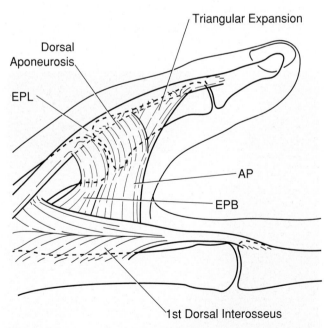

Figure 4–4:
Medial aspect of the thumb metacarpophalangeal joint. Shown in the figure are extensor pollicis longus (EPL), adductor pollicis (AP), dorsal aponeurosis, triangular expansion, first dorsal interosseus, extensor pollicis brevis (EPB).

- Dislocations can be defined as simple (reducible) or complex (irreducible).
- Most dorsal MCP dislocations are reducible by closed means, although a significant number are irreducible.
- In a large series of 132 dislocations reported by McLaughlin,[1] 17% were irreducible.
- Closed reduction is easier if the insertions of the intrinsic muscles in the sesamoids are intact, because these muscles guide the volar plate back into position.
- Radiographs that show significant hyperextension of the joint are predictive of reducibility. If the proximal phalanx is positioned in a more parallel position with regard to the metacarpal, the injury likely is complex. The volar plate, sesamoids, or flexor pollicis longus tendons may become entrapped, preventing reduction. The radiographic appearance of the sesamoids entrapped within the MCP joint is pathognomonic of a complex dislocation (Box 4–2).
- Pure dorsal dislocations rarely lead to collateral ligament instability.
- If there is evidence of volar plate rupture through or distal to the sesamoids, surgical repair performed in order to regain active restraint to hyperextension is indicated. This injury may be difficult to diagnose and may be confirmed by arthrography.
- After reduction of a simple MCP dislocation, the thumb should be immobilized in 20 degrees of flexion for 4 weeks.
- If closed reduction is not successful, repeated attempts are contraindicated.
- Open reduction should be performed in order to disengage the head of the metacarpal from a buttonhole slit in the anterior capsule and from the flexor pollicis brevis muscle (Figure 4–5).
- The approach can be either dorsal or radiopalmar. The dorsal approach is more straightforward and helps to prevent digital nerve injury. The volar plate can be split

| **Box 4–2** | **Thumb Metacarpophalangeal Joint Closed Reduction Technique** |

- A careful closed reduction maneuver must be performed to avoid transforming a simple dislocation into a complex one.
- The thumb must be maintained in adduction to relax its intrinsic muscles. Minimal distraction, if any, is applied.
- The metacarpophalangeal joint is hyperextended, and the proximal end of the proximal phalanx is pushed over the end of the metacarpal head. This action tends to diminish the buttonhole effect on the metacarpal neck that is accentuated by traction.
- It may be helpful to flex the wrist and the thumb interphalangeal joint in order to relax the flexor pollicis longus.
- After reduction, the collateral ligaments should be checked for stability.

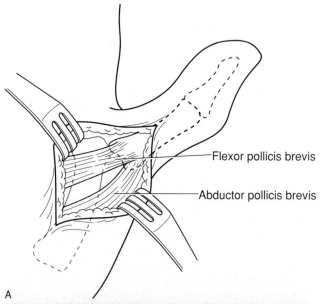

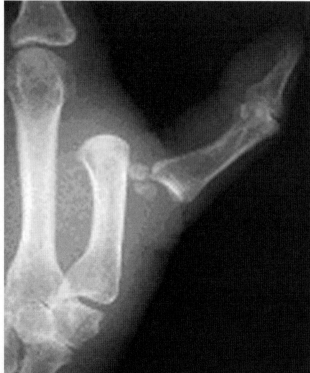

A

B

Figure 4–5:
A, Complex dislocation of metacarpophalangeal (MCP) joint of the thumb. B, Metacarpal head has penetrated the joint capsule with interposition of the volar plate. Sesamoids within the MCP joint are pathognomonic of a complex dislocation that is irreducible by closed means.

longitudinally to facilitate reduction. The MCP joint usually is stable after open reduction, and an immobilization period of only 2 to 3 weeks is required.

- Hyperextension injuries may result in a "locked" MCP joint, associated with a sesamoid fracture. In this injury, both active and passive flexion are lost with extension preserved and must be compared to the contralateral thumb. The injury occurs when a band composed of the accessory collateral ligament, sesamoid, and volar plate ruptures at its proximal attachment. This band becomes entrapped between the metacarpal's radial condyle and the proximal phalanx. These injury patterns require surgical release of the entrapped band of tissue.

## Ulnar Collateral Ligament Injuries

- Injuries to the ulnar collateral are common in skiers and ball-handling athletes.
- Ulnar collateral ligament (UCL) injuries have been noted to be 10 times more common than radial collateral injuries.
- The mechanism is an abrupt, forced radial deviation of the thumb. This condition may result from a fall onto an outstretched hand with an abducted thumb.
- Distal tears of the UCL at its insertion are more common than proximal tears. Avulsion fractures of the ulnar base of the proximal phalanx also may occur (Figure 4–6) but typically are small. However, larger fractures, especially those involving greater than 10% of the articular surface and displaced, may lead to joint incongruity.
- A Stener lesion may occur with complete UCL disruption when the adductor aponeurosis becomes interposed between the distally avulsed ligament and its insertion on the proximal phalanx (Figure 4–7). This interposition does not occur with partial tears.

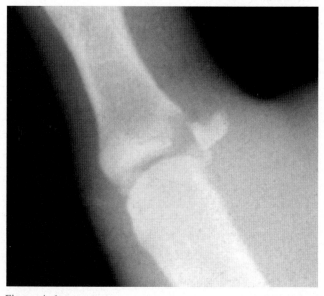

Figure 4–6:
Ulnar collateral ligament avulsion fracture requiring reduction and fixation.

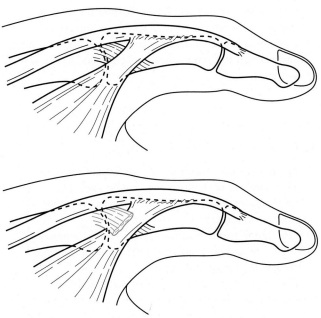

Figure 4–7:

**Stener lesion occurs when the proximal portion of the torn proper collateral ligament on the ulnar side of the thumb metacarpophalangeal joint comes to lie dorsal to the leading edge of the adductor aponeurosis.**

- Differentiating complete from partial tears may be difficult. The physical findings include tenderness, ecchymoses, and swelling along the ulnar border of the joint. With partial tears a definite endpoint may be present on stress testing.
- Stress testing should be performed in extension and 30 degrees of flexion to isolate the UCL and relax the volar plate. Laxity of 30 degrees or more when compared to the contralateral thumb is considered diagnostic. Some authors have suggested that 35 degrees of laxity in full extension is indicative of a complete tear of the proper and accessory collateral ligaments.
- Although the diagnosis of a UCL tear typically is a clinical diagnosis, imaging studies are a useful adjunct. Stress x-ray films may be helpful, and arthrograms have been recommended to demonstrate a leak and the torn end of the collateral. Magnetic resonance imaging and ultrasound studies have received more recent attention. In the hands of experienced examiners, these two modalities have demonstrated high sensitivity and specificity in determining a Stener lesion. Ultimately, they may be most useful in situations where the diagnosis is unclear.

### Nonoperative Treatment

- There is consensus that partial tears can be treated conservatively.
- Partial tears are effectively treated by a 4-week period of continuous immobilization, followed by a 2-week period of splint protection and active range of motion exercises. Strenuous activity is avoided for 3 months post injury.
- There is some controversy regarding the management of acute complete UCL ruptures. Some authors advise immobilization, and others advise operative treatment only if a palpable mass is present adjacent to the metacarpal head, suggestive of a Stener lesion.
- Bony avulsions without significant displacement traditionally have treated with cast immobilization.

### Operative Treatment

- The majority of authors believe that nonoperative treatment of complete UCL ruptures is unpredictable and therefore recommend surgical exploration and repair.
- Repair of the ligament may be direct suture of the ligament to the periosteum or reattachment to bone via bone anchors.
- A small series has reported successful results with arthroscopic reduction of Stener lesion and no suture repair, but with joint reduction maintained by K-wire fixation.
- Chronic instability of the UCL may directly result from failure of acute treatment or failure to recognize a Stener lesion. These injuries should be treated with ligament reconstruction. Options include using a remnant of scarred capsule, extensor indicis proprius tendon, extensor pollicis brevis tendon, adductor pollicis transfer, free tendon transfer, or finally MCP arthrodesis.

## Radial Collateral Ligament Injuries

- As already noted, radial collateral ligament (RCL) injuries are significantly less common than UCL injuries but may be equally as debilitating.
- The abductor aponeurosis is broad and covers most of the radial side of the MCP joint. As a result, interposition almost never occurs with RCL tears.
- The mechanism is forced adduction or torsion on a flexed MCP joint.
- Tears occur with equal frequency both proximally and distally.
- There may be some rotational deformity of the MCP joint where the proximal phalanx shifts volarly on the radial side. There may be dorsoradial prominence of the metacarpal head.
- Partial and complete tears are differentiated by the presence of a definite endpoint.
- Laxity greater than 30 degrees compared to the contralateral thumb is diagnostic (Figure 4–8).

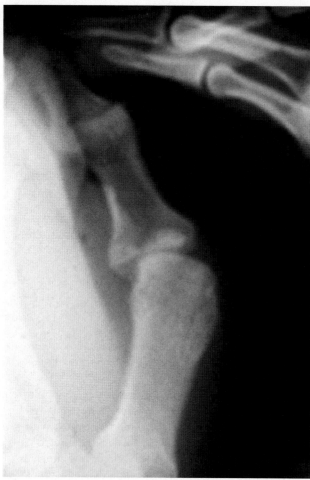

Figure 4–8:
**Stress radiograph reveals evident radial collateral ligament disruption.**

## Nonoperative Treatment

- Partial tears are treated similarly to partial tears of the UCL. However, there is no real consensus on treatment of complete tears. Options range from immobilization to operative repair.

## Operative Treatment

- Direct repair of the RCL is indicated when volar subluxation of the MCP joint occurs, which indicates a tear of the RCL as well as the dorsal capsule.

# Thumb Metacarpal Shaft Fractures

- Shaft fractures are relatively uncommon.
- The diaphyseal bone is quite strong compared to its cancellous, base and stresses usually are well tolerated.

- Metacarpal fractures usually result from direct trauma and often are associated with soft tissue injury.
- Unstable metacarpal shaft fractures may require surgical intervention to prevent shortening and adduction at the fracture site.

# Carpometacarpal Injuries

## Anatomy and Biomechanics

- The base of the thumb metacarpal articulates with the trapezium in the form of a saddle joint. This configuration allows the thumb metacarpal a wide range of motion.
- The thumb metacarpal moves in a conical range of motion from full extension in the plane of the hand toward the palmar surface.
- The most important function of the thumb is opposition, whereby the thumb moves toward the tip of the little finger. This motion can occur because of the ability of the thumb metacarpal to move in abduction and pronation at the trapeziometacarpal (TMC) joint.
- Large loads are imparted to the TMC joint. Axial and bending loads are applied to the joint during pinch and grasp.
- The trapezium is inherently unstable because of its anatomic location at the radial aspect of the wrist and its bony architecture. The basal articulation of the trapezium with the mobile scaphoid also contributes to its potential for instability.
- The stability of the TMC joint results from the stout surrounding ligamentous complex (Figure 4–9).
- The dorsoradial and deep anterior oblique ligaments (dAOL) play the most substantial role in stabilizing the TMC joint.
- The dAOL functions as a pivot for the first metacarpal during palmar abduction to allow pronation. The dAOL statically guides the first metacarpal into pronation, whereas the thenar muscles work in concert to produce abduction and flexion.
- The superficial anterior oblique ligament (SAOL) inserts distal to the articular margins of the TMC joint and allows laxity within the joint. This laxity is essential for pronation to occur during opposition.

## Radiographs

- Accurate evaluation of the injury depends on adequate radiographic examination.
- A true lateral view of the TMC joint must be obtained. The palmar surface of the hand is placed flat on the plate, and the hand and wrist are pronated 15 to 35 degrees. The beam is then directed obliquely 15 degrees in a distal to proximal direction centered over the joint (Figure 4–10).

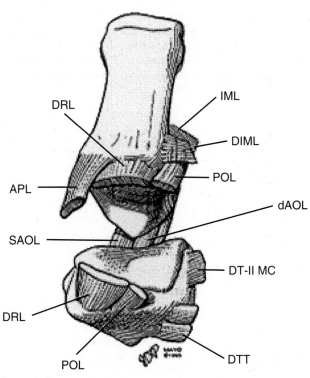

**Figure 4–9:**
The trapeziometacarpal joint has been hinged open from the dorsum to reveal the deep anterior oblique ligament (*dAOL;* beak ligament) lying within the joint just ulnar to the volar tubercle of the metacarpal. *APL,* Abductor pollicis longus; *DIML,* dorsal intermetacarpal ligament; *DRL,* dorsoradial ligament; *DT-II MC,* dorsal trapezio-second metacarpal ligament; *DTT,* dorsal trapeziotrapezoid ligament; *IML,* intermetacarpal ligament; *POL,* posterior oblique ligament; *SAOL,* superficial anterior oblique ligament. (From Bettinger PC, Linscheid RL, Berger RA, Cooney WP, An KN: An anatomic study of the stabilizing ligaments of the trapezium and trapeziometacarpal joint. *J Hand Surg* 24A:786-798, 1999.)

- A traction radiograph may be useful in assessing the effect of traction on fracture reduction.

# Thumb Metacarpal Base Fractures

- Fractures of the thumb metacarpal occur most frequently at the base and are subdivided into intraarticular and extraarticular types.
- The mechanism of injury of metacarpal base fractures is an axially directed force through the metacarpal shaft.

## Extraarticular Metacarpal Base Fractures

- Extraarticular fractures occur in transverse and oblique fracture patterns.

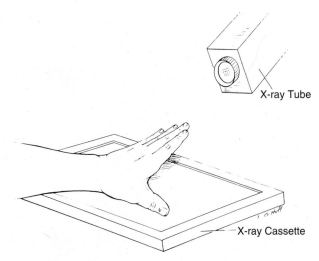

**Figure 4–10:**
True lateral radiograph of the trapeziometacarpal joint. (From Browner BD, Jupiter JB, Levine AM, Trafton PG: *Skeletal trauma.* Philadelphia, 1998, WB Saunders.)

### Nonsurgical Management

- Extraarticular fractures usually can be managed with closed reduction.
- The fracture pattern is apex-dorsal, with the distal fragment in an adducted, flexed, and supinated position.
- The reduction maneuver includes traction, downward pressure at the fracture, and pronation of the distal fragment (Figure 4–11).
- If the reduction is stable, the injury can be managed with a thumb spica cast for 4 weeks.
- Angulation of up to 30 degrees may be accepted because of the mobility of the TMC joint.

### Surgical Management

- If the fracture is unstable and closed reduction cannot be maintained, percutaneous pinning usually is sufficient to stabilize the reduction.
- The pins can be placed directly across the fracture in oblique patterns or transarticular in transverse patterns.
- Open reduction rarely is necessary. Extremely comminuted extraarticular fractures may require internal or external fixation to maintain the length of the metacarpal.

### Intraarticular Metacarpal Base Fractures

- Intraarticular fractures are further subdivided into (1) Bennett, (2) Rolando, and (3) severely comminuted fractures.
- In Bennett and Rolando fractures, the strong deep anterior oblique (beak) ligament remains intact and prevents displacement of the volar fragment.

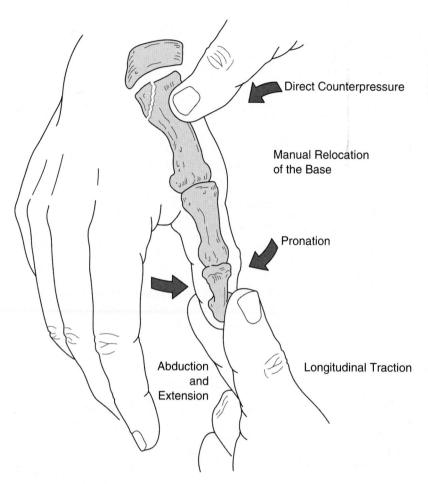

Figure 4–11:

Closed reduction maneuver for extraarticular thumb metacarpal base fractures. (From Browner BD, Jupiter JB, Levine AM, Trafton PG: *Skeletal trauma,* ed 3. Philadelphia, 1998, WB Saunders.)

Direct Counterpressure

Manual Relocation of the Base

Pronation

Abduction and Extension

Longitudinal Traction

- The dorsal fragment and metacarpal are displaced radially and dorsally by the pull of the abductor pollicis longus and the adductor pollicis longus.

### Bennett Fractures

- The Bennett fracture pattern includes a variably sized fragment of the volar-ulnar aspect of the metacarpal base. This is referred to as the *Bennett fragment* and is held in anatomic position by the dAOL, which attaches to both this fragment and the trapezium.
- To adequately treat the fracture, the metacarpal base must be reduced to the Bennett fragment in order to restore articular congruity. A cadaveric study by Cullen et al.[2] reported on contact pressures at the region of articular step-off in a simulated Bennett fracture. It was concluded that there was no biomechanical basis for predisposition to posttraumatic osteoarthritis after the fracture with a small palmar-beak component and a residual 2-mm articular step-off, provided the fragments of the shaft and the beak heal in close apposition. This finding suggests that Bennett fractures that can be reduced with articular incongruity of no more than 2 mm may be treated satisfactorily with closed reduction and percutaneous

pinning without the need for open reduction and internal fixation.

### Nonsurgical Management

- A review of the literature supports the use of the closed reduction and casting, provided a stable reduction with less than 1-mm displacement is maintained. Anatomic reduction of the Bennett fracture is of paramount importance and is closely correlated with long-term outcome.
- Although cast treatment is an option, surgical treatment is more likely to produce reliable results.

### Surgical Management

- Many different surgical techniques have been advocated for treatment of Bennett fractures. The techniques include closed reduction and percutaneous pinning, oblique traction, open reduction and internal fixation with K-wires or Herbert screws, and external fixation. Percutaneous pinning is the most popular. We prefer a single 0.062 K-wire placed through the metacarpal shaft and into the trapezium. It is not necessary to capture the volar-ulnar fragment. Stability then is assessed, and additional K-wires are added only if necessary. Arthroscopic-assisted reduction has been introduced as an adjunct to percutaneous pinning to allow direct visualization of the articular reduction.

- If closed reduction is inadequate, open reduction is performed. The joint is approached dorsally through the Wagner approach in the interval between the abductor pollicis longus and the thenar muscles (Figure 4–12). The fracture is exposed, and fixation is obtained using K-wires, a lag screw, or Herbert screw, depending on the fragment size. The thumb then is immobilized in a spica cast for 4 weeks, after which the pins may be removed.

- External fixation may be necessary in the presence of associated soft tissue injury and loss. Contraindications to open reduction include severe edema, tissue maceration, and deep contamination. The fixator is applied in a triangular configuration by placing pins in the first metacarpal, distal radius, and second metacarpal. The fixator is removed in 4 to 6 weeks.

- In a study comparing open and closed reduction, osteoarthritis was found to correlate with the quality of reduction of the fracture but had developed in all cases even after exact reduction. Anatomic reduction, by open or closed means, is the key to optimal clinical outcome (Box 4–3).

## Rolando Fractures

- T- or Y-shaped thumb metacarpal base fracture. In addition to the volar-ulnar fragment, there is also a large dorsal fragment. All comminuted metacarpal base fractures are commonly referred to in this category.

- Treatment requires both restoration of length and articular congruity. These fractures are difficult to manage and may be destined to development of posttraumatic arthritis and instability despite surgical intervention. Various open surgical techniques have been described, including the use of multiple K-wires, tension bands, and plates. Other options include Thoren traction and external fixation with limited open reduction.

## Surgical Management

- Open reduction can be obtained when the fracture fragments are relatively large. The approach is the same as for a Bennett fracture. Provisional fixation is obtained,

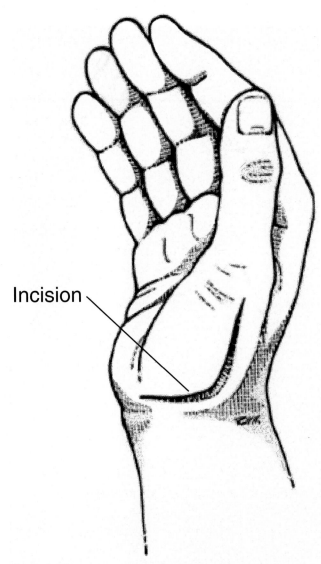

Incision

**Figure 4–12:**
The trapeziometacarpal joint is approached dorsally through the Wagner approach in the interval between the abductor pollicis longus and the thenar muscles. (From Canale ST: *Campbell's operative orthopaedics,* ed 9. St. Louis, 1998, Mosby.)

| Box 4–3 | **Surgical Technique: Closed Reduction and Percutaneous Fixation of Bennett Fractures** |
|---|---|

- Closed reduction can be obtained by longitudinal traction, abduction, and pronation while pressure is applied over the dorsoradial aspect of the metacarpal base.
- If manual reduction is not adequate, additional control may be gained by percutaneous joystick manipulation with K-wires or pointed reduction forceps.
- Various methods of pin fixation have been described, including intermetacarpal pinning between the first and second metacarpals, pinning the first metacarpal shaft to the fragment, and transarticular TMC pins.
- It is not necessary to pin the Bennett fragment but rather to restore the relationship of the metacarpal base to the trapezium (Figure 4–13).

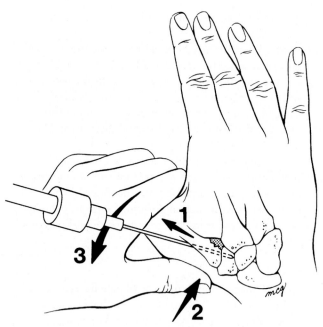

Figure 4–13:
Percutaneous pin fixation of Bennett fracture. Reduction is performed by *(1)* longitudinal traction, *(2)* pressure at the thumb metacarpal base, and *(3)* pronation. The pin is passed from the metacarpal to the trapezium. It is unnecessary to pin the Bennett fragment. (From Green DP, Hotchkiss RN, Pederson WC: *Green's operative hand surgery,* ed 4. New York, 1998, Churchill Livingstone.)

and the fracture then can may be fixed with a small T-plate (Figure 4–14). Percutaneous pins can be added to augment fixation.

- If the fracture is extremely comminuted, restoration of the anatomy of the articular surface may not be possible without extensive devitalization of the fracture fragments. These fractures may be more amenable to Thoren traction or external fixation. Thoren traction (Figure 4–15) uses an oblique pin placed in the metacarpal shaft in such a way as to counteract the forces of the abductor pollicis longus and adductor pollicis. The traction is applied through a banjo outrigger.

## Trapeziometacarpal Dislocations

- Traumatic dislocations of the TMC joint without fracture are uncommon.
- The injury results from a severe abduction force that produces a dorsal dislocation. There is some controversy regarding which ligaments are damaged during the injury, although it is generally believed to involve the deep anterior oblique ligament.

- The major deforming forces after dislocation are the pull of the abductor pollicis longus and the adductor pollicis.
- This dislocation usually can be reduced by closed means without difficulty but generally is unstable. The stability of the reduction can be assessed by passively flexing and adducting the thumb.

### Nonsurgical Management

- If the reduction is stable, the patient can be placed in a thumb spica cast for a minimum of 6 weeks. In the usual case of an unstable reduction, the injury is best treated by surgical stabilization.

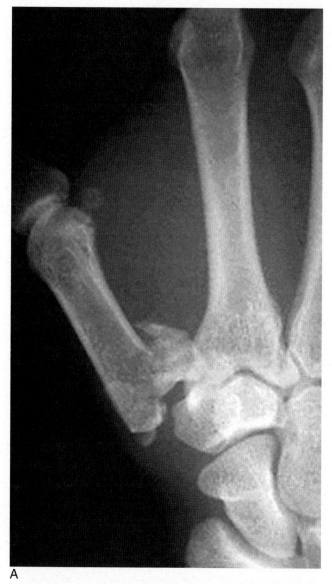

**A**

Figure 4–14:

A, Comminuted metacarpal base fracture.

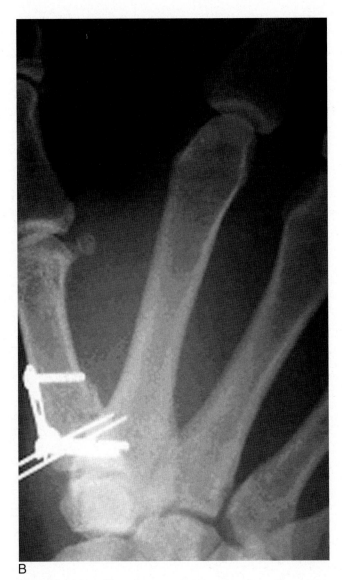

**B**

Figure 4–14: cont'd

B, Operative treatment with open reduction and internal fixation. Percutaneous pins are used for additional stability.

## Surgical Management

- Surgical options include closed reduction and pinning or early ligamentous reconstruction, in which the flexor carpi radialis tendon is used to reconstruct the TMC joint ligamentous support. In a series reported by Simonian and Trumble[3] comparing patients treated surgically, the group of patients treated with early ligamentous reconstruction had a decreased incidence of recurrent instability and joint degeneration. In the closed reduction and pinning group, four of the nine patients treated had unsatisfactory results because of joint instability and degenerative arthritis and underwent reconstructive surgery (Box 4–4).

- Ligamentous reconstruction often is reserved for patients with symptomatic instability after mobilization.

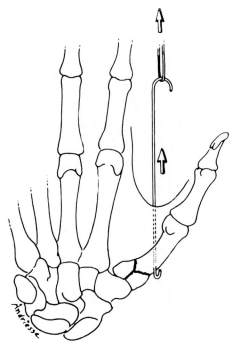

Figure 4–15:

Thoren traction. Oblique pin through the first metacarpal is attached to a banjo outrigger. The net force vector is constructed to correct fracture shortening and varus angulation. (From Breen TF, Gelberman RH, Jupiter JB: Intra-articular fractures of the basilar joint of the thumb. *Hand Clin* 4:491-501, 1988.)

| Box 4–4 | Surgical Technique: TMC Joint Ligamentous Reconstruction as Described by Eaton and Littler[4] |
|---|---|

- TMC joint is exposed through an incision along the radial border of the metacarpal.
- The thenar muscles are reflected extraperiosteally from the metacarpal and volar aspects of the trapezium and the FCR tendon is exposed.
- Any small cartilage fragments or remnants of ligament interposed in the joint space are removed.
- Two transverse incisions are made to harvest the FCR tendon slip, 3 and 6 cm proximal to the wrist crease.
- A strip composed of half its width is split away radially and tunneled to emerge beyond the wrist crease.
- The trapezium is held in a reduced position. The harvested tendon is directed through a channel at the beak of the thumb metacarpal, then dorsal/deep to the APL tendon, and sutured to the FCR insertion site at the base of the second metacarpal (Figure 4–16)

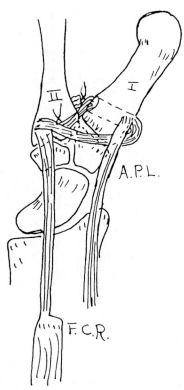

Figure 4–16:

**Diagram of trapeziometacarpal joint reconstruction using flexor carpi radialis (FCR) tendon. *APL, Abductor pollicis longus; I,* 1st metacarpal, *II,* 2nd metacarpal.**

# References

1.  McLaughlin HL: Complex "locked" dislocation of the metacarpophalangeal joints. *J Trauma* 6:683-688, 1965.

2.  Cullen JP, Parentis MA, Chinchilli VM, Pellegrini VD: Simulated Bennett fracture treated with closed reduction and percutaneous pinning: a biomechanical analysis of residual incongruity of the joint. *J Bone Joint Surg Am* 3:413-420, 1997.
    There is no biomechanical basis for predisposition to posttraumatic osteoarthritis after a Bennett fracture with a small palmar-beak component and a residual 2-mm articular step-off, provided the fragments of the shaft and the beak heal in close apposition.

3.  Simonian PT, Trumble TE: Traumatic dislocation of the thumb carpometacarpal joint: early ligamentous reconstruction versus closed reduction and pinning. *J Hand Surg Am* 21:802-806, 1996.
    Early ligamentous reconstruction of the trapeziometacarpal joint after traumatic dislocation, when instability is present, may decrease the incidence of recurrent instability and posttraumatic joint degeneration compared to closed reduction and pinning.

4.  Eaton RG, Littler JW: Ligament reconstruction for the painful thumb carpometacarpal joint. *J Bone Joint Surg* 55A:1655-1666, 1973.

# Thumb Reconstruction

Alexander D. Mih

MD, Associate Professor, Department of Orthopaedic Surgery, Indiana University School of Medicine; The Indiana Hand Center, Indianapolis, IN

## Introduction

- Functional disability from thumb loss is largely dependent on the level of amputation and may vary greatly depending on the individual's needs. Successful reconstruction of a damaged, shortened thumb requires restoration of adequate length, mobility, stability, strength, and sensibility. Various reconstructive procedures producing satisfactory results have been described, with the patient's needs influencing the selection of a specific technique. A stable, mobile, and functional carpometacarpal (CMC) joint is the cornerstone of thumb restoration and is more important than motion preservation at the more distal joints. Thumb amputations are generally divided into those occurring through the distal, middle, and proximal third of the thumb. Appropriate reconstruction for each of these levels is considered in this chapter.

## History

- Severe impairment to hand function caused by thumb loss has been recognized throughout history. A societal recognition of the devastating nature of these injuries is found in Roman and early English legal documents and literature. Current standards recognize complete loss of the thumb as a 50% impairment of the hand. The search for methods to restore thumb function has spanned more than 100 years, including various procedures such as Nicoladoni's description of a toe-to-hand transfer performed as a pedicle flap. Subsequent efforts focused on bone transfer and soft tissue flaps, pollicization, and osteoplastic reconstruction. The birth of the microsurgical era in the early 1960s made replantation of the amputated thumb a possibility and led to numerous elective microsurgical techniques that used all or a portion of the great or lesser toes and other tissues. Efforts have focused on improving the survival, function, and appearance of the thumb reconstructed by conventional or microsurgical methods.

## Classification of Thumb Injuries

- The four main categories of thumb amputation are based on the level of loss. Most types are successfully addressed by more than one type of reconstruction (Figure 5–1).[1]
- *Type A* amputations occur through the interphalangeal (IP) joint, *type B* from IP joint to proximal phalangeal base, *type C* from proximal phalangeal base to midmetacarpal, and *type D* include proximal metacarpal to trapezial level amputations (Table 5–1).

## Level A Amputations: Distal Tip Amputations and Soft Tissue Loss

- Thumb tip amputations allowed to heal by secondary intention follow a predictable and simple course of recovery. This method of treatment is indicated for tip injuries with minimal or no bone exposure. Studies have shown that this method provides excellent long-term results and prevents many of the problems found with

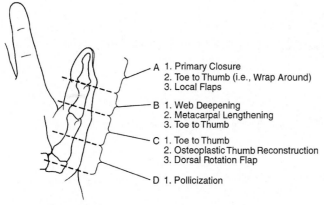

A 1. Primary Closure
2. Toe to Thumb (i.e., Wrap Around)
3. Local Flaps

B 1. Web Deepening
2. Metacarpal Lengthening
3. Toe to Thumb

C 1. Toe to Thumb
2. Osteoplastic Thumb Reconstruction
3. Dorsal Rotation Flap

D 1. Pollicization

Figure 5–1:

**Levels of thumb amputation with corresponding options for reconstruction. (From Thumb reconstruction. In Trumble TT, editor: *Principles of hand surgery and therapy.* Philadelphia, 2000, WB Saunders.)**

local advancement flaps (e.g., V-Y advancement) such as tip hypersensitivity, soft tissue atrophy, and cold intolerance.

- In cases of bone exposure, a rongeur can be used to remove small amounts of distal phalanx, allowing secondary intention healing. More elaborate methods of soft tissue coverage (described later) may be required in cases of significant bone exposure, when primary closure requires significant shortening.

## Palmar Advancement Flap

- The advancement flap described by Moberg allows coverage of wounds involving up to 50% of the palmar aspect of the distal phalanx. Innervated palmar thumb skin may be advanced to cover the palmar surface and tip, providing sensate and durable coverage.

- In this technique, the flap is created by making incisions along the midaxial line of the thumb (Figure 5–2, *top*). The palmar skin is elevated on both the radial and ulnar neurovascular pedicles and is extended to the level of the proximal palmar flexion crease of the thumb.

- This flap is elevated without disturbance of the flexor tendon sheath and is advanced to cover the thumb tip. Advancement is aided by flexion of both the metacarpophalangeal (MP) and interphalangeal (IP) joints, which may be pinned in position. Although flexion of these joints prevents tension on the advanced flap, it may predispose patients to contracture of these joints and should be performed with great caution in older patients.

- A modification of the palmar advancement flap has been described that includes use of a relaxing palmar incision (see Figure 5–2, *bottom*). In this technique, the palmar flap

## Table 5–1: Types of Thumb Amputations

| LEVEL AMPUTATION | TREATMENT | ADVANTAGES | DISADVANTAGES |
|---|---|---|---|
| A (distal to IP joint) | Secondary intention | Simple, few complications | May require bone shortening |
| | Advancement flap (Moberg) | Provides innervated, durable coverage from local source | Prone-to-flexion contracture, coverage area limited to 50% of thumb palmar surface |
| | Cross-finger flap (index) | Large coverage area | Requires harvest from normal digit, potential index and first web contracture, skin color mismatch in dark-skinned patients, transfers hair-bearing skin |
| | Radial forearm flap (circumferential injury) | Very large coverage area | Bulky coverage as fasciocutaneous flap, donor site problems with healing, appearance, adhesion |
| | Index finger flap | Dorsal side coverage | Creates two donor sites, first web contracture |
| | Great toe wraparound flap | Composite tissue restoration | Remote donor site, requires microsurgical techniques, potentially difficult harvest |
| B (proximal phalangeal level) (Z-plasty or dorsal rotational flap) | Web space deepening, +/− metacarpal lengthening | Uses local tissues with distraction lengthening | Provides no additional motion, prolonged external fixator use |
| | Toe-to-thumb transfer | Restores length, stability | Remote donor site, requires microsurgical techniques, potentially difficult harvest |
| C (midmetacarpal level) | Osteoplastic reconstruction | Restores bulk, sensation | Requires attached groin flap or radial forearm flap, sacrifice of sensation from another digit |
| D (proximal metacarpal level | Pollicization | Local donor tissue, restores length and motion, uses digit often bypassed | Sacrifice of digit, first web contracture, stiffness |

Figure 5–2:
*Top,* Palmar advancement flap as described by Moberg. *Bottom,* Proximal transverse incision allows flap mobilization and with skin graft placement reduces joint contracture formation. (From Thumb reconstruction. In Trumble TT, editor: *Principles of hand surgery and therapy.* Philadelphia, 2000, WB Saunders.)

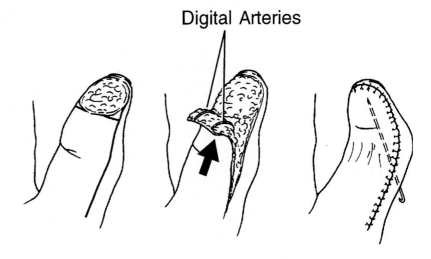

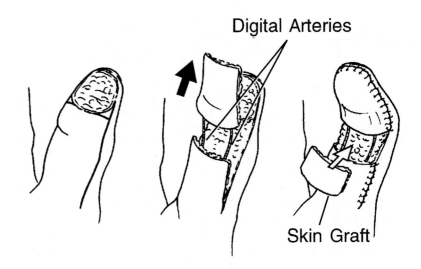

is isolated on its neurovascular pedicles, with creation of a palmar transverse incision to allow advancement of the flap without the need for joint flexion. A full-thickness skin graft is placed into the proximal palmar defect that in most cases lies directly over the proximal phalanx. Use of the proximal release incision and skin graft may be especially beneficial for older patients who are prone to MP and IP joint flexion deformity. Reports have documented the usefulness of this flap in preserving length with minimal morbidity.[1,2,3,4,5]

## Postoperative Rehabilitation

- If nonabsorbable sutures are used, they are removed after 10 to 14 days, and the patient proceeds with active and passive range of motion. If the soft tissues allow, dynamic splinting of the thumb helps reduce IP stiffness.

## Advantages and Disadvantages

- Advantages include sensate coverage from a local source.
- Disadvantages include joint contractures and limitations in areas of coverage to 50% of the palmar surface distal to the IP joint.

## Cross-Finger Flap

- When more than 50% of the palmar surface of the distal phalanx is devoid of soft tissue coverage, the palmar advancement flap may provide inadequate coverage. For injuries that include this larger area, cross-finger flaps may be beneficial.
- In this technique, the skin over the dorsal radial aspect of the index finger is elevated to allow coverage of the palmar surface of the thumb (Figure 5–3). The base of the

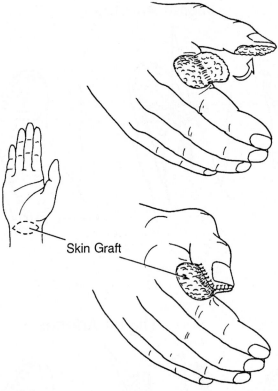

Figure 5–3:

**Cross-finger flap from index provides greater coverage than does palmar advancement flap. (From Thumb reconstruction. In Trumble TT, editor: *Principles of hand surgery and therapy*. Philadelphia, 2000, WB Saunders.)**

flap should extend palmar to the midaxial line to allow for flap rotation to the thumb defect. The area of flap elevation should exceed the defect size by 15% to 20% because of flap shrinkage after elevation.

- The peritenon is left undisturbed. A full-thickness skin graft harvested from the wrist or hypothenar region is inset over this area of the index finger. As with other cross-finger flaps, separation is performed at 2 to 3 weeks. At the time of separation, the soft tissues borders may be primarily closed or allowed to heal by secondary intention. This technique has been useful in terms of restoring soft tissue coverage with adequate sensory return from peripheral nerve fiber ingrowth.

### Postoperative Rehabilitation

- Following separation of the cross-finger flap, a vigorous program of stretching, range of motion, and splinting is required to prevent persistent tightness of the first web and thumb IP joint. The index is prone to flexion deformity during the attached phase and also requires individual stretching and splint use to prevent contracture.

### Advantages and Disadvantages

- This procedure offers greater coverage than the Moberg palmar advancement flap.

- This flap has the disadvantages of requiring a donor site from a normal index finger; the need for skin graft; potential stiffness of the index, thumb, and first web; and the need for a secondary operation.

## Massive Palmar and Circumferential Soft Tissue Loss

- For larger palmar defects and those involving the circumference of the thumb, distant sources of tissue for coverage are required. An attached groin flap and various pedicled and free flaps all are suitable for achieving coverage and are described elsewhere in this book.
- Use of a radial forearm flap as described in the section on dorsal thumb coverage also can be used for palmar defects.

## Radial Forearm Flap for Dorsal Soft Tissue Loss

- In cases of dorsal soft tissue loss about the thumb, coverage can be achieved and length preserved by forming a reversed cross-finger flap from the index finger or the elevation of a radial forearm flap. In most cases, use of a radial forearm flap is preferable because the first web space width and pliability may be maintained.
- The radial forearm flap is elevated as a pedicle flap based on the radial artery and accompanying veins. It may include a branch of the lateral antebrachial cutaneous nerve for a source of innervation and portions of the palmaris longus or flexor carpi radialis for tendon grafts. The arterial flow into this flap is retrograde and requires the presence of a complete carpal arch (Figure 5–4).
- Small bone defects can be addressed simultaneously with inclusion of a portion of the radius within the flap. Because the entire palmar skin of the forearm is usually supplied by the radial artery, ample soft tissue can be harvested for thumb coverage.
- Elevation of this flap requires identification of the radial artery within the fascial septum between the brachioradialis and flexor carpi radialis. Perforators emanate from this artery supplying the forearm fascia and, in turn, the skin.
- The axis of the flap is along the course of the radial artery. The local of the skin paddle should be located proximally to a point long enough to allow the flap to pivot to the thumb defect area without tension after elevation and should allow for approximately 15% shrinkage.
- Dissection must be performed with great care in the middle third of the forearm. In this area, septal perforating branches are less common than in the proximal and distal regions and are often intimately applied to the deep surface of the brachioradialis tendon before coursing along its ulnar border. If these branches

Figure 5–4:
**Presence of complete carpal arch provides retrograde flow to the radial forearm flap. (From Thumb reconstruction. In Trumble TT, editor:** *Principles of hand surgery and therapy.* **Philadelphia, 2000, WB Saunders.)**

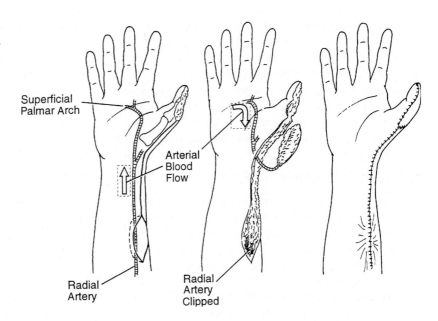

are difficult to identify, inclusion of a portion of the brachioradialis tendon ensures their preservation.

- In most cases, use of a fascial flap provides more satisfactory coverage than a fasciocutaneous flap because of the extreme thickness of the latter type of flap. Elevation of the fascia on the vascularized pedicle provides appropriate coverage. A skin graft applied to the fascia prevents the problems of hypermobile skin and excessive bulk. The skin and dermis are elevated from the underlying fascia and are retracted. The fascia is incised as a flap centered about the course of the radial artery. Dissection is most easily started on the ulnar side of the radial artery where the fascia is elevated from the underlying flexor muscle bellies. Flap dimension should exceed the thumb defect area by 15% to 20% to adjust for shrinkage.

- The radial artery and its accompanying vena comitantes are ligated proximal to the fascial flap. Dissection then proceeds in a proximal to distal fashion, dividing the numerous muscular perforators. Care is taken to prevent devascularization of the flap by preserving the palmar, radial, and ulnar fascial perforators. The radial artery is freed along its dorsal border.

- The flap is rotated into the area of the thumb requiring coverage, and skin graft is applied. Absorbable sutures are recommended to affix the skin graft to avoid interference with its adherence. Alternatively, the flap can be harvested as a fasciocutaneous flap, although in most cases there will be excessive bulk. If used as a fasciocutaneous flap, donor site defects wider than 6 cm will require skin grafting.

- A report has described use of the radial forearm flap combined with the radial thenar flap elevated as a large radial soft tissue sleeve.[6] Advancement of both the radial forearm and thenar soft tissues based on the radial artery may provide circumferential soft tissue coverage for the thumb and may be especially useful in large degloving type injuries.

## Postoperative Rehabilitation

- The limb is elevated and splinted to protect the soft tissues. Anticoagulants are not required. Although the thumb requires immobilization until skin graft stability at 3 weeks, the other digits should be subjected to a range of motion program as much as possible with use of an interval safe position splint.

## Advantages and Disadvantages

- The radial forearm flap offers the advantage of a large area of donor tissue from the involved extremity with the potential for inclusion of bone, nerve, and tendon grafts. Microvascular anastomosis is not required, and, when performed as a fascial flap with onlay skin graft, this flap supplies coverage of appropriate thickness. Sacrifice of the radial artery has not been associated with significant patient symptoms.

- The main disadvantages of this flap are related to its use as a fasciocutaneous flap. In this form, it results in bulky coverage with potentially unstable skin and is associated with a high rate of patient donor site complaints.

## Index Finger Flap for Dorsal Thumb Defects

- An island flap from the dorsum of the index finger based on the dorsal intermetacarpal artery from the first web space offers soft tissue coverage for dorsal thumb defects, preventing the need for bone shortening in the common injuries.

- The flap is elevated from the dorsum of the index finger and may extend from the level of the proximal interphalangeal (PIP) joint to the metacarpophalangeal

(MCP) joint, depending on the size of defect requiring coverage. The skin over the proximal phalanx is elevated along with the subcutaneous fat in a distal to proximal fashion, avoiding the epitenon (Figure 5–5).

- The flap is rotated to the dorsum of the thumb, without twisting of the base to avoid vascular compromise, and sewn in place. Full-thickness skin is harvested to cover the donor site of the index finger. The flap is separated at 2 to 3 weeks.

## Great Toe Wraparound Flap

- The principles of these operations are described in this chapter, but a detailed description of microsurgical reconstructive procedures is given in Chapter 9.
- Use of a filleted composite tissue flap of skin, neurovascular pedicle, nail, and distal phalanx was described by Morrison et al.[7] in 1980. Although this technique originally was described for amputations distal to the MCP joint, it since has been used with iliac crest graft at amputation levels proximal to the MCP joint.[8]
- Dissection of the vascular system is similar to that for the great toe harvest (see later). This flap is often used in cases of thumb loss distal to the proximal phalangeal level and is associated with minimal donor site morbidity because the toe proximal phalanx is preserved.

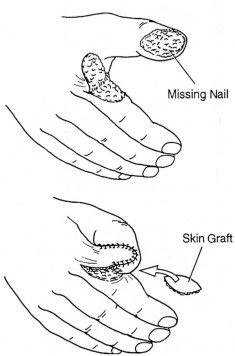

Figure 5–5:
**A rotational flap from the index finger can be used to cover dorsal tissue loss on the thumb. The donor site is covered with a full-thickness skin graft. (From Thumb reconstruction. In Trumble TT, editor: *Principles of hand surgery and therapy.* Philadelphia, 2000, WB Saunders.)**

- A variation of the wraparound flap, the trim-toe flap, has been used in situations where the great toe is much larger than the thumb. In this technique, longitudinal osteotomy of the phalanx is performed to reduce the size of the transferred toe. Measurement of the unaffected thumb is used as a guide to the amount of great toe to be harvested.[9]

## Level B Amputations: Amputations Through the Proximal Phalanx of Thumb

- Amputations at this level include those through the proximal portion of the proximal phalanx. Patients suffering this level of injury have significant complaints in terms of functional loss, especially at the more proximal level, and note difficulty in tasks involving use of the thumb and index finger.
- Functional improvement can be achieved by increasing the relative length of the thumb remnant. This may be effectively achieved by web space deepening, metacarpal lengthening, or a combination of the two procedures. Actual restoration of thumb length can be achieved with microvascular transfer of a portion of the toe.

### Web Space Deepening

- Web space deepening can be performed as an isolated procedure in conjunction with techniques of metacarpal lengthening. Either a two- or four-flap Z-plasty can be performed, with a two-flap Z-plasty creating a deeper web and a four-flap Z-plasty a broader web.
- The two-flap Z-plasty is generally performed using angles measuring 60 degrees. The four-flap Z-plasty is performed using angles of 120 degrees that then are bisected for interdigitation. To prevent tenting of the first web space skin and improve the independent function of the thumb remnant, a portion of the first dorsal interosseous and adductor fascia should be recessed. An external fixator or K-wire is useful in maintaining maximum first web space breadth. Z-plasty can be performed in conjunction with metacarpal lengthening (Figure 5–6).

### Dorsal Rotation Flap

- A dorsal rotation flap can be useful in deepening the first web. The skin and subcutaneous tissues overlying the index and long finger can be elevated in a proximally based flap. This soft tissue elevation should be performed beyond the level of the MCP joints of the index and long finger. The extensor peritenon should be preserved. The flap then can be advanced into the first web to help create supple soft tissue coverage. This flap may be especially useful when more proximal levels of

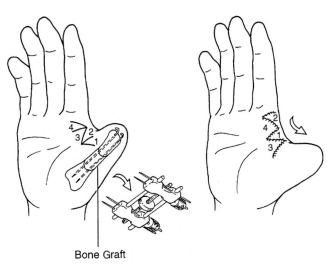

Figure 5–6:
Four-flap Z-plasty can be used alone or in conjunction with metacarpal lengthening for web reconstruction. (From Thumb reconstruction. In Trumble TT, editor: *Principles of hand surgery and therapy.* Philadelphia, 2000, WB Saunders.)

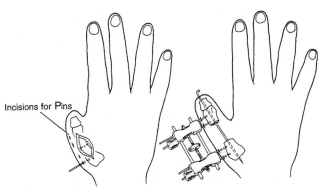

Figure 5–7:
Distracting external fixator used across the osteotomy site to achieve lengthening. (From Thumb reconstruction. In Trumble TT, editor: *Principles of hand surgery and therapy.* Philadelphia, 2000, WB Saunders.)

amputation have occurred and when first web space contracture has developed.
- The first web also can be deepened using skin and subcutaneous tissue elevated from the index finger. In this technique, the flap is elevated from the dorsoradial aspect of the index finger as a proximally based flap, with the proximal and radial pivot point located along the radial margin of the proximal palmar flexion crease. The flap then is advanced along the course of the proximal palmar flexion crease, and a full-thickness skin graft is applied to the donor site overlying the index finger if necessary.

### Postoperative Rehabilitation

- With all methods of web space deepening or coverage, prolonged splinting is required to maintain the breadth of the first web. This commences with the immediate application of a splint with the postoperative dressing and should be continued for several weeks after suture removal with use of a thermomold orthosis.

## Metacarpal Lengthening

- Restoration of effective thumb length can be achieved by metacarpal lengthening osteoplasty. In this technique, the periosteum is incised and elevated as a sleeve, an osteotomy is performed at the middle portion of the metacarpal, and a distracting external fixator is applied spanning the osteotomy site (Figure 5–7).
- Gradual distraction of 1 mm is performed twice per day beginning 3 to 5 days after osteotomy and is continued until 2 to 3 cm of length have been obtained. The process usually takes 3 to 4 weeks. Care must be taken to prevent

thumb adduction contracture, which is common as the lengthening progresses.
- The site of osteotomy is monitored closely by radiography for evidence of consolidation. Whereas in younger patients primary bone consolidation usually occurs, in adults supplementary bone grafting is required once the appropriate distraction length has been achieved. Once appropriate length has been reached with consolidation of bone, web space deepening is performed as previously described.

## Toe-to-Thumb Transfer

- Use of a toe-to-thumb transfer for B and C level amputations can provide excellent restoration of length and stability. The principles of these procedures are described in this section. Microvascular reconstruction of thumb amputations has been performed since the 1960s using a portion or all of the great or second toe.[10] Detailed descriptions of the vascular anatomy have improved the reliability of these microvascular transfers.[11]
- Microvascular transfer may be indicated for all levels of amputation from the level of the distal phalanx to the metacarpal shaft. An adequate soft tissue bed must be present prior to performance of a microvascular transfer. For cases with significant proximal soft tissue loss, pedicled or free vascularized soft tissue transfer may be required to provide coverage before toe-to-hand transfer consideration. An essential prerequisite for free tissue reconstruction is for the patient to completely refrain from smoking or chewing tobacco for at least one month prior to surgery.
- Reconstruction of the amputated thumb by transfer of a portion or all of the great toe or second toe may be performed. In general, the great toe has a better aesthetic appearance than the second toe, but donor site morbidity

is more significant with great toe harvest and may include significant aesthetic and functional disturbance of foot function. Use of the second toe creates minimal donor site morbidity or gait disturbance but provides a thumb post that is of notably reduced size.[12]

- Arterial supply to the foot is conveyed through both a dorsal system from the dorsalis pedis artery and a plantar system based on the posterior tibial artery. The great and second toes both are supplied by the first dorsal metatarsal artery, which is an extension of the dorsalis pedis (Figure 5–8). Several variations of the first metatarsal artery have been described, including an artery that is dorsal to the interosseous muscles (1A), an artery that is intramuscular (1B), a duplicate artery bracketing the interosseous muscle (2A), and a single vascular branch deep to the interosseous muscle (2B). The type 3 variation shows either an absent or a hypoplastic first dorsal metatarsal artery. Although in most cases dissection is performed based on the dorsal arch, these variations necessitate the surgeon's familiarity with the plantar anatomy. When palmar variations are encountered, either the toe harvest must be performed based on the plantar system or anastomosis of a plantar branch to the dorsal circulation must be performed.

- Because of significant variations in arterial supply to the great and second toe, preoperative evaluation should include Doppler ultrasonography or arteriography. In most cases, the vascular anastomosis is performed at the level of the radial artery near the anatomic snuffbox.

- The digital nerves and the terminal branch of the deep peroneal nerve are harvested with the composite graft. The latter nerve is found accompanying the first dorsal metatarsal artery.

## Great Toe Transfer

- The great toe is most often transferred in patients with thumb amputations at or about the level of the MCP joint who desire maximum thumb size. Anatomic studies have shown that the ipsilateral great toe is preferable over the contralateral great toe because of its angulation toward the digits.

- Because of the great toe's primary extension arc of motion, an osteotomy through the metatarsal head in the dorsal-proximal and plantar-distal orientations is required to prevent hyperextension of the newly created metatarsophalangeal joint. Skeletal length can be further augmented using iliac crest bone graft.[13]

- In cases of a plantar dominant circulation pattern, the incision must be performed more proximally on the plantar surface. Donor tendons are harvested with the great toe for transfer with the abductor hallucis used for opposition, the flexor pollicis longus attached to the flexor hallucis longus, the extensor pollicis longus attached to the extensor hallucis longus, and the abductor pollicis attached to the metatarsal head level.

- Although success rates for transfer viability are approximately 90%, use of the transferred great toe may be limited because of poor sensation, malposition, contracture, and poor joint motion.

## Second Toe Transfer

- Second toe transfer is used in cases of metacarpal level amputation. This transfer is associated with less donor site morbidity, albeit with a less satisfactory appearance. Because the second toe is a triphalangeal joint, fusion of the distal interphalangeal joint is recommended to prevent instability with pinch and grasp.

- The best results from transfer of the second toe have been reported with amputations at or distal to the metacarpal neck. More proximal level transfers have yielded only fair results.

- Microvascular transfers can be combined with other procedures, such as web space deepening or pedicle flap coverage. Reports now document significantly improved

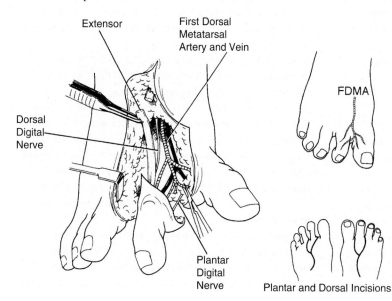

Figure 5–8:
Vascularity of great and second toes provided in most patients by the first dorsal metatarsal artery. (From Thumb reconstruction. In Trumble TT, editor: *Principles of hand surgery and therapy.* Philadelphia, 2000, WB Saunders.)

Extensor

First Dorsal Metatarsal Artery and Vein

Dorsal Digital Nerve

FDMA

Plantar Digital Nerve

Plantar and Dorsal Incisions

function in patients undergoing microvascular reconstruction compared to patients not undergoing reconstruction.[14]

# Level C Amputations: Amputations Through the Midportion of the Thumb Metacarpal

- Level C amputations occurring at the metacarpal level can be successfully treated by osteoplastic reconstruction, dorsal rotational flap, and toe-to-hand transfer.

## Osteoplastic Thumb Reconstruction

- Before the advent of microvascular surgery, the combination of soft tissue coverage, bone grafting, and innervation with a neurovascular island flap was used to restore thumb function and remains an excellent option for many patients. This type of reconstruction can be performed either in multiple stages or as a single procedure, depending on the type of soft tissue coverage used.
- Numerous sources of bone graft and pedicle flap have been described, with most authors preferring the use of iliac crest and the groin flap. Similar types of procedures have been performed using an osteocutaneous radial forearm flap or a free osteocutaneous iliac crest transfer, both of which can be performed as a single-stage reconstruction.

## Groin Flap

- Use of a groin flap based on the superficial circumflex iliac artery (SCIA) has been popular as a source of soft tissue coverage for several decades. The SCIA arises from the femoral artery and pierces the sartorius fascia before dividing into its deep and superficial branches. The flap is outlined to provide an appropriate amount of soft tissue and usually is harvested as an ellipse.
- Flexing the hip and pinching together the skin margins of the inguinal crease give the limits of flap width. With the patient supine, a line is drawn along the inguinal ligament from pubic tubercle to anterior superior iliac spine (ASIS). The path of the SCIA, and therefore the axis of the groin flap, parallels the inguinal ligament 2 cm distal to its course.
- The skin and subcutaneous tissues are elevated from lateral to medial, to the level of the ASIS, centered on the SCIA path. Medial to the ASIS, the dissection must incorporate the full thickness of the subcutaneous fat and the fascia overlying the sartorius muscle to ensure inclusion of the deep branch of the SCIA. The lateral femoral cutaneous nerve is identified in the groove between the sartorius and tensor fascia lata and is preserved by limiting the plane of dissection to a level superficial to this nerve.
- Medial dissection and skin release are required to allow for flap tube creation. Iliac crest bone graft can be harvested and incorporated at the time of flap elevation or delayed until after flap separation and maturation (Figure 5–9).
- With the groin flap attached to the patient's upper extremity, it is critical to secure the position of the limb, especially in the immediate postoperative period. Whereas some have advocated the routine use of external fixation from the iliac crest to the radius, this technique should only be used in children because of its association with upper extremity stiffness. Initial control of the arm and flap may be achieved by use of bulky

**Figure 5–9:**
Iliac crest graft used to add length of thumb at the time of groin flap performance or as a secondary procedure. (From Thumb reconstruction. In Trumble TT, editor: *Principles of hand surgery and therapy.* Philadelphia, 2000, WB Saunders.)

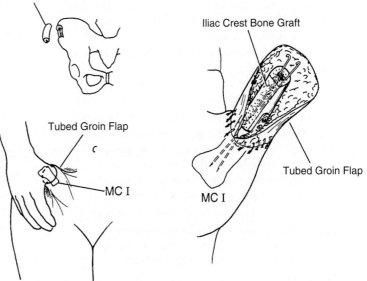

bandages between the arm and body, with the arm secured with taping or circumferential wrapping around the arm and torso to prevent kinking of the flap base or avulsion of the limb from the groin. Once the patient emerges from anesthesia and heavy analgesics, the restraints can be removed, and the patient is instructed on joint mobilization. With depression of the shoulder and bending of the torso, the elbow can be flexed beyond 90 degrees. Opposite shoulder and trunk maneuvers allow for elbow extension.

- While attached, the patient is instructed to perform range of motion exercises as much as possible to prevent upper extremity joint stiffness. The flap is detached from its base at the groin 3 weeks following elevation.

- Secondary bone grafting following complete flap healing prevents exposure of the bone graft to the frequently encountered problems of necrotic wound edges and drainage. The flap is incised and defatted enough to allow for iliac crest bone graft placement. A tricortical nonvascularized graft of appropriate size is harvested from the iliac crest and is affixed to the bony remnant of the thumb, which usually is at the distal metacarpal level.

- Because the groin flap/iliac crest graft construct is devoid of innervation, a neurovascular island flap is combined with this reconstruction as a tertiary procedure.

## Neurovascular Island Pedicle Flaps

- Sensory loss in the palmar surface of the thumb secondary to digital nerve injury may require use of a neurovascular island flap. Original reports of the neurovascular island pedicle flap indicated various sensory disturbances. Modifications of this flap have included division of the nerve of the transferred island flap with a suture repair of this nerve to one of the digital nerves of the thumb.[15]

- The neurovascular island flap is outlined along the ulnar border of the middle finger and is elevated to correspond to the area of the thumb to be covered, with allowance for flap shrinkage (Figure 5–10). Proximal dissection to the palm is performed using zigzag incisions, following the course of the common digital artery between the middle and ring fingers.

- Sacrifice of the corresponding radial branch of the common digital artery to the ring finger is required for proper mobilization of the flap. The flap can be passed under a skin bridge or through a connecting incision made to the thumb to prevent pedicle occlusion.

- Division and secondary repair of the digital nerve innervating this flap has been shown to improve its sensory characteristics and should be performed if a recipient nerve is available. A full-thickness skin graft is harvested to provide coverage to the donor site. Complications include vascular compromise, flap necrosis, and stiffness of both recipient and donor digits.

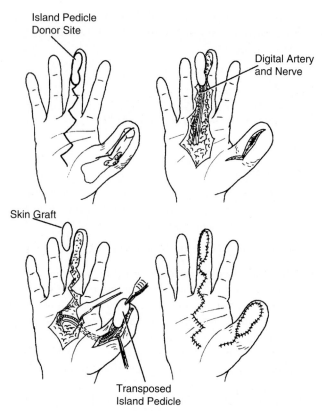

Figure 5–10:
**Neurovascular island flap elevation from long finger with transposition to thumb defect. (From Thumb reconstruction. In Trumble TT, editor:** *Principles of hand surgery and therapy.* **Philadelphia, 2000, WB Saunders.)**

## Single-Stage Osteoplastic Thumb Reconstruction Using Radial Forearm Flap

- In this technique, the bony column can be reconstructed using either iliac crest or a portion of the radius. In most cases, iliac crest is harvested and soft tissue coverage performed using either a radial forearm fasciocutaneous or a fascial flap with applied skin graft as described earlier.

- The radial forearm flap can be harvested with a corticocancellous portion of the radius (Figure 5–11). Simultaneous performance of a neurovascular island flap as previously described provides sensation to reconstructed thumb.

### Advantages and Disadvantages

- Use of a tissue source from the involved extremity obviates the need for microsurgical anastomosis.

- Disadvantages include the requirement for a complete carpal vascular arch and limitations of flap size. Donor site problems with regard to appearance, healing, and tendon adherence have been reported in up to 30% of patients undergoing radial forearm flap procedures. Reports of

Figure 5–11:

**Single-stage osteoplastic reconstruction with pedicled radial forearm harvested with cortico-cancellous segment of radial bone. (From Thumb reconstruction. In Trumble TT, editor: *Principles of hand surgery and therapy.* Philadelphia, 2000, WB Saunders.)**

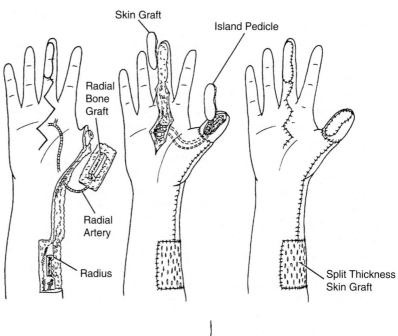

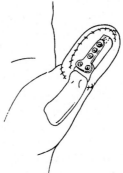

radius fracture following flap harvest indicate the need for postoperative immobilization and protection.

# Level D Amputation: Amputations Through the Proximal Portion of the First Ray

- With loss of the thumb proximal to the midmetacarpal, complete thumb reconstruction is necessary. Amputations at this level require treatment providing greater length than that achieved by web space deepening or metacarpal lengthening.
- Whereas amputations occurring at the level of the metacarpal neck can be reconstructed with the use of toe-to-thumb transfer, amputations proximal to this region usually require pollicization of another digit.

## Pollicization

- Pollicization can be performed using either a normal or an injured digit. With pollicization, thumb post restoration can be performed in a single stage with excellent vascular supply and sensation. Although the index finger is most commonly pollicized, the ring finger is the second choice digit for this procedure. Use of the long finger for pollicization has been described but has the problems of excessive length and difficult soft tissue balancing.
- Creation of an appropriate pollicized digit requires shortening for pinch and opposition. This can be achieved by either segmental resection of a portion of the metacarpal distal to wrist tendon insertions or amputation of the distal phalanx. Metacarpal shortening allows preservation of the nail but provides a digit that is much narrower than the normal thumb. Flexor and extensor tendons are redundant and may require shortening. Intrinsic muscle balancing may be difficult. Therefore, some authors have advocated a pollicization technique that retains metacarpal length but includes distal phalangeal amputation.[16] Whichever technique is selected, the goal of pollicization is the creation of a stable sensate post that is capable of opposition and pinch to the other digits.

## Surgical Technique

- Numerous incisions that provide the rotational skin flaps required for pollicization have been described.[17,18] Whichever type is selected, creation of a supple first web space with adequate coverage is essential for use. The description by Riordan[17] provides an excellent technique for reconstruction and is described with minor modifications.
- A dorsal V-shaped incision is made from the midproximal phalangeal level, with the distal limbs extending along the radial and ulnar midaxial lines. The proximal apex extends to the midmetacarpal region of the index finger. The flap is elevated to include the fat and subcutaneous tissue to the level of the extensor tendon. Preservation of any radial side veins ensures venous outflow (Figure 5–12).
- The midaxial incisions are connected along the palmar surface midway between the digital and PIP crease, and the radial side incision is carried proximally as an S shape that represents the border of the thenar eminence. The palmar flap is elevated along with most of the subcutaneous fat, with only a thin layer left on the neurovascular bundles, and provides the tissue for coverage of the first web space.
- The common digital artery of the index and long finger is dissected, and the radial digital vessels to the long finger are ligated (Figure 5–13). The ulnar digital nerve to the index is separated gently from the radial digital nerve to the long finger and mobilized into the palm.
- The A1 and A2 pulleys are divided to allow the flexor tendons to bowstring and more closely follow the flexor

pollicis longus (FPL) vector of pull. The deep transverse intermetacarpal ligament is divided to allow mobilization and rotation of the index finger.
- The tendons are identified, and the extensor digitorum communis (EDC) tendon to the index is divided at the MCP level with the extensor indicis proprius (EIP) tendon divided 1 cm proximal to this joint. The dorsal and palmar interossei are elevated from the shaft of the metacarpal and from their proximal phalangeal level attachments.
- With the metacarpal shaft exposed, a segment of bone is resected from just distal to the insertion of the extensor carpi radialis longus (ECRL) tendon to the metacarpal neck. Inadequate resection leaves the pollicized digit excessively long, with both cosmetic and functional problems.
- The MCP joint is maximally hyperextended to prevent retropulsion of the joint with pinch and is stabilized with several nonabsorbable sutures or K-wires. The metacarpal head is translated proximally and placed anterior to the metacarpal base so that its alignment is not in the plane of the palm (Figure 5–14). Once positioned anterior to the metacarpal base, the metacarpal head is pronated 120 degrees, palmarly abducted 40 degrees, and extended 20 degrees with its position maintained by K-wires placed through the metacarpal head into the carpus (Figure 5–15)
- Once bony stabilization is achieved, the tendons are attached. The first dorsal interosseous is advanced distally to the radial lateral band forming the thumb abductor. The first palmar interosseous is advanced to the lateral band at the PIP level to create the thumb adductor. The

Figure 5–12:
**Incisions to provide first web and radial side coverage after rotation as described by Riordan.**

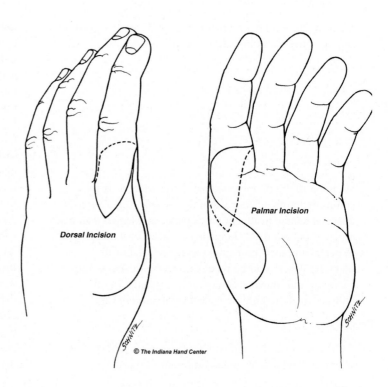

Dorsal Incision

Palmar Incision

© The Indiana Hand Center

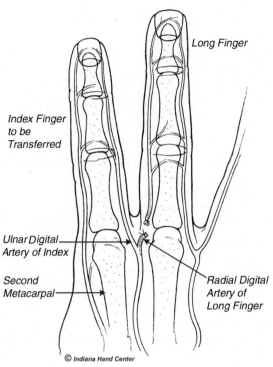

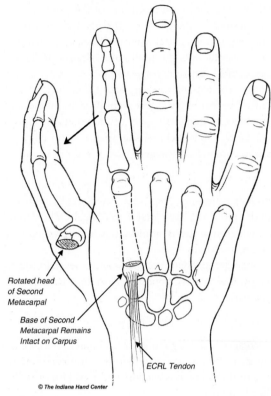

Figure 5–13:
Division of radial digital vascular bundle to long finger is required for index pollicization.

Figure 5–14:
Resection of metacarpal segment from insertion of extensor carpi radiolis longus (ECRL) tendon to metacarpal neck.

Figure 5–15:
The second metacarpal head is positioned volar to the second metacarpal base and affixed with K-wires.

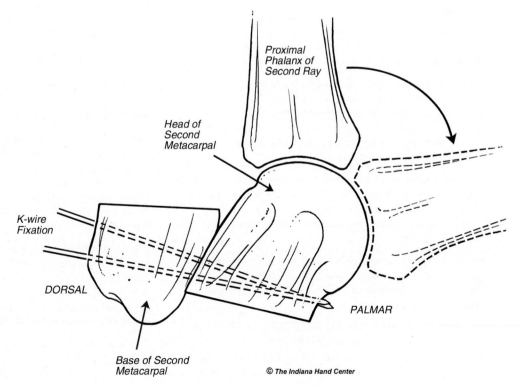
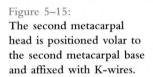

EDC is repaired to the radial side of the extensor mechanism over the proximal phalanx and the EIP is reattached to the central extensor tendon, restoring abductor pollicis longus (APL) and extensor pollicis longus (EPL) function, respectively.

- Flaps are rotated and interdigitated for closure, with the palmar flap forming the first web space and the dorsal flap covering the radial aspect of the pollicized digit. In some cases, a full-thickness skin graft is required to achieve complete coverage.

## Postoperative Rehabilitation

- The bulky dressing is removed 2 to 3 weeks after surgery, and the pin is removed after 4 to 6 weeks. The patient is maintained in a thermomold splint, and active range of motion is started.
- Maximal independent use may require several months of therapy. A secondary opponensplasty may be required in some patients.

## Advantages and Disadvantages

- Advantages include good grasp and pinch, use of a donor digit that often is otherwise bypassed following other types of thumb reconstruction, and lack of morbidity to other body parts.
- Disadvantages of this technique include inadequate first web creation, digital stiffness, and lack of opposition strength, all of which may require secondary reconstruction.[19]

# References

1. Lister GD: The choice of procedure following thumb amputation. *Clin Orthop* 195:45-51, 1985.
   In this classic review, the author outlines the types of reconstructive procedures available for the various levels of thumb loss.

2. Foucher G, Delacre O, Citron N, Molderez A: Long-term outcome of neurovascular palmar advancement flaps for distal thumb injuries. *Br J Plast Surg* 52:64-68, 1999.
   In this study, patients were followed for more than 6 years to evaluate their function following neurovascular palmar advancement flaps for distal thumb injury.

3. Baumeister S, Menke H, Wittemann M, Germann G: Functional outcome after the Moberg advancement flap in the thumb. *J Hand Surg [Am]* 27:105-114, 2002.
   In this study, the excellent results of the Moberg advancement flap are described.

4. Hynes DE: Neurovascular pedicle and advancement flaps for palmar thumb defects. *Hand Clin* 13:207-216, 1997.
   Various palmar, advancement, and pedicle flaps are described in detail by the authors.

5. Keim HA, Grantham SA: Volar flap advancement for thumb and fingertip injuries. *Clin Orthop* 66:109-112, 1969.
   A classic article describing coverage techniques for thumb and fingertip injuries in which the authors credit Dr. Erik Moberg

6. Omokawa S, Mizumoto S, Fukui A et al: Innervated radial thenar flap combined with radial forearm flap transfer for thumb reconstruction. *Plast Reconstr Surg* 107:152-154, 2001.
   This innovative extension of the radial forearm flap describes the elevation and advancement of the radial thenar and forearm combined flap to cover degloving injuries of the thumb.

7. Morrison WA, O'Brien BM, MacLeod AM: Thumb reconstruction with a free neurovascular wraparound flap from the big toe. *J Hand Surg* 5:575, 1980.
   This classic article of the microsurgery literature describes in detail the use of the wraparound flap from the great toe.

8. Lee KS, Park JW, Chung WK: Thumb reconstruction with a wraparound free flap according to the level of amputation. *J Hand Surg [Am]* 25:644-650, 2000.
   This study describes the use of a wraparound flap combined with iliac crest bone graft.

9. Woo SH, Kim JS, Kim HH, Seul JH: Microsurgical reconstruction of partial thumb defects. *J Hand Surg [Br]* 24B:161-169, 1999.
   The authors treated partial thumb defects with free vascularized grafts taken most often from the great toe.

10. O'Brien BM, MacLeod AM, Sykes PJ, Donahoe S: Hallux-to-hand transfer. *Hand* 7:128, 1975.
    This short description of great toe-to-hand transfer is one of the early reports of microvascular thumb reconstruction.

11. Gu Y-D, Zhang G-M, Chen D-S, et al: Vascular anatomic variations in second toe transfers. *J Hand Surg [Am]* 25A: 277-281, 2000.
    In this exhaustive anatomic study of more than 300 second toe transfers, the authors document the variations in the first dorsometatarsal artery.

12. Shin AY, Bishop AT, Berger RA: Microvascular reconstruction of the traumatized thumb. *Hand Clin* 15:347-371, 1999.
    This review article describes the numerous great and second toe anatomic variations. Detailed surgical descriptions of each type of flap are well outlined.

13. Foucher G, Chabaud M: The bipolar lengthening technique: a modified partial toe transfer for thumb reconstruction. *Plast Reconstr Surg* 102:1981-1987, 1998.
    In this small series of patients, a technique of thumb reconstruction using a combination of first web space deepening and digital lengthening with a vascularized partial great toe transfer is described.

14. Chung KC, Wei FC: An outcome study of thumb reconstruction using microvascular toe transfer. *J Hand Surg [Am]* 25:651-658, 2000.
    A battery of outcomes questionnaires found that function of the amputated thumb reconstructed with toe transfer was markedly greater than that of the unreconstructed thumb.

15. Oka Y: Sensory function of the neurovascular island flap in thumb reconstruction—comparison of original and modified procedures. *J Hand Surg [Am]* 25:637-643, 2000.

for developing the palmar advancement flap for thumb coverage.

Sensory function using a neurovascular island flap for thumb reconstruction may be improved by dividing the nerve of the transferred island flap and suturing it to a nerve from the thumb.

16. Brunelli GA, Brunelli GR: Reconstruction of traumatic absence of the thumb in the adult by pollicization. *Hand Clin* 8:41-55, 1992.
    The authors review the history and technical details of pollicization, with description of operative techniques.

17. Riordan D: Pollicization. In Spinner M, editor: *Kaplan's functional and surgical anatomy of the hand,* ed 3. Philadelphia, 1984, JB Lippincott.
    A truly classic article by one of the masters of thumb reconstruction in which the author gives a detailed description of his pollicization technique.

18. Buck-Gramcko D: Pollicization of the index finger. Method and results in aplasia and hypoplasia of the thumb. *J Bone Joint Surg Am* 53:1605-1617, 1971.
    A landmark article reporting on the technique and outcome of numerous pollicizations for congenital thumb hypoplasia.

19. Stern PJ, Lister GD: Pollicization after traumatic amputation of the thumb. *Clin Orthop* 155:85-94, 1981.
    A long-term study of 19 patients undergoing pollicization for traumatic thumb loss showed superior results when nondamaged digits were used compared to previously traumatized ones.

# Distal Radius Fractures

John A. Jiuliano* and Jesse Jupiter†

*MD, MS, BS, Fellow, Department of Hand and Upper Extremity, Massachusetts General Hospital, Boston, MA; Staff Orthopaedic Surgeon, Washington Hospital Healthcare System, Fremont, CA

†MD, Hansjörg Wyss/AD Professor, Harvard Medical School; Director, Orthopaedic Hand Surgery, Massachusetts General Hospital, Boston, MA

## Introduction

- Distal radius fractures account for one sixth of all fractures that are seen and treated in the emergency room.[1]
- There is no consensus regarding the description of the condition, the appropriate treatment, or even the anticipated outcome.[1]
- Goal of treatment is a functional wrist and hand.
- Fractures of the distal end of the radius may be part of a spectrum of injuries that include the distal radioulnar joint (DRUJ), distal ulna, and fracture-dislocations of the carpus.
- Distal radius fractures are more common in women, increase in incidence in both sexes with advancing age, and result more frequently from falls from level ground than from higher-energy trauma (Box 6–1).

## Classification

- To be effective, a classification system must accurately depict the type and severity of the fracture and serve as a basis for both treatment and evaluation of treatment outcome.[2]
- Eponymic descriptions no longer are effective in delineating the individual characteristics of specific fractures.[2]
- There are many historic and contemporary classifications.
  - Frykman Classification (1967)
    - Classification identified individual involvement of the radiocarpal and radioulnar joints and the presence or absence of a fracture of the ulnar styloid process[2]
    - Does not account for quantification of the extent or direction of the initial fracture displacement, degree of comminution, or shortening of the distal fragment[2]
  - Fernandez Classification
    - Emphasizes the mechanism of injury rather than the more traditional radiologic characteristics[2]
    - Divides the types of distal radius fractures into five major groups[2] (Box 6–2 and Figure 6–1)
  - Distal Radioulnar Joint Classification
    - Centers upon the presence or absence of either DRUJ subluxation or dislocation of the ulnar head caused by concomitant rupture of the triangular fibrocartilage complex and capsular ligaments and the degree of joint surface involvement[2]
    - Three basic types of DRUJ lesions have been established, depending upon the residual stability of the DRUJ after the fracture of the distal radius has been reduced and stabilized[2] (Box 6–3)

### Box 6–1    Risk Factors for Distal Radius Fractures

- Development of postmenopausal osteoporosis has been implicated as a critical risk factor.
- The pattern of distal radius fractures is consistent with the pattern of falling in the aging population.[2]
- Postural instability may be more of a risk factor than osteoporosis in women.

| Box 6–2 | Fernandez Classification[2] |
|---|---|
| Type I | Bending fractures: Thin metaphyseal cortex fails because of tensile stresses with the opposite cortex |
| Type II | Shearing fractures of the joint surface |
| Type III | Compression fractures of the joint surface: Articular surfaces are disrupted, with impaction of the subchondral and metaphyseal cancellous bone |
| Type IV | Avulsion fractures: Fractures associated with ligamentous attachments |
| Type V | Combined fractures: Combinations of bending, compression, shearing, or avulsion mechanisms; usually high-velocity injuries |

- AO (Arbeitsgemeinschaft für Osteosynthesefragen) System
  - The most detailed classification, organized in order of increasing severity of the osseous and articular lesions[1]
  - Divides fractures into extraarticular (type A), partial articular (type B), and complete articular (type C) (Figure 6–2)

## Functional Anatomy

- The metaphyseal flare of the distal end of the radius has a large biconcave surface for articulation with the proximal part of the carpel row.[1]
- The distal end of the radius articulates with the convex articular surface of the distal end of the ulna at the sigmoid notch[1] (Figure 6–3).
- The radius and hand rotate about the fixed ulna.[1]
- Experimental data by Palmer have suggested that approximately 80 percent of axial loads are supported by the distal end of the radius and 20 percent by the triangular fibrocartilage and the distal end of the ulna.[1]
- In mechanical studies, Short et al. noted a considerable transfer of load onto the ulna, with progressive dorsal angulation of the distal end of the radius.[1]
- Clinically, this may result in pain at the radiocarpal articulation and limited grip strength if the angulation is not reduced.[1]
- In some patients, especially those younger than 25 years, a pattern of midcarpal instability has been described in association with loss of normal palmar tilt.[1]
- Pain, decreased grip strength, and a midcarpal instability pattern that is seen on lateral radiographs are the hallmarks of this dynamic intercarpal instability, which can be corrected through a corrective osteotomy.[1]
- Malalignment when associated with shortening of the distal end of the radius may result in dysfunction of the DRUJ, manifested by limited rotation of the forearm and impingement of the ulna and the radius.[1]
- The palmar surface of the distal end of the radius is relatively flat, extending volarly in a gentle curve.[2]

- The dorsal aspect of the radius is convex. The anatomic relationships of the extensor retinaculum, six dorsal extensor compartments, and dorsal radial cortex are of extreme importance in the surgical approaches and in as the placement of internal fixation on the dorsum of the radius.[2]
- The articular end of the radius slopes in an ulnar and palmar direction, and the natural tendency for the carpus to slide in an ulnar direction is resisted by the intracapsular and interosseous carpal ligaments.[2]
- Movements of the carpal bones on the distal radius occur in two axes that include flexion and extension in the transverse plane and adduction and abduction in the horizontal plane.[2]
- The combination of these movements permits the hand to pass in a conical dimension described by Kapandji as the "cone of circumduction."[2]
- At the ulnar aspect of the lunate facet arises the triangular fibrocartilage, which extends out to the base of the ulnar styloid process, functioning as an important stabilizer of the DRUJ.[2]
- Additional ("secondary") stabilizers of the DRUJ include the interosseous membrane of the forearm, the pronator quadratus muscle, and the tendons and sheaths of the extensor and flexor carpi ulnaris muscles.[2]
- Several investigators have suggested that the distal radius and ulna can be viewed in terms of bony and articular "columns."[3]
- These concepts have added substantially to our understanding of methods for achieving operative stability of complex fractures and the development of new implants specifically oriented to the structural anatomy of the columns.[3]
- Rikli and Regazzoni divided the distal metaphyseal and articular regions into three columns[3]:
  1. A medial column consisting of the distal ulna, triangular fibrocartilage, and DRUJ
  2. An intermediate column including the medial part of the distal radius with its lunate fossa and sigmoid notch
  3. A lateral column consisting of the scaphoid fossa and radial styloid process (Figure 6–4)
- Medoff suggested that the architecture be viewed in terms of the components of injury and that fractures be viewed in terms of cortical fracture components: the radial column, the dorsal ulnar cortical wall, the volar rim, and the intraarticular and dorsal ulnar split[3] (Figure 6–5).

## Radiographic Anatomy

- In the frontal view, the slope or inclination of the distal end of the radius is represented by the angle formed by a line drawn from the tip of the radial styloid process to the ulnar corner of the articular surface of the distal end of the radius and a line drawn perpendicular to the

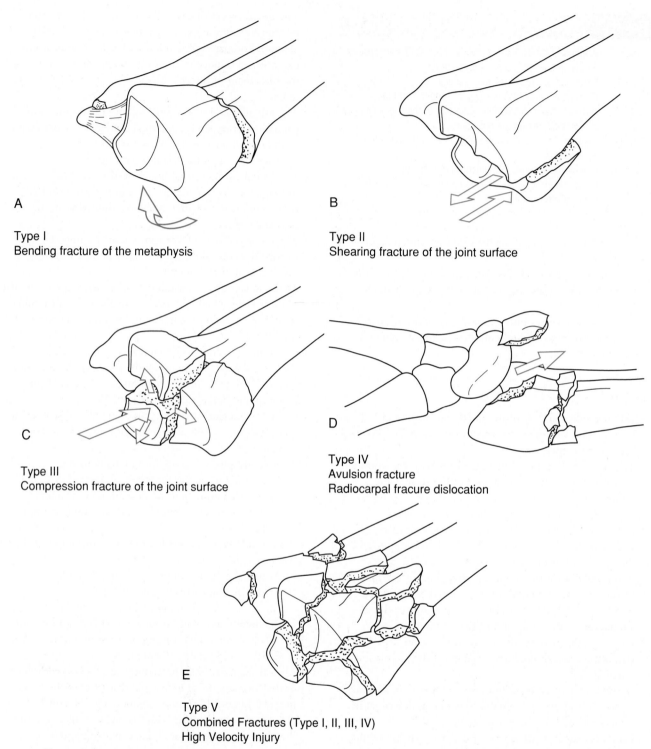

A

Type I
Bending fracture of the metaphysis

B

Type II
Shearing fracture of the joint surface

C

Type III
Compression fracture of the joint surface

D

Type IV
Avulsion fracture
Radiocarpal fracure dislocation

E

Type V
Combined Fractures (Type I, II, III, IV)
High Velocity Injury

Figure 6–1:

**Fernandez classification emphasizes the mechanism of injury rather than the more traditional radiologic characteristics. It classifies fractures into five types: type I bending (A), type II shearing (B), type III compression (C), type IV avulsion (D), and type V combined (E).**

longitudinal axis of the radius. The average inclination is 21 to 23 degrees[3] (Figure 6–6).

- The palmar inclination is obtained by a line drawn connecting the distal most point of the dorsal and volar cortical rims. The angle this line creates with a line drawn perpendicular to the longitudinal axis of the radius

reflects the palmar inclination. The average is 11 to 12 degrees[3] (Figures 6–7 and 6–8).

- The radial length, as measured on the anteroposterior radiograph, represents the distance between a line drawn from the tip of the styloid process perpendicular to the axis of the radius and a second perpendicular line at the

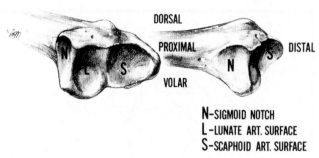

**N**-SIGMOID NOTCH
**L**-LUNATE ART. SURFACE
**S**-SCAPHOID ART. SURFACE

Figure 6–3:
Anatomy of the distal radius depicting the sigmoid notch and scaphoid and lunate facets.

level of the distal articular surface of ulnar head. A normal value is 11 to 12 mm.[3]

• The vertical distance between a line parallel to the proximal surface of the lunate facet of the distal radius and a line parallel to the articular surface of the ulnar head has been referred to as the *ulnar variance*[1] (Figure 6–9).

• Comparison radiographs with the uninjured wrist ideally taken in the same manner with the shoulder abducted 90 degrees and elbow flexed 90 degrees are necessary to determine normal length on an individual basis.[1]

• With fracture displacement, the ulnar head will commonly be in a distal relationship (positive variance), and this measurement can be used to judge loss of radial length or height.[1]

• The articular surfaces of the carpal bones should be parallel and the joint surfaces of similar width

(Figure 6–10). A broken "arc" as described by Gilula is highly suggestive of injury to the supporting ligaments, the carpal bones, or both.[1]

• The initial prereduction radiographs show the extent of the direction of the initial displacement.[4]

• Traction radiographs assist in determining the type of fracture and the reduction.[4]

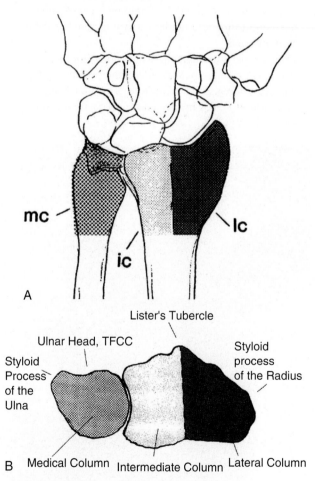

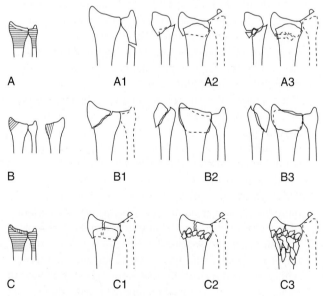

Figure 6–2:
AO/ASIF (Arbeitsgemeinschaft für Osteosynthesefragen/Association for the Study of Internal Fixation) classification of distal radius fractures.
A, Extraarticular fracture. B, Simple articular fracture (partial).
C, Complex articular fracture (multifragmented).

Figure 6–4:
Structural anatomy of the distal radius is divided into three columns by Rikli and Regazzoni. A, Anterior projection demonstrates the medial column *(mc)*, intermediate column *(ic)*, and lateral column *(lc)*. B, Coronal projection of the orientation of the structural columns. TFCC, triangular fibro-cartilage complex.

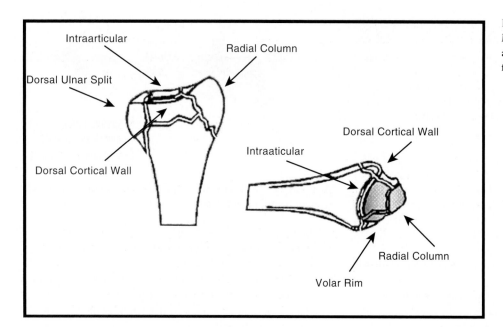

Figure 6–5:
Medoff divided the structural anatomy of the distal radius into five cortical fracture components.

- Repeat radiographic views should be obtained after reduction to identify residual deformity and the degree of comminution.[4]
- Computerized tomography (CT) allows improved assessment of the articular surface and provides additional information regarding the degree of comminution, detection of DRUJ involvement, and quantification of articular gapping.[5]

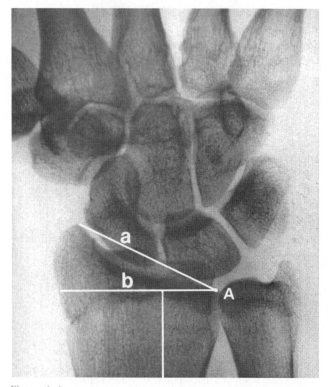

Figure 6–6:
In the frontal plane, the average ulnar inclination is 21 to 23 degrees. a to A, inclination; A to B, perpendicular to long axis of radius.

- CT scanning provides useful information for preoperative planning of intraarticular distal radius fractures[5] and fracture patterns difficult to visualize on plain radiographs.
- Three-dimensional CT image reconstruction has supplemented trispiral tomography and CT as the study of choice (if available) to define the fracture pattern[3] (see Figure 6–18B).
- Reduction of fractures of the distal radius in most cases is obtained by applying the force opposite to that which produced the injury.[3]
- Understanding the mechanism of injury proves useful when deciding on the appropriate reduction maneuvers.[3]
- Dorsal bending-type fractures exhibit increased dorsal angulation, shortening, and radial deviation and supination of the distal fragment. These conditions are reduced by applying longitudinal traction, palmar flexion, ulnar deviation, and pronation.[3]
- The principle of reduction is based on applying tension on the soft tissue hinge located on the concavity of the angulation.
- One problems with longitudinal traction, particularly in comminuted fractures, is the failure to restore the anatomic palmar tilt of the distal articular surface. Although extreme palmar flexion is effective in reproducing palmar tilt, it cannot be maintained because of the adverse effects on hand function and the risk of median nerve compression.[3]
- Impacted compression-type articular fractures and those with extreme displacement may not respond to reduction by ligamentotaxis and may require open reduction.[3]

## Fracture Stability

- Lafontaine et al. studied 112 consecutive fractures of the distal radius treated conservatively and suggested seven

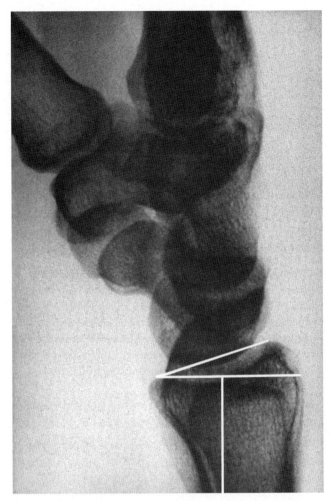

Figure 6–7:

**In the sagittal plane, the normal palmar tilt averages 11 to 12 degrees.**

factors possibly related to instability following fracture reduction[3] (Box 6–4):

1. Initial dorsal (or palmar) angulation greater than 20 degrees
2. Dorsal metaphyseal comminution

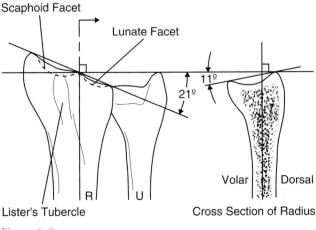

Figure 6–8:

**Schematic drawings of the average inclination and palmar tilt of the distal radius.**

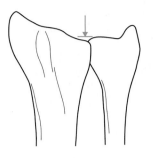 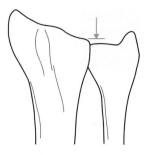

Positive variance        Negative variance

Figure 6–9:

**Ulnar variance of the distal radius.**

3. Intraarticular radiocarpal fracture
4. Associated ulnar fractures
5. Patient age older than 60 years (osteoporosis)
6. More than 5 mm of shortening
7. Displacement more that two thirds the width of the shaft in any direction

- They noted that fractures associated with three or more factors were unstable following closed reduction and plaster immobilization.[3]
- These factors were further defined as radiographic findings that had been determined to be predictive of a poor functional outcome and included the following:
  1. A fracture with a dorsal tilt of the distal radial articular surface of more than 20 degrees[6]
  2. A fracture with articular displacement of more than 2 mm[6]

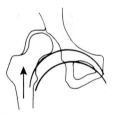 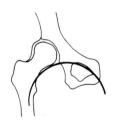

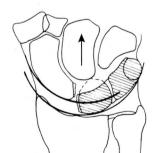 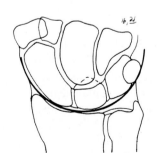

Figure 6–10:

**Scapholunate diastasis may accompany compression fractures of the distal radius. A, Uniform radiographic arc of the proximal carpal row is a sign of intercarpal stability, as is the nondisrupted Shenton-Menard arc for stable hip. B, When traction is applied to the wrist with a scapholunate tear, the scaphoid shifts distally.[3]**

| Box 6–4 | Unstable Fracture Patterns: Radiographic Findings on Initial Injury X-Ray Films |
|---|---|

- Greater than 20 degrees of dorsal or palmar angulation
- Displacement of more than two thirds of the width of the shaft in any direction
- Metaphyseal comminution
- More than 5 mm of shortening
- Intraarticular component
- Associated ulnar fracture
- Osteoporosis

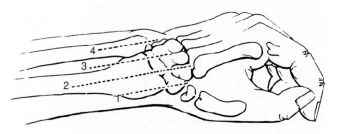

Figure 6–11:

The most common dorsal extensile approaches are illustrated. 1, Interval between 1st and 2nd extensor compartment; 2, interval between 2nd and 4th extensor compartments; 3, interval between 4th and 5th extensor compartments; and 4, interval between 5th and 6th extensor compartments.

3. A displaced fracture with either
   A. A fixed carpal malalignment (a lunate with more than 25 degrees more dorsal angulation than that in the contralateral uninvolved wrist, as seen on lateral radiograph)
   B. Incongruity of the DRUJ (with complete disassociation of the distal ulna from the sigmoid notch of the distal radius as a result of shortening or angulation)
   C. Subluxation of the radiocarpal joint associated with a displaced intraarticular fracture of the distal radius[6]

- Stable fractures do not displace at the time of presentation or following manipulative reduction.[3]
- Abbaszadegan et al. defined stable fractures as bending fractures presenting with minimal displacement, having dorsal angulation less than 5 degrees, and axial shortening less than 2 mm.[3]

## Surgical Approaches to the Distal Radius

- As a general rule, the approach should be extensile, offer sufficient exposure to accomplish the surgical goals, and heal with a limited degree of scarring.[3]

### Dorsal Approaches

- Dorsal exposures involve extensile longitudinal incisions because the mobility and elasticity of the skin limit the potential for scar contracture.[7] Cutaneous nerves should be identified and preserved to prevent a painful neuroma, and large veins should be preserved to limit edema formation.[7] Place the skin incision directly over the interval of intended exposure.[7]

### Between the First and Second Extensor Compartments[7]

- See Figure 6–11, incision 1.
- This interval provides exposure of the dorsoradial aspect of the radius. The radial sensory nerve is at risk.

The first and second compartments are elevated. The articular surface can be visualized to ensure an anatomic reduction through either an arthroscope or an incision in the dorsal wrist capsule. A more distal dissection is required to expose the wrist capsule, and the radial artery and its dorsal carpal branch are at risk as they course from palmar to dorsal through the snuffbox.[7]

### Between the Second and Fourth Extensor Compartments[7]

- See Figure 6–11, incision 2.
- A dorsal longitudinal skin incision is centered over Lister's tubercle. The extensor retinaculum is incised over the radial aspect of the third compartment to preserve an ulnarly based retinacular flap for later placement beneath the second compartment to protect the radial wrist extensor tendons from underlying implants. The extensor pollicis longus tendon is mobilized and retracted radially; it can be left permanently in a subcutaneous position with favorable results. The dorsal surface of the distal radius is exposed through the third extensor compartment. To limit adhesions and tendon irritation, the fourth compartment is subperiosteally elevated, leaving the floor of its compartment intact. The dorsal wrist capsule is incised to allow inspection of the distal radial articular surface and carpus. This arthrotomy may be longitudinal, oblique, or transverse along the margin of the distal radius. A dorsal ligament-sparing capsulotomy can be used when subtotal exposure of the radiocarpal joint is sufficient.

### Ulnar Dorsal Exposures[7]

- See Figure 6–11, incisions 3 and 4.
- Exposures between the fourth and fifth or between the fifth and sixth extensor compartments are straightforward and require identification and preservation of the branches of the dorsal ulnar sensory nerve.[7]

## Volar Exposures

### Henry Radial Volar Exposure

- See Figure 6–12.
- A longitudinal incision is made between the flexor carpi radialis tendon and the radial artery. Any distal extension that crosses the distal palmar wrist crease must do so at an oblique angle. The flexor carpi radialis sheath is incised, and the tendon is retracted ulnarly. The radial artery is retracted radially. Dissection is carried deeply to the pronator quadratus muscle, which is exposed and divided along its most radial aspect, leaving a small cuff of tissue for reattachment. More proximal exposure of the radius is achieved by similarly mobilizing the flexor pollicis longus muscle from its origin on the radius.

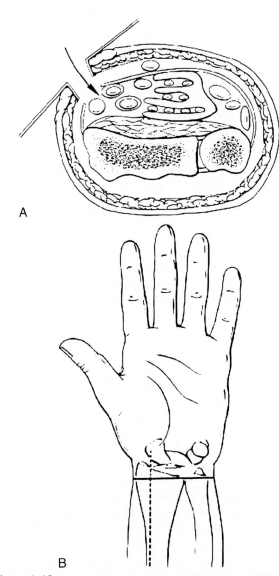

Figure 6–12:
**Distal part of the Henry approach between the tendon of the flexor carpi radialis and the radial artery. The *transverse line* corresponds to the level of the cross-section.**

### Ulnar Volar Exposure

- See Figure 6–13.
- A standard carpal tunnel incision is extended obliquely in an ulnar direction across the distal volar wrist crease and over the ulnar forearm to create a broad, radially based skin flap. This flap should ensure coverage of the carpal canal in case excessive swelling prevents complete wound closure. Deep dissection proceeds through the interval between the ulnar neurovascular bundle and the digital flexor tendons. The transverse carpal ligament is incised to allow mobilization of the flexor tendons and median nerve if an acute carpal tunnel syndrome is suspected. The distal pronator quadratus muscle is incised as it crosses the DRUJ. An incision of the volar wrist capsule may lead to carpal instability and should be avoided. During closure in younger individuals, the transverse carpal ligament may be repaired by a Z-lengthening technique.

### Dorsal Exposure of the Distal Ulna

- Exposure of the ulna on its dorsal or ulnar aspect is straightforward. A straight longitudinal incision is made in the interval between the extensor digiti quinti and extensor carpi ulnaris tendons or over its subcutaneous crest in the interval between the extensor and flexor carpi ulnaris tendons. Branches of the dorsal cutaneous branch of the ulnar nerve should be identified and protected.

## Treatment

- Local factors, including the quality of the bone, associated comminution, extent of displacement of fracture, and energy of the injury, must be taken considered when formulating a plan of treatment.
- Factors associated with the individual patient, such as lifestyle, psychological outlook, associated medical conditions, and compliance, must be considered.[1]

### Extraarticular Fractures of the Distal Radius

- Conservative treatment of distal radius fractures in adults is recommended:
  - Nondisplaced extraarticular fractures
  - Displaced fractures that remain stable following closed reduction
  - Unstable fractures in the elderly, in which the surgeon and patient accept an asymptomatic, well-functioning malunion (Box 6–4)
- Stable fractures may not require a full 6 weeks of immobilization and, because of adequate healing, require a short 3- to 4-week period of immobilization followed by a removable wrist splint until the patient feels comfortable, usually by 5 to 6 weeks following injury.
- Closed reduction is indicated for displaced fractures in which radiographic evidence indicates a stable

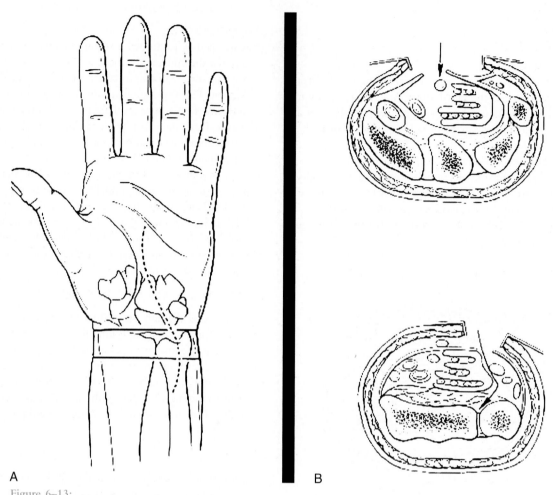

A      B

Figure 6–13:

Extensile approach to the ulnar side of the distal radius and carpal tunnel. A, The level of the approach is demonstrated at the proximal margin of the carpal tunnel. The flexor tendons and median nerve are retracted radially. B, The approach at the level of the ulnar side of the distal radius demonstrates retraction of the flexor tendons and median nerve radially, providing direct exposure to the volar ulnar side of the radius.[3]

realignment of the fracture fragments can be achieved and controlled with meticulous casting technique.

- Adequate anesthesia is imperative.
- Manipulative reduction is performed by
  › Disimpacting the fracture by increasing the initial deformity by extending the distal fragment. These are very unstable and rarely have satius factor outcomes with cost treatment.
  › Reduction is accomplished through traction combined with volar displacement and pronation of the distal fragment.
  › Volar angulated fractures (Smith fractures) require extension and supination of the distal fragments. These are very unstable and rarely have satisfactory outcomes with cast teatment.
- Longitudinal traction with finger traps and a counterweight uses the principle of ligamentotaxis for disimpaction and fragment realignment. Length and ulnar inclination are achieved, but restoration of palmar tilt requires an additional palmarly directed force.

## Immobilization

- Three-point casting technique of Charnley: two points of contact proximally and distally to the fracture on the side of the concavity of the initial angulation, and a counterpoint of contact at the fracture level on the convexity. A slight bend to the splint or cast (10–15 degrees) places the soft tissue bridge (periosteum and overlying tendons) under tension, provided the opposite cortex has good contact (tension-band principle), and maintains stable reduction.
- Dorsally angulated fractures (Colles fractures) are immobilized initially in no more than 15 degrees of palmar flexion and slight pronation (25 degrees) the first 2 weeks in a sugar tong splint. Volarly angulated fractures (Smith fractures) require 30 degrees of dorsal flexion and 40 degrees of supination. Excessive palmar flexion increase the risk of carpal tunnel syndrome, reflex sympathetic dystrophy, and permanent hand stiffness.

- Follow up x-rays films are obtained every week for the first 3 weeks to detect early loss of reduction. Additional x-ray films are taken 4 and 6 weeks after the reduction to detect any late loss of reduction.
- During the first 2 weeks, the initial splint should be adapted and remolded as soon as soft tissue swelling decreases.
- At 2 weeks, the splint is changed to a short forearm cast with a three-point mold for 3 to 4 weeks.
- Closed reduction and casting works best in bending fractures with a moderate amount of angulation (15–20 degrees of dorsal tilt; some authors recommend less than 10 degrees of dorsal angulation[4]), moderate metaphyseal comminution on the concave side of the angulation, and a single transverse fracture of the opposite cortex and adequate bone quality. Some authors recommend less than 50% comminution or involvement of only one cortex.[4] If the single cortical noncomminuted fracture is well reduced without overlapping of the fracture edges (palmar cortex in a Colles fracture) and the soft tissue hinge is maintained under tension, the chances of secondary displacement are minimal.
- Osteoporosis can lead to secondary settling and shortening that may occur up to 3 months after injury.

## Unstable Fractures

- Numerous options for treatment may offset the loss of reduction in an unstable fracture.[3]
  - Percutaneous pinning
  - Intrafocal pinning
  - Arthroscopic assisted fixation
  - External fixation to include nonbridging external fixation
  - Open reduction and internal fixation with or without bone grafting

## Percutaneous Pinning

- Percutaneous pins are combined with either a plaster cast or an external fixator.
- A variety of different techniques of percutaneous pinning of unstable distal radius fractures have been described.
- With unstable extraarticular bending fractures, one method is to place the pins either through the radial styloid alone or in combination with an additional pin directed through the dorsoulnar aspect of the radius.
- With the fracture reduced and wire placement confirmed on radiographic control, the tips of the wire are bent and left just outside the skin. Pins generally are removed between 6 and 8 weeks later (Figure 6–14).

## Intrafocal Pinning (Kapandji)

- Kapandji described a technique whereby Kirschner wire directed into the fracture site (intrafocal) are used to lever the displaced distal radius fracture into anatomic alignment (Figure 6–15).[8]

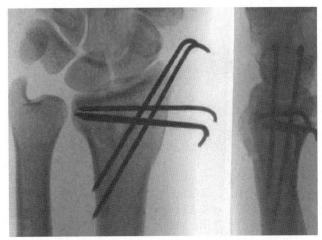

Figure 6–14:
**Example of percutaneous pinning.**

- Contraindications including osteoporotic bone and fractures with severe comminution.

## Arthroscopic-Assisted Fixation

- Small-diameter arthroscope allows manipulation of articular fracture fragments under direct vision.
- Before arthroscopy, a compressive elastic bandage is wrapped around the forearm to retard fluid extravasation into the muscle compartments.
- Small incision with blunt dissection to the wrist capsule is recommended to avoid cutaneous nerve injury.
- The entire joint, including the distal radius, triangular fibrocartilage, and intracapsular and intracarpal ligaments, should be inspected for associated injuries. Scapholunate dissociation is not uncommon with radial styloid fractures, and midcarpal arthroscopy can be useful in visualizing scapholunate and lunotriquetral instability and ligament tears.[9]
- Each fragment to be reduced is manipulated under direct vision with percutaneous insertion of a smooth Kirschner wire introduced into the fragment proximal to the level of the joint.

## External Skeletal Fixation

- External skeletal fixation remains an important tactic in the management of fractures of the distal end of the radius.
- Transarticular frames are applied with pins in the distal radial diaphysis crossing the wrist to pins into the second and sometimes third metacarpal.
- Fractures without comminution can be stabilized with a nonbridging external fixator.[2]
- Used during distal radial osteotomies and reduction of complex fractures.
- May act as a joint distractor, neutralization frame, or buttress, or even for fracture compression.
- With joint distraction, the device has two roles.

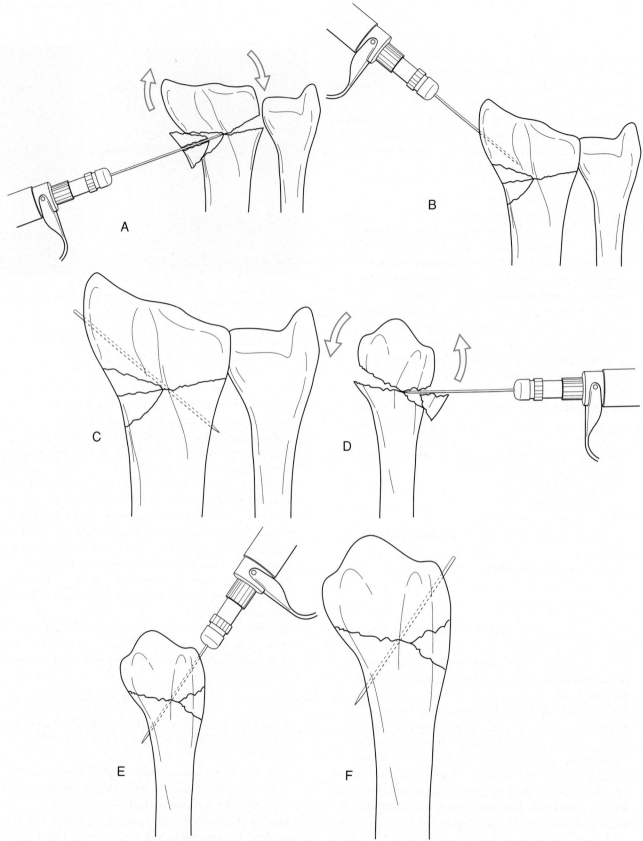

Figure 6–15:

A, To correct the loss of radial tilt, the Kirschner wire is inserted into the fracture plane on the radial side.[9] B, The Kirschner wire is used as a lever to correct the rotation of the distal radius.[9] C, After correcting the radial inclination, the Kirschner wire is driven into the proximal cortex to act as a buttress and support for the fracture.[9] D, The dorsal tilt of the fracture can be corrected by inserting a Kirschner wire along the lines of the fracture.[9] E, The Kirschner wire is used as a lever to correct dorsal rotation.[9] F, To buttress and stabilize the dorsal rotation of the fracture, the Kirschner wire is driven into the proximal and volar cortex.[9]

○ Indirect reduction of comminuted intraarticular fractures through tension on the capsuloligamentous attachments and through a change in the intracapsular joint pressure because of distraction.

○ Maintain fracture fragment alignment when the device is statically locked.[2]

• Neutralization device:

○ Unload and protect a fracture that has internal fixation.

○ A second situation is the protection of bending, torsional, and shearing forces acting upon a realigned extraarticular bending fracture[2] (Box 6–5).

• The fixator should be adjusted to keep the hand and wrist in a neutral position.

• The stability of the external frame and pins can be increased by

1. Predrilling holes prior to pin placement
2. Creating a radial preload with the smooth shank of the pin filling the near cortex hole
3. Increasing the pin-to-pin distance on the same side of the fracture and decreasing the pin-to-pin distance across the fracture
4. Placing the connecting rod closer to the arm and hand

• The external fixator pins are wrapped with sterile gauze, and a volar splint is applied for support and comfort.

• The external fixator allows free motion of the digits and forearm rotation.

## Open Reduction and Internal Fixation of Fractures of the Distal Radius

• Residual deformity after fracture of the distal radius adversely affects wrist and hand function by interfering with the mechanical advantage of the extrinsic hand musculature.[10]

• Residual deformity after fracture may cause pain, limitation of forearm motion, and decreased grip strength as a result of arthrosis of the radiocarpal and distal radioulnar joints, incongruity of the DRUJ, ulnocarpal impingement, and carpal malalignment (Box 6–6).[10]

---

**Box 6–5** | **External Skeletal Fixation: Application Technique[2]**

• Prior to application, the distal radius fracture should be reduced.
• One method of application:
  • Place two pins into the second metacarpal (one at the base and one in the shaft). At risk are the first dorsal interosseous muscle, extensor tendons, and branches of the radial sensory nerve.
  • Pins are placed approximately 45 degrees from the transverse axis of the palm in a converging fashion, creating an angle of 45 to 60 degrees between the two pins in the metacarpal.
  • Place two pins in the radius 10 to 12 cm proximal to the radial styloid, preferably proximal to the muscle bellies of the abductor pollicis longus and extensor pollicis brevis. At risk are overlying tendons, muscle bellies, and especially branches of the radial sensory nerve.

---

**Box 6–6** | **Fracture Patterns Best Treated Surgically[10]**

• Oblique or comminuted palmar bending (Smith) fractures
• Shearing fractures of the articular surface that require buttress plate fixation
• Comminuted or impacted fractures that require direct visualization of the articular surface
• Compression articular fractures in which the lunate facet is split in the coronal plane and the volar fragment is malrotated
• Radiocarpal fracture-dislocation
• Fractures associated with complex soft tissue injury

## Palmar Bending Fractures (Smith's)

• Characterized by an oblique fracture line or metaphyseal comminution (Figure 6–16).
• Fixation is achieved with a volarly applied plate.
• Henry radial volar exposure is used in most cases of palmar bending fractures and, when used in combination with volar fixed-angle locking plates, has been adopted for use in some dorsal bending fractures.

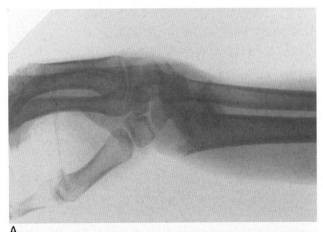
A

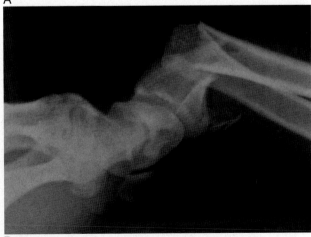
B

Figure 6–16:
**Extraarticular bending fractures. The lateral radiographs demonstrate displacement and metaphyseal comminution.**

- Ulnar volar exposure should be used with extensive soft tissue injury, especially if carpal tunnel and/or ulnar tunnel syndrome is a concern.
- Plate fixation is relatively well tolerated on the volar surface of the radius, and the plate only rarely must be removed.

## Shearing Fractures of the Radial Styloid

- Require anatomic reduction because of their intraarticular nature and ligamentous attachments.
- Fixation can be accomplished using smooth Kirschner wires, screws, or cannulated screws.
- Open exposure of the articular surface is through a dorsal radial incision between the first and second dorsal compartments. The radial artery is protected as dissection proceeds distally within the radial "snuffbox." A capsulotomy is required if the fracture is comminuted.
- Arthroscopy can be used to verify articular reduction and evaluate the scapholunate interosseous ligament.
- If complete tear of this ligament is detected, open repair with either suture anchors or drill holes through the scaphoid is recommended. Partial tears can be treated with percutaneous pin fixation.[10]

## Shearing Fractures of the Dorsal Lunate Facet

- Closed reduction often is difficult because of impaction of the metaphyseal bone.
- Exposure between the fourth and fifth extensor compartments allows reduction and stabilization, and the fragment can be stabilized with percutaneous Kirschner wires. Fixation should be protected against axial load with either external fixation or a cast.

## Dorsal Marginal Shearing Fractures (Dorsal Barton Fractures)

- Dorsal exposure between the second and fourth compartments is often needed.
- Dorsal capsulotomy may be needed to evaluate the articular reduction.
- Fixation can be accomplished with a low-profile plate design.

## Volar Marginal Shearing Fractures (Volar Barton Fractures)

- Require open reduction and support with a volar buttress plate.[10]
- Reduction is achieved by hyperextending the wrist over a rolled towel. Provisional fixation with a 0.045-inch Kirschner wire facilitates placement of a buttress plate.
- Undercontouring of a plate results in compression of the fracture fragments to the intact radius as the screws are tightened sequentially from proximal to distal (Figure 6–17).

## Complex Articular Fractures

- Approach is dependent on both the fracture morphology and any associated soft tissue injury (Figure 6–18).
- Fractures of the articular surface require open exposure through a dorsal capsulotomy.
- Malrotated volar lunate facet fragment requires a separate volar exposure.
- Metaphyseal defects should be grafted with autogenous cancellous bone to provide support for the articular reduction and enhance healing.
- Newer plate designs with fixed-angle constructs provide more support for fractures with extensive comminution or severe osteopenia.

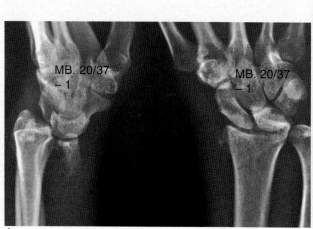 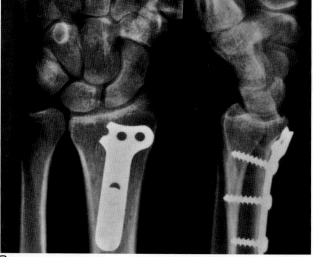

A                                              B

Figure 6–17:
**Anterior marginal shearing fracture of the distal radius with stable internal fixation.**

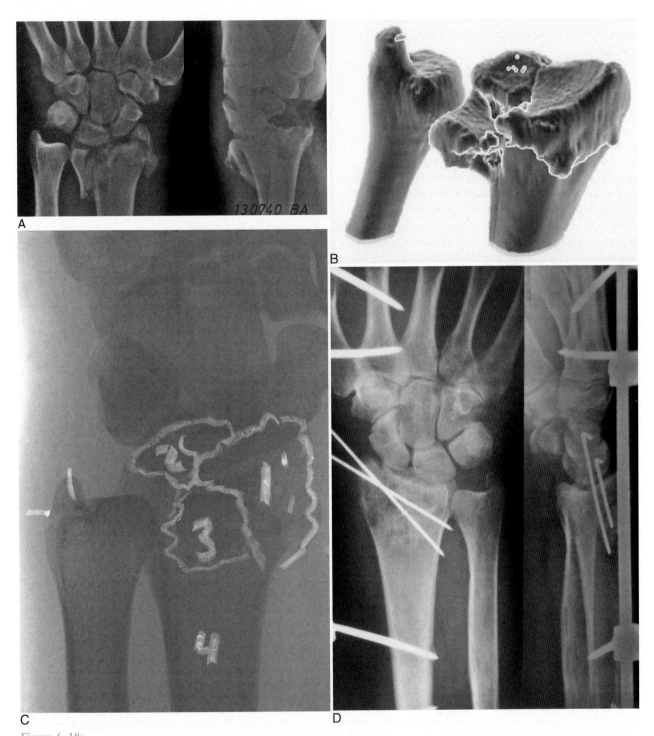

Figure 6–18:
Complex compression articular fracture (A, C). Three-dimensional CT scan demonstrates involvement of the lunate and scaphoid facets (B). Stable fixation was achieved with Kirschner wires and external fixation (D).

## Radiocarpal Fracture-Dislocation

- Using longitudinal traction and rotation of the hand and wrist, the carpus can be relocated onto the distal end of the radius.
- An external fixator is applied and used as a distractor to facilitate surgical repositioning and repair of the radiocarpal ligaments and their avulsion fractures.
- If clinically indicated, the median and ulnar nerves are decompressed.
- Radial styloid, ulnar styloid, and volar articular rim fracture fragments are reattached using other screws or K-wires and occasionally a tension-band wire.
- The volar capsule is repaired back to the distal radius through drill holes or using suture anchors.
- Associated injury to the carpal interosseous ligaments may require concomitant volar exposure to allow ligament repair.
- The external fixator should remain in place for 6 to 8 weeks to protect the repair.
- If there is concern regarding injury to the soft tissue stabilizers of the DRUJ, the forearm should be immobilized in midsupination with a sugar tong splint for 3 to 4 weeks.

## Nascent Malunion

- Traditionally, malaligned fractures in which early healing prevents closed manipulation have been managed expectantly with osteotomy performed at a time remote from the fracture and only after extensive attempts at rehabilitation through therapy.
- Malalignment leads to contracture of the soft tissue structures, arthrosis of the radiocarpal and distal radioulnar joints, and compensatory malalignment of the midcarpal joint.
- Some surgeons are undertaking early open reduction and internal fixation of the malaligned fractures in the nascent stage, based on evidence that greater than 20 degree dorsal tilt of the distal radial articular surface, greater than 15 degrees of dorsal tilt of the lunate, greater than 2 mm of articular incongruity, and radiocarpal subluxation lead to disability in active patients.[10]
- Articular malunion can also be addressed.
- Through the metaphyseal fracture line, the fracture is manipulated out to length and the appropriate alignments of the articular surface are restored.
- Cancellous autograft bone is harvested and placed in the metaphyseal bone defect.
- Stable plate fixation is then applied.[10]

## Grafts

- Both extraarticular and intraarticular distal radial fractures often involve substantial cortical comminution and loss of cancellous bone in the metaphyseal region.

- During the healing process, collapse of the distal fragments into the cancellous defects in the metaphyseal and subchondral regions can lead to secondary displacement and loss of reduction.
- Bone grafting provides mechanical internal support of articular fragments, accelerates bone healing, and provides osteoinductive and osteoconductive potential to the remaining partially devitalized bone.
- Coralline hydroxyapatite has been effective as a bone graft substitute in maintaining articular surface reduction when used in combination with external fixation and Kirschner wires. It has a safety profile comparable with other forms of treatment.[9]
- Injectable bone graft have been developed to fill fracture voids and maintain internal fixation in stable fractures and in displaced fractures that are reducible and stable. This bone grout consists of powdered calcium phosphate and calcium carbonate, and structural characteristics that are very similar to those of bone. It provides significant structural support for cancellous bone in compression but is weak in torsion and shear.[11] Cancellous allograft bone graft has been shown to be safe and effective without the problems of intra-articular extrusion of the graft.

## Associated Injuries

### Ulnar Styloid Fractures

- Ulnar styloid fractures have been reported in up to 50% of distal radius fractures.[9]
- The vast majority heal with fibrous union and remains asymptomatic.[9]
- When the ulnar styloid is fractured below its base and associated with DRUJ instability, fixation can be achieved through an exposure between the extensor digiti quinti and extensor carpi ulnaris tendons.[12,13]
- A tension-band wire can be passed through the proximal ulnar fragment and either around or through the ulnar styloid fragment, with a small Kirschner wire used to fix the fragment to the shaft. Alternatively, bone anchors or cannulated screws can regain this nonunion with implants that minimize soft tissue irritation.
- The forearm should be immobilized in neutral rotation for 6 weeks.[12]

### Distal Radioulnar Joint Disorders

- After satisfactory restoration of radial length, tilt, inclination, and articular congruity, imaging should be performed to be certain the relationship at the DRUJ is anatomic.
- DRUJ stability is assessed by ballottement of the distal ulna relative to the distal radius (Box 6–7 and Table 6–1).
- Supination splinting is the mainstay of postoperative management.
- The forearm is held in full supination for 4 weeks.

| Box 6–7 | **DRUJ Disorders Associated with Distal Radius Fractures** |
|---|---|

- DRUJ is reduced and stable.
  - This is the most common situation. No specific treatment is required.
- DRUJ is reducible but unstable.
  - Usually the DRUJ is stable in full supination. The forearm is splinted in full supination for 4 weeks and continued at night for 3 months.
  - If no stable position is found, the DRUJ ligaments are repaired or the DRUJ is stabilized with a radioulnar pin. The pin is passed just proximal to the radioulnar joint and left in place for 3 weeks.
- DRUJ is not reducible.
  - This is uncommon. The usual cause of an irreducible DRUJ is either malreduction of the radius or soft tissue interposition in the joint. Assuming the reduction of the radius is acceptable, open reduction of the DRUJ is required.

- At 4 weeks, a program of active forearm rotation is started.
- Passive assisted motion is started 6 weeks following surgery.
- Resistive exercises are avoided until a near-normal range of active motion is recovered.
- Night splinting is maintained for 3 months.
- Inadequate treatment of injuries of the DRUJ in association with intraarticular fractures of the distal radius can lead to DRUJ instability, painful impingement, and joint incongruity.

## Functional Aftercare

- Begin active and passive motion of the digits, elbow, shoulder, and rotation of the forearm within 24 hours following surgery.
- Early motion decreases tendon adhesion, reduces soft tissue swelling, and prevents stiffness of the digits.
- Splints and casts must allow full range of motion of the metacarpophalangeal joints by not extending beyond the distal palmar crease.

### Table 6–1: Distal Radioulnar Joint Disorders

| TYPE | JOINT SURFACE INVOLVEMENT |
|---|---|
| *I:* Stable (following reduction of the radius, the distal radioulnar joint is congruous and stable) | None |
| *II:* Unstable (subluxation or dislocation of the ulnar head present) | None |
| *III:* Potentially unstable (subluxation possible) | Present |

Three basic types of distal radioulnar joint (DRUJ) lesions have been established, depending on the residual stability of the DRUJ after the distal radius fracture has been reduced and stabilized.

- Wrist immobilization in a splint, cast, or external fixator may be necessary for 4 to 8 weeks.
- Wrist mobilization may be possible within 2 weeks of injury when surgical fixation with a plate results in a stable construct, such as a volar locking plate.
- In some instances, the metaphyseal and articular comminution is extensive, requiring splint support from 4 to 6 weeks.
- If motion is limited, dynamic pronation-supination or flexion-extension splints should be considered. Generally, 3.5 to 4 months are required until the patient can resume full activity and 1 year until maximum medical improvement and range of motion are reached.

## Outcome and Prognosis

- The final outcome of distal radius fractures depends on the amount of radial shortening, residual extraarticular angulation, articular incongruity of both the radiocarpal and radioulnar joints, presence of ulnar styloid fracture, and associated soft tissue complications.[9]
- Residual increased dorsal tilt is related to loss of palmar flexion, and radial shortening over 4 mm has been associated with decreased forearm rotation.[9]
- Knirk and Jupiter[14] found diminished grip strength was associated with extreme loss of radial length.
- Porter and Stockley found that when the dorsal angle exceeded 20 degrees or the radial angle fell below 10 degrees, grip strength was reduced.[9]
- Short and associates found that increased residual dorsal tilt leads to overloading of the dorsal radiocarpal joint, possibly leading to wrist arthrosis.[9]
- Knirk and Jupiter[14] found that if a fracture healed with greater than 2 mm of residual articular incongruity, 100% of the patients had radiographic evidence of arthritis. Two thirds of these patients were symptomatic and one third were asymptomatic.[14] Even with over 1.0 mm of articular incongruity, degenerative arthritis occured in 90% of cases.[4,12,14]

## Complications

- Median nerve injury is one of the most commonly observed complications.
- A thorough prereduction neurovascular examination must be performed.
- Mild sensory impairment usually can be followed clinically.
- When acute carpal tunnel syndrome is severe and unchanged after reduction, then immediate release is recommended.
- When a patient who required operative intervention for the fracture has a nerve deficit, a carpal tunnel release is indicated.[15]

- Mild forms of reflex sympathetic dystrophy are common with distal radial fractures.
- Patients with increasing pain, swelling, joint stiffness, and paraesthesias during fracture healing require early attention.
- Tendon ruptures resulting from irritation over a plate occur infrequently.
- The extensor pollicis longus tendon is most commonly affected.
- Rupture most often occurs after minimally or nondisplaced fractures, suggesting an ischemic rather than mechanical etiology of the rupture.
- Infection and nonunion occur rarely.
- Malunion of the distal and of the radius is the most common complication following a distal radial fracture The deformity may be extraarticular, intraarticular, or a combination of both.[15]
- Impairment of function rather than radiographic deformity is the reason to treat a distal radial malunion.
- Pathologic biomechanics in the wrist lead to pain, decreased range of motion, and/or midcarpal instability.[15]
- Subsequent traumatic osteoarthritis can develop even in patients with an excellent reduction.

## New Concepts

- The ability to secure both large extraarticular fragments and smaller intraarticular fragments is necessary in many complex fractures.
- Some newer designs provide smaller screws or pins in the transverse distal segment of the plate, which facilitates fixation of smaller articular fragments.[16]
- Soft tissue complications associated with a dorsal plate, including extensor tendon irritation and late rupture, have been attributed to the prominence of the plate and/or screw heads.[15]
- Newer designs have minimized these complications because they incorporate precontouring by the manufacturer, allow ease of further contouring by the surgeon, and use a plate and screw heads with a low profile.[17]
- When the dorsal approach is used, transposition of the extensor pollicis longus tendon at closure can reduce irritation and adhesions, preventing loss of motion and possible later rupture.
- Clinical and biomechanical studies have shown that stable fixation can be achieved with small implants aligned in an orthogonal fashion.
- This technique, described by Swigert and Wolfe, has been advocated to reduce the soft tissue dissection at surgery and to allow early mobilization of the wrist, which may lead to improved outcomes and fewer soft tissue complications.[16]
- Improved implant designs that use fixed-angle screws have led to stable internal fixation of some dorsally

displaced distal radius fractures through a volar approach.[17]

## References

1. Jupiter JB: Current concepts review: fractures of the distal end of the radius. *J Bone Joint Surg* 73A:461-469, 1991.
   An excellent review of distal radius fractures.

2. Fernandez DL, Jupiter JB: *Fractures of the distal radius: a practical approach to management.* New York, 1996, Springer-Verlag.
   A comprehensive source of information on distal radius fractures, their management, and the treatment of complications.

3. Fernandez DL, Jupiter JB: *Fractures of the distal radius: a practical approach to management,* ed 2. New York, 2002, Springer-Verlag.
   This update discusses newer concepts, including modern bone grafting options, radiocarpal fracture-dislocations, malunions, and DRUJ injuries and their treatment.

4. Trumble TE: *Principles of hand surgery and therapy.* Philadelphia, 2000, WB Saunders.
   Chapter 7 is an excellent overview of distal radius fractures and describes their rehabilitation. It concludes with a discussion of malunions and their treatment.

5. Katz MA, Beredjiklian PK, Bozentka DJ, Steinberg DR: Computed tomography scanning of intra-articular distal radius fractures: does it influence treatment? *J Hand Surg* 26A:415-421, 2001.
   Compared to plain x-ray films, CT scanning resulted in increased accuracy and interobserver reliability in fracture assessment, leading to changes in proposed treatment plans.

6. Jupiter JB, Ring D: A comparison of early and late reconstruction of malunited fractures of the distal end of the radius. *J Bone Joint Surg* 78A:739-748, 1996.
   The results of early and late reconstruction of distal radius malunions are comparable. Early reconstruction is technically easier and reduces the overall period of disability.

7. Ring D, Jupiter JB: Operative exposure of fractures of the distal radius. *Techniques Hand Upper Extremity Surg* 3:259-264, 1999.
   An excellent technique guide for exposures of the distal radius.

8. Trumble TE, Wagner W, Hanel DP, et al: Intrafocal (Kapandji) pinning of distal radius fractures with and without external fixation. *J Hand Surg [Am]* 23:381-394, 1998.
   When two or more sides of the radial metaphysis were comminuted, patients with external fixation and pinning had better results than patients with intrafocal pinning alone.

9. Gellmen H: Fractures of the distal radius. In Gellman H, editor: *Fractures of the distal radius.* American Academy of Orthopaedic Surgeons Homograph Series, 1-36, 1998.
   A general overview of distal radius fractures. It also discusses outcome and prognosis and describes complications of the injury.

10. Jupiter JB, Ring D: Open reduction and internal fixation of fractures of the distal radius. In Gellman H, editor: *Fractures of the distal radius.* American Academy of Orthopaedic Surgeons Monograph Series, 37-53, 1998.

Summarizes the indications for and surgical approaches to the distal radius. It describes fracture types, their treatment, postoperative rehabilitation, and complications.

11. Ladd AL, Pliam NB: Use of bone-graft substitutes in distal radius fractures. *J Am Acad Orthop Surg* 7:279-290, 1999.
This study describes the present bone graft substitutes available for distal radius fractures. It describes each product's indications for use and its composition.

12. Trumble TE, Culp RW, Hanel DP, et al: Intra-articular fractures of the distal aspect of the radius. Instructional course lecture of the American Academy of Orthopaedic Surgeons. *J Bone Joint Surg* 80:582-600, 1998.
A comprehensive discussion of intraarticular distal radius fractures.

13. Jupiter JB, Fernandez DL, Whipple TL, Richards RR: Intra-articular fractures of the distal radius: contemporary perspectives. In Cannon, WB Jr, editor: *Instructional course lectures 47.* Rosemont, 1998, American Academy of Orthopaedic Surgeons.
A discussion of the treatment of distal radius fractures based upon the classification of Fernandez. DRUJ disorders also are addressed.

14. Knirk JL, Jupiter JB: Intra-articular fractures of the distal end of the radius in young adults. *J Bone Joint Surg* 68A:647-659, 1986.
Accurate articular restoration was the most critical factor in achieving a successful result. Arthritis was noted in 91% that healed with residual incongruity of the radiocarpal joint. Arthritis developed in only 11% that healed with a congruous joint.

15. Jupiter JB, Fernandez DL: Complications following distal radial fractures. *J Bone Joint Surg* 83A8:1244-1265, 2001.
Malunion and osteotomy of the distal radius is described. A superb discussion covers the management of associated DRUJ disorders in detail.

16. Simic PM, Weiland JA: Fractures of the distal aspect of the radius: changes in treatment over the past two decades. *J Bone Joint Surg* 85A:552-564, 2003.
Reviews significant advances in the treatment of distal radius fractures of the last 20 years. Treatment options and complications are covered.

17. Orbay JL, Fernandez DL: Volar fixation for dorsally displaced fractures of the distal radius: a preliminary report. *J Hand Surg* 27A:205-215, 2002.
The combination of stable internal fixation with preservation of the dorsal soft tissues resulted in rapid fracture healing, reduced need for bone grafting, and a low incidence of tendon problems.

# Distal Radioulnar Joint and Triangular Fibrocartilage Complex

Pamela E. Glennon[*] and Brian D. Adams[†]

[*]MD, Hand Surgery Fellow, Department of Orthopaedic Surgery, University of Iowa, Iowa City, IA
[†]MD, Professor of Orthopaedic Surgery and Biomedical Engineering, Department of Orthopaedic Surgery and Biomedical Engineering, University of Iowa, Iowa City, IA

## Introduction

- Ulnar-sided wrist pain occurs in all age groups. It can be caused by acute trauma, instability, or chronic degenerative processes. The anatomy and biomechanics of the ulnar side of the wrist are complex. There are numerous potential causes for dysfunction and pain. The key to accurate diagnosis is a careful history and detailed physical examination, supported by imaging studies targeted at probable causes. As opposed to ablative or salvage procedures, optimal treatment aims to restore anatomy and function (Box 7–1).

## Anatomy

- Congruence between the sigmoid notch of the distal radius and the ulna head is poor, with the sigmoid notch having a larger radius of curvature than the ulna. Although the notch is shallow, the dorsal and volar rims of the sigmoid notch contribute substantially to joint stability.
- The fovea is a depression on the distal surface of the ulnar head near the base of the ulna styloid. It is an important attachment site for ligaments. Fractures through the styloid base may be associated with ligament injury and distal radioulnar joint (DRUJ) instability.
- Triangular fibrocartilage complex (TFCC), a term popularized by Palmer, refers to the confluence of soft tissues structures spanning the DRUJ.[1] The components

---

**Box 7–1  Causes of Ulnar-Sided Wrist Pain**

1. Fractures or nonunions
   A. Ulnar styloid
   B. Hook of hamate
   C. Pisiform
   D. Triquetrum
2. TFCC tears
   A. Traumatic tears
   B. Degenerative tears (ulna impaction syndrome)
3. Lunotriquetral interosseous ligament and/or meniscal homologue tear
4. DRUJ instability
   A. Acute Galeazzi fracture-dislocation
   B. Acute or chronic Essex-Lopresti injury
   C. Chronic TFCC tear (including ulnar styloid nonunion)
   D. Distal radius malunion
5. ECU tendon conditions
   A. Tendonitis
   B. Subluxation (ECU sheath tear)
6. Arthritis
   A. DRUJ
   B. Pisotriquetral joint

ECU, Extensor carpi ulnaris; DRUJ, distal radioulnar joint; TFCC, triangular fibrocartilage complex.

---

of the TFCC are the triangular fibrocartilage (disc), dorsal and volar radioulnar ligaments, ulnotriquetral and ulnolunate ligaments, extensor carpi ulnaris (ECU) sheath, and meniscus homologue (Figure 7–1). The

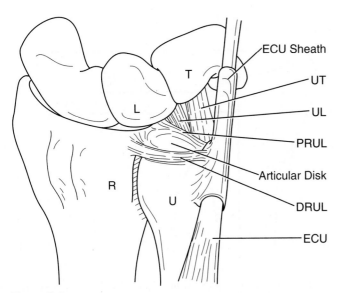

Figure 7–1:

**Anatomy of the triangular fibrocartilage complex as seen looking toward the ulna from the radius.** *DRUL,* dorsal radioulnar ligament; *ECU,* extensor carpi ulnaris; *L,* lunate; *PRUL,* palmar radioulnar ligament, *R,* radius; *T,* triquetrum; *U,* ulna; *UL,* ulnolunate ligament; *UT,* ulnotriquetral ligament.

fibrocartilage disc attaches to the fovea at the base of the ulna styloid and to the ulnar edge of the distal radius at the DRUJ. It blends peripherally with the radioulnar ligaments. The radioulnar ligaments extend from the distal corners of the sigmoid notch, merge ulnarly, and then pass to dual insertions at the fovea and base of the ulnar styloid. The ulnotriquetral and ulnolunate ligaments originate from the volar distal radioulnar ligament and insert on the volar aspects of their respective carpal bones. The ligaments support the carpus and DRUJ. The meniscus homologue is a variable structure, likely derived from synovial tissue, whose function is unknown. In 10% of individuals it has a broad distal insertion on the triquetrum and lunotriquetral ligament, which obscures arthroscopic visualization. If torn, it can be a source of pain from repeated irritation.[1–3] Blood supply to the TFCC derives primarily from the anterior interosseous artery and ulnar artery through vascular channels at the fovea and the base of the ulnar styloid.

- The primary functions of the TFCC are to extend the articular surface of the radius for the carpus, absorb and transmit axial force across the ulnocarpal joint, support the carpus, and provide a flexible connection between the radius and ulna.
- The soft tissue stabilizers of the DRUJ are its capsule, dorsal and volar radioulnar ligaments, other components of the triangular fibrocartilage, interosseous membrane (particularly its central band), and pronator quadratus, with the radioulnar ligaments being the most important.[4–9]

## Biomechanics

- Approximately 20% of axial load transmitted across the wrist passes through the ulnocarpal joint to the ulna.[7] The load varies with wrist position, increasing with ulnar deviation and pronation by up to 150%.[9]
- *Ulnar variance* is the term used to relate the difference in lengths of the radius and ulna, with ulna plus and ulna minus describing the ulna as longer or shorter than the radius, respectively. In a radiographic study of 120 asymptomatic caucasian subjects, ulnar variance averaged −0.9 mm, ranging from −4.2 mm to +2.3 mm, with no differences between genders.[10]
- Changes in ulnar variance and TFCC integrity affect ulnocarpal load transmission. Shortening the ulna by 2.5 mm decreases the load to 4%, whereas increasing ulnar length by 2.5 mm increases the load to 42%.[11] Removal of two thirds or more of the disc reduces ulnar load to as little as 3%.[12]
- The relative contributions of the volar and dorsal radioulnar ligaments to DRUJ stability in different positions of forearm rotation remain controversial despite numerous investigations.[8,13] However, both ligaments are necessary for normal stability and kinematics. Severe instability most often results from detachment of their combined insertion on the ulna.

## Physical Examination

- Inspect for swelling about the DRUJ, ECU sheath, and carpus.
- ECU subluxation is most apparent when the forearm and wrist are in supination and ulnar deviation. The tendon typically subluxates ulnarly.
- Localizing tenderness is a key to an accurate diagnosis of ulnar-sided wrist pain. Palpate the hook of hamate, pisiform, lunate, triquetrum, ulnar styloid, DRUJ, ECU sheath, and ulnocarpal joint. Tenderness in the soft depression proximal to the triquetrum and between the flexor carpi ulnaris (FCU) tendon and ulna styloid suggests a TFCC injury.
- Pain and crepitus with compression of the pisiform against the triquetrum suggest pisotriquetral arthritis.
- Reduced grip strength strongly suggests intraarticular pathology.
- Measure active and passive motion of the wrist and DRUJ and compare them to the opposite side. Decreased forearm rotation associated with crepitus suggests DRUJ arthritis.
- Increased anteroposterior translation of the ulna with passive manipulation of the ulna ("piano key" sign) is evidence of DRUJ instability. Because joint translation varies among individuals and with forearm position, the

test is performed in all forearm positions and compared to the opposite side.[14]

- The modified "press test" is performed by asking the patient to press down on the examination table with the palms of both hands simultaneously. Excessive volar translation of the ulna head on the symptomatic side indicates DRUJ instability.[15]

- The ulnocarpal stress test is used for diagnosing TFCC tears and ulna impaction. With the elbow on the examination table and the forearm vertical, the examiner first grasps the hand and applies an axial load to the wrist. The wrist then is passively moved from radial to ulnar deviation. Testing is repeated in pronation, neutral, and supination. Alternatively, the forearm is rotated while maintaining the wrist in ulnar deviation and under an axial load. Reproduction of pain and clicking are evidence of intraarticular damage.[16,17] Greater loading of the disc's center and the ulnar dome is achieved while performing the ulnocarpal stress test by depressing the ulnar head volarly with the index and long fingers and simultaneously elevating the carpus by pushing the pisiform dorsally with the thumb. The wrist then is moved from radial to ulnar deviation under an axial load.

- The lunotriquetral joint is assessed with the shear test. The lunate and triquetrum are held individually with the thumb and index finger of each hand. The bones are translated relative to each other to assess pain and excessive motion compared to the opposite side.

## Radiographic Evaluation

- A true posteroanterior (PA) view is obtained by positioning the forearm in neutral rotation, with the elbow flexed 90 degrees and the shoulder abducted 90 degrees. The ulna styloid is located at the far ulnar border.

- Ulnar variance is measured on the PA view. A line is drawn through the ulnar edge of the proximal sclerotic line of the distal radius in a direction perpendicular to the long axis of the radial shaft. Variance is the distance between this line and the distal cortical rim of the ulnar dome (Figure 7–2).[18]

- Ulnar variance may be dynamic in some individuals, becoming more positive with pronation and grip. In pronation, the radius is shorter than the ulna as a result of its oblique course from the elbow to the wrist. Thus, if a comparison x-ray film is obtained, forearm position must be the same. Slight proximal migration of the radius may occur during grip as a result of muscle forces, which may replicate the wrist condition causing the symptoms.[18–20]

- A true lateral view is obtained by positioning the forearm in neutral rotation, with the elbow flexed 90 degrees and the shoulder adducted to the patient's side. The third metacarpal, capitate, lunate, and radius are colinear. The pisiform's palmar surface will be midway between the palmar surfaces of the distal pole of the scaphoid and the capitate or the midpoint of the hook of hamate.

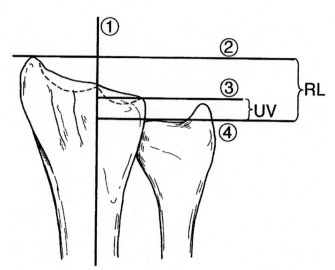

Figure 7–2:
The relative length (RL) of the radius and ulna can be determined by measuring the distance from the tip of the radial styloid *(line 2)* drawn perpendicular to the long axis of the radius *(line 1)* and the distal end of the ulnar articular surface *(line 4)*. The ulna variance (UV) is measured as the distance between *line 4* and *line 3*, the dense cortical line along the ulnar border of the distal radius articular surface. (From: Trumble TE: Distal radioulnar joint and triangular fibrocartilage complex. In Trumble TE, editor. *Principles of hand surgery and therapy*. Philadelphia, 2000, WB Saunders.)

- The lateral view is imprecise for diagnosing DRUJ subluxation if positioning is not exact. With as little as 10 degrees of supination from the neutral position, a dorsal dislocation appears only subluxated and a dorsal subluxation appears reduced.

- Semipronated and semisupinated views may be helpful to evaluate fractures involving the distal ulna and sigmoid notch.

- The carpal tunnel view is useful for diagnosing hook of hamate and pisiform fractures and pisotriquetral arthritis. The view can be obtained with the wrist maximally extended and the x-ray beam directed 15 degrees off the plane of the palm.

- Arthrography is not frequently used because of the high incidence of false-positive and false-negative findings compared to arthroscopy.

- Computed tomography (CT) is useful for evaluating fractures and arthritis, particularly of the sigmoid notch and ulnar head. CT is the standard imaging method for assessing DRUJ instability. Both wrists must be evaluated in identical forearm positions, aligned in the axis of the gantry, and imaged in neutral rotation, supination, and pronation.

- Magnetic resonance imaging (MRI) is useful for assessing the TFCC if proper equipment and expertise are available.[21] Gadolinium or saline injection improves sensitivity. In general, sensitivity in detecting peripheral TFCC tears is less than for disc tears.[21,22] However techniques are rapidly improving, making MRI a more reliable diagnostic tool for ulnar-sided wrist pain, especially when combined with a simultaneous arthrogram.

## Diagnostic Arthroscopy

- Arthroscopy is sensitive for identifying acute tears or degeneration in the central portion of the disc, chondromalacia, and ulnocarpal ligament injuries. Lunotriquetral interosseous ligament (LTIL) tears and a meniscus homologue can be identified. Arthroscopy was more sensitive and accurate than noninvasive imaging modalities in several studies.[23] Incomplete peripheral TFCC tears are more difficult to detect and assess for severity. Lack of resiliency and excessive laxity of the TFCC demonstrated by depressing its distal surface with a probe during arthroscopy (so-called trampoline effect) are indicative of an unstable TFCC because of a peripheral tear.[24]

## Fractures

- Ulnar styloid fractures frequently are associated with distal radius fractures, but most do not require special treatment. Tip of ulnar styloid fractures are common and do not denote DRUJ instability. A painless fibrous union is common. Fractures at the base of the ulnar styloid are potentially more problematic, because they may be associated with disruption of the radioulnar ligaments, resulting in DRUJ instability. Styloid fracture displacement associated with DRUJ widening indicates a higher probability of DRUJ instability.
- Ulnar head fractures almost always occur in conjunction with distal radius fractures and are most common in the elderly or in patients with high-energy injuries. Open reduction internal fixation (ORIF) may be indicated to restore DRUJ congruency, motion, and stability.
- Displaced fractures of the sigmoid notch involving its rims or a substantial portion of the articular surface may require ORIF to restore joint stability and reduce the risk of arthritis.
- Fractures of the hook of the hamate or the pisiform usually result from a blow on the palm of the hand. Nondisplaced fractures through the base of the hamate hook, hamate body, or pisiform usually heal with nonoperative management. Displaced or comminuted fractures and nonunions of the hamate hook or pisiform may be best treated by excision of the hook or the entire pisiform.
- Small dorsal fractures of the triquetrum typically are ligament avulsion injuries that can be managed by

immobilization. Fractures through the body of the triquetrum result from impaction on the distal ulna or are part of a perilunate dislocation. Open reduction with fracture and joint fixation is indicated for fracture displacement or carpal malalignment.

# Triangular Fibrocartilage Complex Conditions

- See Figure 7–3.

## Traumatic Triangular Fibrocartilage Complex Tears

### Class 1A

- A class 1A tear presents with ulnar-sided wrist pain and occasional clicking that is aggravated by power grip and forearm rotation, especially when combined with ulnar deviation. It is a common injury, but it does not cause DRUJ instability and does not require acute operative treatment.
- Conservative management includes rest, immobilization, antiinflammatory medications, and local steroid injections. Patients with ulnar positive wrists may be less likely to respond to conservative management. Arthroscopic tear debridement is the treatment most preferred when symptoms persist.

### Class 1B

- A class 1B tear is a partial or complete avulsion of the TFCC from its ulnar attachments, with or without an ulnar styloid fracture. It may produce DRUJ instability.
- A fracture through the base of the styloid predicts a destabilizing TFCC tear more than a tip fracture. However, the radioulnar ligaments also have substantial attachments at the fovea, which may remain intact and preserve DRUJ stability.
- Symptoms and physical findings of this injury are similar to those of a class 1A tear, but a click usually is absent, and pain and tenderness are more ulnar. Stressing the joint by passive dorsal and volar translation may produce pain even if the DRUJ is stable.
- Because these tears destabilize the TFCC and potentially destabilize the DRUJ, they should be treated initially by immobilization and then activity limitation for 4 to 6 weeks. Most of these injuries respond to conservative measures. Surgery is indicated for persistent symptoms or instability.
- Arthroscopic treatment of peripheral TFCC tears has evolved rapidly over the last few years. Peripheral tears can be sutured to the capsule using various arthroscopic techniques (Box 7–2, and Figures 7–4, 7–5, and 7–6). An open repair is considered for chronic injuries, especially in the presence of an ulnar styloid nonunion or DRUJ instability.

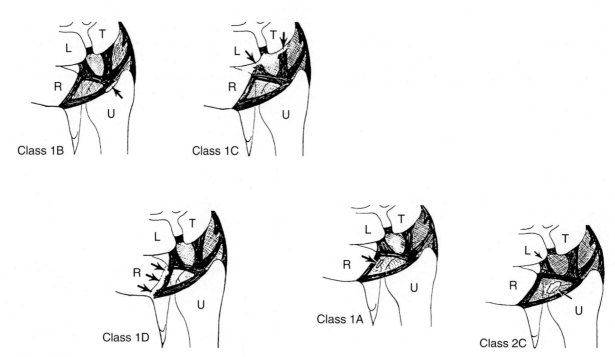

**Figure 7–3:**
Repairable lesions of the triangular fibrocartilage complex include class 1B, 1C, and 1D lesions. Class 2 lesions of the fibrocartilage complex with attrition of the central portion and class 1A lesions that have a tear adjacent to the triangular fibrocartilage complex attachment into the sigmoid notch are not repairable lesions. *L,* lunate; *R,* radius; *T,* triquetrum; *U,* ulna. (From Palmer AK: Triangular fibrocartilage complex lesions: a classification. *J Hand Surg* 14A:594-606, 1989.)

## Class 1C

- A class 1C tear is a partial or complete tear of the ulnocarpal ligaments, either midsubstance or from their attachments to the lunate and triquetrum. It is commonly associated with class 1B tears and lunotriquetral ligament tears.[25] A class 1C tear is less frequently identified than other TFCC injuries, probably because it is more difficult to diagnose and perhaps because it heals more reliably as a result of the rich vascularity in this region. The most obvious sign of a severe injury is volar "sag" of the carpus relative to the ulna on a lateral radiograph.
- In general, these injuries should be managed conservatively for an extended period unless mechanical instability is present early. Open repair has been performed in a few cases.[26] The procedure described by Hui and Linscheid[27] (see chronic DRUJ instability) may be appropriate for a chronic injury.

## Class 1D

- A class 1D tear is a partial or complete traumatic avulsion of the TFCC directly from the radius, with or without a bone fragment, involving one or both radioulnar ligaments. Class 1D injuries frequently are associated with distal radius fractures and usually respond to accurate fracture reduction of the radius. Only in rare cases do these tears by themselves cause DRUJ instability. In the absence of DRUJ instability, symptoms and physical

findings are the same as with other types of traumatic TFCC injury.
- Open repair is indicated for large displaced fractures involving the rim of the sigmoid notch because this injury results in loss of both the bony and ligament restraints. Repair of the disc and dorsal radioulnar ligament to the rim of the radius using both open and arthroscopic techniques has been described.[26,28]

## Degenerative Triangular Fibrocartilage Complex Tears and Ulna Impaction

- Degenerative tears are caused by chronic excessive loading between the ulna and carpus. In a cadaver study, 73% of ulnar neutral or positive wrists had TFCC perforations, whereas only 17% of ulnar negative wrists had perforations.[1] Ulnar positive wrists are associated with a thinner disc, which may be more susceptible to degeneration.[29]
- Symptoms of ulna impaction include ulnar-sided wrist pain exacerbated by rotation and ulnar deviation, particularly with pronation and grip. Physical examination demonstrates pain with the ulnocarpal stress test described earlier in this chapter. Radiographs demonstrate ulna positive variance and sclerosis or subchondral cyst formation in the ulnar corner of the lunate and ulna

| Box 7–2 | Arthroscopic Treatment of Triangular Fibrocartilage Tears |
|---|---|

- Many TFCC tears can be treated arthroscopically. The patient is placed in a wrist traction tower with 15 lb of distraction force. The joint is distended with 5 cc of sterile saline. A standard 3-4 portal (between the third and fourth extensor compartments) is used for visualization and classification of the tear using a 2.7-mm camera, with a probe placed into the 4-5 portal (between the fourth and fifth extensor compartments). The scapholunate and lunotriquetral ligaments also are evaluated. Accessory portals include the 6R (radial to the ECU), 6U (ulnar to the ECU), and 4-5. A 2.5-mm full radius shaver is used to debride central type 1A tears, a torn meniscal homologue, or the attachment sites for ulnar- or radial-sided tears. For ulnar-sided tears (types 1B and 1C), the camera is moved to the 6R portal and the shaver is placed in the 3-4 portal to debride any synovitis. An incision is made longitudinally in line with the 6U portal through skin but not through the capsule. A cannula is used in the 3-4 portal to pass 2-0 Maxon meniscal repair sutures (Davis & Geck, Manati, PA) from the 3-4 portal into the TFCC and out through the capsule ulnarly into the 6U incision. The sutures are tied down over the capsule, taking care not to entrap any branches of the dorsal sensory nerve. Correct tensioning is verified through the arthroscope as the sutures are tied (Figure 7–4). Conversely, the sutures are placed into the TFCC from "outside in" using 18-gauge needles through the 6U portal, passing the suture through the TFCC, grasping the suture end with a suture grasper through the 6U portal, and tying it over the capsular bridge created (Figure 7–5). Radial-sided tears can be treated similarly. The edge of the radius is debrided with the shaver to cancellous bone, then several 2-0 Maxon repair sutures are placed from the 6U portal through a cannula and driven on power through the radius to exit between the first and second extensor compartments. The skin between the compartments is incised and tendons retracted so that the sutures can be tied down to capsule with arthroscopic vision verifying appropriate tension (Figure 7–6).

ECU, Extensor carpi ulnaris; TFCC, triangular fibrocartilage complex.

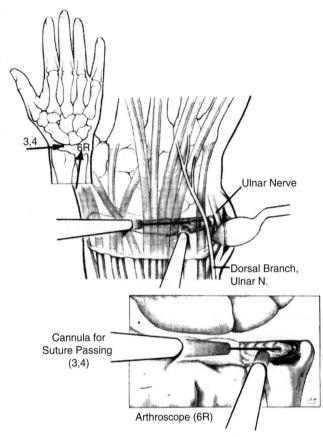

Figure 7–4:

**Peripheral tears of the triangular fibrocartilage complex can be repaired with an inside-out technique by passing the sutures through a cannula in the 3-4 portal while the arthroscope is in the 4-5 portal. (From Trumble TE, Gilbert M, Vedder N: Isolated tears of the triangular fibrocartilage: management by early arthroscopic repair.** *J Hand Surg* **22A:57-65, 1997.)**

head. MRI may show increased signal in the ulnar corner of the lunate. This entity is distinguished from Kienböck's disease in two ways: (1) ulnar variance usually is negative in Kienböck's disease, and (2) radiographic changes and MRI abnormalities typically are diffuse in Kienböck's disease.

- Severity and progression of degenerative changes in the disc of the TFCC, lunate, triquetrum, and ulnar head vary in this condition (Box 7–3). Treatment options include modification of activities to avoid repetitive loading, antiinflammatory medications, wrist splinting, and cortisone injection into the ulnocarpal joint.
- Surgery is indicated for patients with clinical findings and radiographic changes who do not respond to conservative measures. The goal of surgery is to reduce ulnocarpal loading. Arthroscopic debridement of the TFCC disc,

articular surfaces, and lunotriquetral ligament repair or debridement without ulnar shortening is appropriate in ulna-neutral and ulna–negative wrists.

- Partial resection of the ulnar head dome or ulnar shortening via a shaft osteotomy is indicated for wrists that are ulna positive, dynamic ulna positive, or neutral variance.
- Partial resection of the ulnar head dome, known widely as the "wafer" resection as described by Feldon, can be performed arthroscopically or with open technique.[30,31] The resection must not violate the DRUJ or destabilize the ligament attachments at the fovea (Figure 7–7).
- Ulnar shortening osteotomy typically is performed using an oblique saw cut through the shaft of the ulna. An interfragmentary lag screw and dynamic compression plate are used for fixation. Although shortening osteotomy preserves the articular surface of the ulnar head, its effect

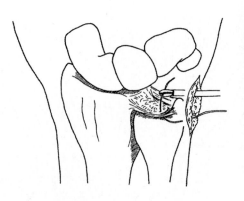
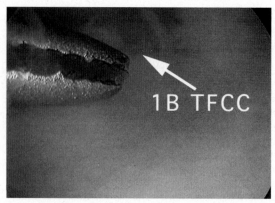

Figure 7–5:

**A,** Using the arthroscopic grasping forceps, the suture is passed from the 4-5 portal and back out through the 6U portal so that the suture can be tied over the 6U portal site, taking care to avoid injury to the dorsal sensory branch of the ulnar nerve. The triangular fibrocartilage complex of the suture can be brought out directly through the 6U portal. **B,** The grasping forceps or the wire loop grasping tool can be used to retrieve the repair suture during arthroscopy. (From Trumble TE: Distal radioulnar joint and triangular fibrocartilage complex. In Trumble TE, editor. *Principles of hand surgery and therapy.* Philadelphia, 2000, WB Saunders.)

on DRUJ congruity is difficult to predict. Typically 2 to 3 mm of bone is resected to level or create a slightly ulnar negative variance, avoiding overshortening.

- Ulnar shortening osteotomy is particularly useful in patients with acquired ulna positive variance secondary to a malunited distal radius fracture, not only because the procedure restores neutral variance but also because it may tighten the ulnocarpal ligaments, which can improve associated lunotriquetral or DRUJ instability.[32]

## Lunotriquetral Interosseous Ligament and Meniscal Homologue Injuries

- Small tears of the LTIL do not cause carpal or DRUJ instability. Acute destabilizing LTIL tears can be reduced and immobilized by lunotriquetral pinning under arthroscopic guidance. Treatment of chronic injuries is

Radial Nerve, Superficial Branch

Arthroscope in 3,4 Portal

Cannula Inserted on Ulnar Border of Wrist

Meniscal Repair Needle Exiting Between 1st and 2nd Dorsal Compartment Tendons

Figure 7–6:

With an arthroscope placed in the 4-5 portal and the suture passing cannula in the 6U portal, class 1D repairs of the triangular fibrocartilage complex can be made. (From Trumble TE, Glibert M, Vedder N: Isolated tears of the triangular fibrocartilage: management by early arthroscopic repair. *J Hand Surg* 22A:57-65, 1997.)

| **Box 7–3** | **Classification by Palmer** |
| --- | --- |

- Class 1: Traumatic
  A. Central perforation
  B. Ulnar avulsion
    - With styloid fracture
    - Without styloid fracture
  C. Distal avulsion (from carpus)
  D. Radial avulsion
    - With sigmoid notch fracture
    - Without sigmoid notch fracture
- Class 2: Degenerative (ulnar impaction syndrome)
  A. TFCC wear
  B. TFCC wear
    - +Lunate and/or ulnar head chondromalacia
  C. TFCC perforation
    - +Lunate and/or ulnar head chondromalacia
  D. TFCC perforation
    - +Lunate and/or ulnar head chondromalacia
    - +LTIL perforation
  E. TFCC perforation
    - +Lunate and/or ulnar head chondromalacia
    - +LTIL perforation
    - +Ulnocarpal arthritis

LTIL, Lunotriquetral interosseous ligament; TFCC, triangular fibrocartilage complex.

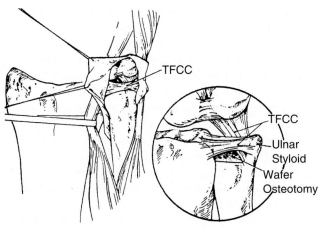

**Figure 7–7:**
The wafer technique of resection of the distal portion of the ulna has been reported for treatment of symptoms of ulnar impaction. TFCC, triangular fibrocartilage complex. (From Feldon P, Terrono AL, Belsky MR: Wafer distal ulna resection for triangular fibrocartilage tears and/or ulna impaction syndrome. *J Hand Surg* 17A:731-737, 1992.)

controversial; both ligament reconstruction and arthrodesis have been used with varying success. The diagnosis and treatment of this condition are covered in Chapter 10.

- The meniscal homologue, when present, can tear because of impingement against the carpus, resulting in pain and swelling. Arthroscopic debridement usually is effective.[3]

# Distal Radioulnar Joint Instability (Box 7–4)

## Simple Dislocations

- By convention, DRUJ dislocations are described by the position of the ulnar head relative to the radius. Most DRUJ dislocations are dorsal and caused by hyperpronation and wrist extension. Volar dislocations occur in the supinated forearm or from a direct blow to the ulnar aspect of the forearm.
- In a dislocation resulting from a pure ligament injury, reduction is uncomplicated unless there is interposed soft tissue, such as the ECU tendon. Under conscious sedation in the emergency department, gentle pressure is applied over the ulnar head while the radius is rotated toward the prominent ulna to reverse the mechanism of injury.
- After reduction, the joint is tested over the full range of forearm rotation to determine the stable arc. Typically, a dorsal dislocation is most stable in supination and a palmar dislocation in pronation. If the joint is stable in an acceptable position of forearm rotation, it is treated in a long arm cast for 3 to 4 weeks, followed by a well-molded short arm cast for 2 to 3 weeks.

---

**Box 7–4**   **Author's Classification of Distal Radioulnar Joint Instability**

- Ligament injury, including ulnar styloid fracture
  - TFCC tear (radioulnar ligaments) from ulna
    - No fractures
    - Fleck fracture from fovea of ulnar head
    - Basilar ulnar styloid fracture (displaced or mobile nonunion)
  - TFCC tear (radioulnar ligaments) from radius
    - No fractures
    - Avulsion fracture of rim(s) of sigmoid notch
- Extraarticular fractures, malunions, or developmental deformities of radius and ulna
  - Angular, rotational, or displaced fractures or malunions
    - Distal radius
    - Ulnar neck
    - Radius shaft (includes Galeazzi fracture)
    - Ulnar shaft
  - Length deficiencies (traumatic and developmental)
    - Radial head injury or absence (includes Essex-Lopresti injury)
    - Distal radius growth arrest (includes Madelung deformity)
    - Distal ulnar growth arrest
    - Defect in radius or ulnar shaft
- Intraarticular fractures or skeletal deformities of DRUJ
  - Sigmoid notch fracture or deficiency
    - Palmar rim
    - Dorsal rim
    - Both palmar and dorsal rims
  - Ulnar head deficiency
    - Displaced fractures
    - Malunion
    - Previous partial or complete resection

DRUJ, Distal radioulnar joint; TFCC, triangular fibrocartilage complex.

---

- If the joint is stable only in extreme pronation or supination, additional treatment should be considered, such as radioulnar pinning in the neutral position or TFCC repair and DRUJ ligament. Radioulnar pinning should be done proximal to the DRUJ, using two large Steinmann pins to avoid breakage with attempts at rotation. The pins can be driven all the way across the radius so that they can be removed from either end should breakage occur. The pins can be further protected by immobilizing the patient in a long arm cast for 6 weeks.

## Distal Radioulnar Joint Instability Associated with Fractures

- In distal radius fractures, initial wide displacement of the DRUJ and severe radial shortening are the most important risk factors for persistent DRUJ instability. The radioulnar ligaments can tolerate no more than 5 to 7 mm of radial shortening before one or both ligaments tear.[33] Displaced fractures through the base of the ulna styloid may disrupt the TFCC and radioulnar ligaments.

Although fracture union is not consistently achieved with any technique, sound fibrous healing in good position can be compatible with resolution of symptoms and DRUJ stability.[34]

- Fracture reduction and maintenance of alignment of the radius are the most important factors for DRUJ stability. The DRUJ should be tested after fixation of the radius. If instability remains after radius fracture reduction, surgical options include pinning the ulna to the radius proximal to the DRUJ (see technique discussed earlier), ulnar styloid fixation, or open repair of the TFCC (Figure 7–8).

- A distal radius malunion with greater than 20 to 30 degrees of angulation creates marked incongruity, alters DRUJ kinematics, distorts the TFCC, and induces palmar DRUJ instability.[33,35] Intraarticular ulnar head fractures and sigmoid notch fractures can cause DRUJ incongruity, instability, and arthrosis.

- Symptoms of chronic instability include pain, weakness, and a joint clunk during active motion. The distal ulna may remain tender and appear prominent. In mild instability, pain and weakness often occur only with activities that require power rotation of the forearm while gripping, for example, when using a screwdriver. Chronic instability rarely improves spontaneously but symptoms may lessen and become tolerable in mild cases. Whether instability predisposes to wrist arthritis is unknown. A 4-week trial of wrist splinting and antiinflammatory medications is indicated for mild instability.

- Chronic instability that is not amenable to conservative treatment is appropriate for surgical intervention. When planning operative treatment, it is important to identify the structures at fault (TFCC, other stabilizers, malunion) and whether arthrosis is present.

- If the instability is purely ligamentous, then repair of the TFCC or reconstruction of the radioulnar ligaments is appropriate (Box 7–5 and Figure 7–9). If instability is caused by a distal radius malunion, corrective osteotomy is required. An osteotomy usually restores DRUJ stability; however, radioulnar length discrepancy also must be corrected. A trapezoidal graft to the radius can correct both angulation and length discrepancy simultaneously. In cases of severe radial shortening, combined osteotomy of the radius and shortening of the ulna may be a more technically feasible option. If bony realignment does not

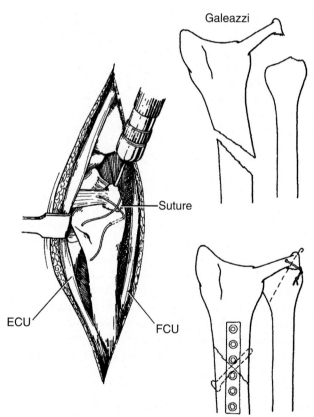

**Figure 7–8:**
Plate fixation of the distal radius restores the length of the forearm following a Galeazzi fracture. Unstable lesions with avulsions of the entire portion of the ulnar styloid require open reduction and internal fixation to restore stability of the distal radioulnar joint. *ECU*, extensor carpi ulnaris; *FCU*, flexor carpi ulnaris. (From Trmble TE: Distal radioulnar joint and triangular fibrocartilage complex. In Trumble TE, editor. *Principles of hand surgery and therapy*. Philadelphia, 2000, WB Saunders.)

---

| **Box 7–5** | **Triangular Fibrocartilage Complex Open Repair (Class 1B Tear)** |

- A 5-cm incision is made between the fifth and sixth extensors and centered over the ulnar head. The EDQ[AU13] sheath is opened except for its most distal part, and the tendon is retracted. The DRUJ is exposed through an L-shaped capsulotomy. The longitudinal limb begins at the ulnar neck and extends to the distal edge of the sigmoid notch, taking care not to cut the dorsal radioulnar ligament. The transverse limb is made along the proximal edge of the dorsal radioulnar ligament and extends to, but not into, the ECU sheath. If the TFCC is suitable for repair, its distal surface is exposed through a transverse ulnocarpal capsulotomy made along the distal edge of the dorsal radioulnar ligament. Using a 0.045-inch Kirschner wire, holes are created in the distal ulna extending from the dorsal aspect of the ulnar neck to the fovea. Two horizontal mattress sutures (2-0 absorbable monofilament) are passed from distal to proximal through the ulnar periphery of the TFCC and then through the bone holes. The sutures are tied with the joint reduced and the forearm in neutral rotation. The dorsal DRUJ capsule and retinaculum are closed but should not be excessively imbricated to avoid loss of pronation. A long arm splint is applied with the forearm rotated 45 degrees toward the most stable joint position. At 2 weeks, the splint is converted to a long arm cast for 4 weeks, followed by a well-molded short arm cast for another 2 to 3 weeks. A removable splint then is used for 4 weeks while motion is regained. Strengthening and resumption of activities are delayed until near painless motion is achieved (Figure 7–9).

---

EDQ, Extensor digiti quinti; DRUJ, distal radioulnar joint; TFCC, triangular fibrocartilage complex.

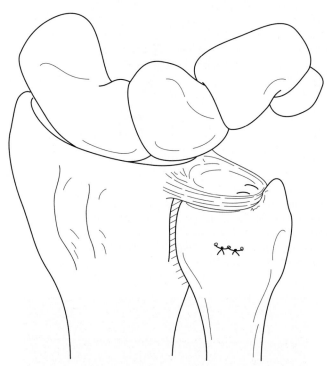

Figure 7–9:
**Open repair of a class IB tear is performed through a dorsal approach, with horizontal mattress transosseous sutures through the ulnar neck.**

restore stability, TFCC repair or a soft tissue stabilization procedure also will be necessary (Figure 7–10).[15,27]

- Distal ulnar arthroplasty is indicated when DRUJ instability is associated with arthrosis or ulnar impaction syndrome. In cases of significant arthrosis, a metal prosthetic replacement[62] or hemiresection-interposition (HIT)[57] for the ulnar head may be used. In cases of ulnar impaction, a wafer resection[42,43] or ulnar shortening[44] is performed in

addition to the stabilization. (These are discussed further in the section on DRUJ arthritis and ulnar impaction.

## Extensor Carpi Ulnaris Tendonitis and Subluxation

- Tendonitis and subluxation of the ECU tendon at the wrist can cause ulnar-sided wrist pain and should be included in the differential diagnosis of TFCC pathology. The anatomy, evaluation, and treatment of these conditions of the ECU tendon are discussed in detail in Chapter 14.

## Distal Radioulnar Joint Arthritis

- Arthritis can be posttraumatic, degenerative, or inflammatory. Pain, swelling, decreased grip strength, and stiffness are the most common symptoms. Tenderness is generally diffuse about the ulnar head. Joint pain is exacerbated by forearm rotation, especially when the joint is manually compressed.
- Differentiating between DRUJ arthritis and ulna impaction syndrome is important because their primary treatments differ. When the two conditions are present, a combined treatment is planned. Radiographs help to localize the area of involvement. In DRUJ arthritis, the proximal margin of the ulnar head typically is the first site demonstrating osteophytes.
- Surgical options include debridement of the joint, a partial resection of the ulnar head, a Darrach procedure, the Sauve-Kapandji procedure, or implant replacement of the ulna head. Arthrodesis of the DRUJ or creation of a one-bone forearm by proximal radioulnar arthrodesis or radius to ulna transfer are the ultimate salvage options.

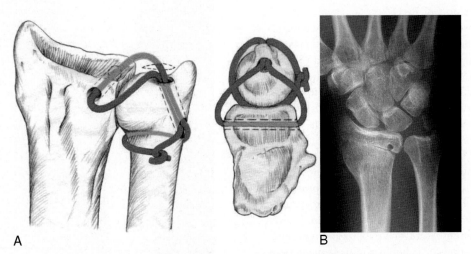

A                                                          B

Figure 7–10:
**A, Method for reconstructing both distal radioulnar ligaments that uses a palmaris longus tendon graft passed through bone tunnels in the distal radius and ulnar head. Location of bone tunnels and route of tendon graft are shown. B, Posteroanterior view of the wrist after distal radius corrective osteotomy and distal radioulnar ligament reconstruction through bone tunnels with palmaris longus graft.**

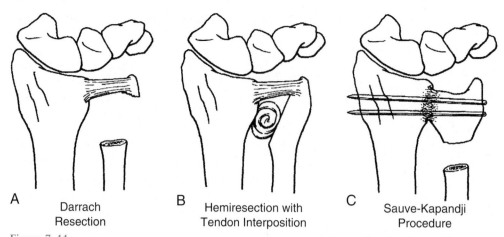

A — Darrach Resection

B — Hemiresection with Tendon Interposition

C — Sauve-Kapandji Procedure

Figure 7–11:
Methods for treating arthritis of the distal radial ulnar joint include excision of the distal ulna (Darrach resection) **(A)**, hemiresection of the distal ulna with tendon graft interposition **(B)**, and a distal radioulnar joint arthrodesis with proximal pseudoarthrosis Sauve-Kapandji technique **(C)**. (From Trumble TE: Distal radioulnar joint and triangular fibrocartilage complex. In Trumble TE, editor. *Principles of hand surgery and therapy.* Philadelphia, 2000, WB Saunders.)

- Joint debridement for limited arthritis has theoretical merit, but clinical experience is limited. The hemiresection interposition technique described by Bowers consists of a partial resection of the ulnar head that eliminates its articular surface with the sigmoid notch combined with a soft tissue interposition intended to prevent radioulnar impingement. If positive ulna variance is present, hemiresection is combined with a shortening osteotomy that typically is performed through the head–neck region.[36]

- The Darrach procedure consists of excision of the distal ulna through its neck. The ulnar styloid and its soft tissue attachments can be retained to preserve some TFCC function. The primary complication is instability of the ulnar stump and radioulnar convergence resulting in impingement against the radius. Thus, the procedure often is combined with a soft tissue stabilization procedure such as a tenodesis to the ulnar stump using a strip of the FCU and/or ECU.[37]

- The Sauve-Kapandji procedure retains the distal ulna, fuses the ulnar head to the sigmoid notch, and creates a pseudarthrosis at the ulnar neck. It is intended to provide better support for the carpus, thus reducing the risk of weakness and ulnar translation of the carpus. Instability of the ulnar stump may develop similar to the Darrach procedure; soft tissue stabilization may help this problem. Spontaneous fusion of the pseudarthrosis also can occur, resulting in lost motion (Figure 7–11).[38]

- Radioulnar impingement after one of these procedures is extremely difficult to treat. Bieber et al.[39] reported that patients who did not respond to a Darrach procedure continued to do poorly despite undergoing up to seven additional operations. Soft tissue stabilization with interposition is an option for radioulnar impingement, particularly if one was not performed in the index operation.

- The ultimate salvage is creation of a one-bone forearm. Creating a one-bone forearm provides stability and can eliminate pain, but it sacrifices all rotation. Preoperative

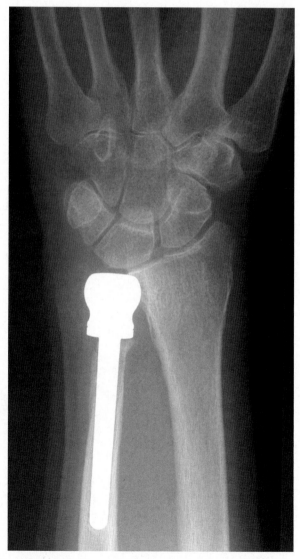

Figure 7–12:
Radiograph of a distal ulna implant arthroplasty (uHead, Avanta Orthopedics, San Diego, CA) for treatment of radioulnar impingement.

immobilization of the forearm allows the patient to decide whether the procedure is appropriate.

- Distal ulna implant arthroplasty is a promising newer option. Distal ulna implant arthroplasty is an attractive concept for the initial treatment of arthritis, because it could better preserve DRUJ kinematics. A functional ulnar head implant also could be useful to alleviate radioulnar impingement and to restore some load transmission after a failed distal ulna resection. Although promising early results have been reported, experience with these implants is limited (Figure 7–12).[40]

## Conclusions

- There are many causes of ulnar-sided wrist pain. Acute trauma can result in fractures, joint instability, tendon dislocations, or TFCC tears. Common causes of chronic pain in the absence of preceding trauma are joint instability, tendonitis, TFCC degeneration, DRUJ arthritis, and ulna impaction syndrome.
- Focused physical examination and appropriate imaging studies are keys to an accurate diagnosis. Wrist arthroscopy is a useful adjunct, because many disorders of the TFCC can be both diagnosed and treated arthroscopically.
- Treatment should be directed at restoring or reconstructing normal anatomy and function whenever possible before proceeding to therapies that resect, ablate, or compromise function.

## References

1. Palmer AK, Werner FW: The triangular fibrocartilage complex of the wrist: anatomy and function. *J Hand Surg [Am]* 6:153-162, 1981.
   This now classic work describes the anatomy and function of the TFCC through anatomic dissection and biomechanical testing of cadavers.

2. Nishikawa S, Toh S: Anatomical study of the carpal attachment of the triangular fibrocartilage complex. *J Bone Joint Surg Br* 84:1062-1065, 2002.
   This anatomic study of cadavers describes the TFCC attachments to the triquetrum, the meniscal homologue.

3. Nishikawa S, Toh S, Miura H, Arai K: The carpal detachment injury of the triangular fibrocartilage complex. *J Hand Surg [Br]* 27:86-89, 2002.
   This article describes symptomatic meniscal homologue tears diagnosed at arthroscopy and treated successfully with debridement in 22 wrists.

4. DiTano O, Trumble TE, Tender AF: Biomechanical function of the distal radioulnar and ulnocarpal wrist ligaments. *J Hand Surg [Am]* 28:622-627, 2003.
   This cadaveric study describes relative tension in DRUJ ligaments in different positions of forearm rotation.

5. Gupta R, Allaire RB, Fornalski S et al: Kinematic analysis of the distal radioulnar joint after simulated progressive ulnar-sided wrist injury. *J Hand Surg [Am]* 27:854-862, 2002.
   Kinematic analysis and serial sectioning found that the TFCC and ECU subsheath were more important than the ulnocarpal ligaments in stabilizing the DRUJ.

6. Kihara H, Short WH, Werner FW et al: The stabilizing mechanism of the distal radioulnar joint pronation and supination. *J Hand Surg [Am]* 20:930-936, 1995.
   A biomechanical, serial sectioning, cadaver study found that the dorsal and palmar radioulnar ligaments, the pronator quadratus, and the interosseous membrane contributed to DRUJ stability.

7. Palmer AK, Werner FW: Biomechanics of the distal radioulnar joint. *Clin Orthop* 187:26-35, 1984.
   The authors describe the anatomy and mechanics of the DRUJ.

8. Stuart PR, Berger RA, Linscheid RL, An KN: The dorsopalmar stability of the distal radioulnar joint. *J Hand Surg [Am]* 25:689-699, 2000.
   A biomechanical study demonstrated relative contributions of the radioulnar ligaments, articular geometry, interosseus membrane, and ECU subsheath to DRUJ stability.

9. Ekenstam F, Palmer AK, Glisson RR: The load on the radius and ulna in different positions of the wrist and forearm. A cadaver study. *Acta Orthop Scand* 55:363-365, 1984.
   In a biomechanical study testing the load along the radius and ulna in different wrist and forearm positions in nine cadaver specimens, relative load along the radius was lowest in a position of wrist flexion, ulnar deviation, and full forearm pronation.

10. Schuind F, Linscheid RL, An KN, Chao EY: A normal data base of posteroanterior roentgenographic measurements of the wrist. *J Bone Joint Surg Br* 74:1418-1429, 1992.
    In 120 adults, the authors establish norms for ulnar variance, carpal height, radial inclination, and distal radioulnar distance as functions of age and gender.

11. Werner FW, Glisson RR, Murphy DJ, Palmer AK: Force transmission through the distal radioulnar carpal joint: effect of ulnar lengthening and shortening. *Handchir Mikrochir Plast Chir* 18:304-308, 1986.
    This biomechanical study demonstrates dramatic alterations in load transmission across the wrist with relatively small (2.5 mm) changes in ulnar length and following removal of the articular disc portion of the triangular fibrocartilage complex.

12. Palmer AK, Werner FW, Glisson RR, Murphy DJ: Partial excision of the triangular fibrocartilage complex. *J Hand Surg [Am]* 13:391-394, 1988.
    In a cadaver model, excision of less than two thirds of the horizontal portion of the TFCC had no statistical effect experimentally on forearm axial load transmission.

13. Bowers WH: Instability of the distal radioulnar articulation. *Hand Clin* 7:311-327, 1991.
    Experimental data and clinical observations are combined to provide a theoretical rationale for understanding DRUJ instability.

14. Morrissy RT, Nalebuff EA: Dislocation of the distal radioulnar joint: anatomy and clues to prompt diagnosis. *Clin Orthop* 144:154-158, 1979.

This article describes injury to the DRUJ and clinical findings.

15. Adams BD, Berger RA: An anatomic reconstruction of the distal radioulnar ligaments for posttraumatic distal radioulnar joint instability. *J Hand Surg [Am]* 27:243-251, 2002.
    Fourteen patients with posttraumatic DRUJ instability were treated with an anatomic reconstruction of the distal radioulnar ligaments, with symptomatic relief in 12.

16. Friedman SL, Palmer AK: The ulnar impaction syndrome. *Hand Clin* 7:295-310, 1991.
    This review describes ulnar impaction, the various treatments, and their indications.

17. Nakamura R, Horii E, Imaeda T et al: The ulnocarpal stress test in the diagnosis of ulnar-sided wrist pain. *J Hand Surg [Br]* 22:719-723, 1997.
    The authors describe the ulnocarpal stress test and review a cohort of 45 patients with positive tests and pathologic findings at arthroscopy.

18. Palmer AK, Glisson RR, Werner FW: Ulnar variance determination. *J Hand Surg [Am]* 7:376-379, 1982.
    This article describes a simple, accurate, and reproducible method of measuring ulnar variance from standard PA radiographs of the wrist.

19. Tomaino MM: The importance of the pronated grip x-ray view in evaluating ulnar variance. *J Hand Surg [Am]* 18:713-716, 2000.
    The authors demonstrate increases in ulnar variance with pronated grip positioning for radiographs and urge inclusion of this view in assessment of ulnocarpal impaction.

20. Friedman SL, Palmer AK, Short WH et al: The change in ulnar variance with grip. *J Hand Surg [Am]* 18:713-716, 1993.
    A study of 66 wrists in symptom-free volunteers revealed that a statistically significant relative increase in ulnar variance occurs with grip.

21. Blazar PE, Chan PS, Kneeland JB et al: The effect of observer experience on magnetic resonance imaging interpretation and localization of triangular fibrocartilage of the wrist. *J Hand Surg [Am]* 26:742-748, 2001.
    The overall accuracy rates for prediction of a TFCC lesion and its location on MRI were 69% and 37%, respectively, with accuracy differing between an experienced and a less experienced observer.

22. Haims AH, Schweitzer ME, Morrison WB et al: Limitations of MR imaging in the diagnosis of peripheral tears of the triangular fibrocartilage of the wrist. *AJR Am J Roentgenol* 178:419-422, 2002.
    The sensitivity MRI for evaluation of the peripheral triangular fibrocartilage complex tear was 17%, with a specificity of 79% and an accuracy of 64%. Weighted kappa values revealed only fair agreement among the three observers.

23. Pederzini L, Luchetti R, Sorgani O: Evaluation of the triangular fibrocartilage complex tears by arthroscopy, arthrography, and magnetic resonance imaging. *Arthroscopy* 8:191-197, 1992.
    Arthroscopy was more sensitive and specific for TFCC and articular pathology than arthrographic and MRI results in 11 symptomatic patients undergoing all three procedures.

24. Hermansdorfer JD, Kleinman WB: Management of chronic peripheral tears of the triangular fibrocartilage complex. *J Hand Surg [Am]* 16:340-346, 1991.
    Open repair of traumatic ulnar-peripheral tears of the TFCC to the fovea of the ulnar head is described. Results were good if no other pathologic conditions coexisted.

25. Melone CP, Nathan R: Traumatic disruption of the triangular fibrocartilage complex. *Clin Orthop* 275:65-73, 1992.
    In a series of destabilizing TFCC tears, there was a spectrum of associated injuries involving the extensor carpi ulnaris sheath, ulnocarpal ligaments, and the peritriquetral ligaments.

26. Cooney WP, Linscheid RL, Dobyns JH: Triangular fibrocartilage tears. *J Hand Surg [Am]* 19:143-154, 1994.
    Using a dorsal approach, open repair of radial and ulnar peripheral tears of the TFCC, combined with ulnar recession, produced generally good results in patients without DRUJ instability.

27. Hui FC, Linscheid RL: Ulnotriquetral augmentation tenodesis: a reconstructive procedure for dorsal subluxation of the distal radioulnar joint. *J Hand Surg [Am]* 7:230-236, 1982.
    A tenodesis procedure using a slip of flexor carpi ulnaris for treatment of posttraumatic dorsal DRUJ or ulnocarpal instability is described.

28. Trumble TE, Gilbert M, Vedder N: Isolated tears of the triangular fibrocartilage: management by early arthroscopic repair. *J Hand Surg [Am]* 22:57-65, 1997.
    Short-term functional outcome after arthroscopic repair of the TFCC was excellent in 24 patients.

29. Palmer AK, Glisson RR, Werner FW: Relationship between ulnar variance and triangular fibrocartilage complex thickness. *J Hand Surg [Am]* 9:681-682, 1984.
    An inverse relationship was found between positive ulnar variance and TFCC thickness.

30. Feldon P, Terrono AL, Belsky MR: Wafer distal ulna resection for triangular fibrocartilage tears and/or ulna impaction syndrome. *J Hand Surg [Am]* 17:731-737, 1992.
    The authors describe partial resection (distal 2-4 mm) of the ulnar dome (wafer resection) for symptomatic tears of the triangular fibrocartilage complex or mild ulna impaction syndrome.

31. Tomaino MM, Weiser RW: Combined arthroscopic TFCC debridement and wafer resection of the distal ulna in wrists with triangular fibrocartilage complex tears and positive ulnar variance. *J Hand Surg [Am]* 26:1047-1052, 2001.
    Short-term follow-up of 12 patients with TFCC tears and ulnar positive wrists who underwent TFCC debridement and wafer resection revealed good pain relief and improved grip strength.

32. Chun S, Palmer AK: The ulnar impaction syndrome: follow-up of ulnar shortening osteotomy. *J Hand Surg [Am]* 18:46-53, 1993.
    Good results were reported following ulnar shortening osteotomy for treatment of ulnar impaction syndrome.

33. Adams BD: Effects of radial deformity on distal radioulnar joint mechanics. *J Hand Surg [Am]* 18:492-498, 1993.

A cadaver experiment found that radial shortening caused the greatest disturbance in kinematics and the most distortion of the triangular fibrocartilage.

34. Mikic ZD: Treatment of acute injuries of the triangular fibrocartilage complex associated with distal radioulnar joint instability. *J Hand Surg [Am]* 20:319-323, 1995.
One hundred thirty patients who had a TFCC injury with DRUJ instability were treated operatively by various techniques.

35. Kihara H, Palmer AK, Werner FW et al: The effect of dorsally angulated distal radius fractures on distal radioulnar joint congruency and forearm rotation. *J Hand Surg [Am]* 21:40-47, 1996.
A biomechanical cadaver study found that DRUJ congruity and stability decreased with dorsal radial angulation greater than 20 degrees and following sectioning of both the TFCC and interosseus membrane.

36. Bowers WH: Distal radioulnar joint arthroplasty: the hemiresection-interposition technique. *J Hand Surg [Am]* 10:169-178, 1985.
This classic article describes partial removal of the ulnar head for arthrosis of the DRUJ that preserves some attachments of the TFCC.

37. Breen TF, Jupiter JB: Extensor carpi ulnaris and flexor carpi ulnaris tenodesis of the unstable distal ulna. *J Hand Surg [Am]* 14:612-617, 1989.
A tenodesis procedure is described to stabilize the resected distal ulna using a distally based slip of flexor carpi ulnaris and a proximally based slip of extensor carpi.

38. Kapandji IA: The Kapandji-Sauve procedure. *J Hand Surg [Br]* 17:125-126, 1992.
This article describes the Sauve-Kapandji procedure.

39. Bieber EJ, Linscheid RL, Dobyns JH, Beckenbaugh RD: Failed distal ulna resections. *J Hand Surg [Am]* 13:193-200, 1988.
This study of patients undergoing the Darrach procedure demonstrated that patients who did not obtain relief from this operation had an average of 2.2 additional operations, with up to seven procedures per patient.

40. van Schoonhoven J, Fernandez DL, Bowers WH, Herbert TJ: Salvage of failed resection arthroplasties of the distal radioulnar joint using a new ulnar head prosthesis. *J Hand Surg [Am]* 25:438-446, 2000.
An ulnar head prosthesis was used to treat painful instability following failed total or partial resection of the ulnar head because of radioulnar impingement. Stability and marked symptomatic improvement were routinely achieved.

# Scaphoid Fractures and Nonunions

Victoria D. Knoll[*] and Thomas E. Trumble[†]

[*]MD, Associated Orthopaedics and Sports Medicine, Plano, TX
[†]MD, Professor and Chief, Hand and Upper Extremity Surgery Service, Department of Orthopaedics, University of Washington School of Medicine, Seattle, WA

## Introduction

- Scaphoid fractures are the most common carpal fracture, followed by fractures of the triquetrum. In the United States, approximately 345,000 scaphoid fractures occur every year.[1] Scaphoid fractures usually result from a fall on an outstretched hand or high-energy trauma and most commonly involve the waist.[2] Fractures of the scaphoid in children are rare, usually involve the distal pole or tubercle, and heal uneventfully with cast immobilization. The retrograde blood supply to the scaphoid can delay healing or result in avascular necrosis (AVN) of the proximal pole. With early diagnosis and treatment, 90% of scaphoid fractures heal.[3] Scaphoid fractures are best identified early so that appropriate treatment can be given to prevent the development of a nonunion that can be challenging to treat. Scaphoid nonunions can present as a persistent "wrist sprain" that does not resolve or new-onset wrist pain without recollection of a specific traumatic event. The goal of treating scaphoid nonunions is to not only consolidate the nonunion but to correct any carpal malalignment. Therefore, scaphoid collapse or significant comminution should be addressed with bone grafting. Avascularity of the proximal pole of the scaphoid may require vascularized bone grafting. Scaphoid nonunions with AVN and comminution are a difficult problem. Untreated scaphoid nonunions lead to a predictable pattern of wrist arthritis for which treatment

can be challenging. For that reason, acute scaphoid fractures and scaphoid nonunions should be diagnosed and appropriately treated early.

## Anatomy and Biomechanics

### Osseous Anatomy

- Scaphoid means "boat" in Greek. The scaphoid is concave in both the ulnar and palmar directions. The scaphoid anatomically can be divided into thirds: distal pole, waist, and proximal pole. The scaphoid tubercle is the distal palmar and radial prominence of the bone. The anatomic "snuffbox" is outlined by the extensor pollicis longus (EPL) and extensor pollicis brevis (EPB) tendons. Tenderness in the "snuffbox" may be indicative of a scaphoid fracture.

### Vascular Anatomy

- A segment of the radial artery runs through the "snuffbox" as it passes from volar to dorsal around the base of the first metacarpal. Dorsal branches from the radial artery supply 70% to 80% of the blood flow to the scaphoid. Vessels that enter volarly supply 20% to 30% of the scaphoid (Figure 8–1).[4] The vessels perforate the distal third of the scaphoid and supply the remaining proximal bone via retrograde blood flow. Proximal pole fractures are slower to heal and can result in AVN because of the retrograde blood flow.

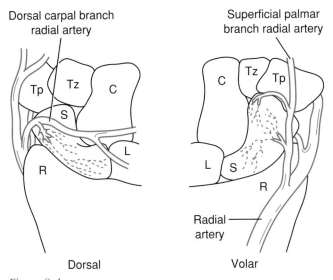

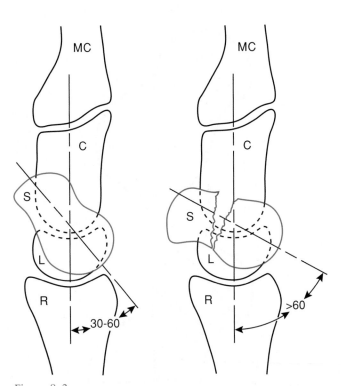

Figure 8–1:
**Dorsal and volar blood supply to the scaphoid from branches of the radial artery.** *C*, Capitate; *L*, lunate; *R*, radius; *S*, scaphoid; *Tp*, trapezium; *Tz*, trapezoid.

Figure 8–2:
**A**, Normal scapholunate angle (SL) is 30 to 60 degrees. A normal capitolunate angle (CL) is (0±15) degrees. **B**, Displaced scaphoid fracture leads to dorsal intercalated segmental instability (SL angle >60 degrees) through internal angulation and humpback deformity. *C*, Capitate; *MC*, metacarpal; *L*, lunate; *R*, radius; *S*, scaphoid.

## Carpal Alignment

- Alignment of the scaphoid is 45 degrees (30–60 degrees) of palmar tilt (on a lateral projection) and 45 degrees radial tilt (on a posteroanterior [PA] projection) measured along the long axis of the scaphoid and the long axis of the radius. The average scapholunate angle is 45 degrees (30–60 degrees) measured between the long axis of the scaphoid and a line bisecting the lunate on a lateral radiograph (Figure 8–2). The normal capitolunate angle is 0 degrees measured between the long axis of the capitate and a line bisecting the lunate on a lateral radiograph. A line drawn parallel with the long axis of the radius should bisect the lunate and pass through the capitate and middle finger metacarpal. The lateral intrascaphoid angle is the intersection of two lines drawn perpendicular to the diameters of the proximal and distal poles (Figure 8–3). The intrascaphoid angle is less than 35 degrees measured on a sagittal view of the scaphoid. If the intrascaphoid angle greatly exceeds 35 degrees, a "humpback" deformity exists. This deformity develops only in fractures distal to the apex of the dorsal ridge. The intraobserver and interobserver reliability are poor for the intrascaphoid angle and much better for the height-to-length ratio. The height-to-length ratio of the scaphoid is measured on a sagittal view. A ratio greater than 0.65 indicates collapse (Figure 8–4).[5] The study by Bain and Bennett,[5] however, did not clinically correlate collapse with management.

## Carpal Mechanics

- The scaphoid is considered vitally important to carpal stability because it links the proximal and distal rows. Scaphoid rotation affects rotation of the entire proximal row.[6] The scapholunate ligament allows the lunate to move with the scaphoid. The ligament is divided into three parts (dorsal, membranous, palmar), with the dorsal portion being the strongest.[7] The scaphoid and lunate flex as the wrist radially deviates. The scaphoid extends as the wrist ulnarly deviates and the lunate tilts dorsally.

## Ligaments

- The dorsal wrist ligaments are weaker than the palmar wrist ligaments (see Figure 1–6). Palmar carpal ligaments form an upside-down V, leaving a weak center portion, called the *space of Poirier,* through which the lunate can dislocate (see Figure 1–5). Displaced scaphoid fractures may induce carpal instability and allow the lunate to extend (dorsal intercalated segmental instability [DISI]) (see Figure 8–2). Through the intact scapholunate ligament, extension of the lunate may extend the proximal scaphoid fragment. This extension of the proximal fragment, coupled with flexion of the distal fragment, has been referred to as a *humpback deformity.* A scapholunate angle greater than 60 degrees is indicative of carpal collapse and a DISI malalignment. The flexion forces on the carpus through the scaphotrapezium and scaphocapitate ligaments can cause the scaphoid to flex over the radioscaphocapitate (RSC) ligament. The

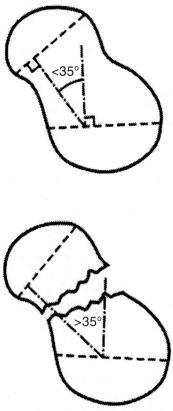

Figure 8–3:
Normal intrascaphoid angle is less than 35 degrees measured on a sagittal view of the scaphoid. An angle greater than 35 degrees is a "humpback" deformity. (From *Hand surgery update 3, scaphoid fractures and nonunions,* 2003, American Society for Surgery of the Hand.)

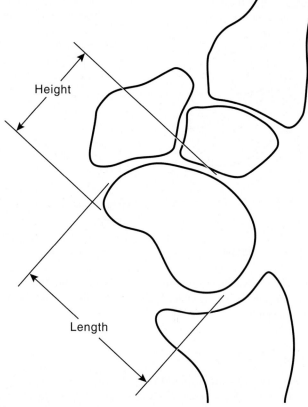

Figure 8–4:
Sagittal view of the scaphoid can be used to measure the height-to-length ratio, which should average less than 0.65. A ratio greater then 0.65 indicates scaphoid collapse.

radioscapholunate ligament, also known as the *ligament of Testut,* attaches to the proximal scaphoid but mainly serves as a neurovascular conduit containing branches from the anterior interosseous artery and nerve.[7]

# Mechanism of Injury

- The most common mechanism of injury is a fall on an outstretched hand with the wrist extended. In this position, the scaphoid is vertical. Scaphoid fractures also occur with the wrist in a neutral or slightly flexed position. One cadaveric study found that a load applied to a hyperextended wrist in radial deviation fractures the scaphoid.[8] Another cadaveric study revealed that a scaphoid fracture occurs when a load is applied to a hyperextended wrist in ulnar deviation.[9] The "puncher's" scaphoid fracture occurs as an axial force travels through the index metacarpal then trapezoid, forcing the distal pole into flexion.[10] In multitrauma patients, the mechanism or position of the wrist often is unknown. The incidence of concomitant distal radius and scaphoid fractures is approximately 5%.[11]

# Diagnosis and Evaluation
## Physical Examination

- A thorough systematic examination is of utmost importance. In a multitrauma patient, every extremity should be palpated, ranged, and examined for pain, crepitus, instability, swelling, hematoma, and ecchymosis. Normally, the anatomic snuffbox is concave. Swelling and loss of concavity in this area are suspicious for a scaphoid or scapholunate ligament injury. Pain may be elicited with range of motion, palpation in the "snuffbox," or palpation over the dorsal wrist. Pain may be elicited by axial load of first metacarpal compressing the scaphoid, palpation in the snuffbox or on the tubercle, or with radial and ulnar deviation of the wrist. When not acute, patients may report a vague aching in the wrist with a loss in motion or strength.

## Radiographs

- PA, lateral, and oblique (45–60 degrees of pronation) radiographs of the wrist are needed to assess osseous architecture and alignment. A "scaphoid" or "clenched fist" view is a PA view taken with the wrist in ulnar deviation (Figure 8–5). This position places the scaphoid in a more vertical position and can accentuate any scapholunate interval widening.[12] It is important to assess all carpal bones and alignment. Widening between carpal bones may indicate ligamentous injury. However, it is uncommon to sustain an associated scapholunate ligament tear with a scaphoid fracture. Nondisplaced fractures are not always evident initially until resorption has occurred at the fracture site, which can take 2 to 3 weeks.

## Bone Scintigraphy

- Fractures usually have increased uptake within 24 hours. In patients with negative radiographs and clinical signs of fracture, a positive bone scan indicates an acute fracture.[13] Increased activity can be nonspecific. Focal uptake indicates an acute fracture or an area of arthrosis. Diffuse uptake may indicate synovitis. Reduced uptake may indicate early bone ischemia or necrosis. Bone scans do not assess bony deformity or soft tissue injury.

## Computed Tomography

- Computed tomographic (CT) scans may currently be the optimal study for assessing bony anatomy.

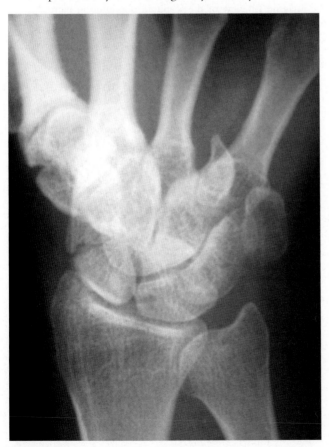

Figure 8–5:
"Scaphoid" or "clenched fist" view of a 40-year-old woman with wrist pain. A scaphoid waist fracture is easily seen.

Two-millimeter-thick cuts every 1 mm are ideal for evaluating the scaphoid. Sagittal images parallel to the long axis of the scaphoid best define collapse or "humpback" deformity at the fracture site.[14] CT scans can more precisely define both the lateral intrascaphoid angle (see Figure 8–3) and height-to-length ratio (see Figure 8–4). CT scans can assess cortical bridging if evaluating the fracture healing is difficult.

## Magnetic Resonance Imaging

- Magnetic resonance imaging (MRI) can assess osseous blood supply and soft tissue integrity (Figure 8–6). Prospective studies have proven MRI is more sensitive and specific than bone scintigraphy in detecting occult scaphoid fractures.[15] Low signal intensity (dark) on T1 indicates bone necrosis. Early AVN has a high signal (bright) that develops into a low signal (dark) on T2 images. High signal intensity (bright) on T2 indicates soft tissue edema. An acute scaphoid fracture exhibits a low-signal line at the fracture site, with high signal intensity in the surrounding bone marrow on T2 images. AVN develops later and is evident as dark signal intensity on T1 and T2 images in the proximal pole of the scaphoid (Figure 8–7).

## Classification

- Various classifications exist describing location and/or stability of a scaphoid fracture. Most involve the waist (75%), then the proximal pole (20%) and least commonly the distal pole or tubercle (5%). Classifications are interesting, but they have not been proven to correlate with treatment. Most commonly, fractures are described as involving the distal pole or tubercle, waist, or proximal pole (Figure 8–8).
- Other classification systems include the following:
  - Russe: Horizontal oblique, transverse, vertical oblique (Figure 8–9)
  - Herbert: Stable acute, unstable acute, delayed union, nonunion (Figure 8–10)

## Acute Scaphoid Fractures

### Emergency Department Management

- If a scaphoid fracture is identified or suspected, the patient should be placed in a protective thumb spica splint. Disagreement exists whether a long arm thumb spica provides better stabilization than a short arm thumb spica.[16] However, if the patient has associated upper extremity injuries, it may be best to place the patient in a long arm thumb spica splint. There should be no weight bearing through the wrist. If a fracture is not seen on initial radiographs but is suspected, the patient should be placed in a splint. Then the patient can return in 2 weeks for repeat radiographs, at which time repeat films may

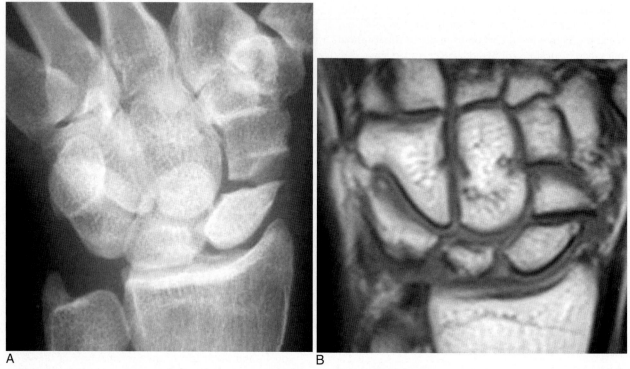

A                                                    B

Figure 8–6:

**A,** Radiograph of a scaphoid nonunion in a 38-year-old man. Avascular necrosis of the proximal pole was suspected because of the dense appearance on the radiograph. **B,** Magnetic resonance imaging T1 view of the scaphoid nonunion in panel A shows normal marrow signal of the proximal pole of the scaphoid. There is no avascular necrosis of the proximal pole.

better delineate a fracture or further diagnostic studies can be ordered. The disadvantage of serial radiographs is the delayed treatment of an unstable fracture or unnecessary immobilization, which can be costly to a patient who cannot return to work. Cost analysis has determined that frequent office visits for repeat radiographs and cast changes is of equal financial cost

as performing MRI to evaluate suspected scaphoid fractures.[17,18]

## Nonoperative Management of Acute Scaphoid Fractures

• Many factors must be considered when treating the patient. Comminution or collapse of the scaphoid may need to be addressed with bone grafting. Although most distal pole or tubercle fractures heal with immobilization, significantly displaced fractures may need internal fixation. Acute nondisplaced (≤1 mm displacement)

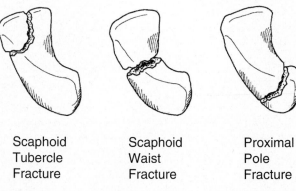

| Scaphoid Tubercle Fracture | Scaphoid Waist Fracture | Proximal Pole Fracture |

Figure 8–8:
Scaphoid fractures can be simply described as involving the distal pole or tubercle, waist, or proximal pole. (From Trumble TE: Fractures and dislocations of the carpus. In: *Principles of hand surgery and therapy,* Philadelphia, 2000, WB Saunders.)

Figure 8–7:
Avascular necrosis of the proximal pole of the scaphoid indicated by the low signal intensity *(dark)* of the proximal pole. AVN indicated by the *arrow.*

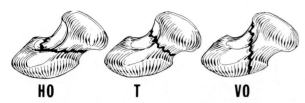

**Figure 8–9:**

Russe classification of scaphoid fractures in reference to the longitudinal axis of the scaphoid. *HO*, Horizontal oblique; *T*, transverse; *VO*, vertical oblique. (From Taleisnik J: *The Wrist.* New York, 1985, Churchill Livingstone, © Elizabeth Roselius.)

scaphoid fractures of the tubercle or the waist are considered stable and can be treated nonoperatively. Such fractures achieve union in the majority of cases.[19] Distal or tubercle fractures often heal with adequate cast immobilization. Pediatric scaphoid fractures occur less often and heal in less time than in adults.[20] A long or short arm thumb spica cast should be utilized until osseous union. Disagreement exists whether a long arm thumb spica provides better stabilization than a short arm thumb spica.[16] CT scans can help evaluate bony bridging across the fracture site. Figure 8–11 outlines a generalized treatment algorithm for acute scaphoid fractures.

## Operative Management of Acute Scaphoid Fractures

- Surgical treatment of scaphoid fractures to prevent nonunions is indicated in the following:
  1. Fracture displacement ≥1.0 mm
  2. Comminution
  3. Proximal pole fracture
  4. Delay in diagnosis and treatment
  5. Intrascaphoid angle greater than 35 degrees
  6. Height-to-length ratio greater than 0.65
  7. Fractures associated with perilunate injuries
- Ideally, fractures should be fixed within 2 weeks of injury when the fracture can still be manipulated easily. Because osseous healing may require 3 to 6 months and nondisplaced fractures can displace over time, many surgeons advocate internal fixation.[21] Many people can return to work or sports faster with operative fixation. Because of the poor healing of proximal pole fractures and the difficulty in treating a nonunion, surgical treatment of proximal pole fractures should be strongly considered.[16] Specially designed headless screws with differential pitch have been developed for fixation of the scaphoid. The differential pitch allows compression at the fracture site, and the screws can be placed beneath the subchondral bone. Cannulated screws allow central placement in the scaphoid, correction of alignment, and stability for fracture healing.[22] Acute fractures with minimal to no comminution can be internally fixed without bone grafting.[23] Occasionally, comminution resulting in a "humpback" deformity requires bone grafting along with internal fixation.

- Percutaneous fixation of fractures has been described for nondisplaced or minimally displaced scaphoid fractures (Figure 8–12).[24] Arthroscopy can be utilized during the percutaneous technique to assess fracture reduction. Percutaneous fixation of the scaphoid can be performed dorsally or volarly. The dorsal approach is preferred for proximal fractures because it provides better fixation of the proximal fragment.[25,26] The percutaneous technique avoids damage to important stabilizing ligaments and blood vessels.
- Open techniques for internal fixation can be performed through a volar or dorsal approach. A volar approach to the scaphoid is preferred for waist and distal fractures. This approach preserves any dorsal blood supply. A dorsal approach is preferred for proximal fractures. This approach allows easier central placement of the screw in the proximal fragment, which is biomechanically advantageous to the stability of the fracture.[27] Also, a small proximal fragment can be displaced when attempting retrograde screw fixation. A short arm thumb spica splint is applied after surgery. Two weeks after surgery, the sutures are removed, and the patient can be placed in a removable thumb spica splint or a short arm cast until healing, depending on the stability of fixation at surgery and reliability of the patient.

# Scaphoid Nonunions

- Proximal pole fractures have an increased chance of nonunion because of tenuous vascularity (Figure 8–13). A delay in diagnosis and treatment can contribute to the development of a nonunion.[28] Other factors that can contribute to nonunions include insufficient immobilization, fracture comminution, fracture displacement, and poor patient compliance. Patients may present with chronic wrist pain and decreased motion and do not recall a specific traumatic event, but they have a scaphoid nonunion. Delayed treatment of scaphoid nonunions decreases the success of treatment.[29]

## Treatment Factors in Treating Scaphoid Nonunions

- Factors to consider when treating scaphoid nonunions include collapse and deformity of the scaphoid, presence of AVN, loss of carpal alignment, and presence of wrist arthrosis. Radiographs should be closely examined for any evidence of arthrosis or carpal malalignment. MRI with intravenous contrast is effective in assessing the degree of bone necrosis. CT sagittal images best define the degree of scaphoid deformity, that is, "humpback" deformity.[14] Scaphoid nonunions without collapse or deformity can be treated successfully with percutaneous fixation without bone grafting.[30] Degree of collapse, need for vascularized bone grafting, and location of fracture determine whether a dorsal or volar open approach is preferred

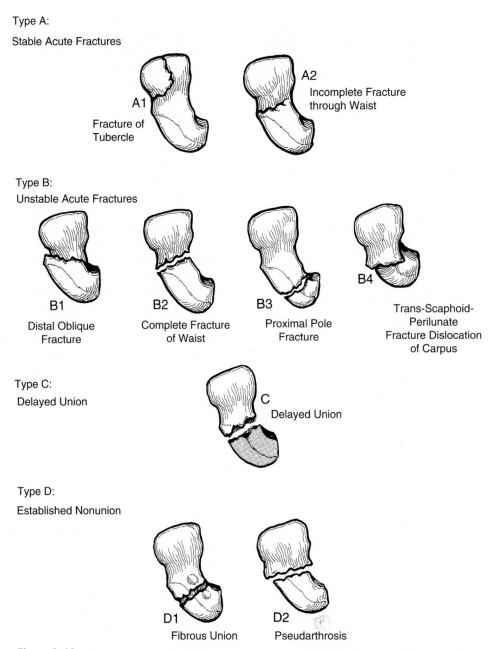

Type A:

Stable Acute Fractures

A1

Fracture of
Tubercle

A2

Incomplete Fracture
through Waist

Type B:
Unstable Acute Fractures

B1

Distal Oblique
Fracture

B2

Complete Fracture
of Waist

B3

Proximal Pole
Fracture

B4

Trans-Scaphoid-
Perilunate
Fracture Dislocation
of Carpus

Type C:
Delayed Union

C

Delayed Union

Type D:
Established Nonunion

D1

Fibrous Union

D2

Pseudarthrosis

Figure 8–10:

Herbert classification of scaphoid fractures. (From Amadio PC, Taleisnik J: Fractures of the carpal bones. In Green DP, editor: *Operative hand surgery*, ed 3. New York, 1999, Churchill Livingstone.)

(Figure 8–14). Nonunions without proximal pole necrosis can be treated successfully with internal fixation and cancellous autograft. Vascularized graft is indicated in nonunions with proximal pole necrosis. Scaphoid waist nonunions are better approached volarly, whereas proximal pole nonunions are better approached dorsally.[31] Scaphoid nonunions with a "humpback" deformity and a viable proximal pole should be approached volarly so that correction of the deformity can be performed with an intercalary wedge bone graft and internal fixation.[4] Bone graft can be harvested from the distal radius or the iliac crest (Figure 8–15).

## Operative Management of Scaphoid Nonunions

- A dorsal approach allows better visualization and central screw fixation of the proximal pole. Revascularization of the scaphoid using the second dorsal intrametacarpal artery implanted into a corticocancellous bone graft has been described.[32,33] However, the most reliable and widely used procedure is the vascularized bone graft of Zaidemberg harvested from the dorsoradial distal radius supplied by a vessel that lies between the first and second dorsal compartments, referred to as the *1,2 intercompartmental*

**Treatment Algorithm for Acute Scaphoid Fractures**

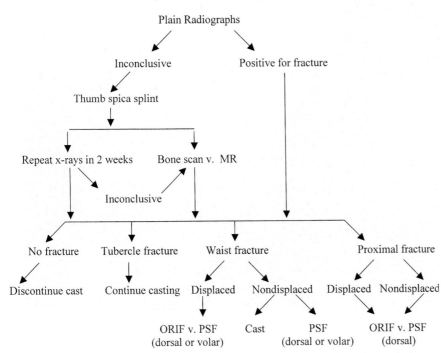

Figure 8–11:
Generalized treatment algorithm for treatment of scaphoid fractures. Many factors must be considered when treating the patient. Comminution or collapse of the scaphoid may need to be addressed with bone grafting. Although most distal pole or tubercle fractures heal with immobilization, significantly displaced fractures may need internal fixation. *ORIF,* Open reduction internal fixation; *PSF,* percutaneous screw fixation.

*supraretinacular artery* (ICSRA) (Figure 8–16).[34] The presence of bone graft and arterial blood flow make this graft reliable, especially if combined with excision of the radial styloid. The 2,3 ICSRA also supplies a portion of the distal radius that can be harvested.[35] Both the 1,2 ICSRA

and the 2,3 ICSRA provide blood flow to the distal radius in a retrograde fashion, allowing rotation to graft the scaphoid. A vascularized graft based on the first dorsal metacarpal artery supplying the index metacarpal has been described.[36]

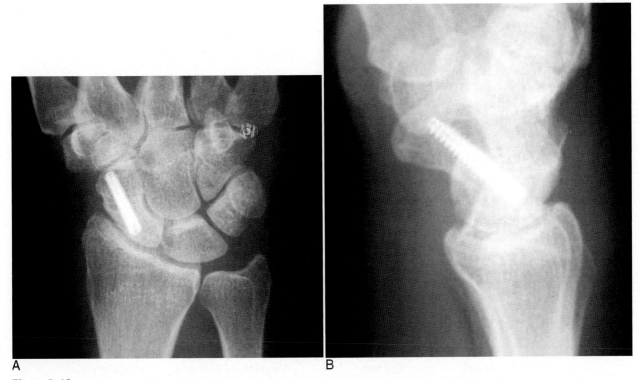

A        B

Figure 8–12:
Posteroanterior **(A)** and lateral **(B)** radiographs of a nondisplaced scaphoid fracture (as demonstrated in Figure 8–5) fixed with a dorsal percutaneous technique.

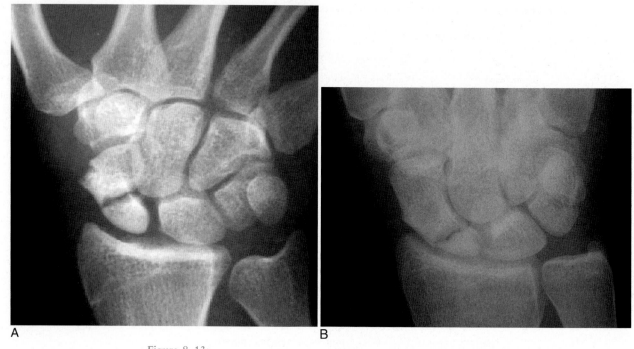

Figure 8–13:
**A,** Scaphoid waist nonunion. **B,** Scaphoid proximal pole nonunion.

• The challenging situation is the scaphoid nonunion with a "humpback" deformity and an avascular proximal pole. Possible solutions include the following[4]:
1. Dorsal approach with attempts at placing the graft as volar as possible. A radial styloidectomy may help in volar placement, and a longer pedicle is found with the index metacarpal graft.
2. Volar approach to correct the deformity and a dorsal approach for a vascularized graft.
3. Volar vascularized bone graft.
• Screw fixation provides more stability at the nonunion site than Kirschner (K) wires.[37] However, K-wires can be used to achieve preliminary fixation of the graft and help prevent rotation of the fracture fragments. Central screw placement in scaphoid nonunions has been shown to decrease time to union.[38] When a scaphoid nonunion is not treated, a predictable pattern of wrist arthritis called *scaphoid nonunion advanced collapse* (SNAC) develops.[39] Salvage procedures for treating advanced arthritis in the wrist caused by scaphoid nonunions include radial styloidectomy, proximal row carpectomy, and intercarpal fusions.

## Surgical Techniques
### Dorsal Percutaneous Scaphoid Fixation

• Percutaneous fixation of fractures has been described for nondisplaced and even minimally displaced scaphoid

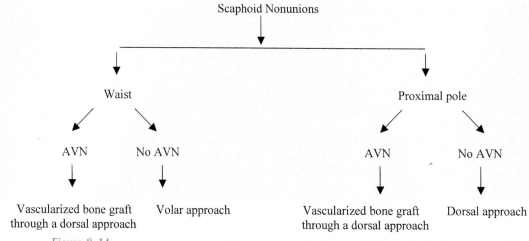

Figure 8–14:
**Generalized algorithm for treatment of scaphoid nonunions.** *AVN,* Avascular necrosis.

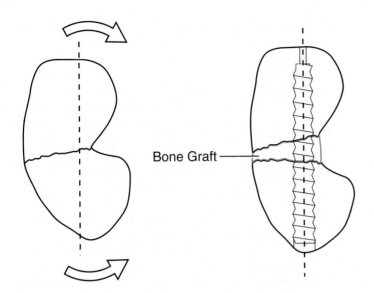

Figure 8–15:
Volar wedge bone graft to correct scaphoid collapse.

Bone Graft

Scaphoid Fracture with
a "Humpback" Deformity

Scaphoid Repaired with
a Volar Wedge Bone
Graft Correcting the
"Humpback" Deformity

fractures. This technique can be performed with the aid of arthroscopy.[24] Percutaneous fixation without bone grafting also has been reported to successfully treat scaphoid nonunions without collapse or deformity.[30] As with open techniques, the dorsal approach allows central placement of the screw in the proximal fragment. A mini-fluoroscope or regular fluoroscope must be available. The wrist is pronated and flexed so that the fluoroscope can visualize the longitudinal axis of the scaphoid, known as the *ring sign*.[25]

- A 0.045-inch guidewire is placed down the central axis of the scaphoid from dorsal to volar (Figure 8–17). After fluoroscopic verification of fracture reduction, carpal alignment, and central screw placement, the screw length is measured off the guidewire using another wire of equal length. Usually, the actual screw length is at least 2 to 4 mm shorter than the measurement.[25] The wire then can be advanced out of the skin at the base of the thumb and clamped with a hemostat to prevent displacement during drilling (Figure 8–18). The pin can be advanced distal to

Figure 8–16:
Dorsal and volar blood supply to the distal radius. Arteries: *1,* radial; *2,* ulnar; *3,* anterior interosseous; *4,* posterior interosseous; *5,* anterior branch of anterior interosseous; *6,* posterior of anterior interosseous; *7,* dorsal intercarpal arch; *8,* 1,2 intercompartmental supraretinacular artery; *9,* 2,3 intercompartmental supraretinacular artery; *10,* dorsal supraretinacular arch; *11,* ulnar branch of palmar radiocarpal arch; *12,* radial branch of palmar radiocarpal arch; *13,* palmar metaphyseal arch.

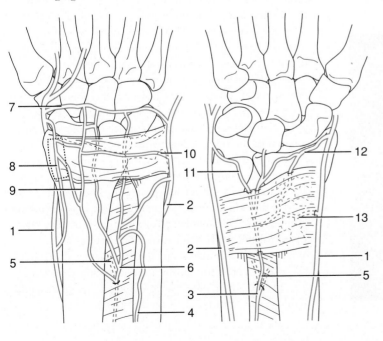

Dorsal          Volar

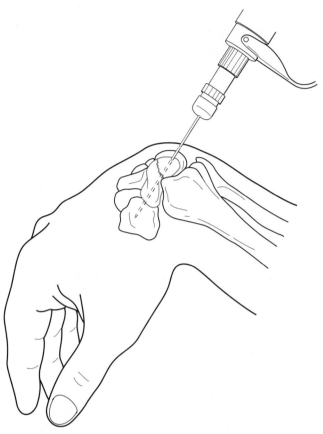

Figure 8–17:
Dorsal percutaneous technique. The guidewire is inserted with the wrist flexed.

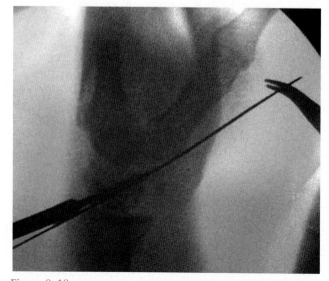

Figure 8–18:
Fluoroscopic image of a dorsal percutaneous technique. The K-wire has been advanced out of the skin at the base of the thumb and clamped with a hemostat to prevent displacement of the wire with drilling.

the radiocarpal joint so that the wrist can extended without bending the wire. Additional fluoroscopic views then can be performed to assess placement and reduction.

- If the fracture is minimally displaced, the guidewire can be advanced out the distal fracture fragment. Additional K-wires are placed into the distal and proximal fragments for manipulation. Once reduction is achieved, the initial guidewire is advanced retrograde into the proximal fragment. Smaller screws require smaller guidewires, which can bend during drilling. To avoid this technical pitfall, a 0.045-inch guidewire can be used to drill the guide hole. This wire then is replaced with the smaller guidewire, over which the screw is inserted.

- Wrist arthroscopy can be performed to assess fracture reduction and intercarpal ligament integrity. A small incision is made around the guidewire, and a hemostat is used to separate any soft tissue. A cannulated hand reamer is used. Screw placement should be monitored under fluoroscopy because fracture distraction can occur with excessive advancement of the screw. Thumb spica splint immobilization occurs for the first 2 weeks, then removable splinting can commence with gentle active wrist range of motion.

## Volar Percutaneous Scaphoid Fixation

- Minimally displaced scaphoid fractures with slight collapse can be treated successfully with a volar percutaneous technique. Extending the wrist often can correct minimal collapse. A small incision is made at the scaphotrapezial joint in line with the thumb metacarpal. Soft tissue is carefully dissected until the scaphoid tubercle can be safely drilled with the guidewire. With the use of fluoroscopy, the wrist is extended, and a 0.045-inch guidewire is placed down the central axis of the scaphoid from the volar distal pole aiming proximal and dorsal. There is no significant difference between the volar and dorsal approach in reference to central screw placement of waist fractures; however, the dorsal approach has proved better in centralizing the screw in the distal pole.[40] An additional wire can be placed to prevent any rotation of the fracture fragments. Once adequate position of the wire is achieved, a depth gauge or another wire of equal length is used to measure the screw length. The actual screw length will be at least 2 to 4 mm shorter than the measured length to allow countersinking of the screw.[25] A cannulated hand reamer is used to ream a path for the screw. Screw placement should be monitored under fluoroscopy for any fracture distraction that may occur. A thumb spica splint is applied for the first 2 weeks, then a removable splint can be applied and gentle active wrist range of motion initiated.

## Dorsal Approach to the Scaphoid

- A dorsal approach is preferred for proximal fractures. This approach allows easier central placement of the screw in the proximal fragment. Also, a small proximal fragment can be displaced when attempting retrograde screw fixation. A dorsal incision is made between the third and fourth dorsal compartments over the radiocarpal joint. The EPL tendon is released from its sheath and retracted radially. A longitudinal incision is made in the wrist capsule, exposing the scapholunate joint. To preserve blood flow to the scaphoid, the tissue attaching to the waist of the scaphoid should be protected. Acutely, the fracture should be easily reduced and provisionally held with K-wires. In nonunions, the fracture site should be cleaned of fibrous debris and necrotic bone. The insertion site for the screw is adjacent to the scapholunate ligament, best seen with the wrist in flexion.[4] After fluoroscopic verification of fracture reduction, carpal alignment, and central screw

placement, the screw length is measured off the guidewire. The wire then can be advanced into the trapezium to prevent displacement during drilling.

## Dorsal Approach to the Scaphoid with Vascularized Bone Graft

- A vascularized bone graft can be harvested from the dorsoradial distal radius supplied by a vessel that lies between the first and second dorsal compartments, that is, the 1,2 ICSRA (Figure 8–19).[34]
- The vessel can be better seen during the procedure if the arm is not exsanguinated. Instead, elevation of the arm with inflation of the tourniquet is preferred.[3]
  A curvilinear dorsal incision is made distally between the

Figure 8–19:
Dorsal vascularized bone graft to the scaphoid using the 1,2 intercompartmental supraretinacular artery (ICSRA). A radial styloidectomy was performed.

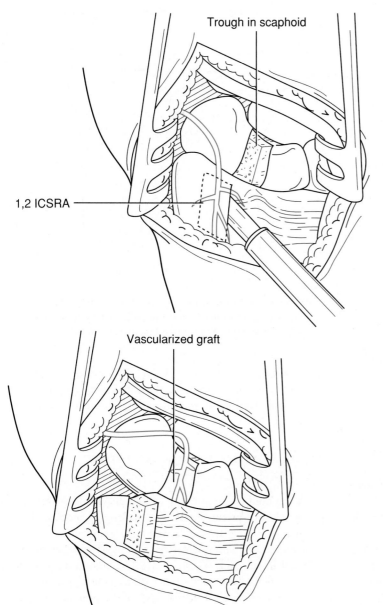

Trough in scaphoid

1,2 ICSRA

Vascularized graft

third and fourth dorsal compartments over the radiocarpal joint and extends proximally over the first and second dorsal wrist compartments. The EPL tendon is released from its sheath and retracted radially. A longitudinal incision is made in the wrist capsule, exposing the scaphoid.

- The nonunion site is debrided of fibrous debris and necrotic bone. An area is prepared to receive the graft. The 1,2 ICSRA should be visualized between the first and second compartments on the extensor retinaculum.[3] The first and second compartments should be minimally released to allow harvest of an adequate cuff of tissue. An elliptical or rectangular shaped graft is outlined with the surrounding vascular cuff of tissue. The graft is elevated using osteotomes. After the pedicle is carefully dissected, the graft is rotated and placed into the prepared nonunion site. Internal fixation is performed carefully so that the vascular pedicle is not damaged.

## Volar Approach to the Scaphoid

- A volar approach to the scaphoid is preferred for waist and distal fractures. This approach preserves the dorsal blood supply and can help reduce waist fractures as the wrist is extended during the procedure. An incision is made along the radial border of the thenar eminence and proximally along the radial aspect of the flexor carpi radialis (FCR) tendon (Figure 8–20). The sheath of the FCR is incised so that it can be retracted ulnarly. Retraction should protect the palmar cutaneous branch of the median nerve. A longitudinal incision is made in the floor of the FCR sheath enough to expose the distal pole of the scaphoid and the waist if necessary. As much of the RSC ligament is left intact when a cannulated system is used. The RSC ligament must be incised proximally when a noncannulated Herbert screw with the Huene device is used. The Huene device compresses the fracture and guides placement of the screw. Because the screw is placed retrograde, the scaphotrapeziotrapezoid joint is sharply dissected to allow distal guidewire and screw insertion.
- In the presence of comminution or "humpback" deformity, bone graft can be placed at the fracture site. Acutely, the fracture should easily reduce and can be provisionally reduced with K-wires. In nonunions, the fracture site should be debrided of any fibrous tissue or sclerotic bone using curettes or a burr. Use of an osteotome or dental pick may be needed to correct any deformity. Again, K-wires can help stabilize the bone. A small portion of the trapezium adjacent to the scaphoid can be removed to aid in central placement of the guidewire or screw. Ideal placement of the screw is along the longitudinal axis of the scaphoid.[22] Intraoperative fluoroscopy is crucial for assessing fracture reduction, carpal alignment, and central screw placement. With a

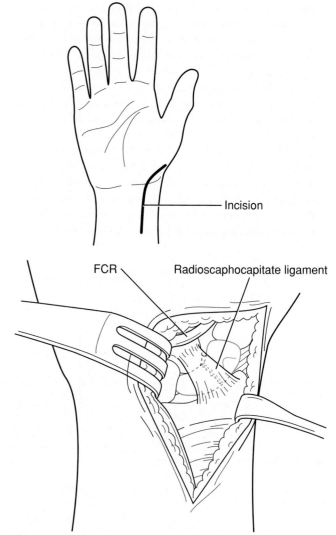

Figure 8–20:
**Volar exposure to the scaphoid. The flexor carpi radialis (FCR) is retracted ulnarly, and the radial artery is retracted radially. The radioscaphocapitate ligament is protected.**

cannulated system, the screw length is measured off the guidewire. Once measured, the wire can be advanced into the distal radius to prevent displacement during drilling.[4]

## Volar Approach to the Scaphoid with Vascularized Bone Graft

- A scaphoid nonunion with a "humpback" deformity and an avascular proximal pole is a challenging problem. In such cases, a volar vascularized bone graft can be performed.[41] The vascularized graft is obtained from the ulnar distal radius (Figure 8–21). The blood supply comes from the radial branch of the palmar radiocarpal arch, which runs along the distal edge of the pronator

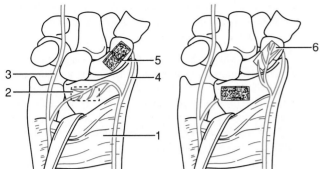

Figure 8–21:

**Volar vascularized bone graft for scaphoid nonunion.**
*1,* Pronator quadratus; *2,* palmar radiocarpal arch; *3,* ulnar artery; *4,* radial artery; *5,* scaphoid nonunion; *6,* vascularized graft.

quadratus (see Figure 8–16). An incision is made along the radial border of the thenar eminence and proximally along the radial aspect of the FCR (see Figure 8–20). The sheath of the FCR is incised so that it can be retracted ulnarly. Retraction should protect the palmar cutaneous branch of the median nerve. A longitudinal incision is made in the floor of the FCR sheath enough to expose the distal pole and waist of the scaphoid and the distal radius. The bone graft is elevated from the ulnar aspect of the distal radius and rotated into the nonunion site. The graft should be obtained as a wedge if needed to correct a "humpback" deformity.

## Conclusion

- Scaphoid fractures are common carpal fractures. When diagnosis and treatment occur early, patients can have an excellent outcome. However, when diagnosis is delayed or treatment is inadequate, delayed union, nonunion, or advanced arthritis can develop, making treatment more challenging. Surgeons should be familiar with both dorsal and volar approaches to the scaphoid. Location of the fracture, comminution, collapse, associated injuries, and presence of AVN all are factors that determine which approach is most appropriate. Advances in compressive screws, radiologic imaging, and surgical techniques have greatly improved the ability to diagnose and treat scaphoid fractures and nonunions.

## References

1. Osterman AL, Mikulics M: Scaphoid nonunion. *Hand Clin* 4:437-455, 1988.
   The natural history of scaphoid nonunion is one of progressive arthritis. Attempts at obtaining bony healing are recommended.

2. Knoll V, Trumble T: *Hand surgery update* 3. American Society for Surgery of the Hand, 2003.

3. Bishop AT: Vascularized bone grafts. In Green DG, Hotchkiss R, Pederson W, editors: *Green's operative hand surgery*. New York, 1999, Churchill Livingstone.

4. Trumble T, Salas P, Barthel T, Robert KQ III: Management of scaphoid nonunions. *JAAOS* 11:380-391, 2003.
   This article discusses the etiology, prevention, and imaging of scaphoid nonunions. Surgical approaches are described.

5. Bain GI, Bennett JD, MacDermid JC, et al: Measurement of the scaphoid humpback deformity using longitudinal computed tomography: intra- and interobserver variability using various measurement techniques. *J Hand Surg [Am]* 23:76-81, 1998.
   The height-to-length ratio is the most reproducible method for assessing the humpback deformity.

6. Trumble T: *Principles of hand surgery and therapy*. Philadelphia, 2000, WB Saunders.

7. Berger R: The gross and histologic anatomy of the scapholunate interosseous ligament. *J Hand Surg [Am]* 21:170-178, 1996.
   The scapholunate interosseous ligament is consistently divisible into three anatomic regions: dorsal, proximal, and palmar. The dorsal region is thick and strongest.

8. Weber ER, Chao EY: An experimental approach to the mechanism of scaphoid waist fractures. *J Hand Surg [Am]* 3:142-148, 1978.

9. Mayfield JK: Mechanism of carpal injuries. *Clin Orthop* 149:45-54, 1980.
   Carpal dislocations result from extension, ulnar deviation, and intercarpal supination. Scaphoid fractures are produced by extension and fracture against the dorsal rim of the radius. The four stages of carpal instability are discussed.

10. Horii E, Nakamura R, Watanabe K, Tsunoda K: Scaphoid fracture as a "puncher's fracture." *J Orthop Trauma* 8:107-110, 1994.
    We investigated 18 scaphoid fractures induced by punching. The wrist position while punching was neutral to slight palmar flexion. Despite the differences in mechanism, the location of the fracture was similar to fractures caused by wrist extension injuries.

11. Hove LM: Simultaneous scaphoid and distal radial fractures. *J Hand Surg [Br]* 19:384-388, 1994.
    Simultaneous fractures of the distal radius and scaphoid are uncommon. Only a small proportion of these injuries represent a more serious disruption with carpal instability.

12. Tiel-van Buul MM, Bos KE, Dijkstra PF, et al: Carpal instability, the missed diagnosis in patients with clinically suspected scaphoid fracture. *Injury* 24:257-262, 1993.
    Bone scans were not useful for detection or exclusion of instability.

13. Tiel-van Buul MM, Roolker W, Broekhuizen AH, Van Beek EJ: The diagnostic management of suspected scaphoid fracture. *Injury* 28:1-8, 1997.
In patients with negative initial radiographs, a normal bone scan excludes scaphoid fracture, and a positive bone scan confirms the presence of a fracture.

14. Sanders WE: Evaluation of the humpback scaphoid by computed tomography in the longitudinal axial plane of the scaphoid. *J Hand Surg [Am]* 13:182-187, 1988.
CT scans in the true longitudinal axis of the scaphoid demonstrate the anatomy, fracture, humpback deformity, and shape of the scaphoid following grafting.

15. Fowler C, Sullivan B, et al: A comparison of bone scintigraphy and MRI in the early diagnosis of the occult scaphoid waist fracture. *Skeletal Radiol* 27:683-687, 1998.
In 40 patients, there was agreement between the bone scintigraphy and MRI findings. In three cases, MRI was more sensitive and specific.

16. Burge P: Closed cast treatment of scaphoid fractures. *Hand Clin* 17:541-552, 2001.
Cast immobilization of the wrist remains the treatment of choice for stable fractures of the waist and distal pole of the scaphoid. Immobilization of the thumb confers no advantage and restricts function unnecessarily. Internal fixation can be considered routinely for proximal pole fractures, regardless of the degree of displacement.

17. Saxena P, McDonald R, Gull S, Hyder N: Diagnostic scanning for suspected scaphoid fractures: an economic evaluation based on cost-minimization models. *Injury* 34:503-511, 2003.
Compares protocols based on diagnostic scanning for suspected scaphoid fractures to protocols that do not rely on scanning techniques.

18. Dorsay TA, Major NM, Helms CA: Cost-effectiveness of immediate MR imaging versus traditional follow-up for revealing radiographically occult scaphoid fractures. *AJR Am J Roentgenol* 177:1257-1263, 2001.
Cost analysis suggests the two protocols are nearly equivalent from a financial standpoint. The loss of productivity from unnecessary immobilization may be substantial.

19. Kozin SH: Internal fixation of scaphoid fractures. *Hand Clin* 13:573-586, 1997.
Scaphoid fracture fixation is indicated in certain acute situations and for scaphoid nonunion.

20. Fabre O, De Boeck H, Haentjens P: Fractures and nonunions of the carpal scaphoid in children. *Acta Orthop Belg* 67:121-125, 2001.
Scaphoid fractures in children are more often located in the distal third, incomplete, and nondisplaced. Nonunion is rare and can be treated by cast immobilization in a child who has never been immobilized. Surgery is indicated if healing has not occurred after 3 months.

21. Rettig ME, Raskin KB: Retrograde compression screw fixation of acute proximal pole scaphoid fractures. *J Hand Surg [Am]* 24:1206-1210, 1999.
Seventeen consecutive patients with acute unstable proximal pole scaphoid fractures were successfully managed with open reduction internal fixation via a dorsal approach, radius bone grafting, and freehand retrograde Herbert compression screw fixation. All fractures healed within 13 weeks.

22. Trumble TE, Gilbert M, Murray LW, et al: Displaced scaphoid fractures treated with open reduction and internal fixation with a cannulated screw. *J Bone Joint Surg Am* 82:633-641, 2000.
Both the Herbert-Whipple cannulated and the AO/ASIF cannulated screws significantly improved the alignment of the scaphoid and decreased carpal collapse, which were correlated with an increase wrist range of motion.

23. Amadio PC, Taleisnik J: Fractures of the carpal bones. In Green D, Hotchkiss R, Pederson W, editors: *Green's operative hand surgery.* New York, 1999, Churchill Livingstone.

24. Slade JF 3rd, Gutow AP, Geissler WB: Percutaneous internal fixation of scaphoid fractures via an arthroscopically assisted dorsal approach. *J Bone Joint Surg Am* 84A(suppl 2):21-36, 2002.
Percutaneous screw fixation allows more predictable union and less morbidity than casting or open reduction internal fixation, with a 100% union rate in 27 fractures at an average of 12 weeks.

25. Slade JF 3rd, Grauer JN, Mahoney JD: Arthroscopic reduction and percutaneous fixation of scaphoid fractures with a novel dorsal technique. *Orthop Clin North Am* 32:247-261, 2001.
Technical description of the dorsal technique of arthroscopic reduction and percutaneous fixation of scaphoid fractures.

26. Haddad FS, Goddard NJ: Acute percutaneous scaphoid fixation using a cannulated screw. *Chir Main* 17:119-126, 1998.
Fifty patients were treated acutely with percutaneous fixation and immediate postoperative mobilization. Union was obtained in all cases after an average of 55 days.

27. McCallister WV, Knight J, Kaliappan R, Trumble TE: Central placement of the screw in simulated fractures of the scaphoid waist: a biomechanical study. *J Bone Joint Surg Am* 85A:72-77, 2003.
Central placement of the screw demonstrated 43% greater stiffness, 113% greater load at 2 mm of displacement, and 39% greater load at failure over noncentral placement.

28. Langhoff O, Andersen JL: Consequences of late immobilization of scaphoid fractures. *J Hand Surg [Br]* 13:77-89, 1998.
No delay in union or increase in nonunion resulted from a delay in immobilization less than 4 weeks, but when the delay exceeded 4 weeks, most fractures had healing complications.

29. Mack GR, Bosse MJ, Gelberman RH, Yu E: The natural history of scaphoid non-union. *J Bone Joint Surg Am* 66:504-509, 1984.
Because few of the 47 nonunions were undisplaced, stable, or free of arthritis after 10 years, a recommendation for reduction and grafting of all displaced ununited scaphoid fractures is made, regardless of symptoms, before degenerative changes occur.

30. Slade JF 3rd, Geissler WB, Gutow AP, Merrell GA: Percutaneous internal fixation of selected scaphoid nonunions with an arthroscopically assisted dorsal approach. *J Bone Joint Surg Am* 85A(suppl 4):20-32, 2003.
A series of 15 patients with fibrous union or nonunion of a scaphoid fracture were treated with a dorsal percutaneous screw. Union occurred in all patients at an average of 14 weeks.

31. Raskin KB, Parisi D, Baker J, Rettig ME: Dorsal open repair of proximal pole scaphoid fractures. *Hand Clin* 17:601-610, ix, 2001.
Proximal pole fractures of the scaphoid are well suited for screw fixation through a dorsal approach. Bone grafting can also be achieved through the same incision.

32. Fernandez DL, Eggli S: Non-union of the scaphoid. Revascularization of the proximal pole with implantation of a vascular bundle and bone-grafting. *J Bone Joint Surg Am* 77:883-893, 1995.
Union was achieved in 10 of 11 patients at an average of 10 weeks following inlay corticocancellous iliac crest bone graft with implantation of the second dorsal intermetacarpal artery for scaphoid nonunion with AVN.

33. Hori Y, Tamai S, Okuda H, et al: Blood vessel transplantation to bone. *J Hand Surg [Am]* 4:23-33, 1979.
A canine study showed active proliferation of new blood vessels and formation of new bone occurring when a vascular bundle was transplanted into intact bone, isolated bone segments, necrotized bone, and homografts of bone.

34. Zaidemberg C, Siebert JW, Angrigiani C: A new vascularized bone graft for scaphoid nonunion. *J Hand Surg [Am]* 16:474-478, 1991.
Description of a consistent vascularized bone graft source from the distal dorsal radius for treatment of long-standing scaphoid nonunions.

35. Sheetz KK, Bishop AT, Berger RA: The arterial blood supply of the distal radius and ulna and its potential use in vascularized pedicled bone grafts. *J Hand Surg [Am]* 20:902-914, 1995.
Investigation of the extraossesous and intraosseous blood supply of the distal radius and ulna, with emphasis on defining potential vascularized pedicled bone grafts to the carpal bones.

36. Mathoulin C, Brunelli F: Further experience with the index metacarpal vascularized bone graft. *J Hand Surg [Br]* 23:311-317, 1998.
A vascularized bone graft from the head of the second metacarpal led to healing of 14 of 15 scaphoid nonunions following failure of other techniques. However, the functional results were acceptable in only 10 cases because of previously unnoticed degenerative lesions.

37. Christodoulou LS, Kitsis CK, Chamberlain ST: Internal fixation of scaphoid non-union: a comparative study of three methods. *Injury* 32:625-630, 2001.
There was no significant difference between the AO and Herbert screws in obtaining union. K-wire fixation produced inferior results and required prolonged immobilization.

38. Trumble TE, Clarke T, Kreder HJ: Non-union of the scaphoid. Treatment with cannulated screws compared with treatment with Herbert screws. *J Bone Joint Surg Am* 78:1829-1837, 1996.
The 3.5-mm cannulated AO/ASIF screw led to quicker healing of scaphoid nonunions compared to the Herbert screw. However, 17 of the 18 cannulated screws had been placed centrally, compared with 7 of 16 Herbert screws (p < 0.01). For both screws, the time to union was significantly shorter when the screw was placed in the central third of the scaphoid.

39. Watson HK, Ballet FL: The SLAC wrist: scapholunate advanced collapse pattern of degenerative arthritis. *J Hand Surg [Am]* 9:358-365, 1984.
A classic article on the SLAC pattern of wrist arthritis.

40. Chan KW, McAdams TR: Central screw placement in percutaneous screw scaphoid fixation: a cadaveric comparison of proximal and distal techniques. *J Hand Surg [Am]* 29:74-79, 2004.
Central screw placement within the scaphoid appears to be an important factor for successful fixation, with the proximal/dorsal approach allowing more central placement in the distal pole during percutaneous screw fixation of waist fractures.

41. Kuhlmann JN, Mimoun M, Boabighi A, Baux S: Vascularized bone graft pedicled on the volar carpal artery for non-union of the scaphoid. *J Hand Surg [Br]* 12:203-210, 1987.
A bone graft taken from the medial part of the radial epiphysis can be pedicled on the radial branch of the volar carpal arch and transferred into the proximal row of the carpus.

# CHAPTER 9

# Carpal Bone Fractures Excluding the Scaphoid

Khemarin R. Seng* and Philip E. Blazar†

*MD, Resident, Department of Orthopaedic Surgery, Massachusetts General Hospital, Boston, MA
†MD, Assistant Professor, Department of Orthopaedics, Harvard Medical School; Brigham and Women's Hospital, Boston, MA

## Introduction

- Diagnosis is a challenge. Complex anatomy combined with difficult radiographic interpretation requires a high index of suspicion, thorough history including mechanism of injury, precise physical examination, and specific radiographic imaging.
- The incidence of carpal fractures reported in the literature varies. In general, the order of frequency is as follows: scaphoid, triquetrum, trapezium, hamate, lunate, pisiform, capitate, and trapezoid.[1–3]

## Mechanism of Injury

- Fall on an outstretched hand with a hyperextension moment and varying degrees of radial or ulnar deviation
- Direct impact or crush
- Indirect ligamentous avulsion

## Triquetrum

- Most common carpal fracture second to scaphoid.
- Pyramid shaped. Distal articulation with hamate bone. Proximal articulation with triangular fibrocartilage complex (TFCC). Palmar articulation with pisiform.
- Fracture patterns include dorsal rim chip fractures and triquetral body fractures (Table 9–1).[4]
  - Chip fractures may represent an avulsion of the dorsal radiotriquetral ligament. Other theories include compression against the ulnar styloid.

- Body fractures can be divided into medial tuberosity, sagittal, transverse proximal pole, transverse body, palmar radial, and comminuted.[5]
  - Medial tuberosity fractures are associated with direct blows to the ulnar border of the wrist.
  - Sagittal fractures are associated with axial dislocation and severe crush injury.
  - Proximal pole fractures are associated with perilunate/greater arc injury.
  - Transverse body fractures are associated with scaphoid injury.

## History/Examination

- Dorsal hand and wrist edema usually are present. Wrist flexion tends to be more painful than extension.[6]
- Tenderness just distal to ulnar styloid with hand in radial deviation is noted.

## Imaging

- Oblique and lateral radiographic views (Figure 9–1).
- Computed tomography (CT) or bone scan may be necessary to make the diagnosis.

## Treatment

- Cast immobilization for 4 to 6 weeks. Tender nonunited fragments may require excision. Body fractures with displacement of greater arc injuries typically are treated with open reduction internal fixation (ORIF).

## Table 9–1:  Carpal Fracture Patterns

| BONE (NORMAL RIGHT POSTERIOANTERIOR AND LATERAL) | FRACTURE TYPES | MOST COMMON TREATMENT | COMMON ASSOCIATED INJURIES | TREATMENT PEARLS |
|---|---|---|---|---|
| **Lunate** | 1. Palmar pole<br>2. Osteochondral (chip)<br>3. Dorsal pole<br>4. Sagittal oblique<br>5. Coronal split | 1. Closed treatment and casting for 4–6 weeks if minimally displaced or small fragments.<br>2. ORIF for intraarticular incongruity or associated instability. | 1. Lunotriquetral or radiolunate ligament tears.<br>2. Kienböck's disease. | 1. Beware Kienböck's disease if fracture present independent of significant trauma.<br>2. Consider MRI for evaluation of vascularity.<br>3. Injury may suggest carpal instability pattern. |
| **Triquetrum** | 1. Dorsal rim chip fractures<br>2. Body fractures<br> a. Medial tuberosity<br> b. Sagittal<br> c. Transverse proximal pole<br> d. Transverse body<br> e. Palmar radial<br> f. Comminuted | 1. Closed treatment with casting for 4–6 weeks if small chip (Type 1) or minimally displaced.<br>2. If large Type 1 or significantly displaced body type may require ORIF. | 1. Dorsal avulsion may represent avulsion from DRC and DIC Ligament.<br>2. Triquetrum and lunate may secondarily flex if DRC Ligament torn.<br>3. Ulnar impaction/TFCC injury may accompany body fracture | 1. Stabilization of DRC and DIC ligament may be required if large dorsal avulsion.<br>2. Arthroscopy may be necessary to evaluate ulnar/TFCC injury after healing of body fracture. |
| **Trapezium** | 1. Vertical transarticular<br>2. Horizontal<br>3. Dorsoradial tuberosity<br>4. Anteromedial ridge<br>5. Comminuted | 1. Thumb spica casting 4–6 weeks for minimally displaced fractures.<br>2. Spanning ex-fix if comminuted.<br>3. ORIF vs. K-wires for displaced intraarticular.<br>4. Ridge excision for symptomatic type 4.<br>5. Trapezium excision or CMC fusion for late arthrosis. | 1. First MC fractures common.<br>2. Ridge fractures may secondarily cause CTS.<br>3. Late first CMC arthritis may develop after intraarticular (IA) injury.<br>4. FCR/FPL rupture possible if medial irregularity | 1. Anatomic reduction for intraarticular fractures.<br>2. May consider primary fusion for combined trapezium and proximal first MC intraarticular fractures. |
| **Trapezoid** | 1. Dorsal rim<br>2. Body | 1. Cast immobilization for 4–6 weeks for minimally displaced fractures.<br>2. May require closed reduction of fracture or second MC and pinning for stabilization.<br>3. ORIF rarely necessary. | 1. Unusual as an isolated injury.<br>2. Usually associated with second MC dorsal dislocation. | 1. Often requires CT or MRI to diagnose.<br>2. Recurrence of posterior subluxation of second MC must be carefully followed.<br>3. Fusion of trapezoid-second MC may be necessary for late arthrosis and pain. |

Continued

## Table 9–1:

| BONE (NORMAL RIGHT POSTERIOANTERIOR AND LATERAL) | FRACTURE TYPES | MOST COMMON TREATMENT | COMMON ASSOCIATED INJURIES | TREATMENT PEARLS |
|---|---|---|---|---|
| **Capitate**<br> | 1. Transverse (axial) body<br>2. Transverse proximal pole<br>3. Coronal oblique<br>4. Parasagittal | 1. Cast immobilization for 4–6 weeks for minimally displaced fractures.<br>2. Closed reduction and K-wires for extraarticular reducible fractures.<br>3. ORIF for irreducible displaced, intraarticular, or proximal pole fractures. | 1. "Scaphocapitate syndrome"—including scaphoid fracture and lunotriquetral ligament injury.<br>2. Avascular necrosis (late) of proximal capitate. | 1. Proximal capitate is mostly intraarticular—leading to poor vascular supply.<br>2. Urgent ORIF of displaced or rotated proximal pole fractures.<br>3. Beware associated (but not apparent) scaphoid fracture, lunotriquetral ligament injury, or other peri-ilunate injury. |
| **Hamate**<br> | 1. Hook<br>  a. Avulsion (tip)<br>  b. Waist<br>  c. Base<br>2. Body<br>  a. Proximal pole<br>  b. Medial tuberosity<br>  c. Sagittal oblique<br>  d. Dorsal coronal fractures | 1. Cast immobilization for 4–6 weeks for minimally displaced fractures.<br>2. Hamate hook excision if continued pain after period of immobilization.<br>3. Rest, equipment adaptation, and immobilization for stress or repetitive injury fracture.<br>4. ORIF of displaced body or intraarticular fractures. | 1. Irritation and eventual rupture of ulnar finger flexors may occur with displaced hook fracture.<br>2. May be associated with fourth or fifth MC dislocation.<br>3. May occur with avulsion of FCU. | 1. Cast immobilization in slight radial deviation will minimize the deforming force of the ulnar finger flexors.<br>2. Hamate hook provides mechanical advantage of ulnar finger flexors.<br>3. Hook has watershed blood supply at waist with feeding vessels through tip and base.<br>4. Consider hamate hook lateral or carpal tunnel view radiograph for visualization. |
| **Pisiform**<br> | 1. Transverse (common)<br>2. Parasagittal<br>3. Comminuted<br>4. Pisotriquetral impaction | 1. Immobilization for 2–4 weeks for minimally displaced or comminuted fractures.<br>2. Consider ORIF or excision and tendon reconstruction if FCU disrupted.<br>3. Excision and tendon reconstruction arthrosis related to healed (or unhealed) fracture. | 1. FCU disruption (partial or complete).<br>2. Triquetral or hamate impaction injury related to mechanism. | 1. Best visualized on lateral radiograph.<br>2. Fibrous union may be well tolerated if FCU in continuity. |

From Putnam MD, Meyer NJ: Carpal fractures excluding the scaphoid. In Trumble TE, editor: *Hand surgery update 3*. Rosemont, Illinois, 2003, American Society for Surgery of the Hand, Table 1. *CMC*, carpometacarpal; *CT*, computed tomography; *CTS*, carpal tunnel syndrome; *DIC*, dorsal intercarpal ligament; *DRC*, dorsal radiocarpal ligament; *FCR*, flexor carpi radialis; *FCU*, flexor carpi ulnaris; *FPL*, flexor pollicis longus; *IA*, intraarticular; *MC*, metacarpal; *MRI*, magnetic resonance imaging; *ORIF*, open reduction internal fixation; *TFCC*, triangular fibrocartilage complex.

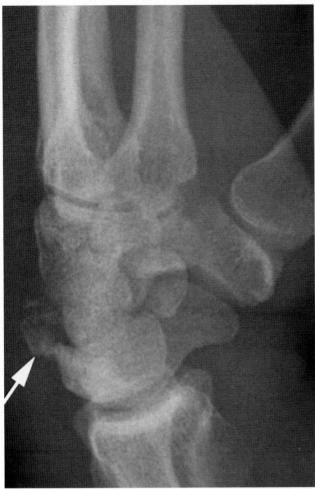

Figure 9–1:
Lateral radiograph of comminuted triquetral fracture. (From Fractures and dislocation of the carpus. In Trumble TT, editor: *Principles of hand surgery and therapy*. Philadelphia, 2000, WB Saunders.)

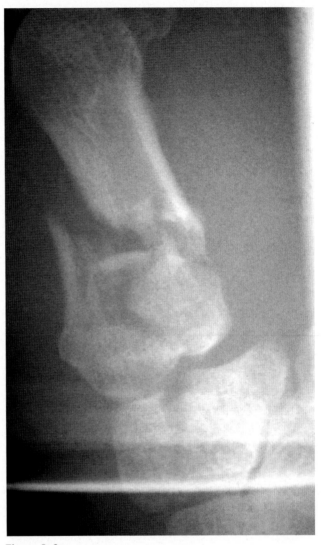

Figure 9–2:
VERTICAL split fracture of trapezium (with associated thumb metacarpal fracture). (From Fractures and dislocation of the carpus. In Trumble TT, editor: *Principles of hand surgery and therapy*. Philadelphia, 2000, WB Saunders.)

## Trapezium

- Isolated trapezium fractures are uncommon. Usually occur in association with first metacarpal or distal radius fracture (Figure 9–2).
- Five patterns: vertical transarticular, dorsoradial tuberosity, horizontal, anteromedial trapezial ridge, and comminuted[2] (see Table 9–1).
  - Dorsoradial fractures occur as a result from compression between the first metacarpal and radius. Compression of the first web space (i.e., handle bar injury) may create this force.
  - Trapezial ridge fractures may occur as a result of dorsopalmar crush and flattening of the transverse carpal ligament and resultant avulsion. Look for associated hook of hamate fracture in this mechanism.

## History/Examination

- Palpate distal to snuffbox. Thumb flexion and extension may produce pain. Resisted wrist flexion produces pain. Weak or painful pinch. Median nerve compressive symptoms occur occasionally.[1]

## Imaging

- Standard anteroposterior (AP)/lateral radiographs.
- Betts view: Semipronated hand with ulnar palm resting on plate and x-ray beam centered on scaphotrapeziotrapezoid (STT) joint.
- Carpal tunnel views needed to see trapezial ridge fracture.[7]
- CT scan may be useful.

## Treatment

- Thumb spica immobilization for 4 to 6 weeks. Excision of fragment if painful.
- Carpal tunnel release for median nerve symptoms.[7]

## Hamate

- Patterns include hook of hamate and body fractures (see Table 9–1).
- Hook of hamate fractures classically occur with stick handling sports. Direct and forceful impact with the end of a golf club, hockey stick, or repetitive trauma with the handle of a tennis racket.
- Ulnar nerve and artery pass ulnar to hamate; therefore, ulnar nerve symptoms may occur.[8]
- Vascularity of the hamate includes a palmar and dorsal pedicle with intraosseous communication. The watershed occurs at the waist, making waist fractures more susceptible to nonunion and osteonecrosis.
- Body fractures can be divided into proximal pole, medial tuberosity, sagittal oblique, and dorsal coronal. Proximal pole fracture can end up as loose intraarticular bodies. Medial tuberosity fractures can result from a direct blow to the ulnar wrist. Sagittal oblique fractures result from dorsopalmar crush. Coronal fractures result from axial compression, as in a fist fight (in association with fifth metacarpal base subluxation/dislocation).[9]

## History/Examination

- Considering all hamate fractures, the hook of hamate fracture is the most common and is discussed in detail here.
- Typical presentation for hook of hamate fractures is a weak or painful grasp and hypothenar tenderness. Pain with resisted little finger flexion. Pain with axial loading of fourth and fifth metacarpal. Ulnar and median nerve symptoms may or may not be present.

## Imaging

- Carpal tunnel radiographic views. Oblique views may be helpful.
- CT scan may be appropriate (Figure 9–3).
- Bone scan may be appropriate.

## Treatment

- For nondisplaced hook of hamate fractures, we prefer using an ulnar gutter cast extending beyond the metacarpophalangeal (MP) joints to the ring and little fingers for 3 weeks. At 3 weeks, the MP joints are mobilized, and the wrist is immobilized for an additional 2 to 3 weeks in a splint or cast. Displaced fractures or associated instability patterns may warrant operative reduction and stabilization procedures.

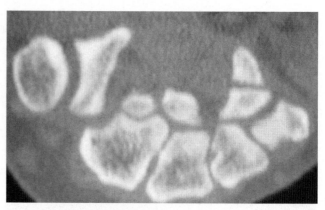

Figure 9–3:
Sagittal computed tomographic scan of hook of hamate fracture. (From Fractures and dislocation of the carpus. In Trumble TT, editor: *Principles of hand surgery and therapy*. Philadelphia, 2000, WB Saunders.)

- Excision may be indicated for a painful hook fragment but is not without pitfalls. Flexor power of the little finger may be decreased because the hook acts as a moment arm, and an excision may result in shortening of the moment arm and decreased power.[5]

## Lunate

- Controversy exists as to whether Kienböck's disease (osteonecrosis of the lunate) should be included in the total incidence of lunate fractures. Regardless, acute trauma can result in isolated lunate fractures.
- Five patterns: frontal palmar pole, proximal osteochondral fractures, frontal dorsal pole, sagittal oblique, and coronal split (see Table 9–1).
  - Dorsal chip fractures of the lunate may exist but often are confused with dorsal chip fractures of triquetrum by plain radiographs.
  - Transverse fractures are associated with Kienböck's disease.

## History/Examination

- Tenderness just distal/ulnar to Lister's tubercle

## Imaging

- AP/lateral views

## Treatment

- Cast immobilization for 4 to 6 weeks. Occasional body fractures with large fragments with displacement may be treated with ORIF.

## Pisiform

- Functions as a sesamoid bone in the flexor carpi ulnaris tendon. Pisiform fractures may disrupt the continuity of this tendon.
- Forms the medial border of Guyon canal.
- Four patterns: transverse, parasagittal, comminuted, and impaction[5] (see Table 9–1).
  - Transverse fractures are the most common, resulting from a direct blow or sudden flexor carpi ulnaris contraction against a fixed pisiform, as in a fall on the palm of the hand.

### History/Examination

- Tenderness to palpation at the hypothenar eminence. Painful little finger flexion.

### Imaging

- AP/lateral views (Figure 9–4).
- Oblique and carpal tunnel views commonly required.
- CT or bone scan may be necessary.

### Treatment

- Cast immobilization for 4 to 6 weeks. Pisotriquetral incongruity is a complication that can lead to degenerative arthritis and may warrant pisiform excision.

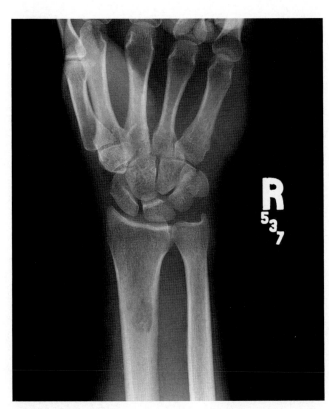

Figure 9–4:
**Anteroposterior radiograph of pisiform fracture.**

A painful pisiform fragment may warrant surgical excision. Excision usually does not compromise the strength of wrist flexion.[1]

## Capitate

- Isolated fractures are rare. Capitate fractures usually occur in the setting of carpal instability. They may occur with scaphoid fractures in what is known as *scaphocapitate fracture syndrome,* a variant of a perilunar dislocation. The proposed mechanism for this syndrome is fall on a dorsiflexed, radially deviated wrist. The scaphoid is fractured, with concomitant transverse capitate fracture.
- Four patterns: transverse proximal pole, transverse body or waist fractures, coronal oblique (verticofrontal), and parasagittal[5] (see Table 9–1).
  - Transverse is the most common and may end up 180 degrees rotated, with the fracture plane pointed proximally leading to nonunion and osteonecrosis.
  - Cyclists are prone to fractures of the dorsal body.

### History/Examination

- Tenderness proximal to base of third metacarpal
- Decreased grip strength

### Imaging

- AP/lateral views.
- Transverse CT may be useful.

## Trapezoid

- Lies in a very guarded position. Isolated fractures are extremely rare. Look for associated second metacarpal/carpometacarpal joint injury. Fracture patterns include dorsal rim and body fractures (see Table 9–1).

### Treatment

- Early diagnosis is key. The general goal is to maintain normal anatomic alignment and prevent arthrosis.
- Early immobilization with splint/cast is standard care, usually for 4 to 6 weeks. Reduction rarely is necessary.
- Be aware of fracture patterns that require operative reduction and fixation to prevent nonunion or osteonecrosis.[2-4,9]

## References

1. Amadio PC, Taleisnik J: Fractures of the carpal bones. In Green OP, Hotchkiss RN, Pederson WC: *Green's operative hand surgery.* New York, 1999, Churchill Livingstone.
   A general reference on carpal fractures excluding the scaphoid.

2. Bryan RS, Dobyns JH: Fractures of the carpal bones other than the lunate and navicular. *Clin Orthop* 149:107-111, 1980.
   A general review on several carpal fractures and their presentation and treatment.

3. Cooney WP: Isolated carpal fractures. In Linscheid RL, Dobyns JH, editors: *The wrist,* vol 1. St. Louis, 1998, Mosby.
   A general reference on carpal fractures, excluding the scaphoid, from a textbook devoted exclusively to the wrist. Excellent detail and illustrations for select fractures.

4. DeBeer JD, Hudson DA: Fractures of the triquetrum. *J Hand Surg* 12B:52-53, 1987.
   Fractures of the triquetrum are discussed, emphasizing their common misdiagnosis as lunate injuries and their frequently subtle radiographic nature.

5. Garcias-Elias M: Carpal bone fractures (excluding the scaphoid). In Watson HK, Weinzweig J, editors: *The wrist.* Philadelphia, 2001, Lippincott William & Wilkins.
   A general reference on carpal fractures excluding the scaphoid.

6. Hocker K, Menschik A: Chip fractures of the triquetrum: mechanism, classification and results. *J Hand Surg* 19B:584-588, 1994.
   A large series of a relatively common carpal bone fracture.
   A mechanism of injury is proposed, and management is discussed.

7. Palmer AK: Trapezial ridge fractures. *J Hand Surg* 6:561-564, 1981.
   A small series is discussed. The fracture is difficult to demonstrate on standard radiographs. Oblique radiographs and the required technique are presented.

8. Torisu T: Fracture of the hook of the hamate by a golfswing. *Clin Orthop* 83:91-94, 1972.
   A relatively unusual fracture, a particular mechanism, and treatment are discussed.

9. Bowen TL: Injuries of the hamate bone. *Hand* 5:235-237, 1973.
   Fractures of the hook, body, and dorsal hamate are discussed and treatment options outlined.

10. Rand JA, Linscheid RL, Dobyn JH: Capitate fractures. *Clin Orthop* 165:209-216, 1982.
    Discusses treatment with anatomic reduction by closed or open means. A high union rate is noted despite relative avascularity (as opposed to the scaphoid).

# Carpal Instability Including Dislocations

Alexander Y. Shin* and Steven L. Moran†

*MD, Associate Professor of Orthopedic Surgery, Mayo Clinic College of
Medicine; Consultant, Department of Orthopedic Surgery, Mayo Clinic, Rochester, MN
†MD, Assistant Professor of Plastic Surgery, Mayo Clinic College of Medicine;
Consultant, Department of Orthopedic Surgery and Division of Plastic Surgery,
Mayo Clinic, Rochester, MN

## Introduction

- Understanding of the wrist and its disorders often is a complex and lifelong pursuit secondary to its complex anatomic and biomechanical intricacies, its abundant pathology, and the widely varied approaches to treatment of its disorders.
- The seminal event in the history of carpal instability occurred in 1972, when Linscheid et al.[1] reported their experience with carpal instability and introduced the terms *dorsal intercalated segmental instability* (DISI) and *volar intercalated segmental instability* (VISI).
- Between 1972 and 1994, further refinement of the definitions of carpal instability and of a variety of types of instability were reported and defined, including midcarpal instability, nondissociative instability, and axial carpal instability.[2–29]
- Despite the explosion of interest in carpal instability and the research efforts into increasing our understanding of these instabilities, many significant questions remain unanswered.

## Anatomy

### Osseous Anatomy of the Wrist

- The wrist is the link between the forearm and the hand.

- Fifteen bones, excluding sesamoid and supranumerary bones
  - Distal radius and ulna
  - Two carpal rows
    - Proximal carpal row: scaphoid, lunate, triquetrum, pisiform
      - Pisiform considered by many a sesamoid bone but provides an important lever arm for the flexor carpi ulnaris tendon
    - Distal carpal row: trapezium, trapezoid, capitate, hamate
  - Base of the five metacarpals
- Joints
  - Radiocarpal joint: two parts
    - Distal articular surface of the radius and the triangular fibrocartilage complex
      - Distal articular surface of the radius has two separate articular facets: scaphoid and lunate facet
    - Proximal carpal row: convex articular facet of the proximal carpal row
  - Midcarpal joint
    - Combination of three types of articulations
      - Lateral: scaphoid trapezium trapezoid (STT) articular
      - Central: scapholunate (SL) and capitate

- Medial: hamate-triquetrum articulation, helicoid shaped
  - Carpometacarpal joint
    - Index, middle carpometacarpal joint highly interlocked with little motion
    - Ring and small carpometacarpal less restrained, greater degree of motion
    - Thumb carpometacarpal, saddle joint, most unconstrained, greatest degree of motion

## Ligamentous

- All ligaments of the wrist are intracapsular, except for three ligaments[30–34]: transverse carpal (flexor retinaculum), pisohamate, and pisometacarpal.
- All ligaments are contained within capsular sheaths of loose connective tissue and fat.[30–34]
  - Difficult to visualize individual ligaments when approaching the carpal joints surgically
  - Within the joint themselves, the ligaments can be viewed as distinct entities (i.e., during arthroscopy of the wrist or when visualizing the volar ligaments via a dorsal approach between the carpal bones)
- Two general categories of ligaments:
  - Intrinsic: have their origin and insertions within the carpus proper (Figure 10–1).
    - Large area of insertion onto cartilage rather than bone and much less elastic fibers compared to extrinsic ligaments
    - Tend to avulse from insertion or origin rather than rupture
      - Proximal carpal row intrinsic ligaments: scapholunate interosseous ligament (SLIL) and lunotriquetral interosseous ligament (LTIL)

- Distal carpal row ligaments: trapezium trapezoid, trapezoid capitate, and capitohamate
- Dorsal intercarpal ligament: scaphotriquetral ligament
- Palmar intercarpal ligaments: STT and triquetral-hamate-capitate
- Extrinsic: typically connect forearm bones to the carpal bones (see Figures 1-5 and 1-6).
  - Stiffer with lower ultimate yield compared to intrinsic ligaments
  - Tend to rupture midsubstance rather than avulse from origin or insertion
  - Volar extrinsic ligaments: mirror configuration of two V-shaped ligamentous bands and include radioscaphocapitate, long radiolunate, short radiolunate, ulnolunate, ulnolunocapitate, and ulnotriquetralcapitate
    - Dorsal extrinsic ligaments: dorsal radiotriquetral

# Biomechanics of the Wrist

## History

- Most authors agree that the SL ligament is the most important factor in the spatial coherence of the carpus.[35–38]

## Mechanics

- The distal carpal row has very little interosseous motion and can be thought of biomechanically as one unit in conjunction with the second and third metacarpals.[33,36]
- The proximal carpal row has no direct tendinous attachments and is described as an *intercalated segment*.

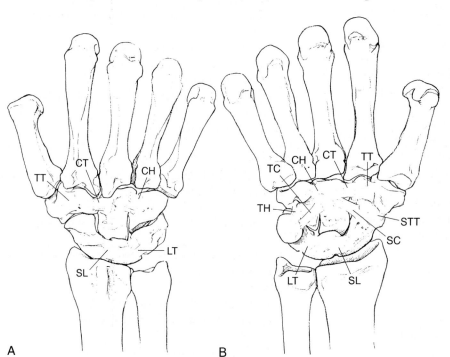

Figure 10–1:

**Intrinsic ligaments of the wrist are ligaments that both originate and insert among the carpal bones. A,** Dorsal view of the wrist demonstrates the scapholunate *(SL)*, lunotriquetral *(LT)*, trapezium trapezoid *(TT)*, capitotrapezoid *(CT)*, and capitohamate *(CH)* intrinsic ligaments. **B,** Volar view of the wrist illustrates the volar aspect of the same ligaments and the scaphoid trapezium trapezoid *(STT)*, scaphocapitate *(SC)*, triquetrocapitate *(TC)*, and triquetrohamate *(TH)* ligaments. (Copyright Mayo Clinic. Reproduced with permission of the Mayo Foundation.)

A                    B

- Its motion is dictated by the push and pull of the flexor and extensor tendons inserting onto the metacarpals.
- During wrist flexion the distal carpal row flexes and deviates ulnarly. With ulnar deviation the distal carpal row flexes, moves ulnarly, and pronates.
- With extension the distal carpal row extends and moves radially. With radial deviation the distal carpal row extends deviates radially and supinates.[39]
- During flexion the proximal carpal row flexes with the distal carpal row. The proximal row extends with the distal carpal row during wrist extension.
- Unlike the distal carpal row, the proximal carpal row does not function as a single unit during wrist motion. Motion between the scaphoid, lunate, and triquetrum differs significantly.[36–38,40–45]
- In radial and ulnar deviation the motion of the proximal carpal row is the inverse of the distal carpal row (Figure 10–2).
  - In radial deviation the distal carpal row moves radially, extends, and supinates, while the proximal carpal row flexes and translates ulnarly. This action results because the scaphoid must flex to make room for the distal carpal row.
  - In ulnar deviation the distal carpal moves ulnarly, flexes, and pronates while the proximal carpal row extends and translates radially.[43,46,47]

## Proximal Row Mechanics

- The scaphoid has a tendency to flex because of the push through the trapezium and capitate. The triquetrum tends to extend because of its helicoid articulation with the hamate.[1]
- Because of the lunate's ligamentous attachments to the scaphoid and triquetrum through the SLIL and the LTIL, the lunate tends to remain balanced and in a neutral position on lateral imaging.
  - During radial deviation, as the scaphoid is pushed into flexion by the distal carpal row, the scaphoid pulls the lunate and triquetrum into flexion through the linkage created through the SLIL and LTIL.
  - In contrast, during ulnar deviation the hamate is pushed into the articular surface of the triquetrum, creating an extension force on the triquetrum that pulls the rest of the proximal carpal row into extension.[48]
  - Several theories on the mechanics of the carpus have arisen. One theory is the role of the scaphoid in linking the proximal and distal rows. This theory maintains that the scaphoid provides a cross link across the rows preventing carpal collapse.[49] Another theory, called the *oval ring theory,* describes a link between the two rows at the radial and ulnar aspects of the wrist (Figure 10–3).

## Axial Force Distribution

- At the radiocarpal level, approximately 80% of the axial joint compressive force is directed through the scaphoid

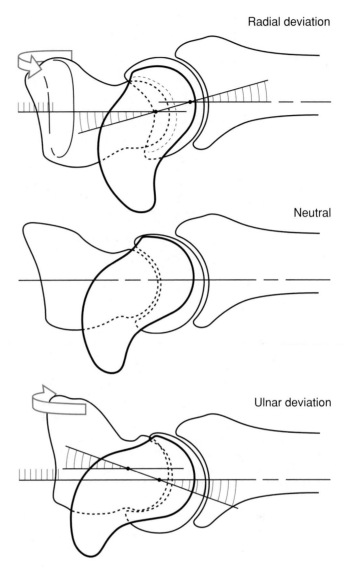

Radial deviation

Neutral

Ulnar deviation

Figure 10–2:
**With radial and ulnar deviation, the motion of the proximal carpal row is the inverse of the distal carpal row. In radial deviation, the scaphoid is pushed ulnarly and into flexion. The helicoidal surface of the triquetrohamate joint produces an extension force on the triquetrum that helps to pull the proximal row into extension.**

and lunate into the distal radius; the remaining 20% is directed through the ulnocarpal joint.[50]
- When forces are measured directly in the radiocarpal joint, 60% of axial force is directed through the scaphoid fossa and 40% is directed through the lunate fossa.[51]

# Biomechanical Properties of the Wrist Ligaments

## Radial Wrist and Scaphoid Stabilizers

- SLIL is as the primary stabilizer of the SL joint.

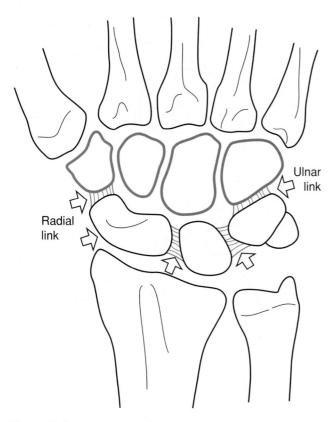

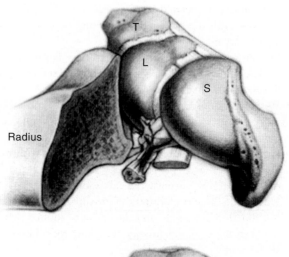

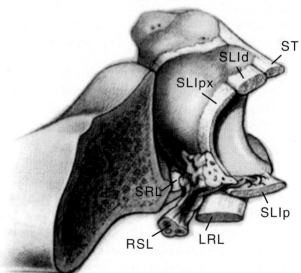

Figure 10–3:
In the oval theory proposed by Lichtman, the carpus is described as an oval connected at the most radial and ulnar aspect. This connection links the two rows together and provides stability of the carpus.

Figure 10–4:
The three components of the scapholunate interosseous ligament are the palmar (SLIp), dorsal (SLId), and proximal (SLIpx) portions. The palmar portion is thought to act as a rotational constraint and the dorsal portion as a translational constraint. *L,* lunate; *LRL,* long radiolunate ligament; *S,* scaphoid, *RSL,* radioscapholunate ligament; *SRL,* short radiolunate ligament; *ST,* scaphotriquetral ligament; *T,* triquetrium.

- SLIL has a failure force of 300 N.[52]
- SLIL is composed of three distinct portions[53] (Figure 10–4):
  ○ Proximal or membranous portion
  ○ Dorsal portion: the strongest portion that prevents translation
  ○ Palmar portion: acts as a rotational constraint
- Distal scaphoid stabilizers include the scaphotrapezial interosseous ligaments (STIL).[54]
- Radioscapholunate ligament (ligament of Testut) is a neurovascular structure and provides little mechanical stability.
- Palmer stabilizers: radioscaphocapitate ligament (RSC), long radiolunate ligament, and short radiolunate ligament (SRL) have properties similar to other ligaments throughout the body, with a failure force of 100 to 200 N.[52,55] These ligaments all are thought to be a secondary stabilizer of scaphoid.

- Dorsal stabilizers: dorsal radiotriquetral ligament, dorsal intercarpal ligament.

## Carpal Instability

### Definition of Carpal Instability

- *Instability* initially was considered analogous to malalignment, which often referred to a static alteration in the normal alignment of the wrist as seen on radiographs. However, the concept of the asymptomatic wrist that is grossly malaligned (as in congenitally hyperlax wrists) or symptomatic wrists that had normal alignment) confused the definition of "instability."

- Based on the collaboration of many wrist surgeons and investigators, the definition of instability of the wrist consists of not only abnormal transfers of load across the wrist (dyskinetics) but also abnormal motion (dyskinematic) within the wrist.

## Classification of Carpal Instability

- Carpal instability is extremely difficult to classify and many classification schemes exist, each with advantages and disadvantages.

- Classification scheme should be a tool to assist the surgeon in understanding the pathoanatomy and guiding treatment.

- One such guide is that developed by Larsen et al. that takes into account six key factors in guiding treatment.[56,57] (Box 10–1)

---

**Box 10–1  Classification of Carpal Instability**

- Chronicity
  - Acute: 1 week after injury
  - Subacute: 1–6 weeks after injury
  - Chronic: >6 weeks after injury
- Constancy
  - Predynamic: no malalignment, sporadic symptomatic dysfunction
  - Dynamic malalignment under stress
  - Static permanent alteration of alignment
- Etiology
  - Traumatic
  - Nontraumatic
- Location
  - Proximal carpal row
  - Distal carpal row
  - Multilevel
- Direction of lunate
  - Dorsal intercalated segmental instability (DISI)
  - Volar intercalated segmental instability (VISI)
  - Ulnar translocation
  - Dorsal translocation
- Pattern of injury
  - Carpal instability dissociative (CID)
    - Dissociation within row
    - Scapholunate, lunotriquetral
  - Carpal instability nondissociative (CIND)
    - Instability between carpal rows
    - Midcarpal instability, capitolunate instability, ulnar translocation
  - Carpal instability complex (CIC)
    - Feature of CID and CIND
    - Perilunar injuries, axial carpal dislocations
  - Carpal instability adaptive (CIA)
    - Extrinsic to wrist
    - Dorsal malunion of the distal radius that causes CIND

---

- Chronicity
  - Acute: within a week of injury
  - Subacute: 1 to 6 weeks after injury
  - Chronic: more than 6 weeks after injury
- Constancy: described by Watson et al.[58] to grade the severity of instability
  - Predynamic instabilities: no malalignment, only sporadic symptomatic dysfunction
  - Dynamic instabilities: malalignment demonstrated under stress
  - Static instabilities: permanent alteration in carpal alignment
- Etiology
  - Traumatic: especially if diagnosed acutely and treated, outcome better than if performed late
  - Nontraumatic: chronic conditions, such as rheumatoid arthritis, that result in carpal instabilities had significantly different treatment than traumatic conditions
- Location
  - Proximal carpal row
  - Distal carpal row
  - Multilevel dysfunction
- Direction: description of the abnormal stance of the carpus regardless of etiology
  - DISI: lunate is abnormally extended (Figure 10–5B)[1]
  - VISI: abnormal lunate flexion[1] (see Figure 10–36C)
  - Ulnar translocation: wrist or portions of the wrist are abnormally displaced ulnarward (Figure 10–6)
  - Dorsal translocation: carpus is unnaturally displaced dorsally (i.e., malunited and dorsally angulated distal radius fracture)
- Pattern: described by the Mayo Clinic Group[4,5,16,29,59,60]
  - Carpal instability dissociative (CID): instability within a row (i.e., proximal or distal row) (Figure 10–7).
    - Examples include SL, lunotriquetral (LT), and capitohamate dissociations.
  - Carpal instability nondissociative (CIND): instability between rows of the carpus or the distal radius (i.e., proximal carpal row and distal radius or proximal and distal carpal rows). There is no injury to the ligaments within the rows (Figure 10–8).
    - Examples include "midcarpal" instability, capitolunate instability pattern (CLIP), and ulnar translocation of the carpus.
  - Carpal instability complex (CIC): wrists that have features of both CID and CIND (Figure 10–9).
    - Examples include perilunate dislocations, ulnar translocation with a SL dissociation, and axial carpal instabilities.
  - Carpal instability adaptive (CIA): implies instability originates not in the wrist but somewhere proximal (distal radius) or distal (metacarpals) to it (Figure 10–10).

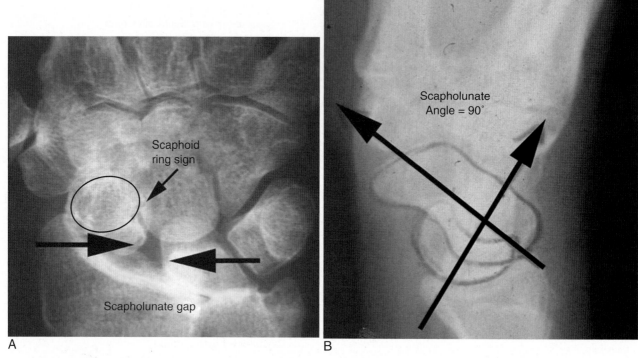

Figure 10–5:

**A,** In patients with a dorsal intercalated segment instability (DISI) pattern injury, the scaphoid can rotate so that the distal pole tilts toward the palm, producing a scaphoid ring sign on posteroanterior radiographs and a gapping between the scaphoid and lunate greater than 2 mm. **B,** The scapholunate angle increases in patients with DISI pattern injuries greater than 60 degrees. (From Fractures and dislocation of the carpus. In Trumble TE, editor: *Principles of hand surgery and therapy.* Philadelphia, 2000, WB Saunders.)

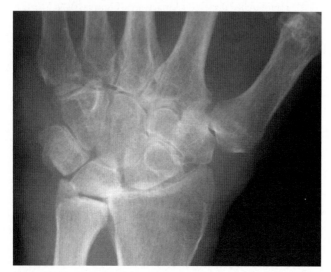

Figure 10–6:

Radiographic example of a patient with rheumatoid arthritis demonstrating ulnar translocation of the entire carpus.

- Wrist alignment is altered secondary to pathology extrinsic to the wrist.
- Examples include distal radius malunion with carpal instability.

## Pathomechanics

### Direct Mechanisms of Injury

- Force directly applied to wrist causing malalignment and derangement of the wrist.
- Common examples of a direct mechanism:
  - Wringer or crush injury to the wrist that results in an axial carpal dislocation[61]
  - Blast injuries
  - Forceful impact, for example, from a hammer, ball, or other object to the wrist

### Indirect Mechanisms of Injury

- Deforming force initially applied at a distance from the wrist resulting in injury to the wrist secondary to the tensile forces applied to the ligaments and compressive forces applied to the articular surfaces.
- Majority of wrist injuries occur secondary to indirect mechanisms and a multitude of combinations of positions of the wrist.
- To understand the injury patterns, Mayfield, Johnson, and Kilcoyne[62] performed cadaveric studies to ascertain the sequence of wrist ligament injuries and progression of ligament injury about the wrist (Figure 10–11). In their model, they studied wrists that sustained a hyperextension/volar radial wrist load injury and

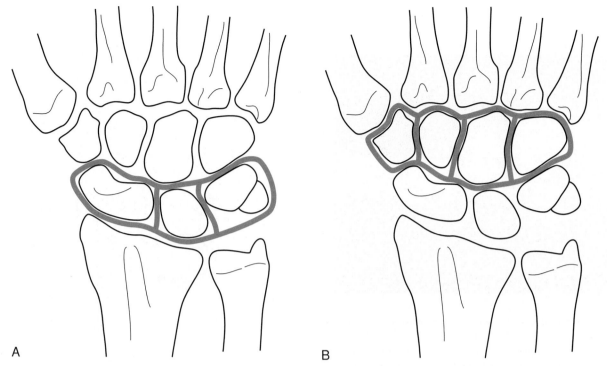

A

B

Figure 10–7:
Carpal instability dissociative results when there is dissociation between elements of a single carpal row. Within the proximal carpal row, there can be a scapholunate or lunotriquetral ligament dissociation. Additionally, fractures can result in a dissociation within a row, that is, scaphoid fracture (**A**). Within the distal carpal row, any of the interosseous ligaments can be dissociated, resulting in CID of the distal carpal row (**B**).

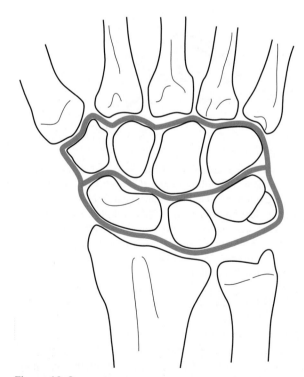

Figure 10–8:
Carpal instability nondissociative results when there is abnormal motion between rows of the carpus or the proximal carpal row and the distal radius. The elements within each row are normal, but the articulation between rows and/or the distal radius is abnormal.

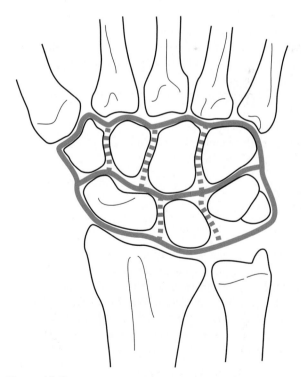

Figure 10–9:
When there is a combination of both dissociative *(dotted lines)* and nondissociative *(solid lines)* elements, the instability pattern is called *carpal instability complex*. This pattern is best illustrated by perilunate dislocations or axial carpal dislocations of the wrist.

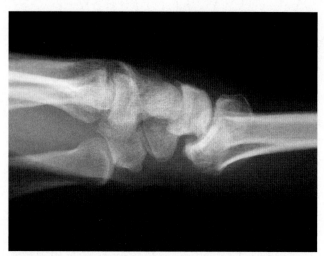

Figure 10–10:

Lateral radiograph of a malunited distal radius fracture with carpal instability adaptive. The patient reported pain with motion at the radiocarpal joint secondary to the carpal instability that developed at the distal radius and proximal carpal row.

described the classic four stages of progressive perilunar instability of the wrist.

- Stage I: SL dissociation or scaphoid fracture
- Stage II: capitolunate dislocation
- Stage III: LT dissociation or triquetral fracture
- Stage IV: lunate dislocation
- Reverse perilunar instability also has been described and suggested by several authors as a mechanism of isolated LT ligament injury.[26,63,64]
  - Three stages of reverse perilunar instability (Figure 10–12)[63]
    - Stage I: LT dissociation
    - Stage II: capitolunate dislocation
    - Stage III: SL dissociation

# Diagnosis

## History

- Patients presenting with wrist instability have a wide range of complaints, symptoms, and disabilities. It is essential to differentiate the mechanisms of injury, chronicity, location of pain, work-related issues, and quality of pain. As such, history is an important part of the diagnosis of wrist instability and should not be overlooked.

## Examination of the Wrist

- Examine the normal wrist first to serve as a baseline of normality for the patient.
  - Assess overall ligamentous laxity (thumb laxity, elbow laxity, shoulder laxity).

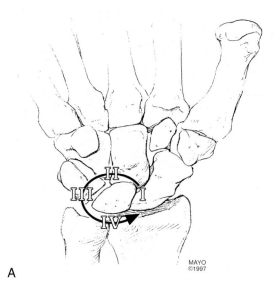

A

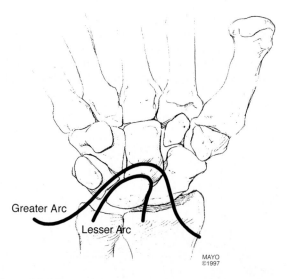

Greater Arc

Lesser Arc

Figure 10–11:

Progressive perilunar instability of the wrist was defined and presented by Mayfield, Johnson, and Kilcoyne.[62] **A,** Stages of progressive perilunar instability of the wrist. The description of each stage is elaborated in text. **B,** When injury occurs in this manner, a pure ligamentous injury can occur (lesser arc injury) or injury that results in a fracture-dislocation pattern (greater arc injury). (Copyright Mayo Clinic. Reproduced with permission of the Mayo Foundation.)

- Range of motion.
- Grip strengths.
- Palpation of the wrist.
  - Nearly every ligament and osseous structure can be palpated by a thorough examination. A methodical and systematic palpation of volar and dorsal structures is essential.
- Joint manipulation.
  - Test and assess range of motion and compare to the contralateral wrist.

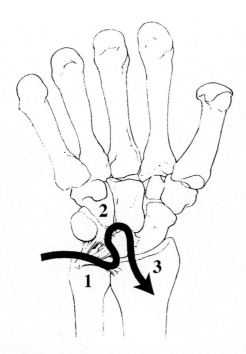

Figure 10–12:
Reverse perilunar instability of the wrist has been proposed as a mechanism of sustaining isolated lunotriquetral ligament injuries. Injury that begins on the ulnar aspect of the wrist follows a predictable pattern and has three stages. (Copyright Mayo Clinic. Reproduced with permission of the Mayo Foundation.)

- Note any crepitation, clicks, clunks, or abnormal motion and determine if pain can be elicited similar to the pain causing the complaint.
- Strength testing.
  - *Pearl:* Grip strength and pinch strength can elicit dynamic instabilities and serve as a baseline for diagnostic anesthetic injections.
  - Diagnostic injections into the radiocarpal, midcarpal or distal radioulnar spaces of the wrist that are associated with relief of pain and improvement of grip strength correlate highly with potential carpal pathology.
- Specific examination findings.
  - A multitude of special tests elicit specific ligament injuries. These tests are detailed in their respective ligament injury section.

## Plain Radiographs and Fluoroscopy

- Posteroanterior (PA), lateral, and oblique films are mandatory for all suspected wrist injuries. Initial evaluation includes assessment of all carpal bones for fractures. The following measurements can be used to assess ligamentous stability:
  - Gilula's lines
    - Gilula described three parallel arcs observed on PA radiographs: one arc corresponds to the proximal articular surface of the proximal row, the second arc corresponds to the distal articular surface of the

proximal row, and the third arc represents the proximal articular surface of the distal carpal row (Figure 10–13). Disruption of one of these arcs suggests a carpal fracture or ligamentous injury.[65]
- Carpal height ratio
  - This ratio is calculated by dividing the carpal height by the length of the third metacarpal (Figure 10–14). The normal ratio is $0.54 \pm 0.03$.
    - In disease processes such as SL dissociation, scapholunate advanced collapse (SLAC) wrist, and Kienböck's disease, collapse of the midcarpal joint decreases this ratio.
- Intercarpal angles
  - Significant deviation from normal values can indicate a disruption of the SLIL or LTIL (Figures 10–15 and 10–16).
  - SL angle
    - Mean 45 degrees.
    - Less than 30 degrees or greater than 60 degrees is considered abnormal (see Figure 10–15).
  - Radiolunate angle
    - Mean zero degrees.
    - Greater than 15 degrees dorsal or palmar is abnormal.
    - Greater than 15 degrees palmar suggests VISI deformity.

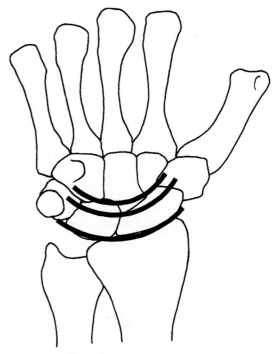

Figure 10–13:
Gilula provided a good screening technique for carpal instability by noting that the radial carpal and midcarpal joints form three sets of concentric lines. (From Fractures and dislocation of the carpus. In Trumble TE, editor: *Principles of hand surgery and therapy.* Philadelphia, 2000, WB Saunders.)

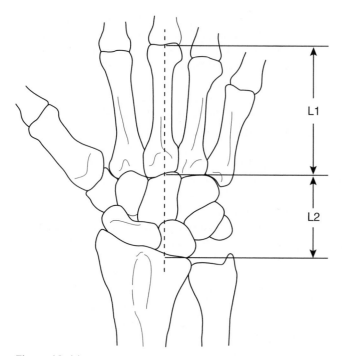

**Figure 10–14:**
**The carpal height ratio is determined by dividing the height of the carpus *(L2)* by the height of the long finger metacarpal *(L1)*. Normal is 0.54 ± 0.03.**

- Greater than 15 degrees dorsal suggests DISI deformity (see Figure 10–15).
  ○ Capitolunate angle
    - Mean zero.
    - Range 30 degrees dorsal to 30 degrees palmar.
  • Intercarpal distance
    ○ Increased distance or diastasis between the scaphoid and lunate or lunate and triquetrum may indicate SLIL or LTIL injury.
      - Greater than 2 mm between scaphoid and lunate is considered abnormal (see Figure 10–5A).

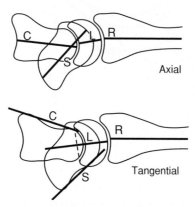

**Figure 10–15:**
**Intercarpal angles can be determined by drawing lines tangential to the contour of the carpal bones or axially through the bones. *C*, capitate; *L*, lunate; *R*, radius; *S*, scaphoid.**

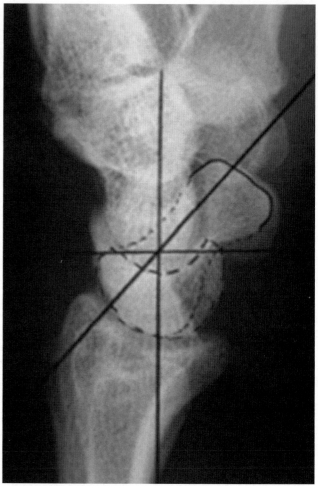

**Figure 10–16:**
**Radiograph showing placement of scaphoid and lunate lines that can be used to determine carpal angles.**

- *Pearl:* Early ligamentous injuries may produce no abnormalities on plain radiographs. If the mechanism and physical examination suggest ligamentous injury, proceed with further studies.

## Computed Tomography

- Computed tomography (CT) provides information about the bony anatomy and may aid in identifying small avulsion fractures.

## Bone Scintigraphy

- Technetium Tc 99m bone scans identify varying degrees of bone remodeling and accesses blood flow within the carpus.
- These studies are most helpful in identifying occult fractures, although they also identify areas of increased blood flow, as in cases of arthritis.
- Studies are sensitive but not specific.

## Arthrography

- Historically the gold standard for diagnosis of ligamentous injuries.

- Contrast medium can be injected into the midcarpal, radiocarpal, and radioulnar joints. Dye flows between any of the compartments indicates a tear.
  - Unless real-time fluoroscopy is used to visualize the origin of the dye leak, arthrography lacks specificity.
    - Attritional changes seen with advancing age may lead to spurious findings.[66-69]
    - Arthrography mostly has been replaced by diagnostic arthroscopy.

### Magnetic Resonance Imaging

- Magnetic resonance imaging (MRI) can provide diagnostic information about the intrinsic and extrinsic ligaments and carpal bones.
- Sensitivity for identifying interosseous ligament injuries has not been clearly established.

## Carpal Instability Dissociative

- When carpal instability is caused by dissociation between bones of the same carpal row, the instability is termed *dissociative* or *carpal instability dissociative* (CID). Distal carpal row CID is very rare and has been reported as case reports.[70] Proximal CIDs are much more common and are the focus of this section.

### Scapholunate Ligament Injuries

#### Introduction

- SL instability is the most common form of carpal instability.
- Disruption in the SL relationship can lead to
  - Unopposed extension forces on the lunate imparted by the triquetrum
    - Leading to a DISI deformity.
  - Abnormal scaphoid motion and dorsal subluxation of the scaphoid from the radial fossa during wrist flexion
    - Leading to eventual wrist arthritis.
  - Migration of the capitate proximally between the scaphoid and capitate
    - Leading to stage III SLAC arthritis.

#### Diagnosis

##### Physical Examination

- Patients may have pain dorsally over the SLIL.
  - The SLIL can be palpated by flexing the wrist and pressing 1cm distal to Lister tubercle.
- Positive scaphoid shift test or Watson maneuver (Figures 10-17 and 10-18).
  - The wrist is moved from ulnar to radial deviation, with the examiner's thumb pressing against the scaphoid tubercle. Patients with partial tears have increased pain dorsally over SL articulation. In complete tears an audible clunk may be heard as the scaphoid is actively subluxed with dorsal pressure and spontaneously

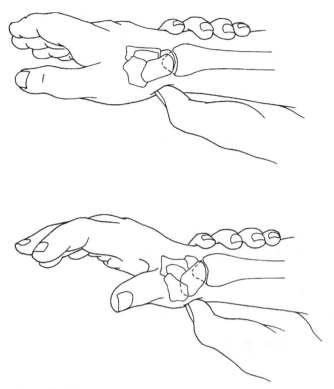

Figure 10-17:
Watson maneuver is performed by applying pressure over the scaphoid tubercle and bringing the wrist from ulnar deviation **(top)** into radial deviation **(bottom)**. (From Fractures and dislocation of the carpus. In Trumble TE, editor: *Principles of hand surgery and therapy.* Philadelphia, 2000, WB Saunders.)

reduces into the radial fossa when the thumb is removed.[27,58,71]

- The scaphoid shift test may give a false-positive result in up to one third of individuals because of ligamentous laxity without injury. Therefore, remember to always check both sides.[72]

#### Imaging Studies

##### Radiographs

- PA and lateral views may show
  - Increased SL angle
    - 45 degrees is normal; greater than 60 degrees is considered abnormal (see Figure 10-5B).
  - Diastasis between the scaphoid and lunate
    - Greater than 2 mm is abnormal (see Figure 10-5A).
  - "Ring sign"
    - As the scaphoid flexes, its distal pole appears as a ring in PA radiographs (see Figure 10-5A).
  - Increased radiolunate angle
    - Greater than 15 degrees dorsal indicates a DISI deformity.
  - Disruption of Gilula lines
    - With advanced carpal instability the capitate migrates into the proximal carpal row, causing disruption of Gilula lines and a change in the carpal height ratio.

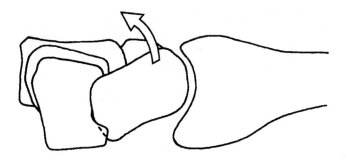

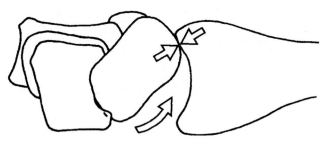

**Figure 10–18:**

In the normal wrist, the intact scapholunate interosseous ligament (SLIL) maintains the scaphoid in alignment with the lunate despite the dorsal pressure. When the SLIL ligament has been disrupted, the scaphoid is no longer stabilized to the lunate and the proximal poles displace dorsally to abut the dorsal rim of the radius, producing an audible clunk. (From Fractures and dislocation of the carpus. In Trumble TE, editor: *Principles of hand surgery and therapy.* Philadelphia, 2000, WB Saunders.)

- "Clenched fist" views
  - May show early SLIL changes (dynamic instability) with widening of the SL interval or increased SL angle as the capitate is driven down into the SL interspace.
- Remember that partial and even complete division of the SLIL does not always produce an abnormality on plain films because of the substantial numbers of secondary stabilizers of the scaphoid in addition to the SLIL.[73]

## Arthrography

- May show communication between the midcarpal and radiocarpal joint, with a dye leak seen at the SLIL indicating a tear.

## Computed Tomography

- Not very accurate for assessing ligamentous injuries.

## Magnetic Resonance Imaging

- Can often identify SLIL injuries but is not 100% sensitive.

## Arthroscopy

- Now the gold standard for diagnosis of "dynamic" instability patterns. Allows for direct inspection of SLIL

and evaluation of supporting extrinsic ligaments (Figure 10–19).
- Arthroscopic instability is graded by the Geissler classification[74]:
  - Grade I: attenuation or hemorrhage of the interosseous ligament as seen from the radiocarpal space. No incongruency of carpal alignment in the midcarpal space.
  - Grade II: attenuation or hemorrhage of interosseous ligament as seen from the radiocarpal space. Incongruency or step-off of carpal space. There may be slight gap (less than width of probe) between carpal bones.
  - Grade III: incongruency or step-off of carpal alignment as seen from both the radiocarpal and midcarpal spaces. Probe can be passed through gap between carpal bones.
  - Grade IV: incongruency or step-off of carpal alignment as seen from both radiocarpal and midcarpal spaces. There is gross instability with manipulation. A 2.7-mm arthroscope can be passed through gap between carpal bones.
- Midcarpal arthroscopy is the key to assessing the stability of the SL joint. From the midcarpal perspective, the normal SL joint is smooth without a step-off or diastasis.

## Stages of Scapholunate Instability

- It is important to distinguish between dynamic and static SLIL instability. SLIL is a spectrum of disease beginning with partial volar tears to total disruption of the SLIL with adaptive changes throughout the carpus.[72]
- Occult or predynamic instability[58,75]

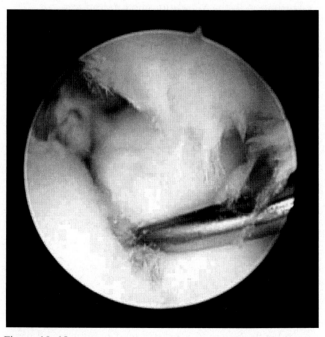

**Figure 10–19:**

Midcarpal arthroscopy shows evidence of a Geissler type III pattern, indicating scapholunate instability. The probe can be inserted between the scaphoid and lunate and rotated freely.

- Partial tear or attenuation of SLIL
- Radiographs normal
- Possible abnormalities with fluoroscopy
- Dynamic
  - Partial or complete tear of SLIL
  - Stress radiographs abnormal
  - Arthroscopy abnormal (Geissler II or III)
- Static
  - Complete SLIL tear with attenuation or attrition of supporting wrist ligaments
  - Radiographs positive for scaphoid changes.
    - SL gap greater than 3 mm, SL angle greater than 60 degrees
    - Arthroscopic findings reveal a Geissler type IV pattern[76,77]
  - With time the lunate extends because of unopposed extension force of the intact LTIL. The lunate becomes fixed in dorsiflexion, visualized as a DISI deformity on lateral x-ray films, (radiolunate angle >15 degrees).
- SLAC
  - With longstanding abnormal positioning of the carpal bones, arthritic changes occur. Arthritic changes are first seen at the scaphoid and move to the midcarpal joint in a standard progression (Figure 10–20).
    - Stage 1: arthritis noted at radial styloid
    - Stage 2: arthritis noted at radiocarpal joint
    - Stage 3: arthritis noted at capitolunate interface

## Treatment

### Acute Injuries

- Cast immobilization
  - Few long term studies to justify effectiveness in cases of confirmed SLIL rupture.
  - Open repair.
    - *Technique:* The carpus is approached through a dorsal midline incision. Retinacular flaps are elevated from the third dorsal compartment to the second compartment radially and from the third dorsal compartment to the fifth ulnarly. A ligament sparing

capsulotomy is made as described by Berger, Bishop, and Bettinger[78] (see Figure 10–39B). This capsulotomy is lined with the fibers of the dorsal intercarpal and dorsal radiotriquetral ligaments. The carpus then is evaluated. The SLIL usually is torn off the scaphoid. The SL relationship is reestablished by placing joysticks into the lunate and scaphoid. The SLIL then is repaired with the aid of drill holes through the scaphoid or with bone anchors. The sutures are passed but not tied until internal fixation has stabilized and reduced the scaphoid to the lunate. The SL interface is reduced and the bones are held with two to three Kirschner (K)-wires or a lag screw. The midcarpal joint also can be pinned for greater stabilization. K-wires are left for 8 to 10 weeks, and patients are protected from full loading for an additional 4 to 6 weeks.[79]

### Chronic Injuries (Dynamic or Static)

- Open repair
  - Open repair of the SLIL can be considered in cases of chronic injury if
    - There is satisfactory ligament remaining for repair.
    - The scaphoid and lunate remain easily reducible.
    - There is no degenerative changes within the carpus.[79]
- Soft tissue procedures (Best for dynamic instability)
  - Dorsal capsulodesis: Procedures that utilize a portion of the dorsal wrist capsule to tether the scaphoid and prevent it from subluxing from the radial fossa.[77,80,81]
    - Blatt: A 1-cm broad flap of wrist capsule is elevated off the ulnar side of the carpal incision. The flap is released from its distal insertion. After derotation of the scaphoid and reduction of the lunate, the capsular flap is attached to the dorsal distal surface of the scaphoid through a drill hole and pullout stitch or with the use of a suture anchor.[81] A transverse trough is created in the scaphoid to assist in capsular ingrowth. The dorsal capsular tissue is imbricated into the capsular flap at the time of closure. The wrist is immobilized for 8 weeks in a long arm thumb spica

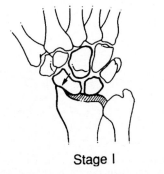 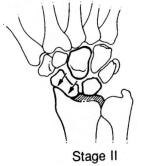 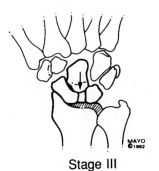

Stage I          Stage II          Stage III

Figure 10–20:
Stages of scapholunate advanced collapse. With advancing carpal collapse, the capitate may migrate proximally, resulting in midcarpal arthritis and disruption of the Gilula lines. (Copyright Mayo Clinic. Reproduced with permission of the Mayo Foundation.)

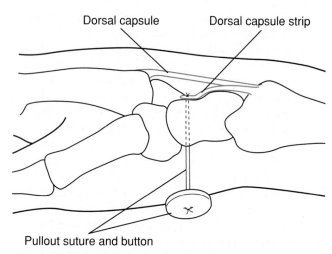

**Figure 10–21:**
Blatt capsulodesis uses a proximally based flap of wrist capsule that is inserted into the distal pole of the scaphoid. This procedure restrains abnormal scaphoid flexion.

cast. Full loading of the wrist is delayed for up to 6 months (Figure 10–21).

○ Mayo: The Mayo capsulodesis begins with a ligament-sparing capsulotomy. The proximal strip of the dorsal intercarpal ligament is rotated and attached to the lunate. This capsulodesis avoids crossing the radiocarpal joint and reestablishes the SL relationship. SL repair is performed using previously described techniques[82] (Figure 10–22).

○ Szabo: This technique advances the scaphotrapezial origin of the dorsal intercarpal ligament onto the radial aspect of the scaphoid in order to control

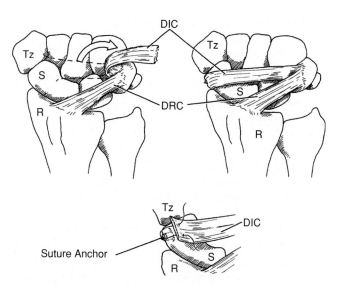

**Figure 10–23:**
Advancing the dorsal intercarpal ligament *(DIC)* along the radial surface of the scaphoid *(S)* controls palmar rotation of the scaphoid and scapholunate gapping. *DRC,* dorsal radiocarpal ligament; *R,* radius; *Tz,* trapezium. (From Fractures and dislocation of the carpus. In Trumble TE, editor: *Principles of hand surgery and therapy.* Philadelphia, 2000, WB Saunders.)

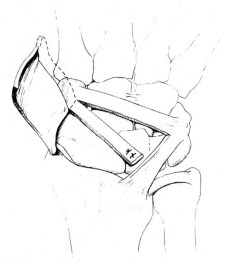

**Figure 10–22:**
Mayo capsulodesis uses the proximal portion of the dorsal intercarpal ligament to tether scaphoid and limit palmar rotation. (Copyright Mayo Clinic. Reproduced with permission of the Mayo Foundation.)

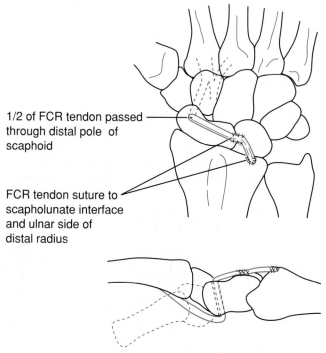

1/2 of FCR tendon passed through distal pole of scaphoid

FCR tendon suture to scapholunate interface and ulnar side of distal radius

**Figure 10–24:**
Brunelli tendon reconstruction. A portion of the flexor carpi radialis *(FCR)* is brought through the distal portion of the scaphoid and then anchored to the dorsal scapholunate ligament and the distal radius.

scaphoid rotation and prevent scaphoid gapping (Figure 10–23).[83,84]

- Tenodesis: These techniques attempt to reestablish the SLIL and SL relationship through the use of varying tendon weaves.
  - Brunelli procedure: Uses a strip of the flexor carpi radialis (FCR) brought palmarly through a bone tunnel in the distal scaphoid. The tendon is brought dorsally and proximally and attached to the distal radius in an attempt to limit scaphoid flexion and stabilize the SLIL and STIL. Modification involves attaching the FCR to the lunate (Figure 10–24).[85]
    - *Technique:* The wrist is approach through standard longitudinal or ligament sparing capsulotomy. The SL ligament is visualized. The scaphoid and lunate are reduced with K-wires. A separate palmar Russe-type incision is made over the distal portion of the FCR. Half of the FCR is harvested, leaving it attached distally to the second metacarpal. This portion of FCR is passed through a bone tunnel in the distal scaphoid. The tunnel is made parallel to the distal articular surface of the scaphoid. The bone tunnel can be made with a cannulated drill passed over a K-wire. The tendon is passed through the tunnel and brought dorsal and proximal to the radiocarpal joint. It is sewn to the dorsum of the SLIL and to the dorsal distal lip of the radius. K-wires are removed at 6 weeks, and range of motion therapy is initiated at 8 weeks.
- Ligament reconstruction
  - Attempts have been made to reconstruct the SLIL with bone ligament–bone constructs from the carpus, foot, and extensor retinaculum (Figure 10–25).[86,87]
- Arthrodesis

- Scaphotrapezial: Watson recommended partial wrist arthrodesis with a fusion of the scaphoid, trapezium, and trapezoid (STT or triscaphe fusion) (Figure 10–26).[88,89] This fusion decreases the flexion extension by 30% and decreases radial to ulnar deviation by 40%. Load distribution is altered at the radial fossa.
  - *Technique:* A transverse or longitudinal incision can be used over the STT joint, allowing visualization of the second and third extensor compartments. The articular cartilage is removed down to bleeding cancellous bone. Three K-wires are driven from the trapezium and trapezoid into the STT joint to confirm position. Bone graft is packed into the defect. Compression is achieved by forcing the scaphoid tubercle dorsally and placing the wrist in some radial deviation. Ideally the scaphoid is placed into mild flexion, to aid in radial deviation and wrist flexion postoperatively. The patient is placed into a long arm cast for 4 weeks, followed by a short arm cast until fusion is achieved.
    - STT fusion has a long track record; however, some complications, including nonunion, have

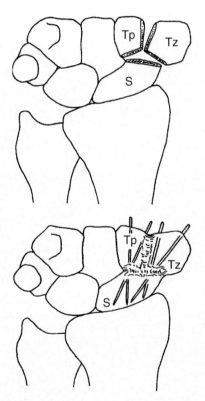

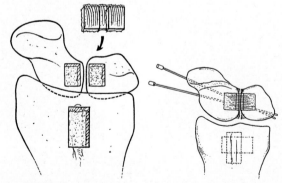

Figure 10–25:
Reconstruction of the scapholunate interosseous ligament can be performed using a bone-ligament-bone block with a portion of the retinaculum that is attached to Lister tubercle.
A bone–ligament-bone block from Lister tubercle is removed with small osteotomes and fashioned to fit into the scaphoid and lunate. A rongeur is used to remove the bone from the middle of the block so that only ligament spans the thin area between the blocks. A burr is used to prepare small bony troughs on the dorsum of the scaphoid and lunate. (From Weiss AP: *J Hand Surg Am* 23:205–215, 1998.)

Figure 10–26:
Scaphoid-trapezial-trapezoid (STT) arthrodesis is stabilized with several Kirschner wires to stabilize the trapezoid (Tp) and trapezium (Tz) to the scaphoid *(S)*. (From Fractures and dislocation of the carpus. In Trumble TE, editor: *Principles of hand surgery and therapy.* Philadelphia, 2000, WB Saunders.)

been reported. Meticulous technique is essential for excellent results.[88–93]

○ SL fusion
  ■ Attempts to fuse these two bones have resulted in high failure rates.[94]
○ Scaphocapitate fusion
  ■ Scaphocapitate arthrodesis is biomechanically very similar to STT arthrodesis.[95]
- Chronic injuries with arthritis (SLAC changes)
  - Stage I
    ○ Early arthritic changes only present at radial styloid.
      ■ STT fusion: Combine procedure with radial styloidectomy for pain relief.
    ○ Scaphocapitate fusion
  - Stage II (Figure 10–27)
    ○ At this point, arthritis already is present in the radial fossa, and attempts at preserving the scaphoid often are futile.
      ■ Four corner fusion: The scaphoid is excised and the midcarpal joint is fused to create one bone block that articulates on the lunate fossa.
        • *Technique:* A longitudinal dorsal exposure to the wrist is used. The scaphoid is excised piecemeal. The opposing surfaces of the lunate, capitate, triquetrum, and hamate are prepared for arthrodesis. A palmar cortical shell of bone is left

to maintain proper spacing between the bones. At this point, any DISI deformity is corrected by flexing the lunate back to a neutral position, often using a K-wire in the lunte as a 'joystick.' The bones are held with three to four K-wires and cancellous bone graft is packed into the intercarpal spaces. Final fixation can be obtained using K-wires, screws, plates and screws, or staples (Figure 10–28). Patients are immobilized in a short arm cast until union (6–8 weeks).

○ *Pearl:* The lunate must be placed into a neutral position prior to pin or screw placement to maximize postoperative motion.
○ Advantage
  ■ Preserves natural lunate radius articulation
○ Disadvantages
  ■ Requires meticulous technique to prevent complications
  ■ Requires 4 to 6 weeks of immobilization
○ Proximal row carpectomy
  ■ Removal of the entire proximal carpal row allows the capitate to articulate with the radius in lunate fossa. The lunate fossa of the radius usually is always preserved in SLAC arthritis. This procedure can be

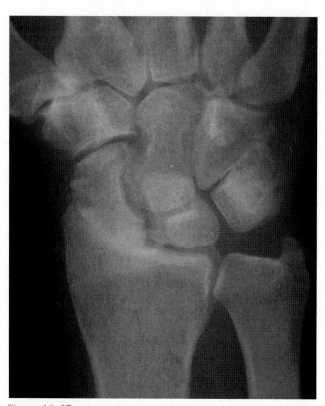

**Figure 10–27:**
Radiograph depicting stage II scapholunate advanced collapse changes with arthritis changes seen at the radial styloid and radioscaphoid fossa.

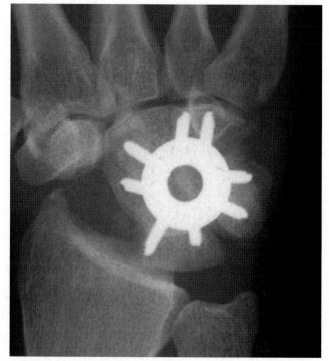

**Figure 10–28:**
Four corner fusion and scaphoidectomy using a circular plate and screws. The capitolunate, capitohamate, and triquetrohamate articulations are solidly arthrodesed. The lunotriquetral joint was not arthrodesed. It is the authors' opinion that as long as the other articulations fuse, there is no difference in the outcome.

performed openly or arthroscopically (Figure 10–29).

- *Technique:* Either a transverse or longitudinal dorsal wrist incision can be used. The extensor retinaculum is incised over the extensor pollicis longus, and flaps are created. We routinely excise the terminal portion of the posterior interosseous nerve just proximal to the wrist because entrapment of this purely sensory portion of the nerve (to the wrist capsule) has been implicated as a possible cause of postoperative pain. The nerve can be found at the most radial margin of the fourth dorsal compartment, just deep to the extensor digitorum communis tendons and alongside the 3-4 intercompartmental septum. A 2- to 3-cm segment is removed just proximal to the articular surface of the radius. The wrist capsule is incised longitudinally, along the third metacarpal axis. Alternatively, a ligament-splitting approach can be used. The lunate and triquetrum are removed, usually in this order. The scaphoid can be excised in its entirety, although we prefer to leave its distal portion attached to the trapezium and trapezoid for additional support of the thumb ray. Carpal impingement on the radial styloid in radial deviation can be managed by limited styloidectomy, but it is important to not destabilize the wrist by removing the radioscaphocapitate ligament in continuity with the resected styloid. The proximal pole of the capitate is seated into the lunate concavity of the radius. If stability is questionable, bone anchors can be used to tension the dorsal flap of the capsule or a temporary K-wire can be used for 3 to 4 weeks to maintain this position. The pisiform is not excised. Closure is performed in layers and includes the extensor retinaculum. The wrist is immobilized in a bulky conforming plaster dressing for 4 to 6 days and then converted to a short arm cast for 3 weeks. Gradual increased motion is permitted using a removable splint for 2 to 4 weeks or until the patient can freely use the wrist.
  - Advantages
    - Easy technical procedure
    - Requires only 3 weeks of immobilization
  - Disadvantages
    - Degenerative changes can be expected at the capitate–radius interface; however, arthritic changes at the capitate–radius interface do not always correlate with clinical symptoms.
  - Ongoing debate exists as to the benefits of four corner fusion over proximal row carpectomy and vice versa; however, no studies to date clearly show superiority of one procedure over the other.
- Stage III (Figure 10–30)
- At this stage the capitate may be too arthritic to allow for proximal row carpectomy. Options may be limited to
- Four corner fusion
- Total wrist fusion
- Total wrist arthroplasty

## Lunotriquetral Ligament Injuries

### Introduction

- Although prior reports of LT injury have been reported,[96–98] it was not until 1984 that Reagan, Linscheid, and Dobyns[64] recognized and reported on the role of the LT ligament in the development of proximal carpal row VISI deformity.
- Although LT ligament dissociation with attenuation of secondary ligamentous restraints resulted in a VISI deformity, not all VISI deformities result from LT ligament injury. VISI deformities appear to have a final common pathway that occurs by multiple mechanisms, all of which depend on LT ligament attenuation.
- In describing injuries of the LT ligament, distinguishing between dynamic and static instability is imperative.[99–101]

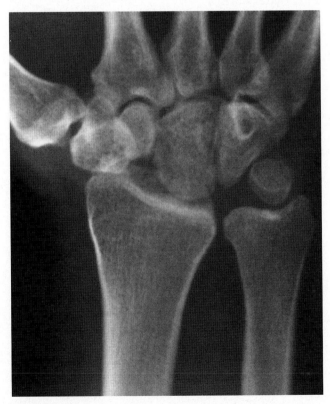

Figure 10–29:
**Proximal row carpectomy.**

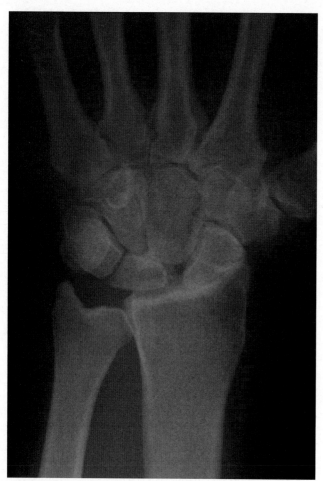

Figure 10–30:
Radiograph depicting stage III scapholunate advanced collapse changes with arthritis changes seen at the radioscaphoid interface and capitate.

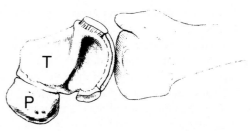

Figure 10–31:
Similar to the scapholunate ligament, the lunotriquetral ligament is a C-shaped ligament with a true dorsal and volar ligament and a membranous portion proximally. Unlike the scapholunate ligament, the volar portion of the lunotriquetral ligament is stronger and more stout compared to the dorsal portion of the ligament. *P*, pisiform; *T*, triquetrum. (Copyright Mayo Clinic. Reproduced with permission of the Mayo Foundation.)

- LT ligament injuries with normal conventional radiographs and dynamic instability (present only under load or in certain positions) are classified as *LT tears.*
- Fixed carpal collapse (VISI) on conventional radiographs represents static instability and is classified as *LT ligament dissociation.*

## Anatomy of the Lunotriquetral Ligament

- Like the SL ligament, the LTILs are C-shaped ligaments that span the dorsal, proximal, and palmar edges of the joint surfaces (Figure 10–31).
- Microscopically, there are true ligaments in the dorsal and palmar subregions and a proximal fibrocartilaginous subregion, known as the *membranous portion.*
- In a study of the ligament properties of the LT ligament, Ritt et al.[102] demonstrated that the palmar region of the LT was the thickest and strongest region. These findings support the "balanced lunate" concept, which proposes that the lunate is torque suspended between the scaphoid, exerting a flexion

moment through the SL ligament and the triquetrum, exerting an extension moment through the LT ligament.

- The dorsal LT ligament region was most important in rotational constraint, whereas the palmar region of the LT ligament was the strongest and transmitted the extension moment of the triquetrum as it engaged the hamate. The membranous proximal portion of the LT ligament complex was of little significance with respect to constraining rotation, translation, or distraction.[103]

## Pathomechanics

- In an uninjured wrist, the scaphoid imparts a flexion moment to the proximal carpal row, while the triquetrum imparts an extension moment, secondary to the midcarpal contact forces. These opposing moments are balanced by their ligamentous attachment to the lunate.
  - With loss of the integrity of the SL ligament, the scaphoid tends to flex, while the lunate and triquetrum tend to extend, imparting a DISI stance.
  - With loss of integrity of the LT ligament, the triquetrum tends to extend, while the scaphoid and lunate rotate in flexion.
- A complete LT ligament dissociation is not sufficient to cause a static carpal collapse into a VISI stance.
  - Sectioning of volar and dorsal subregions of the LT ligament results in a slight divergence of the triquetrum and lunate at extremes of wrist flexion and radial deviation but no collapse, unless considerable compressive forces are applied.[64]
  - Additional tear or attenuation of secondary restraints is necessary to create static carpal instability. Both palmar and dorsal carpal ligaments may play roles as secondary restraints. Two anatomic studies have implicated palmar ligament injury in the development of VISI in LT dissociation. Trumble et al.[104] created dynamic carpal collapse with division of the LTIL and ulnar arcuate ligament (lunocapitate) and static with division of the dorsal radiotriquetral, whereas Horii et al.[40]

demonstrated that sectioning of the dorsal radiotriquetral (dorsal radiocarpal) and dorsal scaphotriquetral (dorsal intercarpal) ligament also produced static VISI following LT ligament injury.

- Loss of dorsal ligament integrity allows the lunate to flex more easily, in part by shifting the point of capitate contact palmar to the lunate axis of rotation (Figure 10–32).

## Physical Examination

- Ulnar deviation with pronation and axial compression elicits dynamic instability with a painful snap if a nondissociative midcarpal joint or LT ligament injury is present.
- Palpation always demonstrates point tenderness at the LT joint.[64] A palpable wrist click occasionally is significant, particularly if it occurs with pain and radioulnar deviation. Provocative tests that demonstrate LT laxity, crepitus, and pain are helpful for accurately localizing the site of pathology. Three useful tests include LT ballottement, shear (Kleinman) test, and compression test.[64,105,106]
  - Ballottement of the triquetrum, described by Reagan, Linscheid, and Dobyns,[64] is performed by grasping the pisotriquetral unit between the thumb and index finger of one hand and the lunate between the thumb and index of the other. If positive, pain and increased anteroposterior laxity are noted during manipulation of the joint (Figure 10–33).

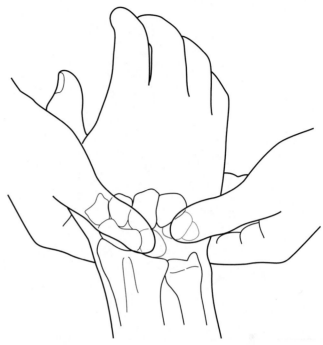

**Figure 10–33:**
Lunotriquetral ballottement test or Reagan test is performed by holding the lunate in the examiner's one hand and the triquetrum/pisiform complex in the examiner's other hand. A dorsal and volar translation is stressed onto the lunotriquetral ligament complex. A positive examination is defined as pain associated with the maneuver in addition to laxity that is increased compared to the uninjured contralateral wrist.

- The shear test, described by Kleinman,[106] is performed with the forearm in neutral rotation and the elbow on the examination table. The examiner's contralateral fingers are placed over the dorsum of the lunate. With the lunate supported, the examiner's ipsilateral thumb loads the pisotriquetral joint from the palmar aspect, creating a shear force at the LT joint (Figure 10–34).
- Pressure on the triquetrum in the "ulnar snuffbox" creates a radially directed compressive force against the triquetrum. Pain elicited with this maneuver may be of LT origin but also may arise from the triquetrohamate joint or triangular fibrocartilage complex pathology.[105] These tests are considered positive when pain, crepitance, and abnormal mobility of the LT joint are demonstrable (Figure 10–35).
- A nondissociative instability pattern secondary to midcarpal laxity at the triquetrohamate joint should be ruled out because the symptoms may be similar. The possibility of injury at both levels should be considered.[107,108]
- Selective midcarpal injection of local anesthetic is useful as a diagnostic tool. Resolution of pain with increased grip strength following injection in patients with LT injuries has been a reliable predictor of satisfactory outcome in our experience. A poor

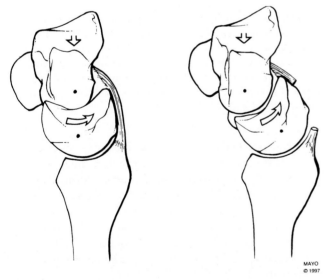

MAYO
© 1997

**Figure 10–32:**
Injury to the lunotriquetral ligament alone is insufficient to produce a volar intercalated segmental instability (VISI). The integrity of the dorsal radiotriquetral (dorsal radiocarpal ligament) must be violated for the lunate to obtain the VISI pattern. Without loss of integrity of the dorsal radiocarpal ligament, the lunate maintains a normal stance. (Copyright Mayo Clinic. Reproduced with permission of the Mayo Foundation.)

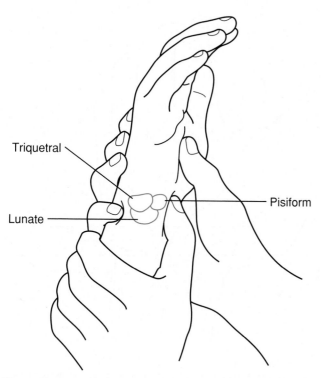

Figure 10–34:
The Kleinman test is performed when the examiner's thumb is placed on the volar aspect over the pisiform and the examiner's other hand stabilizes the wrist. The examiner pushes the pisiform dorsally with the thumb. If dorsal pain is elicited, then the test is considered positive.

response to injection implies an extraarticular cause of the patient's symptoms.

## Radiographic Evaluation

- Radiographs with LT ligament tears often are normal.
- LT dissociation results in a disruption of the smooth arcs formed by the proximal and distal joint surfaces of the proximal carpal row (Gilula arcs 1 and 2) and the proximal joint surfaces of the distal carpal row (Gilula arc 3) (Figure 10–36).
- LT dissociation results in proximal translation of the triquetrum and/or LT overlap.[64,109] Unlike SL injuries, no LT gap occurs (see Figure 10–36).
- Motion studies, including deviation and clenched fist anteroposterior views, are helpful.
  - In LT dissociation, the normal reciprocal motion of scaphoid, lunate, and distal row is accentuated in deviation while triquetral motion is diminished.[105]
  - The increased palmar flexion of the scaphoid and lunate in radial deviation without change of the triquetrum is a manifestation of the loss of proximal row integrity in the normal wrist.[64]
- Careful evaluation of the lunate and triquetrum on lateral radiographs may reveal a malalignment in the absence of frank carpal collapse. The perimeters of the triquetrum and lunate can be traced and their relationship assessed.[64]

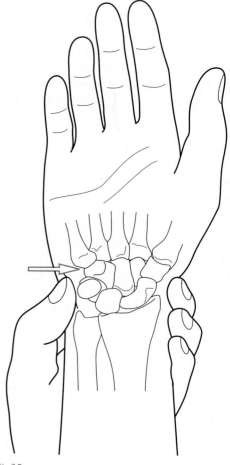

Figure 10–35:
Lunotriquetral compression test uses the helicoid nature of the triquetrohamate articulation to stress the lunotriquetral ligament. By direct radial pressure on the triquetrum, the triquetrum is forced by the hamate articular surface to extend. This action imparts a translation to the lunotriquetral ligament. If pain is elicited, then the test is considered positive for lunotriquetral ligament injury.

- The longitudinal axis of the triquetrum, defined as a line passing through the distal triquetral angle and bisecting the proximal articular surface, forms a 14 degree angle (range +31 degrees to −3 degrees) with the lunate longitudinal axis, defined as a line passing perpendicular to a line drawn from the distal dorsal and volar edges of the lunate. LT dissociation results in a negative angle (mean value −16 degrees) (Figure 10–37).[64]
- If a VISI deformity is present with LT dissociation, the SL and capitolunate angles are altered. The SL angle may be diminished from its normal 47 to 40 degrees or less but often is normal.[1] The lunate and capitate, which normally are colinear, collapse in a zigzag fashion, resulting in an angle greater than 10 degrees.
- Arthrography is valuable, demonstrating leakage or pooling of dye at the LT interspace. However, age-related

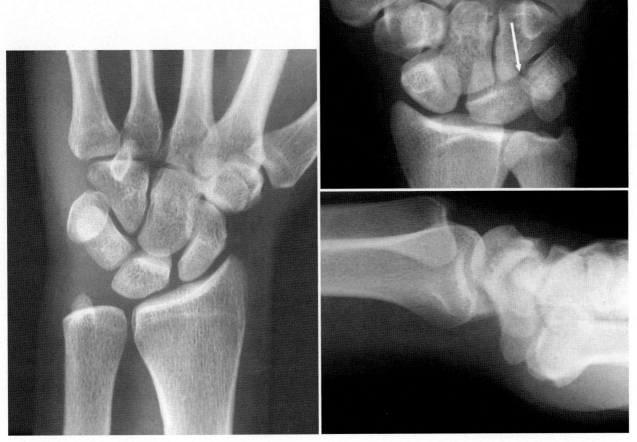

Figure 10–36:
Radiographs of lunotriquetral (LT) ligament instabilities are often very subtle and normal. Occasionally, a small step-off may be noticed at the LT interval and accentuated with a distraction view of the carpus. In this case, there is distal translation of the triquetrum compared to the lunate, which is firmly anchored to the radius via the short radiolunate ligament (**A**). Gross disruption of the LT ligament and rupture of the dorsal intercarpal ligament result in the radiographic appearance shown in panels **B** and **C**. The *arrow* shows the incongruity of the LT interval, and the lateral (**C**) demonstrates the volar intercalated segmental instability deformity. Because of the marked flexion of the scaphoid and lunate, a pseudogap at the scapholunate articulation is seen on the anteroposterior view. This pseudogap occurs because the scapholunate joint has a hourglass-shaped joint space, with the volar and dorsal portions slightly wider than the central portion. When viewed in flexion, the dorsal portion of the joint is seen and gives the illusion of a widened joint space.

LT membrane perforations, other communications between the radiocarpal and midcarpal joints, and asymptomatic LT tears on arthrography of normal wrists have been reported. Therefore, the results of arthrography must be correlated with clinical examination findings.

- A videotaped arthrogram with motion sequences in flexion-extension and radioulnar deviation can further confirm the presence of an LT injury by demonstrating abnormal pooling of the dye column and abnormal proximal row kinematics as previously described.

- Videofluoroscopy is useful for demonstrating the site of a "clunk" that occurs with deviation. In LT sprains, this occurs with a sudden "catch-up" of the triquetrum into extension as the wrist moves into maximal ulnar deviation.

- Technetium Tc 99m-methylene diphosphonate (MDP) bone scans can help identify the site of acute injury but are less specific than arthrography.[109] They may prove helpful in cases where standard films and motion studies are negative.

- MRI technology is not yet reliable for LT ligament imaging but continues to improve and soon may supplant arthrography and bone scans.

### Treatment

- Wrist arthroscopy is both diagnostic and therapeutic. Wrist arthroscopy provides a means to directly inspect the integrity of the LT ligaments and allows for identification and treatment of any associated pathology (Figure 10–38).

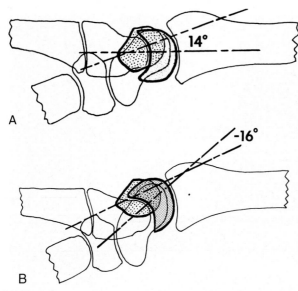

Figure 10–37:

**A,** The normal lunotriquetral angle averages +14 degrees. **B,** In lunotriquetral dissociation with loss of integrity of the dorsal intercarpal ligament, the average lunotriquetral angle averages decreases to −16 degrees. (Copyright Mayo Clinic. Reproduced with permission of the Mayo Foundation.)

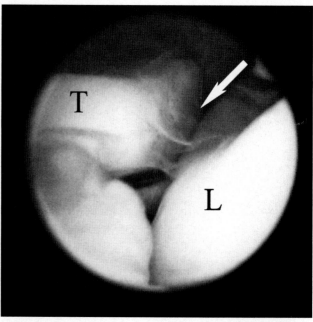

Figure 10–38:

Arthroscopy is the gold standard for diagnosis of lunotriquetral ligament instability. View from the midcarpal joint is the best way to assess the stability of the lunotriquetral ligament complex. Midcarpal arthroscopy shows the step-off between the lunate *(L)* and the triquetrum *(T)* and the placement of a probe through the articulation. *Arrow* points to the joint.

- In our experience, arthroscopy has provided the most accurate means of diagnosis of LT pathology and may replace all other diagnostic studies.
- Carpal instability can be assessed by direct visualization and probing of the carpal joint articulations. Additionally, provocative maneuvers can be performed while directly visualizing the carpal joint articulations.
- Arthroscopic instability is graded by the Geissler classification.[74]
- Midcarpal arthroscopy is the key to assessing the stability of the LT joint. From the midcarpal perspective, the normal LT joint is smooth without a step-off or diastasis.
- Surgical reconstruction
  - In acute and chronic dissociations that demonstrate a VISI collapse and chronic tears unresponsive to conservative management, operative treatment is indicated.
  - The goal of surgical intervention is realignment of the lunocapitate axis and reestablishment of the rotational integrity of the proximal carpal row.
  - Performed via a dorsal ligament-sparing capsulotomy (described in SL dissociation section).
  - A variety of procedures have been described, including LT arthrodesis, ligament repair, and ligament reconstruction (Figure 10–39). If concomitant ulnar negative or positive variance or midcarpal or radiocarpal arthrosis is present, additional procedures, such as ulnar lengthening or shortening, midcarpal arthrodesis, or proximal row carpectomy, may be indicated. Total wrist

arthrodesis may be indicated when degenerative changes make other salvage procedures impossible.
- LT ligament repair
  - LTIL is reattached to the site of its avulsion, generally from the triquetrum.
  - The technique is demanding, requiring use of multiple sutures passed through drill holes or suture anchors placed in the site of the avulsion.
  - Because the strong volar ligament also is disrupted, a combined dorsal and volar approach and augmentation of the repair by plication of the dorsal radiotriquetral and dorsal scaphotriquetral ligaments may be of some value.
  - Protracted immobilization is necessary (10–12 weeks).
  - Patients with strenuous pursuits, chronic instability, or poor-quality LT ligament may be best managed by ligament reconstruction.
- LT ligament reconstruction
  - Ligament reconstruction with a distally based strip of extensor carpi ulnaris tendon graft is the authors' recommended surgery for LT dissociation.
  - Unlike SL ligament reconstruction, this technique, although demanding, yielded uniformly good results in two studies.[64,99–101]
  - Reconstruction preserves LT motion and provides the optimal chance for restoration of normal carpal interactions, unlike LT arthrodesis.

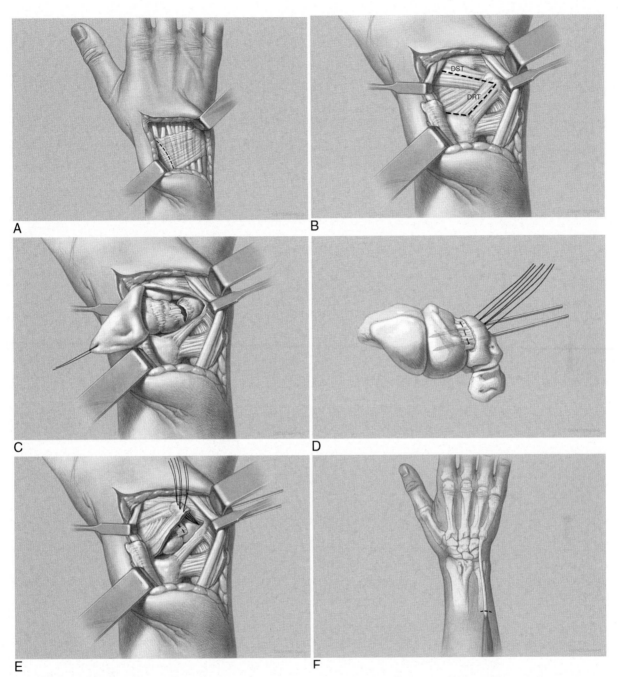

Figure 10–39:

Treatment of lunotriquetral (LT) ligament instability includes repair, reconstruction, or arthrodesis. A curvilinear or longitudinal dorsal incision is made, and the third extensor compartment is released and a ulnar-based retinacular flap is created by dividing the septations between the 3-4 and 4-5 extensor compartments **(A)**. The extensor tendons are retracted, and a dorsal ligament sparing capsulotomy is made along the lines of the dorsal intercarpal (dorsal scaphotriquetral [DST]) and dorsal radiocarpal ligaments (dorsal radiotriquetral [DRT]), extending over the radioscaphoid interval **(B)**. The ulnar-based flap is created, carefully elevating it from the lunotriquetral ligament, which is intimate to the dorsal radiocarpal ligament **(C)**. The LT joint integrity can be evaluated from the midcarpal joint. If the dorsal ligament is attenuated or avulsed, a ligament repair can be performed. The site of the avulsion is prepared with either drill holes or with suture anchors (authors' preference) **(D)**. The LT joint is reduced and pinned with two Kirschner wires **(D)**. The ligament is repaired, and the ligament-sparing capsulotomy is closed down using the same suture anchors, followed by repair of the remainder of the capsulotomy **(E)**. If the LT joint is grossly lax, demonstrating complete instability, LT reconstruction is recommended. A distally based strip of extensor carpi ulnaris (ECU) tendon is harvested using a few transverse incisions over the ECU tendon **(F)**. A 2-0 surgical steel wire is used to hold half of the ECU tendon approximately 8 cm proximal to the wrist. It is passed distally in the ECU sheath and brought out at the level of the dorsal wrist exposure. The wire is pulled, creating a distally based strip of ECU tendon

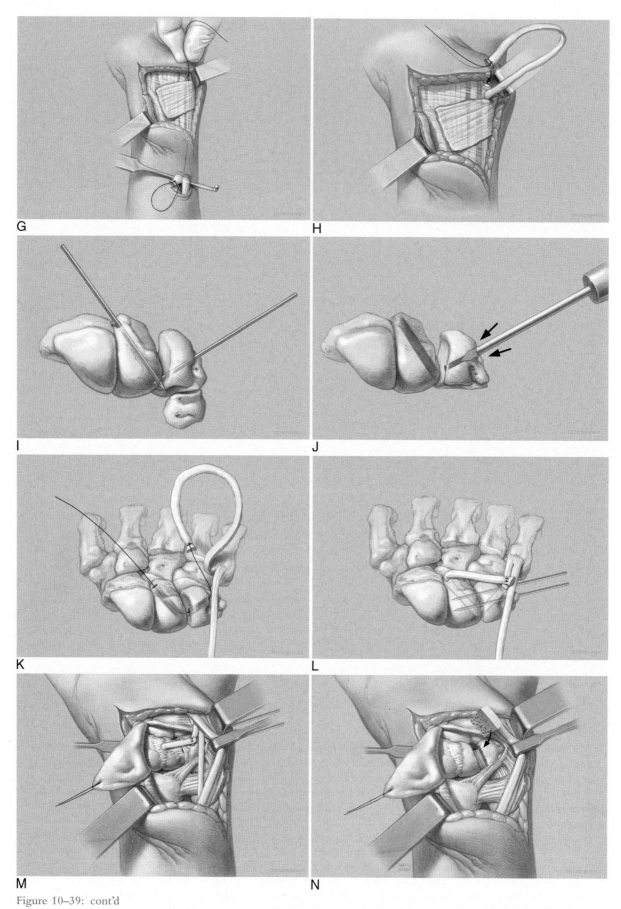

Figure 10–39: cont'd

(G). The tendon strip is passed into the carpus (H). K-wires are placed in the lunate and triquetrum so that they meet at the volar aspect of the joint (I). Bone tunnels are prepared by hand drilling over the K-wires (J). The ECU tendon strip is passed into the triquetrum, volarly through the lunate, and tightened dorsally (K). Two K-wires are used to secure the reduced lunate and triquetrum, and the tendon graft is tied to itself (L, M). If arthrodesis is chosen, the articular cartilage is removed, leaving a rim of articular cartilage intact to maintain the spacing between the lunate and triquetrum (N).

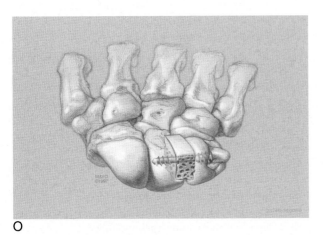

O

Figure 10–39: cont'd
Bone graft is placed into the space, and a cannulated screw is used to compress the arthrodesis site **(O)**. (Copyright Mayo Clinic. Reproduced with permission of the Mayo Foundation.)

- LT arthrodesis
  - Technically less demanding than ligament reconstruction or repair and has become the technique of choice of many authors. However, the method is not without substantial problems.[64]
  - Reported nonunion rate varies from 0% to 57%.[64,110–115]
  - Use of K-wires has resulted in an unacceptably high nonunion rate of 47%.[113] Use of compression screws may improve results, but nonunion remains a significant problem. A 9% nonunion rate was reported with the Herbert screw, and conventional cortical screws may exhibit nonunion rates as high as 57%.[113–115]
  - Ulnocarpal impingement required additional surgery in 14% of LT arthrodesis patients.[110]
  - A variety of techniques exist. The authors prefer denuding the articular cartilage while maintaining a rim of articular cartilage to preserve the normal LT width. Cancellous bone graft (iliac crest or distal radius bone graft) is impacted into the defect, and a cannulated compression screw is placed from the ulnar to radial direction.
- Outcomes and comparative studies
  - Comparison of results and outcomes following arthrodesis, ligament repair, and reconstruction has demonstrated superior results with LT ligament repair or reconstruction.[101]
    - Fifty-seven patients with 57 isolated LT injuries treated by arthrodesis, direct ligament repair, or ligament reconstruction were compared.
    - Average follow-up was 9.5 years (range 2–22).

- The probability of remaining free of complications at 5 years was 68.6% for reconstruction, 13.5% for repair, and less than 1% for arthrodesis.
- Among the LT arthrodeses, 40.9% developed nonunion and 22.7% developed ulnocarpal impaction.
- The probability of remaining free of subsequent surgery at 5 years was 68.6% for reconstruction, 23.3% for repair, and 21.8% for arthrodesis.
- Objective improvements in strength and motion and subjective measures of pain relief and satisfaction were significantly higher in the LT repair and reconstruction groups than in the arthrodesis group.
- Attritional LT instability secondary to ulnar positive variance
  - Refers to LT instability secondary to a long ulna that chronically impacts the triquetrum, resulting in an LT tear with instability. Often associated with a degenerative nonrepairable triangular fibrocartilage tear.
  - Ulnar shortening is an attractive alternative in these cases (Figure 10–40).

## Carpal Instability Nondissociative

- When a normal relationship exists between the components of the distal and proximal rows (i.e., no dissociative instability findings) and abnormal motion or dysfunction occurs between the radius and proximal carpal row or between the proximal and distal rows, the wrist is considered to have a nondissociative carpal instability.

### Radiocarpal

- Nondissociative instabilities of the radiocarpal group included patients with incompetent or insufficient radiocarpal ligaments.
  - Chronic
    - Rheumatoid arthritis secondary to the laxity of the radiocarpal ligaments
    - Developmental deformities
      - Madelung deformity
  - Acute

### Radiocarpal Dislocations

- Ulnar translocation
  - First described by Dobyns et al.[116] in 1975
  - Further redefined by Taleisnik[117,118] into two types (Figure 10–41):
    - Type I: entire carpus, including the scaphoid, is displaced, and the distance between the radial styloid and the scaphoid is widened.
      - Represents a pure CIND

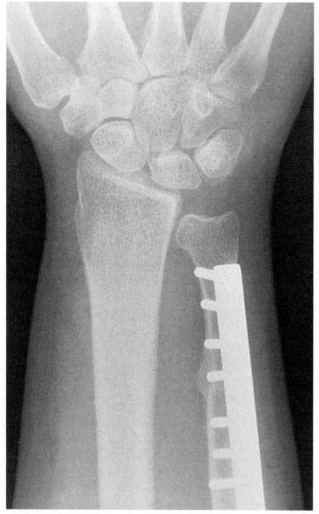

Figure 10–40:

**Degenerative lunotriquetral instability can occur in the face of ulnar positive variance. Treatment of degenerative lunotrique-tral instability secondary to positive ulnar variance is best addressed with a ulnar shortening procedure.**

○ Type II: radius, scaphoid, and distal carpal row relationships are normal; however, the SL space is widened and the lunate and triquetrum are ulnarly translocated.
  ■ Combination of CIND and CID (SL dissociation), making it a CIC
● Treatment
  ○ Only a single series of eight patients with these injuries was reported from the Mayo Clinic.[119]
    ■ Difficult problem to treat effectively
● Disappointing results
● Recommended radiolunate arthrodesis
● Pure radiocarpal dislocations
  ● Exceedingly rare, with 11 cases reported in 1995.[120]
  ● Dumontier et al.[121] reported on 27 radiocarpal dislocations (most associated with radiostyloid fractures)

seen over a 23-year period. Seven radiocarpal dislocations were considered "pure."
  ○ Recommended open reattachment of volar carpal ligaments in pure dislocation through a volar approach to obtain best outcome

## Midcarpal

● Historically, *midcarpal instability* was the term used to describe any instability that occurred in the wrist without a dissociative component. Technically, the dysfunction occurred at either the radiocarpal or midcarpal joint but predominated at the midcarpal joint.
  ● First description by Lichtman et al.[12] in 1981, when they described ulnar midcarpal instability.
    ○ Described characteristic VISI pattern
    ○ Symptoms included pain and spontaneous wrist clunk/click with ulnar deviation
    ○ Attributed to failure of the ulnar limb of the volar ulnar arcuate ligament
  ● Taleisnik and Watson[23] in 1984 described the concept of extrinsic midcarpal instabilities·
    ○ Patients who have a painful snapping/clunking of their wrist with ulnar to radial deviation
    ○ Attribute the lesion to extraarticular injury, in this series a distal radius malunion

## Pathomechanics

● In radial and ulnar deviation of the normal wrist, a smooth transition occurs with a synchronous reciprocal motion between the proximal and distal carpal rows.
● In the pathologic state, the smooth synchronous reciprocal motion is disrupted.
● The stout triquetrohamate and triquetrocapitate (ulnar arcuate) ligaments are necessary to prevent midcarpal collapse during radial and ulnar deviation but also allow for the smooth progressive transition of the proximal row from flexion to extension as the wrist ulnarly deviates.
● The helicoids articulation between the hamate and triquetrum assist in the smooth transition.
● Failure or laxity in the triquetrohamate and triquetrocapitate ligaments results in inadequate prevention of midcarpal collapse (development of VISI deformity), and extension of the proximal row is hampered. This results in the sudden and painful clunk when the wrist is ulnarly deviated, and the triquetrum suddenly follows the hamate surface (Figure 10–42).

## Classification

● Proposed by Lichtman et al.[14] in 1993 based on their experiences and previous reports.

### Palmar Midcarpal Instability

● Acute or chronic VISI malalignment secondary to attenuation or rupture of palmar midcarpal ligaments

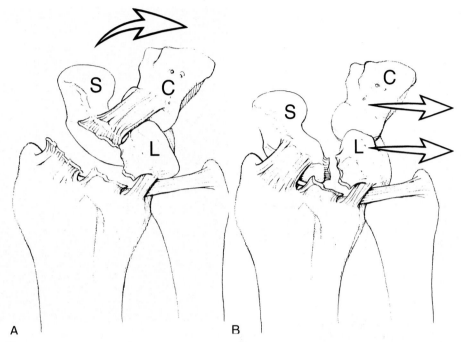

Figure 10–41:
Ulnar translocation has been classified into two types. **A,** Type I is a complete ulnar translocation of the entire carpus *(C)*. **B,** Type II represents the ulnar translocation of the carpus, leaving the scaphoid *(S)* in it normal location. *L,* lunate. (Copyright Mayo Clinic, reproduced with permission of the Mayo Foundation.)

- Medial sided: triquetral hamate capitate ligaments
- Lateal sided: scaphoid capitate trapezoid trapezium ligaments

## Dorsal Midcarpal Instability

- Young patients with bilateral hypermobile wrists
- Secondary to excessive attenuation from trauma or chronic injury
- Symptoms secondary to disruption or attenuation of radiocapitate ligament
  - CLIP: dorsal subluxation of the capitate compared to the lunate[11,122]

## Combined Dorsal and Palmar Midcarpal Instability

- Secondary to laxity of both midcarpal and radiocarpal ligaments
- Includes the proximal carpal row instabilities described by Wright et al.[29]

## Extrinsic Midcarpal Instability

- In patients with chronic dorsal angulated malunited distal radius fractures secondary to stretching of the volar carpal ligaments
- Included in the CIA category

## Diagnosis

- Patients often demonstrate painful clunk maneuver, which often involves ulnar deviation and pronation of the wrist (Figure 10–42).
- Wrist may present with a sag in the midcarpal joint, with limited range of motion and impaired grip strength.
- Circumduction test (axial load and ulnar-dorsal rotation of the wrist) may reproduce the clunk and pain, as does axial loading of the wrist with radioulnar deviation.
- Real-time fluoroscopy examination often is the most useful tool for diagnosis.
  - Normal synchronous motion in radial and ulnar deviation is lost.
  - While ulnarly deviating the wrist from maximal radial deviation, the proximal carpal row suddenly snaps into an extended position, with a dramatic, sometimes audible, and painful clunk.
  - Dorsal and volar stress on the carpus may demonstrate the CLIP.

## Treatment

- All patients are initially treated with nonoperative measures, which include immobilization, nonsteroidal antiinflammatory medications, activity modifications, and corticosteroid intraarticular injections.[29]
- Operative options include

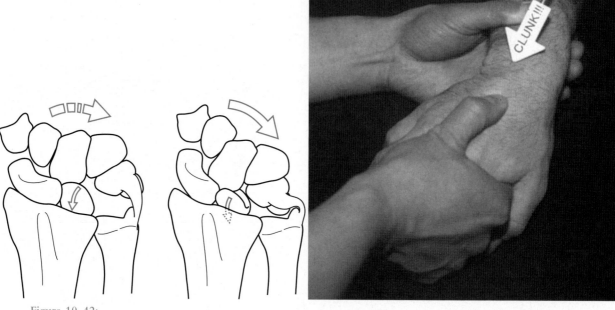

Figure 10–42:

**A,** In nondissociative midcarpal instability, radial and ulnar deviation often results in a *catch-up clunk.* With axial compression and deviation of the wrist from radial to ulnar, nonsynchronous motion occurs such that the proximal carpal row appears to jump from palmar flexion **(left)** to a dorsal extension position **(right)** with a clunk. This clunk represents the proximal carpal row catching up to the distal carpal row during ulnar deviation. **B,** Clinical example of the radioulnar deviation clunk. (From Fractures and dislocation of the carpus. In Trumble TE, editor: *Principles of hand surgery and therapy.* Philadelphia, 2000, WB Saunders.)

- Soft tissue reconstructions[11,14,29,123]
  - Volarly the space of Poirier is obliterated.[11]
    - A volar extended carpal tunnel release is performed, and sutures are placed between the radioscaphocapitate and the long radiolunate ligament radially and between the ulnotriquetrocapitate and ulnolunate ligament ulnarly. The sutures are tightened, thus obliterating the space of Poirier.
  - Dorsally the dorsal intercarpal and radiocarpal ligaments are imbricated.
- Limited intercarpal arthrodesis
  - Triquetrohamate arthrodesis[14]
  - Four corner arthrodesis[14,124]
  - Radiolunate arthrodesis[125]

## Carpal Instability Adaptive

- Concept introduced in 1982 by Allieu, Brahin, and Ascencio.[47]
- Taleisnik and Watson[23] in 1984 reported on 13 patients with dorsally malunited distal radius fractures with secondary midcarpal malalignment.
  - DISI deformity secondary to fracture malunion (see Figure 10–10).

- Progressive pain, tenderness in midcarpal joint, occasional painful clunk.
- Corrective osteotomy consistently resulted in excellent resolution of pain and symptoms.

## Complex Instability of the Carpus

- Combination of CID and CIND in the same wrist is called carpus instability complex. All carpal dislocations except for pure radiocarpal dislocations belong in this category. Five groups of dislocations fall in this category:
- Dorsal perilunate dislocations
- Dorsal perilunate fracture-dislocations
- Palmar perilunate fracture-dislocations
- Axial carpal dislocations
- Isolated carpal dislocations

### Perilunar

- Rare injury patterns that usually are associated with significant trauma (e.g., fall from a height).
  - Diagnosis can be delayed because some radiographic findings may be subtle to the untrained eye. Herzberg et al.[126] reported that 25% of these injuries are missed during initial presentation.

- Lunate often remains bound to the distal radius by stout radiolunate ligaments but carpus dislocates around it, hence the name *perilunar injury*. Capitate may move dorsally, causing dorsal perilunate dislocation, or palmarly, causing palmar perilunate dislocation (Figure 10–43).
- Lunate dislocation occurs when the lunate dislocates from radial fossa palmarly (palmar lunate dislocation) (Figure 10–44) or dorsally (dorsal lunate dislocation).
- Fractures may pass through any bone found within the greater arc of the wrist and include the distal radius, scaphoid, trapezium, capitate, hamate, and triquetrum.
- Lesser arc injuries pass only through ligamentous structures with no corresponding fractures (Figure 10–45).

## Diagnosis

### Physical Examination

- Physical examination may reveal significant swelling, ecchymosis, and decreased range of motion.
- Up to 25% chance of acute carpal tunnel syndrome.[126]

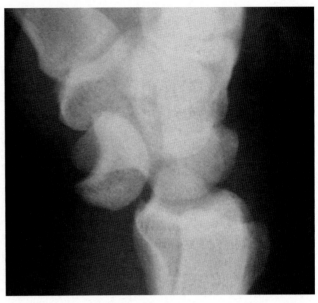

Figure 10–44:
On lateral radiograph, the lunate is displaced volarly while the capitate is articulating with the radius. (From Fractures and dislocation of the carpus. In Trumble TE, editor: *Principles of hand surgery and therapy.* Philadelphia, 2000, WB Saunders.)

### Imaging

#### *Plain Films*

- PA films show disruption of Gilula lines and gapping between carpal bones.
- Lateral films show dislocation of capitate or lunate.

#### *Computed Tomography, Bone Scan, and Magnetic Resonance Imaging*

- CT, bone scan, and MRI usually are not required to make the diagnosis.

### Treatment

#### Acute Presentation

- Closed reduction may be performed initially for pain relief, but surgery is the *definitive treatment.*

#### Technique for Open Repair

- The carpus is opened dorsally with a longitudinal incision over the third and fourth compartments. The retinaculum is released over the third compartment, and retinacular flaps are elevated radially to the second compartment and ulnarly to the fifth compartment. A longitudinal or ligament-sparing capsulotomy is created, and the carpus is exposed. The lunate is initially reduced and held in place with a longitudinal K-wire. This becomes the foundation for carpal reduction. The triquetrum and scaphoid are reduced and held in place with two to three K-wires. SLIL and LTIL repairs are performed with suture anchors or bone tunnels.

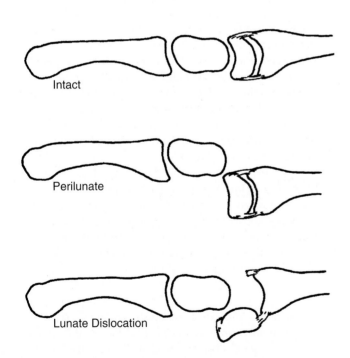

Intact

Perilunate

Lunate Dislocation

Figure 10–43:
In a perilunate dislocation, the capitate is initially displaced dorsal to the lunate. In the final stages of injuries of this spectrum, the capitate reduces into the fossa of the radius, displacing the lunate toward the palm. Perilunate dislocations and lunate dislocations represent two points on the spectrum of carpal fracture-dislocation. (From Fractures and dislocation of the carpus. In Trumble TE, editor: *Principles of hand surgery and therapy.* Philadelphia, 2000, WB Saunders.)

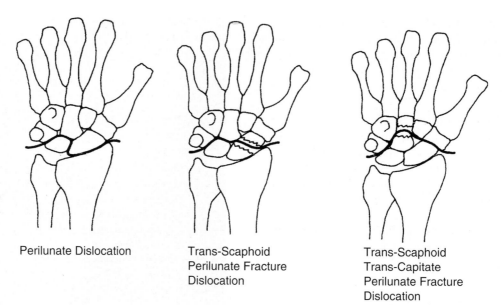

Perilunate Dislocation

Trans-Scaphoid
Perilunate Fracture
Dislocation

Trans-Scaphoid
Trans-Capitate
Perilunate Fracture
Dislocation

Figure 10–45:
Perilunate fracture-dislocations can occur with disruption of the scapholunate interosseous ligament, fracture of the scaphoid, or fracture of the scaphoid and capitate, depending on the path of injury. (From Fractures and dislocation of the carpus. In Trumble TE, editor: *Principles of hand surgery and therapy.* Philadelphia, 2000, WB Saunders.)

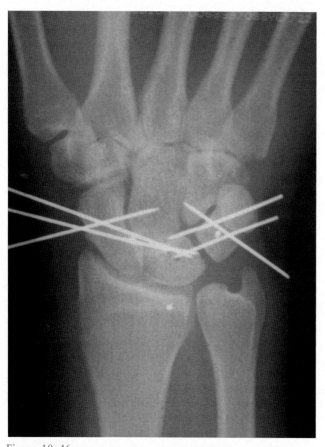

Figure 10–46:
Repair of perilunate dislocation using bone anchors and K-wires. Scapholunate and lunotriquetral ligaments were repaired using suture anchors via a dorsal approach.

Intraoperative fluoroscopy is essential to verify adequate reduction of the proximal carpal row. We reduce the midcarpal joint with two K-wires through the scaphoid into the capitate and an additional two wires from the triquetrum into the hamate and capitate. Once the carpus is reduced, the initial lunate wire may be removed to prevent immobilization across the radiocarpal joint. The wrist is turned palmarly, and an extended carpal tunnel incision is made to view the palmar ligaments. A large rent may be seen in cases of palmar lunate dislocations, or the palmar ligaments may be avulsed from the bone. Ligament repair is performed with heavy suture, wire or screw, and anchor fixation in cases of frank avulsion. Patients are immobilized for 8 to 10 weeks. Radiocarpal motion is allowed at 8 to 10 weeks. K-wires remain for 10 to 12 weeks (Figure 10–46).

## Lunate Dislocations

- These dislocations usually require an extended carpal tunnel approach initially for lunate reduction if the lunate cannot be reduced by closed means (Figure 10–47).

## Delayed Presentation

- Outcomes worse than dislocations repaired acutely.

## Treatment

- Open reduction internal fixation
- Proximal row carpectomy
- Total wrist fusion

- Two studies examining patients treated a minimum of 6 weeks after injury both concluded that open reduction internal fixation provided the most reliable improvement in function and pain.[127,128]

## Axial Carpal

- Axial carpal dissociation of the carpus consists of a traumatic longitudinal disruption, in which the carpus is longitudinally split and displaced.[61,129–131]
- These injuries typically result from severe trauma, such as blast or crush injuries, resulting in fracture-dislocations with loss of the normal architecture of the distal transverse (metacarpal) and proximal (carpal) arch.
- The normal convex relationship between the metacarpal heads is lost, the palm is flattened, rotational deformities of the fingers occur, and the carpometacarpal area is widened.[132,133]
- The spectrum of axial carpal instability ranges from acute, gross traumatic fracture-dislocations with severe soft tissue trauma to chronic dynamic instability between the axial components of the carpus.[70,134] Although a majority of axial carpal instability has been reported as gross traumatic injuries, the concept of axial carpal sprains, with longitudinal dynamic derangement, was described in a case report.[70,134]

## Classification

- After reviewing 40 cases reported in the literature and adding 16 other cases from their retrospective review, Garcia-Elias et al.[61] classified axial dislocations of the carpus into three groups according to the direction of instability (Figure 10–48):
  - Axial-ulnar disruption: carpus splits into two columns, in which the radial column is stable with respect to the radius, and the ulnar column (with the metacarpals) displaces ulnarly and proximally
  - Axial-radial disruption: disruption in which the ulnar column is stable with respect to the radius, and the radial column (including the metacarpals) displaces proximally and radially
  - Combined axial-radial-ulnar disruptions: combination of ulnar and radial displacement of the columns

## Demographics of Injury

- The estimated incidence of axial carpal disruptions is between 1.4% and 2.08% of patients with carpal fracture-dislocations or subluxations.[61,132,135]
- In a retrospective review of patients treated for axial carpal disruptions at the Mayo Clinic over a 15-year

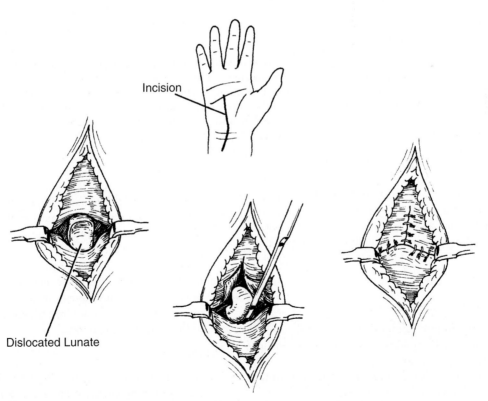

Figure 10–47:
Extended carpal tunnel release incision provides exposure to reduce the volarly displaced lunate. A small elevator is used to reduce the lunate, and the rent in the palmar capsule is repaired with sutures. (From Fractures and dislocation of the carpus. In Trumble TE, editor: *Principles of hand surgery and therapy.* Philadelphia, 2000, WB Saunders.)

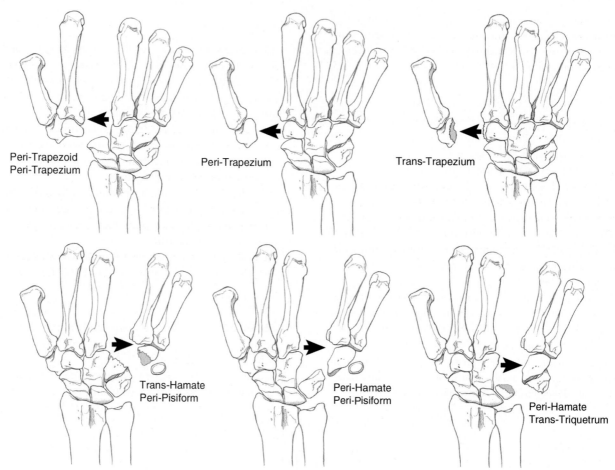

Peri-Trapezoid
Peri-Trapezium

Peri-Trapezium

Trans-Trapezium

Trans-Hamate
Peri-Pisiform

Peri-Hamate
Peri-Pisiform

Peri-Hamate
Trans-Triquetrum

Figure 10–48:
There are three types of axial carpal dislocations: (1) axial-radial dislocations, where the radial part of the carpus is dislocated and unstable; (2) axial-ulnar dislocations, where the ulnar part of the carpus is dislocated and unstable; and (3) a combined axial-radial-ulnar dislocation, in which both types of dislocation coexist in the same wrist. Of the axial-radial dislocations, several patterns of dislocation/fractures exist **(top row)**. Similarly, a variety of patterns of axial-ulnar dislocation/fractures also exist **(bottom row)**. (Copyright Mayo Clinic. Reproduced with permission of the Mayo Foundation.)

period, Garcia-Elias et al.[61] identified 16 patients of 1140 patients with carpal injuries (1.4%).

- With the increasing awareness of axial carpal disruptions and the increasing frequency of industrial accidents, the reported frequency of axial disruptions of the carpus has increased.

## Mechanism of Injuries

- The typical mechanism of injury of axial carpal disruptions is a crush (molding press, roller press, wringer machine), twisting, or blast injury.
- As such, a majority of axial dislocation of the carpus have been industrial injuries.[61,132,135]
- The most common mechanism of injury has resulted from a dorsopalmar compression or crush of the wrist.[9,61,132,136,137]

- With sufficient dorsopalmar force applied to the entire wrist, the bones involved in axial carpal disruption either dislocate or sustain sagittal fractures, depending on the obliquity of the force applied and the plane of the intercarpal joints. The more parallel the intercarpal joint to the direction of force, the increased likelihood for dislocation. With increasing obliquity of the intercarpal joint to the direction of force, the likelihood of fracture in the sagittal plane increases.

## Diagnosis

- A majority of axial carpal dislocations result from high-energy injuries and often present with significant associated soft tissue damage. The severity of associated injuries is directly related to the mechanism of injury and degree of energy imparted.

- The spectrum of soft tissue injury can range from swelling with tenderness to total denudation of the hand.
- Typically, axial disruptions of the carpus have with a dramatic appearance, with massive swelling and tenderness over the entire hand and wrist.
  - With increasing severity of injury, thenar and intrinsic muscles often are severely damaged, flexor and extensor tendons are disrupted, and neurovascular injuries often are present.
  - Vascular injures, with disruption of the radial, ulnar, or both arteries, are not frequent.
  - Nerve injuries are common and can range from transient neuropraxia to axonotmesis. Acute carpal tunnel syndrome is infrequent and most likely is secondary to the traumatic decompression of the carpal canal that occurs with discontinuity of the flexor retinaculum.
  - Associated fractures of the metacarpals, carpometacarpal joint, carpals, and distal radius and ulna frequently are associated with axial dislocation.
- Axial carpal sprains are injuries to the intercarpal ligaments along the longitudinal axis of the carpus and often present as chronic wrist pain. The hallmark of axial carpal dynamic instability of the capitohamate articulation is the arthroscopic finding of diastasis between the capitate and hamate. Normally this articulation does not allow placement of an arthroscopic probe between the capitate and hamate.

## Treatment

- Surgical treatment of axial carpal dislocations often is directed toward treatment of the soft tissues that result from the high-energy crush or blast (Figure 10–49).
- Initial evaluation of these injures must include a thorough assessment of the neurovascular and musculotendinous status of the extremity.
- Early and accurate diagnosis of the soft tissue and bony injuries are essential, because delayed treatment because of inaccurate diagnosis is much less successful compared to early treatment.
- Fasciotomies of the intrinsic and/or forearm compartments should be performed if compartment syndrome is suspected or present.
- Closed reduction with percutaneous fixation of the dislocated and/or fractured carpal bones may be successful; however, interposed soft tissue or bone fragments often preclude an anatomic reduction. In such cases, open reduction is indicated.
- Surgical treatment should be directed at debridement of devitalized tissue, open reduction and percutaneous fixation with K-wires, primary repair or grafting of damaged tendons and/or neurovascular structures, and

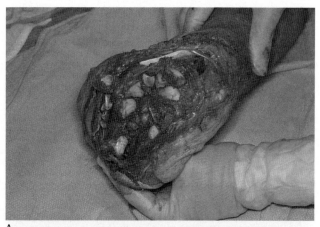

A

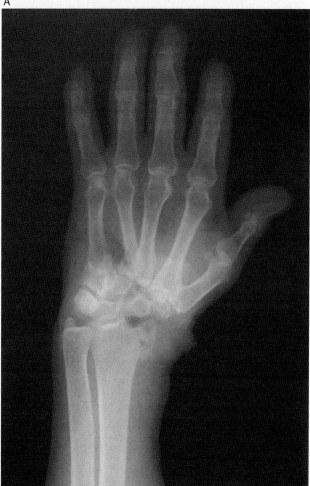

B

Figure 10–49:

High-energy crush injuries result in axial carpal dislocations and fractures and often are open injuries. **A,** Clinical photograph of the injury demonstrates the high-energy trauma that resulted in complete dissociation of the carpometacarpal joints and intercarpal ligaments. **B,** Posteroanterior radiograph of the open axial carpal dislocation. (Copyright Mayo Foundation 2003.)

immediate skin coverage with the local tissues or with local or free tissue flaps.

- A dorsal longitudinal approach is used for direct carpal reduction, and a palmar extended approach is used to evaluated the soft tissues.
- Carpal alignment should be obtained via the dorsal approach, and K-wires are used to stabilize the dislocation.
- Intercarpal ligament repair is seldom possible secondary to the severe damage but occasionally can be performed. In these cases, use of suture anchors is preferred rather than drill holes to minimize trauma to the carpus.
- The volar approach allows for evaluation of the neurovascular and musculotendinous structures and of the carpal canal. If not already decompressed traumatically, a prophylactic carpal tunnel release can be performed. Primary repair or grafting of all damages structures is recommended, followed by immediate wound coverage with loosely sutured skin or with local or distant flaps.
- The ultimate outcome and functional results of treatment depend more on the associated injuries than on the carpal disruption.[61] Lower-energy injuries with fewer associated injuries had better functional outcome than did the high-energy injuries with significant soft tissue damage.
  - In the Mayo Clinic series,[61] more severe soft tissue injuries were present, and only four of 13 patients had a good result, five had a fair result, and four had a poor result. Nerve injury was the most predictable factor in determining outcome, as was an axial-ulnar type of injury.

## Isolated Carpal Bone Dislocations

- Isolated carpal bone dislocations are relatively rare and typically are caused by localized direct or indirect concentrated force over a singe area of the wrist. Reports for each carpal bone exist, and detailing each one is beyond the scope of this chapter.[138–152] With the exception of the lunate and scaphoid, removal of the dislocated bone does not cause significant carpal dysfunction and is well tolerated.

## References

1. Linscheid RL, Dobyns JH, Beabout JW et al: Traumatic instability of the wrist. Diagnosis, classification and pathomechanics. *J Bone Joint Surg* 54A:1612-1632, 1972.
   This article is the first to define DISI and VISI of the wrist. The article helps establish the scaphoid as a mechanical link that stabilizes the intercarpal joints during motion of the wrist.

2. Brown DE, Lichtman DM: Midcarpal instability. *Hand Clin* 3:135-140, 1987.

3. Brown IW: Volar intercalary carpal instability following a seemingly innocent wrist fracture. *J Hand Surg [Br]* 12:54-56, 1987.

4. Cooney WPd, Linscheid RL, Dobyns JH: Carpal instability: treatment of ligament injuries of the wrist. *Instr Course Lect* 41:33-44, 1992.

5. Cooney WP, Dobyns JH, Linscheid RL: Arthroscopy of the wrist: anatomy and classification of carpal instability. *Arthroscopy* 6:133-140, 1990.

6. Culver JE: Instabilities of the wrist. *Clin Sports Med* 5:725-740, 1986.

7. Doig SG, Rao SG, Carvell JE: Late carpal instability associated with dorsal distal radial fracture. *Injury* 22:486-488, 1991.

8. Dunn AW: Fractures and dislocations of the carpus. *Surg Clin North Am* 52:1513-1538, 1972.

9. Garcia-Elias M, Bishop AT, Dobyns JH et al: Transcarpal carpometacarpal dislocations, excluding the thumb. *J Hand Surg [Am]* 15:531-540, 1990.

10. Howard FM, Lichtman DM, Taleisnik J et al: Symposium on carpal instability. *Contemp Orthop* 4:107-144, 1982.

11. Johnson RP, Carrera GF: Chronic capitolunate instability. *J Bone Joint Surg [Am]* 68:1164-1176, 1986.

12. Lichtman DM, Schneider JR, Swafford AR et al: Ulnar midcarpal instability: clinical and laboratory analysis. *J Hand Surg* 6A:516-523, 1981.

13. Lichtman DM, Noble WH, Alexander CE: Dynamic triquetrolunate instability: case report. *J Hand Surg* 9A:185-187, 1984.

14. Lichtman DM, Bruckner JD, Culp RW et al: Palmar midcarpal instability: results of surgical reconstruction. *J Hand Surg [Am]* 18:307-315, 1993.

15. Linscheid RL, Dobyns JH, Beckenbaugh RD et al: Instability patterns of the wrist. *J Hand Surg [Am]* 8:682-686, 1983.
    Explains why DISI and VISI collapse patterns occur. The scaphoid tends to flex, which pulls the lunate with it if the LT ligament has been interrupted. Conversely, the lunate and triquetrum extend if the SL ligament has been disrupted.

16. Linscheid RL, Dobyns JH: The unified concept of carpal injuries. *Ann Chir Main* 3:35-42, 1984.
    A spectrum of intercarpal ligamentous injuries is explained using a unified concept of carpal collapse following ligamentous and bony injury.

17. Linscheid RL, Dobyns JH: Athletic injuries of the wrist. *Clin Orthop* 198:141-151, 1985.

18. Logan SE, Nowak MD: Intrinsic and extrinsic wrist ligaments: biomechanical and functional differences. *ISA Trans* 27:37-41, 1988.

19. Louis DS, Hankin FM, Bowers WH: Capitate-radius arthrodesis: an alternative method of radiocarpal arthrodesis. *J Hand Surg [Am]* 9:365-369, 1984.

20. Mayfield JK: Patterns of injury to carpal ligaments: a spectrum. *Clin Orthop* 187:36-42, 1984.

21. Taleisnik J, Malerich M, Prietto M: Palmar carpal instability secondary to dislocation of scaphoid and lunate: report of

case and review of the literature. *J Hand Surg* 7A:606-612, 1982.

22. Taleisnik J: Triquetrohamate and triquetrolunate instabilities (medial carpal instability). *Ann Chir Main* 3:331-343, 1984.

23. Taleisnik J, Watson HK: Midcarpal instability caused by malunited fractures of the distal radius. *J Hand Surg [Am]* 9:350-357, 1984.

24. Taleisnik J: Current concepts review. Carpal instability. *J Bone Joint Surg [Am]* 70:1262-1268, 1988.

25. Taleisnik J, Linscheid RL: Scapholunate instability. In Cooney WP, Linscheid RL, Dobyns JH, editors: The wrist: diagnosis and operative treatment, vol 1. St. Louis, 1998, Mosby.

26. Viegas SF, Patterson RM, Peterson PD et al: Ulnar sided perilunate instability: an anatomic and biomechanic study. *J Hand Surg* 15A:268-278, 1990.

27. Watson HK, Black DM: Instabilities of the wrist. *Hand Clin* 3:103-111, 1987.

28. Weber ERA: Wrist mechanics and its association with ligamentous instability. In Lichtman DM, editor: *The wrist and its disorders.* Philadelphia, 1988, WB Saunders.

29. Wright TW, Dobyns JH, Linscheid RL et al: Carpal instability non-dissociative. *J Hand Surg [Br]* 19:763-773, 1994.

30. Berger RA, Landsmeer JM: The palmar radiocarpal ligaments: a study of adult and fetal human wrist joints. *J Hand Surg [Am]* 15:847-854, 1990.

31. Berger RA: The anatomy of the ligaments of the wrist and distal radioulnar joints. *Clin Orthop* 383: 32-40, 2001.

32. Berger RA: The ligaments of the wrist. A current overview of anatomy with considerations of their potential functions. *Hand Clin* 13:63-82, 1997.

33. Ritt MJ, Berger RA, Kauer JM: The gross and histologic anatomy of the ligaments of the capitohamate joint. *J Hand Surg [Am]* 21:1022-1028, 1996.

34. Berger RA: The anatomy and basic biomechanics of the wrist joint. *J Hand Ther* 9:84-93, 1996.

35. Landsmeer JM: Studies in the anatomy of the carpus and its bearing on some surgical problem. *Acta Morphol Neederl-Scand* 3:304-321, 1960.

36. Berger RA, Crowninshield RD, Flatt AE: The three-dimensional rotational behavior of the carpal bones. *Clin Orthop* 167:303-310, 1982.

37. de Lange A, Kauer JM, Huiskes R: Kinematic behavior of the human wrist joint: a roentgen-stereophotogrammetric analysis. *J Orthop Res* 3:56-64, 1985.

38. Savelberg HH, Kooloos JG, de Lange A et al: Human carpal ligament recruitment and three dimensional carpal motion. *J Orthop Res* 9:693-704, 1991.

39. Kauer JM: The mechanics of the carpal joint. *Clin Orthop* 202:16-26, 1986.

40. Horii E, Garcia Elias M, An KN et al: A kinematic study of luno-triquetral dissociations. *J Hand Surg* 16A:355-362, 1991.

41. Ruby LK, Cooney WP, An KN et al: Relative motion of selected carpal bones: a kinematic analysis of the normal wrist. *J Hand Surg* 13:1-10, 1988.

42. Sennwald GR, Zdravkovic V, Jacob HA et al: Kinematic analysis of relative motion within the proximal carpal row. *J Hand Surg [Br]* 18:609-612, 1993.

43. Garcia Elias M, Cooney WP, An KN et al: Wrist kinematics after limited intercarpal arthrodesis. *J Hand Surg* 14:791-799, 1989.

44. Sarrafian SK, Melamed JL, Goshgarian GM: Study of wrist motion in flexion and extension. *Clin Orthop* 126:153-159, 1977.

45. Wolfe SW, Neu CP, Crisco JJ: In vivo scaphoid, lunate and capitate kinematics in wrist flexion and extension. *J Hand Surg* 25:860-869, 2000.

46. Brahin B, Allieu Y: [Compensatory carpal malalignments]. *Ann Chir Main* 3:357-363, 1984.

47. Allieu Y, Brahin B, Ascencio G: Carpal instabilities: Radiological and clinico-pathological classification. *Ann Radiol* 25: 275-287, 1982.

48. Cooney WP, Linscheid RL, Dobyns JH: Fractures and dislocations of the wrist. In Rockwood CA, Green DP, Bucholz RW, et al., editors: *Rockwood and Green's fractures in adults,* ed 4. Philadelphia, 1996, Lippincott-Raven.

49. Gilford WW, Bolton RH, Lambrinudi C: The mechanism of the wrist joint with special reference to fractures of the scaphoid. *Gu's Hosp Rep* 92:52-59, 1943.

50. Palmer AK, Werner RW: Biomechanics of the distal radioulnar joint. *Clin Orthop* 187:26-35, 1984.

51. Viegas SF, Patterson R, Todd PD et al: Load mechanics of the midcarpal joint. *J Hand Surg* 18:14-28, 1993.

52. Nowalk MD, Logan SE: Distinguishing biomechanical properties of intrinsic and extrinsic human wrist ligaments. *J Biomech Eng* 113:85-93, 1991.

53. Berger RA: The gross and histologic anatomy of the scapholunate interosseous ligament. *J Hand Surg* 21A:170-178, 1996.
This article provides a detailed analysis of the SL ligament. The ligament can be divided into three parts; the thickest portion is dorsal.

54. Drewniany JJ, Palmer AK, Flatt AE: The scaphotrapezial ligament complex: an anatomic and biomechanical study. *J Hand Surg* 10:492-498, 1985.

55. Mayfield JK, Williams WJ, Erdman AG et al: Biomechanical properties of human carpal ligaments. *Orthop Trans* 3:143-144, 1979.

56. Hodge JC, Gilula LA, Larsen CF et al: Analysis of carpal instability: II. Clinical applications. *J Hand Surg [Am]* 20:765-776; discussion 20:777, 1995.

57. Larsen CF, Amadio PC, Gilula LA et al: Analysis of carpal instability: I. Description of the scheme. *J Hand Surg [Am]* 20:757-764, 1995.

58. Watson H, Ottoni L, Pitts EC et al: Rotary subluxation of the scaphoid: a spectrum of instability. *J Hand Surg [Br]* 18:62-64, 1993.
Rotary subluxation of the scaphoid is not an "all or nothing" phenomenon but a spectrum of instability. Twenty-one percent of normal subjects were found to have an abnormal difference in mobility between their scaphoids.

59. Amadio PC: Carpal kinematics and instability: a clinical and anatomic primer. *Clin Anat* 4:1-12, 1991.

60. Dobyns JH, Cooney WP: Classification of carpal instability. In Cooney WP, Linscheid RL, Dobyns JH, editors: *The wrist: diagnosis and operative treatment,* vol I. St. Louis, 1997, Mosby.

61. Garcia-Elias M, Dobyns JH, Cooney WP, 3rd et al: Traumatic axial dislocations of the carpus. *J Hand Surg [Am]* 14:446-457, 1989.

62. Mayfield JK, Johnson RP, Kilcoyne RK: Pathomechanics and progressive perilunar instability. *J Hand Surg* 5A:226-241, 1980.
This classic cadaver study attempts to identify the pathomechanics involved in perilunate and lunate dislocations. The mechanism of injury identified was extension, ulnar deviation, and intercarpal supination. The stages of perilunar instability were defined.

63. Palmer CG, Murray PM, Snearly WN: The mechanism of ulnar-sided perilunar instability of the wrist (abstr CS 24). American Society for Surgery of the Hand 53rd Annual Meeting, Minneapolis, Minnesota.

64. Reagan DS, Linscheid RL, Dobyns JH: Lunotriquetral sprains. *J Hand Surg* 9A:502-514, 1984.

65. Gilula LA: Carpal injuries: analytic approach and case exercises. *AJR Am J Roentgenol* 133:503-517, 1979.

66. Metz VM, Mann FA, Gilula LA: Lack of correlation between site of wrist pain and location of noncommunicating defects shown by three-compartment wrist arthrography. *AJR Am J Roentgenol* 160:1239-1243, 1993.

67. Metz VM, Mann FA, Gilula LA: Three-compartment wrist arthrography: correlation of pain site with location of uni- and bidirectional communications. *AJR Am J Roentgenol* 160:819-822, 1993.

68. Kirschenbaum D, Sieler S, Solonick D et al: Arthrography of the wrist. Assessment of the integrity of the ligaments in young asymptomatic adults. *J Bone Joint Surg* 77A:1207-1209, 1995.

69. Yin YM, Evanoff B, Gilula LA et al: Evaluation of selective wrist arthography of contralateral asymptomatic wrists for symmetric ligamentous defects. *AJR Am J Roentgenol* 166:1067-1073, 1996.

70. Shin AY, Glowacki KA, Bishop AT: Dynamic axial carpal instability: a case report. *J Hand Surg [Am]* 24:781-785, 1999.

71. Watson HK, Ashmead DT, Makhlouf MV: Examination of the scaphoid. *J Hand Surg* 13:657-660, 1988.
A review of the anatomic basis, performance, interpretation, and utility of the "scaphoid shift" in assessing scaphoid pathology.

72. Wolfe SW: Scapholunate instability. *J Am Soc Surg Hand* 1:45-60, 2001.

73. Meade TD, Schneider LH, Cherry K: Radiographic analysis of selective ligament sectioning at the carpal scaphoid: a cadaver study. *J Hand Surg* 15:855-862, 1990.

74. Geissler WB, Freeland AE, Savoie FH et al: Intracarpal soft-tissue lesions associated with an intra-articular fracture of the distal end of the radius. *J Bone Joint Surg Am* 78:357-365, 1996.

75. Nathan R, Blatt G: Rotary subluxation of the scaphoid revisited. *Hand Clin* 16:417-431, 2000.

76. Stanley JK, Saffar P: Abnormal findings. In Stanley JK, Saffar P, editors: *Wrist arthroscopy.* London, 1994, Martin Dunitz.

77. Deshmukh SC, Givissis P, Belloso D et al: Blatt's capsulodesis for chronic scapholunate dissociation. *J Hand Surg [Br]* 24:215-220, 1999.

78. Berger RA, Bishop AT, Bettinger PC: New dorsal capsulotomy for the surgical exposure of the wrist. *Ann Plast Surg* 35:54-59, 1995.

79. Lavernia CJ, Cohen MS, Taleisnik J: Treatment of scapholunate dissociation by ligamentous repair and capsulodesis. *J Hand Surg [Am]* 17:354-359, 1992.

80. Wintman BI, Gelberman RH, Katz JN: Dynamic scapholunate instability: results of operative treatment with dorsal capsulodesis. *J Hand Surg [Am]* 20:971-979, 1995.

81. Blatt G: Capsulodesis in reconstructive hand surgery. Dorsal capsulodesis for the unstable scaphoid and volar capsulodesis following excision of the distal ulna. *Hand Clin* 3:81-102, 1987.

82. Walsh JJ, Berger RA, Cooney WP: Current status of scapholunate interosseous ligament injuries. *J Am Acad Orthop Surg* 10:32-42, 2002.

83. Slater RR, Szabo RM, Bay BK et al: Dorsal intercarpal ligament capsulodesis for scapholunate dissociation: biomechanical analysis in a cadaver model. *J Hand Surg [Am]* 24A, 1999.
Dorsal intercarpal ligament capsulodesis reduced SL gap formation more than the Blatt capsulodesis and may provide improved motion because it does not cross the radiocarpal joint.

84. Szabo RM, Slater RR, Palumbo CF et al: Dorsal intercarpal ligament capsulodesis for chronic, static scapholunate dissociation: clinical results. *J Hand Surg [Am]* 27A:978-984, 2002.

85. Brunelli GA, Brunelli GR: A new technique to correct carpal instability with scaphoid rotary subluxation: a preliminary report. *J Hand Surg [Am]* 20:S82-85, 1995.

86. Wolf JM, Weiss AP: Bone-retinaculum-bone reconstruction of scapholunate ligament injuries. *Orthop Clin North Am* 32:241-246, 2001.

87. Weiss AP: Scapholunate ligament reconstruction using a bone-retinaculum-bone autograft. *J Hand Surg* 23:205-215, 1998.

Reports 13 of 19 patients were completely satisfied at 3.6-year follow-up after SL ligament reconstruction using an autogenous bone-retinaculum-bone graft.

88. Watson HK, Hempton RF: Limited wrist arthrodeses. I. The triscaphoid joint. *J Hand Surg [Am]* 5:320-327, 1980. The author reviews his first 36 limited wrist arthrodeses. Fourteen of these procedures were "triscaphe" arthrodeses.

89. Watson HK, Ryu J, Akelman E: Limited triscaphoid intercarpal arthrodesis for rotary subluxation of the scaphoid. *J Bone Joint Surg Am* 68A:345-349, 1986.

90. Watson HK, Belniak R, Garcia-Elias M: Treatment of scapholunate dissociation: preferred treatment—STT fusion vs other methods. *Orthopedics* 14:365-368; discussion 14:368-370, 1991.

91. Kleinman WB, Steichen JB, Strickland JW: Management of chronic rotary subluxation of the scaphoid by scapho-trapezio-trapezoid arthrodesis. *J Hand Surg [Am]* 7:125-136, 1982.

92. Kleinman WB: Long-term study of chronic scapho-lunate instability treated by scapho-trapezio-trapezoid arthrodesis. *J Hand Surg [Am]* 14:429-445, 1989.

93. Kleinman WB, Carroll C: Scapho-trapezio-trapezoid arthrodesis for treatment of chronic static and dynamic scapho-lunate instability: a 10-year perspective on pitfalls and complications. *J Hand Surg [Am]* 15:408-414, 1990.

94. Hom S, Ruby LK: Attempted scapholunate arthrodesis for chronic scapholunate dissociation. *J Hand Surg [Am]* 16:334-339, 1991.

95. Ambrose L, Posner MA, Green SM, et al: The effects of scaphoid intercarpal stabilization on wrist mechanics: An experimental study. *J Hand Surg* 17:429-437, 1992. Scaphoid fusion performed with the scaphoid in a vertical position resulted in decreased wrist flexion and ulnar deviation. Fusion of the scaphoid in a horizontal position decreased wrist extension and radial deviation. With the scaphoid in its anatomic position, both STT and SC stabilizations resulted in similar motion.

96. Chaput, Vaillant: Etude radiographique sur les traumatismes du carpe. *Rev Orthop* 4:227, 1913.

97. von Mayersbach L: Ein seltener Fall von Luxation Intercarpea. *Dtsch Z Chir* 123:179, 1913.

98. Hessert W: Dislocation of the individual carpal bones, with report of a case of luxation of the scaphoid and semilunar. *Ann Surg* 37:402-413, 1903.

99. Shin AY, Bishop AT: Treatment options for lunotriquetral dissociation. *Tech Hand Upper Extremity Surg* 2:2-17, 1998.

100. Shin AY, Battaglia MJ, Bishop AT: Lunotriquetral instability: diagnosis and treatment. *J Am Acad Orthop Surg* 8:170-179, 2000.

101. Shin AY, Weinstein LP, Berger RA, Bishop AT: Treatment of isolated injuries of the lunotriquetral ligament. A comparison of arthrodesis, ligament reconstruction and ligament repair. *J Bone Joint Surg Br* 83:1023-1028, 2001.

The probability of remaining free from complications at 5 years was 68.6% for reconstruction, 13.5% for repair, and less than 1% for arthrodesis. Of the lunotriquetral arthrodeses, 40.9% developed nonunion and 22.7% developed ulnocarpal impaction. Results were significantly better for lunotriquetral repair and reconstruction compared to arthrodesis.

102. Ritt MJPF, Bishop AT, Berger RA et al: Lunotriquetral ligament properties: a comparison of three anatomic subregions. *J Hand Surg* 23A:425-431, 1998.

103. Ritt MJPF, Linscheid RL, Cooney WP et al: The lunotriquetral joint: kinematic effects of sequential ligament sectioning, ligament repair and arthrodesis. *J Hand Surg* 23A:432-445, 1998.

104. Trumble TE, Bour CJ, Smith RJ et al: Kinematics of the ulnar carpus related to the volar intercalated segment instability pattern. *J Hand Surg* 15A:384-392, 1990.

105. Beckenbaugh RD: Accurate evaluation and management of the painful wrist following injury. *Othop Clin* 15:289-306, 1984.

106. Kleinman WB: Diagnostic exams for ligamentous injuries. American Society for Surgery of the Hand, Correspondence Club Newsletter No. 51, 1985.

107. Trumble T, Bour CJ, Smith RJ et al: Intercarpal arthrodesis for static and dynamic volar intercalated segment instability. *J Hand Surg* 13A:384-390, 1988.

108. Alexander CE, Lichtman DM: Ulnar carpal instabilities. *Orthop Clin North Am* 15:307-320, 1984.

109. Gilula LA, Weeks PM: Post-traumatic ligamentous instabilities of the wrist. *Radiology* 129:641-651, 1978.

110. Favero KJ, Bishop AT, Linscheid RL: Lunotriquetral ligament disruption: A comparative study of treatment methods (abstract SS-80). American Society for Surgery of the Hand. 46th Annual Meeting, Orlando, Florida.

111. Kirschenbaum D, Coyle MP, Leddy JP: Chronic lunotriquetral instability: diagnosis and treatment. *J Hand Surg* 18A:1107-1112, 1993.

112. McAuliffe JA, Dell PC, Jaffe R: Complications of intercarpal arthrodesis. *J Hand Surg* 18A:1121-1128, 1993.

113. Nelson DL, Manske PR, Pruitt DL et al: Lunotriquetral arthrodesis. *J Hand Surg* 18A:1113-1120, 1993.

114. Martini AK, Cotta H: [Instability of the wrist joint—diagnosis and therapy]. *Aktuelle Traumatol* 19:287-293, 1989.

115. Sennwald GR, Fischer M, Mondi P: Lunotriquetral arthrodesis. A controversial procedure. *J Hand Surg* 20B:755-760, 1995.

116. Dobyns JH, Linscheid RL, Chao EY et al: Traumatic instability of the wrist. *Instr Course Lect* 24:189-199, 1975.

117. Taleisnik J: *The wrist*. New York, 1985, Churchill Livingstone.

118. Taleisnik J: Wrist: anatomy, function, injury. *Instr Course Lect* 27:61-68, 1978.

119. Rayhack JM, Linscheid RL Dobyns JH et al: Posttraumatic ulnar translation of the carpus. *J Hand Surg [Am]* 12:180-189, 1987.

120. Dumontier C, Lenoble E, Saffar P: Radiocarpal dislocations and fracture-dislocations. In Saffar P, Cooney WP, editors: *Fractures of the distal radius.* London, 1995, Martin Dunitz.

121. Dumontier C, Meyer zu Reckendorf G, Sautet A et al: Radiocarpal dislocations: classification and proposal for treatment. A review of twenty-seven cases. *J Bone Joint Surg Am* 83-A:212-218, 2001.

122. Louis DS, Hankin FM, Greene TL et al: Central carpal instability-capitate lunate instability pattern. Diagnosis by dynamic displacement. *Orthopedics* 7:1693-1696, 1984.

123. Hankin FM, Amadio PC, Wojtys EM et al: Carpal instability with volar flexion of the proximal row associated with injury to the scapho-trapezial ligament: report of two cases. *J Hand Surg [Br]* 13:298-302, 1988.

124. Garth WP, Jr., Hofammann DY, Rooks MD: Volar intercalated segment instability secondary to medial carpal ligamental laxity. *Clin Orthop* 201:94-105, 1985.

125. Taleisnik J: Radiolunate arthrodesis. In Blair WF, editor: *Techniques in hand surgery.* Baltimore, 1996, Williams & Wilkins.

126. Herzberg G, Comtet JJ, Linscheid RL et al: Perilunate dislocations and fracture-dislocations: a multicenter study. *J Hand Surg Am* 18:768-779, 1993.
Open injuries and a delay in treatment resulted in poorer outcomes. The incidence of posttraumatic arthritis was 56%. The best radiographic results were observed after open reduction internal fixation.

127. Siegert J, Frassica FJ, Amadio PC: Treatment of chronic perilunate dislocations. *J Hand Surg* 13:206-212, 1988.

128. Inoue G, Shionoya K: Late treatment of unreduced perilunate dislocations. *J Hand Surg Br* 24:221-225, 1999.

129. Norbeck DE Jr, Larson B, Blair SJ et al: Traumatic longitudinal disruption of the carpus. *J Hand Surg [Am]* 12:509-514, 1987.

130. Cooney WP, Bussey R, Dobyns JH, Linscheid RL: Difficult wrist fractures. Perilunate fracture-dislocations of the wrist. *Clin Orthop* 214:136-147, 1987.

131. Green DP, O'Brien ET: Open reduction of carpal dislocations: indications and operative techniques. *J Hand Surg [Am]* 3:250-265, 1978.

132. Garcia-Elias M, Abanco J, Salvador E et al: Crush injury of the carpus. *J Bone Joint Surg Br* 67:286-289, 1985.

133. Primiano GA, Reef TC: Disruption of the proximal carpal arch of the hand. *J Bone Joint Surg Am* 56:328-332, 1974.

134. Shin AY, Glowacki KA, Bishop AT: Dynamic axial carpal instability. *J Hand Surg [Am]* 25:371-372, 2000.

135. Chow SP, So YC, Pun WK et al: Thenar crush injuries. *J Bone Joint Surg Br* 70:135-139, 1988.

136. Garcia-Elias M, An KN, Cooney WP, 3rd et al: Stability of the transverse carpal arch: an experimental study. *J Hand Surg [Am]* 14:277-282, 1989.

137. Garcia-Elias M, An KN, Cooney WP et al: Transverse stability of the carpus. An analytical study. *J Orthop Res* 7:738-743, 1989.

138. Cherif MR, Ben Ghozlen R, Chehimi A et al: [Isolated dislocation of the carpal scaphoid. A case report with review of the literature]. *Chir Main* 21:305-308, 2002.

139. Kubiak R, Slongo T, Tschappeler H: Isolated dislocation of the pisiform: an unusual injury during a cartwheel maneuver. *J Trauma* 51:788-789, 2001.

140. Zieren J, Agnes A, Muller JM: Isolated dislocation of the hamate bone. Case report and review of the literature. *Arch Orthop Trauma Surg* 120:535-537, 2000.

141. Yasuda T: Isolated dislocation of the carpal scaphoid: a case report. *Nippon Geka Hokan* 66:59-65, 1997.

142. Cuenod P, Della Santa DR: Open dislocation of the trapezoid. *J Hand Surg [Br]* 20:185-188, 1995.

143. Frix JM, Levine MI: Isolated dorsal dislocation of the trapezoid. *Orthop Rev* 22:1329-1331, 1993.

144. Demartin F, Quinto O: Isolated dislocation of the pisiform. A case report. *Chir Organi Mov* 78:121-123, 1993.

145. De Tullio V, Celenza M: Isolated palmar dislocation of the trapezoid. *Int Orthop* 16:53-54, 1992.

146. Inoue G, Maeda N: Isolated dorsal dislocation of the scaphoid. *J Hand Surg [Br]* 15:368-369, 1990.

147. McKie LD, Rocke LG, Taylor TC: Isolated dislocation of the trapezium. *Arch Emerg Med* 5:38-40, 1988.

148. Arnaud JP, Girou P, Mabit C et al: [Luxation of the hamate bone. Apropos of a case with review of the literature]. *Ann Chir Main* 6:222-224, 1987.

149. Amamilo SC, Uppal R, Samuel AW: Isolated dislocation of carpal scaphoid. *J Hand Surg [Br]* 10:385-388, 1985.

150. Kopp JR: Isolated palmar dislocation of the trapezoid. *J Hand Surg [Am]* 10:91-93, 1985.

151. Meyn MA, Jr., Roth AM: Isolated dislocation of the trapezoid bone. *J Hand Surg [Am]* 5:602-604, 1980.

152. Sundaram M, Shively R, Patel B et al: Isolated dislocation of the pisiform. *Br J Radiol* 53:911-912, 1980.

# Osteonecrosis of the Carpus

Christopher Allan

MD, Assistant Professor, Hand and Microvascular Surgery, Department of Orthopaedics,
University of Washington; Attending, Harborview Medical Center, Department of
Orthopaedics, Seattle, WA

## Introduction

- Osteonecrosis, or avascular necrosis (AVN), of the carpal bones without a known cause (idiopathic) is rare.
- Lunate AVN (Kienböck's disease) is the most common type of idiopathic carpal AVN.
- Scaphoid AVN not related to fracture (Preiser's disease) is much less common.[1] Idiopathic AVN of the remaining carpal bones is even more rare. Principles described here for the lunate are generally applicable to AVN of other carpal bones.
- The etiology of carpal AVN often is unclear. Trauma may be involved but usually is not obvious.
- Disease progression involves fragmentation and collapse of the affected carpal bones, loss of carpal height, and progression of arthritis eventually involving the entire wrist. Treatment is based on the patient's symptoms and the stage of the disease and attempts (in early stages) to revascularize the bone or (in later stages) to arrest progression of carpal collapse.

## Etiology

- Kienböck's disease occurs most commonly in individuals aged 20 to 40 years and is more frequent in males.[2] It is rarely bilateral. A history of trauma is frequently present. Symptoms include pain over the dorsum of the wrist in the region of the lunate, increasing reactive synovitis and swelling, weakness of grip, pain with motion and eventually at rest, and progressive limitation of wrist motion.

- Isolated or repetitive trauma to a lunate predisposed to injury because of any of several factors (bony geometry, vascularity) may lead to a fracture or vascular compromise. Bone necrosis resulting from diminished blood supply results in trabecular fractures, sclerosis, fragmentation, and collapse of the lunate. Carpal height decreases, the capitate migrates proximally, and the scaphoid hyperflexes, leading to degenerative changes in the radiocarpal joint and throughout the wrist.
- The etiology of Kienböck's disease probably is multifactorial. Abnormalities in blood supply may be a primary factor. The majority of cadaveric specimens receive multiple contributions from both dorsal and palmar branches. However, the lunate was supplied by only a single palmar artery in 7% of wrists in one study and 26% in another study. In addition, intraosseous branching patterns vary; 31% of specimens show a single path through the bone without significant arborization (Figure 11–1).[3]
- A lunate with a single vessel and minimal branching may be at greater risk for AVN following hyperflexion or hyperextension injuries or perhaps following a minimally displaced fracture.
- Severe injuries such as lunate dislocation result in only a transient appearance of AVN, probably because the lunate usually dislocates palmarly, with a flap of vascularized palmar tissue still attached.
- Venous stasis may be a factor. In one study, in vitro intraosseous pressure measurements within normal and

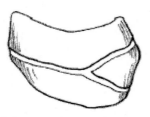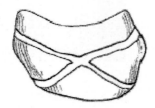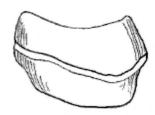

Figure 11–1:

**Three types of vascular branching patterns within lunate. (From Allan CH, Trumble TE: Kienböck's disease. In Trumble TE, editor: *Principles of hand surgery and therapy.* Philadelphia, 2000, WB Saunders.)**

necrotic lunates showed markedly increased pressure in the necrotic bones.[4]

- The geometry of the lunate itself and of surrounding bones may play a role in AVN. Some, but not all, studies have shown negative ulnar variance predisposes to lunate AVN. Negative ulnar variance then may predispose certain patients to development of lunate AVN but likely is not the sole factor.
- Other studies have suggested that a flatter than normal radial inclination predisposes to Kienböck's disease.[5,6] One investigator also noted a tendency toward a smaller lunate in patients with Kienböck's disease.[5]
- Acute trauma is another possible cause of Kienböck disease. An isolated event, such as a fall on the outstretched hand, can compress the lunate between the capitate and the distal radius. Concomitant soft tissue injury may include disruption of the vascular inflow or outflow of the bone.
- Repetitive lesser trauma or multiple cycles of loading may act cumulatively to cause AVN.

## Presentation

- Patients occasionally relate a remote history of trauma, either isolated or repetitive. Symptoms vary depending upon the stage of the disease at presentation and may range from mild discomfort to constant, debilitating pain and a dramatically reduced range of motion.
- Symptoms in stage I resemble intermittent wrist sprains and early nonspecific synovitis, with pain associated with motion, and mild swelling.
- Clinical findings in stage II can include more frequent and severe swelling and discomfort with motion.
- Clinical findings in stage III include progressive stiffness and loss of motion. In stage IIIB, these findings are combined with painful radial instability resulting from flexion malposition of the scaphoid.
- Symptoms in stage IV are similar to those of degenerative arthritis of the wrist, with constant pain either with motion or at rest, chronic swelling, significantly diminished range of motion, and reduced grip strength.

## Physical Examination

- Inspection of the wrist with Kienböck's disease may reveal obvious swelling dorsally.
- Range of motion tends to decrease with increasing stage of Kienböck's disease, first because of swelling and pain and later because of lunate collapse, scaphoid rotation, and arthritic changes.
- As noted in the discussion on presentation, grip strength may be markedly reduced. Swelling over the carpus is common and may occur palmarly and dorsally. Tenderness over the dorsum of the lunate is a frequent finding.
- Pain specifically associated with the scaphoid shift maneuver may be present, beginning with stage IIIa disease, as the scaphoid rotates palmarly.
- Kienböck's disease in its early stages can be difficult to diagnose. Findings of otherwise unexplained mid-dorsal wrist pain, particularly in the younger patient, should suggest further evaluation with magnetic resonance imaging (MRI).

## Radiographic Evaluation and Staging

- Plain x-ray films are obtained if physical examination suggests Kienböck's disease.
- The Lichtman classification uses radiographic criteria to describe disease stage (Box 11–1).
- In stage I Kienböck's disease, plain radiographs either are normal or demonstrate a linear compression fracture without sclerosis or collapse of the lunate (Figure 11–2).
- MRI in stage I disease is suggestive of AVN when uniformly decreased signal intensity (reduced vascularity of the lunate) is noted on T1-weighted images in comparison with the surrounding normal bones (Figure 11–3).
- Partial T1 signal loss also may be seen with ulnar abutment, fractures, enchondromas, and osteoid osteoma. Ulnar

| Box 11–1 | Stages of Kienböck's Disease |
|---|---|
| Stage I | Normal radiographs or linear fracture, abnormal but nonspecific bone scan, diagnostic magnetic resonance appearance (lunate shows low signal intensity on T1-weighted images; lunate may show high or low signal intensity on T2-weighted images, depending on extent of disease process) |
| Stage II | Lunate sclerosis, one or more fracture lines with possible early collapse of lunate on radial border |
| Stage III | Lunate collapse |
| IIIA | Normal carpal alignment and height |
| IIIB | Fixed scaphoid rotation (ring sign), carpal height decreased, capitate migrates proximally |
| Stage IV | Severe lunate collapse with intraarticular degenerative changes at midcarpal joint, radiocarpal joint, or both |

From Allan CH, Joshi A, Lichtman DM: Kienböck's disease: diagnosis and treatment. *J Am Acad Orthop Surg* 9:128-136, 2001.

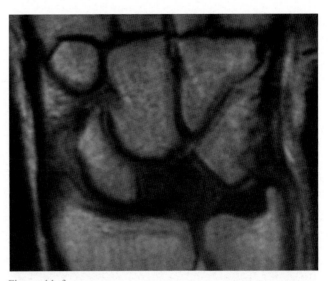

Figure 11–3:
**T1-weighted magnetic resonance image of carpus revealing decreased signal within lunate.**

abutment should be distinguished from Kienböck's disease by the focal proximal and ulnar changes in the lunate resulting from mechanical forces applied to the lunate by the relatively long ulna.

- T2-weighted images typically show low signal intensity in Kienböck's disease but show increased signal in the presence of revascularization.[7] If radiographs are not diagnostic, particularly in stage I, MRI is obtained.
- Stage II Kienböck's disease shows increased radiodensity of the lunate, often with one or more fracture lines (Figure 11–4).
- Lunate height is preserved in stage II disease. Density changes in the lunate often are best appreciated on the lateral plain radiograph (Figure 11–5).
- Stage III is divided into two subcategories. In stage IIIA, lunate collapse has occurred but carpal height is relatively unchanged (Figure 11–6). In stage IIIB, in addition to collapse of the lunate, carpal collapse is apparent, with proximal migration of the capitate and/or fixed hyperflexion of the scaphoid (Figure 11–7). Carpal height is decreased (Figure 11–8).
- Lateral radiographs in stage III disease demonstrate a widened anteroposterior dimension of the lunate and an increased scapholunate angle (Figures 11–9 and 11–10).
- Once the lunate has collapsed, computed tomography (CT) can outline the geometry of the bone for surgical planning.
- Stage IV Kienböck's disease has the findings of stage IIIB disease and degenerative arthritic changes throughout the radiocarpal and/or midcarpal joints.

## Treatment (Box 11–2)

### Stage I

- A trial of immobilization (cast or external fixator) for up to 3 months is appropriate as the first treatment

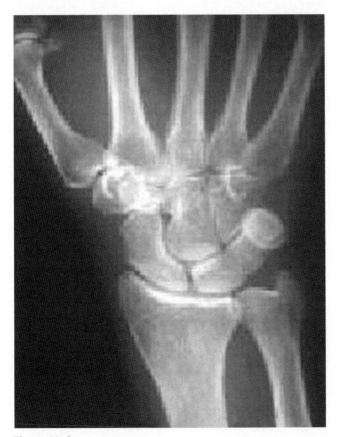

Figure 11–2:
**Stage I Kienböck's disease.**

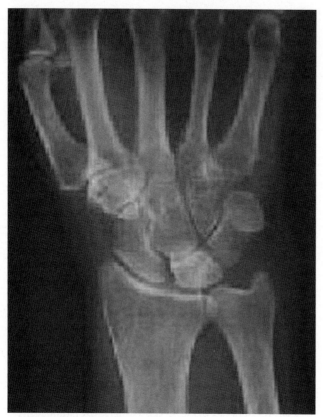

Figure 11–4:
**Stage II Kienböck's disease.**

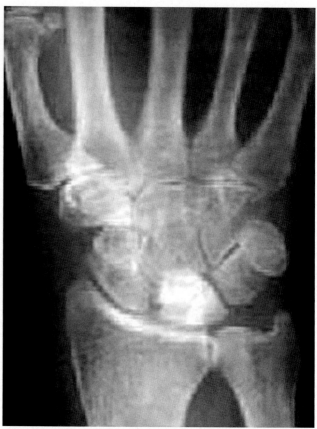

Figure 11–6:
**Stage IIIA Kienböck's disease.**

option in stage I Kienböck's disease. This treatment should allow restoration of vascularity in cases of transient AVN of the lunate. Often, however, the disease progresses.

- In an early series of 22 cases of Kienböck's disease of various stages treated conservatively,[2] 17 showed progression and five showed no improvement.

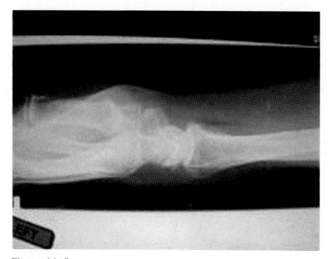

Figure 11–5:
**Stage II Kienböck's disease, lateral view.**

## Stage II or IIIA with Positive Ulnar Variance

- In stage II, lunate avascularity has developed, but the bone has not collapsed, as in stage IIIA. Carpal height is normal. Revascularization procedures (restoring blood supply to the lunate) are most successful in stage II.
- Revascularization can be either direct (via insertion of a vascularized pedicle bone graft into the lunate) or indirect (via unloading of forces across the lunate, through shortening of the capitate or the radius). Direct and indirect methods often are combined.
- Vascularized bone grafts useful in operative procedures to treat lunate AVN can be taken from either the dorsal distal radius or the base of the second or third metacarpal.

## Surgical Technique for Vascularized Bone Graft from the Base of the Second or Third Metacarpal

- This technique takes advantage of the distal vascular arcade or rete over the carpus and allows harvest of a

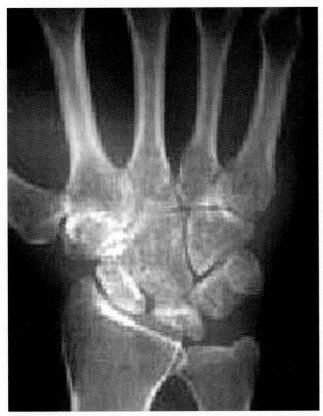

Figure 11–7:
Stage IIIB Kienböck's disease.

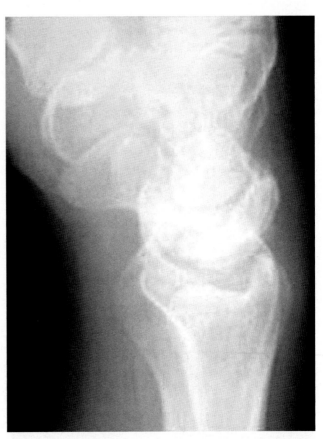

Figure 11–9:
Stage IIIB Kienböck's disease, lateral view.

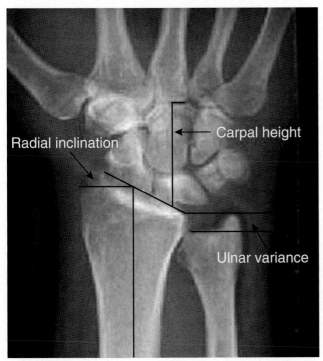

Figure 11–8:
Normal wrist: carpal height, radial inclination, and ulnar variance. (From Allan et al., JAAOS 2001.)

vascularized bone graft and procedures on the carpus (e.g., capitate shortening) through a single midline incision (Figure 11–11).

- Releasing the distal portion of the fourth dorsal compartment exposes the distal vascular arcade. The pedicle can be mobilized to either the ulnar or the radial direction to achieve sufficient length to reach the lunate. The bone graft can be harvested from the base of either the second or third metacarpal, depending on where the artery has the greatest area of contact. The periosteum is incised and included with the bone. A segment of bone several millimeters on a side is harvested from the metacarpal using an osteotome and inserted into a cavity prepared in the lunate using a high-speed burr to perforate the nonarticular surface of the lunate and remove the necrotic bone. The procedure can easily be combined with an unloading procedure such as the capitate shortening procedure.

## Surgical Technique for Vascularized Bone Graft from the Radius

- The incision curves from the dorsal wrist centered over the lunate to the radial border of the distal forearm. The

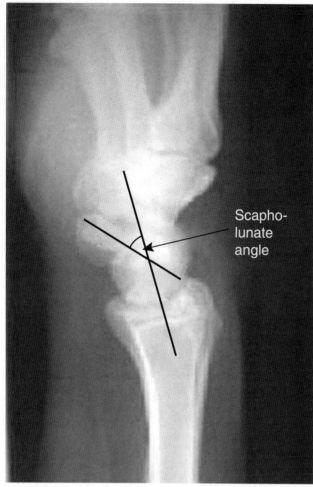

**Figure 11–10:**
**Normal wrist: scapholunate angle measurement. (From Allan CH, Joshi A, Lichtman DM: Kienböck's disease: diagnosis and treatment.** *J Am Acad Orthop Surg* **9:128-136, 2001.)**

| Box 11–2 | Options for Treatment of Kienböck's Disease |
|---|---|

| Stage of Disease | Treatment |
|---|---|
| I | Immobilization (3 months) |
| II or IIIA with negative or neutral ulnar variance | Radius shortening osteotomy, ulnar lengthening, capitate shortening |
| II and IIIA with positive ulnar variance | Direct revascularization and external fixation or temporary scaphotrapeziotrapezoid pinning (stage II only), radial wedge or dome osteotomy, capitate shortening with or without capitohamate fusion, combination of joint leveling and direct revascularization procedures |
| IIIB | Scaphotrapeziotrapezoid or scaphocapitate fusion with or without lunate excision with palmaris longus autograft, radius-shortening osteotomy, proximal row carpectomy |
| IV | Proximal row carpectomy, wrist arthrodesis, wrist denervation |

From Allan CH, Joshi A, Lichtman DM: Kienböck's disease: diagnosis and treatment. *J Am Acad Orthop Surg* 9:128-136, 2001.

- Approximately 50% to 75% of patients treated with direct revascularization procedures show evidence of revascularization of the lunate.[8] Carpal collapse continues to occur in approximately 20% of cases.
- Additional or alternative treatment options in stage II or IIIA with positive ulnar variance include radial closing wedge osteotomy or capitate shortening.[6,9]

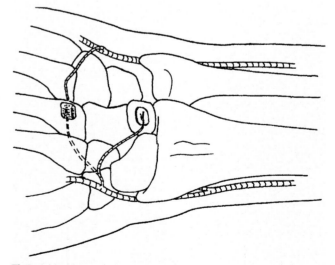

**Figure 11–11:**
**Vascularized bone graft from base of third metacarpal. (From Allan CH, Trumble TE: Kienböck's disease. In Trumble TE, editor:** *Principles of hand surgery and therapy.* **Philadelphia, 2000, WB Saunders.)**

branch of the radial artery between the first and second dorsal compartments, referred to as the *1,2 intercompartmental supraretinacular artery,* is identified and traced distally to the radial artery by releasing the distal portion of the first compartment. The 1,2 intercompartmental supraretinacular artery joins the distal radius after traveling beneath the tendons of the first dorsal compartment. Once the artery has been traced out, a vessel loop is used to measure the length of the pedicle needed for the bone graft to reach the lunate dorsally. Bipolar cautery is used to cauterize the vessel proximal to the planned site of bone graft harvest. The retinaculum between the first and second dorsal compartments is incised and harvested with the bone graft to protect the perforating vessels entering the distal radius. The bone graft is elevated with an osteotome. The vascularized bone graft is placed into the lunate cavity with the pedicle draped distally to prevent impingement against the dorsal lip of the radius.

## Surgical Technique for Capitate Shortening

- The capitate is approached using a dorsal incision. The tendons of the fourth compartment are retracted to the ulnar side, and the capsule overlying the capitate is incised longitudinally. The osteotomy site is planned to pass through the waist of the capitate and is confirmed with fluoroscopy. With a fine oscillating saw, a 2- to 3-mm wafer of bone is resected from the capitate (Figure 11–12). The saw cuts are completed with small osteotomes to prevent injury to the flexor tendons on the palmar surface of the capitate. The bone surfaces of the capitate are compressed manually and stabilized using crossed Kirschner wires or countersunk screws. Capitohamate arthrodesis can be performed using a small burr to denude the cartilage between the carpal bones, and the bone from the capitate osteotomy is packed in the space. Transverse Kirschner wires or cannulated screws are inserted percutaneously from the ulnar border of the hand. There usually is little motion between these bones, and we often omit this portion of the procedure. If Kirschner wires are used, the ends are cut off and buried beneath the skin.
- A biomechanical study of capitate shortening with capitohamate fusion showed significantly decreased resultant load across the radiolunate articulation.[10] This procedure is technically easier than procedures involving the radius and is my preference.

## Stage II or IIIA with Negative or Neutral Ulnar Variance

- In the patient with stage II or IIIA Kienböck's disease and significant negative ulnar variance, shortening osteotomy of the radius may be performed to reduce load on the lunate (Figure 11–13).

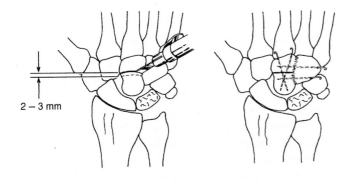

Capitate Shortening

**Figure 11–12:**
**Capitate shortening. (From Allan CH, Trumble TE: Kienböck's disease. In Trumble TE, editor:** *Principles of hand surgery and therapy.* **Philadelphia, 2000, WB Saunders.)**

2 – 3 mm

## Radial Shortening

- This technique is used in symptomatic patients with stage I, II, or IIIA Kienböck's disease and negative ulnar variance. The procedure aims to achieve joint leveling, leaving an ulnar neutral to 1-mm ulnar positive variance. This technique can be combined with a revascularization procedure as described in the section on stage II or IIA with positive ulnar variance.
- The distal radius can be approached either dorsally or palmarly. The dorsal approach is more straightforward, but meticulous attention must be paid to the volar structures when performing the osteotomy. A straight dorsal incision is made just ulnar to Lister's tubercle, from the level of the radiocarpal joint to a point 10 cm proximal. The extensor pollicis longus (EPL) tendon is identified and released from its compartment. The extensor digitorum communis (EDC) tendons and muscle bellies are dissected ulnarward, and the dorsal distal radius is exposed between the EPL and EDC. A T plate or seven-hole dynamic compression plate is applied to the bone. Lister's tubercle usually is removed with an osteotome or rongeur to allow plate application. The T plate allows for a more distally based osteotomy in metaphyseal bone to facilitate healing at the osteosynthesis site. When a dynamic compression plate is used, the most distal two screw holes are drilled, measured, and tapped, and the screws are placed. The second most distal screw then is removed and the plate rotated out of the way on the last screw. The osteotomy is planned at the level of the fourth, or middle, screw hole in the plate. Preoperative planning using radiographs allows estimation of the amount of bone to be removed with the osteotomy. Removal of a wedge of bone sufficient to leave ulnar neutral or 1-mm ulnar positive variance is planned, which generally amounts to 2 to 4 mm of radius. The osteotomy site is marked with two transverse light saw cuts separated by the planned width of bone resection. The distal cut is made partway through, protecting volar structures with retractors. The proximal cut is begun using a free blade fitted into the distal cut as a guide to ensure the cuts are parallel. The proximal cut is completed, and then the distal cut is made. The plate is rotated back into position and the screw replaced in the next-to-last hole. The proximal screws are applied in compression mode. The wound is irrigated and closed in layers, and a sugar tong splint is applied. Removal of the plate at a later date may be advisable if extensor tendon irritation develops.
- Sufficient bone should be removed to result in neutral to 1-mm positive ulnar variance. Positive ulnar variance greater than 1 mm risks abutment of the ulna upon the lunate or triquetrum, with persistent or worsening ulnar-sided symptoms after surgery.

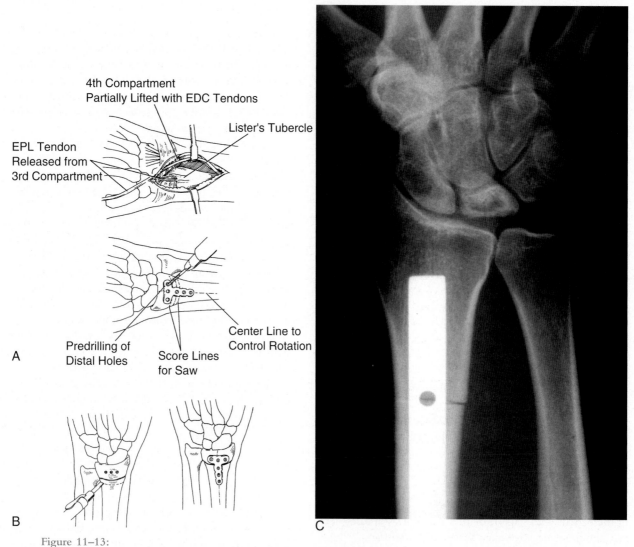

**Figure 11–13:**

**A, B:** Radial shortening. **C:** Postoperative image after radial shortening. (From Allan CH, Trumble TE: Kienböck's disease. In Trumble TE, editor: *Principles of hand surgery and therapy.* Philadelphia, 2000, WB Saunders.)

• A report on radial shortening demonstrated diminished pain in 93% of cases, with radiographic signs of lunate revascularization in one third of patients.[11] Range of motion was improved in 52% but worsened in 19%. Grip strength improved in 74%.

## Stage IIIB

• Stage IIIB Kienböck's disease includes radiographic signs of lunate collapse and loss of carpal height because of hyperflexion of the scaphoid.

• Correcting the scaphoid to its normal posture of 45 degrees of flexion followed by fusion to either the trapezium and trapezoid (scaphoid trapezium trapezoid [STT] fusion) or to the capitate (scaphocapitate [SC] fusion) decreases load across the radiolunate joint and prevents further carpal collapse, although wrist flexion and extension are decreased.[2,12]

## Surgical Technique for Scaphoid Trapezium Trapezoid Arthrodesis

• An incision is made along the dorsoradial aspect of the wrist beginning approximately 1 cm proximal to the base of the thumb metacarpal (Figure 11–14). The EPL tendon is identified and its sheath partially released with that of the extensor carpi radialis longus and brevis tendons so that they can be retracted radially while the EDC tendons are retracted ulnarly. A small fat pad overlying the STT joint must be bluntly dissected. Care should be taken to avoid injuring the branch of the sensory radial nerve. The capsule of the STT joint is incised transversely, and there typically is an overhanging prominence of the trapezoid blocking the surgeon's view. This prominence can be removed with a small osteotome. The surfaces are denuded with a rongeur, and two or three 0.0625-inch Kirschner

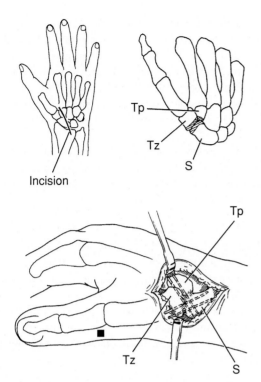

**Figure 11–14:**
Scaphoid trapezium trapezoid arthrodesis. (From Allan CH, Trumble TE: Kienböck's disease. In Trumble TE, editor: *Principles of hand surgery and therapy.* Philadelphia, 2000, WB Saunders.)

wires are driven in a dorsal to palmar direction. The dorsal distal to palmar proximal direction ensures the Kirschner wires will cross the STT joint to stabilize the scaphoid. Bone graft can be harvested from the distal radius and is packed into the space produced by removal of the STT joint cartilage, particularly in the palmar depths of the wound where substantial contact occurs. Placing pressure against the scaphoid tubercle and bringing the wrist into slight radial deviation causes a tight coaptation of the scaphoid and trapezoid surfaces. The Kirschner wires are driven into the scaphoid. A styloidectomy of the radius should be performed at the same time as the STT joint arthrodesis.

- Postoperatively, the patient is immobilized in a cast with the index and middle fingers flexed 90 degrees at the metacarpophalangeal joint and the thumb included in the cast. The cast is maintained for 6 weeks, and then a short arm thumb spica is used for another 2 weeks. The Kirschner wires are removed at this time. Radiographs should be obtained to confirm a solid arthrodesis.

## Surgical Technique for Scaphocapitate Arthrodesis

- This technique can be used as an alternative to STT fusion in stage IIIB Kienböck's disease, and the objectives

are the same. The incision and approach are as described for STT fusion, with retraction of the second and third dorsal compartment tendons radially and the fourth compartment ulnarly. Alternatively a straight dorsal incision as described for the vascular pedicle harvest from the second or third metacarpal base can be used. The wrist capsule is opened longitudinally and the scaphoid, capitate, and lunate identified. The articular surfaces at the scaphoid-capitate interface are denuded of bone with a rongeur or a burr. The very most palmar cartilage and subchondral bone can be left in place to maintain appropriate spacing of the bones.

- Cancellous bone graft is obtained either from a cortical window in the dorsum of the distal radius just proximal to Lister tubercle or via a radial styloidectomy. Alternatively, the iliac crest can be used as the donor site. The scaphoid is manually reduced from its hyperflexed position into approximately 45 degrees of flexion, and two 1.6-mm Kirschner wires are driven from the radial side of the scaphoid into and through both cortices of the capitate (Figure 11–15). These wires should be introduced at an angle, rather than parallel, to one another to reduce motion between the bones. After confirming their position on plain radiographs, the pins are cut short beneath the skin. The cancellous bone graft is packed into the cavity between the scaphoid and the capitate. The capsule is closed, followed by wound closure in layers and application of a sugar tong thumb spica splint. This splint is converted to a short arm thumb spica cast, which is worn until radiographic signs of union are apparent, usually at 8 to 10 weeks.

- In a three-dimensional theoretical wrist model, Iwasaki et al.[12] demonstrated reduced force across the radiolunate joint after STT or SC fusion.

- If significant synovitis is present in stage IIIB disease, excision of the lunate may be performed in addition to the fusion or other procedure. Silicone prostheses are no longer used due to high rates of particulate synovitis (2).

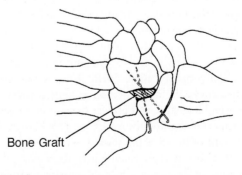

**Figure 11–15:**
Scaphocapitate arthrodesis. (From Allan CH, Trumble TE: Kienböck's disease. In Trumble TE, editor: *Principles of hand surgery and therapy.* Philadelphia, 2000, WB Saunders.)

## Stage IV

- In stage IV Kienböck's disease, generalized degenerative changes are seen throughout the midcarpal joint, radiocarpal joint, or both. Lunate collapse and fixed scaphoid rotation with loss of carpal height are still present.
- Attempts to revascularize or decompress the lunate that do not address the arthritic process fail.
- Treatment options include proximal row carpectomy (PRC) and wrist fusion.
- PRC preserves most of the already limited motion of a wrist with stage IV disease, is simple to perform, and leaves open the possibility for wrist fusion at a later date if required.

## Technique for Proximal Row Carpectomy

- This procedure removes the scaphoid, lunate, and triquetrum, allowing the capitate to settle into the lunate fossa. Motion then occurs through this joint. Preoperative evaluation must include careful assessment of articular wear in the radiolunate joint, which risks early failure of this procedure. Mild wear encountered at surgery can be addressed by interposing dorsal capsule between the capitate head and the lunate fossa. More extensive wear may leave total wrist arthrodesis as the procedure of choice.
- A straight midline incision is made just ulnar to Lister tubercle and centered over the carpus from distal radial articular surface to the level of the metacarpal bases. The EDC tendons are retracted ulnarly and the wrist extensors radially. The wrist capsule is incised longitudinally (if interposition of a flap in the lunate fossa is planned, this is constructed now) and the carpus exposed. Often the collapsed lunate is difficult to identify, and the capitate head is found first. Careful exposure of the entire proximal row is performed. Small Hohmann retractors can be helpful in keeping the capsule edges from obscuring the surgeon's view. The scaphoid, lunate, and triquetrum are removed. Volar flexion of the scaphoid can make this bone particularly challenging to excise completely but is recommended to prevent impingement of retained distal pole fragments on the radial styloid. Using a large K-wire or small Steinmann pin as a joystick can simplify this procedure. Small, sharp osteotomes and curettes can be useful in addition to knife dissection. It is important to identify and protect the radioscaphocapitate ligament, running from proximal and radial across the volar waist of the scaphoid toward the center of the capitate. Injury to this structure may allow excessive ulnar translation of the carpus. Once the proximal row is removed, the capitate is approximated within the lunate fossa (interposing a flap of dorsal capsule, if mild arthritic

wear is present) and the wound closed in layers. A final check is performed to ensure the capitate is located; if it is not, temporary Kirschner wires are used to maintain the capitate in its reduced position within the lunate fossa. A sugar tong splint is applied, and 2 weeks postoperatively the sutures are removed, a removable splint provided, and gentle active range of motion started.
- A 1-cm segment of the posterior interosseous nerve is excised within the fourth dorsal compartment when performing PRC to minimize postoperative pain.

## Kienböck's Disease in Children

- AVN of the lunate in the pediatric population is rare.
- Treatment has ranged from observation alone to temporary pinning of the scaphotrapezial joint or formal radial shortening.[13,14]
- A review article collected data from reports on 32 patients, most treated operatively, and noted significant potential for revascularization of the lunate in children.[15]

## Preiser's Disease

### Etiology

- The factors leading to development of Preiser's disease, or AVN of the scaphoid, are not known with certainty but probably include some form of trauma in the majority of cases. One report found that all of Preiser's original cases and three of seven subsequent reported cases occurred after fracture or other injury.[1] Other suggested factors have included alcoholism, corticosteroids, chemotherapy, systemic lupus erythematosus, and progressive systemic sclerosis.[16] Ulnar positive variance has been present in some cases,[1] but a large series found no such association.[16]

### Presentation

- In a multicenter retrospective series of 19 patients diagnosed with Preiser's disease, the average patient age at presentation was approximately 45 years. Women outnumbered men by approximately 3 to 1. The dominant wrist was affected in approximately two thirds of patients.

### Physical Examination

- Pain was present in the dorsoradial aspect of the involved wrist in all cases, whereas swelling was present in only five of the patients. Of interest, nine patients were diagnosed with concomitant carpal tunnel syndrome at some point during the disease course.

## Radiographic Evaluation

* In this large series, two patterns of scaphoid involvement were identified in Preiser's disease. Cases where the entire scaphoid bone showed MRI signal changes of necrosis and/or ischemia were classified as type I, and those displaying MRI signal changes involving 50% or less of the bone were classified as type 2 (Figure 11–16).

## Staging

* A four-stage classification system for scaphoid necrosis originally was described by Herbert and Lanzetta[1] and modified by Kalainov et al.[16] In stage 1, plain radiographs are normal but MRI reveals signal changes of necrosis. In stage 2 scaphoid sclerosis, lucencies and fissuring are found on plain radiographs. Stage 3 is defined by radiographic fragmentation of the scaphoid. In stage 4, fragmentation and collapse of the scaphoid and periscaphoid arthritis are present.

## Treatment

* As with Kienböck's disease, the optimal treatment of Preiser's disease is not known. A similar array of therapies have been used, ranging from cast immobilization or external fixation to curettage, vascularized bone grafting, scaphoid excision with or without intercarpal fusion, PRC, and total wrist arthrodesis.

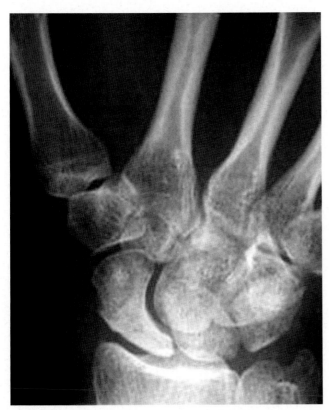

Figure 11–16:
**Preiser's disease involving the proximal scaphoid pole.**

## References

1. Herbert TJ, Lanzetta M: Idiopathic avascular necrosis of the scaphoid. *J Hand Surg [Br]* 19:174-182, 1994.
   In this article, the authors report on a study of eight patients with idiopathic avascular necrosis affecting only the proximal pole of the scaphoid, with proposed classification and treatment.

2. Alexander C, Alexander A, Lichtman D: Kienböck's disease. In Lichtman D, editor: *The wrist and its disorders,* ed 2. Philadelphia, 1997, WB Saunders.
   This chapter addresses in exhaustive fashion much of what is known regarding the etiology, presentation, radiographic staging, and treatment options for Kienböck's disease.

3. Panagis JS, Gelberman RH, Taleisnik J, Baumgaertner M: The arterial anatomy of the human carpus. Part II: the intraosseous vascularity. *J Hand Surg [Am]* 8:375-382, 1983.
   The intraosseous vascular anatomy of the carpal bones of 25 fresh cadaver limbs was studied by injection and Spälteholz clearing techniques, with resultant grouping of bones into three types.

4. Schiltenwolf M, Martini A, Mau H et al: Further investigations of the intraosseous pressure characteristics in necrotic lunates (Kienböck's disease). *J Hand Surg [Am]* 21:754-758, 1996.
   The authors measured intraosseous pressure in 12 normal and 12 necrotic lunates in various positions to test the hypothesis that impairment of venous drainage plays a role in lunate necrosis.

5. Tsuge S, Nakamura R: Anatomical risk factors for Kienböck's disease. *J Hand Surg [Br]* 18:70-75, 1993.
   Contralateral unaffected wrists from 41 males with Kienböck's disease were compared radiographically with wrists from 66 normal males to find anatomic features predisposing to lunate necrosis.

6. Watanabe K, Nakamura R, Horri E, Miura T: Biomechanical analysis of radial wedge osteotomy for the treatment of Kienböck's disease. *J Hand Surg [Am]* 18:686-691, 1993.
   A mathematical model was used to support the theoretical unloading of the lunate that follows radial wedge osteotomy.

7. Desser T, McCarthy S, Trumble T: Scaphoid fractures and Kienböck's disease of the lunate: MR imaging with histopathologic correlation. *Magn Reson Imaging* 8:357-361, 1990.
   MRI proved accurate in prospective evaluation of bone viability for both scaphoid fractures and Kienböck's disease when compared to histologic specimens obtained from 13 necrotic carpal bones.

8. Tamai S, Yajima H, Ono H: Revascularization procedures in the treatment of Kienböck's disease. *Hand Clin* 9:455-466, 1993.
   The authors outline the indications and techniques for revascularization procedures for Kienböck's disease.

9. Almquist E: Capitate shortening in the treatment of Kienböck's disease. *Hand Clin* 9:505-512, 1993.

The author reviews the technique and indications for capitate shortening for Kienböck's disease.

10. Viola R, Kiser P, Bach A et al: Biomechanical analysis of capitate hamate fusion in the treatment of Kienböck's disease. *J Hand Surg [Am]* 23:395-401, 1998.
    This biomechanical cadaver model suggests that capitate shortening with capitate-hamate fusion increases radioscaphoid mean pressure and decreases radiolunate mean pressure.

11. Quenzer D, Dobyns J, Linscheid R et al: Radial recession osteotomy for Kienböck's disease. *J Hand Surg [Am]* 22:386-395, 1997.
    The authors report good results in 68 patients who underwent radial recession osteotomy for avascular necrosis of the lunate.

12. Iwasaki N, Genda E, Barrance P et al: Biomechanical analysis of limited intercarpal fusion for the treatment of Kienböck's disease: a three-dimensional theoretical study. *J Orthop Res* 16:256-263, 1998.
    A three-dimensional mathematical model was used to simulate and compare the biomechanical effects of three different intercarpal fusions for Kienböck's disease.

13. Yasuda M, Okuda H, Egi T, Guidera P: Temporary scapho-trapezoidal joint fixation for Kienböck's disease in a 12-year-old girl: a case report. *J Hand Surg [Am]* 23:411-414, 1998.
    Temporary scapho-trapezoidal joint fixation with Kirschner wires was performed for stage IIIB Kienböck's disease in a 12-year-old girl, allowing clinical and radiographic healing.

14. Minami A, Itoga H, Kobayashi M: Kienböck's disease in an eleven-year-old girl. A case report. *Ital J Orthop Traumatol* 18: 547-550, 1992.
    The authors report the case of an 11-year-old girl with Kienböck's disease treated successfully with radial shortening.

15. Ferlic RJ, Lee DH, Lopez-Ben RR: Pediatric Kienböck's disease: case report and review of the literature. *Clin Orthop* 408:237-244, 2003.
    A 13-year-old boy with symptomatic stage III Kienböck's disease was treated successfully with radial shortening.

16. Kalainov DM, Cohen MS, Hendrix RW et al: Preiser's disease: identification of two patterns. *J Hand Surg [Am]* 28:767-778, 2003.
    A large series of patients with Preiser's disease was reviewed and two different categories of this disorder were identified: complete versus partial vascular impairment of the scaphoid bone as determined by MRI.

# CHAPTER 12

# Flexor Tendon Injuries

Mark Rekant

MD, Philadelphia Hand Center, Philadelphia, PA

## History

- In 1922, Sterling Bunnell,[1] the founding father of American hand surgery, wrote, "If flexor tendons are severed in the finger, the usual place opposite the proximal phalanx, one cannot join them together by sutures with success, as the junction will become adherent in the narrow fixed channel and will not slip. It is better to remove the tendons entirely from the finger and graft in new tendons smooth throughout its length." Dr. Bunnell's statement has offered a challenge to surgeons and scientists interested in tendon injury and repair.
- Before 1966, flexor tendon lacerations in the area of the digit were treated with delayed methods of staged tendon reconstruction.
- Today, despite the challenges imparted by flexor tendon and digital anatomy, advances in the basic science of tendon repair, surgical methods of repair, and rehabilitation, reasonable outcomes can be obtained in most of patients with zone II and other flexor tendon injuries.

## Introduction

- Flexor tendon injuries are common. They involve lacerations and/or ruptures and occur predominately in males between 15 and 30 years old.
- Complete tendon injuries *require* repair/reattachment for return of function.
- Zones of tendon injury (Figure 12–1) influence the type of repair and postoperative regimen.

## Differential Diagnosis

- Nerve injury → muscle paralysis
- Paralysis secondary to *pain* (self-splinting)
- Underlying medical condition, such as polio, leprosy, Charcot-Marie-Tooth, spinal muscular atrophy

## Flexor Tendon Anatomy Overview

### Carpal Tunnel

- In the carpal tunnel, the middle and ring finger superficialis tendons lie volar to the small and index finger superficialis tendons (see Figure 1–14).
- A good way to remember the relationship is that 34 is greater than 25.

### Digital Sheath

- Each of the fingers has a deep flexor digitorum profundus (FDP) and a superficial flexor digitorum superficialis (FDS) tendon.
  - *Note:* Approximately 20% of patients are missing an FDS tendon in the little finger.
- The fibroosseous sheath begins at the level of the metacarpal neck.
- The flexor tendon sheath is composed of five annular pulleys (A1–A5) and three cruciate pulleys (C1–C3) (see Figure 1–18).

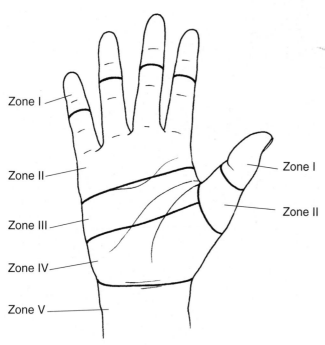

Figure 12–1:

The five flexor tendon zones of injury. (From Trumble TE, Sailer SM: Flexor tendon injuries. In Trumble TE, editor: *Principles of hand surgery and therapy*. Philadelphia, 2000, WB Saunders.)

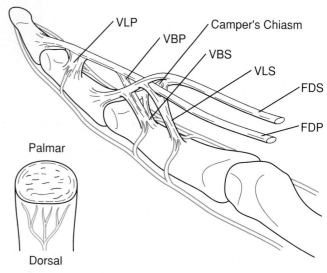

Figure 12–2:

Decussation of the flexor digitorum superficialis produces Camper's chiasm. Both the flexor digitorum superficialis *(FDS)* and flexor digitorum profundus *(FDP)* receive their blood supply via the vinculum longus and brevis. *VBP,* vinculum brevis profundus; *VBS,* vinculum brevis superficialis; *VLP,* vinculum longus profundus; *VLS,* vinculum longus superficialis.

- A2 and A4 are the most important pulleys to preserve in order to prevent bowstringing of the tendon(s).
  - Without pulleys, the tendons can no longer glide juxtaposed to the phalanges. Greater amplitude of muscle contraction is required to obtain the same amount of flexion of the finger.
- Digital artery branches, or vincula, assist with tendon nutrition (Figure 12–2).
- Once in the sheath, the FDS forms *Camper's chiasm* by splitting into two slips that attach on the palmar sides of the middle phalanx.
- The FDP tendon passes through the FDS chiasm and continues on to attach to the volar aspect of the distal phalanx.

## Thumb Sheath (Figure 12–3)

- Only one tendon, the flexor pollicis longus (FPL), provides flexion of the interphalangeal joint.
- The sheath of the FPL is composed of
  - Two annular pulleys
  - Only one oblique pulley, which is the main structure that prevents bowstringing of the tendon
- The FPL has one continuous synovial sheath that begins just proximal to the carpal tunnel and continues the length of the tendon.
  - *Note:* The index, middle, and ring fingers also have a synovial sheath that begins proximal to the carpal tunnel, but the sheath stops at the level of the transverse

intermetacarpal ligaments and resumes within the fibroosseous tunnel. The synovial sheath for the small finger continues on from the palmar bursa to the end of the finger (Figure 12–4).

## Tendon Zones

- **Five** very important zones exist (see Figure 12–1).

## Zone I: Zone of Flexor Digitorum Profundus Avulsion Injuries ("Jersey Finger")

- Region between the middle aspects of the middle phalanx to the fingertip.
  - Contains only one tendon, the FDP.
  - Tendon laceration usually is very close to its insertion
  - Tendon to bone repair usually is required instead of tendon to tendon repair.

## Zone II: "No Man's Land"

- Region from the metacarpal head to the middle of the middle phalanx.
  - Bunnell[1] referred to this area as "no man's land" because the initial results were so poor that he believed no one should attempt primary tendon repairs in this zone.
  - Two flexor tendons: FDS and FDP within the *one* flexor tendon sheath.

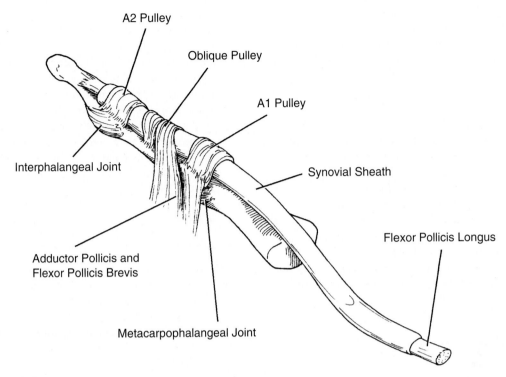

Figure 12–3:
The flexor pollicis longus has two annular pulleys and one oblique pulley. (From Trumble TE, Sailer SM: Flexor tendon injuries. In Trumble TE, editor: *Principles of hand surgery and therapy*. Philadelphia, 2000, WB Saunders.)

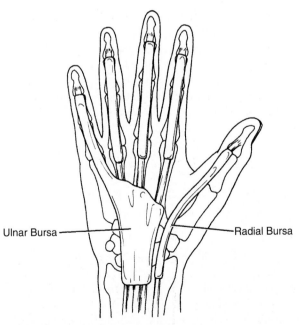

Figure 12–4:
The synovial bursa of the small finger connects with the ulnar bursae in the hand. The index, middle, and ring fingers have digital synovial bursae that are separate from the ulnar bursa. (From Trumble TE, Sailer SM: Flexor tendon injuries. In Trumble TE, editor: *Principles of hand surgery and therapy*. Philadelphia, 2000, WB Saunders.)

- Adhesion formation risk is amplified at the point where the profundus travels through the FDS at the narrow and tight Camper's chiasm (see Figure 12–2).
  - Camper's chiasm can be up to 2 cm long.
- During digit flexion, the two slips of the FDS move toward the midline and compress the profundus tendon.

## Zone III: Distal Palmar Crease

- Region between the transverse carpal ligament and the proximal margin of the tendon sheath formation.
- The lumbrical muscle origins in this zone prevent the profundus tendons from overretracting. Delayed end to end repairs have been successful even several weeks after the initial injury.

## Zone IV: Transverse Carpal Ligament

- This is the region deep to the transverse carpal ligament.
  - Tendon injuries in this zone are rare because of the protection provided by the stout transverse carpal ligament.

## Zone V: Proximal

- Region proximal to the transverse carpal ligament.
  - Distal portion of zone V tendons consists of discrete structures.

- Proximal portion of zone V meets the musculotendinous junction.
  - The junction is a poor site for repair because the tendons become thinner and fan out into fibers that merge with the muscle belly.

## Examination

- Observe the patient from a distance before manipulating the patient who has sustained a painful injury.
- There is a normal arcade to the hand.
  - The index finger demonstrates the least flexion.
  - The little finger displays the greatest flexion.
- If the injured digit demonstrates more extension than the other digits, there is a high likelihood of a tendon laceration that should be evaluated surgically.
- Avoid using a local anesthetic until a careful sensory test has been performed. Determination of a concurrent digital nerve injury is imperative.

### Provocative Testing

#### Testing the Flexor Digitorum Profundus

- Hold the proximal interphalangeal (PIP) joint in extension (blocking the PIP joint) and ask the patient to flex each of the injured digits at the distal interphalangeal (DIP) joint (see Figure 1–16).
- The FDP muscles all fire as a group, except for the index FDP, which can flex independently.

#### Testing the Flexor Digitorum Superficialis

- When the patient holds the other digits in extension, the FDP is blocked from flexing any of the digits except for the index finger (see Figure 1–15).
- The FDS, with independent innervation, can be tested separately.

#### Testing the Thumb

- The FPL can be tested by stabilizing the metacarpophalangeal (MP) joint and asking the patient to flex the interphalangeal (IP) joint (see Figure 1–17).

### Imaging Studies

- The injured hand should be radiographed to exclude any underlying fractures.

## Tendon Structure and Biomechanics

- The overall excursion of the FDS and FDP tendons (wrist and finger motion) is 88 mm and 86 mm, respectively.

- Tendon composition:
  - 78% of type I collagen
  - 19% of type III collagen
  - Remaining 3% includes a wide variety of other collagen types and noncollagen proteins
- Tendons demonstrate a nonlinear viscoelastic property.
  - These properties derive from the tendon's collagen structural deformity, which is time rate dependent. For example, at the bone-tendon interface, a slow loading rate results in an avulsion fracture of bone, whereas a fast loading rate causes tendon failure.

## Tendon Nutrition and Blood Supply

- The nutrition derives from two sources: vascular perfusion (intrinsic) and synovium (extrinsic).
  1. Vascular perfusion (intrinsic):
     - Longitudinal vessels enter the palm and extend down the intratendinous channels.
     - Vessels enter at the level of the proximal synovial fold in the palm.
     - Vincula harbor segmental branches from the digital arteries.
     - Osseous insertions are sources of vascular perfusion.
  2. Direct diffusion (extrinsic) of nutrients from the synovial fluid:
     - Enhanced by the capillary pumping mechanism known as imbibition.
     - Imbibition: Finger flexion provides a pumping mechanism as the tendon glides into the fibroosseous pulleys, which helps draw fluid into the interstices of the tendon through small ridges or conduits.

## Cellular and Biochemical Factors in Tendon Healing

### Physiology of Tendon Injury and Repair (Table 12–1)

- Tendon injuries stimulate a potent chemotactic response.
- Stimulated cells migrate into the zone of injury from either the epitenon or the synovial sheath.
- Cells histologically resembling myofibroblasts synthesize collagen.
- The epitenon is clearly the most active segment of the tendon both for collagen synthesis, with initiation of α-procollagen, and for phagocytosis of collagen debris resulting from the injury.

## Table 12–1: Stages of Intrinsic Repair for Intrasynovial Flexor Tendons

### INFLAMMATORY PHASE (0 TO 14 DAYS)

Fibrin clot forms at the repair site
Macrophage migration and leukocyte migration to the repair site
Phagocytosis of the repair site
Fibronectin production peaks (chemostasis)
bFGF production peaks
Upregulation of integrins
Cells from the epitenon proliferate and migrate to the repair site
   Gliding surface is restored
   Fibrin strands identified in fibroblasts surrounding the repair site
   Immediately after repair, the strength of the repair is related to the strength
     of the suture and the suture method

### Reparative Phase (2 to 6 Weeks)

Intense collagen production, mostly type I
Fibers of collagen are laid down randomly and gradually orient themselves
   along the axis of tensile forces
Cellular ingrowth from the epitenon fills the repair site gap
Neovascularization of the repair site occurs
TGF production peaks
Fibrinous strands of collagen bridge the repair site
DNA content is increased
At 2 weeks after repair, the repair site strength may temporarily decrease, but
   the overall strength increases during this period as collagen deposition
   occurs at the repair site
Repair site strength is still principally related to the strength of the suture and
   the suture material

### Remodeling Phase (>6 Weeks)

Collagen fibers are smooth and uniform in the repair site
Collagen fibers are remodeling to be oriented parallel to the longitudinal axis
   of the tendon
The surface of the tendon is smooth and nonadherent
DNA content remains increased
Decreased rates of cell division
Increase in repair site strength

## Cytokines and Growth Factors

- Platelet-derived growth factor and epidermal growth factor were identified in healing flexor tendons from 3 to 17 days after repair.[2]
- Transforming growth factor-beta was noted in healing tendons and in the tendon sheath.
- Fibroblastic growth factor was absent from the repair process.
- Hyaluronic acid, a normal component of tendon synovial fluid, *did not increase* collagen synthesis and actually depressed cellular proliferation.
- Ascorbic acid at a concentration greater than 50 μg/ml is essential for tendon healing.
- Metalloproteinases assist in regulating collagen synthesis.
- Proteoglycan concentrations are elevated in regions of the tendon and tendon sheath that are subjected to tendon load.

## Tendon Repair Characteristics

- *Repair tendon injuries early.*
  - Most repairs should be performed within the first 2 weeks after injury because the tendon ends and tendon sheaths become scarred, and the musculotendinous units retract.
  - Repairs after 2 weeks may decrease the ultimate mobility of the fingers.
- The strength of the flexor repair and the ability to resist gapping appear to be directly proportional to the number of sutures that cross the repair site.
- Tendon repairs demonstrate a 20% to 40% decrease in tendon strength during the first 3 to 7 days after tendon repair. If repair strength dips below the threshold of the loads produced by active or passive motion, then tendon rupture occurs.
  - Tensile stress on normally repaired flexor tendons is as follows:
    - Passive motion: 500 to 750 g
    - Light grip: 1500 to 2250 g
    - Strong grip: 5000 to 7500 g
    - Tip pinch, index FDP: 9000 to 13,500 g
  - Tendon gapping is the hallmark of tendon failure (gapping of 2 mm or more)
- *Six characteristics of an ideal repair:*
  1. Easy placement of sutures in the tendon (Table 12–2)
  2. Secure suture knots
  3. Smooth juncture of tendon ends
  4. Minimal gapping at the repair site
  5. Minimal interference with tendon vascularity
  6. Sufficient strength throughout healing to permit application of early motion stress to the tendon
  - *Note:* A practical and strong repair allows early active motion without significantly increasing friction with tendon gliding.[3,4]
  - Numerous methods of tendon suture (Figure 12–5) have been advocated in an effort to satisfy the characteristics of an ideal repair.
- *Techniques to minimize gapping*
  - *Place core sutures dorsally.*
    - During digit flexion, the dorsal aspect of the tendon is under the greatest tension. Dorsal placement of core sutures is the best mechanical location for tendon repair.[5]

## Table 12–2: Ideal Core Suture

Material suture properties of sufficient strength to allow early mobilization

Easy material handling when placed into soft tissue

Material durable through the process of tendon repair

Surgical method that is easy to perform and accurately coapts the tendon ends

Surgical method should not interfere with tendon repair

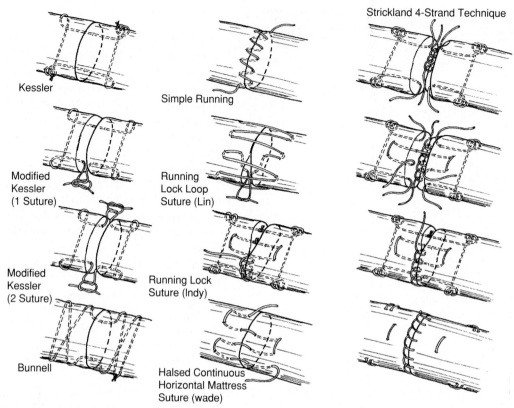

Figure 12–5:

Technique for four-strand repair. **Left column,** Several commonly used core suture techniques. **Middle column,** Different techniques for epitenon sutures. **Right column,** Strickland four-strand repair with epitenon suture. (From Trumble TE, Sailer SM: Flexor tendon injuries. In Trumble TE, editor: *Principles of hand surgery and therapy.* Philadelphia, 2000, WB Saunders.)

○ Dorsal core sutures result in less work of flexion.[6]
  ■ *Note:* Prior conventional wisdom specified that the sutures should be placed in the palmar aspect of the tendon because the blood supply to part of the tendons is via the vincula that are attached to the dorsal surface of the tendon. (Theoretically, sutures placed in the dorsal aspect of the tendon obstruct the blood supply and cause tendon ischemia.) However, later studies of tendon nutrition indicated that imbibition of synovial fluid may be the major pathway for tendon nutrition following tendon injury.
○ *Epitenon sutures improve the strength and quality of tendon repairs.*
  ■ Improves the contour of the repair.
  ■ *Minimizes* gap formation and adds to the ultimate tensile strength of the repair.[7]
○ *No need for tendon sheath repair.*
  ■ Although clinical reports have indicated that repairs of the tendon sheath appear to be safe, a clinical

comparison showed no significant improvement in patients treated with sheath repair compared with patients treated without sheath repair.[8]
  ■ *Note for partial tendon laceration repair:* Lacerations of less than 60% of the cross-sectional area of the tendon should be treated *without* tenorrhaphy and with early mobilization.[9]
  ■ *Note:* It is advantageous to trim frayed or partial lacerations to prevent triggering of the frayed edges.

## Practical Approach: Acute Tendon Repair

● *Exposure:* The skin lacerations often are transverse, making it difficult to extend the incision with a Brunner-type zigzag incision. Longitudinal incisions on opposite sides proximally and distally can provide enough exposure without compromising the skin margins (Figure 12–6).

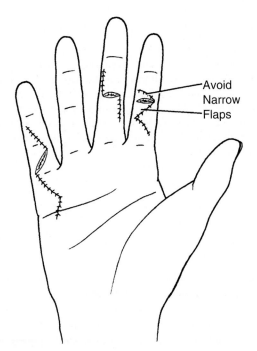

**Figure 12–6:**
Oblique skin incisions can be extended in a Brunner zigzag fashion, but the transverse laceration should be extended with midaxial incisions to prevent skin flaps having too narrow a base to support a viable flap. (From Trumble TE, Sailer SM: Flexor tendon injuries. In Trumble TE, editor: *Principles of hand surgery and therapy.* Philadelphia, 2000, WB Saunders.)

- The level of tendon laceration is defined with the digit fully extended.
- The distal end of the tendon will be distal to the skin and tendon sheath (Figure 12–7) when the tendon is cut with the finger in flexion, as is usually the case.
- If the finger was cut in extension, the tendon laceration is at the same level as the skin laceration.

## Zone I

- As with most tendon lacerations in the digits, the wound must be extended distally and proximally for precise visualization.
- With the proximal tendon retrieved, core sutures are placed in the tendon for subsequent passage with Keith needles. Care is taken to minimize disruption of the important A4 pulley.
- *Tendon fixation:* Keith needles are used to pass the sutures around the distal phalanx exiting through the nail plate dorsally (Figure 12–8). The pullout suture is left in place for 6 to 7 weeks over the nail plate or suture button.
- The repair can be augmented by suturing the remaining distal end of the tendon to the reattached proximal portion of the tendon in a belt and suspenders manner, taking care not to injure (cut) the core sutures with the suture needle.
  - *Note:* Some surgeons prefer to drill the Keith needles through the distal phalanx with a volar to dorsal angle (similar to Figure 12–8) rather than on either side of the bone. Alternatively, mini-suture anchors can be used, although my preference is to use a dorsal suture button.
- FDP avulsion injuries (Jersey finger) (Box 12–1)
  - There are three types of FDP avulsions.[10]
  - In type I avulsions, the tendon has retracted into the *palm.* The tendon should be repaired within 7 days. The blood supply is compromised, and the tendon contracts/shortens.
  - Type II avulsions have retracted to the level of the PIP joint. Blood supply remains. These injuries can be repaired even after a delay of up to several weeks, although an earlier repair is favorable.
  - Type III avulsions usually are attached to a large fracture fragment that prevents the tendon from retracting past the DIP joint. These injuries can be repaired in a delayed fashion similar to type II injuries.

**Figure 12–7:**
The top digit has a laceration of the flexor tendon while the finger is in a flexed position. When the finger extends, the tendon laceration is distal to the site of the skin and tendon sheath laceration. The bottom digit has a laceration of the flexor tendons while the finger is in an extended position. With finger flexion, the tendon ends are easily retrieved from the site of the original laceration. (From Trumble TE, Sailer SM: Flexor tendon injuries. In Trumble TE, editor: *Principles of hand surgery and therapy.* Philadelphia, 2000, WB Saunders.)

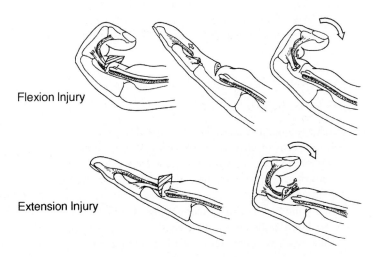

Flexion Injury

Extension Injury

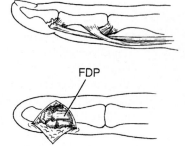

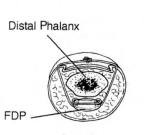

Distal Phalanx

FDP

**D   Typical Cross Section**

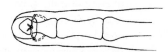

FDP

FDP

Figure 12–8:
A–D, Zone I flexor tendon lacerations are best repaired with a pullout button technique because the lacerations are too distal to obtain a secure suture in the distal end of the tendon. By tying the sutures over the nail, the surgeon can avoid using a pullout button, which often becomes caught on clothing. *FDP,* Flexor digitorum profundus. (From Trumble TE, Sailer SM: Flexor tendon injuries. In Trumble TE, editor: *Principles of hand surgery and therapy.* Philadelphia, 2000, WB Saunders.)

---

### Box 12–1   FDP Avulsion Injuries

**Leddy Classification of FDP Avulsions**

- Type I -Retract into the palm
- Type II – Retract to the level of the PIP joint
- Type III – Level of the DIP joint. Usually are attached to a large fracture fragment that prevents the tendon from further retraction

**Pearls of FDP Avulsions**

- The most commonly injured - Ring finger (IV)
  - The most likely digit to be remaining in a grip, especially during tackling in football (Leddy and Packer, 1977; Trumble et al., 1992).
  - The avulsion occurs when the palyer accelerates while the tackler is still holding the jersey (Figs. 13–35, 13–36, and 13–37).
- The tendon avulsion can occur *with or without* bone.
- When a fracture is present, it does not reliably predict where the tendon end will be because the fracture fragment can be attached to the avulsed volar plate while the tendon has avulsed without a fracture.

---

- *Note: Urgent surgery* is recommended in acute injuries because determination of the type of avulsion from radiographs and clinical examination is inexact.[11]
  - *Note:* Ultrasonography or magnetic resonance imaging can help differentiate the type of injury if necessary.

## Zone II (No Man's Land)

### Repair Technique

- Repair *both* tendon lacerations in zone II.
  - In one retrospective study, 74% of digits with both tendons repaired had good or excellent results compared with 47% of digits with only the profundus tendon repaired.[12]
- Four-strand repair with epitenon repair (see Figure 12–5).
  - Strickland modification of the Kessler repair is performed using two sets of core sutures for the FDP tendon.

- An epitenon suture is placed routinely regardless of vincula attachments or lack thereof.
  - *Note:* By placing the dorsal sutures of the epitenon repair (leaving the 6–0 Prolene suture needle attached loosely to the side to enable completion of this suture) before the core sutures are tied, proper circumferential placement of the epitenon sutures are facilitated, thus ensuring the tendon ends come together evenly without bunching.
- Once the dorsal epitenon sutures are placed, the core sutures are placed. The outer core sutures are tied and then the inner core suture is tied. The remainder of the epitenon repair is completed volarly.
- The slips of the FDS tendon are repaired with simple Kessler sutures or mattress sutures.
- If enlargement of a pulley is desirable, an L-shaped incision can be made in the tendon sheath distally. The sheath will have a funnel shape, which helps accommodate the tendon end.
- If the proximal ends of the tendons have retracted into the tendon sheath and cannot be retrieved, a counter incision is made at the level of the distal palmar crease. In most cases, the tendon can be gently pushed distally with a forceps so that the ends can be retrieved from the incision in the finger.
- If necessary, a no. 5 pediatric feeding tube or silastic tube can be passed from proximal to distal and sutured to the side of the tendon to pass the tendon distally.[3]
- Occasionally, severe retraction of the tendon prevents distal passage of the tendon until a core suture is placed into the tendon as a means of passing the tendon distally.

## Zone III Injuries

- The tendons are repaired using the same suture techniques as described earlier. The exposure of the tendons is much easier and the results are much better because of the absence of the fibroosseous sheath at this level.

## Zone IV Injuries

- The tendons are repaired as described earlier, along with any injuries to the median nerve that is superficial to the tendons.

## Zone V Injuries

- Injuries near the musculotendinous junction can be difficult to repair because the muscle tissue will not hold a suture. Often multiple mattress sutures are necessary if the musculotendinous junction will not hold a core suture.

## Flexor Pollicis Longus Injuries

- These injuries are treated with repairs similar to the finger tendons.
- All efforts are made to preserve the oblique pulley and the A2 pulley.
- To retrieve the FPL tendon if it has retracted proximally, an incision at the level of the wrist (through the flexor carpi radialis sheath) is recommended rather than in the thenar region, where the tendon dives between the thenar muscles. Take care to avoid injuring the thumb's digital nerves, the median, and palmar cutaneous nerves.

# Rehabilitation of Flexor Tendon Injuries

- The key to successful flexor tendon repair is close adherence to a regimented hand therapy rehabilitation program.
- Various protocols following flexor tendon repair are available. Each protocol must consider the stress placed on flexor tendons before and after the repair.
  - Active assisted range of motion.
  - Passive range of motion (Kleinert et al[13] vs. Duran) (Box 12–2).
  - Immobilization is recommended for children younger than 10 years and for patients unable or unwilling to follow a controlled-motion protocol. Immobilize with the wrist in 10 degrees of flexion, MP joints

blocked in 70 degrees flexion, and IP joints neutral for 4 to 6 weeks based on the patient's maturity level and the strength of the initial repair. If the patient is immobilized for only 4 weeks, a removable splint in similar position is used for an additional 2 weeks.
  - Early active motion protocol
    - Early active motion protocols are indicated for intelligent, compliant patients with a solid four-strand repair who can comply with hand therapy on a regular basis for zone I or II injuries.
      - In theory, active motion allows for better overall motion because greater tendon gliding prevents adhesion formation.
      - Concern exists regarding higher rates of tendon rupture with early active motion in noncompliant patients.
  - Passive motion protocol (see Box 12–2)
    - Passive motion protocols are better suited for patients with a two-strand repair and for less compliant patients.
    - Zone III, IV, and V injuries are treated with the passive tendon protocol.

## Passive Flexor Tendon Protocol

### 0–3 Weeks Postoperative Regimen

- No active finger flexion.
- Do not remove the splint except under the supervision of the therapist.
- Do not pick up objects with the injured hand.

### Splinting

- Fabricate a dorsal extension block splint with the wrist in 10 degrees flexion, MP joints blocked in 70 degrees flexion, and IP joints neutral (Figure 12–9).

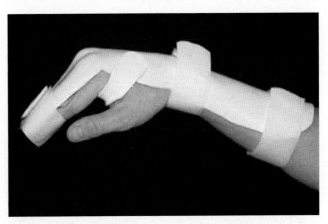

Figure 12–9:
**Dorsal block splint used for protection after flexor tendon repair. (From Trumble TE, Sailer SM: Flexor tendon injuries. In Trumble TE, editor: *Principles of hand surgery and therapy*. Philadelphia, 2000, WB Saunders.)**

---

| **Box 12–2** | **Passive ROM Protocols** |
|---|---|

**Kleinert Technique**

Prevents patients from moving their digits against resistance.
Maintains the digits in a protective position.
Requires that the patient's injured digits be maintained in flexion by using an elastic band that is attached to the level of the wrist.

**Duran Technique**

Uses a protective splint but no elastic bands (Duran and Houser, 1975).
Passive flexion achieved by the therapist or with use of the uninjured hand.
Decreases incidence of flexion contractures at the PIP joint.

Treatment

- Passive flexion using the uninvolved hand, active extension exercises while wearing the splint.
- Passive extension exercises of individual joints performed in guarded positions (all joints flexed except the joint being extended), that is, flex the DIP and MP joints when working on PIP extension.
- Edema management with elevation and compressive wrap (Coban), if needed.

### 3–6 Weeks Postoperative Regimen

Splinting Changes

- Bring the wrist position in the splint to neutral at 3 weeks.
- Can strap the PIP joints into progressively greater extension within the splint if flexion contracture occurs.

Treatment

- Continue passive flexion/active extension exercises in the splint.
- Start "place and hold" exercises by passively placing the injured digit in flexion, then asking the patient to voluntarily contract the muscle in an effort to hold the finger in flexion while releasing the pressure from the hand applying passive flexion.
- Begin gentle soft tissue mobilization for scarred areas.

### 6–9 Weeks Postoperative Regimen

Splinting Changes

- Wean from the dorsal extension block splint as patient reliability permits.

Treatment

- Begin active blocking exercises for DIP and PIP flexion to facilitate differential tendon glide.
- Begin light functional activities (e.g., picking up handfuls of beans or rice, stacking small blocks, picking up lightweight objects of varying sizes requiring different prehension patterns).

### 9–12 Weeks Postoperative Regimen

Treatment

- If stiff, begin static-progressive splinting to correct joint contracture.
- Continue active exercises (full active flexion and extension).
- Continue blocking exercises for DIP and PIP flexion.
- Begin resistive exercises and progress as follows:
  - Light functional activities at 6 weeks (picking up handfuls of beans/rice).
  - Light resistance at 8 to 10 weeks (squeezing soft foam or soft putty).

### 12–16 Weeks Postoperative Regimen

Precautions

- No heavy lifting.

Treatment

- Continue active exercises and blocking exercises, as needed.
- Progress to full resistive activities.
- Work conditioning/hardening, if needed.

### 16 Weeks Postoperative Regimen

Precautions

- None.

Treatment

- Continue for residual deficits until resolved or patient plateaus.

## Early Active Motion Protocol

- *Note:* The following is based on the Indianapolis protocol by Strickland.[3]

### Initial 24–48 Hours Postoperative Regimen

- Postoperative dressing is removed.
- A custom dorsal protective splint is fabricated in the standard position (wrist 10 degrees flexion, MPs 60–70 degrees flexion, IPs neutral) (see Figure 12–9).
- Passive PIP, DIP, and composite joint flexion and extension are started within the dorsal block splint.
- Active extension of the PIP and DIP joints to the limits of the dorsal blocking splint is allowed.
- Compressive wraps or sleeves are used to help decrease edema.

### 24–72 Hours Postoperative to 4 Weeks Postoperative Regimen

- A hinged tenodesis splint is fabricated, permitting wrist position to be varied (wrist motion limited to 30 degrees extension with unrestricted flexion, MPs in 60–70 degrees flexion, IPs neutral).
- Instruction on active "place and hold" exercises in the tenodesis splint:
  - Within the tenodesis splint, the wrist is passively brought into 30 degrees of extension while the fingers are placed into full composite flexion.
  - The patient gently contracts the finger flexors and attempts to hold the flexed position for 5 seconds.
- After each session, the patient returns to the dorsal block splint.

## 4 Weeks Postoperative Regimen

- The same place and hold exercises that were performed in the tenodesis splint are now performed without the guidance of the splint.
  - The fingers are passively flexed with the wrist extended. Flexion of the MP joints with the wrist extended helps decrease the force on finger flexor tendons.[14]
  - Active movement from a full fist, to a hook fist, to a straight fist, to full finger extension is used to facilitate maximum tendon gliding.

## 6 Weeks Postoperative Regimen

- Dorsal blocking splint is discontinued.
- Active finger flexion exercises with joint blocking at both the PIP and DIP joints are added to facilitate tendon gliding.
- Buddy taping can be used to facilitate full flexion.
  - *Note:* Blocking exercises to the small finger are not recommended.

## 8–9 Weeks Postoperative Regimen

- Light strengthening exercises (e.g., squeezing soft foam ball) are initiated.
- Soft putty can be used for strengthening.

## 10–14 Weeks Postoperative Regimen

- Progressive resistive strengthening program is initiated.
- Work simulation and reconditioning may be necessary in cases where severe deconditioning precludes return to work in some occupations.
- Return to full unrestricted activity is allowed at 14 weeks.

## Conclusion

- Successful results require precise surgical technique and strict adherence to a rehabilitation program.

## References

1. Bunnell S: Repair of tendons in the fingers. *Surg Gynecol Obstet* 35: 88-96, 1922.
   Sterling Bunnell further elaborates on his classic article from 1918, discussing atraumatic technique, the need to preserve the pulley system, and the need for postoperative therapy.

2. Duffy FJ Jr, Seiler JG, Gelberman RH, Hergrueter CA: Growth factors and canine flexor tendon healing: Initial studies in uninjured and repair models. *J Hand Surg [Am]* 20:645–649, 1995.
   Growth factors are present in normal canine intrasynovial flexor tendons.

3. Strickland JW: Flexor tendon repair: Indiana method. *Indiana Hand Center News* 1:1-19, 1993.
   The author provides an excellent overview of tendon healing and methods for tendon repair emphasizing a protocol for four-strand repair and early active motion.

4. Thurman RT, Trumble TE, Hanel DP: The two, four and six strand zone II flexor tendon repairs: a standardized in situ biomechanical comparison using the cadaver model. *J Hand Surg* 23A:261-265, 1998.
   Following cyclic loading, two-strand repairs had significantly greater gap formation after cyclic loading than either four-strand or six-strand repairs. The tensile strength of the six-strand repair was significantly greater than either the four-strand or two-strand repair.

5. Soejima O, Diao E, Lotz JC, Hariharan JS: Comparative mechanical analysis of dorsal versus palmar placement of core suture for flexor tendon repairs. *J Hand Surg [Am]* 20:801-807, 1995.
   Dorsal placement of the core suture in tendon repair is stronger than volar suture placement.

6. Aoki M, Manske PR, Pruitt DL, Larson BJ: Work of flexion after flexor tendon repair according to the placement of sutures. *Clin Orthop* 320:205-210, 1995.
   Volar location of suture material significantly increased the work of flexion following tendon repair, compared to a dorsal location.

7. Pruitt DL, Manske PR, Fink B: Cyclic stress analysis of flexor tendon repair. *J Hand Surg [Am]* 16:701-707, 1991.
   A method for evaluating flexor tendon repair techniques with use of cyclic testing is presented.

8. Saldana MJ, Ho PK, Lichtman DM, et al: Flexor tendon repair and rehabilitation in zone II open sheath technique versus closed sheath technique. *J Hand Surg [Am]* 12:1110-1114, 1987.
   There was no significant difference between the results of sheath repair and leaving it open following flexor tendon repair in zone II.

9. Bishop AT, Cooney WP, Wood MB: Treatment of partial flexor tendon lacerations: the effect of tenorrhaphy and early protected mobilization. *J Trauma* 26:301-312, 1986.
   The relative effects of immobilization, early protected mobilization, tenorrhaphy, and no repair of partial flexor tendon lacerations were evaluated in a non–weight-bearing canine model.

10. Leddy JP, Packer JW: Avulsion of the profundus tendon insertion in athletes. *J Hand Surg [Am]* 2:66-69, 1977.
    A discussion of avulsions of the flexor profundus tendon insertion.

11. Trumble TE, Vedder NB, Benirschke SK: Misleading fractures after profundus tendon avulsions: a report of six cases. *J Hand Surg [Am]* 17:902-906, 1992.
    Although the classification of Leddy and Packer is very helpful in determining the prognosis for avulsion fractures of the flexor digitorum profundus, the tendon may pull off the bone and retract farther than suggested by the fracture pattern. Therefore, all flexor digitorum profundus tendon avulsions should be surgically repaired as soon as possible.

12. Tang JB, Shi D: Subdivision of flexor tendon "no man's land" and different treatment methods in each sub-zone. A preliminary report. *Chin Med J Engl* 105:60-68, 1992.

"No man's land" of the flexor tendon system is divided into four subdivisions based on an anatomic study. Comparison of treatment results in each subzone reveals the IIc subzone is the most difficult area for satisfactory functional recovery.

13. Kleinert HE, Kutz JE, Atasoy E, Stormo S: Primary repair of flexor tendons. *Orthop Clin North Am* 4:865-876, 1973.
The authors present their results of early passive rehabilitation following zone II flexor tendon repairs. The authors use elastic bands to passively flex the injured digits.

14. Savage R: The influence of wrist position on the minimum force required for active movement of the interphalangeal joints. *J Hand Surg [Br]* 13:262-268, 1988.
Active and passive muscle tension is discussed in relation to finger flexor and extensor tendons.

# Extensor Tendon Repair and Reconstruction

Lisa L. Lattanza[*] and Emily Anne Hattwick[†]

[*]MD, Assistant Professor, Chief, Elbow Reconstructive Surgery, Department of Orthopaedic Surgery, University of California–San Francisco; Consultant, Shriner's Hospital, Northern California, San Francisco, CA
[†] MD, MPH, Attending Hand Surgeon, Department of Orthopaedics, Children's Hospital National Medical Center, Washington, DC

## Introduction and Anatomy

- The extensor mechanism of the hand and digits is a balance between intrinsic and extrinsic forces and is easily disrupted.
- Two thirds of all acute extensor tendon lacerations are associated with concomitant bone, skin, or joint injuries. Wound debridement, rigid internal fixation, bony healing, repair of neurovascular structures, and skin coverage all take precedence over extensor tendon repair.
- Chronic disruption of the extensor mechanism frequently can be addressed by attempting to rebalance forces that contribute to the extensor mechanism.

### Extrinsic Extensor Anatomy[1]

- All of the extrinsic extensor muscles for wrist, thumb, and finger extension are innervated by the radial nerve. The brachioradialis, extensor carpi radialis longus, and extensor carpi radialis brevis are innervated directly by the radial nerve proper. The rest of the extensors are innervated by a branch of the radial nerve, the posterior interosseous nerve.
- There are six dorsal compartments or fibroosseous tunnels at the wrist created by the extensor retinaculum to prevent bowstringing during wrist extension (see Chapter 1).
- There are two tendons to the index and small fingers. The extensor indicis proprius tendon is usually found ulnar to the EDC tendon in the index finger but variations can occur in this relationship.[2] After loss of

extensor indicus proprius, independent index finger function usually is preserved via the extensor digitorum communis (EDC) tendon. However, the extensor digitorum communis tendon to the small finger is present as a complete structure only 20% of the time. Therefore, loss of extensor digiti minimi (EDM) commonly results in loss of full extension of the small finger.[1]

- Juncturae tendineae interconnect the extensor digitorum tendons and the EDM tendon. These juncturae are important for force redistribution, tendon spacing, and coordination of extension. A laceration to the juncturae can result in subluxation of the extensor tendon over the metacarpophalangeal joint (MCPJ) into the radial or ulnar gutter. Lacerations to EDC tendons can be masked by intact juncturae bridging between tendons. The adjacent intact extensor tendon can extend the finger with a lacerated EDC if the juncturae to the lacerated tendon is intact distal to the laceration (Figure 13–1). Over time the juncturae weaken and an extensor lag can present several weeks after the initial laceration.

### Extensor Mechanism at the Level of the Digits

- The intrinsic muscles of the hand are intricately connected to the extensor mechanism. The sagittal bands at the level of the MCPJ centralize the extensor tendon and attach to the volar plate and periosteum of

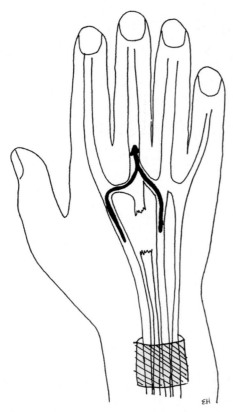

**Figure 13–1:**

**Middle finger zone VI extensor tendon laceration with extension preserved through adjacent juncturae. Examination may be normal, with only slight weakness and pain with resisted extension.**

the proximal phalanx. The lateral bands are the tendinous confluence of the intrinsic muscles on each side of the finger (Figure 13–2). The terminal lateral bands joint are stabilized by the triangular ligament and insert on the distal phalanx to extend the dorsal

interphalangeal joint (DIPJ). The lumbrical and interosseous tendons pass volar as flexors at the MCPJ and dorsal as extensors at the proximal interphalangeal joint (PIPJ) (Figure 13–3).

- The oblique retinacular ligament ([ORL] Landmeer ligament) crosses volar to the PIPJ and dorsal to the DIPJ. When the PIPJ is extended, the ORL tightens, which assists DIPJ extension, that is, coupling PIPJ extension to DIPJ extension (see Figure 13–3).

## Zones of Injury to the Extensor Tendon and Mechanism

- The extensor mechanism is divided into nine zones to facilitate discussion of injury and treatment of acute injuries. Eight zones are commonly used and are discussed here. The odd numbered zones are over joints and the even numbered zones are over bones (Figure 13–4, Table 13–1).
- In zones I through VI, tendon nutrition is via perfusion through the paratenon. In zone VII, a tenosynovium provides tendon nutrition. Zones VIII and IX are fed by small arterial branches from surrounding fascia.

## Evaluation and Diagnosis

- Bony assessment and determination of neurovascular status and flexor tendon function are essential. Thorough wound inspection may reveal joint capsule injury, foreign bodies, and partial tendon lacerations not identified on clinical examination.
- When examining the hand for extensor tendon injury, the wrist should be in neutral position. Examine each finger individually with the adjacent fingers flexed at the MCPJs. This position eliminates the pull of juncturae

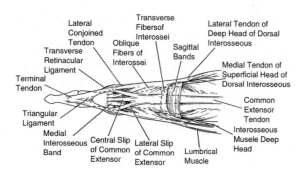

**Figure 13–2:**

**Dorsal depiction of extensor mechanism showing all components. Note the division of the central tendon to contribute to the lateral bands at the proximal interphalangeal joint and its continuation as the central slip attaching to the middle phalanx. Rupture of these central slip of the central tendon leads to boutonnière deformity. (From Trumble TE:** *Principles of hand surgery and therapy.* **Philadelphia, 2000, W.B. Saunders.)**

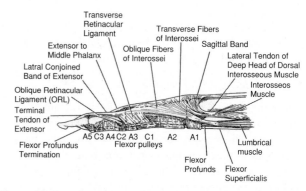

**Figure 13–3:**

**Lateral view of the extensor mechanism. The sagittal bands, transverse and oblique fibers of the interossei, and the lateral bands along with the central tendon compose the extensor hood. The oblique retinacular ligament couples extension of the proximal interphalangeal joint to extension at the distal interphalangeal joint. (From Trumble TE:** *Principles of hand surgery and therapy.* **Philadelphia, 2000, W.B. Saunders.)**

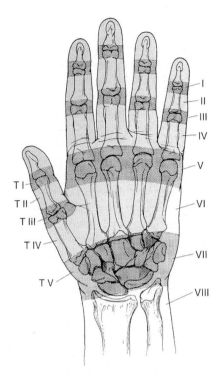

**Figure 13–4:**
**Zones of the extensor tendon system.**

from the adjacent extensor tendons, which could mask an isolated extensor tendon laceration. Other signs of extensor tendon laceration are loss of hyperextension at the MCPJ, extensor lag of the finger, and relative weakness and pain in one finger compared with the other fingers (Box 13–1).

## Suture Technique

- Extensor tendons have less excursion than flexors, so minimal shortening can result in significant loss of motion. Six millimeters of shortening results in a loss of 18 degrees of motion at the MCPJ and PIPJ.[3]
- Ideal suture technique produces minimal shortening, maximum tensile strength, and high load to failure.

Modified Kessler and modified Bunnell techniques provide the best repair strength, minimal gapping, and least loss of motion (Figure 13–5).[4] Nonabsorbable 4-0 or 5-0 sutures are acceptable for zones I through VI. Lacerations through the extensor tendon in zone I can be repaired with a nonabsorbable suture passed through tendon and skin (tenodermodesis). The DIPJ also must follow the mallet finger protocol. Lateral bands should be repaired separately with nonabsorbable 5-0 or 6-0 suture. Zone VI and VII are repaired with 4-0 suture, and zone VIII is repaired with 3-0 suture.

## Zone I Injury: Mallet Finger

- Classic mallet finger involves disruption of the extensor mechanism at the DIPJ. The mechanism is forced flexion of an extended DIPJ. This action can result in tendon rupture, avulsion from its insertion, or bony avulsion (bony mallet). Laceration to the extensor tendon is less common.
- Four types of acute mallet finger deformities have been described (Table 13–2). Treatment depends on patient age, mechanism of injury, associated fractures or osteoarthritis, and chronicity of the injury.
- *Type I* injuries are treated with splinting for 6 to 8 weeks (Table 13–3).
- *Type II* injuries should be primarily repaired at the time of laceration with a figure-of-eight suture of nonabsorbable material. Sutures can incorporate the overlying skin for dermatotenodesis.
- *Type III* injuries require soft tissue coverage of the injury, often a reverse cross-finger graft or other local graft.
- *Types IVa* and *IVb* should be reduced and splinted until the fracture heals. Appropriate reduction implies restoration of joint congruency and realignment of articular surface and contour.
- *Type IVc* with subluxation of the distal phalanx requires open reduction via a dorsal H-shaped incision and internal fixation with a Kirschner wire or 1.0-mm screw. Sometimes a pullout suture or wire provides the best fixation.

| Table 13–1: | Extensor Zones of Injury |
| --- | --- |
| Zone I | Overlies the distal interphalangeal joint, including the terminal insertion of the extensor mechanism or slip |
| Zone II | Includes the middle phalanx and lateral bands; at the thumb it is over the proximal phalanx |
| Zone III | Overlies the proximal interphalangeal joint, where the central slip inserts on the middle phalanx; at the thumb it includes the metacarpophalangeal joint and extensor pollicis brevis insertion |
| Zone IV | Includes the proximal phalanx and extensor mechanism distal to the extensor hood |
| Zone V | Overlies the metacarpophalangeal joint including the extensor hood; this is the area of "fight bite" injuries |
| Zone VI | Over the metacarpals, including juncturae, extensor digitorum communis, extensor indicis proprius, and extensor digiti minimi tendons |
| Zone VII | Dorsal wrist retinaculum with six compartments through which the extrinsic tendons pass from the forearm to the wrist |
| Zone VIII | Just proximal to the retinaculum and distal to the musculotendinous junction |

| Box 13–1 | Clinical Signs of Extensor Tendon Lacerations |
|----------|------------------------------------------------|

- Extensor lag at MCPJ, PIPJ, or DIPJ
- Loss of MCPJ hyperextension with the PIPJ flexed: test of extrinsic extensor
- Pain and weakness of extension against resistance, especially if extension is through juncturae after a complete zone VI laceration

## Therapeutic Regimen

- Type I injuries should be immobilized for 6 to 8 weeks in extension, followed by 6 to 8 weeks of nocturnal splint use and slow daytime weaning from the splint (Figure 13–6). During this time, full active and passive motion of the PIPJ is achieved.[5] If this regimen is interrupted or if deformity recurs, the protocol should be restarted from the beginning. The patient must be reminded that a brief loss of full extension at the DIPJ disrupts whatever healing has begun and restarts the clock for splinting. Attention to the skin on the dorsum of the finger during this splinting period is important because the skin can become macerated and irritated. The best form of splinting is a padded Alumafoam splint contoured to hold the DIPJ in hyperextension. This splint is taped to the dorsum of the finger with cloth tape. For the first few weeks, the patient can return to the clinic for splint changes. The patient should be reminded of the importance of keeping the finger extended 100% of the time and taught how to change the splint and watch for skin breakdown. Stack splints have been used successfully because they hold the finger in hyperextension nicely. Dorsal skin maceration is more problematic with these splints because of direct contact of the plastic on the skin. Another option for maintaining the finger in extension is to place a transarticular K-wire for the first 6 to 8 weeks if compliance or skin irritation is a problem.[6]

Figure 13–5:

**Suture techniques for extensor tendon repair. Modified Kessler and Bunnell core suture techniques using a nonabsorbable 4-0 suture provide greater strength to minimize gapping and failure than simple, figure-of-eight, and mattress sutures.**

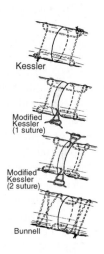

Kessler

Modified Kessler (1 suture)

Modified Kessler (2 suture)

Bunnell

| Table 13–2: Mallet Finger Classification | | |
|------------------------------------------|---|---|
| **MALLET FINGER CLASSIFICATION** | | |
| TYPE I: | TYPE II: | TYPE III: |
| Closed soft tissue disrupting due to hyperflexion injury | Laceration at dorsum of distal interphalangeal joint | Open hyperflexion injury with deep skin abrasion or tissue loss |
| 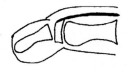 | 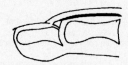 | 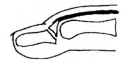 |
| TYPE IVA: | TYPE IVB: | TYPE IVC: |
| Transphyseal injury in skeletally immature digit | Hyperflexion injury involving 20–50% of articular surface | Hyperextension injury involving >50% of articular surface |

*Results in early or late volar subluxation of distal phalanx

| Table 13–3: Mallet Finger Extension Splinting Protocol | |
| --- | --- |
| **MALLET FINGER** | **EXTENSION SPLINTING PROTOCOL (TYPES I, II, III, AND IVB)** |
| First 6–8 weeks | Immobilize DIPJ in full extension/hyperextension, and leave the proximal interphalangeal joint free for active motion. Take care not to move the DIPJ when changing the splint. |
| Second 6–8 weeks | Begin weaning from the splint during the daytime. Continue immobilization at night. |
| After 6–8 weeks | Accept residual deformity up to 15 degrees flexion at the DIPJ. Repeat protocol from beginning if >15 degrees. |
| Splint care and changing splint | Instruct patient to monitor dorsal skin where splint rests for irritation and maceration. When changing splint, the DIPJ must be kept in extension. |
| Other treatments | Type IVa (pediatric) may require transarticular pinning for compliance. Type IVc requires reduction internal fixation. |

DIPJ, Distal interphalangeal joint.

- Chronic mallet fingers up to 3 months old can be treated following the splinting protocol (see Table 13–3).[7] If the deformity persists, tendon advancement is indicated for flexible deformities, and arthrodesis is recommended for rigid deformities.
- Swan-neck deformity develops in chronic mallet fingers because the lateral bands migrate proximally and dorsally, causing hyperextension at the PIPJ (Figure 13–7). The spiral ORL can be used to restore balance or a superficialis tenodesis can be used to prevent hyperextension. Many swan-neck deformities are treated with long-term splinting.

# Zone II Injuries

- Most injuries to the extensor mechanism in zone II result from lacerations and crush injuries. Lacerations distal to the insertion of the central slip result in a mallet deformity. Partial lacerations less than half the width of the tendon can be treated with wound closure and splinting in extension for 7 to 10 days, followed by active range of motion. Lacerations greater than 50% of the

tendon width should be repaired with nonabsorbable suture in running fashion to minimize tendon shortening.

## Therapeutic Considerations

- Zone II injuries can follow the same splinting protocol as zone I injuries (see Table 13–3). Gradual DIPJ flexion exercises begin with 20 to 25 degrees in the first week and progress 10 degrees each week. If the distal joint is tight in extension, the ORL can be stretched by flexing the DIPJ with the PIPJ in extension.

# Zone III Injuries: Boutonnière Deformity

- Disruption of the central slip allows the lateral bands to subluxate volarly and flex the PIPJ while extending the DIPJ (Figure 13–8).
- In the acute setting, the inability to extend the PIPJ against resistance with the joint flexed at 90 degrees

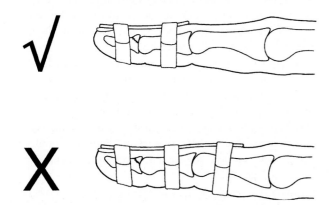

Figure 13–6:
Extension splinting for mallet finger leaves the proximal interphalangeal joint free to flex but keeps the distal interphalangeal joint in full extension. (From Trumble TE: *Priciples of hand surgery and therapy.* Philadelphia, 2000, W.B. Saunders.)

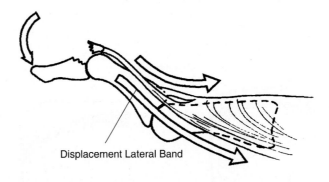

Displacement Lateral Band

Figure 13–7:
Swan-neck deformity from proximal migration of the lateral band complex after disruption of the distal extensor mechanism. The lateral bands move proximally into a more dorsal position and contract, which pulls the proximal interphalangeal joint into extension. (From Trumble TE: *Priciples of hand surgery and therapy.* Philadelphia, 2000, W.B. Saunders.)

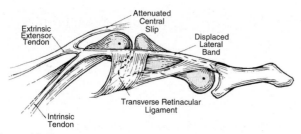

Figure 13–8:

**Boutonnière deformity showing volar migration of lateral bands after disruption of the central slip. As the lateral bands migrate volarly and contract, they produce a flexed posture of the proximal interphalangeal joint but an extended posture of the distal interphalangeal joint.**

suggests central slip avulsion or rupture. Active extension of the DIPJ while in the same position also suggests acute central slip disruption. This test was described by Elson and, if carefully performed, is a reliable way of evaluating an acute boutonnière deformity (Figure 13–9, Box 13–2). Pain may limit patient cooperation, and a digital block improves the success of the test.[8]

- Chronic boutonnière deformities usually involve subluxation of the lateral bands with scarring and adhesions to the underlying capsule. The finger is less supple and the deformity more difficult to passively reduce. Boyes described a test to identify fixed subluxation and adhesions of the lateral bands. The finger is held in extension at the PIPJ, and the patient is asked to flex the DIPJ. When the lateral bands have been in a relatively shortened, volarly subluxated position and are scarred down, PIPJ extension increases the tension in the lateral bands. Therefore, the DIPJ is held tightly in extension, and the patient cannot actively flex this joint (Figure 13–10, Box 13–3).[8]

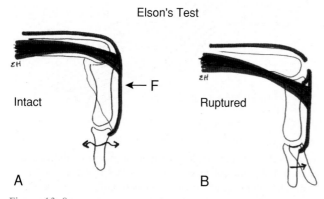

Elson's Test

Intact      ← F      Ruptured

A              B

Figure 13–9:

**Elson test for acute rupture of the central slip. *F,* Static force. (See Box 13–2.)**

---

| Box 13–2 | **Elson Test for Acute Central Slip Rupture (Figure 13–9)** |
|---|---|

- Rest the hand on a table with the finger flexed at the PIPJ over the edge of the table. The examiner holds the PIPJ fixed at 90 degrees while the patient attempts to extend the PIPJ. With an intact central slip and the PIPJ in 90 degrees flexion, the examiner feels extension pressure through the middle phalanx and the DIPJ is flail, that is, not able to actively extend.
- In this same position and with a completely ruptured central slip, the middle phalanx does not exert extension, but the DIPJ is rigid in extension. This result is caused by volar subluxation of the lateral bands when the PIPJ is flexed to 90 degrees. The lateral bands migrate dorsally again when the finger extends in the acute setting.
- A digital block may be required to facilitate patient cooperation with this test in the acute setting.

## Treatment of Acute Boutonnière Deformity[9]

- Closed acute central slip injuries are treated with continuous splinting of the PIPJ in extension for 6 weeks. The DIPJ is left free, and active and passive DIPJ flexion are encouraged to keep the lateral bands and ORL supple.
- Surgical indications for an acute boutonnière deformity are a displaced avulsion fracture of the central slip at the base of the middle phalanx, instability of the PIPJ associated with loss of active or passive extension of the finger, or failed nonoperative treatment. Open central slip injuries require thorough debridement and evaluation of the underlying joint. Both primary closure and healing secondary intention have been described because the central slip tendons do not retract and the scar tissue can bridge the defect if constant splinting is maintained for four to six weeks. Active DIPJ and MCPJ motion is essential while holding the PIPJ in extension during healing. DIPJ motion stretches the lateral bands and keeps them dorsal to the PIPJ. Tension on the lateral bands also reduces the tension on the central slip and facilitates healing.
- Primary suture repair of the central slip to the middle phalanx may be possible; if not, portions of the lateral bands can be sutured together dorsally to recreate a central slip. If the lateral bands cannot be moved dorsally, the Matev procedure, which consists of transecting the lateral bands and suturing one to the remnant central slip tissue and cross suturing the remaining lateral band, can be used (Figure 13–11).

## Treatment of Chronic Boutonnière Deformity[9]

- Treatment is predicated on first restoring passive motion at the DIPJ and PIPJ with therapy and dynamic splinting. Surgical excision of redundant central slip and

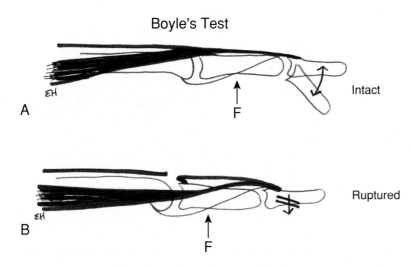

Boyle's Test

A

EH

F

Intact

B

EH

F

Ruptured

Figure 13–10:
Boyes test for chronic rupture of the central slip.
*F,* Static force. (See Box 13–3.)

reconstruction of the slip with appropriate extensor tension then can be achieved. Transarticular K-wires are helpful in maintaining extension at the PIPJ while moving the DIPJ and MCPJ.

- In a supple PIPJ with a Boutonnière deformity, transcription of the central portion of the extensor tendon at the middle phalanx and partially transecting the lateral bands has been described. This procedure allows the extensor mechanism to migrate proximally, moving the lateral bands dorsally and rebalancing the PIPJ. The ORL must be protected during this release to maintain extension at the DIPJ (Figure 13–12).

- When motion cannot be achieved by therapy and splinting, a two-stage procedure can be performed. First, the volar structures are released to allow motion. Then a second procedure is performed to reconstruct the central slip. Tenotomy or partial transection of the distal tendon may allow motion at the DIPJ while leaving contracture at the PIPJ alone. The lateral bands can be partially divided, mobilized dorsally, and attached to the dorsum of the middle phalanx to provide PIPJ extension.

| Box 13–3 | **Boyes Test for Chronic Central Slip Rupture (Figure 13–10)** |
|---|---|

- Hold the PIPJ in extension and have the patient attempt to flex the DIPJ. When the central slip is intact, the patient will be able to flex the DIPJ using the action of the FDP tendon. When the central slip has been ruptured, retracted, and scarred to the proximal tissues, the lateral bands are under more tension with the PIPJ in extension. In this position, the tight lateral bands hold the DIPJ in extension and prevent active flexion of the DIPJ.

- Treatment of boutonnière deformity or central slip rupture relies on extension splinting at the PIPJ to keep the lateral bands in their anatomic dorsal position and active motion at the DIPJ to keep the lateral bands stretched and supple. These actions prevent retraction of the central slip and increased tension in the lateral bands.

## Therapeutic Considerations

- Treatment of closed acute Boutonnière deformities consists of extension splinting of the PIPJ for 6 weeks and repeat splinting if the deformity recurs. The surrounding joints are left free for active full motion during splinting (Figure 13–13).

- After open repair of central slip injuries, the PIPJ is immobilized in extension for 3 to 6 weeks before gradual motion is started. If the lateral bands were not repaired, the DIPJ can be left free to flex and stretch the ORLs.

## Zone IV Injuries

- Partial lacerations are treated with splinting the MCPJ, PIPJ, and DIPJ in extension and the wrist in a neutral position for 3 to 4 weeks. Complete lacerations should be repaired, and associated phalangeal fractures should be internally fixed to allow early active range of motion. Restoration of length and appropriate rotation is important. If proximal phalangeal fractures are allowed to shorten, the extensor mechanism is effectively elongated at the proximal phalanx, leading to an extensor lag at the PIPJ. Dissection should be limited and care taken in handling soft tissues to minimize scarring.

## Therapeutic Considerations

- After repair of zone IV lacerations, tendon-bone adhesions frequently prevent tendon gliding. Traditionally, the MCPJ, PIPJ, and DIPJ are splinted in extension with the wrist in a neutral position for 4 to 6 weeks. To prevent dorsal hood adhesions, an early motion protocol has been suggested.[10] The PIPJ and DIPJ are splinted in extension, except during exercises. The exercises involve flexing the wrist to 30 degrees and the MCPJ is kept at 0 degrees. The PIPJ is slowly actively flexed to 30 degrees and the DIPJ to 20 to 25 degrees for 20 repetitions. This

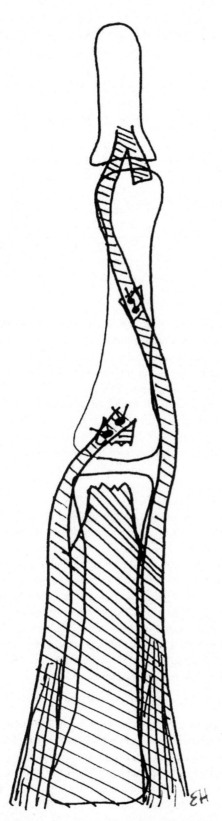

Figure 13–11:
Matev procedure for treatment of boutonnière deformity. One lateral band is divided and sutured to the remnant central slip stump on the middle phalanx. The other lateral band is divided, crossed, and sutured to the opposite lateral band.

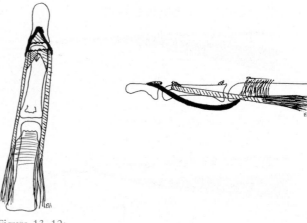

Figure 13–12:
Fowler procedure for chronic boutonnière deformity. The central tendon and lateral bands are divided just proximal to the distal interphalangeal joint, leaving the oblique retinacular ligament intact. This procedure allows the extensor mechanism to migrate proximally, release tension from the lateral bands, and facilitate flexion at the PIPJ.

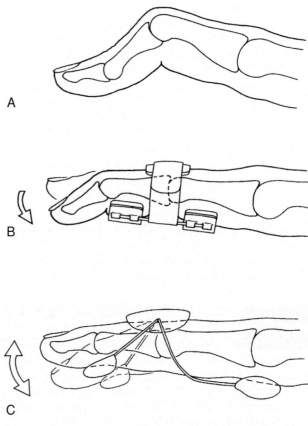

Figure 13–13:
Splinting for boutonnière deformity holds the proximal interphalangeal joint in extension but leaves the distal interphalangeal joint free to flex. The Bunnell rigid extension splint (B) is used for the first 3 to 6 weeks. The patient then can be placed in a Capener dynamic extension splint (C), which allows active proximal interphalangeal joint flexion and passive extension. The patient is weaned to nighttime splint use at 8 to 11 weeks, and then the splint is discontinued.

process may prevent adhesions that ultimately result in poor tendon gliding in zone IV.

## Zone V Injuries

- The "fight bite" is an open wound overlying the MCPJ that occurred with the finger in flexion. The wound can involve the underlying extensor mechanism and even can extend into the joint. Appropriate debridement and assessment of the depth of the wound are imperative to prevent infections such as septic arthritis and osteomyelitis. The wound should be examined with the fingers in the same position when the wound occurred. This action facilitates visualization of the underlying extensor mechanism, joint capsule, and even the joint if the wound extends to that depth. Thorough irrigation of the maximal depth of the wound is required, including intraarticular irrigation if the joint is involved. Wound cultures should be sent, broad-spectrum antibiotics started, and the hand splinted for a few days before starting motion again. If pain persists, operative debridement of the wound and joint may be required.
- Rupture of the sagittal bands presents as a painful snapping at the MCPJ as the extensor tendon subluxates either radially or ulnarly as the finger is brought from full extension into flexion. Splinting in extension with the tendon centralized for 6 weeks usually is sufficient. If the problem presents late or persists after splinting, surgical repair of the sagittal band with a flap of extensor tendon used to reinforce the repair allows early active motion.

### Therapeutic Considerations

- Protocols exist for complete immobilization, early passive motion, and immediate active motion.[12] Clinical studies show that wrist tenodesis exercises with active extensor motion result in greater range of motion without significant rupture rates. With the wrist flexed to approximately 20 degrees, the patient can actively hold the fingers in extension and then actively move the MCPJ from 30 degrees flexion to 0 degrees. Wrist tenodesis exercises are used to allow passive tendon gliding. Ideally, this protocol is started within 24 to 36 hours after surgery.[12] Dynamic splinting with the MCPJ in extension can also be very useful.

## Zone VI Injuries

- Juncturae injuries frequently are missed. Exploration of wounds is the best method for diagnosing and treating these lacerations. Proximal tendon lacerations frequently retract, and repair should be done using four-strand core suture technique (Figure 13–5). Splinting of all of the fingers from DIPJ to wrist in extension protects EDC repairs. Splinting the index finger alone in extension is acceptable after repair of the extensor indicis proprius

(EIP) tendon. Dynamic splinting as in zone V injuries can be very helpful.
- If multiple extensor tendons are injured and there is inadequate length and tendon quality for primary repair, then the more damaged tendons can be repaired end to side to the less injured adjacent tendons. If there is complete loss of tendon and no adjacent tissue is adequate, tendon rods can be placed while the soft tissue bed heals. Then flexor to extensor transfers are used to restore extensor function.

### Therapeutic Considerations

- The controlled active motion protocol for zone V also can be used for zone VI injuries. Immobilized tendons lose strength over time, whereas controlled motion improves the tensile strength of the tendon, improves gliding properties, increases repair-site DNA, and accelerates changes in the surrounding vascularity. Controlled early active tension and motion promotes gliding motion without placing stress at the repair site. Dynamic splints are designed to allow active flexion and thus gliding of the extensor mechanism. Many patients inadvertently actively extend through the slings, which promotes tendon healing.

## Zone VII Injuries

- Laceration to extensor tendons at the level of the retinaculum presents a complex problem. The tendons retract significantly, scar under the retinaculum after repair, and limit finger flexion because of loss of extensor excursion. Partial retinaculum release is required, but complete release results in bowstringing.[13]
- Injuries to the sensory branches of the radial nerve at this level should be addressed with either epineurial repair or resection of the proximal nerve end and burial in surrounding tissue to prevent neuroma formation.

### Therapeutic Considerations

- Immobilization of tendon repair at the wrist leads to scarring and adhesions and should be limited to a short period. The wrist should be immobilized in 10 to 20 degrees extension and early tenodesis exercises started. Active wrist motion from 0 degrees to full extension can begin by 3 to 4 weeks. By 5 to 6 weeks, gradual wrist flexion is started, progressing slowly over the next 2 to 3 weeks to full flexion. When the extensor retinaculum has been disrupted, the extensor tendons bowstrings and increases the work load across the repair site. Slower advances in the protocol may be necessary to protect the repair.[12]

## Zone VIII Injuries

- Wrist and thumb extension should be priorities when sorting out multiple extensor lacerations in zone VIII.

Appropriate incisions and exploration are necessary to identify both proximal and distal tendon ends. Muscle bellies can be repaired with multiple figure-of-eight sutures. Laceration to the posterior interosseous nerve should be repaired because the distance to regenerate to the neuromuscular junction at this level usually is short.

## Therapeutic Considerations

- Splint the wrist in extension and the MCPs in 15 to 20 degrees flexion for 4 to 6 weeks. After immobilization, mobilization is started with both active extension and flexion.

# Extensor Injuries to the Thumb

- Zone T1 injuries are treated similar to mallet injuries in the other fingers by splinting, primary repair in lacerations, and bony fixation with K-wires or screws where more than 50% of the joint is involved.
- Injury to the extensor pollicis brevis is uncommon but is associated with avulsion of the dorsal capsule and radial collateral ligament complex. Cast immobilization is appropriate early, but persistent laxity should be treated surgically.
- Rupture of the extensor pollicis longus (EPL) tendon following a distal radius fracture is well described. Proposed mechanisms of rupture are attritional rupture secondary to fracture fragments, ischemia, or hemorrhages within tendon sheath. Delayed diagnosis is common, with the patient presenting 6 to 8 weeks after fracture with the inability to extend the thumb and resting in an adducted position. Free tendon grafting often is required using an intercalated graft or by transferring EIP to EPL.

## Therapeutic Considerations

- For zone T1 injuries, follow the mallet finger protocol (see Table 13–3). Zones TII to IV, early active tensioning, and motion exercises are recommended. Zone V at the wrist involves the extensor retinaculum and a synovial sheath. Adhesions form if the tendon is immobilized, and early dynamic gliding exercises or controlled active motion is important.

## Complications of Extensor Tendons

- Complex injuries usually include soft tissue damage, tendon injury, nerve injury, and even fractures or other bony injuries. Soft tissue management and fracture care are priorities. Tendon function often is impaired by scarring from associated soft tissue injuries. Early postoperative motion helps decrease adhesions from scarring and improve tendon gliding and function. Tenolysis may be required in more

complex injuries to facilitate better range of motion and function.

# References

### Anatomy

1. von Schroeder HP, Botte MJ: Functional anatomy of the extensor tendons of the digits. *Hand Clin* 13:51-62, 1997.
   The extensor anatomy, including anomalous tendons and multiplicity, is described in detail.

2. Gonzalez MH, Weinzweig N, Kay T, Grindel S: Anatomy of the extensor tendons to the index finger. *J Hand Surg [Am]* 21:988-991, 1996.
   Of 72 cadaver hands, 19% showed anatomic variation from the classic single slip of the EIP lying ulnar to the EDC.

### Suture Technique

3. McCallister W, Cober S, Trumble T: Peripheral nerve defects. J Hand Surg 20: 315-325, 2001.

4. Newport ML, Pollack GR, Williams CD: Biomechanical characteristics of suture techniques in extensor zone IV. *J Hand Surg [Am]* 20:650-656, 1995.
   Biomechanical testing on 16 fresh-frozen cadaver hands found modified Bunnell and modified Kessler techniques superior to the mattress and figure-of-eight techniques used for extensor tendon repairs.

### Mallet Finger

5. Katzman BM, Klein DM, Mesa J, et al: Immobilization of the mallet finger. Effects on the extensor tendon. *J Hand Surg [Br]* 24:80-84, 1999.
   The authors tested 32 cadaveric fingers with open mallet finger lesions and found that joint motion proximal to the DIPJ did not cause a tendon gap.

6. Okafor B, Mbubaegbu C, Munshi I, Williams DJ: Mallet deformity of the finger. Five-year follow-up of conservative treatment. *J Bone Joint Surg Br* 79:544-547, 1997.
   After conservative treatment of 31 patients with mallet finger deformities, patient satisfaction was high, and there was little evidence of functional impairment despite high rates of arthritis and extensor lag.

7. Garberman SF, Diao E, Peimer C: Mallet finger: results of early versus delayed closed treatment. *J Hand Surg [Am]* 19:850-852, 1994.
   This retrospective review found results of conservative treatment of mallet fingers were independent of time from injury to treatment, even up to 8 months.

### Boutonnière Deformity

8. Elson RA: Rupture of the central slip of the extensor hood of the finger: a test for early diagnosis. *J Bone Joint Surg* 68B:229-231, 1986.
   A review of central slip injuries, Boyes test for chronic injury, and a description of a new test for identifying acute central slip injury.

9. Coons MS, Green SM: Boutonnière deformity. *Hand Clin* 11:387-402, 1995.

A treatment algorithm for all types of boutonnière deformities is presented in this in-depth review.

## Rehabilitation

10. Crosby CA, Wehbe MA: Early protected motion after extensor tendon repair. *J Hand Surg [Am]* 24:1061-1070, 1999.
    The authors report good results with an immediate motion and tendon mobilization program with dynamic splinting for extensor tendon repairs.

11. Evans RB: Clinical management of extensor tendon injuries. In Hunter JM, Mackin EJ, Callahan AD, editors. *Rehabilitation of the hand and upper extremity,* ed 5. St. Louis, 2002, Mosby.
    This chapter provides a review of therapeutic regimens and a comparison of outcomes for each regimen. Considerations of specific anatomy, associated injuries and patient factors are included to help guide a complete therapeutic plan.

12. Chester DL, Beale S, Beveridge L, et al: A prospective, controlled, randomized trial comparing early active extension with passive extension using a dynamic splint in the rehabilitation of repaired extensor tendons. *J Hand Surg [Br]* 27:283-288, 2002.
    This randomized, prospective study comparing early active motion with dynamic splinting for extensor tendon repairs in zones IV to VIII found no significant differences between the two groups at final follow-up.

## Zone VII Injury

13. Palmer AK, Skahen JR, Werner FW, Glisson RR: Retinacular release I zone VII injuries leads to bowstringing. *J Hand Surg Br* 10:11-16, 1985.
    Discussion of bowstringing at the wrist after division of the extensor retinaculum.

## Review Articles

Newport ML: Extensor tendon injuries in the hand. *J Am Acad Orthop Surg* 5:59-66, 1997.
This review article covers the basic anatomy, initial evaluation, treatment, surgical technique and rehabilitation of extensor tendon injuries.

Rockwell WB, Butler PN, Byrne BA: Extensor tendon: anatomy, injury, and reconstruction. *Plast Reconstr Surg* 106:1592-1603, 2000; quiz 1604, 1673.
This comprehensive review article describes the anatomy of the extensor tendons, the acute and chronic pathologic conditions affecting the extensor mechanism, the physiology and repair techniques of traumatic injuries, and the reconstructive options for chronic disorders.

# Tenosynovitis: Trigger Finger, de Quervain Syndrome, Flexor Carpi Radialis, and Extensor Carpi Ulnaris

Ioannis Sarris,* Nickolaos A. Darlis,* Douglas Musgrave,† and Dean G. Sotereanos‡

* MD, PhD, Fellow, Upper Extremity Surgery, Department of Orthopaedic Surgery, Allegheny General Hospital, Pittsburgh, PA
† MD, Fellow, Upper Extremity Surgery, Allegheny General Hospital, Pittsburgh, PA
‡ MD, Professor, Orthopaedic Surgery, Drexel University School of Medicine, Philadelphia, PA; Vice Chairman, Department of Orthopaedic Surgery, Allegheny General Hospital, Pittsburgh, PA

## Introduction

- The term *tendonitis* is often used in clinical practice to describe the inflammatory process involving one or more of the numerous tendons that cross the wrist and the hand. Although this term might be accurate in the early stages, with more chronic lesions the synovial sheath of intrasynovial tendons almost invariably is involved, and the term *tenosynovitis* or *tenovaginitis* is more appropriate.
- The synovial sheath is a membranous structure with an inner visceral layer and an outer parietal layer that plays an important role in intrasynovial tendon gliding and nutrition by diffusion. This membranous structure is reinforced locally by outer retinacular components (as are the digital pulleys or the extensor retinaculum) to enhance function. When the membranous sheath becomes inflamed and edematous, the retinacular components prohibit its expansion, and thus the tendons are locally constricted. With chronicity, local ischemia leads to secondary changes to the sheath and tendon. The sheath becomes fibrotic and even can undergo cartilaginous metaplasia, whereas the tendon is locally thinned and fibrotic. These pathologic changes are encountered in the majority of the disorders discussed in this chapter.
- The primary etiology of most of these disorders is still unclear. Repetitive trauma can induce a local inflammatory process, but in most cases an anatomic or intrinsic predisposing factor must exist. Age and gender also are important factors because these conditions are seen more frequently in women in their 50s. Pregnancy is a predisposing factor, and the dominant extremity is more often affected.
- These conditions should be differentiated from more generalized inflammatory processes, as in rheumatoid arthritis. Less commonly, deposits as calcifications, crystals, and amyloid are the primary cause of tendosynovitis. The need to rule out septic tenosynovitis (although its presentation is markedly different than most of these disorders) cannot be overemphasized.

## Trigger Finger

### Anatomy and Pathology

- The digital flexor tendon sheaths are bilayer synovial linings supported and enclosed by a series of five annular and three cruciate pulleys, the so-called *retinacular sheath* (Figure 14–1). The thumb flexor sheath is enclosed by two annular pulleys and one oblique pulley (Figure 14–2).

- The proximal edge of the A1 pulley is near the distal palmar crease for the ring and small fingers, near the

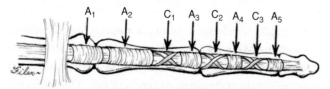

**Figure 14–1:**
The digital flexor tendon sheath is enclosed and supported by a series of five annular and three cruciate pulleys. The A2 and A4 pulleys should be preserved to prevent tendon bowstringing. The A1 pulley is most commonly involved in trigger finger.

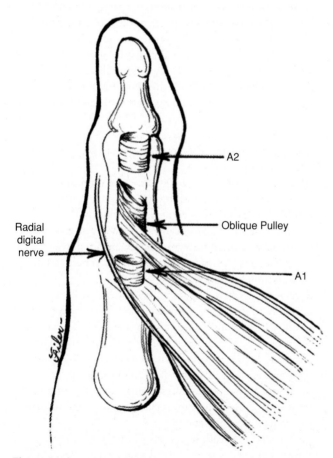

**Figure 14–2:**
The thumb flexor sheath is enclosed and supported by two annular pulleys and one oblique pulley. The A1 pulley is most commonly involved in trigger thumb. The oblique pulley should be preserved to prevent tendon bowstringing. The radial digital nerve obliquely crosses the volar aspect of the thumb and is at risk for injury during trigger thumb release.

proximal palmar crease for the index finger, and midway between the proximal and distal palmar creases for the middle finger. The proximal edge of the first annular pulley of the thumb lies near the metacarpophalangeal (MP) joint flexion crease. The A1 pulleys and the first annular pulley of the thumb arise at the level of the MP joints. The A2 pulleys of the fingers are at the level of the proximal portion of the proximal phalanges and the oblique pulley of the thumb is at the middle region of the proximal phalanx.

- The digital arteries are volar to the digital nerves in the palm but become dorsal to the digital nerves in the fingers. Both structures lie in close proximity to the flexor sheath, paralleling the sheath on both its radial and ulnar borders. The neurovascular bundles are at risk for injury during surgery. The radial neurovascular bundle to the thumb is the most at risk as it passes obliquely across the thenar eminence from ulnar to radial and lies just deep to the dermis at the MP joint flexion crease (see Figure 14–2). It has been reported to be approximately 1 mm anterior to the radial sesamoid and 1 mm deep to the dermis at the thumb MP flexion crease.

- Trigger digits occur because of a disproportion between the digital retinacular sheath and its contents, the flexor tendons and synovial sheath. The first annular (A1) pulley is the usual site of obstruction in trigger fingers. The first annular pulley is the usual source of obstruction in trigger thumbs. The disproportion may be caused by the angular course required by the flexor tendons as they enter the retinacular sheath under the A1 pulley. Authors have proposed that this angular course results in "bunching" of the tendon fibers, leading to an intratendinous nodule. This nodule occurs just distal to the A1 pulley. In diffuse stenosing tenosynovitis resulting from a systemic condition such as rheumatoid arthritis or amyloidosis, the size discrepancy between the retinacular sheath and its contents may extend well distal to the A1 pulley.

- *Histologically*, both the A1 pulley and the flexor tendon in the region of the A1 pulley undergo fibrocartilaginous metaplasia. The normal A1 pulley is composed of an outer vascular layer and an inner gliding layer. In trigger finger, the inner gliding layer hypertrophies, and the cells increase in number, taking on the histologic appearance of chondrocytes. The hypertrophy may progress until the A1 pulley is two to three times its normal thickness. The tendon undergoes fraying and degeneration on its volar, avascular surface in the region where it passes under the A1 pulley. Positive histologic staining for S-100 protein, a protein associated with chondrocytes, indicates the tendon undergoes fibrocartilaginous metaplasia, similar to the A1 pulley.

- The pathologic process in infants usually consists of a nodule *(Notta node)* within the flexor pollicis longus tendon without hypertrophy of the first annular pulley.

## Diagnosis

- Trigger digits, or stenosing tenosynovitis (tenovaginitis) of the digits, are one of the most common causes of hand pain and dysfunction. Primary (idiopathic) trigger finger occurs two to six times more frequently in women than in men and has a peak incidence between the ages of 40 and 60 years as well as being higher in patients with diabetes. Secondary trigger finger is associated with predisposing conditions such as rheumatoid arthritis, diabetes mellitus, gout, amyloidosis, and mucopolysaccharidoses. Multiple digit involvement is not uncommon, nor is bilateral involvement. The ring finger is most commonly involved, followed by the thumb and long finger, the index finger, and then the small finger.
- Patients often notice a painless click in the finger that eventually becomes painful. The pain, when present, frequently localizes to the MP joint and may radiate proximally. The digit may become locked in flexion, with passive extension required to unlock the digit, or locked in extension, with the patient unable to fully flex the finger. Chronic cases of locked trigger digits may result in fixed joint contractures, presenting a diagnostic challenge. Patients frequently attribute the problem to the proximal interphalangeal (PIP) joint.
- Physical examination often reveals a noticeable catching of the digit during active extension from a flexed position. Manipulation by the examiner may be required to extend a locked digit. The flexor sheath should be palpated for a discrete nodule or diffuse tenosynovitis, because this finding may have prognostic and treatment implications. The nodule usually is painful to palpation (Box 14–1).
- Most proposed classification systems divide trigger digits to one of five grades, based on the findings of the physical examination (Box 14–2).
- *Trigger digit in children* is a separate entity from adult trigger digit. Any digit may be affected, but involvement of digits other than the thumb is rare. When digits other than the thumb are involved, spontaneous resolution is more likely. The term *congenital trigger thumb* reflects the belief that the condition is present at birth, but it

| Box 14–1 | Differential Diagnosis of Trigger Finger |
| --- | --- |

- Dupuytren contracture
- PIP joint dislocation
- MP joint dislocation
- MP joint loose body
- Volar plate avulsion with entrapment
- Tendon sheath tumor
- Intrinsic tendon entrapment on an irregular metacarpal head
- Rheumatoid arthritis
- de Quervain disease

| Box 14–2 | Proposed Classification for Trigger Finger |
| --- | --- |
| Grade 0 | Mild crepitus of the flexor sheath without triggering |
| Grade 1 | Abnormal or uneven movement |
| Grade 2 | Clicking or triggering of the digit, but no locking |
| Grade 3 | Locked trigger digit that is passively correctable |
| Grade 4 | Locked digit, possibly with a PIP joint flexion contracture |

frequently is not recognized initially. Others suggest the condition is acquired based on the findings of two large prospective studies in neonates that failed to identify congenital cases of trigger digits.[1,2] Trigger thumb in children is rare, affecting less than 0.05% of children. Bilateral involvement may be present in up to one third of patients overall, and it is even more common in patients with trigger thumb diagnosed at birth. Parents notice that the thumb interphalangeal (IP) joint remains partially flexed. Inability to flex the extended thumb also can be the first manifestation. On physical examination, there usually is a thumb IP joint flexion contracture of 10 to 20 degrees and a palpable nodule near the volar aspect of the MP joint. Trigger thumb in a child must be distinguished from congenital clasped thumb, spasticity, or arthrogryposis. Congenital clasped thumb consists of flexion contractures at both the IP and MP joints, whereas the MP joint is uninvolved in trigger thumb.

## Treatment

- Many primary trigger digits in adults can be successfully treated nonoperatively.
- *Nonoperative treatment* includes activity modification, splinting, ice, massage, nonsteroidal antiinflammatory drugs (NSAIDs), and injections. Many authors recommend corticosteroid injections without splinting as the initial treatment for symptomatic primary trigger digits. Patients who refuse an injection can be treated with immobilization alone.
- Several factors help predict which patients will respond favorably to injections. In one series, 93% of patients with nodular trigger digits treated with one injection remained symptom free at 3 months. Only 48% of patients with diffuse stenosing tenosynovitis were successfully treated with an injection.[3] Patients with multiple digit involvement, symptoms lasting longer than 6 months, or insulin-dependent diabetes mellitus respond less favorably to corticosteroid injections.[4]
- Flexor tendon sheath injections can be performed through either a volar or lateral approach. Through either approach, the tip of a small-gauge needle can be initially placed into the tendon and placement confirmed by asking the patient to flex and extend the digit. The needle is withdrawn slightly such that the flexor sheath can be insufflated with the steroid mixture. Caution should be exercised to avoid intratendinous injections.

Lidocaine injections alone are less efficacious than corticosteroid injections with or without a local anesthetic. Counsel the patient regarding the possibilities of transient elevation of serum glucose (in diabetic patients), skin depigmentation, local subcutaneous fat atrophy or necrosis, and tendon rupture. The patient is instructed to move the finger freely after the injection.

- Many authors recommend a series of up to two corticosteroid injections over the course of 3 weeks for patients with trigger digits resulting from a discrete nodule, a short duration of symptoms (<6 months), and single digit involvement.
- Diffuse stenosing tenosynovitis of short duration can be treated initially with a corticosteroid injection, but repeat injections may not be warranted given the poor response of this form of trigger digits to nonoperative treatment.
- *Open release of the A1 pulley* is the standard surgical treatment for trigger digits. Surgical treatment may be indicated for nodular trigger digits that are unresponsive to a series of two corticosteroid injections or for trigger digits that upon initial presentation are locked, involve multiple digits, result from diffuse stenosing tenosynovitis, or are of long duration (>6 months).
  - Transverse incisions at the proximal edge of the A1 pulley, oblique incisions, Chevron (Bunnell-type) incisions, and longitudinal incisions have been described. Longitudinal incisions that traverse perpendicular to flexor creases may result in flexion contractures.
  - The A1 pulley in adults measures 1.0 to 1.5 cm in length and should be released in its entirety. Preservation of the second annular (A2) pulleys in the fingers, and the oblique pulley in the thumb, is important for prevent bowstringing of the flexor tendons that results in decreased tendon excursion and ultimately to decreased active IP joint flexion. However, the A2 pulley may be continuous with the A1 pulley in approximately 50% of individuals.
  - Care should be taken to protect the neurovascular bundles, acknowledging the radial neurovascular bundle to the thumb takes an oblique ulnar to radial course across the MP joint crease.
  - The procedure is performed with local anesthesia such that the patient can actively flex and extend the digit following A1 pulley release, confirming successful resolution of the triggering.
  - A1 pulley release is not recommended in patients with rheumatoid arthritis and diffused tenosynovitis because of the risk of exacerbating ulnar drift of the digits. Instead, flexor tenosynovectomy should be performed to eliminate the cause of triggering. Some patients with rheumatoid arthritis who have no involvement of flexor tendons respond well to Standard A1 pulley release.

- Partial excision of the FDS with the removal of one slip may be required in some patients with dramatic enlargement of the FDP tendon.
- *Percutaneous A1 pulley release* has been proposed as an alternative technique. Under local anesthesia, the beveled tip of an 18- to 20-gauge needle is inserted into the middle of the A1 pulley. The bevel is oriented parallel to the flexor tendons. A sweeping motion proximally and distally produces a grating sound and results in A1 pulley release. The needle is withdrawn, and the patient flexes and extends the digit to confirm an adequate release. Repeat needle placements may be needed to adequately eliminate the triggering. Percutaneous A1 pulley release usually is performed in conjunction with corticosteroid injection to prevent postoperative painful tenosynovitis without triggering. Some authors recommend not performing percutaneous release in the thumb and possibly the index finger, especially if a PIP joint flexion contracture is present, because the neurovascular bundle may be at increased risk.[5,6]
- Good results can be expected following A1 pulley release. Triggering is eliminated with no complications in approximately 90% of patients undergoing open A1 pulley release. Percutaneous A1 pulley release has been reported to be successful in approximately 93% of patients.[7,8]
- Complications include scar tenderness, mild PIP flexion contractures, neurovascular bundle injuries, ulnar drift of the digit (especially the index finger or any finger in a patient with rheumatoid arthritis), tendon bowstringing, infection, algodystrophy, and recurrence. Complications generally occur in less than 5% of patients, although higher complication rates have been reported. With percutaneous release, concerns remain regarding scoring of the flexor digitorum superficialis tendon, which occurs in many cases; injury to the neurovascular bundles, which lie within 2 to 3 mm of needle tip placement for the index finger and thumb; and potential recurrence from incomplete release.

## Management of Trigger Thumb in Children

- Treatment options include observation, splinting, and open surgical release of the first annular pulley.
- Most authors recommend at least a 6-month period of observation prior to surgical intervention. One third of patients younger than 6 months may have spontaneous resolution of the trigger thumb. Spontaneous resolution after age 6 months is much less common in most series.
- Nonetheless, surgery is required for a significant number of patients. Surgery before age 3 years is generally recommended with open release of the thumb's first annular pulley. The outcome of surgical release in children is generally good. Removal or debulking of the flexor pollicis longus nodule is not recommended.

# de Quervain Syndrome

- de Quervain syndrome is stenosing tenovaginitis of the first dorsal compartment of the wrist, which contains the abductor pollicis longus (APL) and extensor pollicis brevis (EPB) tendons.

## Anatomy

- The anatomy of the first dorsal compartment of the wrist is highly variable. Failure to recognize these anatomic variations can lead to treatment failures in de Quervain syndrome.
  - The EPB tendon is rounder and smaller than the APL and is absent in 5 to 7 percent of individuals. Muscle fibers, if seen within the first dorsal compartment, usually help identify the EPB tendon as the EPB muscle belly extends further distally. Its distal insertion is at the base of the proximal phalanx. The APL usually has two or more tendon slips that may insert onto the trapezium, volar carpal ligament, opponens pollicis, or abductor pollicis brevis and the consistent and functionally important insertion onto the base of the first metacarpal. The most common anatomic variation is one EPB tendon and two APL tendon slips.
  - In up to one third of the general population, the first dorsal compartment is subdivided by a septum into two separate fibroosseous tunnels (Figure 14–3). The ulnar-sided tunnel contains the EPB tendon, and the radial-sided tunnel contains the multiple APL tendon slips. A third deep tunnel containing an anomalous tendon has been reported but is uncommon. A higher incidence of septation of first dorsal compartments is reported in patients with de Quervain syndrome, suggesting that separate fibroosseous tunnels predispose to development of de Quervain syndrome.
  - The deep branch of the radial artery passes through the anatomic snuffbox distal to the radial styloid process and just deep to the first and second dorsal compartments. The artery's location should be recognized, but the artery need not be exposed during first dorsal compartment release.
- Several branches of the superficial radial nerve lie within the subcutaneous fat overlying the first dorsal compartment and should be preserved during surgical approaches (Figure 14–4, A).

## Diagnosis

- The typical patient diagnosed with de Quervain syndrome is a woman (occurs up to six times more frequently than in men) in her 40s or 50s. Association with pregnancy is common but even higher are mothers with infant.
- Patients present with radial-sided wrist pain exacerbated by thumb movements, particularly thumb abduction and/or extension. Pain may radiate distally or proximally along the course of the APL and EPB tendons. By the time of presentation, symptoms usually have been present for weeks to months.
- Physical examination often reveals localized swelling and tenderness over the first dorsal compartment, extending 1 to 2 cm proximal to the radial styloid process. The Finkelstein test involves asking the patient to clasp the thumb into the palm and then applying an ulnar deviation force to the wrist. Rarely, pseudotriggering of the thumb is present and may be related to interference of smooth EPB tendon excursion in its separate fibroosseous tunnel within the first dorsal compartment.
- Intersection syndrome, which involves the junction of the tendons contained in the first and second dorsal compartments, typically presents with symptoms more proximal (4 cm) to the wrist (see Figure 14–4, B). Thumb carpometacarpal joint, radiocarpal, and intercarpal arthritis frequently can be distinguished from de Quervain syndrome based on radiographs and a positive grind test, although the conditions may coexist. Finally, superficial radial nerve neuroma is unlikely without a prior history of local trauma or

Figure 14–3:

The first dorsal compartment often contains a septum that divides the spaces containing the abductor pollicis longus tendon and the extensor pollicis brevis tendon. The most common combination of tendon slips is two abductor pollicis longus tendon slips and one extensor pollicis brevis tendon slip.

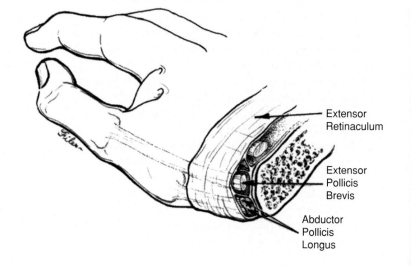

Extensor Retinaculum

Extensor Pollicis Brevis

Abductor Pollicis Longus

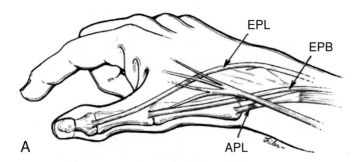

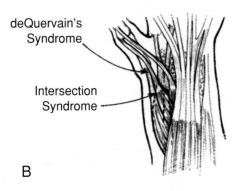

A

deQuervain's
Syndrome

Intersection
Syndrome

B

Figure 14–4:
The radial sensory nerve crosses over the first dorsal compartment and is at risk for injury during first dorsal compartment release (A). The first dorsal compartment tendons (abductor pollicis longus *[APL]* and extensor pollicis brevis *[EPB]*), intersect with the second dorsal compartment tendons (extensor carpi radialis longus and brevis), approximately 4 cm proximal to the wrist (B). *EPL,* Extensor pollicis longus.

surgery and usually can be carefully distinguished using Finkelstein test and seeking a Tinel sign (Box 14–3).

## Treatment

- *Nonoperative treatment* options for de Quervain syndrome include splinting, corticosteroid injections, and various techniques of surgical release of the first dorsal compartment.
  - Splinting alone may be beneficial for acute symptomatic relief but has resulted in a 80% failure rate.[9]
  - Corticosteroid injections into the first dorsal compartment are a moderately effective nonoperative treatment option. A single corticosteroid injection into the first dorsal compartment sheath is successful in alleviating symptoms in approximately 70% of patients. Two injections are successful in approximately 80% of patients.[10] Long-term relief is achieved in approximately 60% of patients.[11] Several studies have documented the high failure rate of injections in patients with a separate EPB fibroosseous tunnel within the first dorsal com-

partment. Corticosteroid injections in patients with diabetes mellitus may be less successful.
- *Surgical treatment* for de Quervain syndrome must adhere to two principles. First, care must be taken to protect and avoid excessive dissection of the superficial radial nerve and its branches. The second principle is to ensure complete release of the first dorsal compartment, especially the separate EPB fibroosseous tunnel.
  - Longitudinal incisions generally lead to fewer superficial nerve incisions than do transverse incisions. Symptoms secondary to superficial radial nerve injury can be far more severe than those resulting from stenosing tenovaginitis of the first dorsal compartment. Transversal incisions have mininized scarring to the tendons and have resulted in a better appearing scar.
  - Release the first dorsal compartment on its dorsal margin, thereby leaving a palmarly based flap of retinaculum to prevent tendon subluxation. It is important to identify both the EPB and all the slips of the APL by placing traction on the tendons. Most authors agree that sheath excision is unnecessary and predisposes the patient to symptomatic volar tendon subluxation. Volar subluxation of the APL and EPB tendons can be addressed with a retinacular sling or a slip of brachioradialis tendon, if symptomatic.
  - Good results have been reported with release of only the EPB fibroosseous tunnel in septated first dorsal compartments, suggesting isolated stenosing tenovaginitis of the EPB sheath is responsible for de Quervain syndrome.[12] Despite this report, most authors

| Box 14–3 | **Differential Diagnosis of de Quervain Syndrome** |
| --- | --- |

- Intersection syndrome
- Thumb carpometacarpal joint arthritis
- Radiocarpal or intercarpal joint arthritis
- Scaphoid fracture
- Superficial radial nerve neuroma

recommend complete release of both fibroosseous tunnels in separated first dorsal compartments.

- Ninety percent of patients can be expected to have a satisfactory outcome following surgical release of the first dorsal compartment for de Quervain syndrome.[13] Preoperative symptoms lasting for more than 10 months reportedly adversely affects prognosis.

# Flexor Carpi Radialis Tendonitis

- Flexor carpi radialis (FCR) tendonitis is a cause of radial pain at the volar side of the wrist. It is rare in comparison with other disorders in the region.

## Anatomy

- The proximity of the FCR tunnel to the radius, trapezium scaphoid, and palmar arch explains the predisposition of the tendon to tenosynovitis with or without trauma.
- The FCR tendon originates from the bipennate flexor carpi radialis muscle approximately 15 cm proximal to the radiocarpal joint. The last 8 cm is completely tendinous.[14] Four to five centimeters proximal to the radiocarpal joint, the tendon is circumferentially covered by the transversely oriented fibers of the antebrachial fascia, which gradually thickens to an average thickness of 3 mm at the level of the trapezial crest.
- Passing the trapezial crest the tendon enters a 17-mm-long fibroosseous tunnel bordered radially by the body of the trapezium, palmarly by the trapezial crest and the transverse carpal ligament, ulnarly by a retinaculum septum that separates the tendon from the carpal tunnel, and dorsally by the insertion of this septum onto the trapezial body. Just proximal to the tunnel, the tendon occupies 60% of the cross-sectional area of the fibrous sheath. Within the tunnel, the tendon occupies 90% of the fibroosseous canal.
- Distal to the tunnel the tendon divides into two slips that attach into the base of the second and third metacarpals (approximately two thirds insert to the second metacarpal and one third to the third metacarpal). The direction of the tendon is collinear with the forearm proximally and deviates approximately 45 degrees within the tunnel and distally.
- Less than 1 mm of soft tissue separates the tendon from the scaphoid tubercle, the scaphoid trapezium trapezoid joint, and the trapezium. Less than 3 mm separates the tendon from the first carpometacarpal joint.[14]

## Pathology

- Primary stenosing tenosynovitis may develop because of overuse or inflammation at the site of the fibroosseous tunnel because of the narrow confines and the deviation of the tendon by 45 degrees from the neutral forearm axis. Tendonitis at the site of insertion also may develop.

- Secondary tendonitis may develop because of pathology from the adjacent structures, including scaphoid fractures, scaphoid cysts, arthritis of the scaphoid trapezium trapezoid joint, or arthritis of the carpometacarpal joint of the thumb.

## Diagnosis

- In primary stenosing tenosynovitis, the patient complains of radiovolar pain at the wrist, often localized to the proximal aspect of the trapezium. Pain occurs with resisted active wrist flexion and radial deviation and with passive extension and ulnar deviation. Pain relief with lidocaine injection into the sheath confirms the diagnosis.
- Secondary tendonitis can result from previous injuries or arthritis of the adjacent structures, making a detailed history of previous injury at the radiovolar aspect of the wrist important.
- Radiographs are essential to recognize pathology from adjacent osseous structures. Magnetic resonance imaging (MRI) may help rule out cysts or ganglia if suspected (Box 14–4).
- Linberg syndrome is an anomalous intertendinous connection between the tendon of the flexor pollicis longus and that of the flexor digitorum profundus.

## Treatment

- *Nonoperative treatment* includes splinting preventing wrist flexion, physical therapy, and corticosteroid injections. Nonoperative treatment usually is effective for primary tendonitis.
  - Splinting in combination with administration of antiinflammatory medications have yielded good results in acute FCR stenosing tenosynovitis.
  - One or two corticosteroid injections are the next step for stenosing tenosynovitis of the FCR tendon. The injection is preferably administered from the volar side over the site of tenderness. Caution should be exercised to avoid intratendinous injections, which increase the rate of spontaneous rupture of the tendon.
  - Ultrasound courses have shown good results as an adjacent measure to the previous nonoperative treatments.
- *Operative treatment* is essential when conservative treatment is unsuccessful or in cases of secondary tendonitis resulting from local pathologic changes.

| Box 14–4 | **Differential Diagnosis of Flexor Carpi Radialis Tendonitis** |
|---|---|

- Osteoarthrosis of the carpometacarpal joint of the thumb
- Scaphoid trapezium trapezoid joint arthritis
- Scaphoid cysts/fracture
- Ganglion cysts
- de Quervain tenosynovitis
- Linberg syndrome

- Operative treatment involves treatment of local lesions (removal of ganglions and osteophytes, bone grafting of cysts, fusion of arthritic joints) and decompression of the tunnel.
- Operative decompression is performed through a volar incision starting proximal to the wrist crease and extending over the proximal thenar eminence.
  - Caution should be exercised to avoid the palmar cutaneous branch of the median nerve, the lateral antebrachial cutaneous nerve, and the superficial radial sensory nerve.
  - The thenar muscle is elevated from the transverse ligament and retracted radially exposing the sheath of the FCR tendon.
  - The tendon sheath and the tunnel are released longitudinally, taking care not to injure the tendon.
  - The tendon is mobilized from the trapezial groove, and the trapezial insertion is released.
- An alternative approach for decompression includes release from within the carpal tunnel if a concomitant carpal tunnel release is performed.
- Good results with operative treatment of FCR tendonitis with a success rate of 90% have been reported in the literature. A history of overuse, cases associated with workers' compensation, long duration of symptoms before treatment, and failure of local anesthetic to ease the symptoms are associated with poor results.

# Extensor Carpi Ulnaris Tendonitis

## Anatomy

- The extensor carpi ulnaris (ECU) is one of the most important stabilizers of the distal radioulnar joint.[15]
- It is the most ulnar extensor of the wrist and originates from the extensor carpi ulnaris muscle approximately 6 to 7 cm proximal to the wrist.
- Although it passes through the extensor retinaculum, a separate deep fibroosseous sheath is formed around it. This fibroosseous deep sheath maintains the tendon in its normal position. The tendon occupies approximately 90% of the space of the fibroosseous sheath. Over the distal ulna it curves ulnarly passing into an ulnar groove on the dorsal surface of the ulna before inserting onto the base of the fifth metacarpal. The narrow space in the fibroosseous sheath and the angulation of the tendon, particularly after voluntary contraction of the muscle, predisposes to tendonitis. The ECU subsheath is part of the triangular fibrocartilage complex of the wrist.
- A few centimeters before insertion, the fibroosseous sheath becomes thinner. Maximum ulnar translocation stress is noted on the tendon and its sheath during ECU muscle contraction with the forearm in supination and

the wrist ulnarly deviated. Rupture of the fibroosseous sheath leading to subluxation or dislocation of the tendon may occur with hypersupination of the forearm and ulnar deviation and flexion of the wrist, with active voluntary contraction of the extensor carpi ulnaris muscle. Division or attenuation of the fibroosseous sheath allows dislocation of the tendon, even with the overlying extensor retinaculum intact.

## Diagnosis

- Usually the patient presents with pain on the ulnar side of the wrist after a single injury or with progressively increased pain.
  - Physical examination reveals pain on the ulnar side of the wrist, pain with palpation over the fibroosseous tunnel and/or the insertion of the tendon to the base of the fifth metacarpal, pain with passive flexion and radial deviation of the wrist, pain with resisted extension and ulnar deviation of the wrist with the forearm in hypersupination, and pain while applying maximum grip strength with resisted ulnar deviation of the wrist. Ulnar nerve dorsal (sensory) branch dysesthesias may coexist.
  - If the fibroosseous sheath is ruptured, the patient may complain of a painful soft snap. Swelling on the dorsal side of the wrist is noted, as is dislocation of the tendon with voluntary contraction of the ECU muscle.
  - Radiographs may be helpful to exclude pathology from the adjacent structures. Diagnosis of ECU tendonitis based on MRI findings alone is not reliable,[16] but MRI is useful in the differential diagnosis of ulnar-sided wrist pain (Box 14–5). Dynamic ultrasound can quickly and accurately make the diagnosis.

## Treatment

- Tendonitis or tenosynovitis of the ECU tendon can be initially treated with *nonoperative* measures such as rest and splinting, antiinflammatory medications, corticosteroid injections, and physical therapy, although the efficacy of a conservative approach has been questioned. Other causes of ulnar-sided wrist pain should be ruled out.
  - Splinting of the wrist in slight extension for 3 weeks and administration of antiinflammatory medications is the first step of the therapy.

| Box 14–5 | Differential Diagnosis of Extensor Carpi Ulnaris Tendonitis |
|---|---|

- Injury of the triangular fibrocartilage complex
- Distal radioulnar joint arthritis
- Fracture, nonunion, or malunion of the ulnar styloid
- Ulnocarpal impaction syndrome
- Calcification of the ECU tendon insertion
- "Snapping" of the ECU tendon

- If pain persists, local injection of corticosteroids is advocated. Caution should be exercised to avoid intratendinous injections.

## Operative Treatment

- If the pain persists or painful subluxation or dislocation is noted, then surgical treatment is warranted.
  - A dorsal incision over the ECU tendon (sixth compartment) is made extending from approximately 2 cm proximally to the wrist to the base of the fifth metacarpal.
    - Caution should be exercised to avoid the dorsal cutaneous branch of the ulnar nerve.
    - The tendon sheath and the tunnel are released longitudinally, taking care not to injure the tendon.
    - Some authors prefer resuturing part of the sheath to prevent subluxation of the tendon and resecting longitudinally part of the tendon. Good results without repair of the sheath have been reported.[17]
    - In cases of *painful ECU tendon subluxation or dislocation,* various techniques for stabilization, including creation of local flaps in chronic cases, hemiresection techniques, and direct repair of the fibroosseous tunnel in acute cases, have been reported. Three different methods for repair of the fibroosseous sheath have been reported, the choice of which depends on the type of lesion.[18]
  - Good results with operative treatment of ECU tendon tendonitis[17,19] and stabilization for painful ECU tendon dislocation have been reported in the literature.[18]

## Conclusions

- For most of the disorders described in this chapter, the initial treatment is conservative. Local steroid injections and/or splinting can control the inflammatory process in its early stages, provided secondary changes in the sheath (fibrosis, cartilaginous metaplasia) do not predominate. The need for splinting after an injection has been challenged for some of these disorders. The role of systematic NSAIDs remains elusive. Proper injection techniques should be followed to prevent complications. Steroid injections in insulin-dependent diabetic patients are not as effective and can interfere with serum glucose control.
- In chronic cases or those unresponsive to conservative treatment, surgical decompression is an excellent option. Common causes of failure in these procedures are incomplete release and nerve injury. Another common pitfall is failure to recognize underlying conditions, such as arthritic osteophytes, ganglion cysts, or coexisting pathology contributing to the patient's symptoms. Although most of these procedures are technically simple, they should not be undertaken lightly.

## References

1. Rodgers WB, Waters PM: Incidence of trigger digits in newborns. *J Hand Surg* 19A:364-368, 1994.

2. Moon WN, Suh SW, Kim IC: Trigger digits in children. *J Hand Surg* 26B:11-12, 2001.
   Combined, these two studies prospectively examined 8746 newborns and failed to identify any case of "congenital" trigger thumb.

3. Freiberg A, Mulholland RS, Levine R: Nonoperative treatment of trigger fingers and thumbs. *J Hand Surg* 14A:553-558, 1989.
   The authors make the clinical distinction of trigger digits into nodular and "diffuse" types, with a higher success rate following injection in the nodular type (93%) compared to the "diffuse" type (48%).

4. Patel MR, Bassini LB: Trigger fingers and thumb: when to splint, inject, or operate. *J Hand Surg* 17A:110-113, 1992.
   In this comparative study of splinting (for an average of 6 weeks) versus injection (with cortisone and lidocaine) in 100 patients, injections were more successful (84% success rate) than splinting (66%).

5. Pope DF, Wolfe SW: Safety and efficacy of percutaneous trigger finger release. *J Hand Surg* 20A:280-283, 1995.
   A cadaveric study of 25 percutaneous A1 pulley releases revealed that 90% of the length of the A1 pulley was successfully released. In five of 13 trigger digits treated percutaneously and subsequently opened, part of the A1 pulley remained intact.

6. Bain GI, Tornbull J, Charles MN, et al: Percutaneous A1 pulley release: a cadaveric study. *J Hand Surg* 20A:781-784, 1995.
   In a cadaveric study, complete percutaneous release of the A1 pulley was noted in 66% of digits.

7. Eastwood DM, Gupta KJ, Johnson DP: Percutaneous release of the trigger finger: an office procedure. *J Hand Surg* 17A:114-117, 1992.
   This pioneering article on percutaneous trigger finger release with a 21-gauge hypodermic needle reported a 94% success rate and no recurrences at a mean follow-up of 13 months.

8. Ha KI, Park MJ, Ha CW: Percutaneous release of trigger digits: a technique and results using a specially designed knife. *J Bone Joint Surg* 83B:75-77, 2001.
   The authors achieved a 93% success rate with percutaneous trigger digit release using a specially designed knife.

9. Weiss AP, Akelman E, Tabatabai M: Treatment of de Quervain's disease. *J Hand Surg* 19A:595-598, 1994.
   In a study comparing treatment of de Quervain disease with injections alone, injections plus splinting, and splinting alone, splinting was found to be of no value.

10. Harvey FJ, Harvey PM, Horsley MW: de Quervain's disease: surgical or nonsurgical treatment. *J Hand Surg* 15A:83-87, 1990.
    Conservative treatment with one or two cortisone and lidocaine injections yielded complete and lasting pain relief in 80% of patients in a study of 79 wrists.

11. Witt J, Pess G, Gelberman RH: Treatment of de Quervain tenosynovitis. *J Bone Joint Surg* 73A:219-222, 1991.

Cortisone and lidocaine injections were successful in 62% when the need for operative release was used as an outcome result for treatment failure in this prospective study of 87 wrists.

12. Yuasa K, Kiyoshige Y: Limited surgical treatment of de Quervain's disease: decompression of only the extensor pollicis brevis subcompartment. *J Hand Surg* 24A:840-843, 1998.
   Sixteen patients underwent surgical release of only the EPB subcompartment for de Quervain disease, and all had relief of symptoms.

13. Ta KT, Eidelman D, Thomson JG: Patient satisfaction and outcomes of surgery for de Quervain's tenosynovitis. *J Hand Surg* 24A:1071-1077, 1999.
   This retrospective study of 43 wrists treated surgically for de Quervain disease reported a complication rate of 9%.

14. Bishop AT, Gabel G, Carmichael SW: Flexor carpi radialis tendinitis. Part I: Operative anatomy. *J Bone Joint Surg* 76A:1009-1014, 1994.
   This is an excellent review of the pertinent anatomy to flexor carpi radialis tendonitis based on the cadaveric dissection of 25 specimens.

15. Spiner M, Kaplan B: Extensor carpi ulnaris: its relationship to the stability of the distal radio-ulnar joint. *Clin Orthop* 68:124-129, 1970.
   This is a classic article on the anatomy and biomechanics of ECU tendon and its fibroosseous sheath.

16. Timins ME, O'Connell SE, Erickson SJ, Oneson SR: MR imaging of the wrist: normal findings that may simulate disease. *Radiographics* 16:987-995, 1996.
   In an MRI study of 26 normal wrists, high signal intensity of the ECU tendon simulating tendonitis was a very common finding.

17. Kip PC, Peimer CA: Release of the sixth dorsal compartment. *J Hand Surg* 19A:599-601, 1994.
   In this report, 12 patients were treated with decompression of the sixth dorsal compartment for ECU tendonitis without an attempt at repair of the ECU sheath, with no resulting distal radioulnar joint or ECU instability.

18. Inoue G, Tamura Y: Surgical treatment for recurrent dislocation of the extensor carpi ulnaris tendon. *J Hand Surg* 26B:6:556-559, 2001.
   This article provides a practical algorithm for treating recurrent dislocation of the ECU tendon by dividing the pathology into three types.

19. Nachinolcar UG, Khanolkar KB: Stenosing tenovaginitis of extensor carpi ulnaris. *J Bone Joint Surg* 70B:842, 1988.
   In this report of 72 patients with ECU tendonitis, local steroids provided long-standing pain relief in only nine patients. The 63 patients treated surgically had uniformly good results.

## Suggested Readings

### Trigger Finger
Thorpe AP: Results of surgery for trigger digit. *J Hand Surg* 13A:199-201, 1988.

This study describes high complication (28%) and failure (40%) rates following open trigger digit release and attributes problems to surgeon inexperience.

Ger E, Kupcha P, Ger D: The management of trigger thumb in children. *J Hand Surg* 16A:944-947, 1991.
In this study, all 53 pediatric trigger thumbs eventually required surgical release, although waiting up to 3 years did not adversely affect the outcome.

Dunsmuir RA, Sherlock DA: The outcome of treatment of trigger thumb in children. *J Bone Joint Surg* 82B:736-738, 2000.
This study reported a 50% rate of spontaneous recovery of trigger thumb in children.

Tan AH, Lam KS, Lee EH: The treatment of trigger thumb in children. *J Pediatr Orthop* 11B:256-259, 2002.
Conservative treatment for trigger thumb in children, including splinting and regular exercises, yielded an overall rate of success of 66%.

### de Quervain Disease
Jackson WT, Veigas SF, Coon TM, et al: Anatomical variations in the first extensor compartment of the wrist. A clinical and anatomical study. *J Bone Joint Surg* 68A:923-926, 1986.
A study of 300 cadaveric wrists and a prospective study of 40 patients who underwent de Quervain tenosynovitis release revealed a significantly higher occurrence of septation of the first dorsal compartment in the population with de Quervain syndrome (67%) than in the cadavers (33%).

### Flexor Carpi Radialis Tenosynovitis
Gabel G, Bishop AT, Wood MB: Flexor carpi radialis tendonitis. Part II: results of operative treatment. *J Bone Joint Surg* 76A:1015-1018, 1994.
In a study of 10 patients who had undergone flexor carpi radialis tunnel release, seven needed additional procedures.

### Extensor Carpi Ulnaris Tenosynovitis
Palmer AK, Skahen JR, Werner FW, Glisson RR: The extensor retinaculum of the wrist: an anatomic and biomechanical study. *J Hand Surg* 10B:11-16, 1985.
This is a classic article on the anatomy and biomechanics of ECU tendon and its fibroosseous sheath.

Hajj AA, Wood MB: Stenosing tenosynovitis of the extensor carpi ulnaris. *J Hand Surg* 11A:519-520, 1986.
This early report discusses surgical technique for release of the ECU compartment.

Rowland SA: Acute traumatic subluxation of the extensor carpi ulnaris tendon at the wrist. *J Hand Surg* 11A:809-811, 1986.
This was the first report of surgical treatment for acute traumatic subluxation of the ECU tendon.

Inoue G, Tamura Y: Recurrent dislocation of the extensor carpi ulnaris tendon. *Br J Sports Med* 32:172-174, 1998.
This article provides a practical algorithm for treating recurrent dislocation of the ECU tendon by dividing the pathology into three types.

# CHAPTER 15

# Nerve Physiology and Repair

Mihye Choi[*] and David T.W. Chiu[†]

[*]MD, Assistant Professor of Surgery, New York University, School of Medicine;
Attending Physician, New York Medical Center, New York, NY
[†]MD, Professor of Plastic Surgery, New York University; Senior Attending,
Director of New York Nerve Center, New York University Medical Center;
Institute of Reconstructive Plastic Surgery, New York, NY

## Introduction

- Although significant advances have been made in the microsurgical repair technology and in our understanding of nerve physiology at the molecular level, restoration of function after a peripheral injury remains a great challenge.
- This chapter aims to elucidate the current understanding of the peripheral nerve's physiology in its normal, injured, and regenerative phases and the basic principles in the treatment of nerve injury.

## Nerve Physiology

### Microanatomy of the Peripheral Nerve

- The neuron is the basic unit of the peripheral nerve. Each neuron consists of a cell body (soma) with cytoplasmic extensions (dendrites and an axon), covered with various synaptic terminals called *boutons* (Figure 15–1).
- The axon is a special cylindrical extension arising from the neuron at the axonal hillock. The function of the axon is twofold: bidirectional axonal transport and electrical impulse conduction.
- For an unmyelinated nerve, each Schwann cell surrounds several small axons. For a myelinated nerve, Schwann cells surround a single axon.
- The myelinated larger axons are wrapped along their entire length by contiguous Schwann cells that are the

glial cells of the peripheral nervous system. The myelinated axon is covered by myelin sheath except for the nodes of Ranvier, which are specialized myelin-free areas that allow ionic exchange and facilitate propagation of electric conduction.
- The myelin sheath is a proteophospholipid, multilayered, compacted cell membrane that maximizes the conduction efficiency and the velocity of action potentials.
- Myelinated axons have four distinctive regions: node of Ranvier, paranode, juxtaparanode, and internode. Each zone is characterized by a specific set of axonal proteins. Voltage-gated sodium channels are clustered at the node of Ranvier, whereas potassium channels are concentrated at juxtaparanodal regions (Box 15–1).

### Connective Tissue Components of the Peripheral Nerve

- The peripheral nerves contain an abundant amount of collagen that makes them strong and resistant to trauma, in contrast to the cranial nerves, which are rich in fiber but have minimal collagen content.
- The cross section of a peripheral nerve contains variable amount of connective tissue (up to 85%) (Figure 15–2).
- The *epineurium,* which is the elongation of the dural sleeve of the spinal nerve roots, can be divided into two layers: external and internal. The external epineurium is the outermost layer surrounding the peripheral nerve and anchors blood vessels entering from the surrounding

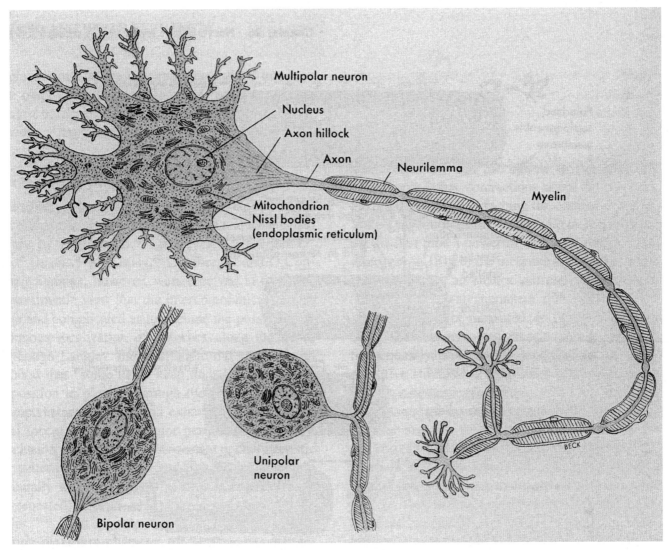

Figure 15–1:
The neuron is the basic unit of the peripheral nerve. Each neuron consists of a cell body (soma) with cytoplasmic extensions (dendrites and an axon) and is covered with various synaptic terminals called *boutons*. The axon is a special cylindrical extension that arises from the neuron at the axonal hillock. (From Anthony CP, Thibodeau GA: *Textbook of anatomy and physiology.* St. Louis, 1983, CV Mosby Co.)

tissue. The internal epineurium fills between fascicles and cushions them from external force.

- The *perineurium* encircles each fascicle and provides the diffusion barrier. It is composed of many layers of flattened cells alternating with collagen fibers. This layer is an extension of the blood-brain barrier and maintains positive pressure within the fascicles. This pressure difference is evident when the cut end of a nerve shows round herniating fascicular ends. This pressure difference is essential for axoplasmic transport and nerve conduction. The perineurium is the strongest component of the nerve trunk and protects nerve fibers from stretch injury.

- The *endoneurium* is the innermost collagen layer surrounding individual axons within the perineurial layer. Larger myelinated axons are wrapped with two layers of endoneurium: the outer longitudinally oriented collagen layer and the inner randomly oriented layer. Smaller myelinated axons have only the outer layer.

| Box 15–1 | Neuron Anatomy and Function |
|---|---|
| Cell body | Protein synthesis |
| Axon | Bidirectional axonal transport and nerve conduction |
| Myelin | Maximizes conduction efficiency |
| Node of Ranvier | Myelin free area for ionic exchange |

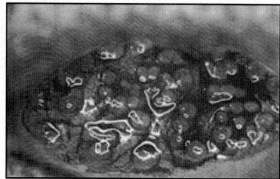

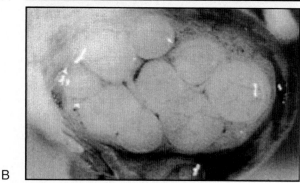

Figure 15–2:

**Fascicular anatomy. The peripheral nerves contain an abundant amount of collagen that makes them strong and resistant to trauma. Each peripheral nerve displays a different fascicular grouping and amount of connective tissue. A, Sciatic nerve. B, Median nerve.** (From Van Beek AL, Pirela-Cruz MA: Microsurgical nerve repairs. In Omer GE, Spinner M, Van Beek AL, editors: *Management of peripheral nerve problems,* ed 2. Philadelphia, 1998, Elsevier.)

- Longitudinal intrinsic blood vessels in the epineurium, perineurium, and endoneurium are interconnected with each other and with extrinsic blood vessels, the arteriae nervora, entering the nerve from surrounding tissue. This rich, longitudinal plexus of blood vessels allows a nerve to be mobilized for a significant distance without ischemic compromise.
- Loose areolar tissue surrounding the peripheral nerve allows longitudinal excursion of the nerve. This is an important feature to prevent traction injury to the nerve crossing a limb joint. Wilgis et al. demonstrated that the median nerve crossing the wrist glides as much as 15.5 mm and the ulnar nerve glides as much as 14.8 mm (Box 15–2).
- The peripheral nerves contain motor, sensory, and autonomic fibers. The motor fibers originate from the motor neurons in the anterior horn of the spinal cord. The sensory fibers originate from the sensory neurons in the dorsal root ganglia. The autonomic fibers are either preganglionic, arising from the neurons in the brainstem/spinal cord, or postganglionic, arising from neurons in paravertebral ganglia.

### Box 15–2 — Connective Tissue Layers of the Peripheral Nerve

| | |
|---|---|
| Epineurium | External: Surrounds the nerve |
| | Internal: Packing material between fascicles |
| Perineurium | Surrounds each fascicle, controls diffusion |
| Endoneurium | Surrounds each axon |
| Arteriae nervosa | Extrinsic and intrinsic blood vessels forming rich longitudinal plexus |
| Loose areolar tissue | Allows longitudinal excursion with joint motion |

- Earlier investigators noted rich plexuses of interconnecting fascicular patterns of proximal nerve trunks and were skeptical of functional repair of the peripheral nerve. Later studies using histochemical analysis and intrafascicular microstimulation in awake patients demonstrated a great degree of topographic localization within the nerve trunk correlating to distal function. Further proximally, motor neurons serving a single muscle are grouped together within the anterior horn of the spinal cord.

## Axoplasmic Transport

- Bidirectional axoplasmic transport can be fast or slow type. Membrane and secretory proteins synthesized in the soma are transported orthograde to the terminal by either a fast or a slow transport system.
- Fast axoplasmic transport moves subcellular organelles, such as synaptic vesicles, down to the nerve ending. This transport requires energy; therefore, it is sensitive to hypoxemia. The reported rates of fast transport are variable, reaching up to 400 mm/day. The fast retrograde transport moves degraded axoplasmic materials, neurotransmitters, and neurotrophic substances ingested at the nerve terminal back to the cell body. Nerve growth factors (NGFs) manufactured by the motor and sensory target organs are transported back to the cell body and are crucial for neuron survival. Retrograde transport also is responsible for carrying pathogens such as herpes simplex virus.
- Slow transport is orthograde only and moves 1 to 4 mm/day, moving components of cytoskeleton such as neurotubules and neurofilaments to the nerve terminal. This speed of transport limits the rate of peripheral nerve regeneration.

## Nerve Conduction

- The neuron has the capability for propagating electric currents. This ability is achieved by the resting potential across the axonal membrane. This negative potential of −60 to −70 mV is maintained by actively partitioning the extracellular sodium and intracellular potassium ions against the concentration gradient.

- Sodium ion gates open when stimulated by an electric impulse and allow sodium ions to rush into the cell following their concentration gradient. This process causes a decrease in the resting membrane potential and represents the rise in the action potential. The sodium channels then close and the voltage-gated potassium channels open, causing potassium ions to diffuse out of the cell, following its concentration gradient. The localized potential thus produced is propagated down the axon, creating the action potential, which is an all-or-none phenomenon. The action potential, once initiated, travels the entire length of the axon without decrement (Figure 15–3).

- In unmyelinated fibers, the longitudinal spread of the electric current occurs with progressive excitation of the adjacent inactive areas. In myelinated fibers, the electric impulse jumps from one node of Ranvier to next the node, in a process called *salutatory conduction.* Therefore, conduction in unmyelinated fibers is slower than in myelinated fibers.

- After each depolarization, a period of recovery is needed to restore the resting potential. The adenosine triphosphatase (ATPase) pump restores the membrane resting potential by actively moving sodium ions out, allowing potassium ions to passively flow back in.

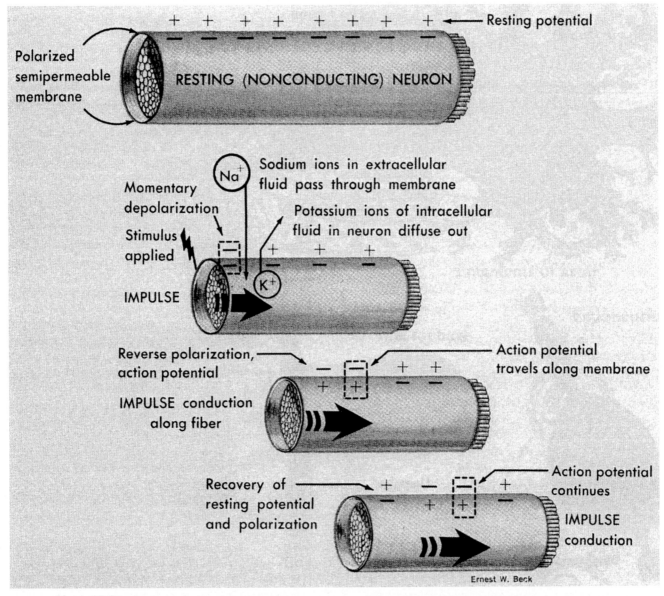

Figure 15–3:
Nerve conduction. Schematic diagram of resting potential, action potential, and repolarization. (From Anthony CP, Thibodeau GA: *Textbook of anatomy and physiology.* St. Louis, 1983, CV Mosby Co.)

- Conduction velocity represents how fast the action potential is propagated to the target organ. Conduction velocity can be increased in two ways: by increasing the diameter of the axon and by decreasing capacitance to the flow. Conduction velocity is proportional to the square of the diameter of the axon. A nerve must be of gigantic size to conduct fast. Schwann cells allow the axon to overcome this problem by surrounding the axon with the high-resistance, low capacitance-insulator myelin. However, the entire nerve cannot be surrounded by a myelin sheath because sodium and potassium ion movements across the axonal membrane would be prevented. Thus, the node of Ranvier, which is a myelin-free segment, plays a crucial role in facilitating ionic exchange and salutatory conduction. Voltage-dependent sodium channels are uniformly distributed along unmyelinated axons but are highly concentrated in the nodes of Ranvier to facilitate salutatory conduction in myelinated axons.

## Neuromuscular Transmission

- Motor axons terminate into several branches, which end in synaptic boutons. The bouton membrane contains voltage-gated calcium channels, which allow influx of calcium ions when stimulated with an impulse. This action triggers the release of synaptic vesicle content: acetylcholine (ACh).
- ACh neurotransmitters cross the synaptic cleft and bind to the receptors in the muscle basement membrane. These receptors are transmitter-gated ion channels that allow passage of sodium ions across the membrane. Sodium influx depolarizes the muscle membrane and results in muscle contraction.
- The smallest unit of this neuromuscular function is the *motor unit,* which represents one motor neuron and the muscle fibers innervated by it. The innervation ratio of the muscle fibers to the motor neuron is 80 to 100 in small muscles, such as the intrinsic muscles in the hand, to 1000 to 2000 in large muscles of the leg.
- Each muscle contains a mixture of the various fiber types: slow fatigable (type I), fast oxidative (type IIA), fast fatigable (type IIB), and fast intermediate (type IIC). Specific nerve fibers innervate different types of muscle fibers: fast fatigable muscle fibers are innervated by large rapidly conducting axons and slow fatigable fibers by smaller, slower axons.
- Botulinum toxins, exotoxins of *Clostridium botulinum,* act at the motor endplates by blocking the release of ACh neurotransmitters. Once feared as the most toxic substance known to man, *Botulinum* toxin enjoys wide popularity in treatments of dystonia and spasticity.

## Sensory Receptors

- The three common types of mechanoreceptors are the Merkel cell complex, Meissner corpuscles, and Pacinian corpuscles (Box 15–3).

| Box 15–3 | Sensory Mechanoreceptors |
| --- | --- |
| Merkel cell complex | Clustered around the sweat duct |
| | 2- to 4-mm receptive field |
| | Slowly adapting |
| | Static two-point discrimination |
| Meissner corpuscle | Located at the sides of the intermediate ridge |
| | Responds to flutter vibration |
| | Rapidly adapting |
| | Moving two-point discrimination |
| Pacinian corpuscle | Located in the subcutaneous tissue |
| | Looks like a grain of rice |
| | Rapidly adapting |
| | Several-centimeter receptive field |
| | Vibration at 250 cps |

# Nerve Injury and Repair

## Classification of Injury

- In 1948, Sir Herbert Seddon devised a classification system of nerve injury based on disrupted internal structures of the peripheral nerve. His system of *neuropraxia, axonotmesis,* and *neurotmesis* is simple and widely used today, because it correlates the degree of nerve injury with the prognosis of functional recovery.[1]
- In 1968, Sir Sydney Sunderland expanded on Seddon's classification system by putting more emphasis on the fascicular layers of the nerve.
- Sunderland's first-degree injury is Seddon's neuropraxia, which is a demyelinating injury with a temporary conduction block that resolves completely in 1 to 2 days.
- The second-degree injury is axonotmesis, where distal degeneration of the injured axon occurs. Regeneration of the axon almost always is complete, because the endoneurial layer is intact and may take up to several weeks, depending on the location of the injury.
- Sunderland's third-degree injury is the less severe of Seddon's neurotmesis category, where the perineurial layer is intact. Regeneration occurs but is not complete because of endoneurial scarring and loss of end-organ specificity within the fascicle.
- Sunderland's fourth-degree injury is more severe, where the axon, endoneurium, and perineurium are disrupted, causing more extensive scarring that blocks axonal regeneration. Spontaneous nerve regeneration often is unsatisfactory in the fourth-degree injury, resulting in neuroma in continuity.
- Sunderland's fifth-degree injury corresponds to severed nerve trunk, and spontaneous regeneration is not possible without surgical coaptation. Sunderland emphasized that any given nerve injury may contain mixed degrees of injury and rarely is pure in classification (Table 15–1).

| **Table 15–1:  Classification of Nerve Injury** | | | |
| SEDDON | SUNDERLAND | INJURY | PROGNOSIS |
| --- | --- | --- | --- |
| Neuropraxia | First degree | Demyelination injury | Temporary conduction block; resolves in 1–2 days |
| Axonotmesis | Second degree | Axonal injury | Regeneration usually is complete; may take several weeks or months |
| Neurotmesis | Third degree | Endoneurium injured | Regeneration occurs but is not satisfactory |
| | Fourth degree | Perineurium injured | Spontaneous regeneration is unsatisfactory; results in neuroma in continuity |
| | Fifth degree | Severed nerve trunk | Spontaneous regeneration is not possible without surgery |

# Degeneration and Regeneration

## Degeneration

- The axon distal to the injury site undergoes a well-described degenerative process known as *Wallerian degeneration,* which involves breaking down the old axon and clearing the myelin debris of the axoplasm (see Figure 15–3). This degenerative process takes at least 1 to 2 weeks; therefore, the electrodiagnostic test performed early may not indicate abnormalities during this period.
- The known key players for Wallerian degeneration are macrophages, Schwann cells, various neurotrophic factors, the injured neuron, and the end organs. They influence each other in an intricate interplay, which is understood only rudimentarily at present.
- Macrophages, in addition to performing phagocytosis, express interleukin (IL)-1, which is a potent stimulator for Schwann cells to produce neurotrophic factors and express neural adhesion molecules.
- The roles of Schwann cells are multiple and crucial. They begin by breaking down myelin, which is followed by proliferation and formation of the band of Bünger within the basal lamina of the original Schwann cell tube. Schwann cells secrete various neurotrophic factors and express neural adhesion molecules. Last, they circumscribe regenerating axons and myelinate them.
- If an axon fails to regenerate immediately, the distal endoneurial tube shrinks irreversibly, making later regeneration of the axon even more difficult. This process appears to be the main reason for the failure to successfully reinnervate muscles following a delayed surgical nerve repair, rather than degeneration of muscle fibers and motor endplates as previously thought.

## Regeneration

- Within hours of injury, the proximal axon begins to regenerate with sprout formation. Collateral sprouts grow from the most distal node of Ranvier proximal to the site of injury. These regeneration sprouts may be fairly close to the injury site in a sharp transection or far in avulsion or crush-type of injury.
- During regeneration, Schwann cells and neurons have an interdependent relationship mediated by neurotrophic factors and neurite outgrowth promoting factors. The neurotrophic factors facilitate bidirectional communication between neurons and Schwann cells. Neurotrophic factors not only act on neurons as previously well described in the literature, but also they exert a vital effect on Schwann cells. Neurite outgrowth promoting factors facilitate attachment of growing axons to other axons and/or Schwann cells, guiding nerve regeneration.

## Neurotrophic Factors

- Neurotrophic factors are a family of peptides essential in neuronal survival after nerve injury. Three major groups of neurotrophic factors are identified: neurotrophins, neurokines, and transforming growth factor (TGF)-β family, including glial-derived neurotrophic factor (GDNF).

### Neurotrophins

- The neurotrophins are small, basic polypeptides, which include NGF, brain-derived neurotrophic factor (BDNF), neurotrophin-3 (NT-3), and neurotrophin-4/5 (NT-4/5).
- NGF is the best known and studied neurotrophic factor since it was first isolated from mouse sarcoma tissue by Levi-Montalcini and Hamburger in 1951. NGF produced by Schwann cells binds to NGF-specific receptors on the axonal membrane. NGF-receptor complex is internalized and transported retrograde to the cell body, which responds with increased synthesis of tubulin, neurofilament, and neurotransmitters. NGF increases survival of sympathetic and sensory neurons but has no significant influence on survival or regeneration of motor neurons. NGF has been proposed for clinical uses, including treatment of Parkinson disease and Alzheimer disease.[2]
- BDNF, NT-3, and NT-4/5 appear to support survival of motor neurons, promote regeneration of the motor neurons, and regulate neuromuscular synapses.

### Neurokines

- The neurokines play a significant role in nerve regeneration. Almost all neurokines of the IL-6 family, except ciliary neurotrophic factor, are up-regulated after nerve injury. Other neurokines, such as leukocyte inhibitory factor and IL-6, are up-regulated in Schwann cells after nerve injury and appear to support motor neurons in vitro.

### Glial-Derived Neurotrophic Factor

- GDNF, which belongs to the TGF-β family, is up-regulated in nerve injury and promotes motor neuron survival. It has a strong trophic effect on Schwann cells, thus implicating its role in nerve regeneration.

## Neurite Outgrowth Promoting Factors

- In addition to producing many neurotrophic factors and their receptors, Schwann cells up-regulate production of neurite outgrowth promoting factors: cell adhesion molecules and extracellular matrix proteins in basement membrane.
- Cell adhesion molecules (CAMs), such as Ng-CAM/L1, N-CAM, and N-cadherin, as well as L2/HNK-1 expressed on the surface of Schwann cells, bind with L1, N-CAM, and with other cell adhesion molecules and integrins on the axonal surface. Interestingly, L2/HNK-1 is expressed only in Schwann cells that line the motor pathways and may play a role in motor neurotropic guidance.
- Extracellular matrix proteins in basement membrane, such as laminin, fibronectin, heparan sulfate proteoglycans, and tenascin, bind to integrins on the surface of growing axons and guide them distally.

## Growth Cone

- The leading edge of each regenerating fiber is called the *growth cone* and contains numerous filopodia that probe into surrounding areas in ameboid fashion. When a suitable surface such as Schwann cell membrane or basement membrane is reached, the filopodium adheres to the surface, the growth cone is pulled forward, and the axon grows in that direction. The growth cone is also active in endocytosis of extrinsic molecules such as neurotrophic factors produced by Schwann cells. These molecules are transported retrograde to the cell body to up-regulate structural protein synthesis and promote further growth.

## Myelination

- When the growing axon reaches the end organ, maturation of the axon progresses proximal to distal. Increase in axonal diameter occurs first, followed by myelination. The final diameter of the mature regenerated axon usually is smaller with a thinner myelin sheath compared to the preinjury status.

- Neurotrophins are key mediators of the peripheral nerve myelination process, both as positive and negative modulators. The myelination program involves numerous intercellular signals, including neuregulins, adenosine triphosphate, and the neurotrophins.

## Reinnervation of the Motor Unit

- When a regenerating motor axon reaches a denervated muscle, reinnervation occurs at the old motor endplates. In normal muscles, there is a random distribution of motor units. In reinnervated muscles, there are clusters of smaller motor units. Even if only a few fibers reach the dennervated muscle, axons sprout to reinnervate many surrounding endplates, forming giant motor units. Schwann cells appear to play an important role in forming motor endplates. Terminal Schwann cells induce and guide regenerating nerve ends into the muscle (Figure 15–4).[3]

## Reinnervation of Sensory Receptors

- When sensory nerve fibers are injured, sensory receptors degenerate much like muscles, the other type of end organ. The Merkel cell-neurite complex degenerates first, followed in a few months by Meissner corpuscles. Pacinian corpuscles appear stable and intact over 1 year.
- Among different sensory modalities, the return of perception, pain, and temperature precedes the return of touch. The touch submodalities recover in an orderly sequence: first the perception of 30 cycles per second (cps) frequency, followed by moving touch, static touch, and finally 256 cps stimulus.[4]

# Clinical Application of Peripheral Nerve Physiology

## Clinical Assessment

- When evaluating a patient with a nerve injury, the hand surgeon must learn the mechanism of injury (stretch, crush, avulsion, sharp, or blunt injury), how much time has elapsed since the injury, the patient's hand dominance, the patient's occupation, and other relevant medical history. Especially crucial is the patient's subjective complaint. Is pain or cold intolerance most debilitating for the patient instead of an obvious dysfunction noted on physical examination?
- The clinical assessment of peripheral nerve function uses tests of both sensibility and motor function. Threshold testing, density testing, and empiric testing are examples of sensory clinical tests (Box 15–4).
- Assessment of motor function can be achieved using subjective muscle grading and quantitative strength testing. As devised by the British Medical Research Council

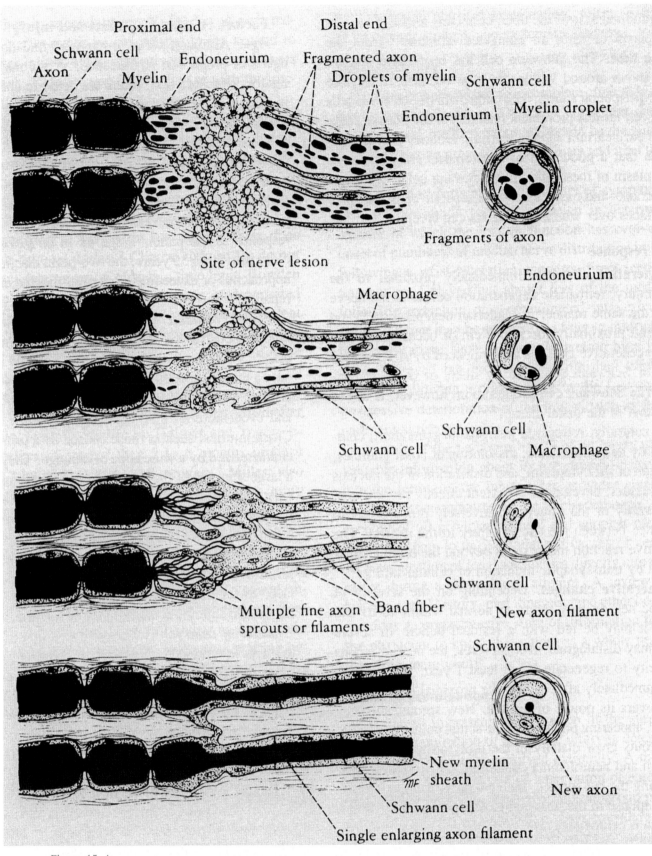

Figure 15–4:
Wallerian degeneration and regeneration. A, Breaking down of axoplasms and cytoskeletons into granular, ovoid debrides. B, Macrophages within the nerve and from circulation are attracted to the injured area in large numbers. By 2 to 3 days, they start to phagocytize these debrides and clear them away. C, Schwann cells start to proliferate with mitosis and form a line known as *Bunger band*. D, Schwann cells wrap around newly regenerating axons and myelinate. (From Snell RS: *Clinical neuroanatomy*, ed 5. Philadelphia, 2001, Williams & Wilkins.)

| Box 15–4 | Sensory Tests | | |
|---|---|---|---|
| | Type | Details | Clinical |
| Threshold test | Semmes-Weinstein monofilament pressure Vibration | Fine filaments with variable stiffness 30–256 cps | Nerve compression syndrome |
| Density test | Static two-point Moving two-point | Tests functioning sensory end organs | Reinnervation and cortical reeducation status |
| Empiric test | British Medical Research Council | Subjective | Qualitative |

(BMRC), subjective staged levels of motor recovery have gained wide clinical acceptance (Box 15–5).

- Quantitative strength testing that relies on measurable data enables the surgeon to compare alternative methods of nerve repair. In quantitative testing, the force of an isolated contracting muscle or muscle group after reinnervation is measured using a load cell, and the result is expressed as a percentage of the contralateral uninjured side. This technique provides more accurate data of the patient's clinical recovery to allow for comparison of results of different methods of nerve repair.
- Based on the evaluation, the hand surgeon determines whether a more proximal or systemic pathology such as cervical radiculopathy or degenerative neuropathy is causing the neurologic deficit, whether a partial or complete nerve injury is present, whether to offer a nonsurgical or surgical treatment option, and the timing of surgical intervention if any is needed. Other laboratory or ancillary tests may help the surgeon in answering some of these questions.

## Ancillary Tests

- Nerve conduction velocity (NCV) studies, electromyography (EMG), somatosensory evoked potentials (SSEP), and magnetic resonance imaging (MRI) are some of the ancillary tests useful for evaluating peripheral nerve function.

## Nerve Conduction Velocity/ Electromyography

- The most sensitive test for detecting nerve compression syndromes with demyelination is the NCV test. EMG, in contrast, is most helpful after a nerve injury that results in denervation with loss of axons.
- To measure NCV, a nerve is stimulated proximally and the response is recorded distally over a fixed distance. The distance between the stimulus and the distal electrode is divided by the latency to calculate the NCV. *Latency* is the measured time interval between the proximal nerve stimulation and distal recording. Electrodes placed in or over muscle detect motor conduction, whereas leads on the digits detect sensory conduction.
- Injuries that cause focal demyelination produce delays in NCV. A decrease in nerve conduction across a localized region indicates compression neuropathy (Box 15–6).
- Various factors such as the nerve being studied, the equipment used and its calibration, the room temperature, and the patient's age influence the results of nerve conduction studies.
- For median nerve motor latency, normal values generally are less than 4.0 ms, whereas sensory latencies are less than 3.6 ms across the wrist.
- For ulnar nerve latency, conduction *velocities* across the elbow average 60 m/s, with the lower limit of normal 50 m/s. In cubital tunnel syndrome, the conduction velocity across the elbow is slowed by at least 10 m/s compared to the forearm segment.
- Normal muscle has no measurable electrical activity in the absence of voluntary contraction, except for a brief burst of insertional activity when the EMG needle is introduced into the muscle. With voluntary muscle contraction, the action potentials form and increase in frequency with increasing intensity of muscle contraction. An injury that disrupts nerve axons produces electromyographic changes such as fibrillations and positive sharp waves in the denervated muscle within 2 to 3 weeks. As reinnervation occurs, the target skeletal muscle begins to demonstrate polyphasic potentials and small voluntary action potentials. Fibrillation patterns can also be detected with severe nerve compression syndromes that produce axonal disruption.

| Box 15–5 | Motor Assessment by the British Medical Research Council |
|---|---|
| 0/5 | No muscle activity |
| 1/5 | Contraction but no movement |
| 2/5 | Movement of extremity but not against gravity |
| 3/5 | Movement against gravity but not resistance |
| 4/5 | Movement against both gravity and resistance with less than normal strength |
| 5/5 | Normal strength |

| Box 15–6 | Nerve Conduction Velocity | |
|---|---|---|
| | Nerve Conduction Velocity | Pathology |
| Peripheral neuropathy | Diffuse slowing of multiple nerves | Diffuse demyelination |
| Compression neuropathy | Focal slowing | Focal demyelination |

## Somatosensory Evoked Potentials

- A peripheral sensory stimulus produces electric signals detectable by electrodes placed on the contralateral scalp. These signals are called *somatosensory evoked potentials*. Any disruption along the sensory pathway results in the failure to detect these signals. The disruption may be either preganglionic or postganglionic. Preganglionic injuries demonstrate abnormal SSEPs but normal conduction velocities because the postganglionic fibers are intact. When ordering the NCV and EMG studies, the surgeon must carefully identify the clinical questions to be answered by these studies.

## Magnetic Resonance Imaging

- MRI technology has advanced significantly in the past 10 years and has been useful in diagnosing nerve lesions early. The MRI axis can be oriented along the course of a peripheral nerve. Experienced neurologists can provide reliable information regarding neuroma formation or spinal nerve root avulsion. Damage to the myelin sheath in neuropraxia may be discerned by the loss of T2-weighted signals.

## Treatment of Nerve Injuries

- For a nerve injury requiring surgical exploration and repair, the surgeon determines whether a primary repair or secondary repair is indicated. The general rule is that the primary coaptation of the severed nerve ends is preferable to a secondary repair using a nerve conduit. It is extremely important for the surgeon to realize that this rule has a limited application. Overcoming a nerve gap by stretching the injured nerve, joint positioning in flexion, or repairing under tension using thick sutures guarantees a suboptimal outcome. Stretching causes a secondary traction injury to the nerve, compromising intraneural blood supply. Joint positioning limits the rehabilitation process and may disrupt the nerve repair site when the patient starts moving the extremity.
- The ideal nerve repair should ensure accurate alignment of each and all fascicles with minimal use of suture material or foreign body. The current state of nerve repair is still evolving, and we have yet to determine the perfect repair technique. In the present era, all nerve repairs should be performed using the operating microscope or at least adequate loupe magnification and microsurgical techniques. Nerve repair sites should be tension free.

## Primary Nerve Repair

- Primary nerve repair includes epineural, group fascicular, and interfascicular repairs. Epineural repair is ideal when the proper alignment of the nerve is apparent in partial nerve injuries, sharp lacerations, or distal nerve injuries (e.g., at the digital nerve level). When a nerve injury includes a crushing component or when the repair is delayed, group fascicular repair is preferred if the group fascicular pattern is distinguishable. Interfascicular repair usually is not performed because of the excessive sutures required at the repair site (such that the suture material potentially prevents regeneration) and the difficulty in aligning the individual fascicles.

## Secondary Nerve Repair

- Secondary repair is used to overcome nerve gaps resulting from segmental nerve loss with crush-type injuries or with delayed repairs. Nerve grafting usually is required for secondary nerve repair. The sural nerve graft is the gold standard for nerve autografts because of the high ratio of axons to connective tissue and the minimal sensory deficit on the lateral aspect of the foot that is generally well tolerated. Digital nerves can be grafted using the lateral or medial antebrachial cutaneous nerves. However, loss of these nerves can lead to significant paresthesias and may not be tolerated well. The small articular branch of the posterior interosseous nerve is a good donor nerve for grafting digital nerves without producing a sensory deficit. Fibrin glue techniques are helpful when using multiple cable grafts to glue them together and for use at the nerve repair site.
- No great substitute presently exists for autogenous nerve grafts; however, research studies are ongoing to find an ideal nerve conduit that will obviate donor site morbidity from nerve graft harvest.
- Sporadic reports on the use of a segment of vessel to bridge a nerve gap have been reported since Bungner's report in a canine model in 1891. Chiu et al. presented histologic and electrophysiologic evidence of nerve regeneration across a venous nerve conduit in rodents. Subsequently, a prospective clinical study comparing sensory recovery in distal peripheral nerves between autogenous vein graft, nerve graft, and direct repair showed comparable results for short nerve gaps (<3 cm) (Figure 15–5).[5]
- Various investigators researched the use of nerve allografts to reduce donor morbidity resulting from autogenous nerve graft harvest.[6] The problems of nerve allografts include the possible transmission of viruses and the need for at least temporary host immunosuppression. Current research studies also focus on using allogenic nerve grafts in conjunction with immunosuppression with minimal side effects or rendering them less antigenic with cryopreservation.
- Other various nonneural conduits have been studied in animals and humans, including polyglycolic acid collagen tubes, silicone tubes, muscle basement membrane, amniotic membrane, and fibronectin mats. When seeded with Schwann cells, these conduits appear more effective in bridging nerve gaps than without Schwann cells in animal studies. Some of these conduits are commercially available, and a few studies show favorable results when

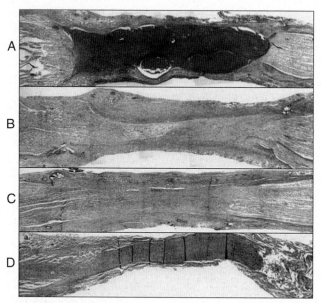

Figure 15–5:
**Autogenous vein conduit.** The autogenous vein nerve conduit undergoes four distinctive but overlapping phases during nerve regeneration. A, Hematoma phase (1–7 days). B, Cellular migration (7–14 days). C, Axonal advancement (11–31 days). D, Myelination and maturation phase.

the conduits are used as an entubulation device in primary neurorrhaphy.

- Nerve transposition is a treatment for injuries of the ulnar nerve near the elbow because of the relative lack of nerve branches near this area. Bone shortening is generally limited to situations in the upper extremity where there is a concurrent fracture.

## Treatment of Neuromas

- Failure of the regenerating nerve fibers to reach distal targets results in either a terminal neuroma or a neuroma in continuity. By definition, every nerve laceration or avulsion that is not repaired results in the formation of a terminal neuroma, and even repaired nerves form a neuroma in continuity.

- Repair of the severed peripheral nerve is the only way to prevent or minimize a terminal neuroma formation. A neuroma located in an area with little soft tissue coverage, such as in the dorsum of the hand or the foot, can be extremely painful. For example, a neuroma involving the sensory branch of the radial nerve may render the patient intolerant of even wearing a long sleeve shirt or a wrist watch. The treatment methods for repairing neuromas include excising the neuroma, burying the neuroma, and capping the neuroma. Excising the neuroma and performing a primary repair or nerve grafting can be an effective treatment if the repair site can be protected under a muscle or soft tissue. When a repair of the severed ends of the nerve is not possible or desirable, resecting the neuroma and burying the proximal end in muscle or even bone can be an effective treatment.

- Treatment of a neuroma in continuity provides another set of challenges because some fibers remain intact and therefore must be protected. The intact fibers may be adherent or traverse within the neuroma. In a mixed nerve with sensory and motor fibers, the surgeon must determine whether the intact fibers are mostly sensory or motor, whether they are worth saving, and, if so, whether a direct separation of the fibers within the neuroma can be avoided. Dissection of the nerve proximal and distal to the neuroma may allow bypassing the neuroma with a nerve graft to the injured group of fascicles, therefore avoiding direct dissection within the neuroma, which may cause further scarring and disruption of the intact nerve fibers. Intraoperative electrical stimulation can be used to help identify the intact motor fibers and protect them during the neuroma resection. Neuromas formed by disrupted motor fibers with intact sensory axons are less symptomatic and, in the upper extremity, can be treated with tendon transfers without the need to explore the neuroma.

## End to Side Neurorrhaphy

- Viterbo et al.[7] demonstrated collateral nerve growth with lateroterminal neurorrhaphy without and with an epineural window in rats, confirming the result with electrophysiologic studies. The clinical application of lateroterminal neurorrhaphy remains experimental because of variable reported results.[8] Donor muscles may become acutely denervated when its innervation is compromised with an end to side neurorrhaphy; however, no long-term deficit has been noted in experimental studies.[9] Subsequent studies of end to side repair have demonstrated that the transected nerve branch sends axons down the outer epineurium of the intact nerve branch receiving the end to side coaptation. Therefore the axons that enter the end to side neurroaphy end up traveling through the outer epineurium of the intact nerve rather than coming from spontaneous budding of axons from an intact nerve.

## Neurotropism

- The concept of purposeful nerve regeneration toward the correct distal pathway and the correct endorgan is called *neurotropism*. Some evidence indicates that tissue specificity exists for regenerating axons by their growing toward nervous tissue rather than other types of tissue. The hypothesis is that axons grow toward a gradient of diffusible substance produced by an appropriate target. Except in the rat sciatic nerve Y-tube model, nerve trunk specificity has not been proven.[11]

- However, increasing evidence suggests that sensory-motor specificity exists. Motor neurons do not preferentially reinnervate motor nerve or muscle rather than sensory neurons. Random reinnervation occurs but motor axons that regenerate into a sensory pathway later become pruned when connected to wrong target organs. After Wallerian degeneration, the motor pathway is different from the sensory later pathway in that carbohydrate epitope L2/HNK-1 is present in the motor pathway.[12]

- No evidence for topographic or end-organ specificity is evident at present, contributing to the great difficulty of mixed nerve reconstructions.

## Conclusions

- Various factors contribute to the outcome following a nerve injury, including the nature of the lesion, presence of axonotmesis or neurotmesis, degree of intraneural scarring, and distance to the target organ. Despite significant advances in neurorrhaphy techniques, the outcomes of nerve repair remain far from ideal.
- Distal nerve pathway deterioration appears to be a primary problem and not muscle atrophy as previously thought. Prolonged denervation causes deterioration in the ability of Schwann cells to guide and promote nerve regeneration. With delayed regeneration, Schwann cells lose $\beta_1$ subunits of the integrins, receptors for laminin, cell adhesion molecules, and p75 low-affinity neurotrophin receptors, all of which are important players in nerve regeneration.
- The last 2 decades have been marked by heightened interest in nerve regeneration. The successes of microscopic neurorrhaphy and autogenous nerve grafting, including interfascicular and cable grafting, have brought enthusiasm. However, the functional result is still far from perfect. Current areas of evolving interests include bridging the nerve gap with nonneural conduits, lateroterminal neurorrhaphy, nerve transfer, immunologic modulation, and deciphering the complexity and interplay at the molecular level of nerve regeneration.

## References

1. Wilgis EFS, Murphy R: The significance of longitudinal excursions in peripheral nerves. *Hand Clin* 2:761–766, 1987.
   The authors demonstrated that longitudinal excursions allow the peripheral nerves to glide across the joints.

2. Drago J, Kilpatrick TJ, Koblar SA, Talman PS: Growth factors: potential therapeutic applications in neurology. *J Neurol Neurosurg Psychiatry* 57:1445-1450, 1994.
   This review article discusses in detail the roles of Schwann cells and various known neurotrophic factors in nerve regeneration.

3. Love FM, Son YJ, Thompson WJ: Activity alters muscle reinnervation and terminal sprouting by reducing the number of Schwann cell pathways that grow to link synaptic sites. *J Neurobiol* 54:566-576, 2003.
   Nerve sprouting in muscle is induced and guided by the processes extended by Schwann cells.

4. Dellon AL: Management of peripheral nerve function in the upper and lower extremities using quantitative sensory testing. *Hand Clin* 15:697-715, 1999.
   Recovery of perception, pain, and temperature precedes the return of touch, and the touch submodalities recover in an orderly sequence.

5. Tseng C, Hu GL, Ambron R, Chiu D: Histologic analysis of Schwann cell migration and peripheral nerve regeneration in the autogenous venous nerve conduit (AVNC). *J Reconstr Microsurg* 19:331, 2003.
   This report shows that the autogenous vein nerve conduit undergoes four distinctive but overlapping phases during nerve regeneration.

6. Easterling KJ, Trumble TE: The treatment of peripheral nerve injuries using irradiated allografts and temporary immunosuppression (in a rat model). *J Reconstr Microsurg* 6:301-307, 1990.
   Irradiation of allografts before transplantation and host immunosuppression with cyclosporin A were studied as a means of lessening rejection of transplanted peripheral nerve tissue.

7. Viterbo F, Trindade JC, Hoshino K, Mazzoni Neto A: End-to-side neurorrhaphy with removal of the epineurial sheath: an experimental study in rats. *Plast Reconstr Surg* 94:1038-1047, 1994.
   This study demonstrates collateral nerve growth with lateroterminal neurorrhaphy without and with epineural window in rats and confirms the result with electrophysiologic studies.

8. al-Qattan MM, al-Thunyan A: Variables affecting axonal regeneration following end-to-side neurorrhaphy. *Br J Plast Surg* 51:238-242, 1998.
   Axonal regeneration following end to side nerve coaptation is more likely to occur when the nerve graft is sutured to the parent nerve using perineurial rather than epineurial sutures.

9. Cederna PS, Kalliainen LK, Urbanchek MG, et al: "Donor" muscle structure and function after end-to-side neurorrhaphy. *Plast Reconstr Surg* 107:789-796, 2001.
   Donor muscle becomes acutely denervated when its innervation is compromised with an end to side neurorrhaphy; however, no long-term deficit is noted.

10. McCallister WV, Tang W, Trumble TE: Is end-to-side neurorrhaphy effective? A study of axonal sprouting stimulated from intact nerves. *J Reconstr Microsurg* 15:597–603, 1999.

11. Chiu DTW, Smahl J, Chen L, Meyer V: Neurotropism revisited. *Neurological Research* 26:381–387, 2004.
    Using a Y-shaped autogenous inferior vena cava graft in a sciatic neve neurotomy model in rodent. The existence of a guiding influence at the distal stump toward the regenerating nerve fibers was demonstrated.

12. Martini R, Schachner M, Brushart TM: The L2/HNK-1 carbohydrate is preferentially expressed by previously motor axon-associated Schwann cells in reinnervated peripheral nerves. *J Neurosci* 14(11 pt 2):7180-7191, 1994.
    Motor neurons preferentially reinnervate motor nerve or muscle rather than sensory neurons. Preferential motor reinnervation appears strong enough to overcome a nerve gap or malalignment.

# Compression Neuropathy

Lee Dellon

MD, Professor, Plastic Surgery and Neurosurgery, Johns Hopkins University, Baltimore, MD;
Clinical Professor of Plastic Surgery, Neurosurgery and Anatomy, University of Arizona,
Tucson, AZ

## Introduction

- Upper extremity chronic nerve compression is a common source of patient sensory and motor complaints. Symptoms present in the hand, forearm, arm, shoulder, or many combinations of these regions.
- Compression neuropathy implies a chronic condition, in contrast to acute compression of a peripheral nerve, as might be seen in trauma.
- Motor symptoms related to chronic compression range from weakness to paralysis.
- Sensory symptoms related to chronic nerve compression include numbness, tingling, and buzzing *but do not include pain.*
- Pain related to the peripheral nerve represents acute nerve compression (with axonal loss), a vascular infarct of a nerve, or a systemic neuropathy.
- With chronic nerve compression, the perceptions of temperature and pain are the *last* to be lost, whereas perceptions related to touch, such as movement, vibration, and pressure, are the *first* to become impaired (Box 16–1).
- Clinical presentations and syndromes related to the upper extremity peripheral nerves are related to the particular sensory and motor territories supplied by the given nerve and the location along that nerve's anatomic pathway at which one or more compression sites occur.

### Box 16–1 Pain Related to the Peripheral Nerve

- Pain most often implies direct nerve trauma.
- Pain can be caused by a vascular infarct of a nerve.
- Pain can be caused by acute nerve compression, e.g., crush.
- *Pain usually is not related to chronic compression.*
- Pain in bilateral extremities may represent neuropathy.
- Pain, bilaterally, with normal two-point discrimination is small-fiber neuropathy.
- Pain and temperature sensation, which are small-fiber perceptions, are the last perceptions to become abnormal in chronic nerve compression. Touch sensations, such as movement and pressure, which are large-fiber perceptions, are the first to become abnormal.
- Absence of pain perception with normal two-point discrimination is a syrinx.
- Absence of pain perception with abnormal two-point discrimination may be leprosy.

## Pathophysiology of Chronic Nerve Compression

- Understanding the pathophysiology of chronic nerve compression permits an appreciation for how the results of physical examination change over time and how patient care must change over time.[1–3]

- Intraneural microvessels have decreased flow with just 20 mm Hg external compression.
- Decreased blood flow causes neural ischemia, the source of paresthesias.
- After approximately 2 months of mild compression, the blood-nerve barrier changes, causing intraneural edema, which increases the pressure upon the microvessels.
- After approximately 6 months of compression, in the rat and subhuman primate models, large nerve fiber demyelination begins (fibers related to perception of touch and motor function).
- After approximately 6 months of compression, perineurial thickening and interfascicular fibrosis begins.
- After approximately 12 months of compression, axonal loss begins in these large fibers.
- With continued external pressure upon a peripheral nerve, progressive structural changes occur that produce predictable clinical symptoms and physical findings.
- Early in chronic nerve compression, symptoms (e.g., paresthesia) related to the sensory nerve occur and change in coordination with the motor nerve, but no physical manifestations are found on physical examination. In contrast, with acute compression, which implies a large increase in pressure upon the nerve over a short time frame, sudden loss of nerve function occurs and is associated with pain and abnormal sensory and motor findings within hours of the onset.
- In the intermediate phase of chronic nerve compression, a combination of ischemic block to axonal transmission and structural changes to the nerve results in weakness of the motor nerve and increased threshold of the sensory nerve.
- In the later phases of chronic nerve compression, there is axonal loss that for the motor system produces muscle wasting and ultimately paralysis and for the sensory nerve produces abnormal two-point discrimination and ultimately anesthesia.
- Based upon the known pathophysiology of chronic nerve compression, a numerical grading system can be constructed to permit staging of nerve compression and to provide an evidence base for clinical decision making (Tables 16–1 to 16–3).

## History Taking

- Listening to the patients' complaints often gives sufficient information to make the correct diagnosis.
- Critical phrases related to upper extremity nerve compressions are given in Box 16–2.
- If the onset of symptoms was sudden or associated with a "cold" or pain episode, consider the cause to be Parsonage-Turner syndrome, a usually self-resolving inflammatory brachial plexopathy, not a nerve compression syndrome.[4]
- If the onset of symptoms was related to a work injury or other form of trauma, obtain the exact description of the

### Table 16–1: Pathophysiologic Basis for Peripheral Nerve Grading Scale

| DEGREE OF SEVERITY | PATHOPHYSIOLOGY | CLINICAL |
|---|---|---|
| Mild | Blood-nerve barrier breakdown | Symptoms, no signs on PEX |
| Moderate | Demyelination abnormal threshold | Symptoms, signs of elevated cutaneous pressure or vibratory thresholds, and/or of weakness |
| Severe | Axonal loss decreased innervation, density | Symptoms, signs of decreased innervation density (abnormal two point discrimination), and/or muscle wasting |

### Table 16–2: Numerical Grading Scale: Median Nerve at the Wrist Level[5]

| NUMERICAL SCORE | | |
|---|---|---|
| SENSORY | MOTOR | DESCRIPTION OF IMPAIRMENT |
| 0 | 0 | None |
| 1 | | Paresthesia, intermittent |
| 2 | | Abnormal pressure threshold (Pressure-Specified Sensory Device) <45 years old ≤3 mm, at 1.0–20 gm/mm$^2$ ≥45 years old ≤4 mm, at 2.2–20 gm/mm$^2$ |
| | 3 | Weakness, thenar muscles |
| 4 | | Abnormal pressure threshold (Pressure-Specified Sensory Device) <45 years old ≤3 mm, at >20.0 gm/mm$^2$ ≥45 years old ≤4 mm, at >20.0 gm/mm$^2$ |
| 5 | | Paresthesias, persistent |
| 6 | | Abnormal innervation density (Pressure-Specified Sensory Device) <45 years old ≥4 mm and <8 mm, at any gm/mm$^2$ ≥45 years old ≥5 mm and <9 mm, at any gm/mm$^2$ |
| | 7 | Muscle wasting (1–2/4) |
| 8 | | Abnormal innervation density (Pressure-Specified Sensory Device) <45 years old ≥8 mm, at any gm/mm$^2$ ≥45 years old ≥9 mm, at any gm/mm$^2$ |
| 9 | | Anesthesia |
| | 10 | Muscle wasting (3–4/4) |

**Table 16–3: Numerical Grading Scale: Ulnar Nerve at the Elbow Level[5]**

| NUMERICAL SCORE | | DESCRIPTION OF IMPAIRMENT |
|---|---|---|
| SENSORY | MOTOR | |
| 0 | 0 | None |
| 1 | | Paresthesia, intermittent |
| | 2 | Weakness |
| | |     Pinch/grip (lb) |
| | |         Female: 10–14/26–39 |
| | |         Male: 13–19/31–59 |
| 3 | | Abnormal pressure threshold |
| | |     (Pressure-Specified Sensory Device) |
| | |         <45 years old |
| | |           $\leq$3 mm, at 1.0–20.0 gm/mm$^2$ |
| | |         $\geq$45 years old |
| | |           $\leq$4 mm, at 1.9–20.0 gm/mm$^2$ |
| | 4 | Weakness |
| | |     Pinch/grip (lb) |
| | |         Female: 6–9/1525 |
| | |         Male: 6–12/15–30 |
| 5 | | Paresthesia, persistent |
| 6 | | Abnormal innervation density |
| | |     (Pressure-Specified Sensory Device) |
| | |         <45 years old |
| | |           $\geq$ 4 mm and <8 mm, at any gm/mm$^2$ |
| | |         $\geq$45 years old |
| | |           $\geq$5 mm and <9 mm, at any gm/mm$^2$ |
| | 7 | Muscle wasting (1–2/4) |
| 8 | | Abnormal innervation density |
| | |     (Pressure-Specified Sensory Device) |
| | |         <45 years old |
| | |           $\geq$8 mm, at any gm/mm$^2$ |
| | |         $\geq$45 years old |
| | |           $\geq$9 mm, at any gm/mm$^2$ |
| 9 | | Anesthesia |
| | 10 | Muscle wasting (3–4/4) |

---

**Box 16–2 History-Taking Critical Phrases**

- Nighttime awakening suggests median nerve compression at the wrist. However, sleeping with the elbow flexed beneath the pillow can cause nocturnal ulnar nerve compression at the elbow.
- "Dropping objects" suggests ulnar nerve compression at the elbow.
- "Clumsiness" suggests ulnar nerve compression at the elbow.
- "Weakness" suggests ulnar nerve compression at the elbow.
- "Fingers going numb while talking on the phone or driving" suggests median nerve compression at the wrist.
- "Thumb and index finger still numb after carpal tunnel decompression" suggests radial sensory nerve compression in the forearm.
- Symptoms extending up the radial side of the arm into shoulder suggest radial nerve compression: radial tunnel, forearm, or both.
- Symptoms that worsen with any activity requiring the arms to be at shoulder level or higher, e.g., "combing hair," suggest brachial plexus compression in the thoracic inlet.

- Observe whether the fingers are positioned normally with respect to their flexion with the hand at rest.
- Observe whether the hand has characteristic appearances of clawing (from ulnar nerve motor loss), a thumb that is flat to the palm (from median nerve motor loss), or both.
- Observe for evidence of loss of pain perception resulting from cuts, scratches, or burn marks about the distal end of the fingers.
- Observe for evidence of sympathetic overactivity or underactivity (e.g., skin color, skin temperature, sweating, dryness).
- Observe for evidence of clothing, jewelry or factitious (rope or rubber bands) causing constriction about the hand, wrist, or forearm.
- Observe if the hand is held in an abnormal posture, such as thumb clenched or all fingers clenched through out the interview.

---

incident and time course of symptoms since the injury or trauma.

- If the symptoms have been present for more than 6 months and are slowly progressing, nerve compression is likely.
- If both feet are involved, the upper extremity complaints must be viewed in the context of a systemic neuropathy, such as diabetic neuropathy.
- The most common causes of nerve compression related to neuropathy in the United States are given in Box 16–3.

## Observation of the Hand with Regard to Nerve Compression

- Observe the appearance of the hand, looking particularly for evidence that the patient has been using the hand at work (e.g., calluses or dirt beneath the fingernails) in order to obtain some idea of hand function.

---

**Box 16–3 Systemic Diseases Predisposing to Nerve Compression in the United States**

- Diabetes
- Thyroid disease
- Collagen vascular disease (vasculitis)
  - Most common: rheumatoid arthritis, lupus erythematosus, scleroderma
- Chemotherapy-induced neuropathy
  - Most common: vincristine, cisplatin (carboplatin), paclitaxel (Taxol), thalidomide
- Alcoholism
- Vitamin deficiency (folate, B$_{12}$, B$_6$)
- Heavy metal toxicity (Pb, Hg, Ar, Cd)
- Lyme disease
- Multiple myeloma (protein immunoelectrophoresis)
- AIDS (secondary to protease inhibitors)

- Observe for unusual or protective clothing over the hand (e.g., a glove).
- Observe for any scars.
- Observe for any skin or joint conditions that may be related to a systemic disease (see Box 16–3).

## Physical Examination Related to Upper Extremity Peripheral Nerves

### Motor

- Examine muscle strength related to a muscle(s) that is(are) unique for a given peripheral nerve (Box 16–4).
- Examine the muscle by manual muscle testing, grading it on a strength scale such as that given in Table 16–4.
- Determine whether the patient is cooperating by giving maximal effort during the examination.
- If possible, specific strength measurements should be made with an instrument, noting dominant and nondominant sides.
  - *Pinch* strength can be measured as either lateral key pinch, which is the preferred method, or between the thumb and one or more fingertips. There is no preferred device, although computer-linked devices that permit data entry directly to a printed report are helpful in reporting results.

| Table 16–4: | Staging Nerve Compression: The British System |
|---|---|
| **SENSORY RECOVERY WITHIN THE AUTONOMOUS ZONE OF THE NERVE** | |
| S0 | Absence of sensibility |
| S1 | Recovery of deep cutaneous pain sensibility |
| S1+ | Recovery of superficial pain sensibility |
| S2 | Return of some degree of superficial pain and tactile sensibility |
| S2+ | As in S2, but with an overresponse |
| S3 | Return of superficial pain and tactile sensibility; no overresponse |
| S3+ | As in S3, but good stimulus localization and some two-point discrimination |
| S4 | Complete recovery |
| **MOTOR RECOVERY OF MUSCLES INNERVATED BY THE NERVE** | |
| M0 | No contraction of any muscle |
| M1 | Perceptible contraction in proximal muscles |
| M2 | Perceptible contraction in proximal and distal muscles |
| M3 | M2 plus all muscles can act against resistance |
| M4 | M3 plus synergistic and isolated movements are possible |
| M5 | Complete recovery |

### Box 16–4   Nerve-Specific Muscle Testing

- Median nerve at wrist
  - Abductor pollicis brevis, opponens pollicis brevis (with other median-innervated muscles being normal)
- Median nerve in forearm
  - Flexor pollicis longus, flexor profundus to index finger, pronator teres, flexor superficialis
- Ulnar nerve at wrist
  - Abductor digiti minimi, first dorsal interosseous (with flexor profundus to little finger being normal)
- Ulnar nerve at elbow
  - Flexor profundus to little finger, flexor carpi ulnaris (with weakness in ulnar innervated intrinsics)
- Radial nerve at elbow
  - Extensors of wrist, thumb, and all fingers
- Radial nerve proximal to elbow
  - Brachioradialis, triceps
- Musculocutaneous nerve
  - Biceps
- Axillary nerve
  - Deltoid
- Suprascapular nerve
  - Supraspinatus, infraspinatus
- Spinal accessory nerve
  - Trapezius
- Long thoracic nerve
  - Serratus anterior (scapular winging)

- *Grip* strength should be measured with the patient seated, the elbow at the side and at 90 degrees, and forearm in a neutral position.
- Hydraulic dynamometers, of the *Jamar*™ type, have interinstrument variability because of fluid loss over time and need to be recalibrated. Their measured force is calculated from the center of their curved handle. A systematic error occurs if there is an absent index finger (strength shifts ulnarly) or an ulnar nerve compression (strength shifts radially). The *Digit-Grip*™ has a straight handle for grasping and records force uniformly across the handle because it has a force transducer at each end of the handle, thus eliminating error. Computer-linked devices are available that print directly for report documentation.

### Sensory

- *Sensibility* implies the neuroanatomy (nerve ending and nerve fiber).[6,7] *Sensation* implies the cortical interpretation of the transmitted nerve impulse.
- By definition, *all testing of sensibility is subjective* because the person being tested must give an interpretation of the test stimulus.
- Measurements of cutaneous thresholds for temperature, vibration, and pressure have been termed in neurology

*quantitative sensory testing.* They have been demonstrated to be reliable and valid because they are reproducible and correlate with patient symptoms. The measurements are also termed *neurosensory testing.*

- The skin territory to be tested should be selected in relation to the unique area innervated by the peripheral nerve being evaluated (Box 16–5).
- The only time testing for *pain* perception with a pin is necessary is if you believe the patient is malingering and states he or she has no feeling in a finger, or if you suspect a syrinx, with involvement of the anterolateral spinothalamic tract (carries pain and temperature perception), in which case there will be diminished pain perception with normal two-point discrimination and intrinsic muscle wasting. *Small-fiber function, like pain perception, is the last to be lost with compression neuropathy.*
- The only time testing for *temperature* perception is necessary is if you believe a small-fiber neuropathy is the source of the pain. Pain symptoms predominate, and large-fiber functions related to touch are normal. Thermal threshold testing is indicated. *Small-fiber function, like temperature perception, is the last to be lost with compression neuropathy.*
- *Perception of* touch, *a large-fiber function, is the first to become involved with compression neuropathy* and includes perception of moving touch, constant touch, and vibration.
- *Vibratory* testing with a tuning fork is indicated in the emergency room setting to evaluate an injured nerve or in the office setting for a quick evaluation or screening of large-fiber function. For example, if the index finger pulp is perceived as "loud or strong" but the little finger pulp is perceived as "soft or weak," then compression of the ulnar nerve is suspected.
- The high-frequency *tuning fork* (256 Hz) evaluates Pacinian corpuscle function. The low-frequency tuning fork (30 Hz) evaluates Meissner corpuscle function. At a sufficient stimulus intensity, any tuning fork evaluates the entire population of quickly adapting large fibers.
- Perception of movement is mediated by the quickly adapting fibers.
- *The disadvantage of using a tuning fork is that the stimulus is a wave.* If the tuning fork is placed at the thumb pulp, the wave traveling proximally stimulates both the radial sensory and the median nerve innervation. Therefore, it is critical in vibratory testing to compare the perception of a piece of skin with its contralateral normal or with some other fingertip with suspected normal sensibility.
- The *vibrometer* changes the qualitative information of the tuning fork into quantitative information, measuring in terms of microns of motion or volts. Vibrometers can be single frequency or multiple frequency but still have the disadvantage that their stimulus input is a wave. Vibratory threshold measurements are valuable for research comparing populations of patients and evaluation of neuropathy related to certain industrial causes, such as vibrating hand-held instruments.
- Perception of constant touch or static touch is mediated by the slowly adapting fibers. These fibers are also large myelinated fibers whose receptors are the Merkel-Cell neurite complex located along the intermediate ridge of the dermal papillae.
- Pressure perception is mediated by the slowly adapting fibers because they vary their frequency of impulse transmission in response to varying stimulus intensity.
- *Measurement of cutaneous pressure threshold is the most critical for evaluation of compression neuropathy* because the stimulus is perceived only through the unique piece of skin tested and because large fiber function is the first to change with compression of a peripheral nerve.
- The *nylon monofilaments,* described by Semmes and Weinstein in 1960, give an estimate of a range for the cutaneous pressure threshold. The number on the monofilament handle is a logarithm of the force in tenths of milligrams. This force must be divided by the cross section of the filament to give pressure. The filaments vary by 10% in their calibration at the time they are purchased and lose up to 10% of their reliability after 100 uses. The filaments are a set, a discontinuous set, and therefore they give an estimate of a range, and not a true measurement. The true measurement is somewhere between two filaments.
- Two-point discrimination requires a high innervation density, that is, a large number of innervated sensory

---

### Box 16–5   Nerve-Specific Sensory Testing

- Median nerve at wrist
  - Index finger pulp (radial sensory can innervate thumb pulp)
- Median nerve in forearm
  - Thenar eminence (palmar cutaneous branch of median nerve arises proximal to carpal tunnel)
- Ulnar nerve at wrist
  - Little finger pulp
- Ulnar nerve at elbow
  - Dorsal ulnar aspect of hand
- Radial sensory nerve in forearm
  - Dorsal radial aspect of hand
- Radial nerve proximal to elbow
  - No unique sensory site
- Musculocutaneous nerve
  - Radial volar forearm (lateral antebrachial cutaneous nerve)
- Axillary nerve
  - Skin overlying deltoid muscle
- Suprascapular nerve
  - No unique sensory site
- Spinal accessory nerve
  - No unique sensory site
- Long thoracic nerve
  - No unique sensory site

corpuscles in a small area of skin. The fingertip pulp and tongue have the highest innervation density (the smallest two-point discrimination), which means the smallest distance at which one from two points can be distinguished. Measurement is achieved with a paper clip and ruler, an engineering gauge with rounded tips, or a *Disk-Criminator*™.

- Two-point discrimination changes late in the course of compression neuropathy because a large number of nerve fibers must have either an ischemic conduction block or axonal degeneration.
- The pressure at which to record two-point discrimination traditionally has been just sufficient to blanch the skin. However, different examiners may press harder because the patient seems to obtain greater input from the higher pressure.
- The *Pressure-Specified Sensory Device*™ is a computer-linked measurement instrument that has a force transducer beneath each of its two hemispheric prongs, permitting documentation of the pressure required to distinguish one from two moving- or static-touch stimuli.
- Measurements from the Pressure-Specified Sensory Device correlate with hand function, identify populations with compression neuropathy (carpal tunnel syndrome, cubital tunnel syndrome, pronator syndrome, brachial plexus compression), and systemic neuropathy.[8,9,10]
- In a blinded, prospective study, neurosensory testing with the Pressure-Specified Sensory Device was as sensitive and specific as electrodiagnostic testing for carpal tunnel syndrome.[11]
- *The pattern of sensory abnormality varies during progressive compression of the peripheral nerve and neural regeneration after nerve decompression* (Box 16–6).

| Box 16–6 | Sequence of Sensory Loss and Recovery |
|---|---|

- Nerve compression
- Pressure required to distinguish one from two static, with distance remaining normal
- Distance for two-point static touch increases
- Same sequence for two-point moving touch
- Pressure threshold for one-point static touch increases
- Pressure threshold for one-point moving touch increases
- Temperature threshold changes
- Nerve regeneration
- One-point moving touch or 30 Hz
- One-point static touch
- 256 Hz
- Two-point moving touch with abnormal pressure and distance
- Two-point static touch with abnormal pressure and distance

## Other Physical Examination Techniques

- *Provocative maneuvers* increase pressure upon the nerve, eliciting symptoms during the office visit, such as flexion (Phalen sign) in carpal tunnel syndrome, elbow flexion for ulnar nerve compression at the elbow, digital pressure upon the median nerve in the forearm for pronator syndrome, and pressure upon the brachial plexus for thoracic outlet syndrome.
- *Tinel sign* originally was defined as distally radiating paresthesias elicited by tapping over a regenerating nerve. Distal progression of the point of maximal response is indicative of nerve regeneration. Today, it is taken as a sign of demyelination or injury to the nerve related to chronic compression at known sites of anatomic narrowing.
- In the *tourniquet test,* application of a tourniquet to the upper arm causes ischemia distally. Ischemia affects the large nerve fibers first because of the longer distance required for oxygen to diffuse into them. If there is a median nerve compression, the first fingers to become symptomatic are the thumb and index finger. If there is an ulnar nerve compression, the first fingers to become numb is the little finger.
- *Each of these tests has important problems with sensitivity and specificity and must be interpreted in the overall clinical context.* Nerve compression can be present in the absence of a positive Tinel sign, and a positive Tinel sign can be present in an individual who is asymptomatic.

## Staging Degree of Nerve Compression

- Clinical decision making regarding treatment must be based upon the degree to which the nerve is compressed.[5,12]
- Traditional descriptive staging is given in Table 16–4.
- Nonoperative treatments are indicated early in nerve compression.
- As pathophysiology progresses and structural changes occur within the nerve and between the nerve and its anatomic relations, the measurements of nerve function change, indicating surgical intervention is necessary and suggesting the time course and potential for clinical improvement (for correlations see Table 16–1).
- Staging of degree of nerve compression can be either descriptive category (e.g., minimal, moderate, severe) or numerical (e.g., on a scale from 0–10).
- Staging of nerve compression should be used for reporting of clinical results.
- Numerical grading scales for the median nerve at the wrist and the ulnar nerve at the elbow are given in Tables 16–2 and 16–3.

# Electrodiagnostic Testing

- *Electrodiagnostic testing* consists of the electrical stimulation of the skin, muscle, or peripheral nerve and the recording of the transmitted neural impulse or muscle contraction in response to that electrical stimulation.
- *Nerve conduction velocity* (NCV) and *electromyography* (EMG) are the traditional tests used for measuring sensory and motor peripheral nerve function.
- When the site being tested is sufficiently distal such that two separate stimulation points cannot be obtained to obtain a velocity (distance/time) measurement, then just the time required to get the response *(distal latency)* is recorded.
- In compressive neuropathy, demyelination slows nerve conduction and increases distal latency. With time, axonal loss causes a decrease in the amplitude of the recorded sensory or motor potential.
- Electrodiagnostic testing is objective because no patient interpretation is needed to obtain the measurement.
- EMG testing is essential for diagnosis of cervical radiculopathy because individual muscle patterns of involvement can be correlated with cervical nerve roots.
- EMG is essential for diagnosis of primary myopathy in patients with diffuse weakness or with diseases of central nervous system origin, such as myasthenia gravis, amyotrophic lateral sclerosis, or spastic hemiplegia.
- Electrodiagnostic testing has been available since the 1950s and is widely accepted for peripheral nerve testing. However, *it has significant problems for upper extremity peripheral nerve surgery.*[13,14]
- To localize a site of compression, the NCV must demonstrate a site of slowing, which implies that more than one site must be stimulated. This is not possible for the brachial plexus or for the median nerve at the wrist. This is compensated by the "inching technique" of Kimura in the palm, but not for the brachial plexus.
- Even for median nerve compression at the wrist, where NCV/EMG is the most specific and most sensitive, a recent meta-analysis demonstrated a 33% false negative rate.[15]
- In the presence of a peripheral neuropathy, like diabetes, NCV/EMG is sufficiently unreliable to demonstrate superimposed nerve compression that reliance upon the physical examination (positive Tinel sign) is recommended.[16]
- NCV/EMG in the postoperative period after nerve decompression is often unreliable because remyelination of the peripheral nerve is usually incomplete.
- Studies of patients who underwent nerve decompression show no difference in outcome regardless of whether the patients had a positive or negative electrodiagnostic study prior to surgery.[17,18]

- If surgery is performed in a patient with a "normal" NCV/EMG and a postoperative complication occurs, a difficult medical legal situation may arise. Abnormal sensory and motor function can be documented with neurosensory and manual motor testing sufficient to indicate the need for surgery.

# Peripheral Nerve Surgery Technical Guidelines

- A series of textbooks related to peripheral nerve surgery is available.
- James Learmonth, MD, who perhaps did the first median nerve decompression at the wrist and the first submuscular transposition of the ulnar nerve at the elbow, can be considered the first peripheral nerve surgeon.[19]
- The American Society for Peripheral Nerve was established in 1990.
- Use of the *tourniquet* in upper extremity surgery to create a bloodless field is essential for appropriate visualization.
- Use of the *bipolar coagulator* is critical for gentle microsurgical technique.
- Using *loupe magnification* is necessary for safety in peripheral nerve surgery.
- Simply removing the external compressive upon a peripheral nerve and separating the peripheral nerve from its adjacent structures is considered a *decompression* or *external neurolysis.*
- Continuing to operate within the peripheral nerve itself, through the epineurium with or without interfascicular neurolysis, called an *internal neurolysis,* remains controversial.
- A meta-analysis of internal neurolysis in median nerve decompression at the wrist demonstrated no significant benefit of internal neurolysis.[20]
- To date, all studies on the benefit of internal neurolysis have used preoperative analysis of staging or randomization; they have not included patients with recurrent nerve compression.
- These studies do not give adequate advice to the surgeon who, during the course of a nerve decompression, identifies a firm, thickened peripheral nerve that has no fascicular pattern. Intraoperative identification of pathology may be sufficient justification for additional intraneural dissection.

# Nerve Compression Syndromes
## CARPAL TUNNEL SYNDROME

- Carpal tunnel syndrome is the most common compression neuropathy in the hand.

- The median nerve is compressed in the carpal tunnel, which has the transverse carpal ligament as the roof. The tunnel contains nine flexor tendons, their synovium, and the median nerve.
- Numbness or paresthesias most commonly occur in the index and middle finger, followed by the thumb. Complaints about the ring finger are uncommon.
- Nighttime awakening is almost universal, as the stronger flexor muscle mass pulls the wrist into flexion during sleep.
- Thenar muscle wasting is a classic sign but is rarely seen today because the medical community and the lay public are so aware of carpal tunnel syndrome symptoms.
- Preserved short flexor function results from ulnar nerve innervation of this muscle.
- Dropping objects and weakness are rare unless median compression is advanced, so these symptoms often reflect a coexisting cubital tunnel syndrome.
- Incidence of carpal tunnel syndrome is 2% in general population, 14% in diabetics, and 30% in diabetics with neuropathy.[16]
- Nonoperative treatment is splinting with the wrist in neutral position. Note that *most shelf splints have the wrist at 20 degrees dorsiflexion and should be bent into the wrist neutral position to reduce pressure on the median nerve.*
- Nonoperative treatment should consist of changes in the activities of daily living and nonsteroidal antiinflammatory medication for 3 months in addition to splinting.
- Cortisone injection into the synovial tissues of the carpal tunnel is appropriate and provides at least temporary relief in up to 80% of patients.[21] Cortisone injection can be done from the proximal to the distal wrist crease and slightly ulna to it (Figure 16–1).
- Nonoperative treatment is indicated in each patient. However, if staging the degree of compression demonstrates the patient is in an advanced category, then the chance of successful nonoperative treatment is small.
- In patients with an advanced degree of compression, surgical decompression of the median nerve is indicated.
- *Surgical decompression of the median nerve at the wrist has a high percentage of good to excellent results, regardless of whether an open or endoscopic decompression technique is used* (Figures 16–2 and 16–3).[22]
- In the open technique, the incision must be made along the radial border of the ring finger to avoid injury to the palmar cutaneous branch of the median nerve. Injury to this nerve causes a painful postoperative scar without radiation to the fingers. It is important to protect the recurrent motor branch of the median nerve. This can be identified using the landmarks described in Figure 16–3. The median nerve can be located by determining the intersection of Kaplan's line and a line bisecting the index-middle finger web space.
- Decompression routinely includes division of the distal antebrachial fascia as it thickens to form the transverse carpal ligament, because this process can compress the median nerve against the volar surface of the radius.

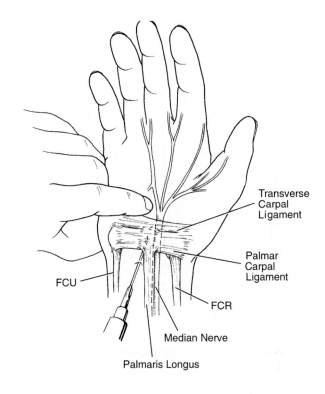

**Median Block**

Figure 16–1:

Steroid injection of the carpal tunnel can be performed with a distally aimed 22 gauge needle inserted at the distal volar wrist crease just ulna to the palmaris longus (PL) tendon, or in the midpoint of the volar wrist when the PL is not present. FCR, flexi carpal radialis; FCU, flexi carpal ulnaris.

- Endoscopic carpal tunnel release has been demonstrated to provide an earlier return to work and a less sensitive scar on the palm than does open release.[23] The two portal technique uses a small transverse incision made at or slightly proximal to the distal palmar crease in the mid-volar aspect of the wrist. The incision is centered on the palmaris longus, if present. The palmaris longus is retracted radially in order to protect the palmar cutaneous branch of the median nerve. The synovium is reflected using a small, specially-designed elevator, and the canal is dilated in order to make room for the endoscopic device. The device is positioned along the axis of the radial border of the ring finger, and is inserted into a maximum depth of approximately 3 cm.
- Postoperative immobilization of the wrist in neutral position for up to 1 week is indicated to prevent bowstringing of the flexor tendons out of the carpal canal.
- Early movement of the fingers to create gliding of the median nerve across the wrist operative site is indicated to minimize adhesions during the healing process.
- Improvement following carpal tunnel decompression is so typical that failure to improve suggests additional problems may be present.
- Steroid cream massaged into the scar from the sixth week to the third month is helpful in minimizing the scar.

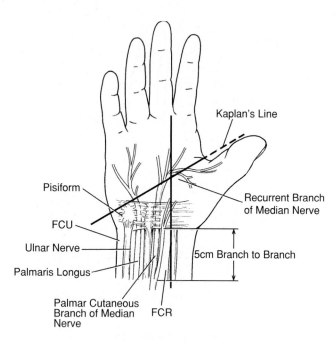

CTS-Important Landmarks

Figure 16–2:

Kaplan's line is drawn along the ulna border of the abducted thumb. The motor branch is identified as the intersection of Kaplan's line in a line drawn longitudinally in the web space of the index and middle fingers.

- Differential diagnosis of the patient who does not improve after carpal tunnel decompression is given in Box 16–7.
- The *double crush concept* applies to carpal tunnel syndrome, in that compression anywhere or at multiple sites along the

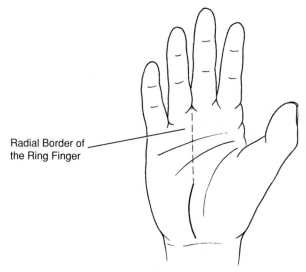

Figure 16–3:

A carpal tunnel incision made along a line drawn proximally from the radial border of the ring finger avoids injury to the recurrent motor branch and the palmar cutaneous motor branch of the median nerve.

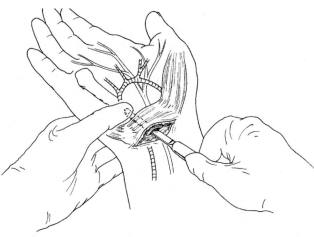

Figure 16–4:

The hamate sound helps dilate the carpal canal to prepare for insertion of the endoscopic device.

axis of C6 can summate to cause symptoms, even though compression at one site alone would not be sufficient to cause symptoms. Carpal tunnel syndrome patients often have symptoms that go into their neck and shoulder. If these symptoms persist after carpal tunnel decompression, a more proximal source of compression exists.

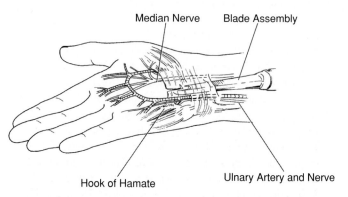

Figure 16–5:

The important anatomic structures to consider when using the single portal endoscopic device include the transverse carpal ligament, the superficial palmar arch, and the ulna border of the median nerve, particularly the common digital nerve to the third web space.

| Box 16–7 | Differential Diagnosis of Failed Carpal Tunnel Surgery |
| --- | --- |

- Recurrent or persistent carpal tunnel syndrome
- Proximal median nerve compression in the forearm
- Radial sensory nerve entrapment in the forearm
- Upper trunk brachial plexus compression
- Cervical radiculopathy (C5/C6)

## MEDIAN NERVE COMPRESSION IN THE FOREARM

- The median nerve at the elbow level contains all the fibers that transverse the carpal tunnel, the motor fibers to the radial wrist flexors, finger flexors (except the flexor profundus to the little and ring fingers), and forearm pronators, and sensory fibers to the palm and volar wrist joints.
- Median nerve compression in the forearm has been subdivided historically into the *anterior interosseous nerve syndrome* and *the pronator syndrome.*
- Proximal median nerve compression is commonly seen in patients whose job requires repetitive flexion and pronation of the forearm.
- Proximal median nerve compression is often seen in association with other compression neuropathies, such as carpal and cubital tunnel syndrome. In the setting of a worker using both hands, proximal median nerve compression may appear as a bilateral problem or a systemic neuropathy.
- Classically, the pronator syndrome has little motor deficit and primarily results in symptoms of numbness in the hand with the median-innervated fingers.[23]
- Classically, the anterior interosseous nerve syndrome results in weakness and/or paralysis of the flexor pollicis longus and the flexor profundus to the index finger and no sensory symptoms.
- The double crush concept applies to the median nerve in the region of the proximal forearm and elbow in that, depending upon the topographic organization of fascicles in the median nerve and the anatomic variables of the muscle origins, many patients have so-called *incomplete* or *mixed syndromes.*
- Although electromyographic studies can identify denervation of the muscles innervated by the median nerve, often there is a combination of forearm flexors and pronator teres abnormalities, or the test is interpreted as normal.
- Neurosensory testing of the thenar eminence with the Pressure-Specified Sensory Device can identify involvement of the palmar cutaneous branch of the median nerve, documenting compression of the proximal median nerve.[24]
- The anatomic structures that can be responsible for compression of the median nerve proximally, and therefore the structures that must be evaluated intraoperatively and divided, are given in Box 16–8.
- The anterior interosseous nerve is at risk for compression if the deep head of the pronator teres is fibrous and if the nerve fascicle originates on the radial side instead of the deep (dorsal) side of the median nerve.[25]
- The terminal branches of the anterior interosseous nerve innervate the volar wrist joint. Therefore, complaints of

| Box 16–8 | Anatomic Structures Causally Related to Median Nerve Compression in the Forearm |
|---|---|

- Ligament of Struthers (humerus to medial humeral epicondyle)
- Lacertus fibrosis
- Deep head of the pronator teres
- Fibrous arch between heads of the superficialis muscles

*volar wrist pain may accompany compression of the median nerve in the forearm.*

- Pain referred to the proximal forearm with resisted middle or ring finger proximal interphalangeal joint flexion indicates the presence of an arch between the superficialis muscles crossing the median nerve. This often is a separate arch or site than is the deep head of the pronator teres.
- The ligament of Struthers is exceedingly rare, whereas the lacertus fibrosis is constant (Figure 16–6).
- Nonoperative management includes changing activities of daily living and, in the work environment, may require an ergonomic evaluation and job rotation.
- Splinting and cortisone injections usually are not helpful.
- Surgical approach should permit exposure from the medial elbow to the midforearm but does not have to incorporate a long zigzag incision, except where crossing the antecubital crease is necessary (Figure 16–7).
- With the surgical approach, care should be taken not to injure either the medial or the lateral antebrachial cutaneous nerve, which can be a source of a painful scar.

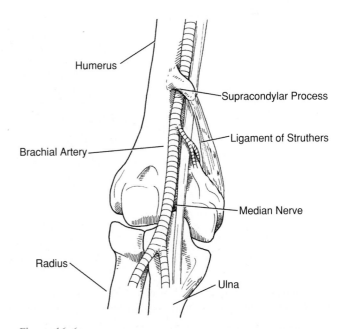

Figure 16–6:
**The ligament of Struthers bridges the supracondylar process of the humerus to the medial epicondyle or the origin of the humeral head of the pronator teres.**

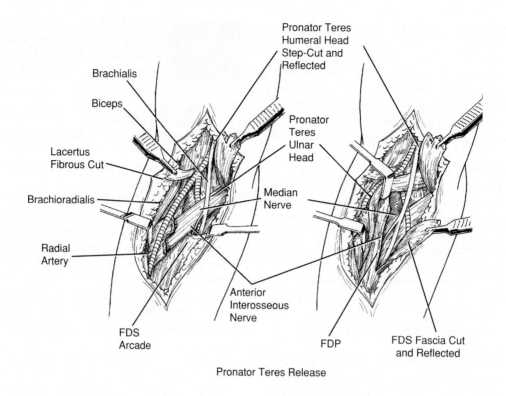

Pronator Teres Release

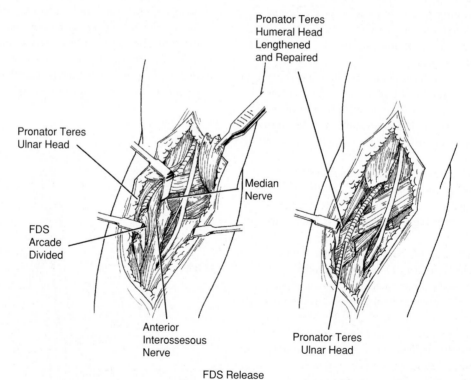

FDS Release

**Figure 16–7:**
Decompression of the proximal median nerve involves release of the lacertus fibrosis, the humeral head of the pronator teres, the vascular leash proximal to the flexor digitorium sublimis (FDS), the FDS and its fascia. FDP, Flexor digitorium profundus.

- Immediate postoperative use of the arm in terms of flexion, pronation, and supination is essential to prevent scarring of the median nerve.
- In the muscular forearm, postoperative muscle bulk contributes to hypertrophic scarring. A steroid cream massaged into the scar for 6 weeks beginning at postoperative week 3 can be effective in minimizing the scar.
- If the surgery is to include an ulnar nerve transposition, then exposure of the lacertus fibrosis and sometimes the deep head of the pronator teres can be accomplished through the medial elbow incision, minimizing the length required for the volar incision.

## Ulnar Nerve Compression at the Wrist

- Ulnar nerve compression at the wrist is termed the *ulnar tunnel syndrome.*
- Ulnar nerve compression at the wrist can accompany carpal tunnel syndrome, as demonstrated by abnormal distal ulnar nerve findings when electrodiagnostic studies are performed for carpal tunnel syndrome.
- The ulnar nerve and ulnar artery plus a collection of fat occupy a space described by Guyon. There is a thin but firm roof bridging from the palmar fascia, the palmaris brevis muscle (present in 20%), and the hamate toward the pisiform. The deep surface of the ulnar tunnel is the pisohamate ligament.[26]

- The shape of the ulnar tunnel in cross section changes from triangular to round and increases in area when the transverse carpal ligament is divided. Therefore, the ulnar tunnel should not be opened routinely during carpal tunnel surgery.
- Symptoms related to ulnar nerve compression at the wrist always include numbness of the little finger pulp and sometimes the ring pulp, but not the dorsum of the hand, and variable degrees of intrinsic muscle weakness or loss of coordination of the fingers.
- The double crush concept suggests that if a patient has cubital tunnel syndrome or a systemic neuropathy, the ulnar nerve may be sufficiently compressed in the ulnar tunnel so as to contribute to ulnar-sided hand symptoms.
- Traditionally, ulnar nerve compression at the wrist occurs distal to the hook of the hamate, causing compression of just the motor branch. Clawing and first dorsal interosseous muscle wasting may occur in the presence of a normal hypothenar muscle mass and function and normal sensibility in the little finger.
- The most common cause of compression of the ulnar nerve at the wrist level is a lipoma or a ganglion. Symptoms of ulnar tunnel syndrome vary, depending on the site of the compression (Figure 16–8).

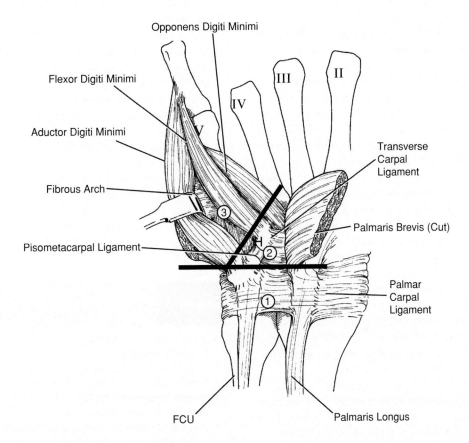

Figure 16–8:
The ulna tunnel can be divided into three sections: Lesions in zone I often produce a combined sensory and motor deficit. Lesions in zone II, cause a pure motor deficit. Lesions in zone III cause pure sensory deficits. (This is from Figure 18–10 on page 330 in the textbook.)

- Twenty-five percent of patients have a fibrous origin of the hypothenar muscles that can cause compression of the deep motor branch.
- Inflammation of the pisotriquetral joint may cause ulnar nerve symptoms, as may occlusion of the ulnar artery or an ulnar artery aneurysm.
- Work conditions (e.g., using a jackhammer) or sports activities (e.g., bicycling) can cause ulnar nerve compression at the wrist.
- Two classic sports injuries—hitting the ground with a golf club or hitting a baseball—can cause fractures of the hook of the hamate with an associated ulnar nerve compression. Special imaging may be required to demonstrate this fracture.
- Surgical decompression of the ulnar nerve at the wrist can be performed through the typical incision for carpal tunnel decompression. Care should be taken to trace out the course of the motor branch to make sure that the decompression is complete.

## Cubital Tunnel Syndrome

- Ulnar nerve compression in the cubital tunnel is the second most common nerve entrapment in the upper extremity.
- The ulnar nerve lies within the postcondylar groove, where it is covered by a relatively fibrous roof going from the medial humeral epicondyle to the olecranon.
- Prior to about 1959, this syndrome almost always was related to fracture or dislocation about the elbow, and the syndrome was called *posttraumatic ulnar palsy*. With improvement in the care of this trauma, so-called *idiopathic ulnar neuritis* continued and was identified by Osborne as the ulnar nerve being compressed beneath the fibrous arch joining the two heads of the flexor carpi ulnaris. He called this syndrome *tardy ulnar palsy*. The name *cubital tunnel syndrome* was given to the symptom complex by Stafford and Feindel in 1973.[27]
- With flexion of the elbow greater than 30 degrees, the shape of the tunnel narrows distally, at Osborne's band, causing pressure upon the ulnar nerve. This pressure increases through 120 degrees of elbow flexion and then increases further with shoulder abduction, as the medial cord origins of the ulnar nerve are stretched.
- The double crush concept applies to the ulnar nerve in that compression of the lower trunk of the brachial plexus in the thoracic outlet syndrome often is present in patients with cubital tunnel syndrome. The C8 potential contribution to these multiple sites of compression along the same nerve is less common than compression at the most distal site, Guyon's canal, at the wrist.
- Sensory symptoms resulting from cubital tunnel syndrome *usually* include numbness in the little and ring finger that worsens with use of the hand requiring elbow flexion but does not occur at night unless the person sleeps with the arm beneath the pillow.
- Motor symptoms include weakness, clumsiness, and dropping objects.
- For musicians, the symptoms are related to difficulty in using the fingers either as fast, or for as long, as they used to, especially for violin, guitar, and piano players. These symptoms in musicians may be mistaken for "spasticity" or "dystrophy." They usually are helped by relaxation techniques and stretching, such as Pilates, and changing the practice schedule. Surgical decompression is rarely required.
- When determining treatment for cubital tunnel syndrome, staging the degree of compression is critical (see Table 16–1).
- Nonoperative treatment consists almost entirely of avoiding elbow flexion beyond 30 degrees for up to 3 months. Such treatment has been demonstrated to result in improvement in 80% of patients with a mild degree of compression but in less than 30% of those with a severe degree of compression.[28] The treatment must be done every night using a towel wrapped around the arm to prevent extreme elbow flexion; however, during the day, critical activities that require elbow flexion are allowed.
- Electrodiagnostic studies that show conduction velocity slowing across the elbow less than 50 m/s or a decrease of more than 10 m/s from the conduction velocity below the elbow or the contralateral side is evidence of cubital tunnel syndrome. However, the false-negative rate is approximately 50%.
- If patients have symptoms of cubital tunnel syndrome after more than 3 months of nonoperative treatment and they have documented neurosensory and motor evidence of abnormal ulnar nerve function and a positive Tinel sign in the postcondylar groove, then surgical decompression is indicated.
- *No single operation for ulnar nerve decompression at the elbow is universally accepted.*
- Box 16–9 lists the five operations commonly used for cubital tunnel syndrome.
- A study measuring intraneural ulnar nerve pressures in fresh cadavers demonstrated that the only technique that decreased the pressure on the ulnar nerve proximal to,

---

| **Box 16–9** | **Operations for Cubital Tunnel Syndrome** |
|---|---|

- In situ (simple) decompression
  - Open or endoscopic
- Medial humeral epicondylectomy
- Anterior subcutaneous transposition
- Anterior intramuscular transposition
- Anterior submuscular transposition
  - Learmonth technique (reattachment of muscle origin in situ)
  - Dellon musculofascial lengthening (Z-lengthening)

across, and distal to the elbow, and for all ranges of motion of the elbow, was the anterior submuscular transposition using the **Z**-lengthening or musculofascial lengthening technique described by Dellon et al.[29]

- No randomized prospective study has identified which procedure has the best outcome in preoperatively staged patients (see Table 16–1).
- Two meta-analyses, one decade apart, arrive at the same conclusion: there is a high percentage of recurrent or failed ulnar nerve decompressions at the elbow, approaching 25% to 33% for the different techniques.[30,31] The best consistent results are achieved for anterior submuscular transposition by the musculofascial lengthening technique.[31]
- The most common anatomic structures responsible for failure of ulnar nerve surgery at the elbow are listed in Table 16–5. Failure to address each of these structures creates a situation in which a new site of increased pressure upon the ulnar nerve can occur postoperatively.

Surgical options include:

- *In situ decompression*: In this technique, the roof of the cubital tunnel and Osborne's fascia is released from just posterior to the medial epicondyle distally through a small curved incision. The goal is to leave the roof of the cubital tunnel proximal to the medial epicondyle intact in order to prevent anterior subluxation during flexion. If the nerve subluxes following this in situ release, a formal anterior transposition should be performed.
- *Medial epicondylectomy*: In this approach, the goal is to remove the medial epicondyle, which forms the anterior wall of the cubital tunnel. Care must be taken to expose the nerve, release the ligament, and identify the medial collateral ligament inserting on the medial epicondyle. Muscle origins of the FCU in pronator teres have to be elevated from the medial epicondyle in order to provide an adequate release and then these are reattached to the adjacent periosteum (Figure 16–9).

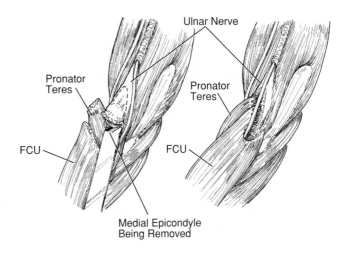

Medial Epicondyletomy

Figure 16–9:
**The medial epicondylectomy is performed with an osteotome. Intra-operative radiographs are required to ensure adequate resection of the medial epicondyle. FCU, flexor carpi ulnaris.**

- *Anterior subcutaneous transposition*: In this technique, the roof of the cubital tunnel and Osborne's ligament are released through a curvilinear incision. Care must be taken to expose and excise the medial intermuscular septum for approximately 10 cm proximal to the medial epicondyle, in order to avoid a secondary site of compression. A neurolysis is performed, and the ulnar nerve is transposed anteriorly onto the fascia of the flexor-pronator mass. In order to prevent the nerve from relocating back into the cubital tunnel, a fascial flap is elevated from the anterior surface of the flexor-pronator mass as demonstrated in Figure 10. This flap is then sutured to the superficial fascia, providing a barrier against relocation (Figures 16–10 and 16–11). The anterior submuscular transposition is performed using a curvilinear incision made just posterior to the cubital tunnel to protect the medial brachial cutaneous nerve. After release of the cubital tunnel ligament, 10 cm intramuscular septum is removed and Osborne's fascia between the two heads of the FCU is incised. A blunt curved clamp is placed under the origin of the FCU to protect the median nerve. The clamp should be placed proximal to the median nerve's first branch, the motor branch to the pronator teres. The FCU origin is divided in a step-cut fashion, leaving a cuff of tendon for reattachment of the muscle origins. All septae under the FCU need to be divided to allow anterior transposition of the ulna nerve parallel to the median nerve. Frequently, the posterior motor branch to the FCU has to be mobilized from the ulna nerve for several centimeters by internal neurolysis to complete the transposition.
- The incision for ulnar nerve decompression almost always crosses a branch of the *medial brachial cutaneous nerve*.

| Table 16–5: | Critical Anatomic Structures that Must be Treated to Prevent Recurrent Ulnar Nerve Compression at the Elbow | |
|---|---|
| **ANATOMIC STRUCTURE** | **INITIAL SURGICAL TREATMENT** |
| Roof of cubital tunnel | Incision of entire length |
| Fascia of flexor carpi ulnaris | Incision of 3-cm length distally |
| Medial intermuscular septum | Excision of 2-cm segment |
| Fascia from medial head of triceps | Incision from medial intermuscular septum |
| Anomalous origins of triceps | Divide medial head if above to ulnar nerve |
| Epitrochlearis anconeus | Divide if this anomalous muscle is present |
| Arcade of Struthers | (There is no arcade of Struthers) |

Figure 16–10:

The anterior subcutaneous transfer of the ulna nerve relies on a fascial sling created from the fascia of the flexor pronator origin to prevent the nerve from returning to the cubital tunnel. FCU, flexor carpi ulnaris.

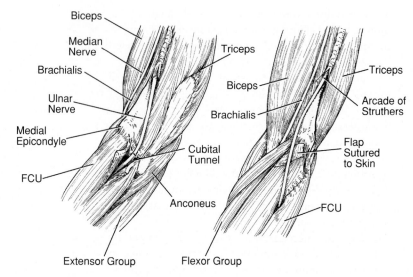

Subcutaneous Transposition of Ulnar Nerve

Direct injury to this nerve, stretching, or adherence to the medial humeral epicondyle after surgery causes a painful scar. Pain posterior to the medial humeral epicondyle may be a neuroma of the medial brachial cutaneous nerve.[32]

- The painful postoperative scar is treated with topical steroid massage into the scar, ultrasound, and, if this fails, resection of the neuroma and implantation of the nerve proximally into the triceps muscle.
- *When evaluating the postoperative patient who complains of pain in the elbow region, remember that the ulnar nerve does not innervate the elbow.* This symptom indicates a neuroma of the medial antebrachial or medial brachial cutaneous nerve. You must find a Tinel sign that radiates to the little finger to diagnose recurrent or failed ulnar nerve compression at the elbow. A painful trigger point or Tinel sign that only hurts at the elbow represents a neuroma in that elbow location.

Figure 16–11:

Medial view of the elbow. The anterior submuscular transposition requires the release of the intermuscular septum, the cubital tunnel, and a division of the flexor pronator origin to transpose the nerve anteriorly. FCU, flexor carpi ulnaris.

## Radial Sensory Nerve Compression

- The original article by *Wartenberg,* translated from the 1932 report in German, described what was believed to be *an inflammation of the radial sensory nerve, not a compression neuropathy.* He described the provocative maneuver of forearm pronation that elicited symptoms and pain in the distribution of this nerve with sudden ulnar deviation of the wrist.
- This syndrome is found in the setting of trauma, with crush injury, or with use of an external fixation device in the forearm.
- The radial sensory nerve is compressed in pronation by the movement of the extensor carpi radialis longus toward the brachioradialis tendon, at the site where the nerve transits from deep to superficial. Sometimes there is a small sheath binding the radial sensory nerve to the deep surface of the brachioradialis. Sometimes the nerve exits through the brachioradialis tendon.

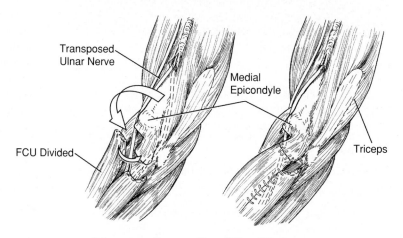

Submuscular Transposition of Ulnar Nerve

- Symptoms are just sensory and consist of a burning, paresthesia, or numbness along the dorsoradial aspect of the hand.
- *These symptoms can be described simply as numbness in the thumb and index finger, leading to a misdiagnosis of carpal tunnel syndrome.*
- Radial sensory nerve crosses the wrist joint while being tethered proximally. Ulnar wrist deviation, especially if the thumb is grasped, causes a shooting dorsoradial pain. *This is similar to the positive Finkelstein sign with de Quervain tenosynovitis and must be distinguished from tendonitis by demonstrating the resisted thumb extension is not painful.*
- The physical examination should identify the Tinel sign just posterior (lateral) to the insertion of the brachioradialis into the radius.
- The compression site is where the radial sensory nerve exits from deep to the fascia that joins the extensor carpi radialis longus to the brachioradialis.
- The surgical technique consists of releasing the fascia from the exit point of the radial sensory nerve as far proximal as necessary so that the nerve is no longer compressed with forearm pronation.
- During the dissection, care should be taken to not injure the overlying lateral antebrachial cutaneous nerve.[33]
- Postoperative care requires immediate mobilization. Allow pronation/supination.

## Radial Nerve Compression at the Elbow

- Traditionally, compression neuropathy of the radial nerve at the elbow is considered two different syndromes: the *posterior interosseous nerve compression* and the *radial tunnel syndrome.*
- The concept of the double crush is important for the radial nerve in the elbow region because the few different anatomic structures that may compress the nerve all lie within 3 to 5 cm of each other, and in any neurolysis of the radial nerve in this location, all structures should be evaluated.
- Anatomic structures that may compress the radial nerve at the elbow are fibrous or muscular connections from the biceps to the brachioradialis that form the roof of the radial tunnel, a fibrous edge to the extensor carpi radialis brevis muscle, and the fibrous covering of the supinator muscle (arcade of Frohse).
- As the radial nerve exits the loose groove between the brachialis and the brachioradialis, it crosses the lateral humeral epicondyle. This area can be tight if there has been previous trauma or external compression, for example, from the splints used for treatment of lateral humeral epicondylitis (tennis elbow).

- Radial tunnel syndrome symptoms consist primarily of aching in the region of the lateral elbow and can be confused with epicondylitis. *The critical difference on physical examination is that with epicondylitis the tender site is at the lateral humeral epicondyle, at the extensor muscle origin, but with compressive neuropathy of the radial nerve the nerve itself is tender approximately 1.5 cm anterior and distal to the epicondyle.*
- Symptoms with radial tunnel syndrome may give a distribution throughout the length of the radial nerve distally, including the forearm and dorsal wrist. A coexisting radial sensory nerve compression must be evaluated.[34]
- Physical examination for radial tunnel syndrome should include resisted middle finger extension. This action forces the extensor carpi radialis brevis to contract to maintain the third metacarpal position, causing pressure on the radial nerve. Pain is referred to the region of the radial tunnel.
- *The symptoms of posterior interosseous nerve "palsy" all are motor, with the exception of aching in the dorsal wrist, because the terminal branches of this nerve innervate the dorsal wrist capsule.*
- The motor symptoms of posterior interosseous nerve palsy range from weakness of grasp to paralysis of individual or all muscles that extend the wrist and fingers.
- Surgical exposure for decompression of the radial nerve can either be anterior or posterior. Our preference is anterior (Figure 16–12).
- For this approach, a curvilinear incision is performed crossing the antecubital fossa. The interval between the brachialis and the brachioradialis is identified and bluntly dissected. The radial nerve is identified and traced distally to the Arcade of Froshe, which is the thickened anterior fascial edge of the supinator muscle. This fascia is split, as is the fascial edge of the extensor carpi radialis brevis, and any constricting vascular leash (see Figure 16–12).
- The posterior approach uses a curved incision along the posterior border of the mobile wad. The interval between the ECRB and EDC is identified and split longitudinally. The Arcade of Froshe, the thickened fascial edge of the supinator muscle, and the fascia over the proximal supinator muscle is identified and released in order to decompress the nerve. Through this approach, it is easier to decompress the nerve from distal to proximal, as branches of the posterior interosseous nerve can be identified exiting distal to the supinator muscle and traced proximally by splitting the muscle (Figure 16–13).
- Postoperatively, immediate mobilization is critical.

## Brachial Plexus Compression (Thoracic Outlet Syndrome)

- Compression of the brachial plexus in the thoracic inlet traditionally was called *scalenus anticus syndrome* but more lately and incorrectly has been called *thoracic outlet syndrome.*

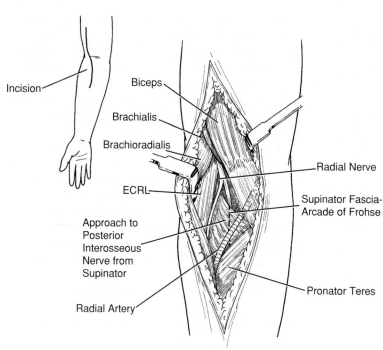

Incision

Biceps

Brachialis

Brachioradialis

ECRL

Approach to Posterior Interosseous Nerve from Supinator

Radial Artery

Radial Nerve

Supinator Fascia-Arcade of Frohse

Pronator Teres

Anterior Approach to Radial Nerve

**Figure 16–12:**
The anterior, or Henry's approach for decompression of the distal portion of the radial nerve and the posterior interosseous nerve first identifies the radial nerve in the interval between the brachialis and the brachioradialis. ECRL, extensor carpi radialis longus.

- The symptoms of brachial plexus compression can be so universal in the neck, shoulder, and entire hand and arm that many neurologists continue to doubt the existence of *neurologic thoracic outlet syndrome*. The "belief" in the existence of this syndrome is worsened by *the inability of electrodiagnostic tests to demonstrate the compression of the plexus*, with the exception of the rare "true neurogenic" type in which the lower trunk of the plexus is involved.[35,36]

- Routine chest x-ray films and cervical oblique x-ray films should be obtained to determine a pulmonary cause of the symptoms, such as a Pancoast tumor, or the presence of a cervical rib.

- Symptoms can extend to facial pain and temporomandibular joint pain, presumably because of secondary effects on the cervical plexus.

**Figure 16–13:**
The posterior approach, or Thompson's approach, uses the interval between the extensor digitorium communis (EDC) and extensor carpi radialis brevis (ECRB). ECRL, extensor carpi radialis longus; APL, abductor pollicis longus.

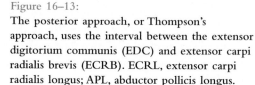

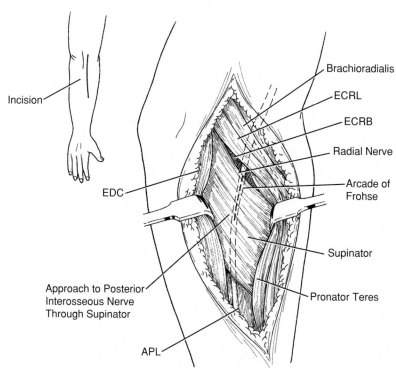

Incision

Brachioradialis

ECRL

ECRB

Radial Nerve

Arcade of Frohse

EDC

Supinator

Pronator Teres

Approach to Posterior Interosseous Nerve Through Supinator

APL

Posterior Approach to Radial Nerve

- Headaches can be a common feature because of tightness in the scalene muscles.
- There usually is a history of trauma, such as whiplash or direct neck/shoulder blunt trauma. Diagnostic studies should include MRI of the cervical spine and the shoulder if these symptoms are present.
- An occupational component may contribute if work involves extensive overhead use of the hands or even work at shoulder level.
- Symptoms of hand swelling reflect compression of the subclavian vein, whereas symptoms of coldness may reflect either lower trunk compression with involvement of the sympathetic inflow or subclavian artery compression. Diagnostic studies should include imaging of these vessels for these symptoms.
- *Congenital anomalies* related to muscles and fibrous bands are common in the thoracic inlet (Table 16–6) and in the presence of trauma may limit excursion of the brachial plexus sufficiently to cause stretch/traction-type problems.
- Physical examination must demonstrate tenderness of the brachial plexus beneath the anterior scalene muscle and a *positive provocative sign (of Roos),* which is onset of symptoms and heaviness in the hands and arms within 1 minute of holding the hands above the head.[37]
- *No surgery should be contemplated until the patient has undergone at least 6 months of special exercises designed to stretch the scalene muscles and strengthen other shoulder muscles.*[38]
- Neurosensory testing can be performed with the hands at rest and after provoking the brachial plexus by elevating the hands
- Thoracic surgeons began treating this problem in 1966 by transaxillary first rib resection. Gaining exposure of the origin of the first rib injures the intercostobrachial nerve in 66% of patients and is associated with risk for pneumothorax and injury to the subclavian artery and the C8 and T1 nerve roots.[37]
- The transaxillary first rib resection is performed through a curved incision. The surgery is performed with the patient in the lateral decubitus position. The curved skin incision is made over the third interspace. The supreme thoracic artery is ligated and the anterior scalene muscle is divided with scissors after being separated from the subclavian vein. The middle scalene muscle is released subperiosteally, in order to avoid injury to the long thoracic nerve. The periosteum is stripped from the first rib during periods when the lung is deflated in order to avoid injury to the pleura. An angled rib cutter is used to divide the anterior and posterior margins of the rib. It is important to check the pleura for leaks, and a chest tube is placed if necessary (16–14). Supracalviacular approach is performed with the patient in a beach chair position. The incision is made 1 cm above and parallel to the clavicle. For any surgery near the great vessels, the patient's blood should be cross-typed and transfusion blood should be readily available in the operating room. The platysma muscle is divided and the external jugular is also ligated and divided. Using a superiosteal dissection, a third of the trapezius a sternocleidomastoid insertions are released from the clavicle. The omohyoid muscle, transverse cervical artery, and suprascapular artery run across the posterior triangle, and they are divided. The phrenic nerve runs along the anterior surface of the anterior scalene muscle, and it should be protected. Any cervical ribs that are present are removed if they impinge on the brachial plexus. The first thoracic rib is identified and the periosteum overlying it is incised. The anterior and middle scalene attachments are elevated subperiosteally. Kerrison rongeurs are used to divide the first rib at the anterior and posterior margins of the wound without injuring the pleura below. Anomalous bands between the scalene muscles and the first thoracic rib are often present and should be released. Once the rib is removed, the wound is filled with saline while the lungs are inflated to identify any pleural leaks that would require a chest tube. The wound is closed in layers.
- Supraclavicular approach offers the surgeon better exposure and therefore the opportunity to minimize operative complications. Transient phrenic palsy

| Table 16–6:    Anatomic Anomalies in the Thoracic Inlet |
| --- |
| Cervical rib |
| Fibrous bands from C7 transverse process |
| Extra origins for scalene muscles |
| Prefixed or postfixed brachial plexus |
| Intraplexus anomalous connections |
| Elevated position of subclavian artery |
| Muscle of Albinus (scalenus minimus) |
| Fibrous edges of scalene muscles |
| Anomalous vessels crossing plexus |
| Sibson fascia crossing T1 nerve root |
| Proximal junction of T1 to C8 |

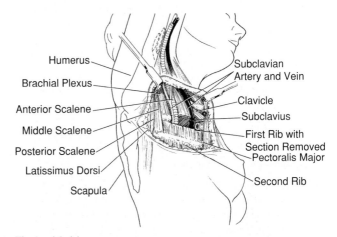

Figure 16–14:
**The transaxillary first rib resection offers a cosmetically appealing approach, but the limited exposure and the potential injury to the intercostobrachial nerve are significant concerns.**

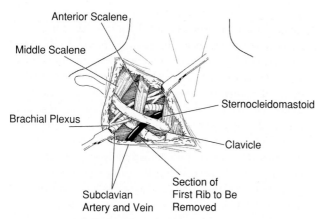

Figure 16–15:

**The supraclavicular approach offers excellent visualization of the structures producing thoracic outlet syndrome.**

reportedly is the most common complication, so avoiding traction on this nerve during plexus neurolysis and scalenectomy must be emphasized.[39]

- Anterior scalenectomy with or without first rib resection is the preferred approach. The same success can be achieved leaving the first rib (Figure 16–15).[40,41]
- Postoperatively the patient should be encouraged to turn the head and shrug the shoulders to encourage gliding of the plexus and prevent recurrence because of scar.

# References

1. Mackinnon SE, Dellon AL, Hudson AR, Hunter D: Chronic nerve compression—an experimental model in the rat. *Ann Plast Surg* 13:112-120, 1984.
   Demonstration that narrowing the diameter of a nerve causes acute degeneration and that a silicon tube the diameter of a nerve takes 6 months to induce compression.

2. Mackinnon SE, Dellon AL, Hudson AR, Hunter DA: A primate model for chronic nerve compression. *J Reconstr Microsurg* 1:185-194, 1985.
   Documentation of a primate model for chronic compression. Confirms rat model.

3. Mackinnon SE, Dellon AL: Experimental study of chronic nerve compression: clinical implications. *Clin Hand Surg* 2:639-650, 1986.
   Pathophysiologic changes from chronic compression imply progressive clinical signs and symptoms and ability to stage degree of nerve compression.

4. Wong L, Dellon AL: Brachial neuritis presenting as anterior interosseous nerve compression—Implications for diagnosis and treatment: a case report. *J Hand Surg* 22A:536-539, 1997.
   Parsonage-Turner syndrome is an inflammatory brachial plexopathy that often presents as anterior interosseous nerve palsy or axillary nerve palsy.

5. Dellon AL: Clinical grading of peripheral nerve problems. *Neurosurg Clin North Am* 12:229-240, 2001.
   Inclusion of computer-assisted neurosensory and motor testing devices into grading scales for upper and lower extremity compression neuropathy.

6. Dellon AL: *Evaluation of sensibility and re-education of sensation in the hand.* Baltimore, 1981, Williams & Wilkins.
   Description of neurophysiology related to sensibility and testing.

7. Dellon AL: *Somatosensory testing and rehabilitation.* Silver Springs, 1997, American Occupational Therapy Association.
   Description of neurosensory testing.

8. Dellon ES, Keller KM, Moratz V, Dellon AL: Validation of cutaneous threshold measurements for the evaluation of hand function. *Ann Plast Surg* 38:485-492, 1997.
   Validation of the Pressure-Specified Sensory Device for measuring sensibility in the hand and prediction of hand function based upon those measurements.

9. Dellon AL, Keller KM: Computer-assisted quantitative sensory testing in carpal and cubital tunnel syndromes. *Ann Plast Surg* 38:493-502, 1997.
   Normative upper extremity values for the Pressure-Specified Sensory Device compared to a population of patients with carpal and cubital tunnels syndrome.

10. Dellon AL: Management of peripheral nerve problems in the upper and lower extremities using quantitative sensory testing. *Hand Clin* 15:697-715, 1999.
    Diagnosis and treatment of compressive neuropathy, nerve injury and reconstruction, and evaluation of neural regeneration.

11. Weber R, Weber RA, Schuchmann JA, Ortiz J: A prospective blinded evaluation of nerve conduction velocity versus pressure-specified sensory testing in carpal tunnel syndrome. *Ann Plast Surg* 45:252-257, 2000.
    The Pressure-Specified Sensory Device was demonstrated to be as sensitive and specific as electrodiagnostic testing with significantly less pain in the diagnosis of carpal tunnel syndrome.

12. Dellon AL: A numerical grading scale for peripheral nerve function. *J Hand Ther* 4:152-160, 1993.
    Introduction of numerical grading scale for evaluating peripheral nerve function.

13. Dellon AL: Pitfalls in electrodiagnosis. In Gelberman RH, editor: *Operative nerve repair and reconstruction.* Philadelphia, 1991, JB Lippincott.
    Problems inherent in electrodiagnosis are reviewed.

14. Dellon AL: WOG syndrome. *Muscle Nerve* 17:1336-1342, 1994.
    Position against routine electrodiagnostic studies for nerve compression.

15. AAEM Quality Assurance Committee: Literature review of the usefulness of nerve conduction studies and electromyography for the evaluation of patients with carpal tunnel syndrome. *Muscle Nerve* 16:1392-1414, 1993.
    A meta-analysis by neurologists showing 33% false-negative NCV/EMG in patients with symptomatic carpal tunnel syndrome.

16. Perkins BA, Olaleye D, Bril V: Carpal tunnel syndrome in patients with diabetic polyneuropathy. *Diabetes Care* 25:565-569, 2002.
Electrodiagnostic testing could not identify those with carpal tunnel syndrome in the presence of diabetic neuropathy, requiring reliance on the history and physical examination.

17. Greenwald D, Moffitt W, Cooper A: Effective surgical treatment of cubital tunnel syndrome based on provocative clinical testing without electrodiagnostics. *Plast Reconstr Surg* 104:210-214, 1994.
Excellent results obtained from decompression of ulnar nerve in the absence of abnormal electrical testing.

18. Le Roux PD, Ensign TD, Burchiel KJ: Surgical decompression without transposition for ulnar neuropathy: factors determining outcome. *Neurosurgery* 27:709-714, 1990.
The relative magnitude of slowing of ulnar nerve conduction velocity across the elbow was not significantly correlated with the success of in situ decompression in relieving symptoms.

19. Dellon AL, Amadio PC, Learmonth JR: The first peripheral nerve surgeon. *J Reconstr Microsurg* 16:213-216, 2000.
Learmonth, a neurosurgeon, probably performed the first carpal tunnel decompression and described the submuscular transposition of the ulnar nerve and much more.

20. Chappell R, Cootes V, Turkelson C: Poor outcomes for neural surgery (epineurotomy or neurolysis) for carpal tunnel syndrome compared with carpal tunnel release alone; a meta-analysis. *Plast Reconstr Surg* 112:983-990, 2003.
This meta-analysis found no evidence that surgery in addition to division of the transverse carpal ligament was helpful for carpal tunnel syndrome and may cause complications.

21. Gerritsen AA, de Krom MC, Stuijs MA, et al: Conservative treatment options for carpal tunnel syndrome: a systematic review. *J Neurol* 249:272-280, 2002.
Only steroid injection into the carpal tunnel demonstrated limited effectiveness. No evidence indicated other nonoperative treatments were effective.

22. Trumble TE, Diao E, Abrams RA, Gilbert-Anderson MM: Single-portal endoscopic carpal tunnel release compared with open release. *J Bone Joint Surg* 84A:1107-1115, 2002.
Good to excellent results from carpal tunnel decompression with both open and endoscopic approaches. Literature is reviewed.

23. Hartz CR, Linscheid RL, Gramse RR, Daube JR: The pronator teres syndrome: compressive neuropathy of the median nerve. *J Bone Joint [Am]* 63:885-890, 1981.
The indications and techniques for surgical decompression and the relevant anatomy are described.

24. Rosenberg D, Conolley J, Dellon AL: Thenar eminence quantitative sensory testing in diagnosis of proximal median nerve compression. *J Hand Ther* 14:258-265, 2001.
Pronator syndrome can be identified by measuring the cutaneous pressure threshold of the thenar eminence using the Pressure-Specified Sensory Device.

25. Dellon AL: Musculotendinous variations about the elbow. *J Hand Surg* 11B:175-181, 1986.
Variations in the origins of the muscles about the elbow are described. Their relationship to treatment of compressive neuropathy is critical.

26. Gross MS, Gelberman RH: The anatomy of the distal ulnar tunnel. *Clin Orthop* 196:238-243, 1985.
The three zones of the ulnar tunnel are described.

27. Mackinnon SE, Dellon AL: Chapter 9, Cubital tunnel syndrome. In *Surgery of the peripheral nerve.* New York, 1988, Thieme.
Approximately 100 pages related to ulnar nerve compression at the elbow.

28. Dellon AL, Hament W, Gittelsohn A: Non-operative management of cubital tunnel syndrome; results of 8 year prospective study. *Neurology* 43:1673-1677, 1993.
A numerical grading system was used to stage cubital tunnel syndrome. Success of nonoperative management was related to the degree of ulnar nerve compression.

29. Dellon AL, Chang ET, Coert JH, Campbell K: Intraneural ulnar nerve pressure changes related to operative techniques. *J Hand Surg* 19A:923-930, 1994.
A cadaveric study comparing in situ decompression, medial epicondylectomy, and anterior subcutaneous, intramuscular, and submuscular transposition. Only the musculofascial lengthening technique decreased intraneural pressure in all locations along the ulnar nerve about the elbow and with all degrees flexion.

30. Dellon AL: Review of treatment results for ulnar nerve compression at the elbow. *J Hand Surg* 14:688-699, 1989.
This meta-analysis noted that anterior submuscular transposition yielded the most excellent results and anterior intramuscular transposition yielded the fewest excellent results. Reports for musculofascial lengthening had not yet been reported.

31. Mowlavi A, Andrews K, Lille S et al: The management of cubital tunnel syndrome: a meta-analysis of clinical studies. *J Hand Surg* 26A:327-334, 2001.
Low recurrence rates were documented for submuscular transposition with the musculofascial lengthening technique of Dellon.

32. Dellon AL, Mackinnon SE: Injury to the medial antebrachial cutaneous nerve during cubital tunnel surgery. *J Hand Surg* 10B:33-36, 1985.
First description of neuroma of the cutaneous nerve that crosses incision used for ulnar nerve decompression surgery at the elbow.

33. Mackinnon SE, Dellon AL: Overlap of lateral antebrachial cutaneous nerve and superficial sensory branch of the radial nerve. *J Hand Surg* 10A:522-526, 1985.
Overlap of radial sensory nerve and lateral antebrachial cutaneous nerves occurs in 75% of patients. During neurolysis of the radial sensory nerve, care should be taken to not injure the lateral antebrachial cutaneous nerve.

34. Peimer CA, Wheeler DR: Radial tunnel syndrome/posterior interosseous nerve compression. In Szabo RM, editor: *Nerve compression syndromes: diagnosis and treatment.* Thorofare, NJ, 1989, Slack.

The spectrum of radial tunnel and posterior interosseous nerve compression and treatment algorithms and surgical approaches are described.

35. Gilliatt RW, LeQuesne PM, Logue V, Sumner AJ: Wasting of the hand associated with a cervical rib or band. *J Neurol Neurosurg Psychiatry* 33:615-619, 1970.
   True, neurogenic "thoracic outlet syndrome" is a rare compression of the lower trunk of the brachial plexus. It can be identified by an EMG positive for median and ulnar innervated intrinsic muscle denervation, decreased ulnar sensory amplitude, and normal amplitude for median sensory action potentials.

36. Wilbourn A, Urschel HC: Evidence for conduction delay in thoracic outlet syndrome is challenged. *N Engl J Med* 310:1052-1053, 1984.
   Emphasis on the inability of electrodiagnostic testing to identify brachial plexus compression in the thoracic inlet.

37. Roos D: Transaxillary approach to the first rib to relieve thoracic outlet syndrome. *Ann Surg* 163:354-358, 1966.
   One of the earliest reports of the transaxillary approach. Discusses techniques and potential complications.

38. Novak CB, Collins ED, Mackinnon SE: Outcome following conservative management of thoracic outlet syndrome. *J Hand Surg* 20A:542-548, 1995.
   An exercise program that stretches the anterior scalenes and strengthens the upper trapezius, rhomboids, and serratus anterior is outlined and demonstrated to provide relief in up to 90% of patients with symptoms of "thoracic outlet syndrome."

39. Hempel GK, Shutze WP, Anderson JF, Bukhari HI: 770 consecutive supraclavicular first rib resections for thoracic outlet syndrome. *Ann Vasc Surg* 10:456-463, 1996.
   Following surgery for thoracic outlet syndrome, good or excellent responses were achieved in 86%.

40. Dellon AL: The results of supraclavicular brachial plexus neurolysis (without first rib resection) in management of post-traumatic "thoracic outlet syndrome." *J Reconstr Microsurg* 9:11-17, 1993.
   Neurolysis of the brachial plexus for compression at the thoracic inlet, preserving the first rib, can give excellent results, with few complications.

41. Sanders RJ: *Thoracic outlet syndrome: a common sequela of neck injuries*. Philadelphia, 1991, JB Lippincott.
   Long-term outcome was similar for treatment of "thoracic outlet syndrome" by supraclavicular plexus neurolysis with preservation or resection of the first rib.

# CHAPTER 17

# Complex Regional Pain Syndrome

Evan D. Collins

MD, Department of Orthopaedic Surgery, Baylor College of Medicine, Houston, TX

## Introduction

- In 1946, Evans[1] first introduced the term *reflex sympathetic dystrophy* (RSD) to describe patients suffering from consistent extremity pain that was relieved with anesthetic blocks. The widespread use of the terms *RSD* and *causalgia* without any clearly defined diagnostic criteria makes reliable, reproducible clinical research impossible. In addition to *RSD* and *causalgia,* physicians historically have used a variety of other terms to describe the same clinical phenomenon, such as Sudeck atrophy, shoulder-hand syndrome, and posttraumatic dystrophy. In an attempt to redefine these nebulous, often confusing pain syndromes, in 1994 the International Association for the Study of Pain (IASP) developed a new nomenclature that replaced the terms *RSD* and *causalgia* with the terms *complex regional pain syndrome* (CRPS) *types I* and *II.*[2] In general, CRPS type I replaces *RSD*, and CRPS type II replaces *causalgia.* The new nomenclature reflects an interest in classifying patients descriptively based on their clinical presentation and a more structured system for classifying patients that will be useful in determining the effectiveness of therapeutic treatments.

## Definitions

- The diagnosis of CRPS is always one of exclusion, regardless of the nomenclature used.
- CRPS type I is defined as a disease that develops from an initial noxious or painful event. Subsequently, pain and dysfunction develop out of proportion to the initial event and cannot be linked to any specifically pathologic process.
- The hallmark of any diagnosis of CRPS is pain out of proportion to the inciting event.
- The specific IASP diagnostic criteria for CRPS are as follows:
  1. It develops after an initial noxious or painful event.
  2. Spontaneous pain or allodynia (pain with light touch) occurs. Hyperesthesia (increased sensitivity to touch) occurs beyond the territory of a single peripheral nerve and is disproportionate to the inciting event.
  3. There is, or has been, evidence of edema skin blood flow changes or abnormalities in the sudomotor activity in that region since the inciting event.
  4. The diagnosis is excluded by the presence of conditions that would otherwise account for the amount of pain and dysfunction present.
- The main diagnostic criteria are the same for CRPS type I and type II, except that type II is associated with an identifiable nerve injury.
- Other terms that require definition are *sympathetically mediated pain* (SMP) and *sympathetically independent pain* (SIP), both of which overlap with CRPS.
- SMP is defined as any pain state that is maintained by sympathetic efferent innervation, circulating catecholamines, or neurochemical action. Patients who have a positive response to any sympathetic blockade can be considered to have SMP.
- *Patients who do not respond* to sympathetic blocks have SIP. The sympathetic status of the pain is independent of CRPS classification into type I or II. Therefore, patients

can be stratified into four groups: SMP CRPS type I, SMP CRPS type II, SIP CRPS type I, and SIP CRPS type II.

## Clinical Presentation

- CRPS is varied and can be divided into stages of progression based on the duration of symptoms.
  - Stage I CRPS occurs after the initial innocuous event and can last up to *3 months.*
    - Patients usually describe a constant burning pain out of proportion to the initial event. Allodynia (pain with light touch) and hyperpathia (pain at rest) predominate the clinical picture. *Edema initially involving the periarticular portion of the extremity usually begins in the distal region and progresses to more proximal involvement of the extremity.*[2] Edema and swelling in this region are the most commonly seen clinical manifestations of the condition.[3] Discoloration of the extremity, notably erythema reflecting alterations in blood flow (autonomic nervous system dysfunction), is present. Hyperhidrosis (excessive sweating) is commonly seen in the early phases of the condition, and the limb is maintained in a protective posture.
  - Progression to stage II or the *dystrophic phase* occurs within *3 to 9 months* of symptoms from the initial event.
    - This phase is characterized by the predominance of pain and by marked stiffness of the extremity. Other changes reflect persistent alterations in blood flow, resulting in *increased warmth followed by cyanosis.* Skin changes become evident, with a lack of skin creases, loss of hair, and decreased moisture on the hand. *Radiographs in this phase often are positive for disuse osteopenia of the involved limb, and clinical muscle wasting often is present.*
  - Stage III occurs *9 to 18 months* after injury and is called the *atrophic stage.*
    - This stage is characterized by decreased pain, with a concomitant increase in overall stiffness and lack of usefulness of the involved limb. Stiffness in joints is not affected by the initial trauma and a hallmark of late phase RSD. In general, the extremity becomes pale, dry, and cool, and the skin develops a glossy appearance with trophic changes.[4]
      - No documentation that each person suffering from CRPS develops all three stages and that these stages progress in a sequential fashion has been reported in the literature. In fact, bone studies suggest that the stages are subtypes of CRPS and are not sequential stages.[5] However, recognizing the predominating complaint and stage often affects treatment of these patients.

## Pathophysiology

- The exact mechanism of CRPS is unknown, but a combination of several factors appears to produce the disease.
- Livingston[6] first described a positive feedback cycle to explain the pathogenesis of RSD (CRPS I). He theorized that activation of nociceptors leads to excitation of a spinal cord-mediated reflex, which increases the activity of the efferent sympathetic system. The subsequent response of vasoconstriction and ischemia stimulates the pain mechanism. Regardless of whether the limb appears cool or warm (because of arteriovenous shunting), much of the pain of CRPS is ischemia related.
  - The sympathetic theory has been revised, suggesting that an unregulated sensitivity of $\alpha$-adrenergic receptors for catecholamines induces RSD.[7]
- Another hypothesis suggests that the primary cause of CRPS is an exaggeration of the peripheral neural inflammatory response to tissue injury.[8]
- A study by Christensen, Jensen, and Noer[9] seems to support this theory by demonstrating the positive effect of corticosteroids on CRPS patients, with a significant decrease in symptoms early on. There also may be a genetic predisposition to developing CRPS. Soucacos et al.[10] reviewed 109 patients with CRPS and found a 3:1 ratio of females to males and an increased risk for individuals with a family member with this condition.

## Diagnosis

- The diagnosis of CRPS is made clinically, after other diagnoses have been eliminated. Radiographs and three-phase bone scans can be used as adjunctive/complementary tests to support the clinical diagnosis.[11,12]
- Radiographs of the extremity may demonstrate periarticular demineralization on plain films, supporting the diagnosis of CRPS.[13] However, this is a late finding because 30% to 50% of calcium stores must be depleted before any change can be detected.
- Bone scans may be more sensitive at an earlier stage.[14] A positive result is diffuse activity in the involved joints in the third (delayed) phase of the scan. The results of bone scan do not diagnose CRPS. In numerous studies, the specificity and sensitivities have varied.
- Factors that increase the reliability of bone scans are patient age over 50 years and symptom duration for at least 6 months. In these patients, negative bone scan suggests the condition is not CRPS.
- Bone scans may be useful for predicting which patients develop CRPS after stroke.[11]
- Thermography,[15] which indirectly measures blood flow in an extremity, has been used for diagnosis of more

subtle cases of CRPS and for defining whether the pain is SIP or SMP. Increased temperature, implying increased blood flow, following a sympathetic block is suggestive of SMP.

- The quantitative sudomotor reflex test attempts to quantify irregularities in the autonomic nervous system by evaluating the amount of resting sweat that occurs on the extremity. An abnormal resting sweat test reflects increased sympathetic activity, which is suggestive of SMP.

## Patients at Risk

- Distal radius fractures are the most common cause. Patients who developed CRPS type I following distal radius fracture had three features in common:
  1. Fractures required manipulation,
  2. Fractures were associated with ulnar styloid injuries, and
  3. Fractures were casted primarily.
- Elevated intracast pressure, potentially predisposed by tight casts and extreme (Cotton-Lodder) positions, seems to be the most common risk factor.
- The reported incidence of CRPS following *spinal cord injury, traumatic brain injury,* or *stroke* is up to 7%.[16] Following strokes resulting in hemiplegia, 75% of patients developed symptoms in the shoulder, usually during the second and third months.
- Risk factors include marked upper extremity weakness for at least 2 weeks after the stroke, visual field deficits, and presence of a subluxated shoulder joint.
- Patients with *a previous history of CRPS who require subsequent surgery* are at risk for recurrence. A retrospective study by Reuben, Rosenthal, and Steinberg[17] found that postoperative stellate ganglion blocks in patients with a history of CRPS reduced the recurrence rate of CRPS. The assumption of the study was that all the patients had SMP. Patients with SIP may not receive the same postoperative benefits.

## Treatment

- Early recognition and an aggressive multidisciplinary treatment approach are paramount to the treatment of patients with CRPS.
  - Soucacos et al.[10] evaluated 105 patients with RSD. In a comparison of patients who sought early treatment (defined as 4 months from onset of symptoms) versus patients who sought treatment late in the course of disease, aggressive treatment and stellate ganglion blocks resulted in very good outcomes in more than 94% of patients treated early. Other studies found similar results, with high rates of treatment success in patients treated very early.

### Occupational and Physical Therapy

- The primary role of occupational and physical therapy in the early stages CRPS is to decrease pain and edema and to prevent the development of stiffness.

- Initial treatment includes immobilization and splinting of the extremity. Elevation and massage both should be incorporated into the treatment algorithm if the patient can tolerate them because they reduce and limit edema. Aggressive passive range of motion exercises should not be attempted in the early phases of the disease because the exercises may only provoke pain and possibly increase inflammation.
- Contrast baths have been used effectively for desensitizing patients and improving blood flow to the extremities. This maneuver should be repeated as often as the patient can tolerate.
- Transcutaneous electrical nerve stimulator (TENS) unit has been demonstrated to have a positive outcome, specifically for patients with CRPS type II.[1]
- A stress-loading program of traction and compression exercises has been shown to be effective. In a study by Watson and Carlson,[18] 41 patients treated with stress loading were evaluated 3 years after treatment. Eighty-eight percent of the patients had pain relief, 95% had improved range of motion, and all had improved strength. Eighty-four percent of patients had returned to their previous occupation.

## Pharmacologic Therapy

- Currently many medications are available, and several have shown some promise in the treatment of patients with CRPS. The literature often is anecdotal and has yet to result in a reliable medical protocol for use in all patients.
  - α-Adrenergic blockers seem to be most effective for patients with SMP.
  - Calcium channel blockers inhibit smooth muscle contraction, thereby relaxing or vasodilating the peripheral arterioles and improving circulation. The advantage of calcium channel blockers is that they do not affect the venous capacitance system, thereby decreasing the risk of orthostatic hypotension. In a study of nifedipine given to 13 patients with CRPS type I, seven patients had complete relief, two had partial relief, and three stopped taking the medication because of headaches.
- Sympathetic interruption can be achieved using local anesthetics, regional blocks, or surgical ablation.
  - Stellate ganglion blocks, using lidocaine or bupivacaine, can be used to confirm the diagnosis and to treat SMP. A positive response is indicated by decreased pain, increased blood flow to the extremity, increased temperature in the extremity, and a clinical *Horner's syndrome* (ptosis, miosis, anhidrosis). The pain relief often lasts well beyond the duration of the block. Initially one or two blocks can be attempted to assess their effectiveness. If pain relief is only temporary, the block can be repeated until pain is controlled for a maximum of 12 blocks. Patients who receive no or only partial pain relief with stellate

ganglion blocks likely have SIP, implying that continued blocks would not be beneficial. Hobelmann and Dellon[19] used indwelling axillary sheath catheters to provide continuous sensory and sympathetic blockage in patients with CRPS. None of the patients had exacerbation of CRPS. Elimination of pain with a continuous block enables occupational therapy to commence earlier than might otherwise be possible.

- Surgical sympathectomy for patients with SMP reportedly resulted in 91% to 100% good or excellent results.[20]
- The role of nonsteroidal antiinflammatory drugs is controversial. Although they may inhibit pain and decrease swelling and edema, Stanton-Hicks et al.[6] found that 60% to 70% of patients had no pain relief.
- Corticosteroids have been used. Christensen, Jensen, and Noer[9] noted decreased edema and pain following administration of high-dose steroids (100 mg/day for several weeks). The risk of complications at such high doses led some researchers to evaluate different dosing patterns for treatment. Kozin[13] and others reported a good response to systemic corticosteroids initially given at high doses (60–80 mg/day in divided doses) and then quickly tapered. The efficacy of a Medrol dose-pack as initial treatment had better overall results and limited side effects when given to patients with CRPS of less than 6 months' duration.
- Tricyclic antidepressants (e.g., amitriptyline [Elavil]) may be effective.
- Gabapentin (Neurontin) is a mild anticonvulsant that has been shown to be highly effective.[21,22] Side effects are relatively mild (dizziness, diplopia, nausea, somnolence).
- Alternative treatments of CRPS include *acupuncture,* with reported success up to 90%. Gellman, Pian-Smith, and Botte[23] also reported acupuncture was effective in treating CRPS recalcitrant to other treatments.

# References

1. Evans JA: Reflex sympathetic dystrophy; report of 57 cases. *Ann Intern Med* 26:417-426, 1947.
   Classic review article on reflex sympathetic dystrophy, including diagnosis and treatment in the author's experience of 57 cases.

2. Stanton-Hicks M, Janig W, Hassenbusch S, et al: Reflex sympathetic dystrophy: changing concepts and taxonomy. *Pain* 63:127-133, 1995.
   This classic article redefined the "taxonomy" of RSD into CRPS (complex regional pain syndrome) type I and type II to help eliminate confusion in the literature. Type I becomes synonymous with RSD and type II with causalgia. The term SMP (sympathetically mediated pain) was also found to be a useful descriptive term.

3. Gellman H, Collins ED: *Complex regional pain syndrome in the upper extremity. Orthopaedics.* St. Louis, 2002, Mosby.

4. Wilson PR: Post-traumatic upper extremity reflex sympathetic dystrophy. Clinical course, staging, and classification of clinical forms. *Hand Clin* 13:367-372, 1997.
   This article focuses on classifying RSD clinically into sympathetically maintained versus sympathetically independent. Sympathetic blockade is found to be useful only in the former. Other treatments are discussed.

5. Bruehl S, Harden RN, Galer BS, et al: Complex regional pain syndrome: are there distinct subtypes and sequential stages of the syndrome? *Pain* 95:119-124, 2002.
   This study suggests three distinct subtypes of CRPS rather than sequential progression.

6. Stanton-Hicks M, Baron R, Boas R, et al: Complex regional pain syndromes: guidelines for therapy. *Clin J Pain.* 14(2):155-266, 1998.
   Describes an algorithm for the treatment of CRPS including self-management techniques, treatment modalities, and functional rehabilitation.

7. Arnold JM, Teasell RW, MacLeod AP, et al: Increased venous alpha-adrenergic response in patients with reflex sympathetic dystrophy. *Ann Intern Med* 118:619-621, 1993.
   This study examined 11 patients with RSD and showed a consistent hypersensitivity in their veins (compared to controls) to adrenergic agonists.

8. Oyen WJ, Arntz IE, Claessens RM, et al: Reflex sympathetic dystrophy of the hand: an excessive inflammatory response? *Pain* 55:151-157, 1993.
   More patients with early RSD had positive indium-111 IgG scintigraphy than patients with late RSD. These findings suggest inflammation was present more often in early RSD and may play a role in its development.

9. Christensen K, Jensen EM, Noer I: The reflex dystrophy syndrome response to treatment with systemic corticosteroids. *Acta Chir Scand* 148:653-655, 1982.
   Randomized study that looks at treating patients with RSD with oral prednisone versus placebo. Among the 13 patients in the study, 75% were clinically improved in the 12-week period versus 20% in the placebo group.

10. Soucacos PN, Diznitsas LA, Beris AE, et al: Reflex sympathetic dystrophy of the upper extremity. *Hand Clin* 13:339-353, 1997.
    This review article discusses the complexity of RSD and outlines five clinical subtypes. Early diagnosis and treatment are emphasized.

11. Gellman H, Nichols D: Reflex sympathetic dystrophy in the upper extremity. *J Am Acad Orthop Surg* 5:313-322, 1997.
    Review article summarizing the various useful diagnostic and therapeutic modalities.

12. MacKinnon SE, Holder LE: The use of 3-phase radionuclide bone scanning in the diagnosis of reflex sympathetic dystrophy. *J Hand Surg* 9A:556-563, 1984.
    Notes diffuse increased tracer uptake in the delayed image (phase III) of bone scans was diagnostic for RSD, with sensitivity of 96% and specificity of 98%.

Summary of CRPS using the new definitions and classification. Diagnosis and treatment are discussed.

13. Kozin F, Ryan LM, Carerra GF, et al: The reflex sympathetic dystrophy syndrome (RSDS) III. Scintigraphy studies, further evidence for the therapeutic efficacy of systemic corticosteroids, and proposed diagnostic criteria. *Am J Med* 1:23-39, 1981.

14. O'Donoghue JP, Powe JE, Mattar AG, et al: Three-phase bone scintigraphy. Asymmetric patterns in the upper extremities of asymptomatic normals and reflex sympathetic dystrophy patients. *Clin Nucl Med* 18:829-836, 1993.
    Three-phase bone scans of 61 asymptomatic patients were randomly mixed with 17 studies of patients previously diagnosed with RSD. The sensitivity for RSD was unacceptably low at 29%.

15. Hendler N, Uematesu S, Long D: Thermographic validation of physical complaints in "psychogenic pain" patients. *Psychosomatics* 23:283, 1982.
    Thermography (as a sympathetic measuring tool) was found to be of value in several cases by providing the diagnosis of a pain syndrome in individuals who had been mislabeled with psychogenic pain.

16. Gellman H, Eckert RR, Botte MJ, et al: Reflex sympathetic dystrophy in cervical spine cord injured patients. *Clin Orthop* 233: 129-131, 1988.
    Ten percent of patients with spinal cord injury were diagnosed with RSD, some of whom were effectively treated with stellate ganglion blocks during rehabilitation.

17. Reuben SS, Rosenthal EA, Steinberg RB: Surgery on the affected upper extremity of patients with a history of complex regional pain syndrome: a retrospective study of 100 patients. *J Hand Surg* 25:1147-1151, 2000.
    This study suggests that a postoperative stellate ganglion block may be beneficial in a patient with a history of prior CRPS undergoing surgery.

18. Watson HK, Carlson L: Treatment of reflex sympathetic dystrophy of the hand with an active "stress loading" program. *J Hand Surg* 12:779-785, 1987.
    The "stress loading" program has been used effectively for treatment of RSD over the past 20 years. The advantages of the program are its effectiveness, simplicity, safety, and noninvasiveness.

19. Hobelmann CF, Dellon AL: Use of prolonged sympathetic blockade as an adjunct to surgery in the patient with sympathetic maintained pain. *Microsurgery* 10:151-153, 1989.
    Use of prolonged sympathetic blockade with an axillary catheter allowed patients with a history of RSD to safely undergo surgery for treatment of an associated nerve injury.

20. Schwartzman RJ, Liu JE, Smullens SN, et al: Long-term outcome following sympathectomy for complex regional pain syndrome type 1 (RSD). *J Neurol Sci* 150:149-152, 1997.
    A retrospective study of 29 patients with CRPS type I (RSD) who underwent endoscopic transthoracic sympathectomies. All seven patients (100%) who had undergone sympathectomy within 12 months of injury, nine of 13 patients (69.2%) who had undergone sympathectomy within 24 months of injury, and only four of nine patients (44.4%) who had undergone sympathectomy more than 24 months after injury achieved permanent (>24 months) symptom relief.

21. Mellick GA, Mellick LB: Reflex sympathetic dystrophy treated with gabapentin. *Arch Phys Med Rehabil* 78:98-105, 1997.
    First clinical study to show efficacy of gabapentin in treating patients with refractory CRPS.

22. Mellick GA, Mellick LB: Gabapentin in the management of reflex sympathetic dystrophy. *J Pain Symptom Manage* 10:265-266, 1995.
    Similar to the 1997 study by the same authors but with a larger cohort of patients.

23. Gellman H, Pian-Smith MC, Botte MJ: Acupuncture: alternative modalities for pain management. *Instr Course Lect* 49:559-563, 2000.
    Acupuncture was effective in treating CRPS refractory to conventional treatment.

# CHAPTER 18

# Tendon Transfers for Peripheral Nerve Injuries

Daniel N. Switlick* and Joseph E. Sheppard†

*MD, Department of Orthopaedic Surgery, University of Arizona Health Sciences Center, Tucson, AZ
†MD, Department of Orthopaedic Surgery, University of Arizona Health Sciences Center, Tucson, AZ

> "Each time a tendon is transferred in a hand, every other muscle and tendon is affected because balance is disturbed."
>
> **Paul W. Brand**

## Introduction

- Peripheral nerve injuries of the upper extremity result in significant functional deficits that may improve with nerve repair or grafting but may require tendon transfer to restore function.
- Hundreds of potential transfers to restore function have been described; however, this chapter presents the most commonly performed transfers that produce the most predictable results.

## General Principles of Tendon Transfers

### Basic Tenets of Tendon Transfers
(Box 18–1)

- *Tissue equilibrium:* Skeletal stability, maximum joint mobility, and skin/subcutaneous maturation are critical prior to tendon transfer surgery.

| Box 18–1 | Basic Tenets of Tendon Transfers |
|---|---|

- Tissue equilibrium
- Joint mobility
- Adequate donor strength
- Adequate donor amplitude
- Expendable donor
- Straight line of pull
- One tendon, one function
- Synergy

- *Joint mobility:* As soon as possible after initial injury, efforts should be directed at maintenance of joint mobility through rehabilitation. If necessary, contracture corrections should be performed prior to tendon transfer surgery.
- *Adequate donor strength:* Transferred muscle-tendon units must have a contractile capacity strong enough to accomplish the desired task of the paralyzed muscle (Table 18–1). Transferred muscles typically lose one grade of motor strength; thus, potential motors must have a motor strength of grade 4 or 5. Motor strength can be improved postoperatively with appropriate rehabilitation. The choice of donor should be individualized based on the specific needs of the patient (e.g., a carpenter may require more strength, but a musician might prefer more excursion). Additional power may be required to overcome the added resistance and shortened moment arm encountered when the tendon passes through a pulley.
- *Adequate donor amplitude:* The surgeon should choose a donor muscle with an excursion equal to or greater to the excursion of the paralyzed muscle-tendon unit, if possible (Table 18–2). Generally, the excursion can be estimated by Smith's 3-5-7 rule: wrist flexors/ extensors = 3 cm, metacarpophalangeal (MCP) extensors = 5 cm, flexor digitorum profundus (FDP) = 7 cm.[1] Excursion of a muscle-tendon unit can be increased to some extent by freeing some of the fascial and bony attachments and by the tenodesis effect if the tendon crosses multiple joints.

| Table 18–1: | Relative Forearm and Hand Muscle Strengths |
|---|---|
| **MUSCLE** | **STRENGTH RELATIVE TO FCR** |
| BR | 2.0 |
| FCU | 2.0 |
| ECRL, ECRB, ECU | 1.0 (each tendon) |
| PT, FPL, FDS, FDP | |
| EDC, EIP, EDQ | 0.5 (each tendon) |
| APL, EPB, PL | 0.5 (each tendon) |
| Interossei | 2.7 (total/combined) |
| Lumbricals | 0.5 (total/combined) |

From Trumble T: *Principles of hand surgery and therapy.* Philadelphia, 2000, WB Saunders Company.

| Table 18–2: | Excursion of Forearm and Hand Muscles |
|---|---|
| **MUSCLE** | **EXCURSION (CM)** |
| BR | 2.0 |
| FDP | 7.0 |
| FDS | 6.5 |
| EPL | 6.0 |
| EDC | 5.0 |
| EIP | 5.0 |
| FPL | 5.0 |
| FCU | 3.0 |
| FCR | 3.0 |
| ECRL | 3.0 |
| ECRB | 3.0 |
| ECU | 3.0 |
| EPB | 3.0 |
| APL | 3.0 |
| Lumbricals | 3.8 |
| Thenar | 3.8 |
| Interossei | 2.0 |

From Trumble T: *Principles of hand surgery and therapy.* Philadelphia, 2000, WB Saunders Company.

- *Expendable donor:* Careful preoperative muscle grading and planning are necessary to prevent further imbalance. If a patient has developed an adaptive functional maneuver using a particular potential donor muscle, transfers using other potential donors should be considered or the patient may experience a net loss of function after transfer.
- *Straight line of pull:* A straight line between the origin and insertion of a muscle maximizes efficiency and power.
- *One tendon, one function:* Transfers that are split to recipient insertions with different excursions will only effectively function to move the joint with the shortest excursion.
- *Synergy:* Transfers using muscles that typically fire in concert with the paralyzed muscle (often a stabilizing antagonist) in a desired function typically are more effective and easier to re-educate.

## Biomechanics

- The insertion point of a tendon creates a compromise between mechanical leverage and the degree of joint motion with contraction of the motor unit.
- Tendon insertion farther from the axis of a joint results in an increased mechanical advantage and thus increased power with contraction, but the joint moves through a relatively shorter arc of motion.
- Tendon insertion close to the axis of a joint results in greater joint range of motion (ROM) with a particular

motor unit contraction. However, because of the short moment arm, greater force is required to flex the joint through that ROM.

- Pulleys hold the tendon closer to the axis of a joint, thus increasing the potential ROM with a set motor unit excursion at the cost of decreasing strength.
- Pulleys are effective at improving fine motor control of a joint distant to the contractile unit.
- To achieve motion only at the terminal joint in a series of joints, an opposing, stabilizing force must be present at each of the proximal joints in the series.
- Motion of a joint is affected by the excursion of the tendon and applied tension of the motor unit and is limited by the applied resistance, which may be compounded by resistance because of scarring of the muscle-tendon unit or of the joint itself.
- Although motion at the MCP and interphalangeal (IP) joints typically occurs in a single plane, joint deformity or loss of normal supporting structures may result in motion of that joint in an abnormal axis.[2]

## Muscle Geometry

- Brand[3] defines important mechanical characteristics as follows:
  - Mean fiber length is fairly constant throughout a muscle.
  - Mean fiber length is proportional to potential excursion.
  - Mass or volume of muscle fibers is proportional to work capacity.
  - Cross-sectional area of all fibers is proportional to maximum tension or force.
- Using these characteristics, Brand further defined the work capacity of various muscles for transfer:
  - Mass fraction is the percentage of total weight comprised by each forearm and hand muscle.
  - Tension fraction is the volume of the muscle (derived from the mass) divided by the mean fiber length. It provides a measure of the contractile tension capacity of a muscle.
- Fridén and Lieber[4] found that muscles are less efficient and less powerful at extremes of the muscle working sarcomere length. Therefore, choosing motor units with appropriate excursion and setting tension within the functional range of the sarcomere is important.[4]

## Surgical Technique

- Transfers should be individualized based on the patient's functional needs, available motors, and extent of tissue injury.
- In progressive diseases with a typical pattern of involvement, do not use donor muscles that likely will be further weakened by the disease process.
- Drapes should be applied above the level of the elbow to allow access to the entire forearm and to allow adequate motion to tension appropriately.

- A leg should be draped separately to allow access for tendon graft if necessary.
- Atraumatic technique should be emphasized with gentle tendon handling.
- Avoid incisions over planned tenorrhaphy sites because the resultant scar may limit excursion.
- Transfer of tendons over a healthy tissue bed is important. Avoid transfers in heavily scarred areas and consider dorsal transfers if extensive volar scarring is present.
- Avoid placing transferred tendon in contact with bone, fascia, or scar, because adhesions to these immobile tissues will increase resistance and limit excursion. Remember, fat is your friend because it provides a smooth gliding surface free of adhesions.
- When transferring a tendon through the interosseous membrane, allowing the muscle belly to lie within the window—rather than the tendon—results in less restriction of motion from scarring.
- End to end tenorrhaphies result in a more linear line of pull and thus a more efficient transfer, with optimization of excursion and minimization of resistance.
- Appropriate tension is critical to achieve optimal tendon excursion, maximize the efficiency of the contractile unit, and place the hand in a functional position.
- Muscle excursion can be increased significantly by partially freeing the muscle from fascial and bony attachments.
- The tenodesis action of the wrist can increase flexion of one joint by extending another, and vice versa; therefore, preserving this effect is crucial in order to maximize potential tendon excursion. This is particularly true for combined median and ulnar palsies, in which wrist extension improves cylindrical grasp, and transfers for radial nerve palsy, which frequently require slight wrist flexion to optimize MCP joint extension.
- The tenodesis effect may allow tendons without an active motor to function passively.
- In patients with multiple nerve injuries and few potential motors, capsulodesis can be used to prevent joint hyperextension and to position joints in a more useful position.
- Tenodesis of several tendons to achieve a functional action, such as tenodesis of thumb and finger flexors to achieve grasp with wrist dorsiflexion, may be effective in patients with limited available motors and multiple nerve injuries.
- Arthrodesis of the wrist should be avoided if possible in order to preserve the tenodesis effect; however, it may be required in cases of severe deformity or pain.
- Failure of a tendon transfer can be attributed to several causes:
  - Failure of motor: poor motor education or inadequate donor motor strength
  - Failure of mobility: scar or preoperative joint contracture
  - Failure of excursion: poor tensioning or inadequate donor amplitude

- Technical failure: rupture of tenorrhaphy
- Combined: inadequate line of pull or use of one motor for multiple functions
- Most transfer failures result from postoperative scarring, especially at the level of tendon juncture.
- If postoperative adhesions are not improved by hand therapy within 12 weeks of initiating therapy, tenolysis should be performed, followed by immediate active and passive motion exercises.

## Preoperative Evaluation and Timing of Tendon Transfers

### Preoperative Evaluation

- Following initial injury, careful patient evaluation should include assessment of (1) degree of function of all muscles of the forearm and hand, (2) muscles without function, (3) degree and pattern of sensibility, (4) degree of bone and soft tissue injury, and (5) joint ROM.
- Muscles should be individually palpated to judge degree of contraction.
- Adaptive functions learned by a patient must be assessed because they impact upon potential muscle donors.
- Patients must be examined when they are trying to accomplish functional tasks rather than when they simply are passing their hand or digits through a ROM, because applied stress may reveal imbalances that will prevent them from accomplishing functions necessary in their daily activities or employment.
- Patients should be queried of their needs and most significant functional deficits in order to individualize the transfers that will prove most functional.
- Brand[5] recommends creating diagrams for each joint affected by paralysis to create a plan for appropriately balanced transfers.
- Smith[1] recommends creating charts for preoperative planning with separate columns identifying what muscles work in a particular patient, what muscles are available for transfer, and what function is needed.
- Goals, expectations, planned procedures, and postoperative plan should be thoroughly discussed with the patient to ensure appropriate understanding of limitations, expected outcomes and rehabilitation process prior to undertaking transfers.
- Contraindications to tendon transfer surgery include: 1) unstable tissue bed (chronic or unhealed wounds, bony nonunion, infection; 2) noncompliant, unreliable or unmotivated patient; 3) untreated progressive disease; 4) significant joint contractures; 5) unilateral extremity involvement with significant sensory deficit (relative).

### Timing of Transfers

- Tendon transfers for muscle or tendon loss can be performed when tissue is stable for transfer.

- Tendon transfers for nerve injury require consideration of the cause of injury and potential for spontaneous recovery.
- Timing of return of function after traumatic nerve injuries may be variable and is dependent on whether the injury is secondary to neuropraxia, axonotmesis, or neurotmesis.
- Nerve palsies associated with lacerations or open fractures should prompt immediate nerve exploration.
- Results of nerve repair or grafting can vary, depending on the level of repair, age of the patient, extent of injury, and whether the nerve is predominantly motor, sensory, or mixed.
- Grabb[6] notes that recovery after nerve repair is slower and less predictable in older patients, high-level nerve injury, and more equal proportion of motor and sensory fibers.
- Ring, Chin, and Jupiter[7] found that primary nerve repair in lacerated radial nerves associated with high-energy open humerus fractures results in persistent deficit, and they recommend delayed nerve grafting.
- Nerve repair or grafting versus early tendon transfers should depend on the potential for nerve recovery.
- Results of nerve repair/grafting are less predictable with nerve grafts longer than 4 cm or significant scarring is present in the region of the nerve.[8]
- After acute nerve exploration, an adequate period of time should be allowed for nerve recovery.
- Generally, after a 30-day latent period, nerve recovery proceeds at a rate of 1 mm/day after nerve repair.
- In addition to assessing for proximally innervated muscle contraction, an advancing Tinel sign may indicate nerve recovery, and the site of Tinel sign should be carefully measured in relation to a bony landmark.
- Omer[9] recommends completing tendon transfers 12 weeks after the time of expected recovery of function in traumatic nerve deficits.
- Muscle re-education typically is easier and better outcomes are achieved if tendon transfers are performed within 1 year after injury.
- Electromyographic (EMG) studies may be helpful in assessing recovery of peripheral nerve injury. A baseline study should be completed 6 weeks after injury in the absence of apparent recovery.
- EMG studies will not provide useful information and may be falsely negative if they are performed within 2 to 4 weeks of injury. They cannot accurately differentiate between axonotmesis and neurotmesis.[10]
- Decreased fibrillation potentials and return of voluntary motor unit potentials on EMG testing herald nerve recovery.[11]
- Nerve conduction studies are especially helpful in the setting of progressive polyneuropathy.[12]

### Early Treatment

- Tendon transfers should not be attempted until tissue equilibrium is achieved.

- Hand therapy should be initiated as soon as possible after injury to maintain or regain joint mobility. Release of joint contractures should be completed as necessary prior to tendon transfer surgery.
- Insertion of silicone rods in the tissue bed in the location of proposed tendon transfers may be indicated in extensive soft tissue injuries to provide a healthy bed for the future transfer.[9,13]
- Tissue expanders with transposition flaps are useful for providing full-thickness skin coverage.
- Bracing may be effective in assisting patients with more functional wrist positioning, especially in the setting of radial nerve palsy.
- While awaiting nerve recovery, some early transfers (internal splinting) may be considered (e.g., pronator teres [PT] to extensor carpi radialis brevis [ECRB] in radial nerve palsy) in order to maintain hand function and facilitate joint motion.

## Radial Nerve Palsy

- Radial nerve injuries can be divided into high (complete) radial nerve injury and low (posterior interosseous nerve [PIN]) injury (Box 18–2).
- Primary deficits in radial nerve palsies, based on the level of injury (Box 18–3), are (1) loss of wrist extension (in complete palsy), (2) loss of finger extension, and (3) loss of thumb extension.

| Box 18–2 | Primary Motor Deficits Associated with Nerve Injuries |
|---|---|

- Complete radial
  - Wrist extension/stabilization
  - Finger extension
  - Thumb extension
- Posterior interosseous nerve
  - Finger extension
  - Thumb extension
- High median
  - Thumb opposition
  - Flexion of index, long, and thumb
- Low median
  - Thumb opposition
- High ulnar
  - Flexion of ring and small
  - Power pinch
  - Power grip
  - Precision movements/fine motor coordination
  - Persistent abducted small
- Low ulnar
  - Power pinch
  - Power grip
  - Precision movements/fine motor coordination
- Persistent abducted small
- Clawing ring and small

| Box 18–3 | Radial Nerve Innervated Muscles |
|---|---|

**Radial nerve**
- Triceps
- BR
- ECRL

**From Radial, Superficial Radial, or PIN**
- ECRB

**PIN**
- Supinator
- EDC
- ECU
- EDQ
- APL
- EPL
- EPB
- EIP

- Sensory loss in radial nerve injuries typically is not clinically significant.
- Biceps function compensates for elbow flexion and forearm supination loss (brachioradialis [BR] and supinator).
- Active wrist extension provides a critical stabilizing force to the wrist and significantly increases grip strength by maintaining the wrist in a position that optimizes finger flexion.
- Preserving at least one wrist flexor in radial nerve palsy tendon transfers improves finger extension via the wrist flexion tenodesis effect.[14]
- Patients with PIN palsy will not require transfer to achieve wrist dorsiflexion, although they typically deviate radially because of extensor carpi ulnaris (ECU) paralysis and therefore may require transfer of extensor carpi radialis longus (ECRL) to ECRB or ECU.
- All common tendon transfers for high radial nerve palsy include transfer of PT to ECRB to provide wrist extension.
- Early end to side transfer of PT to ECRB is advocated by some to provide active wrist extension and improve function while awaiting nerve and muscle recovery. It can be reversed if significant recovery occurs.
- Table 18–3 lists common tendon transfers for radial nerve paralysis.

| Table 18–3: | Tendon Transfers for Radial Nerve Paralysis | | |
|---|---|---|---|
| | BRAND | JONES | MODIFIED BOYES |
| Wrist extension | PT–ECRB | PT–ECRB | PT–ECRB |
| Thumb extension | PL–EPL | PL–EPL | PL–EPL |
| Finger extension | FCR–EDC | FCU–EDC | FDS IV–EDC |

- Flexor carpi ulnaris (FCU) Jones transfer has several theoretical disadvantages: (1) FCU is the most important wrist flexor and only functioning ulnar deviator; (2) normal wrist axis is dorsal radial to palmar ulnar; and (3) FCU is too strong and of too limited excursion.[8,15]
- FCU transfer should not be performed in PIN palsy, otherwise significant radial wrist deviation will occur.
- Flexor carpi radialis (FCR) Brand transfer (Figure 18–1) results in less radial wrist deviation than FCU transfer and provides strong grip strength; however, it may not provide enough excursion to produce finger extension in the absence of the wrist tenodesis effect.
- Flexor digitorum superficialis (FDS) Boyes transfer (Figure 18–2) results in increased excursion. Theoretically, independent wrist and finger extension is possible.
- Use of FDS III versus FDS IV versus both is debated.[8,16,17] We recommend the use of FDS III for the following reasons: (1) FDS III is more powerful than FDS IV, and the FDS IV may be more important in power grip; (2) Lieber et al.[17] showed that the muscle architecture of FDS III more closely resembles that of extensor digitorum communis (EDC) than any other potential transfer to EDC; and (3) FDS III has an independent muscle belly and this may result in better independent motion if transferred.
- Incision placement depends upon transfer combination.
- A strip of periosteum should be harvested with the PT tendon attachment to prolong the tendon.
- The PT tendon is passed superficial to the BR and tunneled subcutaneously to insert at the musculotendinous junction of the ECRB (Figure 18–3).
- The PT tendon should be attached end to side to the intact ECRB musculotendinous unit so that it continues

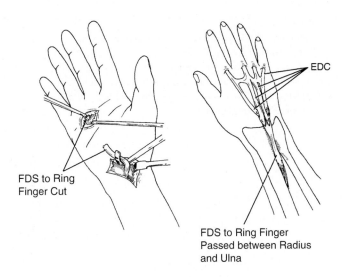

FDS to Ring Finger Cut

FDS to Ring Finger Passed between Radius and Ulna

EDC

### Modified Boyes Transfer

**Figure 18–2:**
**Modified Boyes transfer for radial nerve palsy.** *EDC,* extensor digitorum communis; *FDS,* flexor digitorum superficialis. (From Trumble T: *Principles of hand surgery and therapy.* Philadelphia: WB Saunders Company, 2000, with permission.)

to function as a forearm pronator and provides wrist extension.
- If FCR transfer is performed, a zigzag incision across the wrist crease can be performed to harvest the tendon near the insertion. The palmaris longus (PL) can also be transected near its insertion through this palmar incision.
- If FCU transfer is performed, a palmar ulnar-based longitudinal incision is performed to transect the FCU tendon just proximal to the pisiform, with a transverse limb (hockey stick) at the level of the wrist flexion crease to harvest the PL.
- If FDS transfer is performed, the tendon can be harvested via a transverse incision at the distal palmar crease and can be rerouted through separate incisions to pass through the interosseous membrane or around the radial border.
- The EDC and extensor indicis proprius (EIP) tendons are sutured together and freed from the extensor retinaculum.
- In most cases, the EDC tendons are transected at their musculotendinous juncture to achieve a more direct line of pull.
- Through the proximal rerouting incision, donor muscles are freed of bony attachments as necessary and directed to their attachment on the EDC tendons.
- Most patients lack a separate slip of EDC to the small finger, in which case the EDQ should be included in the transfer to EDC.[8]
- The extensor pollicis longus (EPL) tendon is transected at its musculotendinous junction and transposed out of its

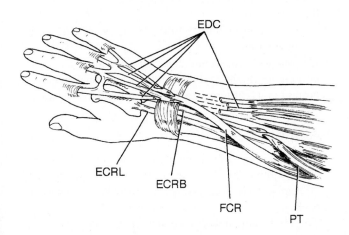

EDC

ECRL

ECRB

FCR

PT

### Brand Transfer

**Figure 18–1:**
**Brand transfer for radial nerve palsy.** *ECRB,* extensor carpi radialis brevis; *ECRL,* extensor carpi radialis longus; *EDC,* extensor digitorum communis; *FCR,* flexor carpi radialis; *PT,* pronator teres. (From Trumble T: *Principles of hand surgery and therapy.* Philadelphia, 2000, WB Saunders Company.)

Figure 18–3:

Pronator teres *(PT)* to extensor carpi radialis brevis *(ECRB)* transfer for radial nerve palsy. *BR,* brachioradialis; *ECRL,* extensor carpi radialis longus; *EDC,* extensor digitorum communis; *R,* radius. (From Trumble T: *Principles of hand surgery and therapy.* Philadelphia, 2000, WB Saunders Company.)

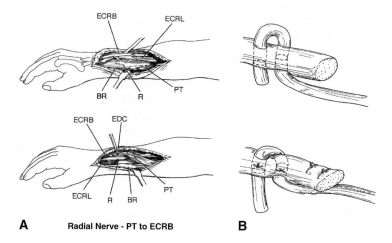

**A**    Radial Nerve - PT to ECRB    **B**

sheath and over the anatomic snuffbox to overlie the first dorsal compartment, where it is attached to the PL (Figure 18–4). In this position, it produces both thumb IP extension and abduction.

- Palmaris longus is absent in 20% of patients. Options for transfer to EPL in these patients include (1) FDS III or IV around the radial border or through the interosseous membrane; (2) BR if preserved (PIN palsy only), although muscle belly attachments must be freed to increase excursion; or (3) original Boyes transfer, which includes FDS III to EPL and EIP, FDS IV to EDC, and FCR to extensor pollicis brevis (EPB) and abductor pollicis longus (APL).[8]

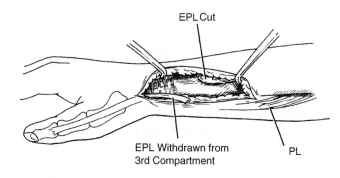

EPL Cut

EPL Withdrawn from 3rd Compartment    PL

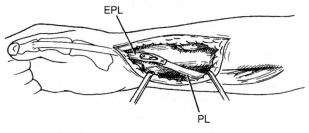

EPL

PL

PL to EPL

Figure 18–4:

Palmaris longus (PL) to extensor pollicis longus *(EPL)* transfer for radial nerve palsy. (From Trumble T: *Principles of hand surgery and therapy.* Philadelphia, 2000, WB Saunders Company.)

- Including the EPL with transfer to EDC in patients devoid of PL does not restore thumb abduction and should be avoided.
- Order of tensioning should be (1) PT to ECRB, (2) FCR, FDS, or FCU to EDC, and (3) PL to EPL.
- The assistant should hold wrist and finger position in extension during suturing.
- 3-0 or 4-0 nonabsorbable suture should be used.
- Tension is set to produce full wrist and finger extension, yet allow full finger flexion in 20 degrees of wrist extension.
- Pronator to ECRB tension is set at maximal stretch of pronator with 45 degrees wrist dorsiflexion.
- In transfer to EDC, tension is applied to the point of 50% maximal stretch of the transferred muscle-tendon unit with the wrist in neutral or slight dorsiflexion and the fingers in full extension. Full finger flexion at all joints should be possible.
- With the wrist in neutral, EPL and PL are secured under maximal tension.
- If a patient has significant radial wrist deviation postoperatively, the ECRB insertion can be split and a portion of it transferred to the base of the third metacarpal.

## Postoperative Care

- All transfers for radial nerve palsy should be immobilized in 90 degrees elbow flexion, neutral forearm rotation, and 30 degrees wrist dorsiflexion with the MCP joints in full extension.
- Thumb is immobilized in abduction, with full MCP and IP joint extension.
- Week 3: dynamic extension outrigger splint with wrist in 30 degrees dorsiflexion and 30 degrees MCP joint flexion block. Increase MCP flexion block weekly.
- Week 5: active wrist and digit ROM with synergistic movements. Resting night splint maintaining wrist dorsiflexion and finger and thumb extension. Initiate biofeedback for muscle re-education.

- Week 6: passive ROM to increase finger flexion. Flexion taping of joints as needed.
- Delay passive ROM if MCP joint extensor lags are greater than 30 degrees. Continue extension splinting at night and between exercises.
- Week 8: progressive strengthening with soft lightweight foam (Nerf) ball and putty. Discontinue splinting. Initiate functional activities.

## Median Nerve Palsy

- Median nerve injuries can be divided into low and high median nerve palsies, with transfers for low median palsy more common primarily because of wrist lacerations, chronic carpal tunnel syndrome, polyneuropathy, and congenital absence of thenar muscles (see Box 18–2).
- Patients must be evaluated for web space contracture preoperatively and appropriate stretching exercises initiated as needed to prevent transfer failure.

## Low Median Nerve Palsy

- Because of loss of innervation of the thenar muscles, the primary motor deficit in low median nerve palsy is loss of thumb opposition (Box 18–4).
- Median nerve palsy results in significant functional deficits because of loss of sensation on the palmar aspect of the thumb, index, and long fingers.
- In the absence of sensation, any function regained by tendon transfers requires direct observation because of lack of sensory feedback, which limits the utility of the transfers.
- If sensory deficits are severe despite nerve repair and grafting, microsurgical digital nerve transfer or neurovascular cutaneous island pedicle flaps can be performed to restore sensibility (Figure 18–5).[18]
- Thumb opposition consists of combined thumb abduction, flexion, and pronation.

---

**Box 18–4   Median Nerve Innervated Muscles**

- Pronator teres
- FCR
- FDP index
- FDP long (partially innervated by ulnar)
- FDS
- FPL
- Pronator quadratus
- Lumbricals to index and long
- Thenar muscles
  - Opponens pollicis
  - Abductor pollicis brevis
  - Flexor pollicis brevis (superficial head)

---

- The abductor pollicis brevis (APB) is the most effective muscle of thumb opposition. Therefore, transfers are inserted near the APB insertion to restore this function.[19]
- Many transfers have been proposed; the most common are listed in Box 18–5.
- Except for the PL transfer, the vector is directed from the pisiform to the APB insertion.
- Selection of donor often is determined by the cause of the opposition deficit.
- PL transfer can be performed concomitantly with carpal tunnel release in chronic carpal tunnel syndrome.
- Lacerations often are associated with significant volar scarring, in which case EIP transfer may be more effective to prevent scarring.
- Congenital absence of thenar muscles often is treated with Huber transfer. The muscle-tendon unit is easier to transfer in children than in adults and provides thenar bulk that is more cosmetically pleasing.
- In the EIP transfer (Figure 18–6), the EIP tendon is brought around the ulnar border, passed through a subcutaneous tunnel across the palm, and inserted at the APB insertion.
- Incisions are made at the dorsum of the index metacarpal for harvest, at the dorsum of the wrist and ulnar border of the forearm for redirection, and over the radial side of the thumb MCP joint for insertion.
- An EIP transfer should include a strip of extensor hood (which then should be carefully repaired) to provide adequate length.
- The junctura tendineae to the index EDC can be released in EIP transfer to improve independent index finger extension.
- The index finger should be splinted in extension postoperatively to prevent extensor lag.
- In the FDS transfer (Figure 18–7), the ring FDS tendon is harvested from a transverse incision in the distal palm between the A1 and A2 pulleys.
- An additional incision is made over the pisiform through which the FDS tendon is rerouted through a window in the palmar fascia radial to the pisiform or through a distally based loop created from a slip of FCU tendon sutured back onto itself.
- The FDS tendon is tunneled subcutaneously to another incision over the APB insertion, where it is sutured.
- Harvesting the FDS from its insertion results in an increased incidence of swan-neck deformity and proximal interphalangeal (PIP) joint flexion contractures[19,20] whereas tendon division proximal to the PIP joint helps to avoid this deformity.
- The PL (Camitz) transfer (Figure 18–8) is performed by extending a carpal tunnel incision to allow mobilization of the PL tendon, including a strip of palmar fascia distally to provide additional length.
- The PL tendon is redirected subcutaneously to another incision over the APB insertion, where it is secured.

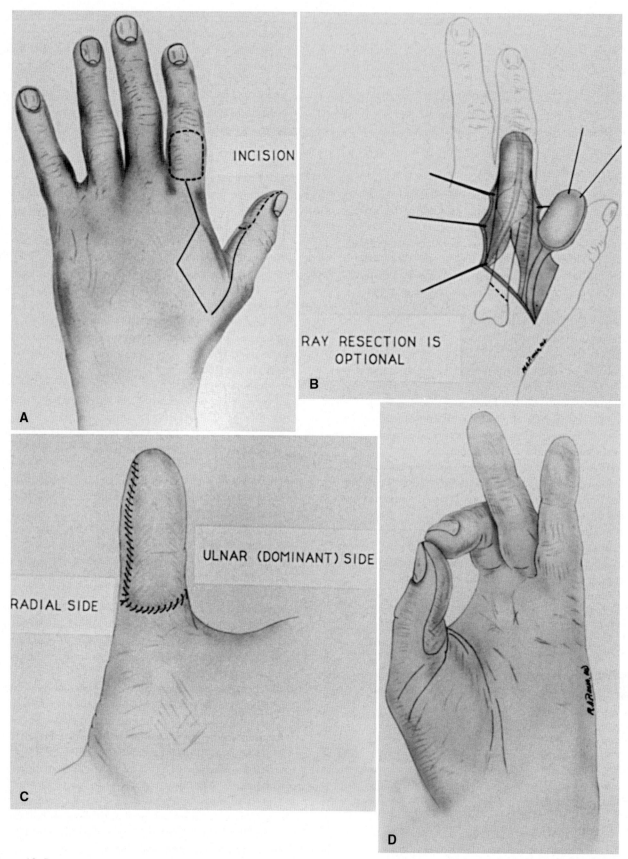

Figure 18–5:

Island pedicle flap for sensation in median nerve palsy. (From Omer GE Jr: Combined nerve palsies. In Green DP, Hotchkiss RN, Pederson WC, editors: *Green's operative hand surgery*. Philadelphia, 1999, Churchill Livingstone.)

| Box 18–5 | Tendon Transfers for Median Nerve Paralysis |
|---|---|

**Low median**

- EIP to APB
- FDS IV to APB
- PL to APB (Camitz)
- ADM to APB (Huber)

**High median**

- Above with the addition of
  - Side to side FDP ring/small to index/long
  - BR to FPL

- The abductor digiti minimi (ADM) Huber transfer (Figure 18–9), like the EIP transfer, is highly restricted in length.
- An incision is made over the ulnar border of the hand to allow mobilization of the ADM muscle, which is detached from its insertion at the base of the proximal phalanx.

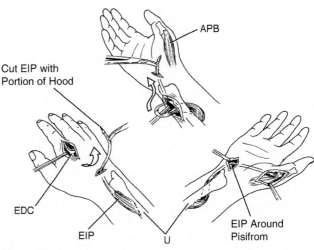

Figure 18–6:

Extensor indicis proprius *(EIP)* to abductor pollicis brevis *(APB)* opponensplasty for median nerve palsy. *EDC,* extensor digitorum communis; *U,* ulnar. (From Trumble T: *Principles of hand surgery and therapy*. Philadelphia, 2000, WB Saunders Company.)

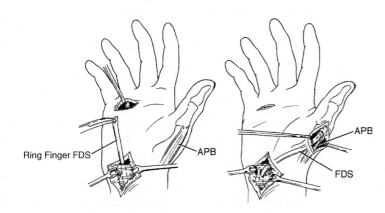

Figure 18–7:

Flexor digitorum superficialis *(FDS)* to abductor pollicis brevis *(APB)* opponensplasty for median nerve palsy. (From Trumble T: *Principles of hand surgery and therapy*. Philadelphia, 2000, WB Saunders Company.)

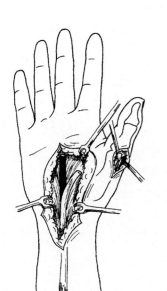
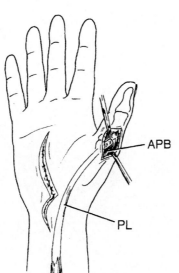

Figure 18–8:

Camitz opponensplasty for median nerve palsy. *APB,* abductor pollicis brevis; *PL,* palmaris longus. (From Trumble T: *Principles of hand surgery and therapy*. Philadelphia, 2000, WB Saunders Company.)

- The ADM is flipped over, hinging on its origin on the pisiform, and tunneled subcutaneously to an additional incision to insert at the APB insertion point.
- All opposition transfers should be tensioned to allow appropriate opposition with wrist dorsiflexion and allow full thumb adduction with wrist flexion.

## Postoperative Care

- Postoperatively the thumb should be splinted for 4 weeks in full opposition, with the wrist extended slightly in the EIP and ADM transfers and flexed slightly in the FDS and PL transfers.
- After week 4, a long opponens splint is used for an additional 4 weeks. The splint is removed to perform active thumb opposition exercises and wrist mobilization.
- Progressive strengthening and stretching exercises are initiated 2 months postoperatively.

## High Median Nerve Palsy

- Primary deficits in high median paralysis include (1) loss of opposition, (2) loss of index finger flexion and weak long finger flexion, (3) loss of thumb IP joint flexion, and (4) sensory loss.
- Opposition and sensory loss are corrected as noted in the Low Median Nerve Palsy Section.
- Side to side transfer of ring and small finger FDP tendons to long and index finger FDP tendons corrects finger flexion deficits (Figure 18–10).
- Tenodesis of the index distal interphalangeal (DIP) joint when performing side to side FDP transfer decreases the number of joints that the transfer must cross, thus increasing flexion at the remaining joints (see Figure 18–10).
- A distal forearm volar longitudinal incision is performed to expose the FDP tendons, which then are tenodesed with two separate transverse locking sutures.

- Transfer of BR to flexor pollicis longus (FPL) restores active thumb flexion (Figure 18–11).
- The first dorsal compartment is released to allow exposure of the BR insertion.
- BR is sharply elevated from the radius and freed from fascial attachments to improve its excursion.
- The FPL tendon, which is transected at the musculotendinous junction, is sutured to the BR using a Pulvertaft weave.
- Tension is set to allow full extension of the IP joint with 20 degrees wrist flexion and sufficient IP joint flexion with passive wrist extension.

## Postoperative Care

- In addition to the protocol listed for the associated thumb opposition transfer, the wrist should be immobilized in neutral or slight flexion.
- MCP and PIP joints should be in flexion with a dorsal block splint.
- Passive digit flexion and active extension exercises should be performed.
- At 3 weeks, place and hold exercises are initiated.
- At 6 weeks, wrist extension and tenodesis exercises are started.
- At 8 weeks, progressive strengthening and stretching exercises are performed.

## Ulnar Nerve Palsy

- Ulnar nerve injuries can be divided into low level (at the wrist) and high level (at the elbow). FDP involvement is the primary distinguishing characteristic (see Box 18–2).
- Patients with ulnar nerve injury have functional deficits resulting from paralysis of most of the hand intrinsic muscles (Box 18–6).

Figure 18–9:

Huber opponensplasty for median nerve palsy. *ADM,* abductor digiti minimi; *APB,* abductor pollicis brevis. (From Trumble T: *Principles of hand surgery and therapy.* Philadelphia, 2000, WB Saunders Company.)

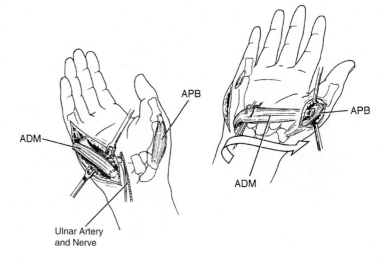

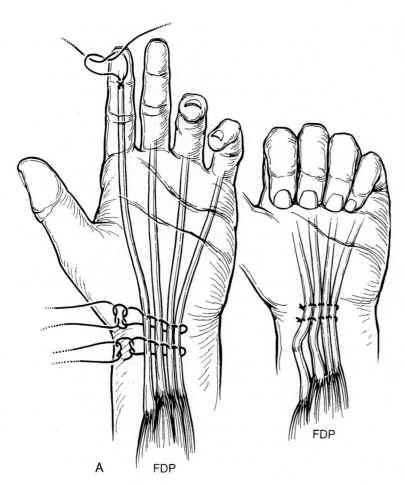

Figure 18–10:
Flexor digitorum profundus *(FDP)* side to side tenodesis with index distal interphalangeal tenodesis for high median nerve palsy. Side to side FDP tenodesis can be performed for high ulnar palsy as well; however, in ulnar palsy the index FDP can be left free to allow independent index flexion. (From Omer GE Jr: Combined nerve palsies. In Green DP, Hotchkiss RN, Pederson WC, editors: *Green's operative hand surgery.* Philadelphia, 1999, Churchill Livingstone.)

- Primary deficits in ulnar nerve palsies are (1) loss of hand fine motor coordination, (2) loss of power pinch, (3) persistent abducted small finger (Wartenberg sign, Table 18–4), (4) loss of power grip and normal transverse metacarpal arch, (5) clawing primarily involving ring and small fingers in low ulnar palsy, (6) lack of clawing, but loss of full flexion of ring and small fingers in high ulnar palsy, and (7) loss of ulnar hand sensation.[21,22]
- Because of variations in innervation pattern (see Box 18–6) and in muscle strength and joint mobility, functional deficits may vary; thus, treatment should be individualized.

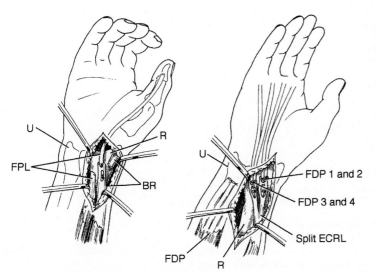

Figure 18–11:
Brachioradialis *(BR)* to flexor pollicis longus *(FPL)* transfer for median nerve palsy and extensor carpi radialis brevis *(ECRB)* to flexor digitorum profundus *(FDP)* for combined high median and ulnar nerve palsies. *R,* radius; *U,* ulna. (From Trumble T: *Principles of hand surgery and therapy.* Philadelphia, 2000, WB Saunders Company.)

| Box 18–6 | Ulnar Nerve Innervated Muscles |
|---|---|

- FCU
- FDP ring and small
- FDP long (partially innervated by median)
- Abductor digiti minimi
- Flexor digiti minimi
- Opponens digiti minimi
- Lumbricals ring and small
- 4 Dorsal interossei
- 3 Palmar interossei
- Adductor pollicis
- Deep head of flexor pollicis brevis

- Clawing is more significant in patients with low ulnar nerve palsy than high ulnar nerve palsy because the FDP, which is a primary component of the imbalance that causes clawing, is paralyzed in high ulnar palsy.

## Low Ulnar Nerve Palsy

- Although loss of interossei function creates deficits in precision hand motion, greater functional deficits exist that must be addressed via transfer of limited available motors.
- Small and ring finger clawing is commonly seen in low ulnar nerve injury because of paralysis of the interossei and lumbricals to these digits.
- Clawing occurs as extrinsic extensors attempt to produce IP extension in place of the paralyzed lumbricals. MCP hyperextension ensues because of lack of a stabilizing flexion force at the MCP joint. Increased tension on the extrinsic finger flexors because of MCP hyperextension results in flexion at the IP joints.[20]

- In addition to the cosmetic deformity, ulnar nerve palsy results in a functional deformity because of loss of sequential flexion of MCP, PIP and DIP joints. This asynchronous "roll-up" flexion deformity (Figure 18–12) limits the capacity to grasp objects of varying diameter.[16,20]
- Loss of power grip and metacarpal arch stability occurs because of paralysis of the interossei and hypothenar muscles.
- Paralysis of the adductor pollicis and first dorsal interosseous muscles results in significant weakness of thumb–index key and tip pinch.
- EPL can provide weak thumb adduction, with further contribution of the FPL resulting in increased power and hyperflexion of the thumb IP joint (Froment sign, see Table 18–4). The FPL helps to make the EPL into a more effective adductor by increasing the tension on the EPL as thumb IP joint flexion increases.
- Small finger hyperabduction occurs as a result of persistent extensor digiti minimi (EDM) tone with paralysis of the small finger palmar interosseous muscle.
- Primary goals of treatment of low ulnar nerve palsy are correction of clawing and the associated roll-up functional deformity, improvement of thumb power pinch, restoration of the metacarpal arch, and correction of persistent small finger abduction. However, individual patients vary in their needs and deficit pattern, so an individualized approach to transfers is necessary in ulnar nerve palsies.
- Table 18–5 lists reconstructive options recommended by Omer for low ulnar nerve palsy.
- Procedures to correct clawing can be divided into static and dynamic transfers.

| Table 18–4: Diagnostic Eponyms in Ulnar Nerve Palsy | |
|---|---|
| Duchenne sign (1867) | Clawing of ring and small fingers |
| Bouvier maneuver (1851) | If MP hyperextension blocked, IP extension can occur |
| Andre-Thomas sign (1917) | Hyperflexion of wrist in an attempt to improve IP extension |
| Pitres-Testut sign (1925) | Inability to abduct the extended long finger in radial and ulnar deviation<br>Inability to bring extended fingertips to a cone |
| Wartenberg sign (1930) | Inability to adduct the extended small finger |
| Jeanne sign (1915) | Thumb MP hyperextension with key pinch or gross grip |
| Froment sign (1915) | Hyperflexion of the thumb IP joint with key pinch |
| Masse sign (1916) | Flattening of the palmar metacarpal arch |
| Pollock sign (1919) | Weakness of DIP flexion of ring and small finger |
| Martin (1763)–Gruber (1870) | Median or anterior interosseus nerve branch to ulnar nerve<br>Communications in proximal forearm carrying motor fiber communications to intrinsics |
| Riche (1897)–Cannieu (1897) | Motor fibers from recurrent motor branch of median nerve<br>Communications to motor branch of ulnar nerve in the palm |

From Sheppard JE: Tendon transfers. In Trumble T, editor: *Hand surgery update 3*. Rosemont, IL, 2003, American Society for Surgery of the Hand.

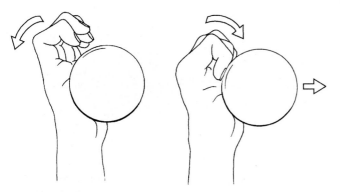

Figure 18–12:

**Roll-up posture in ulnar nerve palsy. (From Trumble T:** *Principles of hand surgery and therapy.* **Philadelphia, 2000, WB Saunders Company.)**

- Brandsma and Hastings note that while static corrective procedures (arthrodesis, capsulodesis and tenodesis) will correct cosmetic deformity, dynamic procedures (tendon transfers) are necessary to correct functional deficits as well as cosmesis.[20,23]
- Brandsma and Brand[20] recommend against using static procedures in patients with only intrinsic paralysis.
- Capsulodesis procedures stretch out over time in patients with strong extrinsic extensors and should be used only in patients with weak or absent extensors, such as patients with combined palsies.
- Although Omer[21] prefers the ECRL transfer to correct clawing, Goldfarb and Stern[24] recommend using a Zancolli lasso or modified Stiles-Bunnell transfer for clawing and provide an excellent description of the most common and reliable transfers for low ulnar nerve palsy.
- The Zancolli lasso procedure (Figure 18–13) transfers the FDS between the A1 and A2 pulleys and sutures it back onto itself.

- The Zancolli lasso procedure is excellent at preventing MCP hyperextension but results in some MCP flexion contracture.
- The modified Stiles-Bunnell procedure (Figure 18–14) also uses the FDS and is elegant in that it allows both MCP flexion and IP joint extension if inserted into the lateral band. However, it does not produce significant grip strength.
- Bouvier maneuver (see Table 18–4) should be performed to determine the existence of extensor lag, in which case the modified Stiles-Bunnell transfer provides additional IP extension and thus improved results.[25]
- Use of a wrist extensor (Brand transfer) (Figure 18–15) may result in stronger grip. However, the procedure, which requires tendon grafting and passage through the intermetacarpal spaces, increases the risk of adhesions and does not restore the metacarpal arch.
- The Brand transfer does not allow use of ECRB for thumb adductorplasty.
- Transfers to correct clawing that pass through the carpal canal also improve the flattened metacarpal arch and are the most mechanically efficient. However, they may not provide as strong of a grip as dorsal transfers.[26]
- Harvesting the FDS tendon may result in swan-neck deformity at the PIP joint. Therefore, Omer[21] harvests only half of the tendon insertion, tenodesing the other half across the PIP joint to prevent hyperextension.
- Brandsma and Brand[20] note that clawing may not be apparent in the index and long fingers at rest. However, with applied functional stress, clawing may occur as the only remaining MCP stabilizing force is the relatively weak lumbricals. Thus, transfers to correct clawing should include slips to the index and long fingers.
- All transfers to correct clawing must pass palmar to the transverse metacarpal ligament.

## Table 18–5: Transfers for Low Ulnar Nerve Palsy

| NEEDED FUNCTION | PREFERRED TRANSFER | ALTERNATIVE TRANSFER |
|---|---|---|
| Thumb adduction for key pinch | ECRB with free tendon graft between 3rd and 4th metacarpals to abductor tubercle of thumb | Long FDS to abductor tubercle of thumb with palmar fascia as the pulley |
| Proximal phalanx power flexion and integration of MCP and IP motion (clawed fingers) | ECRL with four-tailed free tendon graft passed palmar to deep transverse metacarpal ligament to either A2 pulley of flexor sheath or to radial band of dorsal apparatus | FCR (if wrist flexion contracture) with four-tailed free tendon graft to A2 pulley |
| Thumb-index tip pinch | Accessory slip of APL to first dorsal interosseous tendon and arthrodesis of thumb MP joint | EPB to first dorsal interosseous tendon (if thumb MP joint arthrodesed) |
| Metacarpal arch and adduction for the little finger | EDM tendon split and ulnar half transferred palmar to deep transverse metacarpal ligament to proximal phalanx or radial band of dorsal apparatus | If little finger clawed as well as abducted, insert ulnar half EDM into A2 pulley of flexor sheath |
| Volar sensibility for fingers | Proximal median digital nerve translocated to distal ulnar digital nerve | Free or vascularized nerve graft |

From Omer GE Jr: Ulnar nerve palsy. In Green DP, Hotchkiss RN, Pederson WC, editors: *Green's operative hand surgery.* Philadelphia, 1999, Churchill Livingstone.

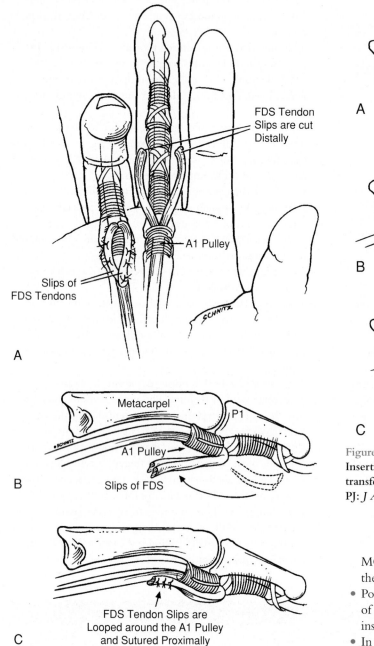

Figure 18–13:
Zancolli lasso procedure to correct claw deformity. *FDS,*
flexor digitorum superficialis. (From Goldfarb CA, Stern PJ:
*J Am Soc Surg Hand* 3:14-26, 2003.)

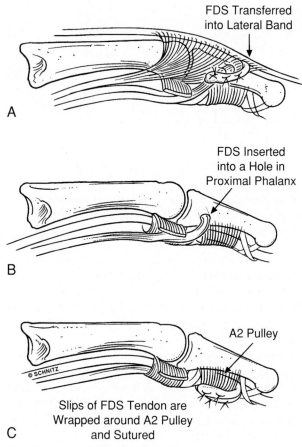

Figure 18–14:
Insertion options for flexor digitorum superficialis *(FDS)*
transfer to correct claw deformity. (From Goldfarb CA, Stern
PJ: *J Am Soc Surg Hand* 3:14-26, 2003.)

- Transfer insertion point in correction of clawing is a
  critical consideration and should be determined based on
  the patient's functional goals.
- Options for insertion point of transfers correcting
  clawing include (1) lateral bands, (2) A2 pulley, and
  (3) bone of proximal phalanx.[24]
- Lee and Rodriguez[26] note that insertion on the
  A2 pulley is the most effective site biomechanically for

MCP flexion; however, lateral band insertion results in
the most effective PIP and DIP extension.
- Power pinch of the thumb is achieved reliably by transfer
  of the ECRB with a tendon graft (Smith transfer) to the
  insertion of the adductor pollicis (Figure 18–16).[27]
- In the Smith transfer, the ECRB is released from its
  insertion and brought out to lie dorsal to the extensor
  retinaculum. A tendon graft then is passed through the
  second intermetacarpal space from an incision at the
  ulnar aspect of the thumb MCP joint using a hemostat.
- The graft is attached to the adductor pollicis insertion
  and woven into the ECRB to allow the thumb to rest
  against the radial border of the index finger in neutral
  wrist flexion, allowing thumb abduction and adduction
  against the index finger with wrist extension and flexion,
  respectively.
- Key pinch also can be achieved by transferring the ring
  FDS through a palmar fascia pulley to the abductor
  tubercle of the thumb (Figure 18–17). However, this
  procedure results in further reduction in grip strength.

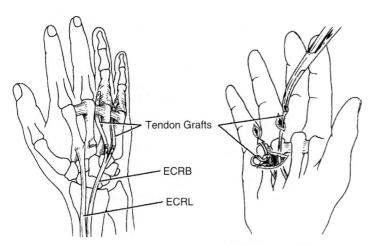

Figure 18–15:
**Brand transfer to correct clawing in ulnar nerve palsy.** *ECRB,* extensor carpi radialis brevis; *ECRL,* extensor carpi radialis longus. (From Trumble T: *Principles of hand surgery and therapy.* Philadelphia, 2000, WB Saunders Company.)

- Omer[21] recommends thumb MCP arthrodesis to improve thumb tip stability during key and tip pinch in patients with instability of these joints.
- Correction of abduction of the small finger can be performed by releasing the ulnar tendon insertion of the

EDM, passing it palmar to the transverse metacarpal ligament, and inserting it onto the radial collateral ligament or A2 pulley on the radial side of the small finger.

## High Ulnar Nerve Palsy

- Patients with high ulnar nerve lesions typically have paralysis of the FDP to the ring and small fingers. They may also have FCU paralysis.
- Clawing typically is not seen in high ulnar nerve palsy because of extrinsic flexor paralysis. However, clawing results when transfers are performed to provide finger flexion, so procedures to correct clawing also must be performed.
- Transfers as noted for low ulnar nerve palsy should be performed in addition to transfer to achieve active finger flexion.
- The ring FDS should not be used for transfers if the ring FDP is paralyzed.

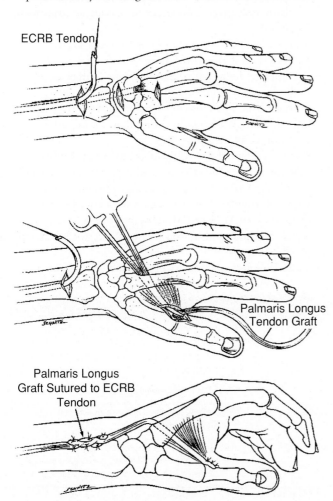

Figure 18–16:
**Extensor carpi radialis brevis** *(ECRB)* **to adductor pollicis** (Smith) transfer for power pinch in ulnar nerve palsy. (From Goldfarb CA, Stern PJ: *J Am Soc Surg Hand* 3:14-26, 2003.)

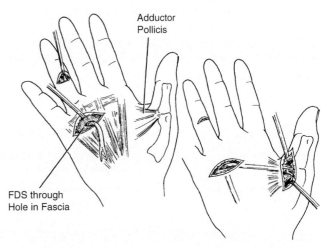

Figure 18–17:
**Flexor digitorum superficialis** *(FDS)* **adductorplasty for power pinch in ulnar nerve palsy.** (From Trumble T: *Principles of hand surgery and therapy.* Philadelphia, 2000, WB Saunders Company.)

- Side to side tenodesis of the ring and small FDPs to the long FDP can improve finger flexion strength, leaving the index FDP free to provide independent index finger flexion.
- Side to side tenodesis should be performed with two separate transverse locking sutures. The small and ring fingers should be place in partial flexion to maximize grip strength with FDP contraction (see Figure 18–10).
- Loss of FCU function typically does not need to be addressed by transfer.
- Loss of sensibility can be addressed as in patients with median nerve palsy. However, patients with complete anesthesia of the small finger may be better served by amputation of the digit.

## Postoperative Care

- Following transfers to correct clawing, the hand is placed in a splint for 3 weeks, maintaining the IP joints in extension and the MCP joints in 70 degrees flexion. If the FDS is used, the wrist is placed in slight flexion. If a wrist extensor is used, the wrist is placed in slight extension.
- After week 3, active ROM is started within a dorsal block splint that maintains MCP joint flexion and IP joint extension. A hand-based protective splint is used between therapy sessions.
- At week 6, active MCP joint extension is initiated.
- At week 8, gentle strengthening and stretching exercises are performed.
- At week 12, unrestricted use is permitted.
- Following transfer to allow power pinch, the thumb is splinted in an adducted position against the index finger.
- The wrist is kept in slight extension if Smith transfer is performed and in slight flexion if FDS transfer is performed.
- At week 4, gentle thumb active ROM exercises are initiated, and a removable hand-based splint maintaining the thumb in adduction is used between therapy sessions.

- At week 8, gentle resistive and tenodesis exercises are started.
- At week 10, strengthening exercises are started.

## Combined Nerve Paralysis

- Because of the significant combined deficit in function and sensory loss, most injuries to multiple nerves result in an extremity that will be used only as a helping hand. However, transfers are critical to provide function to the bilaterally involved individual.
- The loss of sensation and proprioception severely limits function even after tendon transfer. Neurovascular reconstruction should be performed to provide sensibility.
- Because of the limited motors available, careful planning should be performed based on available donors and needed function.
- As noted by Eversmann,[28] efforts to obtain tissue equilibrium are critical in the patient with multiple nerve injuries because soft tissue injury usually is extensive. Use of silastic rods may be necessary to provide an appropriate tissue bed.
- Transfers should be planned so that the transferred tendons do not cross, thus limiting scarring.
- A complete discussion of the treatment of injuries to multiple nerves is beyond the scope of this chapter; however, combined low median and ulnar nerve palsy are discussed briefly because together they are the most common combined palsy.
- Omer[29] presented six requirements for wrist and hand function restoration: (1) improved key pinch, (2) restored thumb abduction, (3) true tip pinch between thumb and index, (4) improved power flexion with coordination or integration of MCP and IP joint motion, (5) restored metacarpal arch, and (6) specific sensibility for key or tip pinch.
- Table 18–6 lists transfers to achieve these requirements.

## Table 18–6: Transfers for Combined Low Median and Ulnar Nerve Palsy

| NEEDED FUNCTION | PREFERRED TRANSFER | ALTERNATIVE TRANSFER |
|---|---|---|
| Thumb adduction | ECRB to abductor tubercle | FDS (long) to abductor tubercle if not bound by palmar scar |
| Thumb opposition | EIP via pulley to APB insertion | PL or FDS if not involved in injury |
| Thumb-index tip pinch | APL with tendon graft to first dorsal interosseous + thumb MCP joint arthrodesis | EPB or PL to first dorsal interosseous + thumb MCP arthrodesis |
| Restoration metacarpal arch | EDM split to radial collateral ligament of small MCP or A2 pulley | FDS (small) deep to transverse metacarpal ligament between fourth and fifth MC or FDS (long or ring) combined for thumb adduction and metacarpal arch |
| Power flexion MCP joint and integration of MCP and IP joint motion | ECRL or BR with four-tailed tendon graft to A2 pulley or lateral bands | FCR with four-tailed tendon graft to A2 pulley or lateral bands |
| Restoration sensibility | Sensory superficial radial nerve translocation | Flag flap or fillet flap from index to volar thumb |

Adapted from Omer GE Jr: Combined nerve palsies. In Green DP, Hotchkiss RN, Pederson WC, editors: *Green's operative hand surgery.* Philadelphia, 1999, Churchill Livingstone.

- Postoperative rehabilitation should follow the course described for each individual transfer. However, because multiple surgical procedures often are necessary, they should be planned to allow similar rehabilitation goals and postoperative splinting requirements.

# References

1. Smith RJ: *Tendon transfers of the hand and forearm.* Boston, 1987, Little, Brown and Company.
   This classic text comprises a complete discussion of all aspects of tendon transfer surgery by one of the key contributors in the field.

2. Brand PW: Biomechanics of tendon transfer. *Orthop Clin North Am* 5:205-230, 1974.
   An excellent discussion of the biomechanical principles of tendon transfers for peripheral neuropathy of the upper extremity.

3. Brand PW, Beach RB, Thompson DE: Relative tension and potential excursion of muscles in the forearm and hand. *J Hand Surg* 6A:209-219, 1981.
   A complete review of key characteristics of forearm muscles and the relationship of these factors to work capacity and potential excursion in tendon transfers.

4. Fridén J, Lieber RL: Tendon transfer surgery: clinical implications of experimental studies. *Clin Orthop* 403S:S163-S170, 2002.
   Discusses the implications of appropriate length-tension relationships during tendon transfers. The concept of muscle adaption in tendon transfers is discussed.

5. Brand PW: Biomechanics of tendon transfers. *Hand Clin* 4:137-154, 1988.
   An updated version of Dr. Brand's concepts with expansion of previous principles.

6. Grabb WC: Management of nerve injuries in the forearm and hand. *Orthop Clin North Am* 1:419-431, 1970.
   A description of the cellular level changes in peripheral nerve injury, with a discussion of factors that affect outcome of nerve repair. Techniques of nerve repair are discussed.

7. Ring D, Chin K, Jupiter JB: Radial nerve palsy associated with high-energy humeral shaft fractures. *J Hand Surg* 29A:144-147, 2004.
   Review of radial nerve palsy following high-energy humeral shaft fracture.

8. Green DP: Radial nerve palsy. In Green DP, Hotchkiss RN, Pederson WC, editors: *Green's operative hand surgery.* Philadelphia, 1999, Churchill Livingstone.
   A discussion of the author's extensive personal experience, including historical vignettes that add to the inherent beauty of a discussion of this subject.

9. Omer GE: Timing of tendon transfers in peripheral nerve injury. *Hand Clin* 4:317-322, 1988.
   Dr. Omer reviews initial patient evaluation, timing of surgery, and general technical aspects of tendon transfer surgery.

10. Iyer VG: Understanding nerve conduction and electromyographic studies. *Hand Clin* 9:273-287, 1993.
    A complete, clear discussion of electrodiagnostic tests with review of definitions, indications, and interpretation.

11. Brumback RA, Bobele GB, Rayan GM: Electrodiagnosis of compressive nerve lesions. *Hand Clin* 8:241-254, 1992.
    A review of nerve and muscle physiology and the role of electrodiagnostic studies in the evaluation of nerve lesions.

12. Mackin GA, Gordon MJ, Neville HE, Ringel SP: Restoring hand function in patients with severe polyneuropathy: the role of electromyography before tendon transfer surgery. *J Hand Surg* 24A:732-742, 1999.
    Discusses the benefits of using preoperative electromyography in patients with functionless hands secondary to slowly progressive polyneuropathies.

13. Grossman JAI, Pomerance J: Staged opposition transfer. *J Hand Surg* 23A:290-295, 1998.
    Use of a staged reconstruction with the initial stage consisting of tendon-rod placement prior to the second stage of tendon transfer is outlined.

14. Zachary RB: Tendon transplantation for radial paralysis. *Br J Surg* 23:358-364, 1946.
    This study emphasizes retention of a strong wrist flexor to retain the tenodesis effect of the wrist when performing tendon transfers for radial nerve palsy.

15. Strickland JW, Kleinman WB: Tendon transfers for radial nerve paralysis. In Strickland JW, editor: *Master techniques in orthopaedic surgery, the hand.* Philadelphia, 1998, Lippincott-Raven Publishers.
    The authors outline current options and the associated factors involved in the final decision for tendon transfers for radial nerve paralysis.

16. Trumble T: *Principles of hand surgery and therapy.* Philadelphia, 2000, WB Saunders Company.
    Dr. Trumble's excellent chapter on tendon transfers includes all of the key elements involved in successful tendon transfers.

17. Lieber RL, Jacobson MD, Fazeli BM et al: Architecture of selected muscles of the arm and forearm: anatomy and implications for tendon transfer. *J Hand Surg* 17A:787-798, 1992.
    This anatomic study evaluates the architecture of the muscles in the forearm and relates the architecture to the contractile properties of potential donor muscles.

18. Omer GE Jr: Tendon transfers for median nerve paralysis. In Strickland JW, editor: *Master techniques in orthopaedic surgery, the hand.* Philadelphia, 1998, Lippincott-Raven Publishers.
    A well-illustrated guide to the surgical techniques of transfers for median nerve palsy.

19. Davis TRC, Barton NJ: Median nerve palsy. In Green DP, Hotchkiss RN, Pederson WC, editors: *Green's operative hand surgery.* Philadelphia, 1999, Churchill Livingstone.
    The authors provide excellent background of the functional deficits associated with median nerve palsy and discuss their impressions and preferences.

20. Brandsma JW, Brand PW: Claw-finger correction: considerations in choice of technique. *J Hand Surg* 17B:615-621, 1992.
An excellent description of the etiology of deformity and disability after ulnar nerve injury, with a discussion of tendon transfer options.

21. Omer GE Jr: Ulnar nerve palsy. In Green DP, Hotchkiss RN, Pederson WC, editors: *Green's operative hand surgery*. Philadelphia, 1999, Churchill Livingstone.
Impeccably written by a surgeon with immense experience with the functional restoration of the intrinsic deficient hand. Extensively referenced and illustrated.

22. Sheppard JE: Tendon transfers. In Trumble T, editor: *Hand surgery update 3*. Rosemont, IL, 2003, American Society for Surgery of the Hand.
A review of key concepts in tendon transfer surgery with complete annotated bibliography.

23. Hastings H II: Ulnar nerve paralysis. In Strickland JW, editor: *Master techniques in orthopaedic surgery, the hand*. Philadelphia, 1998, Lippincott-Raven Publishers.
Dr. Hastings was a fellow of Dr. Richard J. Smith. This well-illustrated chapter outlines the surgical treatment of ulnar nerve palsy.

24. Goldfarb CA, Stern PJ: Low ulnar nerve palsy. *J Am Soc Surg Hand* 3:14-26, 2003.
A discussion of the clinical presentation of patients with intrinsic deficit, with a well-illustrated review of the most reliable transfers for low ulnar nerve palsy.

25. Özkan T, Özer K, Gülgönen A: Three tendon transfer methods in reconstruction of ulnar nerve palsy. *J Hand Surg* 28A:35-43, 2003.
The authors recommend use of Zancolli lasso or ECRL transfer in patients with short-term paralysis who require increased grip strength, whereas modified Stiles-Bunnell transfer was recommended to correct clawing and disability in patients with long-standing paralysis with extensor lag.

26. Lee DH, Rodriguez JA, Jr: Tendon transfers for restoring hand intrinsic muscle function: a biomechanical study. *J Hand Surg* 24A:609-613, 1999.
Notes that the volar route appears to be more efficient than a dorsal intermetacarpal route and that lateral band insertion provides a small but significant increase in PIP and DIP joint extension. The A2 pulley insertion site is the most efficient for achieving MCP flexion.

27. Smith RJ: Extensor carpi radialis brevis tendon transfer for thumb adduction: a study of power pinch. *J Hand Surg* 8:4-15, 1983.
Describes tendon transfer options for restoring power pinch in patients with ulnar nerve deficits.

28. Eversmann WW Jr: Tendon transfers for combined nerve injuries. *Hand Clin* 4:187-199, 1988.
Discusses tendon transfers for combined lesions of peripheral nerves including a unified postoperative rehabilitation program and using dynamic tenodeses.

29. Omer GE Jr: Combined nerve palsies. In Green DP, Hotchkiss RN, Pederson WC, editors: *Green's operative hand surgery*. Philadelphia, 1999, Churchill Livingstone.
Another exceptional chapter on tendon transfers in Green's text. Dr. Omer presents an extensive discussion of options for treating multiple-nerve injured patients.

# CHAPTER 19

# Dupuytren's Disease

## John D. Lubahn

MD, Chairman, Department of Orthopaedic Surgery, Hamot Medical Center, Erie, PA

## Introduction

- Dupuytren's disease is a clinical entity that is commonplace in every hand surgeon's practice and is frequently encountered by any physician who treats patients with maladies of the musculoskeletal system.
- Since Dupuytren's original description and lecture on December 5, 1831, the disease has been treated surgically when severe contractures are present and function is compromised.
- Some of the earliest descriptions of Dupuytren's disease can be found in the book *Observationum in Hominis Affectibus* by Felix Plater,[1] published in 1614.
- Earlier references can be found in the Scandinavian literature, but a comprehensive, accurate, written description of the disease did not appear until 1777, when Cline described Dupuytren's disease as originating in the palmar fascia and performed the first anatomic dissection of the palmar fascia.
- In 1787, Cline proposed, but never performed, fasciectomy. In 1822, his student Sir Astley Cooper performed the first fasciectomy on a patient. In 1831, Dupuytren recommended open limited fasciectomy through transverse incisions, leaving the wound open and splinting the hand in extension.
- These principles of treatment are still applied today by most hand surgeons around the world for the day-to-day treatment of Dupuytren's disease.

## Epidemiology

- Dupuytren's disease is common in people of northern European ancestry. In a study from England, based on medical interviews, Ling[2] found a 16% incidence of Dupuytren's disease when he interviewed patients and obtained a family history. When relatives were examined, the incidence rose to 68%. Based on this study, he concludes that Dupuytren's disease is a mendelian dominant gene.
- Dupuytren's disease has been associated with diabetes, tuberculosis, and AIDS, the latter believed to be related to an alteration in free-radical metabolism.
- Seizure disorders have been associated with Dupuytren's disease, perhaps through abnormal metabolism of scar tissue in the brain or the hand or perhaps through a side effect of various anticonvulsant therapies.
- The disease has been associated with minor trauma and has developed after cuts or closed injury to the palm. However, Zachariae[3] showed that, in Scandinavia, the disease was as common in office workers as it was in factory workers.
- Cytokines, which are hormone-like peptides found in humans, have been shown to be mitogenic in human cells and may be capable of stimulating transformation of human fibroblasts into myofibroblasts (a principle cell type found in Dupuytren's disease).
- Transforming growth factor (TGF-β), platelet-derived growth factor, fibroblast growth factor, and possibly even nerve growth factor may be responsible.

## Normal Anatomy

- Typically the palmar fascia is a triangular-shaped fascial structure with its apex pointed proximally and the base of the triangle at the metacarpophalangeal joints (Figure 19–1). It is composed of four longitudinal bands overlying the rays to each digit and is attached to the skin through fibrous septa and to the underlying intrinsic muscles through the ligaments of Legueu and Juvara. These ligaments are actually fibrous septa that divide the palm into seven canals, with each tendon and neurovascular bundle occupying a canal. More distal and transverse in the palm is the superficial transverse metacarpal ligament. This structure and Cleland's ligament, located dorsally and running obliquely from the bone to the skin, and Grayson's ligament, lying palmar and running transversely from the flexor sheath to the skin, effectively surround the neurovascular bundle (Figure 19–2).

## Pathophysiology/Abnormal Anatomy

- The clinical pathoanatomy of Dupuytren's disease begins as a nodule in the palmar fascia.
- Histologically, in this early stage of the disease, the nodule is filled with an abundance of cells, predominantly fibroblasts and myofibroblasts.
- The collagen surrounding the cells contains an increased amount of type III collagen compared to normal cells,

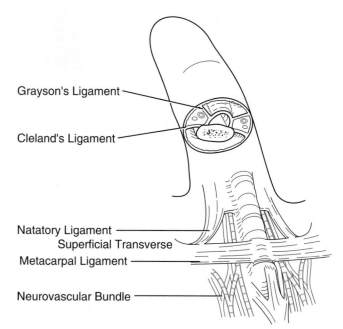

**Figure 19–2:**

**Schematic diagram of the fascial structures of the finger showing Grayson's ligament lying palmar to the neurovascular bundle and running transversely from the flexor sheath to the skin. Lying more dorsally is Cleland's ligament running in a more oblique direction from the phalanx to the skin. The lateral digital sheet of Gosset forms the base of the triangle surrounding the neurovascular bundle.**

which contain primarily type I collagen. Type III collagen is found in greater proportions in scar tissue, is less elastic, and may explain the similar behavior between Dupuytren's tissue and scar tissue.

- One manifestation of the genetic predisposition to the disease in addition to the increased levels of type III collagen may be increased levels of free-radical formation in the palm. This finding has been associated in Great Britain with an increased incidence of the disease in HIV-positive patients. Treatment with free-radical scavengers may hold some promise for these individuals.
- In the palm of the hand, the nodule extends to the longitudinally oriented normal bands of the palmar fascia. Typically, as the disease progresses, the nodule and these bands form a pathologic cord that often causes dimpling of the skin. This cord extends through the fibrous septa of the palm distally to the finger, where the evolution from normal fascial structures to diseased fascia is less clear.
- As the diseased fascia extends from the palm to the finger, it may wrap around the neurovascular bundle, pulling it to a more superficial subcutaneous position. A dimple in the fold with soft pulpy compressible skin in the distal palm as described by Short and Watson[4] should alert the surgeon that the neurovascular bundle may lie in a superficial position. In this case, careful proximal to

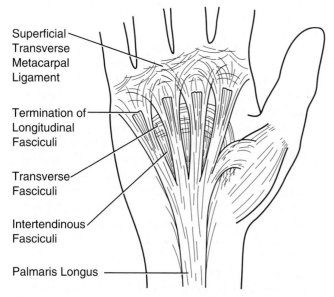

**Figure 19–1:**

**Schematic diagram of the palmar fascia showing longitudinal bands that become cords in the disease state. Running superficially, distally, and transversely is the superficial transverse metacarpal ligament, which does not become involved in Dupuytren's disease.**

distal dissection is necessary to protect the common digital nerve. The surgeon should remember that the nerve almost always is forced toward the midline and into a more superficial position by the cord. This relationship typically is called a *spiral cord* (Figure 19–3).

- The diseased fascia is filled with myofibroblasts, which contain elements of smooth muscle actin.
- The myofibroblasts are attached to each other at areas called *desmosomes*. As the smooth muscle contracts, considerable force can be exerted from one cell to another.[5]
- The diseased fascia in the central cord extends across the metacarpophalangeal joint to the finger. As the cord contracts, the finger is pulled into flexion. The proximal interphalangeal (PIP) joint also may become involved as the diseased palmar fascia extends along the lateral digital sheet and Grayson's ligaments. A spiral cord may exist at this level bringing the neurovascular bundle to a more subcutaneous position on the finger similar to the palm.

## Clinical History

- Patients typically present with a tender nodule in the palm. Pain may vary in intensity, from nearly no pain to quite significant pain.

- Patients often describe a history of trauma, but no clear correlation with injury has been proven. If the disease progresses into a contracture, the metacarpophalangeal joint typically is involved, such that the hand cannot be placed flat on a tabletop.
- The PIP joint also may be involved, limiting finger extension and compromising function.
- Patients often complain of difficulty retrieving objects from a pocket, wearing gloves, and other aspects of personal hygiene.
- Associated clinical findings may include knuckle pads (Garrod) over the dorsum of the PIP joints (Figure 19–4).
- Ledderhose's disease is a similar condition on the plantar fascia of the foot. Patients typically complain of pain associated with long periods of standing and certain types of shoe wear.
- Peyronie's disease involves the penile fascia.
- Carpal tunnel syndrome may be seen in association with Dupuytren's disease. Controversy exists as to whether the carpal tunnel syndrome should be treated first and then the Dupuytren's disease, or whether the two can be treated simultaneously. Nissenbaum and Kleinert[6] believed concomitant carpal tunnel release and palmar fasciectomy could result in postoperative complications such as swelling and complex regional pain syndrome. They suggested treating the more symptomatic condition first. In contrast, Michon[7] believed the two conditions could be treated safely during one surgical setting, as did Gonzalez and Watson.[8]

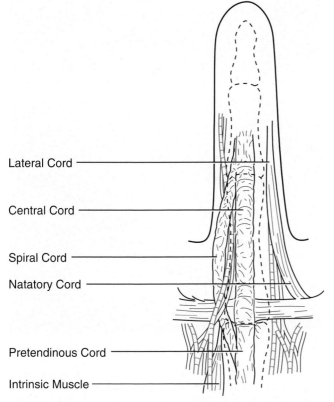

Lateral Cord

Central Cord

Spiral Cord

Natatory Cord

Pretendinous Cord

Intrinsic Muscle

Figure 19–3:
Relationship between the spiral cord and the neurovascular bundle as the spiral cord forces the neurovascular bundle toward the midline.

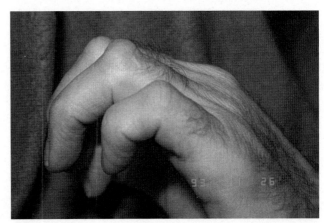

Figure 19–4:
Patient with thickened tissue over the dorsum of the proximal interphalangeal joint of all digits. This accumulation of fibrous tissue is called a *knuckle pad*. Surgical removal often results in an aggressive recurrence. Injection may quell periods of inflammation and pain. Benign neglect may offer the best solution because the knuckle pad usually becomes asymptomatic with time.

- Diabetes may be seen with Dupuytren's disease. Glucose levels should be monitored closely to minimize postoperative complications.
- Seizure disorders are not a contraindication to surgery but should warn the surgeon that the patient may have a more aggressive form of the disease.
- Trigger finger may be seen in association with Dupuytren's disease, and release can be performed simultaneously. One rare indication for removal of a solitary nodule is in association with release of a trigger finger.
- Boutonnière deformity should be differentiated from severe PIP joint flexion contracture. Hyperextension of the distal interphalangeal (DIP) joint should alert the surgeon that a boutonnière is present. When the oblique retinacular ligament test is positive (resistance to passive DIP joint flexion when the PIP joint is held passively extended), the surgeon should recognize that the lateral bands have slipped palmar to the axis of PIP joint flexion, and the central slip of the dorsal apparatus has become attenuated. Successful treatment may consist of splinting the PIP joint in extension postoperatively combined with passive DIP joint flexion. In cases of severe DIP joint extension contracture, tenotomy of the terminal tendon of the dorsal apparatus as described by Fowler may be indicated.

## Nonoperative Treatment

- Multiple nonsurgical treatments have been attempted, including injection with trypsin and/or corticosteroids, such as methylprednisolone (Depo-Medrol). Depo-Medrol injection has proved to be beneficial in patients with early, painful, small nodules and in patients with aggressive recurrence of the disease. From 20 to 40 mg of a mixture of lidocaine and Depo-Medrol is injected into the nodule or an area of inflamed, recurrent disease. Although the condition is not cured, some degree of palliation of the process can be expected.
- Medications that have been attempted include nonsteroidal antiinflammatory drugs, allopurinol, and, in unpublished reports from Great Britain, Viagra.
- In some early contractures involving the metacarpophalangeal joint, injection-using collagenase has been beneficial in correcting the contracture.[9] Unfortunately collagenase is a new and experimental procedure and is not yet approved for general use.

## Surgical Indications

- Removal of the early, tender nodule often can result in a flare-type reaction and may worsen the condition or cause it to return early with more severe involvement. Likewise, areas called *knuckle pads* located over the dorsum of the PIP joint are better treated with local

injection of corticosteroid or nonsteroidal medication. A tender nodule noted early also can be injected. Occasionally these nodules are seen in association with trigger finger and should be injected along with the trigger finger. If the nodules continue to occur or remain symptomatic at the time of trigger finger release, they can be removed and studied histologically.

- Patients with Dupuytren's disease often have few complaints. However, complaints may include difficulty retrieving coins from pockets, wearing gloves, shaking hands, or performing personal hygiene tasks such as washing the face or shaving.
- The so-called table test (Figure 19–5) is an indication for surgical intervention, particularly if the patient's inability to place the hand flat on a tabletop compromises any of the aforementioned activities. Contractures that

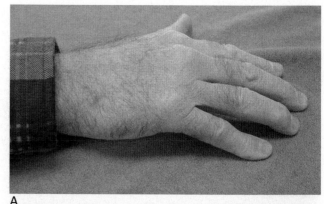

A

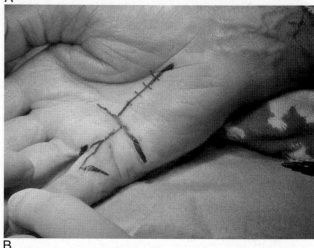

B

Figure 19–5:

**A,** A positive table top test shown here with a metacarpophalangeal joint flexion contracture. When present, the patient cannot place his/her hand flat on the surface. **B,** The incision extends proximally as far as the diseased fascia is located. A transverse incision is made in the distal palm and a longitudinal incision extends onto the involved digit and is broken up by a Z-plasty.

progress significantly over short periods are an indication for surgical treatment. In general, PIP joint contractures of 40 degrees or more are released, noting that the procedure becomes more difficult as the degree of contracture progresses.  A PIP joint contracture of 40 degrees in the ring or small finger may be better tolerated and allow the patient to grip objects more easily than the 40 degree contracture in the long or index finger. While Dupuytren's disease is more common in the ring and small fingers, PIP joint contractures are poorly tolerated in the long and index fingers. Patients with no complaint or true functional loss for their vocational and avocational interests remain best served with nonsurgical treatment.

## Surgical Treatment

- A classic surgical technique in Dupuytren's disease is the open palmar fasciectomy as described by McCash.[10] This technique has been my preferred surgical treatment for 20 years.  The procedure begins by outlining the skin incisions (Figure 19–6). A transverse incision is made in the distal palm. A zigzag incision is extended proximally toward the apex of the palmar fascia. Longitudinal incisions are extended toward each of the involved fingers, outlining 60-degree Z-plasties where appropriate if the PIP is also involved in the contracture. Tourniquet control is important to allow clear visualization of the neurovascular structures and their relationship to the diseased fascia. In cooperative patients with single digit involvement, the procedure usually can be performed with local anesthesia or wrist block combined with intravenous conscious sedation. For more extensive disease, axillary block or general anesthesia is preferred. Bier block has been described but often results in edema in the tissues, compromising the dissection.  Tourniquet pain can become a problem if Bier block anesthesia is used, if the procedure lasts longer than anticipated, or if the disease proves more extensive than it first appeared.

- Dissection is always started proximally, isolating the neurovascular bundles adjacent to the involved longitudinal cord. The neurovascular bundles should be protected under direct vision and can be marked by an encircling small rubber vessel loop. This method becomes particularly helpful in cases of highly recurrent contracture, when a spiral cord is present, or when the contracture is particularly difficult to dissect. Skin hooks are used to apply tension to the skin edge, and a beaver blade is often used, cutting longitudinally at the subcutaneous margin to remove the diseased tissue. Sometimes the skin and diseased fascia are so intimately connected that removal of the diseased fascia results in removal of a small segment of skin. Such defects are rarely a problem and heal uneventfully if left open. If severe recurrent disease is encountered, a large area of skin may need to be removed and a skin graft required for coverage. Particular care is required as the dissection extends across the metacarpophalangeal joint to the base of the finger. The diseased fascia and nerve may spiral around one another but this approach should remain safe as long as the nerve is well visualized throughout the course of the dissection. In general, a knife used to cut longitudinally toward a nerve is safer than scissors. If scissors are used, both tips should be visible at all times. If one of the cutting edges of the scissor is placed behind the cord or any extension of the diseased fascia, the surgeon risks

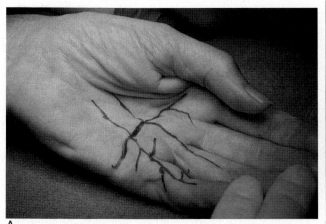
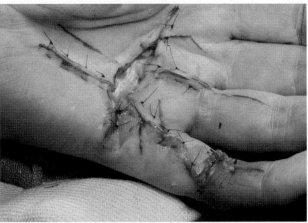

A  B

Figure 19–6:

**A,** Intraoperative photograph of a hand with two digits involved in Dupuytren's disease outlining the incisions. **B,** The same hand following wound closure. The transverse incision in the distal palm and the transverse limbs of the Z-plasties in the fingers are left open for tension-free skin margins.

cutting a common or proper digital nerve or artery that may be located immediately beneath the diseased tissue being removed. Dissection in the distal palm must proceed slowly and carefully, because the nerve may deviate medially almost at a right angle and is subject to injury with longitudinal dissection. If the nerve is well visualized, damage or laceration can be avoided. However, as the surgeon performs an increasing number of surgical procedures for Dupuytren's disease, partial or complete nerve laceration is almost an inevitable complication at some point during surgery on recurrent or primary disease. If damage occurs, the nerve should be repaired at the close of the procedure using an operating microscope or loupe magnification strong enough to allow the surgeon to see the intrafascicular anatomy of the nerve. The patient and/or family should be advised of the complication. They should be reassured that protective sensation or better often returns and that, lacking involvement of a border digit, the patient may remain asymptomatic or minimally bothered by the nerve injury. If a border digit is involved, the best possible nerve repair must be performed and the patient followed closely until protective sensation or better returns.

- In certain instances where identifying the nerve and artery in the palm are difficult, they can be identified in the finger distally. Dissection then proceeds retrograde, from distal to proximal, again "outflanking, surrounding, and capturing" the disease.

- A spiral cord may occur in the finger. Care again must be taken to protect the nerve as it becomes wrapped in the diseased components of the lateral digital sheet and Grayson's ligament. I do not believe a spiral cord develops from a normal structure called a *spiral band*. Rather, the spiral cord develops as a confluence of disease in the fibrous septa in the distal palm, extending to the finger to involve Grayson's ligaments, the lateral digital sheet, and, on the way to the finger, the natatory ligament. As contracture occurs in these structures, the finger is pulled into flexion, much like a lattice closing on itself. The diseased fascia wraps itself around the nerve and draws the nerve toward the midline of the finger.

- When removing a spiral cord from around a nerve or neurovascular bundle, the diseased fascia can be amputated on one side or the other. Alternatively, it can be kept as a solid unit, passed beneath the vessel and nerve toward the finger, and the dissection continued as far as necessary to allow complete removal.

- Once all the diseased tissue has been completely mobilized, with protection of all the remaining normal structures, the last attachment of abnormal to normal tissue is divided. In the case of PIP joint contracture, the diseased fascia often attaches to the flexor sheath or the lateral digital sheet and/or Grayson's ligament. If a PIP joint contracture still exists after removal of the diseased fascia, gentle passive manipulation of the PIP joint into

extension is performed. Care must be taken not to rupture the palmar plate and checkrein ligaments, thereby causing the PIP joint to sublux into hyperextension as noted in the complications section of this chapter. Aggressive surgical release of the checkrein ligaments and palmar plate also can destabilize the PIP joint, causing more disability than a residual 15- or 20-degree flexion contracture.

- At one point in the evolution of the surgical treatment of Dupuytren's disease, radical fasciectomy was proposed, that is, removal of all normal and abnormal fascia to prevent recurrence. However, Skoog[11] in Scandinavia reported that when radical fasciectomy was performed, patients experienced sensitivity in the palm when gripping heavy objects. Manual laborers, in particular, reported difficulty returning to work. Therefore, Skoog performed removal of the diseased fascia only, leading to the term *selective aponeurosectomy*.

- Once all the disease has been excised, the wound is copiously irrigated and closure begun.

- The checkrein ligament is not released. Any residual contracture following regional fasciectomy is accepted to avoid joint instability and/or stiffness.

- Longitudinal incisions on the finger broken into Z-plasties are closed, leaving the transverse component of the Z-plasty open. If no PIP joint contracture is present but diseased tissue is located over the palm, a traditional Brunner-type incision is acceptable. I typically close the wound before deflating the tourniquet. However, in extensive disease where the tourniquet time is approaching 2 hours, it is wise to deflate the tourniquet before closure. Leaving the transverse incision open in the distal palm virtually eliminates the risk of hematoma. A small accumulation of blood in the proximal palm or at the base of a finger still is possible but unlikely to cause pain or compromise circulation to the skin. Leaving the wound open also allows free drainage of lymphatic fluids, thereby minimizing edema and providing tension-free extension of the involved digits.

- Postoperatively, I place the hand in a bulky dressing with a dorsal splint and encourage the patient to flex and extend the fingers as early as possible. Most patients are seen the next day for a dressing change and instructed on an active range of motion program that focuses on flexion and extension. Extension splints usually are worn during the evening, but patients are asked to actively exercise the fingers in flexion during the day to prevent losing flexion. When multiple digits are involved, molded Orthoplast splints are fabricated. In single digit disease, Alumafoam splints usually are sufficient. Therapy is important in patients who are slow to regain motion. Certified hand therapists are important, because they more likely will recognize early signs of complex regional pain syndrome and should be better trained to educate the patient to regain a normal range of motion. In

patients who travel a considerable distance and do not
have a hand therapist near their home, good communication with the closest physical or occupational therapist
is important to ensure that the goals of therapy and the
means for achieving those goals are clear to all concerned
and are in the patients' best interest. Not all patients
require therapy after surgery for Dupuytren's disease, but
when they do, the skill and care of the therapist is as
important as that of the surgeon.

- Wound care involves daily dressing changes with 4 × 4
  gauze and Kling and/or Ace bandage. Peroxide can be
  used to help remove the dressing if it sticks to the open
  area. The peroxide should be diluted to half strength to
  avoid excessive drying of the skin. Using this technique,
  the wound usually heals with a scar. Lister showed this
  healing process was achieved through gradual relaxation
  of the skin edges by tattooing the edges with methylene
  blue and watching the dots approach one another
  (Figure 19–7).
- In younger individuals in whom recurrence rates can be
  expected to be high, fasciectomy alone combined with
  full-thickness skin graft has proved successful in
  preventing disease recurrence.[12]
- Another useful procedure for some surgeons is the
  technique of segmental aponeurectomy as described by
  Moermans.[13] The technique involves removing segments
  of a contracted cord through small incisions to allow the
  finger to be brought into full extension.  The technique
  sounds easier than it is to perform, but it does have a role,
  particularly in unique situations (Figure 19–8). A 70-
  year-old man with Dupuytren's disease of his dominant
  right ring finger sustained a dislocation of the PIP joint
  of the same finger after a fall. Of interest, the PIP joint
  could not be reduced until the patient was taken to the
  operating room and a segmental aponeurectomy was

performed. Following removal of the appropriate amount
of fascia, the PIP joint could be brought into a fully
extended, reduced, stable position (Figure 19–8, *B*). He
then was treated with a program of extension block
splinting, buddy tape, and frequent daily dressing changes
for the transverse wounds that were left open. By 6
weeks, a successful result was obtained.

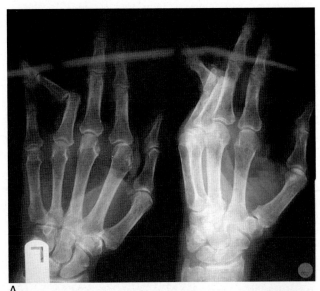

A

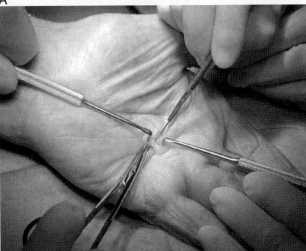

B

Figure 19–8:
**A,** A 70-year-old man with Dupuytren's disease fell on his outstretched right hand and sustained an open proximal interphalangeal (PIP) joint dislocation of the right ring finger. Although
the joint could be reduced, a reduction could not be maintained
because of the severity of preoperative Dupuytren's contracture.
**B,** Operative fasciectomy was required, and given the history of
an open fracture, the decision was made to remove only enough
of the palmar fascia to allow the PIP joint to be maintained in a
stable position. This technique, described by Moermans, worked
well. It allowed full extension as seen during follow-up and a
stable, reduced PIP joint as seen on x-ray film.

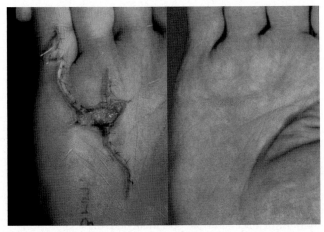

Figure 19–7:
**Wound healing in the open palm technique by gradual relax-
ation of the skin edges as illustrated by tattooing the edges of
the wound with methylene blue and observing the dots coa-
lescing into one.**

- The diseased tissue can be removed through multiple VY-plasties.[14,15] Bedeschi[15] modified the procedure further by shaping the VY-plasties like a honeycomb (Figure 19–9). A 60-degree Z-plasty should increase the length of the contracture by 75%. This finding is true under ideal circumstances; however, I have found that the type III collagen, which dominates Dupuytren's tissue, is somewhat less plastic. This procedure works well, particularly when single digits are involved and the surgeon and patient desire a closed wound.

- The arterial blood supply to the palm is limited. With the skin tethered to the underlying fascia by fibrous septa, any type of large, random rotation flap, as can be easily performed on the dorsum of the hand, is not possible on the palmar side.

- Regardless of the surgical technique selected, certain principles should be followed when removing disease fascia in Dupuytren's disease. Exposure should begin proximally and extend distally. Diseased fascia should be carefully separated from vital normal structures, such as the neurovascular bundles and flexor tendons. As the distal palm is approached, the surgeon should be cognizant of the potential for a so-called spiral cord.

A spiral cord usually is recognized by the presence of a mass of soft pulpy compressible tissue in the palm.[4] As the diseased fascia extends from the palm to the finger, it may wrap around the neurovascular bundle, bringing the nerve toward the midline in a subcutaneous position (Figure 19–10).

# Complications

- Numerous complications are possible after fasciectomy for Dupuytren's disease. The resident or fellow may be unable to list them all on the space provided on a standard operating room consent form, but documenting on the chart that an extensive discussion was held may be key to avoid an angry patient or litigation.

- Recurrent disease is perhaps the most common complication and can be better termed *extension of the disease*. In younger patients with aggressive diathesis, extension of the disease may occur sooner than later after fasciectomy, possibly as soon as 3 or 4 weeks. This early occurrence sometimes is called a *flare reaction* and should alert the surgeon to Dupuytren's diathesis when it occurs in young males. Nonsteroidal antiinflammatory drugs can

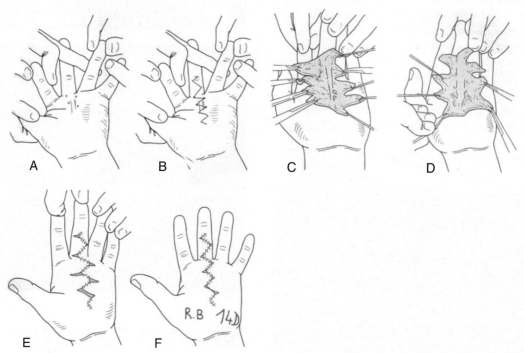

Figure 19–9:

"Honeycomb incision" allowing skin closure with VY-plasty. **A,** First four basic markers for the top angles of the zigzag incision at the palmodigital level. **B,** Incision design. **C, D,** The wide exposure allowed by this technique enables extensive and safe palmar and digital fasciectomy. **E,** At the end of the operation, note the complete correction of the contracture. Only the zigzag incision is sutured. Transverse incisions become small open areas, avoiding tension on wounds and preventing hematomas. **F,** The same patient 14 days later. (Redrawn from Bedeschi P: Various views and techniques. Management of the skin. Part 1: Honeycomb technique. In McFarlane RM, McGrouther DA, Flint MH, editors: *Dupuytren's disease: biology and treatment. The hand and upper limb series, vol 5.* Edinburgh, 1990, Churchill Livingstone. From Lubahn JD: Dupuytren's disease. In Szabo RM, Marder RA, Vince KG, et al, editors: *Chapman's orthopaedic surgery,* vol 2. ed 3. Philadelphia, 2001, Lippincott.)

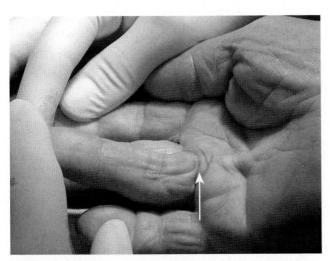

**Figure 19–10:**
**Area of skin dimpling that should alert the surgeons that a spiral cord may exist and that the nerve can be located in the immediate subcutaneous position.**

be given to minimize the inflammation. Referral to a hand therapist for supervision of a gentle range of motion program as described by Ros Evans, CHT (certified hand therapist), with the use of elastomer and Coban to the inflamed area to minimize edema may prove beneficial.[16]

- Skin slough is seen in patients in whom the palm is closed tightly and may lead to infection and the need for antibiotics. Depending on the nature and extent of the disease, the antibiotics can be administered on an inpatient basis with parenteral antibiotic therapy or on an outpatient basis with oral antibiotics.

- Damage to the neurovascular bundle(s) of the affected digit is an unfortunate complication that may occur from extending the PIP joint from a fixed flexion contracture. If a finger has poor capillary filling postoperatively, the splint should be removed and the finger placed in a more flexed position. If color does not return in 10 to 20 minutes, the artery should be explored for a suspected intimal tear. Sometimes the contracture is so severe that passively bringing the PIP joint from 90 degrees or more flexion to an extended position results in a transient neuropraxia.

- The digital nerve or artery can be completely or partially severed during release of the PIP or metacarpophalangeal joint in Dupuytren's disease. When severing occurs, the nerve or artery should be promptly repaired. The artery may require a small vein graft to maintain the PIP joint in full extension. Arterial repair or vein graft reconstruction is necessary only if the circulation is compromised. Such complications should be communicated to the family and the patient during the immediate postoperative period. If well managed, long-term sequelae of these complications can be prevented.

- If a border digit sustains a neurovascular complication, nerve repair does not yield a reasonably sensate digit, and

the contracture recurs to some extent, particularly in the PIP joint of the small finger, the patient may be best treated with an amputation.

- Amputation should be performed with caution in patients with Dupuytren's disease because amputation is not a practical solution for recurrent disease in the remaining digits.

- Finally, if an overzealous PIP joint contracture release is performed and the entire palmar plate is released, the PIP joint may sublux dorsally. In this situation, early recognition and splinting may salvage the PIP joint. However, if dorsal subluxation persists, the standard sublimis tenodesis can be considered. In my experience, PIP joint arthrodesis in a functional position offers the best chance for stabilizing the joint and salvaging the finger.

# References

1. Plater F: *Observationum in Hominis Affectibus, vol 3*. König JL, Brandmyller J, Basel LI, 1614.
   A medical textbook, published in Latin, in which a contracture in the palm and attributes it to a thickening of the palmar fascia is described.

2. Ling RS: The genetic factor in Dupuytren's disease. *J Bone Joint Surg* 45B:709-718, 1963.
   Perhaps the most thorough evaluation of Dupuytren's disease from a genetic standpoint. Sixty-eight percent of patients had relatives affected with Dupuytren's disease, with the conclusion that Dupuytren's disease probably results from a single mendelian dominant gene.

3. Zachariae L: Dupuytren's contracture. The aetiological role of trauma. *Scand J Plast Reconstr Surg* 5:116-119, 1971.
   The author concluded that trauma was unimportant in the etiology or development of Dupuytren's contracture.

4. Short WH, Watson HK: Prediction of the spiral nerve in Dupuytren's contracture. *J Hand Surg* 7A:84-86, 1982.
   Forty of forty-four patients with a spiral nerve had an area of pulpy redundant skin, for a 90% sensitivity in alerting the surgeon as to the presence of a spiral nerve. There was a preoperative mention of this condition in 10 patients in whom no spiral nerve was found, indicating a 4% false-positive rate.

5. Majno G, Gabbiani G, Hirschel BJ, et al: Contraction of granulation tissue in vitro: similarity to smooth muscle. *Science* 173: 548-550, 1971.
   The force of myofibroblast contracture is comparable to that of rabbit skeletal muscle.

6. Nissenbaum M, Kleinert HE: Treatment considerations in carpal tunnel syndrome with coexistent Dupuytren's disease. *J Hand Surg* 5A:544-547, 1980.
   The authors noted a high percentage of unsatisfactory results and reflex sympathetic dystrophy in patients with simultaneous fasciectomy and carpal tunnel release, particularly in women. It was therefore recommended that surgical treatment of these conditions be performed separately.

7. Michon J: Serious postoperative complications in Dupuytren's disease. *J Hand Surg* 2A:238, 1977 (abstract).

Michon believed that carpal tunnel syndrome and Dupuytren's disease can be treated concomitantly.

8. Gonzalez F, Watson HK: Simultaneous carpal tunnel release and Dupuytren's fasciectomy. *J Hand Surg* 16B:175-178, 1991.
The authors note no increased incidence of complications for simultaneous surgical treatment of Dupuytren's disease and carpal tunnel syndrome.

9. Badalamente MA, Hurst LC: Enzyme injection as nonsurgical treatment of Dupuytren's disease. *J Hand Surg* 25A:629-636, 2000.
The authors conclude that collagenase injection may be helpful, safe, and effective to treat Dupuytren's disease and may be a reasonably effective alternative to surgical fasciectomy.

10. McCash CR: The open palm technique in Dupuytren's contracture. *Br J Plast Surg* 17:271-280, 1964.
The author describes the technique of leaving transverse wounds open to allow healing by granulation. Longitudinal incisions are closed with Z-plasties.

11. Skoog T: The transverse elements of the palmar aponeurosis in Dupuytren's contracture. Their pathological and surgical significance. *Scand J Reconstr Surg* 1:51-63, 1967.
The author recommends surgical removal of the diseased fascia only, noting that complete radical palmar fasciectomy often leaves the palm of the hand unprotected. The underlying nerves experience sensitivity and pain with heavy gripping.

12. Hueston JT: The control of recurrent Dupuytren's contracture by skin replacement. *Br J Plast Surg* 22:152-156, 1969.
The author notes that recurrence can be successfully prevented by using a full-thickness skin graft in severe contracture.

Although this procedure requires a period of immobilization and risks stiffness, it may be the only way to successfully prevent recurrence.

13. Moermans JP. Segmental aponeurectomy in Dupuytren's disease. *J Hand Surg* 16B:243-254, 1991.
Segments of diseased tissue measuring approximately 1 cm in length were excised through several small skin incisions. Thorough attempts were made to remove all Dupuytren's tissue, with the goal of achieving "discontinuity." Results were believed to compare favorably with results of more conventional techniques.

14. King EW, Bass DM, Watson HK: Treatment of Dupuytren's contracture by extensive fasciectomy through multiple YV-plasty incisions: short-term evaluation of 170 consecutive operations. *J Hand Surg* 4A:234-241, 1979.

15. Bedeschi P: Various views and techniques. Management of the skin. Part 1: Honeycomb technique. In McFarlane RM, McGrouther DA, Flint MH, editors: *Dupuytren's disease: biology and treatment. The hand and upper limb series, vol 5.* Edinburgh, 1990, Churchill Livingstone.
Researchers from references 14 and 15 note that the disease can be treated surgically with short VY-plasties. Minimal tension should be present on the wound with the fingers held in full extension.

16. Evans RB, Dell PC, Fiolkowski P: A clinical report of the effect of mechanical stress on functional results after fasciectomy for Dupuytren's contracture. *J Hand Ther* 15:331-339, 2002.
This technique of avoiding tension on the suture line to prevent a postoperative flare of fibromatosis should be routine for any therapist treating patients following fasciectomy.

# Fingertip Injuries, Nail Bed Injuries, and Amputations

Owen J. Moy\* and Loretta Coady†

\*MD, Clinical Professor, Orthopaedic Surgery, State University of New York School of Biomedical Sciences at Buffalo; Director, Hand Fellowship Program, Hand Center of Western New York, Buffalo, NY
†Hand Fellow, SUNY at Buffalo School of Biomedical Sciences, Buffalo, NY

## Introduction

- Traumatic injuries to the fingertip and nail are the most common injuries encountered by hand surgeons in an emergency setting. Children and young adults are the age groups that most commonly present with nail injuries. The middle finger is most commonly involved because of its length and exposure, followed by the ring, index, little, and thumb. Common sources of injury to the fingertip include doors, crush injuries between two unyielding objects, and lacerations from power saws, snow blowers, and lawnmowers.

- The distal phalanx, which supports the nail plate, is fractured in half of all fingertip injuries.

- Inadequate, delayed, or inappropriate treatment can lead to functional and aesthetic problems, such as chronic ulceration from inadequate or inappropriate soft tissue coverage, nail deformities (hook nail, split nail, onycholysis), and painful neuromas.

- The treatment plan must consider the patient's age, occupation, reliability, and long-term functional goals.

## Anatomy

- The *fingertip* is considered the region of the distal phalanx distal to the insertion of the flexor and extensor tendon. It includes the perionychium, nail plate, and volar pad.

- The *perionychium* consists of the nail and surrounding structures, including the hyponychium, nail bed, and nail fold.

- The *paronychium* is the fold where the nail meets the skin of the finger on each side of the nail.

- The *eponychium* is the soft tissue proximal on the dorsal surface of the nail.

- The *nail fold* consists of the dorsal roof and ventral roof. The dorsal roof gives the nail its characteristic shine.

- The *nail bed* consists of the germinal matrix and the sterile matrix. The *germinal matrix* is located below the dorsal roof, approximately 2 mm distal to the extensor tendon insertion out to the *lunula* (white half-moon). It is responsible for 90% of nail growth. As the nail cells duplicate, they flatten and are pressed upward and forward. The nuclei are retained in many of these cells, giving the lunula its white color. The *sterile matrix* adds approximately 10% to the nail plate and is mostly responsible for nail plate adherence. It begins at the lunula and extends to the hyponychium.

- The *hyponychium* is the keratinous plug beneath the distal edge of the nail where the nail bed meets the fingertip. This site is abundant in lymphocytes and polymorpholeukocytes and provides a barrier to bacteria and fungi.

- The palmar digital arteries supply the fingertip. The radial vessel usually is larger in the ring and small finger. The ulnar vessel usually is larger in the index, middle finger, and thumb. The artery trifurcates near the distal interphalangeal (DIP) joint with a branch to the volar pulp, a branch parallel to the paronychium, and a branch to the proximal nail fold.

- Venous drainage of the fingertip is supplied by a system of dorsal, palmar, and oblique communicating veins.
- The radial and ulnar digital nerves accompany the volar digital arteries and divide just distal to the DIP joint, sending branches into the pulp of the finger and nail bed.
- Nails grow at a rate of 0.1 mm/day. After injury, growth does not normalize for approximately 100 days. The nail grows fastest from age 4 to 30 years. Nails grow faster on the fingers than on the toes. They grow more rapidly on longer digits. Nails grow more quickly in summer than in winter.

# Nail Bed Injuries

- Radiographs should be taken prior to definitive treatment to identify bony injury. Approximately 50% of nail bed injuries present with an associated distal phalanx fracture. Most are comminuted distal tuft fractures that require only nail bed repair and splinting.
- A digital block frequently is necessary in order to completely examine the extent of the injury.
- The hand from the fingertips to the wrist or distal forearm should be sterilely prepped and draped.
- A 0.5-inch Penrose drain or the open digital portion of a latex glove can be used to exsanguinate the digit and provide a bloodless field by acting as a tourniquet at the base of the finger. *Flag the tourniquet* with either a hemostat or a piece of gauze under the drain as a reminder to remove the tourniquet at the end of the procedure. Failure to do so could result in loss of the digit that was just so painstakingly repaired (Box 20–1).

## Box 20–1    Stepwise Repair of Nail Bed Injuries

- Obtain dedicated finger x-ray films of affected digit(s).
- Administer one dose of intravenous antibiotics and update tetanus.
- Reduce and reimage fracture, if necessary.
- Evaluate motor, vascular, and neurologic status.
- Obtain adequate lighting, assistance, and instruments.
- Administer digital block.
- Prepare and drape hand up to wrist or distal forearm.
- Apply digital tourniquet using Penrose drain or sterile glove.
- Remove nail plate using fine hemostat, freer elevator, or fine scissors.
- Repair sterile and germinal matrix, using 6-0 plain sutures (preferably under magnification vision).
- **Remove tourniquet.**
- Replace nail plate or apply Xeroform to matrix and under nail fold.
- Wrap digit distal to PIP joint in soft bulky dressing or splint.
- Instruct patient to keep hand elevated, give 2 days of prophylactic oral antibiotics, and schedule follow-up appointment.

- Loupe magnification is helpful for identifying and repairing injuries.

## Subungal Hematoma

- The traditional treatment of a hematoma involving less than 50% of the nail is drainage by a sterile heated paperclip, needle, or ophthalmic cautery. The heated instrument instantly cools when it contacts the hematoma. Advantages include less pain and less costly intervention than nail removal. A disadvantage is missing a potentially significant nail bed injury.

## Lacerations

- These are common injuries from low-energy trauma. Patients may present with the nail visibly lacerated or with a large (>50%) subungal hematoma with or without a distal phalanx fracture.
- Following adequate digital anesthesia, surgical preparation, and exsanguination, the nail plate is removed with a small elevator or curved iris scissors, taking care not to damage the underlying nail bed or overlying nail fold. The undersurface of the nail is examined, adherent matrix is harvested from the nail plate, and the nail is soaked in Betadine while the matrix is repaired. The germinal matrix may be better visualized by making 90-degree angle back cuts at each corner of the nail fold (Figure 20–1).
- The lacerations can be repaired with 6-0 or 7-0 plain or chromic sutures. *Never use nonabsorbable sutures.*
- Associated comminuted tuft fractures are treated by repair of the nail bed and splinting. The nail plate can be used to stabilize the fracture. A hole must be placed in the nail plate to provide adequate drainage. The nail plate is repositioned under the nail fold to prevent scar formation between the dorsal roof and ventral floor. A 4-0 or 5-0 nylon suture placed distally through the nail plate and paronychium is used to secure the nail plate.

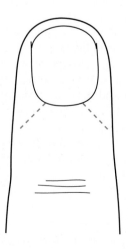

Figure 20–1:

Ninety-degree angle back cuts at each corner of the nail fold. (From Van Beek AL, Kassan MA, Adson MH, Dale V: Management of acute fingernail injuries. Hand Clinic, 6:23–38, 1990.)

- More proximal or displaced fractures must be reduced and pinned to prevent subsequent nail bed deformity. This can be accomplished with two 0.028 to 0.035 K-wires, avoiding the DIP joint, if possible.
- An open physeal fracture *(Seymour fracture)* can present in children as a nail bed injury. The nail plate is avulsed from the nail fold and is found lying superficial to the proximal nail fold. The injury is diagnosed by careful radiologic examination, usually in the lateral view. The fracture is reduced, and the sterile matrix and germinal matrix are repaired. The nail plate is used to help maintain reduction. Pinning is generally avoided unless the fracture is highly unstable. This injury is discussed in more detail in Chapter 29.
- The fingertip is dressed with nonadherent gauze and a splint that immobilizes the DIP joint.
- The dressing is changed 5 to 7 days later. The stay suture through the nail plate is removed at 2 to 3 weeks. The nail plate usually adheres to the sterile matrix for 1 to 3 months until it is pushed off by the new nail.

## Crushing and Avulsion Injuries

- These injuries result from higher-energy traumas. The nail bed may be squeezed between the nail plate and distal phalanx, or the nail plate can be completely ripped from the nail fold, avulsing a portion of the nail bed.
- The initial approach is the same as with less complex lacerations: digital block, surgical preparation, removal of the remaining nail, and inspection of the nail bed. Inspection of the anatomic structures is vital for good outcome. Uniform nail growth is impeded if a portion of the germinal matrix is missing. Nonadherence results if a portion of the sterile matrix is missing (Box 20–2).
- Undermining and advancing the surrounding matrix can repair very small defects in the matrix. Retained nail bed fragments adherent to the undersurface of the avulsed nail plate should be retrieved and applied as a graft with 7-0 chromic sutures.
- Small areas of sterile matrix loss can be replaced by harvesting split-thickness sterile matrix from adjacent matrix using a no. 15 blade scalpel. The blade should be visible through the graft to avoid taking full-thickness

graft. Alternatively, a split-thickness graft can be harvested from an adjacent fingernail bed or from the great toe.
- The germinal matrix that cannot be repaired primarily or retrieved as a graft from the avulsed nail can be replaced with a full-thickness graft from a toe or a digit that is going to be discarded. Unlike the sterile matrix, grafts of germinal matrix must be oriented properly to prevent lateral nail growth. Nail bed grafts should be cut only 1 to 2 mm longer than their recipient area.
- The nail often is missing or too badly injured to allow replacement into the nail fold. Placement of a prosthetic stent, such as Silastic, Xeroform, or suture packing material, between the dorsal and ventral walls can be considered.

### Late Reconstruction

- The nail bed can be explored up to 7 days after injury; however, the risk of infection is greater.
- Nail deformities often occur after injuries are improperly or inadequately treated. Common deformities are hook nail, split nail, and nonadherent nail (onycholysis).
- A hook nail results when the matrix is advanced or pulled distally to obtain coverage of a wound without proper bony support. This situation is corrected by removing the nail and trimming the matrix back to the level of the distal phalanx.
- Split nail and nonadherent nails result from scarring of the matrix. Scars in the nail bed that are 3 mm or more in width cannot be closed with undermining and primary closure. Treatment involves excising the scar and replacing sterile matrix with a split-thickness matrix graft and germinal matrix with a full-thickness matrix graft.
- A more aggressive option involves ablating the nail by complete excision of the remaining matrix and covering the wound with a split-thickness skin graft.

## Fingertip Amputations

- Partial amputation of the fingertip generally involves loss of nail bed, soft tissue, and frequently underlying bony support. Fingertip amputations can occur in various directions: transverse, volar oblique, dorsal oblique, or lateral oblique.
- Treatment goals consider the patient's overall medical condition, age, occupation, expectations, and functional requirements. Options range from conservative treatment involving dressing changes to complex grafts and flaps. The end result should leave the patient with stable skin coverage, good sensibility, minimal morbidity, and early return to work.

### Primary Closure

- This method is recommended when the amount of tissue loss and location of injury allow placement of sutures without excess tension.

---

### Box 20–2 Nail Bed Repair Pearls

- *Do not* forget the x-ray film.
- *Assume* sterile matrix requires drainage or repair when distal phalanx is fractured in a crush injury.
- *Do* remove the tourniquet before applying the dressing.
- *Remember* that 1 cm of soft tissue defects over unexposed bone can be allowed to granulate and reepithelialize.
- *Combine* procedures to obtain coverage (e.g., volar flaps and dressing changes).
- *Use* absorbable sutures.
- *Treat* early for best outcomes.

## Dressing Changes

- Allows closure of the wound by secondary intention. Best used for small wounds (<1 cm) without exposed bone, nerve, vessel, or tendon. Advantages include simplicity, lower health care costs, no donor site morbidity, minimal scarring, and good results in properly selected patients. Disadvantages include prolonged recovery time during the period of wound care (Box 20–3).
- The wound is debrided of necrotic material and irrigated, and dressing changes are started.
- Mennen and Wiese[1] treated 200 patients with weekly "OpSite" dressing changes over an average of 20 days. By the end of 3 months, two-point discrimination averaged 2.5 mm, and fingertip pulp was nearly normal in appearance.
- Allen[2] reviewed 60 fingertip injuries in 50 patients who were treated conservatively, with acceptable results. Injury severity ranged from isolated soft tissue injuries to those that included nail bed and bony injury. The only surgical treatment involved trimming the distal phalanx to allow soft tissue coverage prior to beginning dressing changes. Dressings changes were performed every 4 to 5 days until the wound was healed. The major problem was cold sensitivity and nail dystrophy. Most of the patients had near-normal sensation, pinch, and joint mobility at final assessment 6 months after injury.

## Split-Thickness Skin Graft

- These grafts contain the entire epidermis and a portion of the dermis.
- Advantages include a high rate of take in less than optimal conditions and abundant donor sites. Disadvantages include poor sensibility, lack of durability, contracture, and loss of pigmentation.

## Full-Thickness Skin Graft

- These grafts contain the entire epidermis and dermal layers. Most common donor sources are the ulnar border of the palm; the volar wrist crease; the inner, upper arm; the non–weight-bearing plantar aspect of the foot; and the non–hair-bearing groin crease.
- Advantages relative to split-thickness skin graft are less contracture, more stable coverage, and aesthetically superior wounds. Disadvantages include the need for donor site closure.
- The skin and/or matrix often can be harvested from the amputated part, defatted, and placed on the open wound as a full-thickness graft.
- Schenck and Cheema[3] used full-thickness *hypothenar grafts* to reconstruct 25 digits in 20 patients and followed them for an average of 9.5 months. Eighty-six percent of patients had two-point discrimination of 10 mm or less, with half having two-point discriminations less than 6 mm. No patients complained of hypersensitivity. They concluded that the hypothenar area can provide up to 2 cm × 6 cm of coverage with acceptable cosmetic and functional outcome. Hong et al.[4] used hypothenar composite grafts to reconstruct the fingertip deformities of 15 patients, resulting in an average two-point discrimination of 5.7 mm at an average follow-up of 35 months. This option is appealing because the hypothenar skin is similar to the lost skin (thickness and pigmentation), the donor site is in the same operative field, and the donor site can be closed primarily.
- Rose et al.[5] described the *"cap technique"* for fingertip amputations at the lunula that takes advantage of the periosteal capillary network surrounding the distal phalanx. The distal tuft of bone is removed from the

| Box 20–3 | Coverage Options | | |
|---|---|---|---|
| **Technique** | **Advantages** | | **Disadvantages** |
| Dressing changes | Simple, inexpensive, no donor site, minimal scar | | Prolonged recovery |
| Split-thickness skin graft | Abundant donor tissue, high rate of take | | Not durable, contractures, poor sensation, loss of pigmentation |
| Full-thickness skin graft | More durable, fewer contractures, good color match | | Donor site morbidity |
| "Cap" | Tip appears normal | | Shortened digit |
| Lateral VY flap | Good for oblique, volar, and transverse injuries | | Lateral injuries |
| Triangular volar flap | Good for dorsal, lateral oblique, and transverse injuries | | Volar injuries |
| Cross-finger flap | Good coverage for volar injury with exposed bone or tendon | | Two donor sites needed, donor finger immobilized for 10 days |
| Thenar flap | Durable, good color match | | PIP joint stiffness, age restriction, donor site sensitivity |
| Flag flap | Coverage for adjacent volar or dorsal surfaces | | Donor site needs full-thickness skin graft, not durable, insensate |
| Island flap | Well-vascularized and innervated flap, useful for secondary reconstruction | | Technically challenging, sensory reeducation postoperatively |
| Moberg flap | Full-thickness coverage, good sensation | | Neurovascular bundles at risk during mobilization |
| Kite flap | Can be sensate, if transferred with branch of radial sensory nerve | | Donor site requires full-thickness skin graft |

amputated part. The proximal stump is circumferentially trimmed of its soft tissue for a distance of 6 mm while sparing the proximal 2 mm of germinal matrix. A thin cuff of periosteum and adjacent tissue is retained to preserve the vascular network. The amputated "cap" is inset over the bone peg, giving the illusion of a normal but slightly shortened digit (Figure 20–2).

## Local Flaps

- This type of flap involves mobilization and reposition of adjacent tissue for coverage of the defect.
- The *lateral* **VY** *flap* (Figure 20–3) is used for coverage of transverse and some oblique defects. It is a modification of the original Kutler flap, in which the incision was made only through skin and subcutaneous tissue. The modified lateral **VY** flap is made by creating a **V**-shaped incision twice the length of the defect. The dorsal incision is made through the skin and down to the periosteum parallel and 2 mm lateral to the eponychium. The volar incision is made only through skin, preserving

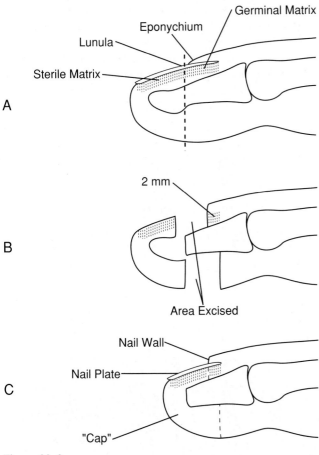

Figure 20–2:
**A,** Amputation through fingertip lunula. **B,** Distal tuft of bone filleted from palmar pulp and distal nail bed. Shaft of phalanx is trimmed circumferentially, leaving 2 mm of germinal matrix on the dorsal surface. **C,** Composite tip reapplied as a "cap" over skeletal bone peg. (Redrawn from Rose EH, Norris MN, Kowalski TA et al: *J Hand Surg* 14A:515, 1989.)

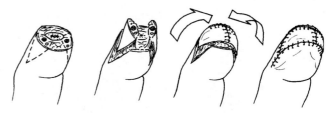

Figure 20–3:
**Kutler flap provides sensate soft tissue coverage for the fingertip in small central defects.** (From Trumble TE, editor: *Principles of hand surgery and therapy*. Philadelphia, 2000, WB Saunders.)

the major neurovascular structures. The flaps are mobilized and joined at the midline, permitting 10 to 14 mm of mobilization on each side.

- The *triangular volar flap* (Figure 20–4), originally described by Atasoy et al.[6] in 1970, can be used to cover transverse and dorsal defects. The flap is based on the volar surface of the fingertip down to the DIP joint and is advanced over the exposed fingertip. This procedure allows local coverage up to 12 to 14 mm; however, subsequent studies have found diminished sensation to two-point testing.
- The lateral **VY** flap is superior to the volar flap when confronted with volar oblique injuries. The volar **VY** flap is most applicable to dorsal oblique and lateral oblique injures. Either technique is suitable to transverse distal fingertip amputations.

## Regional Flaps

- These flaps are tissues transferred from a nonadjacent area of the hand to the injured digit. They provide coverage within the same surgical field as the injury but create a donor site defect, with additional potential morbidity.
- The *cross-finger flap* (Figure 20–5) takes dorsal skin and subcutaneous tissue from the adjacent finger's middle phalanx to cover the injured tip or volar defect. A full-thickness flap based on the side of the injured digit is elevated, taking care to leave the extensor paratendon intact. The flap is turned over to cover the adjacent defect. The injured digit must be flexed to approximate the donor site. A full-thickness skin graft is applied to the donor site. The flap is detached from the donor digit at

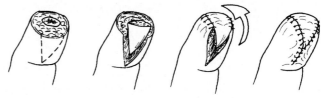

Figure 20–4:
VY flap provides sensate soft tissue coverage for the fingertip in small central defects. (From Trumble TE, editor: *Principles of hand surgery and therapy*. Philadelphia, 2000, WB Saunders.)

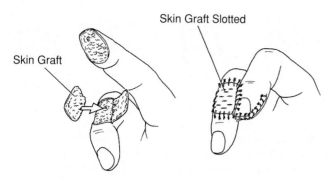

Figure 20–5:

**Cross-finger flap provides soft tissue coverage for the palmar aspect of the adjacent finger or thumb, but a full-thickness skin graft is required for the donor site. (From Trumble TE, editor:** *Principles of hand surgery and therapy*. **Philadelphia, 2000, WB Saunders.)**

approximately 2 weeks. Cold intolerance and stiffness remain problems. Normal (<6 mm) two-point discrimination returns more consistently in a younger patient population.

- The *thenar flap* (Figure 20–6) is indicated for loss of the skin and pulp of the long or ring terminal phalanx. A proximal, radially based full-thickness flap is raised proximal to the metacarpophalangeal (MCP) joint crease of the thumb, taking care to not injure the digital nerves. The flap should be 50% larger than the size of the defect. The injured digit is flexed to meet the elevated graft. The donor defect can be covered with a full-thickness skin graft from the groin or the volar wrist crease. The flap is divided 10 to 14 days later. The advantage is a thick, more durable graft with good color match. The most common criticism of this flap is proximal interphalangeal (PIP) joint contracture and donor site sensitivity. Melone, Beasley, and Carstens[7] refute this criticism by describing 150 applied thenar grafts with residual PIP contractures in 4% of the patients and 3% sensitivity at the donor site

after 1 year. However, this flap is best not used in patients older than 50 years and in those with degenerative joint disease.

- The *flag flap* uses dorsal digital skin over the middle or proximal phalanx to cover either palmar or dorsal soft tissue defects of the same or adjacent digits. The flap is mobilized on a dorsolateral skin pedicle one third the width of the flap. The defect requires a full-thickness skin graft and is limited in durability.
- The *neurovascular island flap* is technically more challenging. Sensate tissue from the less critical ulnar side of the middle or ring finger is elevated on its neurovascular bundle and transferred to the more critical surface of the thumb, radial side of the index, middle, ring, or ulnar side of the little finger. A local neurovascular island flap was described by Cook, Jakab, and Pollock,[8] with two-point discrimination within 2 mm of the adjacent digit in follow-up of 8 to 14 years. The mobilized neurovascular bundle is at risk for injury, and the donor requires full-thickness skin graft coverage.
- *Moberg flap* (Figure 20–7) is commonly used for thumb defects up to 2 cm long. The entire volar surface of the thumb is elevated off the flexor sheath to the level of the MCP joint, preserving the digital neurovascular bundles within the flap. The interphalangeal (IP) joint is flexed up to 30 degrees. Depending on the degree of tension of the advanced flap, mobilization can be started within days.

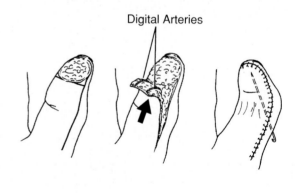

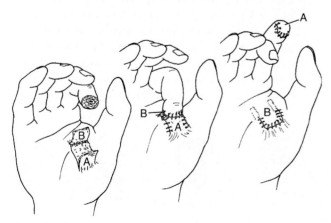

Figure 20–6:

**Thenar flap provides soft tissue coverage for the index and middle fingers without requiring a skin graft for the donor site. (From Trumble TE, editor:** *Principles of hand surgery and therapy*. **Philadelphia, 2000, WB Saunders.)**

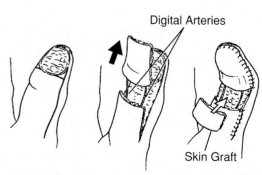

Figure 20–7:

**Moberg flap provides sensate soft tissue coverage for the palmar aspect of the thumb tip. (From Trumble TE, editor:** *Principles of hand surgery and therapy*. **Philadelphia, 2000, WB Saunders.)**

The thumb has a consistent dorsal vascular supply from the first dorsal metacarpal artery and the princeps pollicis, preventing necrosis of the dorsal skin during mobilization. Baumeister et al.[9] found 74% normal sensitivity at 27 months with no flexion contractures at the IP joint. Cold sensitivity was the most common complaint.

- The kite flap, or *first dorsal metacarpal artery flap,* can reconstruct thumb defects. It is based on the first dorsal metacarpal artery and provides skin from the dorsal aspect of the proximal phalanx of the index finger. It includes a branch of the radial sensory nerve. The pedicle is dissected proximally to allow repositioning without tension on the neurovascular bundle. The donor site is covered with a full-thickness skin graft. Trankle et al.[10] found no age-related difference in sensitivity of the island flap and minimal donor site morbidity.

- Many of these procedures can be performed under local anesthesia in the emergency room setting, provided the patient is willing to cooperate, lighting and visualization are adequate, sterile technique can be maintained, and appropriate instruments are available. Hematoma drainage, repair of nail bed lacerations, fracture reductions, volar and lateral **VY** flaps, flag flap, hypothenar grafts, the "cap" technique, and cross-finger flaps are procedures that potentially can be performed safely in the emergency room. Repairs and reconstructions that require avoidance or visualization of adjacent neurovascular structures should be done in the operating room and include the Moberg flap, neurovascular island flap, thenar flap, and metacarpal artery flap.

## Proximal Amputations

- Amputations *through the DIP joint* are treated by shortening and rounding the condyles of the middle phalanx to provide a smooth bony stump without a square, bulbous end. The extensor and flexor tendons are transected proximally and allowed to retract. Do *not* attach the opposing tendons to pad the stump or the quadrigia effect will result, impairing finger flexion and grip strength. Distal release of the flexor digitorum profundus tendon may lead to a lumbrical plus deformity. As the profundus and attached lumbricals move proximally, tension on the lateral bands impairs active flexion of the PIP joint (Figure 20–8). This can be treated via distal intrinsic release in the outpatient setting. The digital nerves should be dissected from the surrounding tissue, pulled distally, cut, and allowed to retract proximally to prevent symptomatic neuroma formation (Figure 20–9).

- Amputations *through the middle phalanx* are shortened to allow primary closure while maintaining flexor digitorum superficialis (FDS) attachment. If the amputation is proximal to the FDS attachment, active PIP motion will be lost. The digit can be shortened through the PIP joint

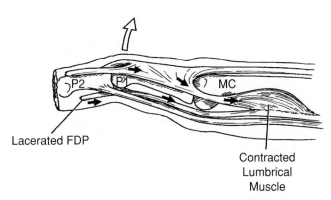

Figure 20–8:
Amputations at the distal interphalangeal joint can result in the lumbrical plus finger as the force of the flexor digitorum profundus *(FDP)* tendon is directed to the central slip via the attached lumbrical to produce paradoxical proximal interphalangeal joint extension while the patient tries to make a fist. *MC,* metacarpal; *P1,* proximal phalanx; *P2,* middle phalanx. (From Trumble TE, editor: *Principles of hand surgery and therapy.* Philadelphia, 2000, WB Saunders.)

to allow primary closure. Pinch usually is transferred to the long finger after amputation to the index proximal to the mid-middle phalanx level.

- *Amputations through the PIP joint* and the *proximal phalanx* are treated by reshaping the condyles of the proximal phalanx, followed by primary closure. The proximal stump is under motor control of the intrinsics and extensor digitorum communis. Active

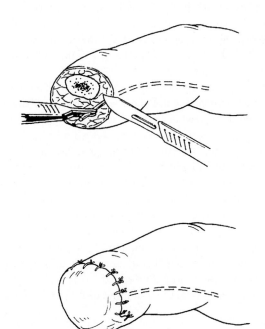

Figure 20–9:
Transecting the nerve ends proximal to the skin edges is an important step in revision amputation. (From Trumble TE, editor: *Principles of hand surgery and therapy.* Philadelphia, 2000, WB Saunders.)

flexion of 45 degrees is possible. A short stump of proximal phalanx in the long and ring fingers leaves a space in the middle of the closed hand. An elective ray amputation or prosthetic replacement closes the residual space, preventing the loss of small objects from the palm.

- Most amputations in adults can be completed in the emergency room under local anesthesia. Intravenous sedation may be helpful in an anxious patient.

## Replantations

- Replantation is the reattachment of a part that has been completely amputated.
- Revascularization is the repair of a part that has been incompletely amputated and requires vascular repair to prevent necrosis of the partially severed body part.
- Consideration must be given to the anticipated function, which should equal or better the function achieved with a revised amputation.
- Referral should be made to an experienced replant center with an available 24-hour replant team.
- Indications include, but are not absolutely limited to, amputations of guillotine-type, multiple digits, thumb, whole hand proximal to MCP joints, distal to FDS insertion, and almost any part of a child. Replanted digits in children tend to have a lower survival rate but superior functional results.
- Relative contraindications are crushed or mangled parts, multiple levels, serious comorbidity (especially arteriosclerosis), prolonged ischemia time (warm >6 hours proximal to the carpus, warm >8 hours for the digits, cold up to 30 hours for the digits), mental instability, and amputation proximal to the FDS insertion in a single-digit injury.
- The proper transport method involves wrapping the part in a cloth moistened with Ringer lactate or normal saline and placing the bundle in a plastic bag or specimen container. The bag or container then is transported over ice.
- The sequence of repair is cleaning and debridement, neurovascular identification in the stump and amputated part, bone shortening and stabilization, extensor tendon repair, flexor tendon repair, arterial anastomosis, venous anastomosis, nerve repair, and soft tissue coverage.
- Common postoperative problems include cold intolerance and tendon adhesions. Cold intolerance tends to improve with time. Tenolysis can be performed after 3 months when motion is limited.
- Replantation is discussed in more detail in Chapter 23.

## References

1. Mennen U, Wiese A: Fingertip injuries management with semi-occlusive dressing. *J Hand Surg* 18B:416-422, 1993.
   The authors managed 200 fingertip injures with weekly OpSite dressing changes, resulting in near-normal two-point discrimination and pulp shape on follow-up.

2. Allen MJ: Conservative management of fingertip injuries in adults. *Hand* 12:257-265, 1980.
   The result of a prospective trial on 60 fingertip injuries treated with debridement and dressing changes is presented.

3. Schenck RR, Cheema TA: Hypothenar skin grafts for fingertip reconstruction. *J Hand Surg* 9A:750-753, 1984.
   The paper describes the results of full-thickness hypothenar grafts used to reconstruct 25 digits in 20 patients.

4. Hong JP, Lee SJ, Lee HB, Chung YK: Reconstruction of fingertip and stump using a composite graft from the hypothenar region. *Ann Plast Surg* 51:57-62, 2003.
   The authors present the results of 15 cases of hypothenar graft application to fingertip injuries.

5. Rose EH, Norris MN, Kowalski TA et al: The "cap" technique: nonmicrosurgical reattachment of fingertip amputations. *J Hand Surg* 14A:513-518, 1989.
   Nonmicrosurgical reattachment of fingertip amputations by shortening the digit and using the periosteal vascular network over the distal phalanx to produce a normal-appearing but slightly shortened digit is described.

6. Atasoy E, Ioakimidis E, Kasdan ML et al: Reconstruction of the amputated fingertip with a triangular volar flap. *J Bone Surg* 52A:921-926, 1970.
   This is the original description of the triangular volar flap, with 64 cases presented.

7. Melone C, Beasley R, Carstens J: The thenar flap—an analysis of its use in 150 cases. *J Hand Surg* 7:291-297, 1982.
   The authors share their experience with 150 thenar flaps and refute the often-quoted complications of interphalangeal joint contractures and donor site tenderness.

8. Cook FW, Jakab E, Pollock MA: Local neurovascular island flap. *J Hand Surg* 15A:798-802, 1990.
   The authors present the results of the local neurovascular island flap in 21 patients.

9. Baumeister S, Menke H, Wittemann M, Germann G: Functional outcome after the Moberg advancement flap in the thumb. *J Hand Surg* 27A:105-114, 2002.
   A Moberg flap was used to reconstruct the thumb pulp in 36 patients.

10. Trankle M, Sauerbier M, Heitmann C, Germann G: Restoration of thumb sensibility with the innervated first dorsal metacarpal artery island flap. *J Hand Surgery* 28:758-766, 2003.
    The authors investigated the quality of sensibility of the innervated first dorsal metacarpal artery island flap to the thumb in 25 patients.

## Suggested Readings

### Anatomy

Zook EG: Anatomy and physiology of the paronychium. *Hand Clin* 18:553-559, 2002.
   This review article provides a detailed description of the anatomy and physiology of the perionychium.

### Nail Bed Injuries

Brown RE: Acute nail bed injuries. *Hand Clin* 18:561-575, 2002.

This review article describes commonly encountered fingertip injuries and detailed management techniques to produce aesthetic and functional results.

Shepard GH: Perionychial grafts in trauma and reconstruction. *Hand Clin* 18:595-614, 2002.
The author describes surgical revision of posttraumatic nail bed deformities using full-thickness and split-thickness nail matrix grafts.

## Fingertip Amputations

Goitz RJ, Westkaemper JG, Tomaino MM, Sotereanos DG: Soft tissue defects of the digits. *Hand Clin* 13:189-205, 1997.
The authors describe common options for coverage of soft tissue defects of the digits, from the simple dressing changes to the more complex regional flaps.

## Local Flaps

Kutler W: A new method for fingertip amputation. *JAMA* 133:29-30, 1947.
The original description of the bilateral VY advancement flap, based on the terminal branches of the digital arteries, is presented.

Tupper J, Miller G: Sensitivity following volar V-Y plasty for fingertip amputations. *J Hand Surg* 10B:183-184, 1985.

Sensitivity outcomes of the volar VY advancement flap on 20 fingertip amputations over an average of 5.9 years are examined.

Shepard GH: The use of lateral V-Y advancement flaps for fingertip reconstruction. *J Hand Surg* 8:254-259, 1983.
The author describes a refinement of the Kutler lateral VY advancement flap, based on anatomic studies of the fibrous septa and neurovascular bundles of the distal phalanx.

## Regional Flaps

Kappel DA, Burech JG: The cross-finger flap. An established reconstructive procedure. *Hand Clin* 1:677-683, 1985.
The authors share their experience with cross-finger flaps in over 200 patients.

Sherif MML First dorsal metacarpal artery flap in hand reconstruction. Clinical application. *J Hand Surg* 19A:32-38, 1994.
The authors used this flap to treat traumatic soft tissue defects in 23 patients.

## Replantations

Soucacos PN: Indications and selection for digital amputation and replantation. *J Hand Surg* 26B:572-578, 2001.
A review article describes selection criteria and general indications for undertaking the delicate process of replantation.

# Soft Tissue Coverage of the Hand

Arshad Muzaffar

MD, Assistant Professor, Department of Plastic Surgery, University of Washington;
Attending Physician, Department of Plastic Surgery, Children's Hospital and Regional
Medical Center, Seattle, WA

## Introduction

- Any method for the reconstruction of soft tissue defects in the hand should preserve or restore function and provide wound coverage.
- Soft tissue coverage in the hand should supply tissue that is thin, pliable, durable and that will allow tendon gliding without creating contractures at joints or web spaces. An ideal reconstruction in the hand should allow for sensation, dynamic function, and restoration of form.
- The "reconstructive ladder"[1] should guide the choice of reconstructive options. In general, the simplest method of closure that fulfills the wound requirements should be selected. The reconstructive ladder progresses from simple to complex, as follows:
  - Primary closure
  - Wound contraction ("secondary intention")
  - Skin graft
  - Flap
    - Local
    - Distant
    - Free
- The choice of graft versus flap coverage depends upon a careful and thorough analysis of the wound and meticulous preparation of the wound before coverage.
- Definitive wound coverage should be undertaken when control of the wound has been achieved, that is, the wound is clean, with healthy granulation tissue. Ideally, wound coverage is achieved within 1 week of the injury.

## Preoperative Assessment and Wound Analysis

- The critical components of the hand should be assessed with a careful physical examination and radiographs. An inventory should be taken with respect to the wound: blood supply, innervation, skeletal stability, muscle-tendon units, skin coverage, and functional joints.
- The essential requirements for a successful initial reconstruction include skeletal stability, blood supply, and soft tissue coverage. Other components of a functional hand, including nerves, muscle-tendon units, and joints, can be treated either primarily or secondarily, depending upon the case.
- Assessment of the wound should consider several factors:
  - Wound location
  - Wound size, including depth
  - Zone of injury
  - Wound contamination or infection
  - Presence of key structures that must be covered (bone, tendon, ligament, nerve, vessel).

## Wound Preparation

- Debridement of the wound may be necessary. Any nonviable tissue must be excised. Longitudinal structures that are intact (tendons, nerves, axial vessels) generally should not be debrided.

- Infected wounds must be treated with surgical debridement and culture-specific antibiotics. Serial debridements may be required before definitive coverage is performed.
- Because such debridement usually produces a wound that is significantly larger than the initial wound, soft tissue coverage should be planned accordingly. The ultimate plan is made after debridement has been completed, yielding a clean, flat, healthy wound bed.

# Methods of Coverage

## Skin Grafts

- Autografts can be either full-thickness skin graft (FTSG) or split-thickness skin graft (STSG). Graft take depends upon contact between the graft and the wound bed to allow for inosculation (ingrowth of vessels into already existing vascular channels) and neovascularization (new vessel formation).
- A healthy, clean wound bed without exposed bone, tendon, or cartilage is required for skin graft application. Generally, grafts do not take over exposed bone or tendon in the absence of periosteum or peritenon, respectively. On the fingertip, a skin graft may take over exposed distal phalanx in a fingertip amputation, although this is not preferred. Moreover, skin grafts do not provide the appropriate gliding envelope for tendons.
- Skin grafts can consist of autograft (from the patient), allograft (from a human skin bank), or xenograft (usually porcine skin). Xenograft is used primarily as a "biologic dressing" and usually does not revascularize. Allograft can revascularize and "take"; however, it is rejected after the first week. It often is used to promote vascular ingrowth into a wound bed and to prepare the wound bed for later autografting. "Take" of an allograft indicates a high likelihood that an autograft will take.
- During the first 24 to 36 hours, the graft must survive on diffusion ("serum imbibition"); however, without revascularization after that point, the graft will not survive. Anything that disturbs the revascularization process, such as hematoma, infection, or shear, will prevent proper graft take. The best way to maintain contact between the graft and wound bed is with multiple staples or sutures, ensuring the grafts are fixed down to the wound bed in irregular areas. A moist compressive dressing or bolster over the graft provides pressure and immobilization. A tie-over bolster of Xeroform gauze often is used as a skin graft dressing. Alternatively, in extremity wounds with complex geometry, the vacuum-assisted closure device is an extremely useful skin graft "bolster." Dressings are left on for 1 week and then removed.
- Because split grafts are thinner, they take better than full-thickness grafts, are more resistant to infection, and do

better with a marginal wound bed. Full-thickness grafts, however, contract less, are more durable and flexible, and have better sensation. Therefore, they are preferred for areas prone to shear and load, such as fingertips, the palm, and areas over joints. In general, FTSGs are better for palmar wounds, whereas STSGs are better for dorsal wounds. Split grafts can be either meshed or unmeshed. Meshed grafts have fewer problems with seroma, hematoma, and infection and, therefore, have better take. However, the appearance of meshed STSGs is less acceptable.
- Donor sites for split grafts include the lateral thigh, hip, buttock, scalp, or nearly anywhere. The medial thigh should be avoided because the skin is much thinner and a full-thickness wound can develop if skin is harvested there. Generally, skin in adults should be harvested at 0.0010- to 0.0012-inch thickness. A no. 15 scalpel can be used to check the set thickness: the blade is approximately 0.001 inch thick, and the thick back part is 0.0015 inch thick. Proper thickness can be confirmed if the blade just fits into the dermatome's opening without undue stress.
- The donor area can be prepared with either mineral oil or saline to allow smooth passage of a Padgett or Zimmer electric dermatome. Tongue depressors can be used to apply tension to facilitate taking the graft. Small donor sites are dressed with an occlusive dressing (e.g., OpSite, Tegaderm), whereas larger donor sites are dressed with Xeroform gauze and a Kerlix gauze roll. The dressing is taken down to the Xeroform layer after 24 to 48 hours, and the Xeroform is left open to air. Heat lamps or blow dryers can be used to dry out the donor site.
- Donor site complications can include infection, hypertrophic scarring, and conversion (donor site becomes a full-thickness wound).
- Full-thickness skin can be harvested from the groin crease (lateral to the hair), abdomen, antecubital crease, proximal medial forearm, or hypothenar aspect of the hand, which provides thick, glabrous skin. The fibular aspect of the great toe also provides good FTSGs and composite grafts for fingertip reconstruction. The volar wrist crease can be used; however, the resulting scar can be a theoretical psychosocial disability because it may be mistaken for scar from a suicide attempt, although in practice this has not been an issue. Full-thickness grafts should be harvested without fat. This is best accomplished using a scalpel, carefully raising the graft off the subcutaneous fat. The donor site usually is closed primarily. Large FTSGs should be pie-crusted with a no. 11 blade scalpel to allow egress of blood and serum. Careful dressing and splint or cast application are critical for good skin graft take. The same dressing principles as discussed for STSG apply for FTSG. In particular, on the digits (e.g., after burn scar contracture release), small FTSGs can be bolstered with custom-cut, layered dressings of Xeroform gauze and

dressing gauze, held in place with Mastisol and Steri-Strips. Care must be taken not to place any circumferential dressings around digits. These dressings should be protected with a cast. In some cases, Kirschner wire immobilization of the grafted digit may be required to protect the graft while it is healing.

- Donor site complications include hypertrophic or keloid scarring.

## Flaps: Basic Principles

- Flaps can be categorized according to their blood supply (random vs. axial), their method of transfer (e.g., pedicled or free flap), and their location (local, regional, or distant). In the digits, location can be further categorized as homodigital and heterodigital.
- *Random flaps* depend on the subdermal or subcutaneous vascular plexus to maintain flap viability. Examples of random flaps include the VY advancement flap for fingertip reconstruction (homodigital), the cross-finger flap (heterodigital and interpolation), the dorsal rotation flap for first web space release (local flap), and the abdominal or chest wall flaps (distant flaps).
- *Axial flaps* are supplied by a named artery. The axial pattern flaps can be divided into (1) cutaneous, (2) fasciocutaneous, and (3) musculocutaneous. The groin flap is an example of a cutaneous axial flap. The radial forearm flap is an example of a fasciocutaneous axial flap. The latissimus dorsi flap can be raised as a musculocutaneous flap. Because axial flaps are better vascularized than random flaps, they can be made larger than random flaps and bring blood supply into the wound. The axial pattern flaps can be raised as a pedicled flap when applied in the same region, or the pedicle can be divided and reattached using a microvascular technique as a free tissue transfer.
- *Pedicled flaps* of the advancement, rotation, or transposition type can be transferred in a single stage. Interpolation flaps, such as the cross-finger or thenar flaps, must be transferred in two stages. These flaps remain attached to their donor sites until the flaps become vascularized by the wound bed. The base of the flaps then can be divided at the second stage procedure, and the insetting of the flaps completed. Usually the period between the two stages is approximately 2 to 3 weeks.
  - Transposition, rotation, and advancement flaps are moved into an adjacent defect, whereas interpolation flaps must cross intervening intact tissue to reach the defect.[1,2]
- The application of flaps in the hand and upper extremity are discussed with respect to the location of the soft tissue defect.

## Digits

- Fingertip injuries are extremely common. For transverse injuries or those with more dorsal than volar tissue loss, a VY advancement flap from the volar pulp provides coverage. This is a random flap. Either a single volar flap or bilateral flaps from the lateral borders of the digits can be used. The VY flap cannot be used for wounds with primarily volar tissue loss. These wounds can be covered with either heterodigital flaps or a local flap.
- The cross-finger flap is a useful heterodigital flap. This flap is a random interpolation flap taken from the dorsum of an adjacent finger and applied to the defect. It must remain attached to the defect for approximately 2 weeks before the flap base can be divided. The flap donor site is skin grafted at the first-stage procedure.[2]
- Alternatively, volar fingertip wounds can be covered with a thenar flap, which is a random, local, interpolation flap. The thenar flap is used for defects of the index and middle fingers. It is raised from the glabrous skin on the thenar eminence. Again, this flap is left attached to its base for 10 to 14 days before the second-stage division and inset. Because of the flexed posture of the finger during this time, the risk of flexion contractures in patients older than 30 years can be significant.[2]
- Defects of the tip of the thumb can be treated with the Moberg advancement flap (Figure 21–1). This is a homodigital, axial flap based upon the radial and ulnar digital arteries of the thumb. The volar soft tissues of the thumb are raised with the neurovascular bundles and advanced into the defect in a single-stage procedure. The flap can be advanced approximately 1.5 cm. Greater advancement can be achieved by dividing the skin proximally and then back grafting the defect. This flap is unique to the thumb because of the thumb's excellent dorsal blood supply and the hyperextensibility of the thumb interphalangeal joint.[3,4] Alternatively, the cross-finger flap can be used for this purpose (Figure 21–2).
- More extensive distal defects of the digits can be covered by a neurovascular island flap from another digit, as described by Littler.[2,5] This flap is particularly useful for restoring sensate tissue to the opposing surface of the thumb or index finger. The neurovascular pedicle is tunneled across the palmar skin so that the flap can reach the defect.
- More proximal defects of the digits can sometimes be covered by a homodigital rotation or transposition flap. Proximal defects on the dorsum of the digits that cannot be covered by such flaps can be covered with a heterodigital reverse cross-finger flap. This flap consists of the fat and fascial layer between the skin and extensor peritenon. The donor site skin is elevated, remaining pedicled on the side of the digit away from the defect, while the flap tissue is pedicled on the side adjacent to the defect. Flap skin coverage is provided with a split-thickness graft, while the skin from the donor site is simply sutured back into place (Figure 21–3). More proximal palmar wounds can be covered by a standard cross-finger flap.[1,2]

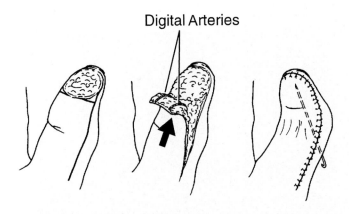

Digital Arteries

Digital Arteries

Skin Graft

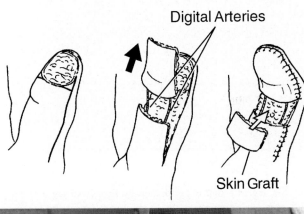

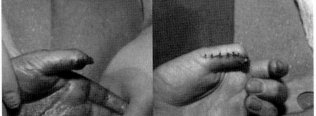

Figure 21–1:
**Moberg advancement flap used for thumb tip coverage. (A,** From Trumble TE, editor: *Principles of hand surgery and therapy.* Philadelphia, 2000, WB Saunders.)

- The *axial flag flap* is useful for coverage of proximal palmar digital defects and more distal defects of the hand proper (i.e., from the metacarpophalangeal [MCP] area proximally), both palmar and dorsal. This axial flap is based upon a dorsal digital artery that takes branches from either the proper digital artery or the dorsal metacarpal artery. This artery is most reliably found in the web space between the index and middle fingers. The flap territory includes the dorsal tissue between the MCP and proximal interphalangeal joints and the midaxial lines of the digit. The axial flag flap can be used as either a homodigital or heterodigital flap. The donor site is skin grafted. Doppler examination is recommended when planning the flap.[2,6]

- Random pedicled flaps from the abdomen or chest wall, although not ideal, can be used when none of the previous options is feasible.

## Hand (Proximal to Metacarpophalangeal Level)

### Local Flaps

- Local flaps to cover dorsal and palmar hand wounds include some that have been mentioned earlier, namely, rotation or transposition flaps, axial flag flaps, and neurovascular island flaps. In addition to these flaps, in cases that require amputation of a digit and have an associated defect in the hand (e.g., gunshot wound), a fillet flap from the amputated digit can provide useful coverage of the wound.

- Another useful local flap is the dorsal metacarpal artery flap. This flap can be used antegrade or retrograde for coverage of dorsal hand or digit wounds. The retrograde flap is based upon vascular connections between the palmar and dorsal circulation that occur at the level of

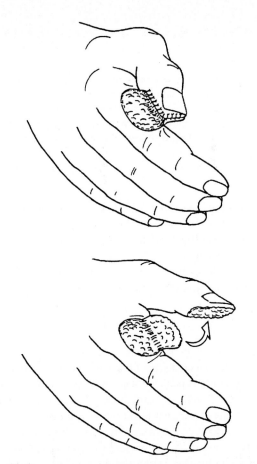

Figure 21–2:
**Cross-finger flap used for larger volar thumb tip defect with donor site skin grafted.** (From Trumble TE, editor: *Principles of hand surgery and therapy.* Philadelphia, 2000, WB Saunders.)

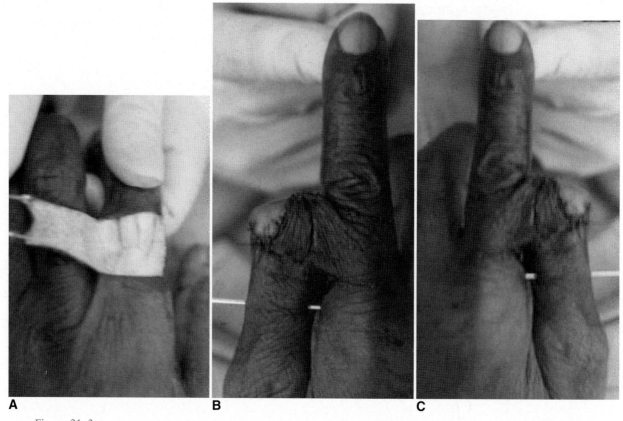

**Figure 21–3:**
**A,** The reverse cross finger flap using the subcutaneous tissue as a separate flap is performed by first elevating a thin flap of skin with the base on the opposite side of the finger requiring coverage. **B,** In the next step of the reverse cross finger flap, a flap of subcutaneous tissue with the volar veins and peritenon is raised and rotated to cover the dorsal defect on the adjacent digit. **C,** In the final step of the reverse cross finger flap, a skin graft is sutured onto the subcutaneous tissue flap on the recipient site.

the metacarpophalangeal (MP) joint (sometimes more proximally) and the level of the web space.[2,6,7] As with the axial flag flap, Doppler examination of the flap is an important step.

- The first dorsal metacarpal artery flap is useful for coverage of wounds of the proximal thumb (Figure 21–4).

### Distant Fascial and Fasciocutaneous Flaps

- When local flaps are not available or are not adequate to cover the defect, distant flaps can be used. As mentioned earlier, random pedicled flaps from the abdomen or chest wall can be used to cover defects on the hand and digits. The abdominal pocket flap is extremely useful for burn or degloving/avulsion injuries when there has been a substantial area of skin loss on the dorsum of the hand. The incision in the abdomen or groin is made, and the skin is undermined in order to allow the hand to be buried into the pocket. Three weeks after the hand has been placed in the pocket, the surgeon has

several options. The hand can be dissected away from the roof of the skin pocket so that the subcutaneous tissue with its vascularized granulation tissue is still attached to the dorsum of the hand. This now makes a good bed for a split in the skin grafts, and the pocket site can be closed primarily. In other cases where additional full-thickness skin is required over the defect, the skin overlying the buried hand can be incised so that the skin and subcutaneous tissue are left still attached to the hand.

### Groin Flap

- An axial pedicled flap can be raised from the lower abdomen. The groin flap is based upon the superficial circumflex iliac artery (SCIA) and provides a large area of skin and subcutaneous fat (Figure 21–5). Extensions of the flap distal to the anterior superior iliac spine are random. The pedicled groin flap is reliable, and the donor defect can be closed directly by flexing the hip and undermining the abdominal skin to produce a scar that is

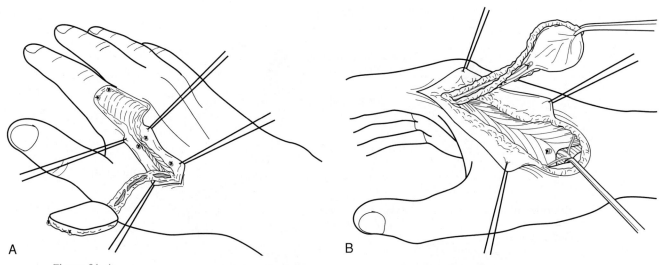

Figure 21–4:

**Proximally based dorsal metacarpal artery flap for dorsal thumb coverage (A) and distally based flap for dorsal digit coverage (B).**

well hidden. However, the groin flap can be bulky, especially in obese patients. The groin flap also can be raised as a free tissue transfer.

- The SCIA takes origin from anterolateral aspect of the femoral artery in most cases, beginning 2 to 3 cm below the inguinal ligament. The SCIA travels laterally superficial

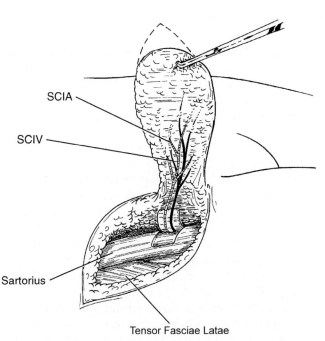

SCIA

SCIV

Sartorius

Tensor Fasciae Latae

Figure 21–5:

Groin flap. *SCIA*, Superficial circumflex iliac artery; *SCIV*, superficial circumflex iliac vein. (From Trumble TE, Vedder NB: Tissue transfer: pedicle and free tissue flaps. In Trumble TE, editor: *Principles of hand surgery and therapy*. Philadelphia, 2000, WB Saunders.)

to the fascia and parallel to the inguinal ligament. At the medial border of the sartorius muscle, the SCIA frequently divides into the two branches, superficial and deep. By elevating the fascia of the sartorius muscle with the flap, the surgeon can include both the deep and superficial branches to maximize flap survival.[1,2,8]

## Radial Forearm Flap

- The radial forearm flap can provide fascial or fasciocutaneous coverage either as a pedicled flap or as a free tissue transfer based on the radial artery. The radial forearm flap can be harvested as a composite flap with a portion of bone from the cortex of the radius. Tendons such as the palmaris longus and flexor carpi radialis can be included with the flap to provide a combined coverage of soft tissue defects and tendon reconstruction.[1,2,9] The flap has been described as a distally based pedicled flap for hand reconstruction.[1,2] In the upper extremity, the forearm flap usually is used based on its vascular pedicle rather than as a free tissue transfer (Figures 21–6 and 21–7).
- The radial forearm flap provides thin, supple tissue that is ideal for coverage in the hand. However, the donor defect can be troublesome, frequently requiring skin grafting directly over the paratenon of the flexor tendons, producing an undesirable donor site appearance. The portion of the bone along the lateral half of the radius between the pronator teres and the pronator quadratus is available for harvesting with the flap as a vascularized bone graft. This provides approximately 10 cm of bone, which is cortical and slightly curved. The bone is vascularized by the periosteal contributions of the radial artery.
- It is important to perform an Allen test to test the patency of the ulnar artery and determine whether the

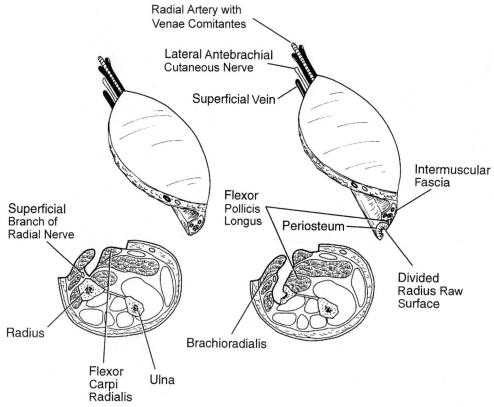

Figure 21–6:
Radial forearm flap. (From Trumble TE, Vedder NB: Tissue transfer: pedicle and free tissue flaps. In: Trumble TE, editor: *Principles of hand surgery and therapy.* Philadelphia, 2000, WB Saunders.)

artery supplies all the digits, including the thumb. Although anatomic variations can occur, in clinical practice, nearly all individuals without prior injuries or vascular disease have the ability to perfuse the thumb and index finger from the ulnar artery alone.[10]

- The cephalic vein usually lies within the territory of the flap and is useful for microvascular anastomosis. When used as a pedicle flap, reverse flow through the venae comitantes usually is adequate, even through flow must proceed against the valves. By performing a venous outflow anastomosis with the cephalic vein, this congestion can be avoided.

## Posterior Interosseous Flap

- The posterior interosseous flap is another thin, pliable flap that can be used for coverage of the hand, either as a fascial or a fasciocutaneous flap. This axial flap is based on the posterior interosseous artery that travels in the septum between the extensor carpi ulnaris and the extensor digiti quinti (i.e., between the fifth and sixth extensor compartments). The flap is used in a retrograde fashion for coverage of the hand. As such, it is important to note the extent of the zone of injury distally, because the pedicle may be unreliable in the setting of a wide zone of

injury or focal injury to the communication between the anterior and posterior interosseous circulations (at the level of the distal radioulnar joint). The flap axis is centered on a line from the lateral epicondyle of the humerus to the distal radioulnar joint.[11,12]

## Lateral Arm Flap

- The lateral arm flap is an axial flap that often can be harvested from the injured limb. A vascularized portion of the humerus can be included with this flap to provide bone and soft tissue reconstruction. The flap can be split either longitudinally or transversely to permit a fold in the flap to cover a wider array of defects. These flaps can be bulky and thick, and they often leave an unattractive donor site defect, particularly when skin grafting is required (Figure 21–8).

- The blood supply to the lateral arm flap is via the posterior radial collateral artery that arises from the profunda brachii artery. The posterior radial collateral artery passes posterior to the origin of the lateral intermuscular septum to supply the periosteum overlying the distal humerus. The posterior radial collateral artery provides branches to the muscles in both anterior and posterior compartments. The main

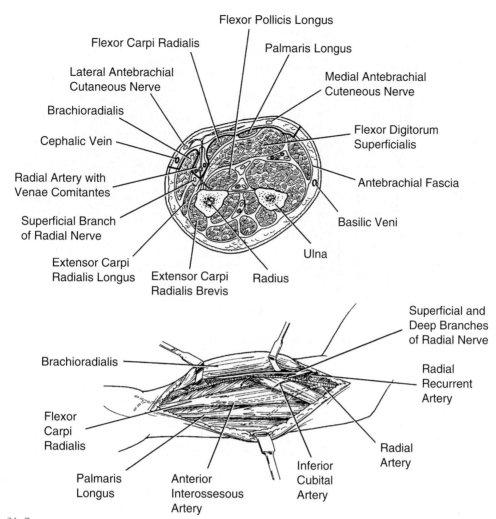

Figure 21–7:
Radial arterial anatomy. (From Trumble TE, Vedder NB: Tissue transfer: pedicle and free tissue flaps. In Trumble TE, editor: *Principles of hand surgery and therapy.* Philadelphia, 2000, WB Saunders.)

branches to the fascia and skin arise between the lower half of the line between the deltoid tubercle and the epicondyle. Ideally, skin flaps are elevated as an elliptical island of skin centered over this line.[1,2,13]

- Other useful distant fasciocutaneous flaps include the scapular flap,[14] which is supplied by the circumflex scapular artery (CSA), and the anterolateral thigh flap, which is supplied by the descending branch of the lateral femoral circumflex artery.[1] These flaps are transferred to the hand as free flaps.

## Scapular Flap

- The scapular flap can provide a fairly large surface area of skin and fascia or fascia alone (Figure 21–9). This axial flap is based on the CSA. The skin has less subcutaneous fat than the groin flap and usually is hairless. The donor site usually can be closed directly; however, a tight closure results in a spreading scar high on the back.

- The CSA is a branch of the subscapular system. The subscapular artery is 3 mm in diameter and takes its origin from the axillary artery. It then branches into the CSA (the first branch), the serratus branch, and the thoracodorsal artery, which supplies the latissimus dorsi. The CSA passes posteriorly to the subscapularis through the muscular triangle bordered by the teres major, teres minor, and long head of the triceps. The artery gives off branches to the subscapularis and teres major and minor during its course. The CSA forms two terminal branches. The terminal descending branch travels deep to the teres major, and the cutaneous branch then splits into the transverse and descending branches. The transverse branch supplies the scapular flap (transverse orientation across the scapula), while the descending branch supplies the parascapular flap (oblique orientation along the lateral border of the scapula). The CSA can provide a pedicle 4 to 8 cm long with an artery that is 2.5 to 3.5 mm in

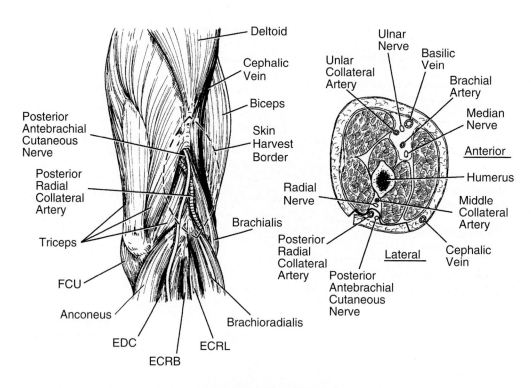

Lateral Arm Flap Harvest

Figure 21–8:

Lateral arm flap. *ECRB,* Extensor carpi radialis brevis; *ECRL,* extensor carpi radialis longus; *EDC,* extensor digitorum communis; *FCU,* flexor carpi ulnaris. (From Trumble TE, Vedder NB: Tissue transfer: pedicle and free tissue flaps. In Trumble TE, editor: *Principles of hand surgery and therapy*. Philadelphia, 2000, WB Saunders.)

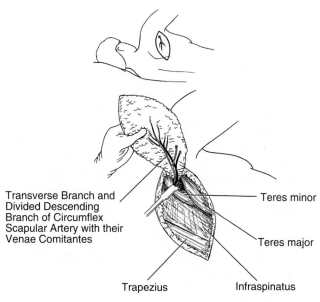

Figure 21–9:

Scapular flap. (From Trumble TE, Vedder NB: Tissue transfer: pedicle and free tissue flaps. In Trumble TE, editor: *Principles of hand surgery and therapy*. Philadelphia, 2000, WB Saunders.)

diameter. The arteries are accompanied by two venae comitantes, which provide adequate drainage for the flap. Although flaps up to 24 cm long have been reported, the standard flap is approximately 15 cm long by 10 cm wide.

## Distant Muscle and Musculocutaneous Flaps

- Useful muscle and musculocutaneous flaps include the latissimus dorsi, serratus anterior, and gracilis flap. The latissimus dorsi, based upon the thoracodorsal artery, is a workhorse flap for coverage of large wounds of the hand and upper extremity. The serratus anterior, based upon the serratus branch from the subscapular artery, is an extremely versatile flap for coverage of wounds with complex contours in the hand.[15,16] The gracilis flap, based upon the medial femoral circumflex artery, can be used not only for soft tissue coverage but also to restore function through the anastomosis of its motor nerve, a branch of the obturator nerve.[1]

## Conclusions

- Adherence to the principles of wound analysis and preparation combined with selection of an appropriate tissue transfer allows for a functionally and aesthetically satisfying result in coverage of soft tissue defects of the hand and upper extremity.

- Wounds with exposed bone, cartilage, tendons, ligaments, nerves, and vessels generally require flap coverage. Otherwise, skin grafts usually suffice. Careful use of dressings, splints, and casts is critical in achieving skin graft "take." Flap choice should be based upon wound requirements, wound location, and available donor sites. In all cases, the reconstructive ladder should serve as a guideline in choosing a method for wound coverage.

# References

1. Mathes SJ, Nahai F: *Reconstructive plastic surgery.* New York, 1997, Churchill-Livingstone.
   The classic text describing the panoply of flaps and the principles of reconstruction.

2. Hentz VR, Chase RA: *Hand surgery: a clinical atlas.* Philadelphia, 2001, WB Saunders.
   An outstanding new atlas of hand surgery, including excellent chapters on "Skin, Soft Tissue, and Amputations" and "Microvascular Surgery."

3. Baumeister S, Manke H, Wittemann M, Germann G: Functional outcome after the Moberg advancement flap in the thumb. *J Hand Surg* 27A:105-114, 2002.
   Notes excellent outcomes for the Moberg advancement flop. All 36 patients survived, normal sensation was achieved in 74%, and no thumb developed a permanent flexion contracture.

4. Foucher G, Delaire O, Citron N, Molderez A: Long-term outcome of neurovascular palmar advancement flaps for distal thumb injuries. *Br J Plast Surg* 52:64-68, 1999.
   The authors believe neurovascular palmal flaps should be the first choice for coverage of 1- to 2-cm thumb tip pulp defects.

5. Littler JW: Neurovascular pedicle transfer of tissue. *J Bone Joint Surg* 38A:917, 1956.
   Littler's original presentation of the sensate flap for digital reconstruction.

6. Yang D, Morris SF: Vascular basis of dorsal digital and metacarpal skin flaps. *J Hand Surg* 26A:142-146, 2001.
   A detailed description of the vascular anatomy and clinical applications for flap design are presented.

7. Okada E, Maruyama Y, Hayashi A: Stepladder dorsal metacarpal flaps for dorsal finger and hand reconstruction. *Ann Plast Surg* 48:48-52, 2002.
   A variation of the dorsal metacarpal artery flap is presented, which may be a useful technique for reconstruction of dorsal finger and hand defects.

8. Ohmori K, Harii K: Free groin flaps: their vascular basis. *Br J Plast Surg* 28:238, 1975.
   This article addresses the vascular anatomy of the groin flap's pedicle, which is variable, and the advantages of using the free groin flap.

9. Song R, Gao Y, Song Y, Yu Y: The forearm flap. *Clin Plast Surg* 9:21, 1982.
   Introduces the radial forearm flap, which is often used as a distally based pedicled flap for coverage of the hand. It also can be used as a free tissue transfer.

10. Ciria-Llorens G, Gomez-Cia T, Talegon-Melendez A: Analysis of flow changes in forearm arteries after raising the radial forearm flap. A prospective study using color duplex imaging. *Br J Plast Reconstr Surg* 52:440-444, 1999.
    Following radial forearm flaps, another "major vascular axis" based on the anterior interosseous artery develops, and overall blood flow to the hand is not compromised.

11. Costa H, Gracia ML, Vranchx J et al: The posterior interosseous flap: a review of 81 clinical cases and 100 anatomical dissections: assessment of its indications in reconstruction of hand defects. *Br J Plast Surg* 54:28-33, 2001.
    Primary indications for this flap include dorsal hand defects up to the metacarpophalangeal joints, reconstruction of the first web space, and extensive lesions of the ulnar border of the hand.

12. Zancolli EA, Angrigiani C: Posterior interosseous island forearm flap. *J Hand Surg* 13B:130-135, 1988.
    The vascular anatomy and surgical technique for the reverse posterior interosseous flap are reviewed.

13. Katsaros J, Schusterman M, Beppu M et al: The lateral upper arm flap: anatomy and clinical application. *Ann Plast Surg* 12:489-500, 1984.
    A discussion of the lateral arm flap, its anatomy, clinical applications, advantages, and disadvantages.

14. Dos Santos LF: The vascular anatomy and dissection of the free scapular flap. *Plast Reconstr Surg* 73:599-604, 1984.
    An anatomic dissection of the scapular flap is presented, carefully describing the circumflex scapular artery pedicle and the use of these flaps to cover forearm defects.

15. Brody GA, Buncke HJ, Alpert BS, Hing DN: Serratus anterior muscle transplantation for treatment of soft tissue defects in the hand. *J Hand Surg* 15A:322-327, 1990.
    The serratus anterior muscle flap is versatile for coverage of hand defects and has a long pedicle of up to 15 cm if the entire subscapular axis length is used.

16. Fassio E, Laulan J, Aboumoussa J et al: Serratus anterior free fascial flap for dorsal hand coverage. *Ann Plast Surg* 43:77-82, 1999.
    Describes another thin, pliable fascial flap for hand reconstruction. It has a long, constant vascular pedicle and the option of harvesting other tissues with the flap.

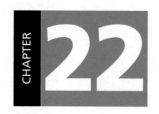

# CHAPTER 22

# Hand Infections

Roger Cornwall

MD, Pediatric Hand and Upper Extremity Surgeon, The Children's Hospital of Philadelphia; Assistant Professor of Orthopaedic Surgery, University of Pennsylvania School of Medicine, Philadelphia, PA

## Introduction

- Infections in the hand and wrist, which can lead to necrosis and fibrosis if not properly and promptly treated, can easily disturb the intricate functional anatomy of the hand.
- Numerous closed spaces exist in the hand and fingers, allowing collections of infection that require surgical drainage despite appropriate antimicrobial treatment.
- The progression from inoculation to clinically relevant infection depends on the virulence of the organism, the quality and viability of local tissue, and the immune status of the host.

## Epidemiology

- Most hand infections result from direct inoculation following punctures, lacerations, open fractures, and bites.
- Cellulitis, paronychias, and felons are the most commonly encountered hand infections and are often treated by primary care practitioners.
- Among serious infections, those caused by human bites are the most common, accounting for up to 50% of cases.
- Septic arthritis, pyogenic flexor tenosynovitis, and abscesses each composes fewer than 10% of cases of hand infections.

## Microbiology and Pharmacology

- Hand infections requiring surgical treatment most often are caused by staphylococcal and streptococcal species but often are polymicrobial.[1]

- The organisms causing hand infections often can be predicted by the mode of inoculation, the pattern of infection, and the immune status of the host (Box 22–1).
- Antibiotic resistance is increasingly common, with *Staphylococcus aureus* resistant to penicillin and cefazolin in 16% of a series of 247 cultures obtained from surgically treated hand infections.[1]
- Methicillin-resistant *S. aureus* (MRSA) can cause community-acquired hand infections even in immunocompetent hosts.[2,3]
- Uncommon organisms such as *Acinetobacter* and *Pseudomonas* spp. are resistant to first-line antimicrobial therapy in nearly all cases.

| Box 22–1 | Microbiology of Hand Infections |
|---|---|
| **Clinical Clues** | **Typical Organism(s)** |
| Acute, suppurative infections | Gram-positive aerobes, such as *Staphylococcus aureus* |
| Chronic, indolent infections | Atypical organisms, such as *Mycobacteria* and fungi |
| Heavily contaminated wounds | Polymicrobial, including gram-negatives and anaerobes |
| Human bites | α-hemolytic and β-hemolytic *Streptococcus*, *Eikenella*, anaerobes |
| Fish spine inoculation | *Vibrio* species |
| Marine water exposure | *Mycobacterium marinum* |
| Rose thorn inoculation | *Sporothrix schenckii* |
| Immunodeficient host | Polymicrobial, including gram-negatives |

## Taking a History

- A complete history (Box 22–2) is of vital importance for several reasons:
  - The mode of inoculation can give important clues to guide empiric antimicrobial therapy while awaiting culture results.
  - The duration of symptoms can guide treatment. Some infections can be treated with intravenous antibiotics early in their course but require urgent surgical drainage late in their course.
  - The time course of progression can differentiate indolent, acute, and rapidly progressive (such as necrotizing fasciitis) infections.
  - The immune status of the host can determine the severity of infection and the likelihood of progression and complications.
  - Response or lack of response to prior treatments can give clues to the nature or severity of infection.

## Physical Examination

- The intricate anatomy of the hand demands a careful and detailed physical examination for suspected infections.
- Erythema can indicate simple cellulitis or accompany a more serious deep infection. Proximal streaking of erythema suggests lymphangitic spread.
- Swelling can be helpful, depending on location.
  - Dorsal hand swelling usually is nonspecific.
  - Palmar swelling suggests infection of the underlying compartment. For example, loss of the concavity of the palm suggests midpalmar space abscess.
  - Fusiform swelling of the finger can represent pyogenic flexor tenosynovitis.
- Fluctuance often is difficult to detect even when an abscess exists, and its absence cannot rule out a deep infection. Dorsal hand fluctuance can be hidden by overlying edema distending the thin, capacious skin. Palmar fluctuance can be masked by the thick, tethered palmar skin.
- The posture of the hand can help localize an infection, because an infection within a compartment forces that part of the hand into a position of maximal volume in order to minimize pressure.

---

**Box 22–2  Essential Components of the History**

- Age and health/immune status of the host
- Occupational/environmental exposures
- Mode of inoculation (laceration, puncture, human bite, etc.)
- Duration and progression of symptoms
- Localization of symptoms
- Systemic symptoms
- Prior treatment(s)

---

  - Pyogenic flexor tenosynovitis causes the finger to rest in a flexed position.
  - Web space infection causes the adjacent fingers to abduct.
- An infected compartment is tender to palpation and to any maneuver that decreases its volume:
  - Pyogenic flexor tenosynovitis causes tenderness to palpation along the entire flexor sheath and pain with passive extension of the involved finger.
  - An infected web space is tender both dorsally and volarly and with passive adduction of the adjacent fingers.
  - An infected joint is tender to palpation circumferentially and to passive range of motion in any direction.
- Neurologic and vascular complications can follow severe infection or infection in immunocompromised or vasculopathic individuals, making a detailed neurovascular examination critical.

## Ancillary Studies for Hand Infections

- Peripheral white blood cell count with differential, erythrocyte sedimentation rate, and C-reactive protein can help judge the severity of an infection but typically are not sufficiently sensitive or specific to make a diagnosis.
- Cultures and sensitivities are important.
  - Cultures should be obtained prior to starting antimicrobial treatment whenever possible.
  - Gram stains can be helpful acutely.
  - Both aerobic and anaerobic cultures should be obtained.
  - If the history suggests atypical organisms (e.g., *Mycobacteria*, fungus, *Sporothrix schenckii*), the laboratory should be notified of the suspected organism so that the appropriate culture media and techniques will be used.
  - *Culture results should always be checked* until finalization by the laboratory, regardless of the clinical course.
- Radiographs can detect foreign bodies, fractures, and late osteomyelitis.
- Magnetic resonance imaging and ultrasonography can detect fluid collections if the physical examination is unreliable or inconclusive.

## Principles of Treatment

- Many infections can be treated with oral or parenteral antimicrobial agents early in their course. Use empiric antibiotics first, narrowing the spectrum later as allowed by culture results.
- Monitor closely the clinical response to antimicrobial treatment. Signs and symptoms of infection that do not resolve within 12 to 24 hours of antimicrobial treatment suggests one of two possibilities:
  - The antimicrobial agent is incorrect or insufficient. Reevaluate the clinical clues, reexamine culture and

sensitivity results, consider broadening the antimicrobial spectrum, and consult an infectious disease specialist if unsure.

- The infection requires surgical treatment. Reexamine the hand, consider ancillary studies if unclear, and proceed to surgical exploration if indicated.
- Surgical treatment of hand infections must allow adequate drainage while minimizing trauma.
  - Incisions should be designed so that vital structures such as nerves, tendons, and vessels are not left exposed and allowed to desiccate if the wound is left open.
  - Incisions should be designed to minimize the functional effects of scar contracture.
  - Local anesthesia often is ineffective in the acidic environment of an infection and may spread infection along tissue planes.
- Formal rehabilitation often is required.
  - Immobilization early during treatment can allow faster resolution of inflammation, but the hand should be immobilized such that stiffness is minimized (wrist slightly extended, metacarpophalangeal (MCP) joints flexed at least 70 degrees, interphalangeal joints extended).
  - Rehabilitation should be started as soon as the acute phase has subsided.
  - The patient should be enlisted as an active participant in rehabilitation from the beginning of treatment.

## The Immunocompromised Host

- Diabetes poses a significant risk for serious infections in the hand.[4,5]
  - Infections are polymicrobial in 50% of cases.
  - Amputations are required for 17% to 40% of deep hand infections.
  - Coexisting renal failure increases the amputation rate and worsens prognosis.
  - Insulin dependence does not seem to affect prognosis.
- Human immunodeficiency virus (HIV) infection may predispose patients to serious hand infections, although the relative causative contributions of immunosuppression and intravenous drug use (often coexistent) have not been clarified in the available literature. Nonetheless, be alert for polymicrobial infections in these patients.
- The immunosuppressive medications required following organ transplantation pose a risk for serious and atypical infections in posttransplant patients. Fungal infections are common.

## Infections According to Mode of Inoculation

### Human Bites

- Human "bites" to the hand result from conflict in nearly all cases. As a result, the patient often does not divulge an accurate history for fear of punitive action. Moreover, many such bites initially appear minor and in the patient's opinion do not seem to warrant urgent attention. Therefore, many patients do not present for medical care until after an infection has become established. A series of 35 human bites found a mean time from injury to presentation of 4 days, with more than half of patients presenting after 2 days.[6]
- A human bite should be suspected in any infected laceration over the finger MCP joints, especially in a young male's dominant hand.
- Assuring the patient complete confidentiality and reminding him or her that grave consequences can result from an untreated or improperly treated infection with oral flora may help in obtaining an accurate history.

### Acute Human Bite Wounds

- All lacerations resulting from contact with a human mouth should be considered contaminated, even if no signs of infection are present at the time of presentation. The wound should be thoroughly irrigated.
- Because most lacerations occur during a punch with a clenched fist, the metacarpophalangeal joints are easily penetrated. A plain radiograph may demonstrate a minute depression of the underlying metacarpal head suggesting impaction by a tooth and thus intraarticular penetration (Figure 22–1). The absence of a depression fracture does not, however, rule out intraarticular penetration.
- Intraarticular penetration can be ascertained by injecting a small amount of normal saline into the MCP joint (Box 22–3). Methylene blue dye also can be used, but it can be difficult to see in a bloody wound, it is messy, and spillage of even one or two drops in the subcutaneous tissue near the wound can confound the test results.

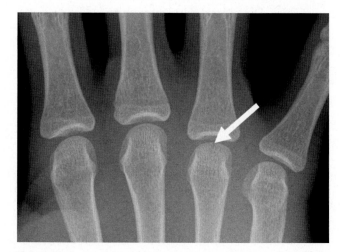

Figure 22–1:

**Metacarpal head depression fracture *(arrow)*. Note the subtle nature of the fracture and the ease with which it can be overlooked by an observer not specifically seeking this finding.**

<table>
<tr><td>

**Box 22–3** | **Diagnosis of Puncture Wounds to the MCP Joint**

- A 20-gauge intravenous catheter is inserted into the dorsoradial or dorsoulnar aspect of the MCP joint, away from the laceration.
- Traction on the affected digit makes intraarticular placement easier.
- Injection of less than 3–5 ml of saline should distend the joint and cause resistance to further injection if the joint capsule is intact.
- If the capsule has been violated by the laceration, saline should flow easily out of the laceration with minimal resistance.
- When in doubt, assume that the injury penetrated the MCP joint and treat accordingly.
- The catheter should be left in place for irrigation of the joint with 500 ml of normal saline.
- The joint should not be irrigated directly through the laceration, even if intraarticular penetration is easily seen, because such irrigation can drive bacteria from the wound deeper into the joint.
</td></tr>
</table>

- A systematic review of randomized controlled trials found prophylactic antibiotics were helpful in preventing infection following human bites.[7] Antibiotics should be chosen to ensure coverage of *Streptococcus viridans*, *Eikenella* spp., and oral anaerobes and should be tailored to the patient's immune status and local microbial resistance patterns.

## Established Human Bite Infections

- Established infections from human bites usually require treatment with parenteral antibiotics and formal surgical debridement.
- The wound should be extended in a longitudinal fashion avoiding the prominence of the metacarpal head to avoid a wound that exposes the extensor tendon gliding over the metacarpal head. The underlying MCP joint, if penetrated, should be opened and copiously irrigated. The adjacent web spaces should be inspected for signs of purulence. The wound should be left open if the extensor tendon is not exposed or partially closed over a drain if the tendon is directly beneath the wound.
- Intravenous antibiotics should be used postoperatively. In this patient population, potential noncompliance with an outpatient antibiotic regimen (63% in one series[6]) should prompt the surgeon to consider using intravenous antibiotics until the infection resolves rather than switching to oral antibiotics early in the postoperative course.

## Animal Bites

- The hand and upper extremity are the most common sites for dog and cat bites. Children and young adults are the individuals most often bitten, and the offending

animal usually is known to the victim. Dog bites more commonly occur in males and cat bites more commonly in females. Dog bites unusually consist of abrasions and lacerations, whereas cat bites usually consist of puncture wounds.
- As with human bites, victims of seemingly minor dog or cat bites often present late for medical attention for fear of punitive action toward their pet. Often the wound appears to warrant medical attention only after an infection becomes apparent.
- A careful history regarding the immunization history of the animal, if known, must be obtained. Rabies vaccination is not routinely necessary.
- The wounds should be carefully irrigated and debrided.
- A systematic review of randomized trials failed to show a benefit of prophylactic antibiotics following uncomplicated dog and cat bites.[7] Nonetheless, infection rates as high as 80% in retrospective series still encourage some to use prophylactic antibiotics. Regardless of the decision to use prophylactic antibiotics, close follow-up must be ensured to detect an infection early if it occurs.
- Cats' teeth are long and slender and can penetrate and inoculate deep spaces despite seemingly innocuous wounds. A deep infection can brew beneath an apparently healed pinhole-sized wound. Deep spaces can include web spaces, joints, flexor tendon sheaths, and palmar spaces. Puncture wounds on opposite sides of the finger or hand commonly occur and should be identified. A careful and thorough examination is required as described in the physical examination section above. If joint penetration is suspected, the joint should be irrigated as described for human bites.
- The incidence of infections after dog and cat bites is difficult to establish because most series of such infections are retrospective in nature and thus are subject to overestimation by selection bias. Infection incidence varies from 2% to 6% in available prospective series.[7]
- The most commonly isolated organisms from dog and cat bite infections are *Streptococcus viridans*, *Pasteurella multocida*, *S. aureus*, and anaerobes.
- Penicillin is the antibiotic of choice for treatment of dog and cat bite infections.

## Posttraumatic Infection

- Hand trauma is common, but infections following uncomplicated lacerations are rare. Prophylactic antibiotics are not required in uncomplicated lacerations.
- Infections follow open hand fractures at a rate of 2% to 5%, which is much lower than the infection rate for open lower extremity fractures.
- Although multiple prospective series have demonstrated a benefit of prophylactic antibiotics in open lower extremity fractures, no such trials have shown a similar

benefit in open hand fractures. Prophylactic antibiotics can be given for open fractures of the hand and fingers, and treatment of the fracture should be dictated by fracture pattern, location, and soft tissue injuries. Surgical debridement of devascularized tissue is important.

- Infections are uncommon following gunshot wounds to the hand, and fear of infection should not delay definitive skeletal stabilization.[8]
- Infections follow flexor tendon repairs at a rate of approximately 2%, and the rate does not appear to be influenced by the use of prophylactic antibiotics.[9]

## Postsurgical Infection

- Infections are uncommon following elective hand surgery. A series of 2337 elective hand and upper extremity surgery cases found a deep infection rate of 0.3%, regardless of the use of prophylactic antibiotics.[10] Similar series found infection rates of less than 1%.
- Although several randomized, prospective trials found prophylactic antibiotics lowered the incidence of infection following major orthopedic procedures, such as long-bone fixation and total joint arthroplasty, no such data exist for hand surgery procedures. The very low rate of infection following hand procedures would require a very large trial to prove an advantage to prophylactic antibiotic use.
- Hand operations lasting more than 45 minutes to 2 hours may be associated with an increased risk for infection, and antibiotic prophylaxis should be considered.[10,11]
- Cefazolin is the currently recommended antibiotic when prophylaxis is believed to be necessary. For patients with serious allergies to β-lactam antibiotics, clindamycin or vancomycin can be used.

# Specific Anatomic Infections

## Onychomycosis

- Onychomycosis is a fungal infection of the nail apparatus. Fingernail onychomycosis is less common than toenail onychomycosis but still impacts quality of life. Onychomycosis typically is chronic, with a history of prolonged or repeated exposure to water. *Trichophyton rubrum* and *Candida* spp. are the most common offending organisms.
- Onychomycosis comes in three types:
  - Subungual, from distal hyponychial invasion
  - Proximal, from eponychial invasion
  - Secondary, from disseminated fungal infection in an immunocompromised host
- Many nail problems, including melanoma, can mimic onychomycosis, making fungal smears/cultures (30%–80% sensitive) and histopathology necessary for diagnosis.
- Topical antifungals can be used for distal onychomycosis. Oral antifungals are reserved for proximal cases.

Terbinafine and itraconazole are the recommended first-line and second-line oral agents, respectively, based on their toxicity profiles. Systemic treatment cures only 75% of cases, making nail removal a necessary adjunct to medical treatment in some cases.

## Paronychia

- Paronychia is an infection of the nail fold. Bacteria enter through a break in the seal between the nail and the nail fold. Thus, frequent manicures and nail biting are risk factors. *S. aureus* is the most common infecting organism, with *Streptococcus* spp. and oral anaerobes the infecting organisms in cases related to nail biting.
- Paronychia presents as pain, swelling, and redness of the nail fold, sometimes with spontaneous drainage of purulent material.
- Paronychias can be treated early by warm soaks and oral cephalosporins, provided an abscess is not present under the nail fold.
- If an abscess is present or if conservative treatment fails to resolve the symptoms, incision and drainage must be undertaken. A simple approach to incising a paronychia is to slide a no. 11 scalpel blade under the lateral nail fold parallel to the nail plate (Figure 22–2). The abscess is adequately drained and no scar remains. Do not, however, slide a blade proximally under the eponychial fold, because injury to the germinal matrix may result. Cultures of the purulent material should be obtained. Antibiotics are started immediately, and warm soaks are started 24 hours after incision.

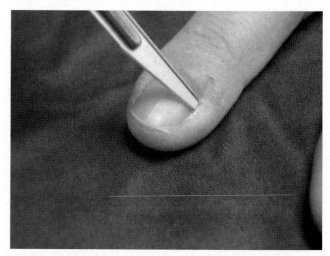

Figure 22–2:

**Approach used for incising an acute paronychia. A no. 11 blade is slid under the lateral nail fold, releasing the purulent material. This approach saves an incision and thus a scar, but it cannot be used when a paronychia is accompanied by a felon or more proximal infection. Avoid sliding the blade proximally and damaging the germinal matrix.**

- Chronic paronychias typically are attributed to *Candida albicans* infection and are associated with repeated water exposure. Antifungal treatment is of limited benefit, and eponychial marsupialization is sometimes required. However, some authors believe chronic paronychia represents an exposure dermatitis rather than infection and have shown good results with topical corticosteroids.[12]

## Felon

- A felon is an abscess of the pulp of the finger or thumb. Felons generally originate from direct inoculation, although a history of penetrating trauma cannot always be elucidated.
- Because of the constrained anatomy of the pulp, with numerous vertical septa separating fat compartments, infection can increase pressure sufficiently to cause necrosis of fat and skin. Presenting symptoms and signs are pain, tense swelling, redness, and warmth at the pulp. A focal area of skin blanching/thinning is sometimes seen.
- Infection of adjacent structures should be ruled out. A felon can spontaneously decompresses into four areas:
  - Into the bone of the distal phalanx, causing osteomyelitis
  - Into the distal interphalangeal joint, causing septic arthritis
  - Into the flexor tendon sheath, causing pyogenic flexor tenosynovitis
  - Out through the skin
- Surgical decompression usually is necessary. A variety of incisions have been described. A fish-mouth incision around the tip of the finger should be avoided because painful scars and nail deformities may result. If the abscess appears about to decompress through the skin volarly, a straight, midline, volar incision through the thinned skin works well. Otherwise, a straight midaxial incision works well (avoiding the radial side of the index finger and the ulnar side of the thumb and small finger) (Figure 22–3). Once the incision is made, all vertical septa must be disrupted bluntly throughout the pulp in order to decompress all fat compartments.
- Purulent material should be cultured and antibiotics started immediately. Warm soaks should be started 24 hours after incision and continued until the wound heals.

## Herpetic Infection

- Herpetic whitlow is an infection of the finger caused by herpes simplex virus (HSV). Oral exposure is a common risk factor, so children (who constantly have their hands in their mouths) and dental workers (who constantly have their hands in other people's mouths) are at highest risk.
- Herpetic whitlow presents as painful vesicles near the tip of the finger, with or without erythema. The pain is substantial and may precede the appearance of vesicles.

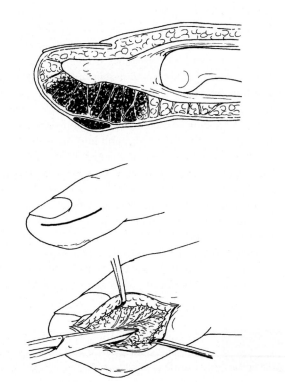

Figure 22–3:
Incising a felon. A lateral incision is used, and all vertical septa are divided by blunt dissection. Avoid the border surfaces of the digits. (From Trumble TE, Hashisaki P. Hand infections. In Trumble TE, editor: *Principles of hand surgery and therapy*. Philadelphia, 2000, WB Saunders.)

Tzanck smear and viral culture of vesicular fluid can confirm the diagnosis if it is not clear clinically.

- Lesions should not be incised and debrided because viremia and bacterial superinfection can result. Therefore, differentiation from paronychia and felon is important.
- Most symptoms resolve spontaneously in immunocompetent individuals, although oral acyclovir usually shortens the duration of symptoms. Acyclovir may be necessary to suppress symptoms or prevent recurrence in individuals with HIV infection or patients on immunosuppressive drugs following transplantation.
- Blistering dactylitis (a superficial bacterial infection of the fingertip) can coexist with herpetic whitlow in children, and antibiotics should be given if symptoms worsen or fail to resolve spontaneously.

## Pyogenic Flexor Tenosynovitis

- Pyogenic flexor tenosynovitis is an infection of the flexor tendon sheath. Infection within this enclosed space can cause scarring and necrosis of the tendons contained within the space, causing severely impaired function. For this reason, early recognition and prompt treatment are important.
- Flexor tenosynovitis may result from direct inoculation or from spread of an adjacent deep infection. Therefore, in

the presence of another deep hand infection, tenosynovitis must be ruled out. However, in a significant number of cases no direct source can be identified.

- The presenting symptoms and signs of flexor sheath infection are well described and include a partially flexed resting posture of the finger, pain with passive extension, fusiform swelling of the entire finger, and volar tenderness along the length of the finger and into the palm. All of these signs may not be present, especially if the infection has progressed enough to cause ischemia or digital nerve dysfunction. Because the small finger and thumb flexor sheaths can communicate, infection of one can lead to infection of the other and result in the so-called horseshoe abscess.

- If symptoms have persisted for less than 24 hours (uncommon), intravenous antibiotics and splinting may resolve the infection. If the signs and symptoms do not

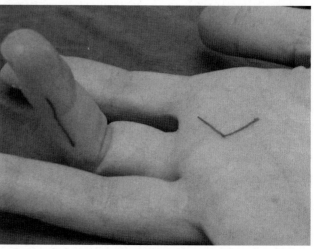

Figure 22–4:

**Examples of incisions used for closed-sheath irrigation of an infected flexor sheath. The catheter is inserted through the proximal incision and irrigation is allowed to drain distally. A variety of proximal incisions can be used, and either a midaxial or palmar distal incision can be used.**

| Box 22–4 | Closed-Sheath Irrigation for Pyogenic Flexor Tenosynovitis (Figure 22–4) |
|---|---|

- An incision is made in the palm at about the level of the distal palmar crease.
- The A1 pulley is incised to gain access to the sheath.
- Purulent fluid should be seen and cultures should be sent.
- A second incision is made at the distal interphalangeal (DIP) joint flexion crease (transverse) or in the midaxial line at DIP joint level (longitudinal).
- The flexor sheath is opened under the distal incision.
- A pediatric feeding tube is modified by cutting several small holes in its side, taking care not to weaken the tube substantially.
- The tube is passed into the flexor sheath through the incision in the palm. Normal saline is irrigated through the tube.
- Ensure that the fluid egresses freely from the distal incision. If the fluid does not flow out easily, sufficient pressure may build up within the finger and cause digital ischemia.
- If fluid does not flow out distally, advance the tube until it protrudes from the distal wound. Irrigation in this fashion relies on the Venturi effect to draw pus out through the tube with the flowing saline.
- Once the sheath is thoroughly irrigated (approximately 500 ml of saline usually is sufficient), the tube can be attached to a large, sterile, saline-filled syringe and left in place for postoperative irrigation.
- Postoperative irrigation can be episodic, irrigating the sheath every few hours with a few milliliters of saline or continuously with a pump at 10 milliliters per hour.
- Continuous irrigation runs the risk of unsupervised pressure buildup within the finger and should be used with caution, if at all.
- Any irrigation tends to be painful, and evidence indicates postoperative irrigation may not be necessary.[14]
- Irrigation can be continued for 24 to 48 hours postoperatively, after which the tube is pulled (ensure the tube is intact) and wounds are left to heal secondarily.

resolve within 12 hours, surgical drainage is warranted. In addition, surgical irrigation should be performed urgently if symptoms have persisted for more than 24 hours prior to presentation.

- Surgical drainage of a flexor sheath infection can be accomplished effectively using closed-sheath irrigation (Box 22–4 and Figure 22–4).[13]

- After resolution of the acute infection, hand therapy should be started as soon as possible in order to restore motion and function.

## Deep Hand Space Infections

- The hand contains several enclosed potential spaces that may house abscesses (Figure 22–5). Deep hand space infections are uncommon with the widespread use of antibiotics for simple hand infections. Nonetheless, the orthopedist should be familiar with the evaluation and treatment of these infections because they can cause significant morbidity.

- Box 22–5 summarizes infections in the deep spaces of the hand (Figure 22–6).

## Septic Arthritis

- Septic arthritis is uncommon in the hand and wrist. Finger joint infections most often occur following direct inoculation, whereas wrist joint infection can follow bacteremia.

- The presenting findings of septic joints in the hand and wrist are similar to those in other joints. Pain and swelling about the joint, with limited range of motion and circumferential tenderness, are the hallmarks. Concomitant infections (web space, flexor sheath, felon, etc.) should be ruled out.

Figure 22–5:
Several enclosed spaces exist in the hand, and infections requiring surgical drainage can involve one or more spaces. (From Trumble TE, Hashisaki P. Hand infections. In Trumble TE, editor: *Principles of hand surgery and therapy*. Philadelphia, 2000, WB Saunders.)

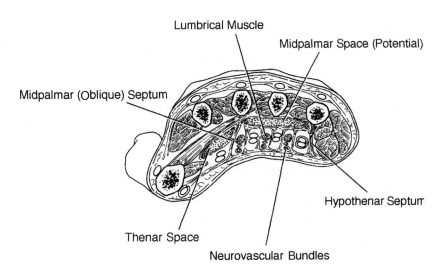

Lumbrical Muscle
Midpalmar Space (Potential)
Midpalmar (Oblique) Septum
Hypothenar Septum
Thenar Space
Neurovascular Bundles

| Box 22–5 | Deep Hand Space Infections |
|---|---|
| **Space** | **Clinical Notes** |
| Midpalmar space | Space contains all long flexor tendons and lumbricals, and arterial arches and branches of ulnar and median nerves. Space may communicate with Parona space anterior to pronator quadratus. When infected, concavity of palm is lost; palm may even be convex. Drain carefully through palmar incision. |
| Web spaces (2, 3, 4) | Spaces contain digital neurovascular bundles. Abscess may exist on volar and dorsal sides of web space ("collar button" abscess). Adjacent fingers typically are abducted. Drain through dorsal and volar incisions (Figure 22–6). |
| Thenar space | Space contains thenar muscles and first dorsal interosseus muscle. Can also have "collar button" (aka "dumbbell" or "pantaloon") abscess of first web space. Drain through volar incision or combined volar and dorsal incisions, taking care not to injure neurovascular bundles to thumb. |
| Subaponeurotic space | Space lies deep to extensor tendons on dorsal surface of hand. Can be difficult to appreciate fluctuance under significant dorsal edema; aspiration or ultrasonography may help. Can be drained through one longitudinal incision or two longitudinal incisions with a wide skin bridge. Do not leave extensor tendons exposed and thus allowed to desiccate. |

- Aspiration is not difficult in the wrist and MCP joints. Fluid obtained should be sent for culture and cell count. Peripheral blood white cell counts and erythrocyte sedimentation rate are not as helpful for diagnosing small joint infections as they are for large joint infections.
- *S. aureus* is the most commonly isolated organism, although infections in immunocompromised individuals or infections resulting from human bites typically are polymicrobial. Gonococcal infection should be suspected in young, sexually active individuals. Mycobacterial infection should be suspected in chronic, indolent infections of the wrist.
- If the patient presents with symptoms of less than 24 hours' duration, intravenous antibiotics alone may

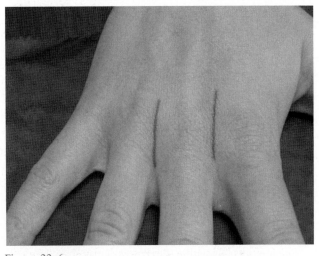

Figure 22–6:
Incisions used for drainage of web space infections. Separate incisions should be used when draining adjacent web spaces so that wounds can be left open without desiccating the extensor tendon of the intervening finger.

eradicate the infection. However, if symptoms do not resolve promptly, if symptoms have been present for more than 24 hours, or if factors such as immunocompromise or mode of inoculation predict aggressive infections, decompression should be performed urgently. Surgical drainage usually is not difficult, although care should be taken not to contaminate adjacent spaces or injure nearby structures. Incisions should be placed so that vital structures will not be exposed if the wound is left open. The proximal interphalangeal and distal interphalangeal joints can be exposed in the midaxial line, the MCP joints can be exposed dorsally or dorsolaterally, and the wrist should be exposed dorsally.

- Outcomes vary following septic arthritis in the hand and wrist, but some degree of joint stiffness is almost inevitable. Proximal interphalangeal joints fare especially poorly, as do patients presenting after several days of symptoms.[15]

- Gout can mimic septic arthritis in the hand. Trauma can precipitate an acute attack. The physical examination can reveal redness, swelling, and circumferential tenderness. If aspiration is difficult or unsuccessful, as can be the case in the proximal interphalangeal joint, surgical exploration may be warranted. The discovery of a pasty, white substance (with crystals on microscopy) and the absence of pus confirm the diagnosis of gout. The wound should not be left open if gout is discovered surgically, because leaving the wound open can allow sinus tract formation. Gout and septic arthritis can coexist. If gout is diagnosed or suspected, ensure that the symptoms resolve promptly with gout medications such as indomethacin.

- Calcium pyrophosphate deposition disease (CPPD; "pseudogout") can mimic septic arthritis of the wrist. The diagnosis of CPPD is suspected when radiographs reveal calcification of the triangular fibrocartilage complex and can be confirmed by isolating crystals in a joint aspirate. Arthritis of inflammatory bowel disease also can mimic wrist joint infection. Joint fluid cultures are negative, and symptoms resolve with treatment of the bowel symptoms.

## Osteomyelitis

- Osteomyelitis is uncommon in the hand and wrist. The distal phalanx is the most commonly infected bone in the hand. The route of inoculation usually is direct trauma or spread from adjacent infection.

- The diagnosis of osteomyelitis should be suspected when a soft tissue wound or infection fails to resolve as expected.

- Radiographs are normal early in the course of osteomyelitis but within 2 to 3 weeks may show bony destruction. Technetium and indium scans allow earlier diagnosis, as does magnetic resonance imaging.

- Treatment usually involves surgical debridement of all infected and necrotic bone. Fractures or nonunions, if present, should be stabilized. Antibiotics should be continued until all signs and symptoms have resolved.

## Necrotizing Fasciitis

- Necrotizing fasciitis is a rapidly progressive, potentially lethal infection of fascia.

- Group A β-hemolytic *Streptococcus* is the most common offending organism, although *S. aureus* and others also may be involved.

- Initial presentation may be similar to cellulitis. Clinical clues to the diagnosis of necrotizing fasciitis are listed in Box 22–6.

- Plain radiographs may show air in soft tissues, but this finding is not necessary for the diagnosis. Magnetic resonance imaging shows increased signal intensity in the fascia on T2-weighted images.

- Initial laboratory evaluation should include markers of infection and measurement of electrolytes, renal function, liver function, and coagulation. The infection may progress to septic shock, acute respiratory distress syndrome, multisystem organ failure, and death within hours to days.

- Most patients present critically ill. Resuscitative measures should be instituted emergently with the aid of critical care specialists. Radical debridement of fascia well beyond the zone of obvious infection should be performed emergently (Figure 22–7). Repeated debridements and amputation may be required. Intravenous antibiotics should be given emergently and should cover streptococcal, staphylococcal, and anaerobic species until culture results allow narrowing the spectrum. Ancillary treatments, including immune globulin and hyperbaric oxygen, have not proved beneficial in randomized trials and should not delay emergent surgical debridement.

- Nearly half of patients with extremity necrotizing fasciitis require amputation and nearly one third die, even young, healthy patients treated aggressively.[16,17]

| Box 22–6 | Clues to the Diagnosis of Necrotizing Fasciitis |
| --- | --- |

- Unusually severe pain
- Rapid spread of symptoms
- Bullae
- Skin anesthesia
- Subcutaneous crepitus
- Systemic toxicity
- Failure to respond to appropriate antibiotics
- Patient's sense of doom

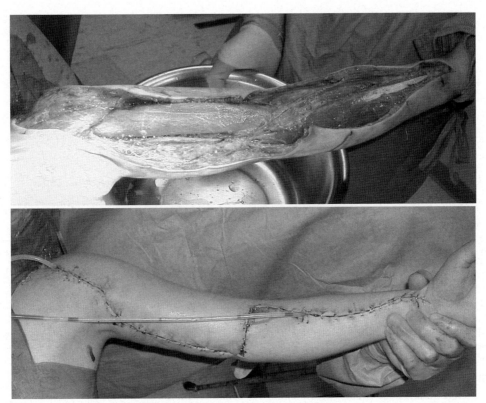

Figure 22–7:
Necrotizing fasciitis of the upper extremity required extensive debridement of fascia. The muscle and skin were not involved in the infection and remained viable, allowing later secondary closure without skin grafts. (From Trumble TE, editor: *Hand surgery update 3*. Rosemont, IL, 2003, American Society for Surgery of the Hand.)

| Box 22–7 | Selected Uncommon Infections in the Hand and Wrist |
|---|---|
| **Organism** | **Clinical Notes** |
| **Fungal** | |
| *Sporothrix schenckii* | • From rose thorn inoculation.<br>• Sporotrichosis consists of granuloma at inoculation site with proximal lymphadenopathy (sometimes draining).<br>• Culture on modified Sabouraud agar at room temperature. |
| *Aspergillus* spp. | • Causes infections in immunocompromised hosts.<br>• Invasive aspergillosis can occur on extremities, with small area of skin necrosis surrounded by erythema.<br>• Diagnosed by fungal smear from border of lesion.<br>• Treatment is wide excision and amphotericin B.<br>• Incisional debridement could allow metastasis of hyphae and result in disseminated infection. |
| *Rhizopus* spp. | • Causes mucormycosis, similar to invasive aspergillosis in presentation.<br>• Fungal hyphae can invade and occlude arteries, causing limb gangrene.<br>• Treatment is early wide excision and amphotericin B. |
| *Coccidioides* spp. | • Can cause extensor or flexor tenosynovitis, and osteomyelitis at the ends of long bones.<br>• Surgical debridement and amphotericin B are required. |
| *Histoplasma* spp. | • Histoplasmosis can present as granulomatous tenosynovitis and cause carpal tunnel syndrome.<br>• Can progress to disseminated infection if not treated.<br>• Debridement and amphotericin B are required. |
| **Mycobacterial** | |
| *M. tuberculosis* | • Can cause dactylitis (in children only, similar to sickle cell dactylitis), tenosynovitis (usually flexor, with "rice bodies" in wrist and palm), osteomyelitis (usually in carpus or distal radius), or arthritis (usually in wrist).<br>• Symptoms are chronic and rarely systemic.<br>• Diagnosis is made by surgical biopsy.<br>• Chemotherapy is started empirically, and surgical debridement often is necessary. |

*(Continued)*

| Box 22–7 | Selected Uncommon Infections in the Hand and Wrist—cont'd |
|---|---|
| *M. marinum* | • Associated with water exposure or fish handling.<br>• Upper extremity is most common site of infection.<br>• Can cause verrucae, subcutaneous granulomata, or deep infections (tenosynovitis, arthritis, osteomyelitis).<br>• Rule out sporotrichosis if water exposure is not part of the history.<br>• Diagnosed by culture of biopsy specimens on Lowenstein-Jensen agar at 30 to 32 degrees Celsius.<br>• Chemotherapy is used routinely, and surgical debulking is necessary for deep infections. |
| **Other**<br>*Vibrio vulnificus* | • Inoculation usually is from puncture by a fish spine.<br>• Infection typically is rapidly progressive, causing extensive skin and soft tissue necrosis.<br>• Can cause necrotizing fasciitis.<br>• Urgent or emergent surgical debridement or amputation often is necessary, despite sensitivity to many antibiotics. |

For these uncommon infections with complex antibiotic treatment regimens, the team of the infectious disease specialists and the hand surgeons will provide the optimal management.

# Uncommon Infections

- A variety of uncommon infections can occur in the hand and wrist, especially in immunocompromised individuals.
- Knowledge of risk factors and clinical presentations should raise sufficient suspicion to prompt accurate and specific culture requests and allow timely and appropriate treatment (Box 22–7).

# References

1. Weinzweig N, Gonzalez M: Surgical infections of the hand and upper extremity: a county hospital experience. *Ann Plast Surg* 49:621-627, 2002.
   The authors reviewed 443 surgically treated hand infections from a 3-year period and identified high prevalences of polymicrobial infections and antibiotic resistance.

2. Connolly B, Johnstone F, Gerlinger T, Puttler E: Methicillin-resistant *Staphylococcus aureus* in a finger felon. *J Hand Surg* 25A:173-175, 2000.
   The authors report a case of methicillin-resistant Staphylococcus aureus infecting the finger of an otherwise healthy, immunocompetent young adult.

3. Karanas YL, Bogdan MA, Chang J: Community acquired methicillin-resistant *Staphylococcus aureus* hand infections: case reports and clinical implications. *J Hand Surg* 25A:760-763, 2000.
   The authors describe four cases of community acquired MRSA hand infections in patients without risk factors such as intravenous drug use, long-term venous access catheters, long-term antibiotic use, or nursing home residence.

4. Gonzalez MH, Bochar S, Novotny J et al: Upper extremity infections in patients with diabetes mellitus. *J Hand Surg* 24A:682-686, 1999.
   The authors retrospectively reviewed 45 patients with diabetes and surgically treated hand infections, of which 39% required amputation, with associated comorbidities predicting risk of amputation.

5. Conner RW, Kimbrough RC, Dabezies EJ: Hand infections in patients with diabetes mellitus. *Orthopedics* 24:1057-1106, 2001.
   The study retrospectively reviewed 50 diabetic patients with hand infections and high rates of polymicrobial infection and amputation.

6. Tonta K, Kimble FW: Human bites of the hand: the Tasmanian experience. *Aust N Z J Surg* 71:467-471, 2001.
   The authors reviewed 35 human bite hand injuries in Australia, of which 34 resulted from conflict and most patients failed to comply with treatment.

7. Medeiros I, Saconato H: Antibiotic prophylaxis for mammalian bites. *Cochrane Database Syst Rev* 1, online, 2003.
   In this systematic review of all randomized, prospective trials on the prophylactic use of antibiotics to prevent infections in uncomplicated human, dog, and cat bites, a conclusive benefit to antibiotic prophylaxis was found for human bites but not for dog or cat bites.

8. Chappell JE, Mitra A, Weinberger J, Walsh L: Gunshot wounds to the hand: management and economic impact. *Ann Plast Surg* 42:418-423, 1999.
   In a review of 90 patients treated for gunshot wounds to the hand, the authors recommend early definitive fracture fixation and prophylactic antibiotics.

9. Stone JF, Davidson JSD: The role of antibiotics and timing of repair in flexor tendon injuries of the hand. *Ann Plast Surg* 40: 7-13, 1998.
   In a retrospective review of 140 patients who underwent zone I to IV flexor tendon repairs, the use of antibiotic prophylaxis and the time from injury to surgery had no effect on occurrence of postoperative infection.

10. Kleinert JM, Hoffman J, Crain GM et al: Postoperative infection in a double-occupancy operating room: a prospective study of two thousand four hundred and fifty-eight procedures on the extremities. *J Bone Joint Surg* 79A:503-513, 1997.
    The authors prospectively followed 2458 elective surgeries performed in double-occupancy operating rooms and found an overall infection rate of 1.4%, with length of operating time greater than 45 minutes predicting infection risk.

11. Hoffman RD, Adams BD: The role of antibiotics in the management of elective and post-traumatic hand surgery. *Hand Clin* 14:657-666, 1998.
    Based on a thorough literature review, the authors do not recommend prophylactic use of antibiotics for clean, elective procedures lasting less than 2 hours.

12. Tosti A, Piraccini BM, Ghetti E, Colombo MD: Topical steroids versus systemic antifungals in the treatment of chronic paronychia: an open, randomized double-blind and double dummy study. *J Am Acad Dermatol* 47:73-76, 2002.
    This randomized, double-blind, double-dummy study reported that topical corticosteroids were more effective than systemic antifungals in treating chronic paronychia.

13. Gutowski KA, Ochoa O, Adams WP Jr: Closed-catheter irrigation is as effective as open drainage for treatment of pyogenic flexor tenosynovitis. *Ann Plast Surg* 49:350-354, 2002.
    The authors retrospectively reviewed 47 patients with pyogenic flexor tenosynovitis. They compared patients treated with closed-catheter irrigation to those treated with open drainage and concluded that closed-catheter irrigation is the treatment of choice.

14. Lille S, Hayakawa T, Neumeister MW et al: Continuous postoperative catheter irrigation is not necessary for the treatment of suppurative flexor tenosynovitis. *J Hand Surg* 25B:304-307, 2000.
    The authors reviewed the records of 75 patients treated for pyogenic flexor tenosynovitis and concluded that postoperative irrigation is unnecessary.

15. Boustred AM, Singer M, Hudson DA, Bolitho GE: Septic arthritis of the metacarpophalangeal and interphalangeal joints of the hand. *Ann Plast Surg* 42:623-629, 1999.
    The study retrospectively reviewed 28 patients with septic arthritis in the hand and showed a high rate of stiffness and poor results.

16. Tang WM, Ho PL, Fung KK et al: Necrotizing fasciitis of a limb. *J Bone Joint Surg* 83B:709-714, 2001.
    The authors retrospectively reviewed 24 patients treated for necrotizing fasciitis of an extremity and reported high mortality and amputation rates.

17. Gonzalez MH, Kay T, Weinzweig N et al: Necrotizing fasciitis of the upper extremity. *J Hand Surg* 21A:689-692, 1996.
    The authors present a series of 12 cases of upper extremity necrotizing fasciitis with no mortalities but three amputations.

## Reviews

Jebson PJL, Louis DS, editors: Hand infections. *Hand Clin* 14: 511-711, 1998.
Together, these articles represent probably the most comprehensive review of hand infections published within the past 5 years.

Wright PE II: Hand infections. In Canale ST, Daugherty K, Jones L, editors: *Campbell's operative orthopaedics*, vol 4, ed 10. Philadelphia, 2003, Mosby.

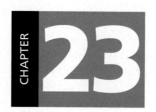
# Replantation

## Michael S. Murphy* and James P. Higgins†

*MD, Department of Orthopaedic Surgery, Johns Hopkins University School of Medicine; Attending Hand Surgeon, Department of Orthopaedic Surgery, The Curtis National Hand Center, Union Memorial Hospital, Baltimore, MD
†MD, Teaching Faculty, Department of Plastic Surgery, Johns Hopkins University School of Medicine; Attending Hand Surgeon, The Curtis National Hand Center, Department of Orthopaedic Surgery, Union Memorial Hospital, Baltimore, MD

## Introduction

- *Replantation,* by definition, is the reattachment by microsurgical means of a completely severed part. In contrast, *revascularization* is the reattachment of a part that has some remaining soft tissue attachment following injury. Usually arterial and/or venous repair is needed to maintain viability.

- Replantation may require vein grafting, but grafting often can be avoided with appropriate skeletal shortening. Typically, shortening is performed to reach an area beyond the zone of initial injury. Various methods of fixation can be used and are dictated by fracture pattern, injury level, and surgeon preference.

- Nerve repairs are performed acutely with the zone of injury estimated. Standard methods of tendon repair are used. Tendon rehabilitation protocols require some modification as a result of the multisystem nature of these injuries. Acute skin grafts may be needed and should be used liberally.

- Success of replantation as a whole requires achievement of several difficult goals: viability, stability, sensation, and function. Initial management of both the amputated part and the patient are critical to the success of the procedure (Box 23–1).

## History

- The first successful replantation was reported by Malt and McKhann in 1962. They replanted a transhumeral level arm amputation in a 12-year-old child. Subsequently, in 1963 Chen Zhong-Wei in China successfully replanted a distal forearm level amputation. The first successful digital replantation was performed in 1968 by Komatsu and Tamai.

### Box 23–1 Replantation: Key Concepts

- Microsurgical replantation is the reattachment of a completely amputated part.
- Arterial and venous repair is required.
- Interposition vein grafting may be needed.
- Nerve repair is performed acutely with the zone of injury estimated.
- Fracture stabilization with skeletal shortening facilitates other necessary repairs.
- Digital replantation requires Zone II flexor tendon repairs. Standard techniques of tendon repaired are utilized.
- Flexor tendon rehabilitation is compromised by fracture protection and concomitant extensor tendon repair.
- Soft tissue is often reperfused after lengthy periods of ischemia.
- Skin grafting is often required.

# Epidemiology/Costs to Society

- Few epidemiologic studies have examined the incidence of amputations and replantations and their impact on society in terms of surgical and hospital costs, workforce costs, and rate of return to previous levels of function. A study from Sweden determined the incidence was 1.9 per 100,000 person-years (males 3.3, females 0.5). Eighty-six percent occurred in males and 9% in children (ages 0–14 years). The majority occur in men aged 45 to 54 years. Factory workers (26%) and carpenters (14%) were the most commonly injured.[1]

# Emergency Management

- From the field to the initial treatment facility, the patient should be appropriately medically stabilized. Tourniquets should not be applied. Bleeding usually is controllable by bulky pressure dressings, elevation, and ice. Antibiotics and tetanus prophylaxis are provided. X-ray films are helpful, but other than initial assessment and stabilization, transfer to the replantation facility should not be delayed.

# Management of Amputated Part

- All parts should be collected in the field, regardless of severity of injury and degree of contamination. Appropriate cooling should be performed. This cooling is best achieved by wrapping the part in a saline-saturated sponge, placing the part in a plastic bag, and placing the bag on a bed of ice. The part should be labeled with patient demographic information.

## Ischemia Time

- Replantation of a digit does not result in reperfusion of muscle; therefore, digits can be replanted after longer periods of ischemia. Of the musculoskeletal system, muscle is the tissue least tolerant to ischemia because of the high oxygen demands of the myocytes. Digits can be replanted after as many as 6 hours of warm ischemia. However, with amputations involving the hand or forearm, even 2 to 3 hours of warm ischemia time can result in substantial muscle necrosis that may produce systemic coagulopathy after reperfusion. The venous outflow from a reperfused extremity contains many toxic compounds, such as oxygen free radicals, which cause tissue damage and vasospasm. Cooling of the amputated part to 4° C dramatically prolongs the time between injury and successful replantation. Cooling below 4° C causes the formation of intracellular crystals and tissue damage that is identical to frostbite. Although properly cooled parts have been replanted up to 36 hours from the time of injury, the survival rate of an amputated part decreases with the delay to replantation (Box 23–2).

**Box 23–2 Principles of "Spare Parts Surgery"**

- In multiple digit amputations, the best preserved parts may be transposed to the most functional location. In the absence of a replantable thumb, for example, an amputated digit can be replanted in the thumb position to maximize the final functional outcome of the hand as a unit. Acute index finger pollicization should be considered in the setting of unreplantable thumb with damaged index digit.
- Nonreplantable digits should be critically inspected for individual parts that may be harvested as free grafts (i.e., skin, nerve, bone, vessel) for other replantable digits.

# Digital Replantation

- A relative indication for digital replantation is a single digit sharp amputation distal to the sublimis insertion. These patients typically gain adequate proximal interphalangeal joint motion and have fewer problems with neuroma pain. Although the technique is criticized as a cosmetic procedure, patient satisfaction often is high (Boxes 23–3 and 23–4).

## Technical Aspects Digital Replantation

- Team approach is best.
- Surgical preparation of the part begins before the patient is anesthetized.
- Axillary block anesthesia using long-acting anesthetics with supplementary general is administered, depending on the length of procedure.
- Indwelling axillary catheters are used postoperatively when significant vasospasm or postoperative pain is anticipated:
  - Smokers
  - Children
  - More proximal levels of amputation: transmetacarpal, forearm

## Methods of Fixation

- Digital replantation requires appropriate skeletal fixation. K-wires, 90-90 wires, miniplate fixation, and

**Box 23–3 Indications for Digital Replantation**

- Multiple digital amputations regardless of level
- Thumb amputations
- Any pediatric digital amputation

**Box 23–4 Contraindications to Digital Replantation**

- Multilevel amputations
- Crush, degloving injuries
- Medically or emotionally unstable patient
- Prolonged warm ischemia

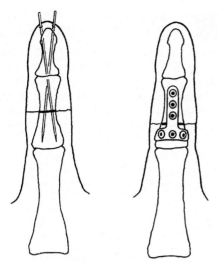

Figure 23–1:
**Kirschner wires or plate and screw fixation provides skeletal stabilization. (From Trumble TE, editor: *Principles of hand surgery and therapy.* Philadelphia, 2000, WB Saunders.)**

intramedullary forms of fixation all have been successfully used (Figure 23–1).

- Digital amputations are most often secured with Kirschner wires or 90-90 wiring. Transmetacarpal amputation requires miniplate fixation. Amputation at the wrist level typically demands shortening and acute wrist arthrodesis. Standard methods of compression plate fixation are used with more proximal amputations such as the distal to midforearm. The method of fixation is selected after consideration is given to amount of soft tissue stripping required, potential for postoperative mobilization, surgical time constraints, and characteristics of the fracture pattern.

## Sequence and Technical Considerations

- Midaxial incisions
- Structure by structure reconstruction (rather than digit by digit)
- Skeletal stabilization
- Flexor and extensor tendon repairs
- Nerve repair
- Anticoagulant therapy
- Tourniquet deflation
- Arterial repair
- Vein repairs
- Skin repair with absorbable materials and skin grafting as needed
- Midaxial incisions can be left open to prevent constrictive closure (Figure 23–2).

## Dressings

- Nonadherent dressings are applied loosely. Cotton dressings soaked with mineral oil are extremely

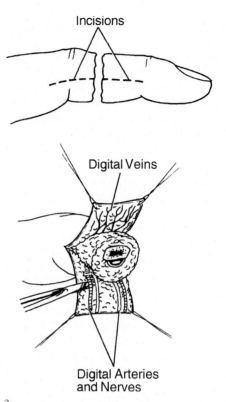

Figure 23–2:
**Midaxial incisions provide excellent exposure of the neurovascular bundles with flaps that are easy to close over the vessel anastomoses. (From Trumble TE, editor: *Principles of hand surgery and therapy.* Philadelphia, 2000, WB Saunders.)**

nonadherent, even in the face of a large amount of bleeding. These materials facilitate dressing changes, minimizing the potential for discomfort that can potentially stimulate vasospasm. Dressings must not be constrictive, which can occur if the dressings become soaked with blood. Such an event can result in venous occlusion with secondary arterial obstruction. Splints are required, maintaining a position of protection.
- Extremity elevation is maintained to prevent venous congestion.

## Results of Digital Replantation[2]

- The survival rate should be greater than 90% in appropriate candidates.
- Females, patients younger than 13 years, and nonsmokers demonstrate improved rates of replantation survival.
- Amputations at the proximal interphalangeal joint demonstrate lower survival rates than amputations distal or proximal to that level.
- Procedures involving two arterial anastomoses improve survival over single artery repairs.[3]
- Those requiring arterial reconstruction with vein grafts have lower survival rates than direct anastomoses.
- Performance of more than one venous conduit greatly improves survival rates.

- The most accurate predictive factor of survival is mechanism of amputation, with crush, avulsion, and degloving injuries faring the worst.
- Alcohol abuse demonstrates no impact on survival rates.

## Major Limb Replantation

- *Major limb amputations* are defined as those occurring proximal to the wrist. More proximal replantations are less technically challenging to perform because the structures (particularly blood vessels) are substantially larger than their counterparts in the hand or digits. Despite the lesser technical challenge, functional outcomes of major limb replantation are poor and can be attributed to the following:
- Intolerance of skeletal muscle tissue to prolonged ischemia. This can be decreased with early, aggressive use of temporary vascular shunts.
- Greater distance of repaired motor and sensory nerves from their target motor endplates and sensory dermatomes.
- Adequate and thorough soft tissue debridement is crucial in amputations proximal to the wrist, because failure to remove all devascularized muscle risks potentially catastrophic postoperative infection, acidosis, and hyperkalemia (reperfusion syndrome) (Box 23–5).

### Treatment Considerations

- The decision to replant limb amputations can be difficult given the great challenge and significant risks of major replantation. Several studies have attempted to provide objective means of estimating outcomes and approaching the initial decision to pursue major limb replantation. One large study demonstrated the functional superiority of replanted limbs over prosthetics.[4] Objective sensibility testing, however, was excluded as a measured outcome. Studies have demonstrated younger age and more distal levels yielded significantly improved functional scores. Mechanism of injury and ischemic time also have been shown to be strongly predictive of functional outcome.[5,6]

## Pediatric Replantation

- Regardless of the mechanism or level of injury, any amputation in a pediatric patient is an indication for attempted replantation.

| Box 23–5 | **Special Sequence Considerations for Major Limb Replantation** |
|---|---|

- Once the patient is prepared for replantation, arterial and venous shunts are used to minimize ischemic time while stabilization is obtained.
- Bone shortening and rigid internal fixation are pursued after debridement if possible.
- Direct arterial and venous anastomoses or vein grafting then is performed.
- Repair of tendons, nerves, and skin follows.

- Replantation distal to the eponychium may require the routine use of controlled bleeding. Replacement of distal tip injuries as composite (not revascularized) grafts demonstrates a 43% to 58% success rate, with children faring better than adults.[7]
- Prolonged episodes of postoperative vasospasm may occur before reperfusion is demonstrated.
- Cold intolerance is reported in greater than 40% of replanted digits.
- Partial or complete physeal arrest may occur. Angular deformity may follow. Longitudinal growth may be only 80% to 90% that of the contralateral side.[8,9]
- The pediatric patient population generally displays superior functional and sensory results compared to the adult population. Studies have documented high patient and parental satisfaction.

## Adjunctive Therapy

- No standard perioperative pharmacologic adjunctive therapy exists. An absence of prospective randomized trials demonstrating the relative efficacy or danger of these agents has resulted in a lack of uniformity in the hand surgery community. The use and timing of antithrombotics, thrombolytics, and topical and systemic vasodilators are guided primarily by the individual experience of particular centers or surgeons.[10] Many surgeons routinely use a combination of daily low-dose aspirin therapy started immediately postoperatively and continued for at least 2 weeks. This therapy can be used in conjunction with a continuous infusion of low-molecular-weight dextran starting 1 hour prior to vascular anastomosis and continuing for 5 days postoperatively. Because of its osmotic effects, dextran is withheld or used with caution in patients with a history of renal insufficiency, coronary artery disease, or pulmonary disorders. A 5-day course of oral allopurinol may limit reperfusion injury and maximize sensory outcomes. The xanthine oxidase inhibitory effects of allopurinol may decrease swelling, pain, and infection by limiting the activation of neutrophils and resultant release of cytotoxic oxidants.[11] Other agents used include dipyridamole, heparin, warfarin (Coumadin), thrombolytics, prostaglandins, chlorpromazine (Thorazine), and other vasodilators.

## Secondary Surgery

- The compound nature of these injuries often leads to unsatisfactory immediate results that require secondary surgical intervention.
- Frequency of secondary surgery ranges from 2.9% to 93.2% of patients and appears to increase as functional expectations increase.[12]
- The largest series of 1018 digital revascularizations (n = 273) or replantations (n = 745) reported a

secondary surgery rate of 35%. The most common reconstructive procedure was tenolysis (54%), followed by staged tendon grafting (29%) and capsulotomy (23%). The factors reported to increase the likelihood of secondary surgery after replantation included more proximal level amputations, crushing mechanism of injury, fewer vascular anastomoses, venous insufficiency, and age over 10 years.[2]

- Secondary procedures are generally performed at least 3 to 4 months after replantation or after functional improvements plateau in hand therapy.
- The order of secondary surgeries is determined by the prerequisites for each tissue type reconstruction. These surgeries are performed in the following logical order to maximize success: skin (grafts, flaps, contracture release/Z-plasty), skeleton (osteotomy, bone grafts), nerve (grafting, neurolysis, neuroma resection), joint (capsulectomy, arthroplasty, arthrodesis), and tendon (tenolysis, tendon grafting/transfer).

## Conclusions

- Since the advent of replantation 40 years ago, the hand surgery community has made tremendous strides in the surgical care of the amputated limb.
- The continued expansion of clinical experience at large centers and the increasingly global nature of our specialty will accelerate our advances.
- With the challenge of achieving viability largely overcome, our society will continue to focus its efforts on maximizing improvements in function and sensibility.

## References

1. Atroshi I, Rosberg HE: Epidemiology of amputations and severe injuries of the hand. Hand Clin 17:343-350, 2001.
   The incidence of amputations over a 9-year period was 1.9 per 100,000 person-years (males 3.3, females 0.5), with most occurring in males in the 45- to 54-year age group.

2. Waikakul S, Sakkarnkosol S, Vanadurongwan V, Un-nanuntana A: Results of 1018 digital replantations in 552 patients. Injury 31:33-40, 2000.
   In an analysis of 1018 digital amputations and devascularizing injuries from a single center, survival rate of the 745 amputations was 93%. Predictive factors are discussed.

3. Lee BI, Chung HY, Kim WK et al: The effects of the number and ratio of repaired arteries and veins on the survival rate in digital replantation. Ann Plast Surg 44:288-294, 2000.
   In a study of 631 consecutive digital replantations, the authors found better survival when at least one vein was repaired for each artery repaired, especially at distal levels.

4. Graham B, Adkins P, Tsai TM et al: Major replantation versus revision amputation and prosthetic fitting in the upper extremity: a late functional outcomes study. J Hand Surg [Am] 23:783-791, 1998.

Twenty-two patients with replantations proximal to the wrist had better functional outcomes as assessed by the modified Carroll test than 22 age- and level-matched amputees fitted with prostheses.

5. Chew WYC, Tsai T: Major upper limb replantation. Hand Clin 17:395-410, 2001.
   In an assessment of 34 cases of major limb replantation, ischemia time and level of amputation were found to be strongest predictors of functional outcome.

6. Waikakul S, Vanadurongwan V, Unnanantana A: Prognostic factors for major limb replantation at both immediate and long-term follow-up. J Bone Joint Surg Br 80B:1024-1030, 1998.
   In a series of 186 major upper limb replantations, 10% of replantations failed, with level and mechanism of amputation predicting outcome.

7. Heistein JB, Cook PA: Factors affecting composite graft survival in digital tip amputations. Ann Plast Surg 50:299-303, 2003.
   This prospective evaluation of 57 digital tip composite grafts revealed a 48% to 53% survival rate, with tobacco use, age greater than 18 years, and alcohol use correlating with failure.

8. Cheng GL, Pan DD, Zhang NP, Fang GR: Digital replantation in children: a long-term follow-up study. J Hand Surg [Am] 23:635-646, 1998.
   This study assesses 26 pediatric (14 months to 12 years) replantations with an average follow-up of 11 years and reports excellent functional results and bone growth.

9. Yildiz M, Sener M, Baki C: Replantation in children. Microsurgery 18:410-413, 1998.
   Thirteen pediatric replantation cases were studied with average 4.2-year follow-up. Survival rate was 84%, and functional results and bone growth were good.

10. Conrad MH, Adams WP: Pharmacologic optimization of microsurgery in the new millennium. Plast Reconstr Surg 108:2088-2096, 2001.
    This excellent review summarizes pharmacologic strategies for microsurgical procedures.

11. Waikakul S, Unnanantana A, Vanadurongwan V: The role of allopurinol in digital replantation. J Hand Surg [Br] 24:325-327, 1999.
    In this randomized controlled trial of 98 patients with thumb amputations and ischemic times of greater than 10 hours, allopurinol decreased infection rate, swelling, and pain and improved sensation compared to controls.

12. Wang H: Secondary surgery after digital replantation: its incidence and sequence. Microsurgery 22:57-61, 2002.
    This review of 19 prior series reports the frequency of secondary surgery after replantation ranges from 2.9% to 93.2%.

## Recent Replantation Review Articles

Lim BH, Tan BK, Peng YP: Digital replantations including fingertip and ring avulsion. Hand Clin 17:419-431, 2001.

Merle M, Dautel G: Advances in digital replantation. Clin Plast Surg 24:87-105, 1997.

# CHAPTER 24

# Osteoarthritis of the Hand and Wrist

Michael E. Leit* and Matthew M. Tomaino†

*MD, MS, Clinical Assistant Professor of Orthopaedic Surgery, University of Rochester School of Medicine, Rochester, NY; Assistant Professor of Surgery, Uniformed Services University, Bethesda, MD; Attending, University of Rochester Medical Center, Rochester, NY; Chief Orthopaedic Surgeon, Lakeside Memorial Hospital, Brockport, NY
†MD, MBA, Professor of Orthopaedic Surgery, University of Rochester School of Medicine; Chief, Division of Hand and Upper Extremity Surgery, University of Rochester Medical Center, Rochester, NY

## Introduction

- The term *osteoarthritis* is commonly used to refer to any degenerative condition of articular cartilage other than the classically described inflammatory arthropathies such as rheumatoid disease and the seronegative spondyloarthropathies. Conditions that result from previous trauma, crystalline deposition diseases, and infection should be described specifically based on their etiology.

- Osteoarthritis best describes the degeneration of articular cartilage that occurs without clear etiology. Some authors believe "primary idiopathic osteoarthritis" is a more descriptive name for this condition. The clinical and radiographic examination of the hand is fundamental to making the diagnosis of primary idiopathic osteoarthritis.

- Idiopathic osteoarthritis and traumatic arthrosis have a substantial amount of overlap. In some cases, it may be impossible to determine whether the origin was idiopathic, as occurs with osteoarthritis, or related to an injury, as occurs in traumatic arthritis. If there is a history of a fracture or ligament disruption, such as a tear of the scapholunate (SL) interosseous ligament, or a scaphoid nonunion, it is appropriate to label those forms of wrist degeneration as traumatic in origin, for which many individuals prefer the term *arthrosis*.

- Patients with osteoarthritis and traumatic arthrosis typically note pain and stiffness, unlike patients with rheumatoid arthritis, in whom deformity may present a larger problem than pain.

- The distal interphalangeal (DIP) joint is the most commonly involved site in all variants of osteoarthritis of the hand on radiographs. The trapeziometacarpal (TM) joint is the next most commonly involved site of disease in the primary generalized form of osteoarthritis. It causes significant functional disability secondary to painful, weakened pinch and grip. The TM joint is the most common site for symptomatic arthritis in the hand.

- Management of osteoarthritis (primary generalized and erosive forms) of the fingers and thumb requires an understanding of functional imperatives, treatment options, and surgical outcomes. This chapter addresses these issues, which can be summarized as follows:

  1. Involvement of the DIP joint (Heberden nodes) requires treatment for symptomatic instability, painful deformity, or mucous cyst and, in most cases, is addressed effectively by arthrodesis.

  2. The incidence of arthritis at the proximal interphalangeal (PIP) joint in primary generalized osteoarthritis is less than at the DIP and TM joints. By contrast, in erosive osteoarthritis the PIP joint is more frequently involved than the TM joint.

3. The PIP joint (Bouchard nodes) is treated by implant arthroplasty or by arthrodesis.
4. Osteoarthritis of the metacarpophalangeal (MCP) joint is rare and generally is posttraumatic. Arthritis of the MCP joints occurs in hemachromatosis, and iron-binding levels should be evaluated.
5. The thumb basal joint is treated with a combination of trapezium excision and ligament reconstruction for advanced disease or alternatively with fusion when scaphotrapezial arthritis is not present. Ligament reconstruction and metacarpal extension osteotomy are options for the symptomatic hypermobile TM joint. Arthritis involving the basal joint can be separated as follows:
   A. Primary carpometacarpal (CMC) joint arthritis
   B. Primary scaphoid trapezium trapezoid joint arthritis
   C. Pantrapezial joint arthritis
6. Primary wrist osteoarthritis is rare, is posttraumatic in nature, and results in pain with wrist movement and gripping.
   A. Primary osteoarthritis and posttraumatic radiocarpal arthrosis
   B. Scapholunate advanced collapse (SLAC) secondary to SL interosseous ligament injury or scaphoid nonunion advanced collapse (SNAC) pattern following scaphoid nonunion

# Pathophysiology of Disease

- Osteoarthritis is the result of an interplay between biomechanical and biochemical factors.
- Cytokines derived from the synovium, such as interleukin-1, activate degradative enzyme synthesis in the chondrocyte, which results in breakdown of the proteoglycan matrix components.
- Neutral proteases and metalloproteoglycanases play a central role in catabolism of the matrix, resulting in decreased hydrophilic properties and a smaller volume of hydration of cartilage. These biochemical events significantly alter the mechanical properties of hyaline cartilage, making it more susceptible to failure under load and less effective in buffering the subchondral trabeculae from impact loading and fracture.
- Further, hyaline cartilage and the surrounding collagenous tissues may be sensitive to estrogen-related compounds, potentially clarifying our understanding of the gender predisposition of this disease.
- Abnormal loading of the joint with increased contact areas as a result of ligamentous injury or attrition, loss of articular cartilage, and articular step-off following trauma all contribute to osteoarthritis.

# Osteoarthritis of the Trapeziometacarpal Joint

- Pellegrini[1] deserves recognition for advancing our understanding of the pathophysiology of osteoarthritis, particularly with respect to clinical disease at the TM joint. Pellegrini's analysis of both surgical and postmortem specimens of the TM joint revealed articular cartilage wear in the dorsal compartment. However, more importantly, the palmar joint surfaces were often found to be polished to eburnated bone.
- Eburnation of the bone always began on the most palmar perimeter of the joint and spread dorsally with progressive disease. Palmar cartilage surface degeneration was closely associated with degeneration of the beak ligament from the articular margin of the metacarpal. Frank detachment of the ligament from its normal position confluent with the joint surface reduced its mechanical efficiency in checking dorsal migration of the metacarpal on trapezium during dynamic flexion-adduction of the thumb.
- Pellegrini also showed that the primary loading areas during lateral pinch are in the same palmar regions of the joint as the eburnated surfaces in diseased joints. Furthermore, division of the beak ligament in specimens with healthy cartilage surfaces altered the contact patterns and reproduced the topography of the eburnated lesions observed in the arthritic joints. Contact patterns in specimens with end-stage arthritic disease were notable for pathologic congruity with total contact of joint surfaces, hypertrophic marginal osteophytes, and diffuse eburnation.
- Biochemical analysis of hyaline cartilage from arthritic TM joints revealed preferential loss of glycosaminoglycan from the extracellular matrix with relative sparing of the collagen framework in the palmar regions of the joint where osteoarthritic lesions first appear.
- Pelligrini has advanced a compelling hypothesis regarding the etiology of TM osteoarthritis.
   1. It begins with initial attrition of the beak ligament and culminates in eventual detachment with destabilization of the thumb metacarpal.
   2. Dorsopalmar metacarpal translation generates increased shear forces in the palmar contact areas of the joint and damages the protective surface layer of the hyaline cartilage. This allows regional access of synovially elaborated inflammatory mediators to the cellular elements in the deeper cartilage layers.
   3. Eventually, a complete loss of the hyaline cartilage results from the combined effects of both abnormal biomechanical forces and biochemical breakdown of the

matrix. Such an etiology of osteoarthritis of the unstable TM joint is consistent with the empirical clinical observations of amelioration of synovitis and retardation of the progression of arthritic disease in young women with symptomatic hypermobile joints following palmar beak ligament reconstruction procedures.

## Osteoarthritic Finger

### Evaluation and Management of the Distal Interphalangeal Joint

- The DIP joint is the most frequently involved as noted on radiography. The indications for intervention are limited to pain, instability, deformity, and the presence of a mucous cyst (Figure 24–1).
- Physical examination reveals swelling, Heberden nodes, occasionally erythema, tenderness to palpation, and decreased range of motion. A mucous cyst, which is actually a ganglion overlying the joint, may be present.
- Radiographs taken in the anteroposterior (AP) and lateral plain views reveal joint space narrowing, subchondral sclerosis, cyst formation, and osteophytes.
- Nonoperative management is limited to activity modification, nonsteroidal antiinflammatory drugs (NSAIDs), and occasionally steroid injections.
- Operative intervention includes arthrodesis versus arthroplasty. Although reports document good results following arthroplasty at the DIP joint, fusion is a more predictable and simpler procedure and is equally effective; hence it is most frequently recommended. When the DIP joint is fused, it is important to remove the overlying osteophytes to improve the aesthetic appearance of the joint following fusion. The joint should be fused in 5 to 10 degrees flexion. This facilitates prehensile activities compared to fusion in an extended position. For this reason, I (M.M.T.) have preferred Kirschner wires for internal fixation rather than a small cannulated screw. The latter holds the joint in more extension than is ideal for prehension. Take note of your own DIP joints in a position of function: they are never in full extension. The cannulated screw is an attractive option nonetheless because of outstanding stability at the outset.
- When a mucous cyst is present and requires excision, the causative osteophyte should be removed. In cases of recurrence or for severe deformity, it is advisable to perform a fusion at the same time in order to address underlying degenerative changes. If relatively painless motion accompanies a mucous cyst, cyst excision alone is recommended.

### Evaluation and Management of the Proximal Interphalangeal Joint

- Similar to the DIP joint, evaluation and treatment of the osteoarthritic PIP joint must take into consideration the patient's subjective complaints, such as pain, dissatisfaction

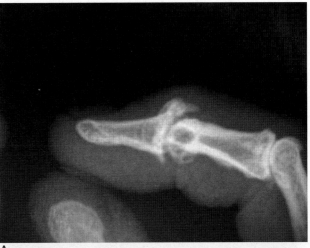

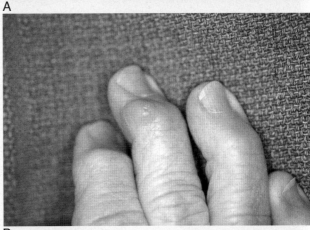

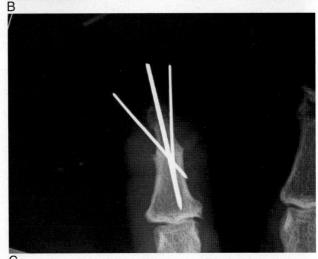

Figure 24–1:
Osteoarthritis of the distal interphalangeal joint. **A,** Lateral x-ray film shows joint degeneration and dorsal osteophyte. **B,** Accompanying mucous cyst. **C,** Anteroposterior x-ray film after fusion.

with appearance, and functional limitations, in addition to objective dysfunction such as stiffness, instability, flexor tendon adherence, and extensor tendon abnormalities (Figure 24–2).

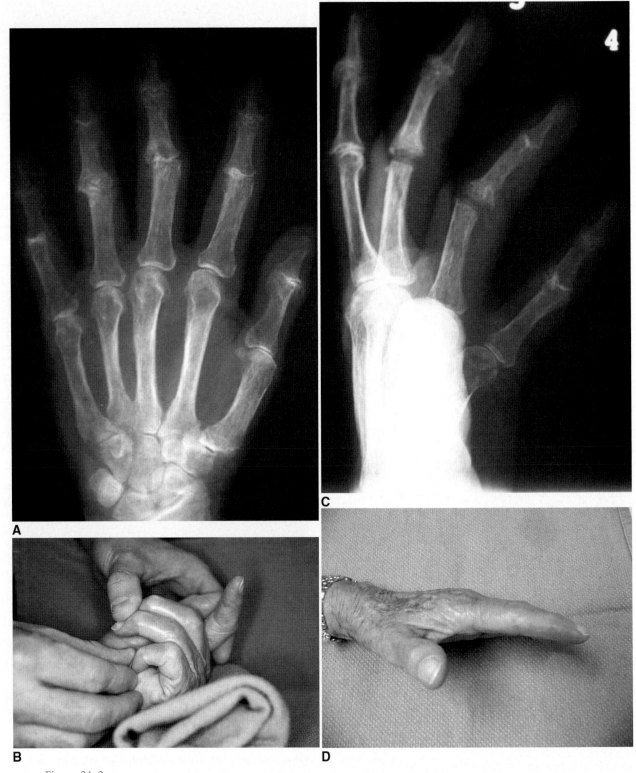

Figure 24–2:
Osteoarthritis of the proximal interphalangeal (PIP) joint. **A,** Anteroposterior x-ray film shows degenerative changes at the PIP joints of each finger. **B,** Clinical picture shows limitation primarily at the long and ring fingers. The other PIP joints were not painful. **C,** X-ray film following ring and long PIP joint implant arthroplasty. **D,** Digital extension.

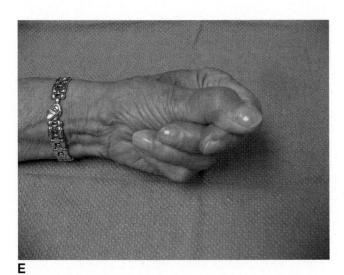

**E**

Figure 24–2: cont'd

**E, Digital flexion.**

- Bone quality, soft tissue envelope, and neurovascular status require evaluation in order to assess the feasibility of surgical intervention.
- Physical examination reveals swelling, Bouchard nodes, occasional erythema, tenderness to palpation, and decreased range of motion.
- Radiographs taken in the AP, lateral, and oblique plain views reveal joint space narrowing, subchondral sclerosis, cyst formation, osteophytes, and occasionally joint subluxation.
- The functional flexion range for the PIP joint occurs within a 60-degree arc of motion. Following implant arthroplasty, the patient generally can achieve approximately 60 degrees of motion. Implant arthroplasty is not recommended for joints in which motion is limited and not expected to improve after surgery, unless the goal of surgery is to redistribute motion into a more useful range, as in the setting of preoperative swan-neck or boutonnière deformity.
- Arthroplasty should *not* be recommended in fingers that function well despite the presence of Bouchard nodes and joint changes. NSAIDs, activity modification, and digital range of motion exercises are the mainstays of nonoperative treatment.
- Surgical intervention for the osteoarthritic PIP joint involves a decision between arthroplasty and arthrodesis. Swanson has acknowledged that the latter provides a more predictable outcome for the index finger, in which the lateral stresses associated with pinch are expected to compromise the stability and durability of the implant. Pelligrini and Burton[2] retrospectively confirmed this recommendation by demonstrating failure patterns after a number of implants were used to reconstruct index finger PIP joints. Their report underscored the difference between the radial digits, which assume primary responsibility for lateral and key pinch, and the

ulnar side of the hand, which participates in power grasp. We recommend arthrodesis of the arthritic index PIP joint and implant arthroplasty in the ulnar three digits.
- Techniques for arthroplasty at the PIP joint include the dorsal approach, which uses the central slip either splitting or sparing techniques. The volar approach has also been described[3] and has the advantages of preserving the extensor tendon insertion while allowing exposure of the flexor tendon apparatus. This latter approach is reasonable in the PIP joint with osteoarthritis or posttraumatic arthrosis because deformity is less common than in the rheumatoid patient, in whom exposure of the extensor tendon apparatus maybe required to correct deformity.
- Patients who have PIP joint disease commonly also have DIP joint involvement. Surgical intervention at the DIP joint follows the principles outlined in the section on osteoarthritic finger.

## Evaluation and Management of the Metacarpophalangeal Joint

- Arthrosis at the MCP joint is relatively common in rheumatoid disease, but idiopathic primary osteoarthritis of the MCP joint is infrequent. Most cases of MCP arthritis are posttraumatic. MCP osteoarthritis is seen in the setting of hemochromatosis.
- Examination is notable for swelling, occasional erythema, tenderness to palpation, and decreased range of motion.
- Radiographs of the hand taken in the AP, lateral, and oblique plain views reveal joint space narrowing, subchondral sclerosis, cyst formation, osteophytes, and occasionally joint subluxation.
- Treatment is similar to the PIP joint. The functional range of motion at the MCP joint averages approximately 60 degrees. Arthroplasty should *not* be recommended in fingers that function well despite radiographic changes. NSAIDs, activity modification, and digital range of motion exercises are the mainstays of nonoperative treatment.
- Before the development of reliable implants, a number of resection arthroplasties were described to avoid arthrodesis. Although good results were reported, these resection arthroplasties are of historical significance only because better correction of ulnar and palmar subluxation of the phalangeal bases and better overall stability result with the use of implants. Newer unconstrained implants may allow collateral ligament retention and improved durability.

## Osteoarthritic Thumb Basal Joint

### Evaluation and Management of the Basal Joint

- Radiographic evidence of osteoarthritis involving the TM joint of the thumb is common and is second only to osteoarthritis at the DIP joint in prevalence. Although decision making for treatment of osteoarthritis at the PIP and DIP joints is fairly straightforward, a number of options have been described for reconstructing the painful thumb TM joint. Most surgical treatment options are of historical interest only. The current mainstay of surgical treatment is trapezium excision and ligament reconstruction.

- Physical examination reveals tenderness along the thumb TM joint. The traditional grind test, performed with axial compression, flexion, extension, and circumduction, causes crepitance and pain. It is important to examine the patient and not to proceed with operative treatment simply based on radiographs. Patients may be asymptomatic despite significant radiographic evidence of joint degeneration. It is important to perform an Allen test if surgery is contemplated, because exposure of the basal joint, if a dorsal approach is elected, involves mobilization of the radial artery and may jeopardize its patency.

- Radiographic evaluation of the arthritic TM joint includes a posteroanterior (PA) stress and lateral view and a Robert (pronated anterior posterior) view.

- Nonoperative treatment includes antiinflammatory medication, intraarticular steroid injection, hand- or forearm-based thumb spica splint immobilization, and thenar muscle isometric conditioning.

- It is critical to evaluate the entire hand for signs and symptoms of carpal tunnel syndrome, stenosing flexor tenosynovitis (trigger finger), de Quervain tenosynovitis, MCP joint instability, and scaphotrapezial and scaphotrapezoidal arthritis. Encroachment on the carpal canal by the subluxed trapezium or swelling following basal joint arthroplasty may exacerbate mild carpal tunnel syndrome, which occurs concomitantly in almost half of patients. Carpal tunnel syndrome, pain secondary to a trigger thumb, or de Quervain tenosynovitis may compromise compliance with postoperative hand therapy. It is important, therefore, to surgically address these entities if they coexist with basal joint arthritis.

## Staging of Disease

- Osteoarthritis may be confined to the TM joint, or it may involve the pantrapezial joint complex. Eaton and Littler[4] described four stages of TM osteoarthritis (Box 24–1).

- Of note, the Eaton staging system neglects any mention of the scaphotrapezoidal joint. Irwin, Maffulli, and Chesney[5] heightened our appreciation of neglected scaphotrapezoidal arthritis as a potential cause of residual pain after the ligament reconstruction tendon interposition (LRTI) arthroplasty. Tomaino, Vogt, and Weiser[6] reported a prevalence of 62% in 37 hands. Because the x-ray sensitivity and specificity for disease at the scaphotrapezoidal joint are only 44% and 86%, respectively, routine intraoperative assessment of the scaphotrapezoidal

| Box 24–1 | **Eaton Stages of Trapeziometacarpal Osteoarthritis** |
|---|---|
| Stage 1 | Normal joint with the exception of possible widening from synovitis |
| Stage 2 | Joint space narrowing with debris and osteophytes <2 mm in size |
| Stage 3 | Joint space narrowing with debris and osteophytes >2 mm in size |
| Stage 4 | Scaphotrapezial joint space involvement in addition to narrowing of the TM joint |

joint is recommended at the time of arthroplasty by pulling on the index and long fingers. When arthritis is present, a 2- to 3-mm excision of the proximal trapezoid is recommended in order to prevent residual pain in the postoperative period following arthroplasty.

## Treatment

- Indications for surgical treatment of basal joint disease of the thumb are almost exclusively pain or deformity that interferes with daily function, including grip and pinch. The treatment options for all stages, with the exception of stage 1, can be lumped together. The current "gold standard" of treatment of all advanced stages is trapezium excision in conjunction with ligament reconstruction, using any one of a number of alternative techniques. Some surgeons preferentially perform a hemitrapeziectomy for stages 2 and 3 disease rather than a complete resection. Pantrapezial involvement contraindicates procedures such as TM arthrodesis[7] or hemitrapeziectomy alone.

## Stage 1 Disease

- Until recently, surgical treatment has centered on reconstruction of the palmar beak ligament with a slip of flexor carpi radialis (FCR) tendon as described by Eaton and Littler[4] (Figure 24–3). However, for this procedure to provide pain relief, the joint surfaces must be free of eburnation and demonstrate only early changes of chondromalacia, at most, in the contact areas of the palmar compartment. The TM joint can be exposed effectively using a modified Wagner approach, with an incision centered over the dorsoradial aspect of the thumb metacarpal. The decision to perform ligament reconstruction without trapezium excision is predicated upon intraoperative confirmation of satisfactory articular surfaces. The surgeon and patient must be prepared to exercise an alternative treatment option if the degenerative changes are more extensive.

- The objective of ligament reconstruction in the treatment of the hypermobile TM joint is restoration of a static restraint to dorsal translation. Eaton et al.[8] reported long-term follow-up on 50 thumbs following the

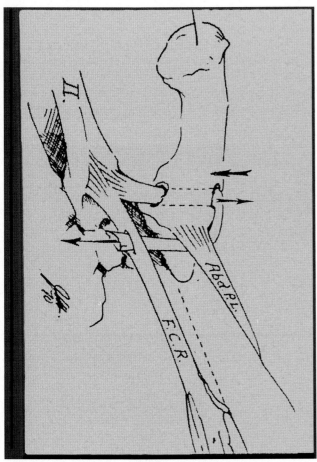

Figure 24–3:
**Eaton ligament reconstruction.** *Abd P.L.,* abductor pollicis longus; *F.C.R.,* flexor carpi radialis.

procedure. For eight thumbs with stage 1 disease and a normal TM joint space, excellent pain relief and complete restoration of pinch strength resulted. Freedman, Eaton, and Glickel[9] showed that ligament reconstruction restored pain-free TM stability and prevented the development of TM osteoarthritis in 15 (65%) of 23 thumbs at an average follow-up of 15 years.

- The biomechanical analysis by Pellegrini et al.[10] of the effect of thumb metacarpal osteotomy inspired Tomaino's[11] prospective investigation of this procedure's efficacy for treatment of stage 1 disease (Figure 24–4). The rationale for thumb metacarpal extension osteotomy involves dorsal load transfer and a shift in force vectors during pinch. A 30-degree closing wedge extension osteotomy effectively unloaded the palmar compartment and shifted the contact areas to the intact dorsal articular cartilage. Tomaino reported on 12 patients enrolled between 1995 and 1998, with an average follow-up of 2.1 years, and showed that all osteotomies healed at an average of 7 weeks, and 11 patients were satisfied with outcome. Grip and pinch strength increased an average of

8.5 and 3 kg, respectively. Thumb metacarpal extension osteotomy is an effective "biomechanical alternative" to ligament reconstruction as treatment for Eaton stage I disease of the TM joint.[10]

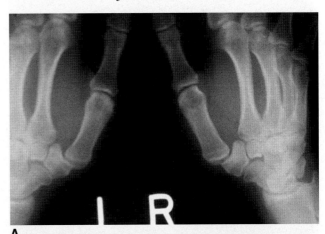

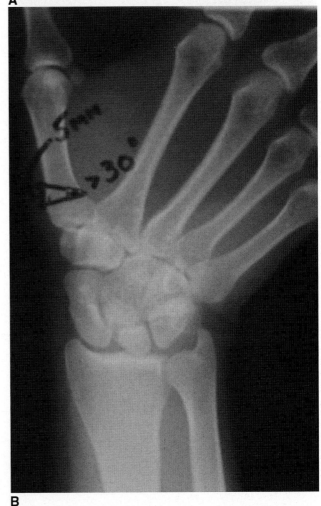

Figure 24–4:
**Stage 1 basal joint disease. A,** Preoperative stress x-ray film demonstrates stage 1 disease (normal trapeziometacarpal joint). **B,** Preoperative lateral x-ray film with the planned 30-degree extension osteotomy.

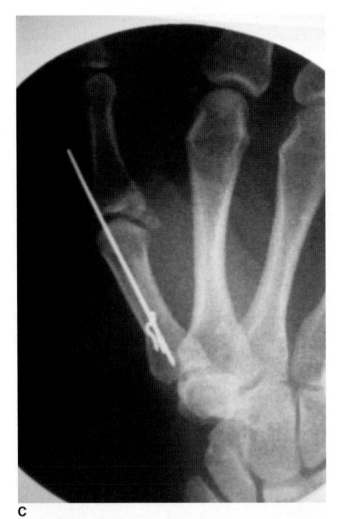

**C**

Figure 24–4: cont'd
**C,** Lateral x-ray film after osteotomy.

- TM arthroscopy arguably is the newest procedure available for treating stage 1 disease. The technical pearls have been published by Berger,[12] and some surgeons advocate arthroscopic synovectomy, ligament thermal shrinkage, and temporary TM pinning. The absence of published reports of outcome justifies a modicum of resistance before adopting this alternative. Hopefully prospective assessment of efficacy are forthcoming (Figure 24–5).

## Advanced Stages: Surgical Treatment Options

- Advanced disease implies end-stage degeneration of the TM joint (stages 2–4), salvageable only by a procedure that removes or replaces the entire articular surface. Although a number of reports have underscored superlative pain relief with TM joint fusion, mobility is limited, and abnormal wear at adjacent unfused joints can develop.[7,13]

- Simple trapezium excision avoids the problems associated with fusion and the complications of material wear and instability associated with implant arthroplasty. Weakness and instability historically have compromised long-term functional results in the absence of concomitant ligament

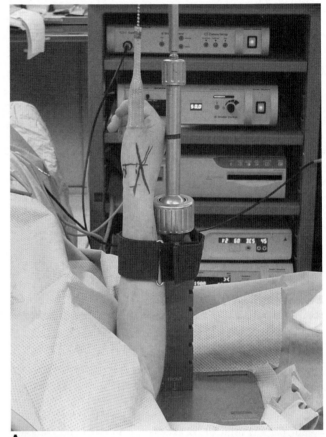

**A**

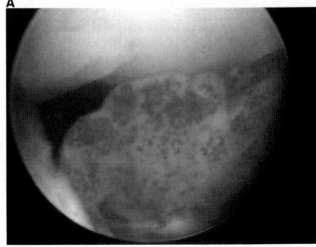

**B**

Figure 24–5:
**Trapeziometacarpal (TM) Arthroscopy. A,** TM arthroscopy setup. **B,** Arthroscopic photo of TM synovitis.

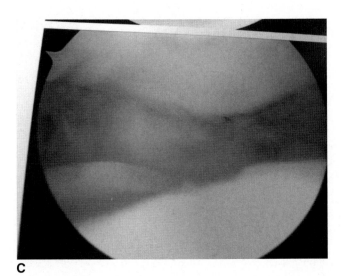

**C**

Figure 24–5: cont'd

**C,** Arthroscopic photo after synovectomy.

reconstruction. Even the addition of fascial or tendon interposition by Froimson,[14] in an effort to improve grip strength and reduce metacarpal shortening, failed to improve long-term results. Simple trapezium excision in conjunction with temporary distraction and pinning has gained popularity—the so-called hematoma-distraction arthroplasty.[15] Long-term follow-up has not yet been reported for this procedure, and the potential for a decline in pinch strength with time seems inevitable, at least in higher-demand thumbs.

- Cemented arthroplasty has been associated with an unacceptably high loosening rate and has fallen from favor. The de la Caffiniere prosthesis has undergone design revisions intended to reduce the incidence of early metacarpal loosening by enlarging the stem diameter, adding a circumferential collar and providing a modular head-neck segment. The polyethylene trapezial component remains unchanged. Meaningful results using this new component design will not be available for several years.

- Hemiarthroplasty is an effective treatment (Figure 24–6 A, B).

- We recommend the LRTI arthroplasty for basal joint reconstruction for pantrapezial involvement. This procedure includes trapezium excision, ligament reconstruction, and tendon interposition. The LRTI, as originally described by Burton and Pellegrini,[16] used half the width of the FCR tendon for ligament reconstruction. Many surgeons, including Burton, altered this procedure to include the entire width of the FCR tendon in order to facilitate harvest and provide a bulkier tendon for interposition. Tomaino and Coleman[17] reported no morbidity following the use of the entire tendon. Passing the entire width of the FCR tendon through a bony channel in the thumb metacarpal is facilitated by tapering the proximal width of the tendon and using a Carrol tendon passer (Figure 24–6 C through F and Box 24–2).

- With respect to LRTI arthroplasty, results seem to improve for several years following the operation, underscoring the protracted time necessary to achieve maximum strength following the procedure. Documentation of durable long-term performance following this procedure[18] contrasts markedly with the long-term outcomes after prosthetic trapezium replacement and trapezium excision with fascial interposition.

- Tissue interposition appears to promote repopulation of the arthroplasty space with denser, less "fatty" scar tissue, theoretically providing a more effective "secondary restraint" to proximal metacarpal migration over time. However, Gerwin et al.[19] and Kriegs-Au et al.[20] demonstrated that tissue interposition probably does not matter, at least in the short term. Furthermore, there appears not to be a correlation between some degree of subsidence and outcome unless scaphometacarpal impingement occurs, which is more likely when no ligament reconstruction has been performed.

- Many surgeons have elected to use alternative methods of suspending the metacarpal, and some have stopped pinning it for 4 weeks. Appreciation of underlying principles and technically sound execution will increase the likelihood of functional improvement, which should be measured against very favorable long-term outcomes reported in 1995 following long-term assessment of the LRTI, regardless of the method.

- Thompson[21] has been credited with describing use of a slip of the abductor pollicis longus (APL) tendon using tunnels through both thumb and index metacarpal bases. Others have avoided using any bony tunnel, simply by weaving a slip of APL around the FCR and sewing it back dorsally to itself and/or periosteum.[22] The world's literature uniformly describes favorable outcome following such suspensionplasties, characterized by excellent pain relief and significantly improved strength.

## Special Considerations

- The status of the thumb MCP joint is of critical importance to the long-term stability of the more proximal basal joint reconstruction. Any propensity for hyperextension in excess of 30 degrees during lateral (key) pinch requires either fusion or volar capsulodesis of the MCP joint. Failure to address a hyperextensile MCP joint may result in the longitudinal collapse of the thumb during pinch. This causes thumb metacarpal flexion and adduction and increases stresses on the ligament reconstruction. Accordingly, if there is more than 30 degrees of hyperextension instability during key pinch, we recommend either arthrodesis in 5 to 10 degrees flexion or volar capsulodesis. If hyperextension stability is less than 30 degrees, temporary stabilization in flexion with a Kirschner wire is used for 4 weeks.

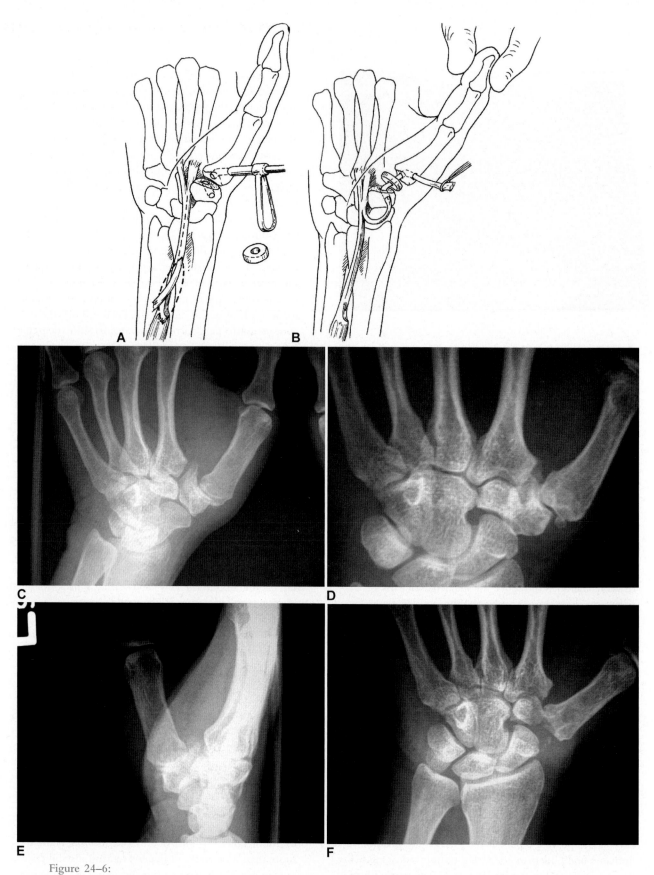

Figure 24–6:

**A,** A drill guide is used to drill a hole in the dorsal radial cortex of the metacarpal. This hole is connected to a drill hole made into the proximal articular surface of the metacarpal base. **B,** Once the desired tension on the flexor carpi radialis (ECR) tendon has been applied with the thumb held in supination, the FCR tendon is secured to the periosteum on the dorsal and radial portion of the thumb metacarpal. Ligament reconstruction tendon interposition (LRTI) for advanced basal joint arthritis. **C,** Preoperative stress x-ray film demonstrates advanced basal joint arthritis. **D,** Preoperative lateral x-ray film. **E,** Preoperative pronated anteroposterior x-ray film. **F,** Postoperative x-ray film after LRTI arthroplasty.

---

### Box 24–2   Fundamentals of LRTI Arthroplasty

- Trapezium excision to remove arthritic joint surfaces
- Palmar oblique ligament reconstruction to restore thumb metacarpal stability and prevent axial shortening
- Fascial interposition to reduce the likelihood of impingement between neighboring bony surfaces

## Salvage

- One cause of unsatisfactory outcome following basal joint arthroplasty revolves around the failure to address scaphotrapezial or scaphotrapezoidal disease. Routine complete excision of the trapezium certainly precludes the former and allows adequate intraoperative observation and treatment of the latter by partial excision of the proximal trapezoid, as previously mentioned.
- Another likely cause of long-term failure is instability at the MCP joint, which has been mentioned. With lateral pinch, hyperextension at that level causes reciprocal deformity more proximally. This leads to metacarpal adduction and stresses the reconstructed ligament. Accordingly, early identification of hyperextension in excess of 30 degrees should prompt stabilization in order to protect the integrity of the basal joint ligament reconstruction. Even with a sound ligament reconstruction and appropriate stabilization of the MCP joint, it is theoretically possible to develop recurrent laxity at the basal joint secondary to stretching of the FCR tendon. However, this finding was not observed among the initial cohort of patients reported in 1995 with this procedure with 10 years follow-up.
- In the absence of a residual FCR tendon, the APL tendon can be used, as described by Thompson,[21] as a salvage procedure for the revision of a failed silicone implant arthroplasty. This option also is useful at the time of an initial basal joint arthroplasty should the FCR tendon be damaged or found incompetent.

## Osteoarthritic Wrist

### Evaluation and Management of the Radiocarpal Joint

- Primary wrist osteoarthritis is rare. Most wrist arthrosis is posttraumatic in nature and results in pain with wrist motion and grip. Causes include intraarticular distal radius fracture, chronic scaphoid nonunion, and chronic SL dissociation. SLAC occurs as a result of SL injury, and SNAC pattern follows scaphoid nonunion (Figure 24–7).
- SL dissociation results in scaphoid flexion, which results in increased contact forces per smaller contact area. A reproducible pattern of radiocarpal and intercarpal degeneration develops.[23] Radioscaphoid and capitolunate changes occur in a predictable sequence, but radiolunate changes are rare in the SLAC wrist because the lunate and lunate fossa remain congruous. A similar pattern occurs with an unstable scaphoid nonunion and results in the SNAC pattern of traumatic arthrosis, which differs from the SLAC pattern because the proximal pole of the scaphoid extends with the lunate. Thus, radioscaphoid changes most typically occur between the styloid and the scaphoid distal pole (Box 24–3).

- Physical examination with direct palpation reveals tenderness over the carpus. The patient often experiences pain even with gentle passive range of motion. Neurovascular examination of the hand is intact.
- Radiographs taken in the AP, lateral and oblique plain views reveal joint space narrowing, subchondral sclerosis, and cyst formation in the carpal bones and distal radius.
- Nonoperative management includes activity modification, NSAIDs, and occasionally steroid injections, which can provide symptomatic relief, particularly in the low-demand patient.
- Indications for surgical treatment of radiocarpal disease is almost exclusively pain or deformity that interferes with daily functions, particularly grip. Correlation between patient symptoms and radiographic appearance frequently is poor, and treatment must be tailored to specific patient complaints. Fassler, Stern, and Kiefhaber[24] reported a number of patients with SLAC arthritis on radiograph with minimal or no pain.

### Surgical Treatment Options

- Surgical options include motion-preserving and motion-sacrificing procedures. The question is arthrodesis versus some form of arthroplasty.[25,26]
- Adequate pain relief is the most critical outcome metric; therefore, the decision between limited and full wrist fusion or proximal row carpectomy (PRC) must take into account patient expectations. Complete wrist fusion typically eliminates all pain, whereas motion-preserving options may not at higher demand levels.
- The risk of performing a partial wrist fusion or PRC over a complete wrist fusion is some residual pain in the remaining portion of the joint. The patient should understand that intraoperative inspection of the articulations influences the final treatment plan. The only real contraindication to complete wrist fusion is the person who requires some motion to perform a vocation or avocation.

### Box 24–3   Stages of SLAC Arthritis

| Stage I | Degenerative change at the scaphoid waist and radial styloid |
|---|---|
| Stage II | Degenerative changes at the proximal pole of the scaphoid and scaphoid fossa of the distal radius |
| Stage III | Degenerative changes at the capitolunate joint |

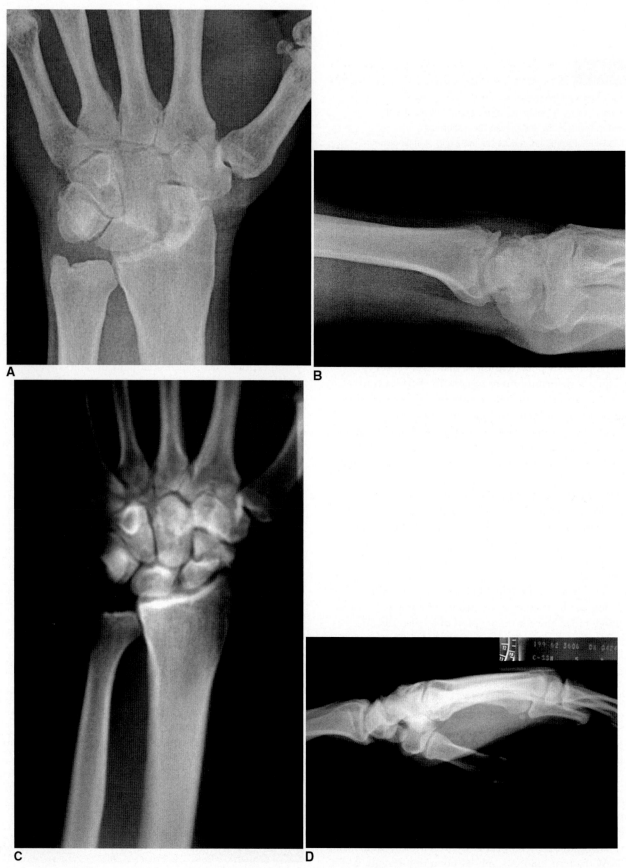

Figure 24–7:
Scapholunate advanced collapse (SLAC) and scaphoid nonunion advanced collapse (SNAC) wrist. **A,**
Anteroposterior (AP) X-ray film of SLAC wrist. **B,** Lateral X-ray film of SLAC wrist. **C,** AP X-ray film of
SNAC wrist. **D,** Lateral X-ray film of SNAC wrist.

- A number of techniques for limited and complete wrist fusion have been described. Notwithstanding, a number of variations in technique—complete arthrodesis and limited arthrodesis—rely on several common principles.

## Surgical Exposure of the Wrist

- A midline, dorsal wrist incision just ulnar to Lister tubercle is used. It is important to elevate full-thickness skin flaps. The third compartment is opened and a midline capsulotomy is performed. The incision is extended distally along the third metacarpal if wrist fusion is performed. The floor of the fourth compartment is exposed so that a posterior interosseous neurectomy can be performed.

## Proximal Row Carpectomy

- PRC is indicated for patients with stage II SLAC wrist arthritis. The PRC is an effective motion-preserving procedure.[27] Although the PRC does not reestablish normal articular contact, long-term studies show that the capitate functions nicely in the lunate fossa as long as the radioscaphocapitate ligament is intact.
- The midcarpal joint is inspected to ensure there is enough sparing of the articular surface of the capitate to perform the PRC instead of a total wrist fusion. The scaphoid is osteotomized at the waist to facilitate removal. The lunate and triquetrum are removed. The capitate is reduced into the lunate fossa of the radius. If the radial deviation is 5 degrees or less, a limited radial styloidectomy should be performed (Figure 24–8).
- Imbriglia and Broudy[28] demonstrated that once degeneration occurs in the midcarpal joint with loss of the articular surface from the capitate, PRC may lead to accelerated arthrosis between the capitate and lunate fossa of the radius. In cases of stage III SLAC, however, dorsal capsular interposition may extend the indications for PRC.
- Wyrick, Stern, and Kiefhaber[29] evaluated 10 patients with PRC and compared them to 17 patient with four-bone fusion and scaphoid excision. Three patients in the four-bone fusion group did not respond compared with no failures in the PRC group. They reported that PRC was their motion-preserving procedure of choice in the absence of advanced capitolunate degenerative changes.

## Four-Bone Fusion

- In active patients who would benefit from a motion-preserving operation, a four-bone fusion including the capitate, lunate, triquetral, and hamate (CLTH) provides stability and allows continued motion at the radiocarpal articulation while removing the painful arthrosis at the radioscaphoid joint.[30] Midcarpal degenerative changes seen in stage III SLAC and SNAC arthritis are an excellent indication for the four-bone fusion, also known as the *four-corner fusion*.

- Minami et al.[31] noted minimal degenerative changes in the radiolunate joint following CLTH fusion. They compared evaluation at an average of 22 months with average follow-up of 89 months in 11 wrists that underwent four-bone fusion. Clinical and radiographic parameters were maintained at long-term follow-up.
- Sauberbier et al.[32] treated 36 patients with stage II and III SLAC and SNAC arthritis with scaphoid excision and midcarpal fusion. At 25-month follow-up, they evaluated patients' range of motion, grip strength, and completed DASH, Krimmer, and Mayo wrist scores. They concluded that four-bone fusion was an excellent operation for reducing pain and restoring function when treating SLAC and SNAC arthritis.
- A midline, dorsal approach is used as previously discussed. The scaphoid is removed. The surfaces between each of the four bones are decorticated, and the capitate, lunate, triquetrum and hamate are stabilized with Kirschner wires. It is important that the lunate be reduced (derotated) out of dorsiflexion and that the capitate be reduced. Otherwise, radiocapitate impaction may limit wrist extension. First, a pin is placed across the lunotriquetral articulation. Then pins are placed into the hamate and capitate with the carpus distracted so that they are directed into the triquetrum and lunate, respectively. Care should be taken to avoid dorsal rotation of the lunate. The patient is placed in a cast until the fusion heals (Figure 24–9). Alternatively, special plate fixation for the four bone fusion can be used to decrease the time of immobilization.

## Total Wrist Fusion

- Patients with painful, pancarpal arthritis affecting activities of daily living and occupational duties are excellent candidates for total wrist fusion. Motion-preserving procedures are relatively contraindicated in heavy laborers with degenerative changes involving radiocarpal and midcarpal joints. Total wrist fusion is the best option for these patients and for patients who have not responded to PRC.
- Autogenous bone graft and dorsal plate fixation is the most common technique of total wrist fusion. The surgical approach is as described in the section on surgical exposure of the wrist. This procedure predictably relieves pain and provides a stable wrist, particularly for manual labor. Grip strength appears to be maximized when the wrist is fused in 10 to 15 degrees extension (Box 24–4 and Figure 24–10).
- Patient satisfaction is high, and most patients have excellent functional status.[33] Houshian and Schroeder[34] reported 40 of 42 patients fused with a contoured plate had good to excellent results. Thirty-nine of the 42 patients fused with one operation. The overall complication rate was approximately 28%. Complications of the procedure include wound dehiscence, infection and extensor tendon irritation, and frank rupture. It is important to remember to

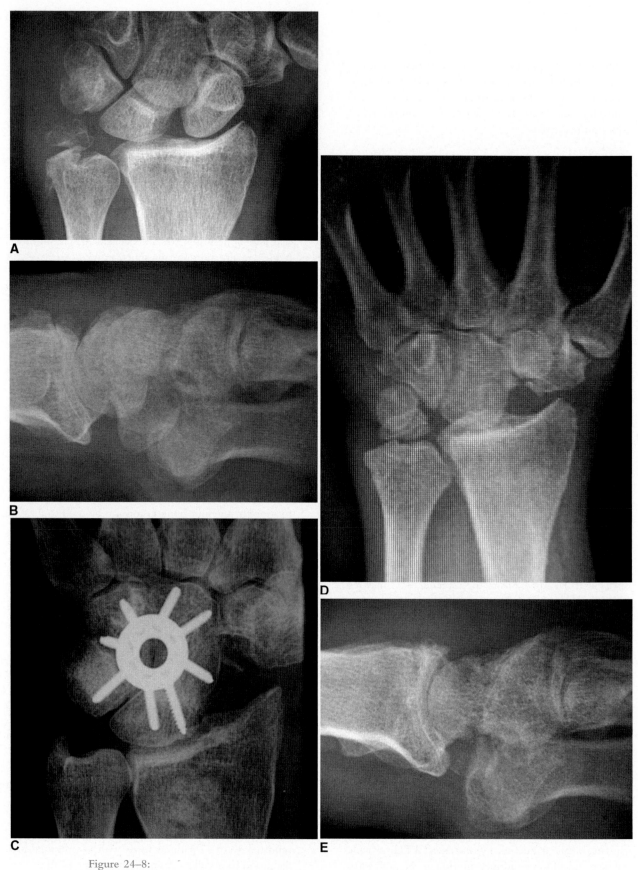

Figure 24–8:

Proximal row carpectomy. **A,** Preoperative anteroposterior (AP) x-ray film of scapholunate advanced collapse (SLAC) wrist. **B,** Preoperative lateral x-ray film of SLAC wrist. **C,** The scaphoid is transected to facilitate removal. **D,** Postoperative AP x-ray film after PRC. **E,** Postoperative lateral x-ray film.

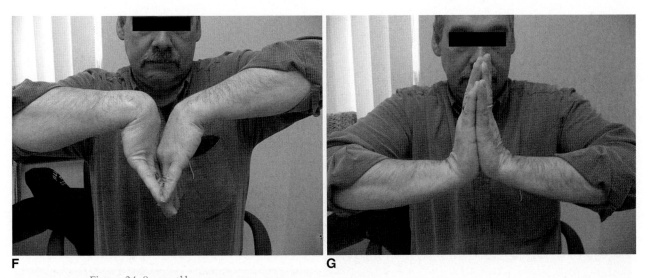

Figure 24–8: cont'd
**F,** Postoperative wrist flexion. **G,** Postoperative wrist extension.

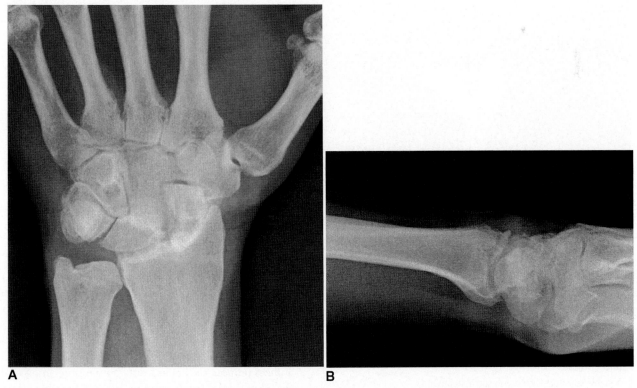

Figure 24–9:
Four-corner fusion. **A,** Preoperative anteroposterior (AP) x-ray film of scapholunate advanced collapse (SLAC) wrist. **B,** Preoperative lateral x-ray film of SLAC wrist.

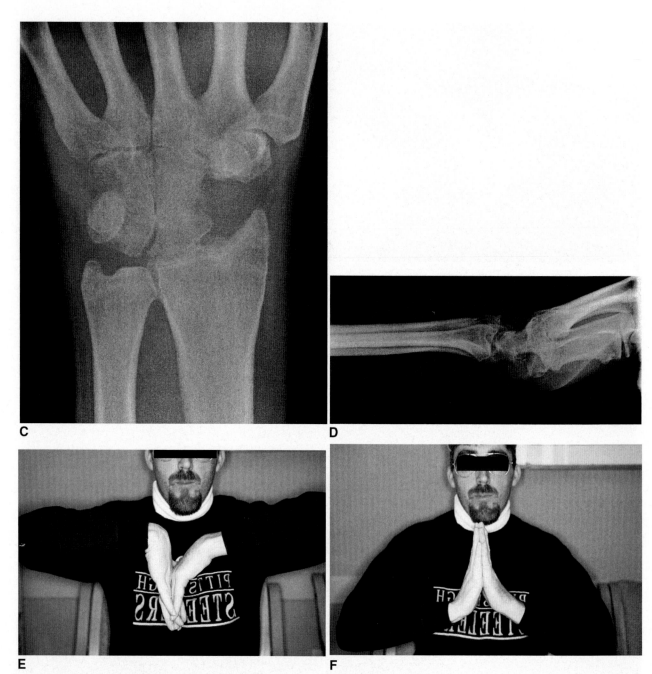

Figure 24–9:  **Cont'd**
**C,** Postoperative AP x-ray film after four-corner fusion and scaphoid excision. **D,** Postoperative lateral film.
**E,** Postoperative flexion. **F,** Postoperative extension.

| **Box 24–4**   **Principles of Wrist Fusion** |
| --- |
| 1. Decortication must be complete. |
| 2. The deformity must be corrected and the wrist optimally positioned for subsequent hand function. |
| 3. Autologous bone graft should accompany decortication in order to expedite union. |
| 4. A stable construct is critical to successful fusion. |
| 5. The status of the distal radioulnar joint (DRUJ) must be evaluated because arthritis of the DRUJ or ulnocarpal abutment may cause persistent painful forearm rotation. |

transpose the extensor pollicis longus during this procedure. Almost half of the surgeries for complications were for plate removal.[35]

- Hartigan, Nagle, and Foley[36] reported on PRC in conjunction with wrist fusion. Seventeen patients all demonstrated fused their wrists using this technique. The authors propose the "radius-distal row fusion" in light of the advantage of fewer joints to fuse and the removal of sclerotic bones that may be hard to fuse. The proximal row can be used as bone graft, obviating the need for

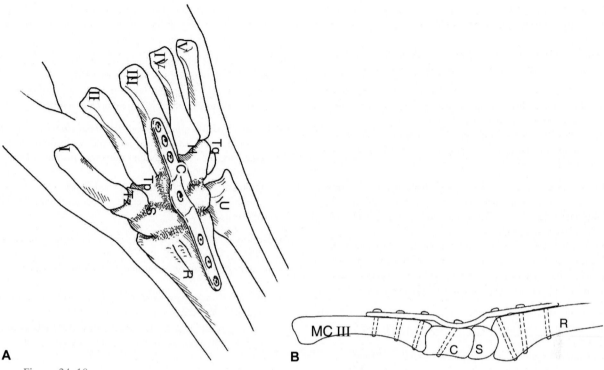

Figure 24–10:

**A,** The AO/ASIF wrist fusion plate provides an ideal means of performing a wrist arthrodesis that allows for wrist extension. **B,** The plate is designed to allow 2.7 mm screws to be placed in the metacarpal and carpus white 3.5 mm screws are placed in the radius. An approach through the third dorsal compartment is performed and a distally based flap of the capsule is elevated.

additional iliac crest bone graft. The outcome scores were good to excellent.

## Total Wrist Arthroplasty

• Limited literature on total wrist arthroplasty in patients with osteoarthritis is available. The procedure has been primarily performed in patients with rheumatoid arthritis. Initial reports of rheumatoid patients show some promise, but long-term follow-up is still lacking. Currently, there are no prospective longitudinal studies involving patients with osteoarthritis. Aseptic loosening, tendon balance, and implant durability are concerns in the higher-demand osteoarthritic patient. Meaningful long-term results using new component design will not be available for years. At present, we recommend one of the aforementioned treatments of SLAC arthritis instead of total wrist arthroplasty.

## Conclusions

• Osteoarthritis of the thumb, fingers, and wrist provides the hand surgeon with an extraordinary opportunity to eradicate pain and improve function. If preoperative assessment is complete, treatment is founded on the principles described in this chapter, and technical

execution is carried out without complication, outcome is favorable in the overwhelming majority of patients.

## References

**Thumb and Fingers**

1. Pellegrini VD: Osteoarthritis of the thumb trapeziometacarpal joint: A study of the pathophysiology of articular cartilage degeneration. II. Articular wear patterns in the osteoarthritic joint. *J Hand Surg* 16A:975-982, 1991.
   Analysis of both surgical and postmortem specimens of the trapeziometacarpal joint revealed typical wear patterns.

2. Pelligrini VD, Burton RI: Osteoarthritis of the proximal interphalangeal joint of the hand: Arthroplasty or fusion? *J Hand Surg* 16A:955-956, 1991.
   The authors report variable results and complications following a variety of surgical procedures for PIP joint arthritis.

3. Lin HH, Wyrick JD, Stern PJ: Proximal interphalangeal joint silicone arthroplasty: clinical results using an anterior approach. *J Hand Surg* 20A:123-132, 1995.
   A review of 69 proximal interphalangeal joint silicone arthroplasties in 36 patients inserted through an anterior approach found good pain relief but variable functional gains.

4. Eaton RG, Littler JW: Ligament reconstruction for the painful thumb carpometacarpal joint. *J Bone Joint Surg* 55A:1655-1666, 1973.
Classic article describing TM joint beak ligament reconstruction for Eaton stage 1 disease using a slip of the FCR.

5. Irwin AS, Maffulli N, Chesney RB: Scapho-trapezoid arthritis. A cause of residual pain after arthroplasty of the trapeziometacarpal joint. *J Hand Surg* 20B:346-352, 1995.
The authors heightened our appreciation of unaddressed scaphotrapezoidal arthritis as a potential cause of residual pain after LRTI arthroplasty.

6. Tomaino MM, Vogt M, Weiser R: Scaphotrapezoid arthritis. Prevalence in thumbs undergoing trapezium excision arthroplasty and efficacy of proximal trapezoid excision. *J Hand Surg* 24A:1220-1224, 1999.
These authors showed that x-ray sensitivity and specificity for disease at the scaphotrapezoidal joint was only 44% and 86%, respectively, and they recommend routine intraoperative assessment of the scaphotrapezoidal joint at the time of arthroplasty.

7. Stern PJ: Trapeziometacarpal joint arthrodesis in primary osteoarthritis: a minimum two-year follow-up. *J Hand Surg* 26A:109-114, 2001.
The authors report their retrospective review of 59 TM arthrodeses with follow-up from 2 to 20 years.

8. Eaton RG, Lane LB, Littler JW, Keyser JJ: Ligament reconstruction for the painful thumb carpometacarpal joint: a long-term assessment. *J Hand Surg* 9A:692-699, 1984.
This study reviews 50 extraarticular ligament reconstructions to stabilize the thumb carpometacarpal joint by routing a portion of the flexor carpi radialis through the base of the thumb metacarpal.

9. Freedman DM, Eaton RG, Glickel SZ: Long-term results of volar ligament reconstruction for symptomatic basal joint laxity. *J Hand Surg* 25A:297-304, 2000.
Ligament reconstruction restored pain-free TM stability and prevented the development of TM osteoarthritis in 15 of 23 lax thumbs at an average follow-up of 15 years.

10. Pellegrini VD Jr, Parentis M, Judkins A, et al: Extension metacarpal osteotomy in the treatment of trapeziometacarpal osteoarthritis: a biomechanical study. *J Hand Surg* 21A:16-23, 1996.
In a biomechanical study, extension metacarpal osteotomy effectively unloaded the palmar contact area in nonarthritic and moderately arthritic specimens, but not in advanced arthritis.

11. Tomaino MM: Treatment of Eaton Stage I trapeziometacarpal disease with metacarpal extension osteotomy. *J Hand Surg* 25A:1100-1106, 2000.
This study prospectively evaluated the efficacy of an extension osteotomy of the metacarpal for Eaton stage I arthritis in 12 patients.

12. Berger RA: A technique for arthroscopic evaluation of the first carpometacarpal joint. *J Hand Surg* 22A:1077-1080, 1997.
This article describes the surgical technique of first CMC arthroscopy with experience in 12 patients.

13. Hartigan BJ, Stern PJ, Kiefhaber TR: Thumb carpometacarpal osteoarthritis: arthrodesis compared with ligament reconstruction and tendon interposition. *J Bone Joint Surg* 83A:1470-1478, 2001.
This study revealed similar results with both fusion and LRTI arthroplasty with regard to pain relief and patient satisfaction but higher complication rates with fusion.

14. Froimson AI: Tendon arthroplasty of the trapeziometacarpal joint. *Clin Orthop Rel Res* 70:191-199, 1970.
Excision of the trapezium with tendon interposition provided good short-term but declining long-term results.

15. Kuhns CA, Emerson ET, Meals RA: Hematoma and distraction arthroplasty for thumb basal joint osteoarthritis: a prospective, single-surgeon study including outcomes measures. *J Hand Surg* 28A:381-389, 2003.
Pinning the metacarpal in a distracted position following trapezial excision led to excellent outcomes despite late proximal metacarpal migration

16. Burton RI, Pellegrini VD: Surgical management of basal joint arthritis of the thumb. Part II. Ligament reconstruction with tendon interposition arthroplasty. *J Hand Surg* 11A:324-332, 1986.
This article describes palmar oblique ligament reconstruction combined with tendon interposition (LRTI) arthroplasty with part of the flexor carpi radialis tendon for advanced osteoarthritis of the thumb basal joint with review of 25 cases.

17. Tomaino MM, Coleman K: Use of the entire width of the flexor carpi radialis tendon for the LRTI arthroplasty does not impair wrist function. *Am J Orthop* 29:283-284, 2000.
There appears to be no morbidity associated with use of the entire width of the FCR tendon at 1 year after LRTI arthroplasty.

18. Tomaino MM, Pellegrini VD Jr, Burton RI: Arthroplasty of the basal joint of the thumb. Long-term follow-up after ligament reconstruction with tendon interposition. *J Bone Joint Surg* 77:346-355, 1995.
The authors report good long-term results following LRTI in 24 thumbs (22 patients) followed an average of 9 years.

19. Gerwin M, Griffith A, Weiland AJ, et al: Ligament reconstruction basal joint arthroplasty without tendon interposition. *Clin Orthop* 342:42-45, 1997.
In this prospective, randomized study, tendon interposition was found not necessary for maintenance of joint space after basal joint resection arthroplasty if ligament reconstruction is performed.

20. Kriegs-Au G, Petje G, Fojtl E, et al: Ligament reconstruction with or without tendon interposition to treat primary thumb carpometacarpal osteoarthritis: a randomized study. *J Bone Joint Surg* 86A:209-218, 2004.
This article shows no advantage of tendon interposition over ligament reconstruction alone for basal joint arthritis.

21. Thompson JS: "Suspensionplasty": Trapeziometacarpal joint reconstruction using abductor pollicis longus. *Op Tech Orthop* 6:98-105, 1996.
Detailed description of the suspensionplasty technique with excellent pearls for performing this procedure.

22. Sigfusson R, Lundborg G: Abductor pollicis longus tendon arthroplasty for treatment of arthrosis in the first car-

pometacarpal joint. *Scand J Plast Reconstr Hand Surg* 25:73-77, 1991.

The authors describe a technique in which a portion of the APL was used in a figure-of-eight fashion around the FCR and remaining portion of the APL.

**Wrist**

23. Watson HK, Ballet FL: The SLAC wrist: scapholunate advanced collapse pattern of degenerative arthritis. *J Hand Surg* 9A:358-365, 1984.
Four thousand wrist x-ray films were reviewed to establish the pattern of sequential changes in degenerative arthritis of the wrist.

24. Fassler PR, Stern PJ, Kiefhaber TR: Asymptomatic SLAC wrist: does it exist? *J Hand Surg* 18A:682-686, 1993.
Twenty-two of 30 wrists with incidental radiographic evidence of SLAC arthritis had no pain.

25. Cohen MS, Kozin SH: Degenerative arthritis of the wrist: proximal row carpectomy versus scaphoid excision and four corner arthrodesis. *J Hand Surg* 26A:94-104, 2001.
Results of four-corner fusion and proximal row carpectomy for SLAC arthritis performed by two different surgeons are compared.

26. Krakauer JD, Bishop AT, Cooney, WP: Surgical treatment of scapholunate advanced collapse. *J Hand Surg* 19A:751-759, 1994.
The outcome of six different procedures for SLAC arthritis was compared in 55 patients.

27. Tomaino MM, Delsignore J, Burton RI: Long term results following proximal row carpectomy. *J Hand Surg* 19A:694-703, 1994.
Twenty-three wrists treated with proximal row carpectomy were evaluated at an average of 6 years follow-up.

28. Imbriglia, JE, Broudy, AS: Proximal row carpectomy: clinical evaluation. *J Hand Surg* 15A:426-430, 1990.
Proximal row carpectomy for treatment of the radiocarpal joint arthritis was studied in 27 patients.

29. Wyrick JD, Stern PJ, Kiefhaber TR: Motion preserving procedures in the treatment of scapholunate advanced collapse wrist: proximal row carpectomy versus four-corner arthrodesis. *J Hand Surg* 20A:965-970, 1995.
Seventeen patients treated with scaphoid excision and four-corner fusion for SLAC wrist were followed for a mean of 27 months.

30. Ashmead D 4th, Watson HK, Damon C, et al: Scapholunate advanced collapse. *J Hand Surg* 19A:741-750, 1994.
The results of 100 cases of scaphoid excision and limited wrist arthrodesis were reviewed at an average of 44 months.

31. Minami A, Kato H, Iwasaki N, Minami M: Limited wrist fusions: comparison of results 22 and 89 months after surgery. *J Hand Surg* 24A:133-137, 1999.
Seventeen wrists with limited wrist arthrodesis (11 intercarpal arthrodesis and four radiocarpal arthrodesis) were evaluated 22 and 89 months after surgery.

32. Sauerbier M, Trankle M, Linsner G, et al: Midcarpal arthrodesis with complete scaphoid excision and interposition bone graft in the treatment of advanced carpal collapse (SNAC/SLAC wrist): operative technique and outcome assessment. *J Hand Surg* 25B:341-345, 2000.
Thirty-six patients with either stage II or III SNAC and SLAC wrists were treated with scaphoid excision and midcarpal fusion.

33. Weiss, AC, Wiederman G Jr: Upper extremity function after wrist arthrodesis. *J Hand Surg* 20A:813-817, 1995.
This study performed a functional evaluation of 23 patients who underwent wrist arthrodesis for post-traumatic conditions.

34. Houshian S, Schroeder HA: Wrist arthrodesis with the AO titanium wrist fusion plate: a consecutive series of 42 cases. *J Hand Surg* 26B:355-359, 2001.
Forty-two wrist fusions were performed using the AO/ASIF wrist fusion plate.

35. Zachary SV, Stern PJ: Complications following AO/ASIF wrist arthrodesis. *J Hand Surg* 20A:339-344, 1995.
Seventy-three wrist arthrodeses (71 patients) using AO/ASIF dorsal plate fixation and iliac crest bone graft were retrospectively reviewed to assess complications.

36. Hartigan BJ, Nagle, Foley MJ: Wrist arthrodesis with excision of the proximal carpal bones using the AO/ASIF wrist fusion plate and local bone graft. *J Hand Surg* 26B:247-251, 2001.
Wrist fusion and PRC were simultaneously performed on 17 patients using the AO/ASIF plate and bone graft from the excised carpal bones.

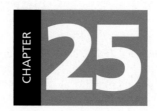

# CHAPTER 25

# Rheumatoid Arthritis—Hand and Wrist: Skeletal Reconstruction

Anthony M. Sestero,[*] Peter J. Stern,[†] and Leigh S. French[‡]

[*]MD, Orthopaedic and Hand Surgeon, Northwest Orthopaedic Specialists, P.S., Spokane, WA
[†]MD, Director and Chairman, Norman S. and Elizabeth C. A. Hill Professor of Orthopaedic Surgery, Department of Orthopaedic Surgery, University of Cincinnati College of Medicine, University of Cincinnati, Cincinnati, OH
[‡]MSPT, Medical College of Virginia/Virginia Commonwealth, Physical Therapy; Staff Physical Therapist, Bethesda Hand Rehabilitation, Cincinnati, OH

## Introduction

- Rheumatoid arthritis (RA) is a chronic, inflammatory, systemic disease that produces its most prominent manifestations in diarthrodial joints.
- It affects approximately 1% of the population, with women affected 2.5 times more often than men.
- It invariably has a progressive course ranging from mild and self-limiting to rapidly progressive with multisystem involvement and significant morbidity and mortality.
- The age of onset usually is between 40 and 70 years. The incidence increases with advancing age.
- It can affect any diarthrodial joint. In the hand and wrist, the radiocarpal, metacarpophalangeal (MCP), and proximal interphalangeal (PIP) joints are commonly affected.[1]

## Diagnostic Tests

- Clinical features of RA vary greatly among patients.
- No laboratory test, histologic finding, or radiographic feature is diagnostic of RA.
- The most common complaints are symmetric peripheral joint pain, stiffness, and swelling. Other clinical features of RA are listed in Table 25–1.[1,2]

### Table 25–1: Clinical Features of RA

**Symptoms**
- Joint swelling
- Pain/stiffness (commonly in the morning and lasting > 1 hour)
- Weakness
- Deformity
- Fatigue
- Malaise
- Fever
- Weight loss
- Depression

**Articular characteristics**
- Palpation tenderness
- Synovial thickening
- Effusion (early)
- Erythema (early)
- Decreased range of motion (later)
- Ankylosis (later)
- Subluxation (later)

**Distribution**
- Symmetrical
- Distal more common than proximal: hand > elbow > shoulder
- PIP, MCP, wrist, and ankle > elbow, knee, shoulder, and hip

Lee DM, Weinblatt ME: Rheumatoid arthritis. *Lancet* 358:903–911, 2001.

- Early diagnosis is important, because it permits early, aggressive medical intervention, which can be more effective in limiting the effects of the disease.[3]
- If diagnosis is delayed until skeletal deformity has developed, the damage to the articular surfaces is irreversible.
- Histologic studies of synovium from asymptomatic patients have shown active synovitis. Therefore, clinical evaluation alone has a poor correlation with predicting disease progression. Laboratory studies may be a better reflection of the disease activity.[1]
- Diagnostic studies near the onset of disease focus on laboratory studies. Radiographs historically have been more useful with more advanced disease. Radiographic evidence of erosions may not appear for several months to more than 1 year after onset of the disease. However, radiographic evidence of disease is present in 70% of patients within the first 2 years. Serologic studies typically become positive within the first few months.[1]
- Magnetic resonance imaging and ultrasound are sensitive to detecting disease earlier. These modalities can identify synovial hypertrophy, bone edema, and erosive changes as early as 4 months after disease onset.[1]

## Laboratory Studies

- No single test can determine RA. Following an accurate history and physical examination, selective use of rheumatologic laboratory studies may help confirm the diagnosis. Indiscriminate testing increases false-positive rates.[4]
  - Erythrocyte sedimentation rate (ESR)
    - Nonspecific indicator of the presence or absence of inflammation.
    - Resolution of an elevated ESR indicates successful treatment in RA.
    - A very high ESR (>100 mm/hr) almost always is associated with pathology.
  - C-reactive protein
    - Nonspecific indicator of presence or absence of inflammation
    - Produced by the liver in response to interleukin (IL)-1 and IL-6
    - Falls rapidly once stimulus is removed
    - Lower false-positive rate than ESR
  - Rheumatoid factor (RF)
    - RF is present in 70% to 90% of patients with RA.
    - RF can be seen in patients without RA. Up to 75% of positive results are false-positive results.
    - Elevated RF levels may be seen in other rheumatologic diseases, chronic infections, pulmonary fibrosis, cirrhosis, and sarcoidosis.
    - RF may take several months to become present.
    - High levels of RF are poor prognostic indicators.
  - Complete blood count with differential
    - Leukocytosis with a normal differential, thrombocytosis, and slight anemia may occur.
  - Antinuclear antibodies
    - Negative in RA
  - $\alpha_2$-globulins and $\alpha_1$-globulins
    - Elevated in RA
  - Serum complement
    - Normal or slightly elevated in RA
  - Arthrocentesis: 5000 to 25,000 leukocytes/mm$^2$ with 85% polymorphonuclear leukocytes
  - Other tests to consider alternative diagnoses include anticardiolipin antibodies, lupus anticoagulant, HLA-B27, uric acid, and Lyme titer.[2,4]

## Pathophysiology

### Genetic

- Etiology of RA is unknown.
- Genetic factors account for 60% of a population's predisposition to develop RA.[1]

### Histology

- The synovium shows angiogenesis, hyperplasia, and leukocyte infiltration.
- The angiogenesis creates an increased number of blood vessels but also changes their characteristics to facilitate transit of leukocytes.
- The synovium normally is created of two cell types: type A (macrophage-like) and type B (fibroblast-like). Hyperplasia increases the number of these cells to create synovial lining of 10 or more cells deep.
- Influx of inflammatory cells includes T cells, B cells, macrophages, and plasma cells.
- Pannus is characteristic of RA. It is a locally aggressive synovial tissue that invades cartilage with its population of mononuclear cells and fibroblasts releasing metalloproteases.
- T cells appear to play an integral role. They account for a part of the mononuclear infiltrate in the synovium and are organized into aggregates similar to those in lymph nodes. There appears to be an abnormality in antigen presentation to the T cells.
- Cytokines are soluble proteins that mediate intercellular interaction affecting immune cell division, differentiation, and chemotaxis. Tumor necrosis factor (TNF)-$\alpha$ and IL-1 are present in large quantities in RA synovium. Both affect synovial cell proliferation, metalloproteinase expression, secretion of other cytokines, and prostaglandin production. In vitro and animal studies have shown that these cytokines produce arthritis. Antibodies to these cytokines have halted the arthritis process in animal models.[1,3,5]

# Medical Management

- Strategy for medical management, and the medications used have changed dramatically in the past decade.
- The previous strategy involved a pyramid therapy approach. This therapy involved initially conservative interventions with nonsteroidal antiinflammatory drugs (NSAIDs) over several years. Disease-modifying antirheumatic drugs (DMARDs) were withheld until clear erosions had occurred.
- The new strategy is one of early and aggressive use of DMARDs. This changed because of studies showing the failure of the previous strategy and increased awareness of the systemic effects of RA and its effect on a patient's quality of life, productivity, and life expectancy.
- Medications are divided into four classes: glucocorticoids, NSAIDs, DMARDs, and analgesics.
- NSAIDs and glucocorticoids are used for their antiinflammatory and analgesic effects. In some patients, these agents adequately suppress symptoms. The side effects of NSAIDs and glucocorticoids have been well described. Limiting these side effects with the use of cyclooxygenase-2 selective inhibitors and limiting the total dose of glucocorticoids have been beneficial.
- DMARDs, by definition, are medications that modify the progression of RA.
- Numerous DMARDs are available (Table 25–2).
- Methotrexate is frequently prescribed for initial treatment in patients with moderate to severe disease. The toxicity appears to be dose related. New medications include leflunomide, etanercept, and infliximab.
- Leflunomide inhibits pyrimidine synthesis and may effect T-cell activation. It has been slightly better than methotrexate in clinical studies and has improved the function and quality of life in the patients tested.
- Etanercept and infliximab act by inhibiting TNF-α. These medications have been highly effective in patients who have not responded to other DMARDs. The effects on disease often are dramatic. The current drawbacks include the need for subcutaneous and intravenous administration, high cost, and concerns over increased susceptibility to infections.
- These new DMARDs give hope to future development of medications that can target the pathophysiology of RA as our understanding of RA increases.[3,5]

# Wrist: Distal Radioulnar Joint Arthritis

## Clinically Relevant Anatomy

- The distal radioulnar joint (DRUJ) is inherently unstable.
- Osseous constraint is limited, with the radius of curvature of the sigmoid notch larger than the radius of curvature of the distal ulna. This position allows approximately 150 degrees of rotation and translation. The ulnar head translates dorsally with pronation and palmarly with supination.
- Stability is conferred by extrinsic soft tissues and the triangular fibrocartilage complex (TFCC).
- The extrinsic stabilizers consist of the extensor carpi ulnaris (ECU) and its subsheath, the pronator quadratus, the interosseous membrane, the dorsal carpal ligament complex, and flexor carpi ulnaris (FCU).
- The TFCC consists of the articular disc or triangular fibrocartilage, the meniscus homologue, the dorsal and volar distal radioulnar ligaments, the ulnocarpal ligaments (volar ulnolunate and ulnotriquetral), and the sheath of the ECU tendon.
- Most strength of the TFCC comes from the dorsal and palmar distal radioulnar ligaments.
- The ulnocarpal ligaments are important in resisting the dorsal subluxation of the ulnar head.
- Rheumatoid synovitis focuses in three main areas of the DRUJ: prestyloid recess, sacciform recess, and along the ECU sheath. Synovitis is most aggressive at the ligament attachments.
- Loss of ligament integrity leads to dorsal subluxation of the ulnar head, carpal supination, ulnar translocation of the carpus, and increased radial deviation of the wrist.[6,7]

## Physical Examination

- Early clinical findings include pain and swelling at the DRUJ and pain at the extremes of forearm rotation.
- Later clinical findings include those described as the *caput ulnae syndrome* when dorsal subluxation of the ulnar head and carpal supination have occurred:
  - Weakness of the hand and wrist
  - Painful range of motion
  - Dorsal displacement of the distal ulna
  - Crepitance of the DRUJ articulation
  - Bulging synovium along the ECU and long extensor tendons

| Table 25–2: | Disease Modifying Anti-Rheumatic Drugs (DMARDS) |
| --- | --- |

- Methotrexate
- Leflunomide
- Sulfasalazine
- Cyclosporine
- Azathioprine
- Gold sodium malate
- D-penicillamine
- Hydroxychloroquine
- Minocycline
- Etanercept
- Infliximab

Pisetsky DS, St. Clair EW: Progress in the treatment of rheumatoid arthritis. *JAMA* 286:2787–2790, 2001.

- The "piano key sign" is passive dorsal subluxation of the ulnar head following removal of pressure from manual reduction.[6,7]
- The caput ulnae syndrome may lead to rupture of the ulnar finger digital extensor tendons, which is known as *Vaughan-Jackson syndrome.*

## Radiographic Examination

- Biplanar radiographs early on may show diffuse osteopenia and soft tissue swelling.
- Intermediate findings may include marginal erosions that usually begin at the distal scaphoid and ulnar styloid. These erosions may progress to the proximal DRUJ and ECU subsheath regions. Splaying of the DRUJ secondary to synovitis may occur.
- "Scallop sign" is pressure erosions at the sigmoid notch and indicates impending extensor tendon rupture.
- The lateral view should be assessed for radioulnar subluxation. A true lateral view should place the anterior cortex of the pisiform midway between the scaphoid tuberosity and the anterior cortex of the capitate.
- Erosions at the ulnar aspect of the distal radius should be identified if surgical intervention is planned. This may predispose the carpus to ulnar translation if the distal end of the ulna is resected.
- Ulnocarpal translocation should be identified as a relative contraindication to distal ulna resection without preceding radiocarpal arthrodesis. Ulnocarpal translocation is defined at greater than 50% of the lunate ulnar to the edge of the distal radius (Figure 25–1).[6,7]

## Nonoperative Management

- Nonoperative management is based on medical management, hand therapy, and injection.
- Hand therapy has a comprehensive approach including education, instructions on maintaining joint protection, functional assessment, exercise, activity modification, and splinting.
- Several hand therapy philosophies can be applied to nonoperative treatment of the rheumatoid hand.
  - Exercises should be administered in a pain-free range to prevent overstretching of the joint structures that often are distended by the inflammatory process. The key to a successful exercise program for RA necessitates the establishment of boundaries to prevent painful exercise.
  - Rest is often a neglected entity but should be considered as an adjunct measure to ensure a balanced program.
  - Fundamental exercises include active range of motion of the elbow, wrist, and shoulder. Hand exercises include gentle flexion and extension of digits and thumb opposition. To prevent proximal joint stiffness, the supine position is beneficial in executing shoulder and elbow exercises.

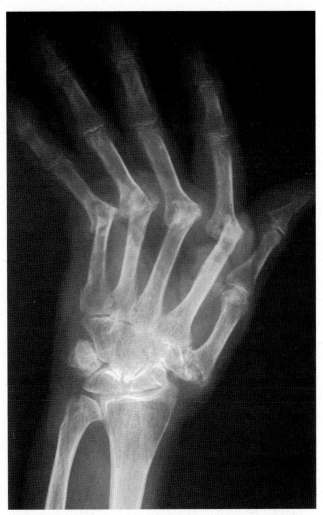

Figure 25–1:

**Radiograph showing distal radioulnar joint arthritis, ulnar translocation of the carpus, radial deviation of the metacarpals, and ulnar deviation and subluxation of the proximal phalanx.**

- Extreme caution and prudent therapy skills dictate the integration of a strengthening program for the RA patient. Therapy exercises should never create deforming forces and joint stability should never be sacrificed in attempts to gain strength. For example, grip strengthening places digits in a position with a strong propensity to increase ulnar deviation. If grip-strengthening activities are used, the MCP joints must be correctly splinted to neutralize the forces and end range flexion may be eliminated.
- Splinting the wrist in neutral may decrease inflammation and compensate for attenuated ligaments.
- Steroid injections may be helpful. However, delivery may be incomplete in distribution and may lead to extensor tendon ruptures.[6,7]

## Operative Management

- Indications for operative intervention in the DRUJ include pain relief, restoration of function (particularly forearm rotation), prevention of further damage, and cosmesis.

## Synovectomy

- Synovectomy in isolation or in concert with other procedures is rarely indicated.
- Operative management depends on the dysfunction and the extent of bony erosions that have occurred. Synovectomy may be indicated in the presence of limited bony involvement and a stable DRUJ.

## Darrach and Sauve-Kapandji Procedures

- These procedures eliminate the DRUJ articulation, increase forearm rotation, and minimize a cause of tendon rupture.
- The Darrach procedure involves resection of the distal aspect of the ulna.
- The Sauve-Kapandji procedure involves fusion of the DRUJ and resection of a segment of ulna proximal to this fusion, creating a pseudoarthrosis.
- Indications for either procedure include pain, limitation of motion, subluxation or dislocation, and extensor tendon synovitis or rupture.
- The Sauve-Kapandji procedure may be more indicated in the setting of ulnocarpal translocation or in the presence of increased radial inclination to offer greater ulnar-sided support to the carpus. However, ligamentous insufficiency in RA is more likely a cause of ulnar translocation and not an inadequate ulnar buttress. In such instances, a radiolunate fusion more likely will be effective as discussed in the section entitled Wrist: Radiocarpal Arthitis.
- Expected outcomes for the Darrach procedure have been reported as 60% to 95% pain relief and less than 10% incidence of recurrence of DRUJ synovitis or distal stump instability.
- Another variation of distal ulnar resection is the hemiresection interposition arthroplasty (HIT). This procedure involves resection of only the articular portion the ulnar head. It preserves the ulnar attachment of the TFCC and includes insertion of a soft tissue interposition (anchovy) at the site of resection. This allows preservation of the distal radioulnar relationship while removing the pathologic articular surface of the distal ulna. This procedure relies on an intact TFCC, which is commonly injured in advanced RA, and therefore may be contraindicated in many patients (Figure 25–2).[6]

## Operative Techniques

- The patient should receive general or regional anesthesia for all these procedures.

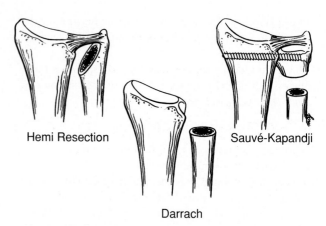

Figure 25–2:
**Surgical interventions on the distal radioulnar joint: hemiresection arthroplasty, Darrach procedure, and Sauve-Kapandji procedure.**

## Darrach Procedure

- *Approach:* Two approaches have been commonly used.
  1. Midlateral approach: Incision carried through the ECU/FCU interval.
  2. Dorsal approach: Incision carried between the fourth and fifth dorsal compartments.
  - *Warning:* The structure at risk during either approach is the dorsal sensory branch of the ulnar nerve. Adequate subcutaneous dissection should be carried out in either approach to visualize and protect this structure.
- *Bone resection:* Recommendations have varied between 1 to 4 cm. However, because instability of the ulnar stump can be a difficult complication, we recommend resection of the ulna just proximal to the ulna articular surface. This leaves the pronator quadratus attached to the ulna. The osteotomy should be performed with a power saw for best control. The cut should be made to prevent irritation to the surrounding soft tissues. Dingman et al. have shown that there is no difference in outcome between subperiosteal or extraperiosteal resection, transverse or oblique osteotomy, or removal or retention of the ulnar styloid.[8] A synovectomy of the DRUJ should be performed prior to closure (Figure 25–3).
- *Closure:* The capsule should be imbricated with the forearm held in supination to reduce distal ulna instability postoperatively.
- *Immobilization:* Well-padded sugar tong splint with forearm supinated.
- *Rehabilitation:* Follow-up at weeks 1, 3, and 6.
- *Therapy:*
  - 10–14 days: Wound and edema management. Fabrication of Muenster splint with forearm supinated.
  - 3 weeks: Fabrication of wrist immobilization splint with the wrist positioned in 15 degrees extension.

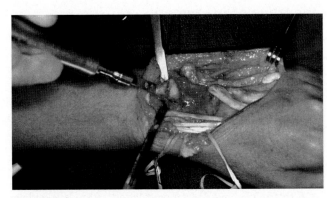

Figure 25–3:
**Intraoperative photograph of the patient shown in Figure 25–1 showing the attritional ruptures of the extensor tendons and a Darrach procedure being performed.**

Edema and scar management. Initiate active and active-assisted exercises to include wrist flexion and extension and forearm rotation.
- 6 weeks: Discontinue splint and initiate gentle strengthening.

## Sauve-Kapandji Procedure

- *Approach:* Dissection is carried through the fifth/sixth dorsal compartment interval and through the DRUJ capsule, taking care to remain proximal to the TFCC. The ulnar head and proximal shaft are exposed subperiosteally.
- *Bone resection:* Articular surfaces of the ulnar head and sigmoid notch are denuded of cartilage to create an opposable bed of cancellous bone. Once this is completed, 10- to 14-mm of ulna is resected just proximal to the DRUJ. Bone from this resection can be used to augment the arthrodesis.
- *Fixation:* Fixation is placed from the ulnar head into the radius. A subcutaneous approach to the ulnar head is created with a small incision between the ECU/FCU. Care must be taken to protect the dorsal branch of the ulnar nerve. A neutral ulnar variance should be confirmed prior to placement of fixation. Fixation may be achieved with Kirschner wires or screws. We prefer two cannulated 3-mm lag screws.
- *Closure:* The periosteum of the ulna and DRUJ capsule. Skin incisions are sutured.
- *Immobilization:* Well-padded sugar tong splint with forearm in neutral to slight supination.
- *Rehabilitation:* Follow-up at weeks 1, 3, 6, and 12.
- *Therapy:*
  - 10–14 days: Wound and edema management. Fabrication of Muenster splint with forearm positioned in neutral.
  - 3 weeks: Scar and edema management. Active and passive range of motion exercises to digits and shoulder.
  - 6 weeks: Active and active-assisted exercises initiated to the wrist and forearm.

- 8 weeks: Passive range of motion exercises and discontinuation of the splint can be initiated once the fusion is confirmed. Gentle progressive strengthening to the hand, wrist, forearm, and elbow.
- 10 weeks: Gentle dynamic splinting can be initiated to the wrist and forearm if necessary.

## Hemiresection Interposition Arthroplasty

- *Approach:* Between the fifth and sixth dorsal compartments. Retinacular and capsular flaps are created upon opening the DRUJ for reconstruction at closure. Care is taken to protect the TFCC.
- *Bone resection:* An oblique osteotome is created from the proximal aspect of the ulnar head articular surface to point radial to the ulnar prestyloid recess so as not to detach the TFCC. The arm should be rotated to confirm that no radioulnar impingement occurs. The defect is filled with an "anchovy" created from the palmaris longus or from a segment of the ECU or FCU.
- *Closure:* The capsule and retinacular flaps should be imbricated as needed to achieve reduction of any dorsal subluxation of the ulnar head.
- *Immobilization:* Well-padded sugar tong splint.
- *Rehabilitation:* Follow-up at weeks 1, 3, and 6.
- *Therapy:*
  - 10–14 days: Wound and edema management. Fabrication of a wrist immobilization splint. Active and gentle passive exercises initiated to wrist and forearm.
  - 3 weeks: Scar and edema management. Upgrade exercise program.
  - 6 weeks: Discontinue splint and initiate progressive strengthening if excessive pain is not present.

# Wrist: Radiocarpal Arthritis

## Clinically Relevant Anatomy

- The radiocarpal and midcarpal articulations are complex and rely on balanced coordination for normal function.
- This coordination occurs through the unique anatomy of each carpal bone, the numerous extrinsic and intrinsic ligaments, and the forces passing through these joints.
- Initial changes in the radiocarpal articulations occur with synovitis and subsequent development of cartilage degeneration, periarticular erosions, and osseous destruction.
- Ligamentous support may be disrupted by attenuation from synovitis or by destruction of their ligamentous attachments to bone.
- Forces crossing the wrist joints are altered with loss of carpal height, ankylosis of surrounding joints, or deviation

of forces from abnormalities in neighboring joints, or loss of force from tendon ruptures.

- The most common pathologic changes in the radiocarpal joint include volar subluxation and carpal supination, ulnar translocation, and scapholunate disruption (see Figure 25–1).
- Deformities at the wrist also have effects on the proximal and distal joints. Carpal volar subluxation and supination lead to caput ulnae syndrome as previously described. Ulnar translocation leads to radial deviation of the metacarpals, ulnar deviation forces at the MCP joints, and swan-neck deformities of the interphalangeal joints.[9]

## Physical Examination

- Inspection of the wrist position reveals most deformities and functional difficulties. Prominence of the ulnar head, circumferential "thickening" of the wrist, radial deviation of the metacarpals, ulnar deviation of the digits, and extensor lag of the ulnar digits all may occur.
- Synovitis of the radiocarpal joint and tenosynovitis of the extensor tendons may be differentiated by several clinical features (Table 25–3).
- A provocative maneuver to assess for volar subluxation and supination of the carpus is placement of dorsally directed pressure on the pisiform to reduce the carpus. Removal of this pressure is followed by immediate subluxation.[9]

## Radiologic Examination

- Posteroanterior and lateral radiographs of the wrist help evaluate for erosions, loss of carpal height, ulnar translocation, integrity of the scapholunate ligament, and subluxation of the radiocarpal joint.[9]

## Nonoperative Management

- Nonoperative management is based on medical management, hand therapy, injections, and splinting.
- Hand therapy has a comprehensive approach that includes education, exercise, activity modification, and splinting.
- Splinting the wrist in neutral may decrease inflammation and compensate for attenuated ligaments. This may help control symptoms and improve function.
- Steroid injections may produce symptomatic relief.[9]

---

### Table 25–3: Clinical Features of Synovitis

**Radiocarpal Synovitis**
- Fusiform swelling with radial and ulnar extension
- Difficult to palpate the boundaries of the swelling
- No motion of the swelling with finger flexion and extension
- Pain with motion, especially at the extremes of passive flexion and extension

**Extensor Tenosynovitis**
- Localized dorsal swelling, occasionally with dumb-bell shape with extension on the proximal and distal aspects of the extensor retinaculum
- Often able to palpate the boundaries of the swelling
- Motion of the swelling with finger flexion and extension

---

## Operative Management

- The choice of operative intervention in the rheumatoid wrist depends on several factors. The primary goals are pain relief, restoration of function, prevention of further damage, and cosmesis. The choice must be made in concert with the patient's goals.
- The options for intervention depend on the stage of disease progression. During the early phase, synovectomy may be appropriate and may dramatically decrease the risk of tendon rupture. However, as articular and skeletal destruction advances, synovectomy alone is inappropriate. With articular and skeletal destruction, arthrodesis (either limited or total) or replacement arthroplasty may be considered.[9]

### Synovectomy

- *Indications:*
  - Persistent synovitis despite at least 6 months of adequate medical management
  - Persistent pain and carpal tenderness
  - Evidence of synovitis at the time of extensor tendon repairs or transfers
  - Evidence of synovitis at the time of limited carpal arthrodesis
  - Larsen radiographic rating of 0 to II[9]
- *Approach:* A dorsal longitudinal skin incision just ulnar to Lister's tubercle is developed. Care must be taken to avoid branches of the superficial radial and ulnar nerves. Full-thickness skin flaps are elevated down to the extensor retinaculum. We prefer to incise the retinaculum over the fourth compartment. Radial and ulnar base flaps expose the second through sixth compartments. This permits extensor tendons synovectomy. The subretinacular layer is incised radially and raised subperiosteally to expose the joint capsule. Capsulotomy can be performed in several ways. Often the capsulotomy is an inverted T. The cross of the T is at the level of the distal radius. Another common approach is through a distal based U-shaped incision.
- Synovium is removed with a rongeur from both the radiocarpal and midcarpal joints.
- *Arthroscopic synovectomy:* This has the advantage of limiting surgical dissection and therefore accelerating rehabilitation. However, associated pathology such as extensor tendon synovitis cannot be treated.
- *Closure:* The retinaculum should be closed deep to the extensor tendons to limit exposure to possible attritional ruptures.
- *Immobilization:* Well-padded short arm splint is applied with the wrist in 20 to 30 degrees extension.
- *Rehabilitation:* Follow-up at weeks 1, 3, and 6.
- *Therapy:*
  - 1 week: Wound and edema management. Fabrication of wrist support splint. Gentle active range of motion exercises of the wrist and digits.

- 2–3 weeks: Wound, scar, and edema management. Advancement of exercise program coupled with gradual weaning of the splint.
- 6 weeks: Wrist splint should be discontinued, with return to normal daily activities using the wrist.

## Limited Radiocarpal Arthrodesis

- The limited radiocarpal arthrodeses most useful in the rheumatoid wrist are the radiolunate and radioscapholunate.
- These procedures were designed to remove painful articulations, prevent or correct ulnar translocation, and preserve some range of motion.
- Postoperative motion averages 30 degrees flexion and 30 degrees extension for a radiolunate arthrodesis, with less following a radioscapholunate arthrodesis.
- *Indications and considerations:*
  - Clinically symptomatic wrist with local carpal tenderness.
  - Larsen grade 0 to IV at the radiocarpal joint and preservation of the midcarpal joint.
  - Ulnar translocation of the carpus.
  - Can be performed at the time of tenosynovectomy, tendon repair or transfers, or MCP arthroplasties.
  - The scaphoid can be added into the fusion if more extensive radiocarpal destruction has occurred, with the understanding that this method leads to greater motion loss.[9]
- *Approach:* See synovectomy approach.
- *Arthrodesis:* The carpus is relocated onto the distal radius to confirm congruous surfaces for the radiocarpal arthrodesis. Under distraction, the midcarpal joint should be inspected to confirm adequate articular cartilage. Once both of these have been achieved, the articular surfaces of the distal radius and lunate are denuded of articular cartilage.
- *Fixation:* The lunate can be held to the distal radius with numerous devices, including staples, Kirschner wires, and fully threaded headless screws. Headless screws have the advantage of being low profile and providing rigid fixation and compression at the arthrodesis site. However, the poor bone quality seen in rheumatoids may necessitate use of the other devices (Figure 25–4).
- *Closure:* See synovectomy closure.
- *Immobilization:* The wrist is placed in a short arm splint.
- *Rehabilitation:* Follow-up at weeks 1, 3, 6, and 12.
- *Therapy:*
  - 10–14 days: Wound and edema management. Fabrication of a wrist support splint. Active and passive range of motion exercises to digits. Emphasis is placed on composite flexion and full extension exercises, including isolated extensor digitorum communis (EDC) exercises.
  - 3 weeks: Scar and edema management.

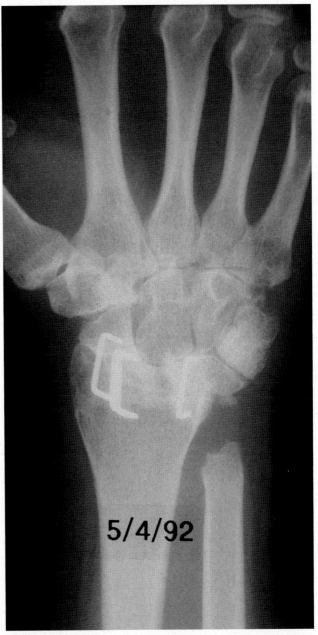

5/4/92

Figure 25–4:
**Radiograph showing a patient after a radioscapholunate fusion and Darrach resection of the distal ulna.**

- 6–8 weeks: Active wrist exercises can commence if radiographs dictate.
- 10 weeks: Active-assisted and gentle passive range of motion exercises initiated to wrist. Gradually wean from splint.
- 12–14 weeks: Gentle strengthening initiated to hand, wrist, and proximal upper extremity.

## Total Wrist Arthrodesis

- This is a reliable procedure that achieves stability and pain relief at the sacrifice of wrist motion.

- Two techniques can be used to achieve arthrodesis. One is the use of rods from the third metacarpal or second and/ or third web space into the distal radius. The other is a dorsal plate and screw construct from the metacarpal to the distal radius.
- Rod fixation must be supplemented with a derotational fixation: a second rod, radiocarpal staples, or a dorsal tension band wire.
- Plate and screw fixation achieves a rigid construct with more extension and greater compression at the arthrodesis site. This decreases the need for postoperative casting and improves grip strength once fusion is achieved. Disadvantages include more soft tissue dissection, the possibility of extensor tendon irritation, and the necessity for plate removal. These constructs also depend on the pullout strength of the screws for fixation. The poor bone quality seen in RA may be insufficient to permit screw and plate fixation.
- *Indications:*
  - Severe instability of the radiocarpal joint
  - Severe articular destruction of the radiocarpal and midcarpal joints
  - Bilateral disease in which the contralateral wrist will be able to retain motion
  - Salvage of a failed previous surgical intervention, including limited arthrodesis or total wrist arthroplasty and/or history of sepsis
  - Anticipated necessity of upper extremities for weight bearing
- *Contraindications:*
  - Lack of adequate soft tissue coverage or tenuous dorsal skin
  - Presence of active infection[10]
- *Approach:* A dorsal approach is used for either method. The skin incision is begun distally between the second and third metacarpals and continued proximally over Lister's tubercle for an additional 2 to 3 cm. The third dorsal compartment is opened. The subretinacular and capsular incision can be carried down to bone along the ulnar aspect of the extensor carpi radialis brevis. The radiocarpal joint can be seen through this incision.
- *Plate fixation:* The skin incision may need to be extended from the distal aspect of the third metacarpal to the outcroppers (abductor pollicis longus and extensor pollicis brevis) to facilitate placement of the plate and screws. The dorsal aspect of the third metacarpal can be exposed with minimal disturbance of the interosseous muscles. With the fourth compartment reflected ulnarly, the dorsal aspect of the radius should be sufficiently exposed for placement of the plate. The remaining cartilage should be denuded at the radiocarpal, midcarpal, carpometacarpal, and all intercarpal joints. We excise the triquetrum and use it for bone graft. The plate most commonly used is the Synthes precontoured wrist fusion

plate. This plate is custom made for wrist arthrodesis, with 2.7-mm screws distally over the metacarpal and 3.5-mm screws proximally over the radius (see Figure 24–11). Placement should be directly dorsal on the radius and metacarpal to prevent rotation. The position of the wrist and the plate should be confirmed by fluoroscopic and gross evaluation prior to screw placement, following a single screw in the proximal and distal aspects, and after final screw placement.
- If Steinmann rod fixation is used, a separate incision will be necessary over the head of the third metacarpal with dissection down to its articular surface. The articular surface is accessed by longitudinally splitting the extensor tendon. Preoperatively, the metacarpal medullary canal should be determined to be of sufficient diameter to accept a large enough rod to provide adequate fixation in the radius. If the medullary canal is prohibitively small, the rod may need to be placed in the second or third web space. However, this placement is at a cost of less rigid fixation. The surfaces to be fused are denuded of articular cartilage. Serially larger Steinmann pins are passed from the metacarpal head into the radius with the wrist held in a reduced position with acceptable coronal angulation. A second pin is used as a tamp to advance the pin sufficiently into the metacarpal so that a future MCP implant can be placed. At the radiocarpal joint, additional fixation should be added to achieve rotational stability. Staples, Kirschner wires, or tension band wires can be used. A tension band can be created by placing a transverse drill hole in the distal radius metaphyseal region, sufficiently deep to the dorsal cortex to prevent the wire from cutting out. A 22-gauge stainless steel wire is passed through this drill hole and around the base of the third metacarpal in a figure-eight pattern. The figure-eight construct then is tightened (Figure 25–5).
- A Darrach procedure usually is done concomitantly.
- *Closure:* The dorsal apparatus must be securely repaired with a nonabsorbable suture. The dorsal wound should have as much capsule and retinaculum closed over the hardware as possible. A drain may be necessary.
- *Immobilization:* Well-padded short arm splint with several days of extremity elevation.
- *Rehabilitation:* Follow-up at weeks 1, 3, 6, and 12.
- *Therapy:*
  - 10–14 days: Wound and edema management. Fabrication of a short arm cast or wrist immobilization splint (clamshell design). Active and passive range of motion exercises are initiated to thumb, digits, forearm, elbow, and shoulder. Isolate extensor indicis proprius, EDC, and extensor pollicis longus (EPL) to prevent dorsal tendon adherence.
  - 3 weeks: Scar and edema management. Emphasis on composite flexion and isolated tendon gliding exercises.

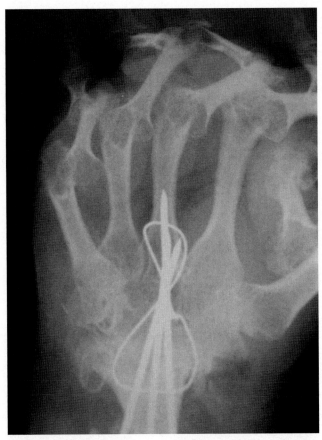

**Figure 25–5:**
**Postoperative radiograph following tension band arthrodesis of the wrist.**

- 6 weeks: With limited passive flexion of digits, composite taping or dynamic flexion splinting of digits may be necessary.
- 8–10 weeks: Progressive strengthening for shoulder and elbow with wrist splint support. A work-conditioning program is recommended for patients returning to the work force. Resistance to supination and pronation should be delayed until 10 to 12 weeks to avoid torsional load to fusion site.
- 12–14 weeks: The wrist support splint can be discontinued if radiographs demonstrate consolidation of the fusion site.

## Total Wrist Arthroplasty

- *Indications:* The ideal candidate is a low-demand patient having bilateral wrist arthritis with relatively good stability and bone stock but who is not a candidate for a less aggressive procedure. This procedure removes the painful articulation, restores carpal height to improve grip strength, and preserves mobility.[11]
- *Designs:* Several designs are available. The limitations on wrist arthroplasty designs are similar to those in other joints. The amount of constraint built into the design seems to be the predictor of the mode of failure. Highly

constrained designs lead to loosening at the bone–implant interface and minimally constrained designs may lead to instability and dislocation. The more current designs seem to have improved performance over the earlier implants. These designs include the biaxial total wrist arthroplasty from Beckenbaugh[12] and the universal total wrist implant from Menon.[13] Both implants have a metal-polyethylene articulation with a transverse oriented axis. The fixation of these implants differ, especially distally. The biaxial design has a porous coated stem that is cemented into the capitate and third metacarpal, producing greater fixation than its predecessors. The universal total wrist arthroplasty added screw fixation on the radial and ulnar aspect of the stem. The addition of these screws appears to have increased the stability of the distal implant.

- *Approach:* Longitudinal skin incision in the midline of the dorsal wrist. The third compartment is opened and the EPL retracted. The distal ulna is approached through the fifth dorsal compartment. Subperiosteally, the distal ulna is circumferentially exposed and resected just proximal to the DRUJ. The approach to the wrist joint is continued through the third dorsal compartment with elevation of the fourth dorsal compartment ulnarly. A T-shaped capsulotomy is performed so that the entire carpus and distal radius are visualized.
- *Bone cuts:* The distal radius articular surface is resected perpendicular to its coronal and sagittal axes. The proximal carpal row is resected and the distal carpal row is fashioned to accept the implant.
- *Implantation:*
  - The medullary canal of the third metacarpal is located with an awl and fluoroscopic confirmation. Great care must be taken to not perforate the third metacarpal shaft.
  - The medullary canal is reamed to a size adequate to accept the distal stem.
  - The distal carpus must be prepared to accept the curvature of the distal implant. This can be prepared by the reamer provided with the set or by manual contouring.
  - The distal trial implant is placed to confirm position and fit.
  - The medullary canal of the distal radius is located with an awl.
  - The radius is sequentially rasped to accept the proximal stem.
  - The proximal trial component is placed to confirm position and fit.
  - Cement fixation is used at the surgeon's discretion (Figures 25–6 and 25–7).
- *Closure:* The wound is closed, with the capsule and retinaculum approximated as tension allows. The skin is closed with staples or sutures. A drain is placed depending on hemostasis at the end of the procedure.
- *Immobilization:* Well-padded short arm splint.

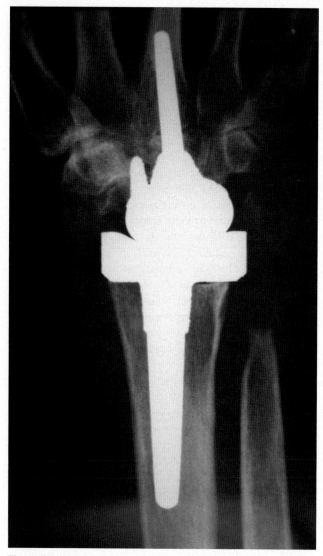

Figure 25–6:
Postoperative posteroanterior radiograph following total wrist arthroplasty.

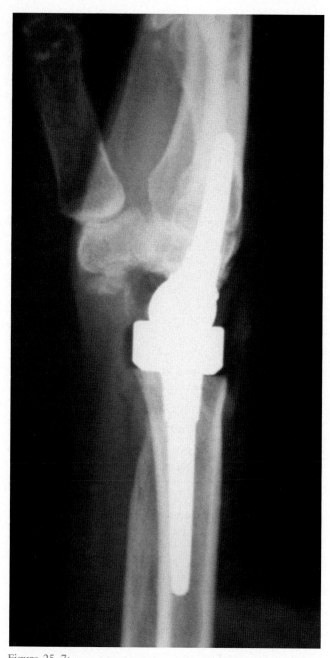

Figure 25–7:
Postoperative lateral radiograph following total wrist arthroplasty.

- *Therapy:*
  - 10–14 days: Wound and edema management. Fabrication of wrist immobilization splint (clamshell design). Active and passive range of motion exercises initiated to digits. Emphasis is placed on composite flexion and extension, including isolated EDC exercises.
  - 3–4 weeks: Scar and edema management. Confirm reestablishment of digital motion. Gentle active motion initiated to wrist.
  - 6 weeks: Discontinuation of wrist immobilization splint. Active-assisted and gentle passive range of motion exercises initiated to wrist.
  - 8 weeks: Gentle strengthening of the wrist and hand. Return to full use with daily activities. Restrictions on weight and contact activities reviewed.

# Metacarpophalangeal Arthritis
## Clinically Relevant Anatomy

- The MCP joint is a diarthrodial, condylar articulation.
- The metacarpal head is asymmetric in the sagittal, axial, and coronal planes. In the sagittal plane the condyle is volar to the midline of the shaft. In the axial plane the volar aspect of the metacarpal head is larger in diameter than the dorsal aspect. These two features produce a cam effect, placing the collateral ligaments in tension when the joint is flexed. In the coronal plane, there is slight

ulnar and proximal angulation, which may contribute to ulnar deviation deformity with advanced RA.

- There are six degrees of freedom to the MCP joint: flexion/extension, radial/ulnar deviation, and rotation. Radial and ulnar deviation occurs with the joint in extension secondary to collateral ligament stability.

- The major static stabilizers of the joint include the collateral ligaments and volar plate. The collateral ligaments course from a dorsal proximal to volar distal direction across the joint but remain dorsal to the flexion axis of rotation. This position prevents volar, radial, and ulnar subluxation. This stabilization becomes greater with increasing flexion. The volar plate passes from the volar metacarpal neck to the volar lip of the proximal phalanx. It is attached to the accessory collateral ligaments at its lateral margins. It prevents dorsal subluxation.[14,15]

- The major dynamic stabilizers of the MCP joint include the extrinsic extensor tendons, flexor tendons, and intrinsic tendons. The extensor tendons attach to the proximal phalangeal base via the sagittal bands, providing dynamic stabilization against volar subluxation. The intrinsic tendons, especially the lumbricals, pass volar to the flexion axis of rotation and therefore prevent dorsal subluxation. These become contracted with the common RA deformity of volar subluxation.[14]

- Asymmetry of the normal joint plays a role in the consistent volar and ulnar subluxation of the MCP joint with RA. These asymmetric structures include slight ulnar slope to the MCP joint, weaker radial sagittal band, and weaker radial collateral ligament.[15]

- Volar subluxation and ulnar deviation seen in RA occur for the following reasons:
  - Radial deviation of the metacarpals associated with ulnar translocation of the carpus.
  - Asymmetric anatomy of the MCP joint, which becomes accentuated with synovial attenuation of static and dynamic stabilizers.
  - Loss of extensor tendon stabilizing force because of rupture or ulnar subluxation. The tendon falls volar to the flexion axis of rotation, potentiating the volar-directed force of the flexor and intrinsic tendons and leading to volar subluxation of the joint with contracture.
  - Attenuation of the volar plate and collateral ligaments leads to volar and ulnar subluxation of the flexor tendon sheath, resulting in further volar and ulnar deforming force.
  - The intrinsic muscles (particularly on the ulnar side) undergo a structural change leading to flexion contracture and increased volar deforming force.
  - The abductor digiti minimi, which inserts on the volar-ulnar base of the small finger proximal phalanx, is responsible for the severe ulnar deviation sometimes seen in the small finger.

- The sequence of these changes is debated. They all play a role in creating the deformity, and preventing any one of these processes would not be sufficient to halt the others.

- The cartilage and periarticular bone is affected with advancing disease. This has been classified by Larsen into six stages (Table 25–4).[14,15]

## Physical Examination

- The examination of each patient with RA must be systematic and systemic. When the hand and wrist are in question, the entire upper extremity must be examined. Assessment of the shoulder, elbow, and cervical spine should precede examination of the hand and wrist.

- Examination of the wrist, as described previously, may reveal pathology about the DRUJ or radiocarpal joint, which will have a direct effect on the mechanics of the MCP joint. Pathology occurring proximal to the MCP joints must be addressed prior to intervention at the MCP joints. The integrity of the flexor and extensor tendons must always be evaluated.

- Examination of the MCP joints should include the following:
  - Inspection for synovitis, ulnar deviation, and volar subluxation of the proximal phalanx with prominent metacarpal heads and subluxed extensor tendons.
  - Measurement of active and passive range of motion (including extensor lag).
  - The presence of intrinsic tightness should be assessed with the Bunnell test, as described in the section entitled Proximal Interphalangeal Arthritis: Physical Examination. Also, determine the possibility of relocation of the joint, and extensor tendons if subluxated.[15]

## Radiographic Examination

- Evaluation should be performed with standard posteroanterior and lateral views (see Table 25–3 and Figure 25–1).

## Nonoperative Management

- Nonoperative management is based on medical management, hand therapy, injections, and splinting.

| Table 25–4: | Larsen Radiographic Classification of MCP Destruction |
|---|---|
| 0: | No changes |
| I: | Slight changes, including periarticular swelling |
| II: | Erosions apparent, mild joint narrowing |
| III: | Medium destructive changes with erosions and joint space poorly defined |
| IV: | Severe destructive changes with collapse and significant erosions |
| V: | Mutilating changes |

Wilson RL, Carlblom ER: The rheumatoid metacarpophalangeal joint. *Hand Clin* 5:223–237, 1989.

- Hand therapy has a comprehensive approach that includes education, exercise, activity modification, splinting, and assistive devices for activities of daily living.
  - Patients exhibiting early swan-neck deformity should be instructed on gentle stretching of the distal interphalangeal (DIP) and PIP joints with the digits held in the hook position to prevent intrinsic contractures (see Figure 1–25).
- Splinting the wrist in neutral may decrease inflammation and compensate for attenuated ligaments. This may help control symptoms and improve function at the MCP level.
- A static forearm based splint holding the wrist in neutral and the MCP joints in extension and slight radial deviation (using dividers) can be worn at night.
- Steroid injections may be helpful in relieving some symptoms but are ineffective in improving function once deformity has occurred.

## Operative Management

### Metacarpophalangeal Arthroplasty

- The most common arthroplasty performed in the hand and wrist for RA is at the MCP joint.
- The most commonly used implants are silicone rubber hinges.
- Metal on polyethylene and pyrolytic carbon implants have been introduced. The silicone implants are used as a spacer, whereas the newer implants resurface the joint surfaces similar to arthroplasties elsewhere in the body.
- *Indications:* In general, this procedure is indicated in patients with RA who have painful deformity with destruction or volar subluxation of the joint and fixed deformity that cannot be treated with soft tissue reconstruction.[14–16] More specific indications include the following:
  - Decreased arc of motion (<40 degrees)
  - Marked flexion contracture with the joint fixed in a poor functional position
  - MCP joint pain with radiographic deformity
  - Ulnar drift (>30 degrees)
- *Contraindications:*
  - Presence of vasculitis, poor skin condition, inadequate bone stock, or infection.

### Technique Silicone Arthroplasty

- *Approach:* A dorsal transverse incision is made at the junction of the metacarpal neck and head. Dorsal veins are preserved. The extensor mechanism is longitudinally incised through its midportion to expose the joint capsule.
  - There are variations on the incision through the extensor mechanism. Some surgeons prefer to incise through the ulnar sagittal band to release this

deforming force. Others prefer to incise through the radial sagittal band to allow for imbrication at the time of closure. The radial collateral ligament is tagged with 4-0 nonabsorbable suture for later reattachment.

- The capsule is incised longitudinally. The origin of the collateral ligaments and ulnar intrinsic tendon insertions are released to allow relocation of the proximal phalanx.
- *Bone cuts:* The metacarpal head is resected with a transverse cut through the metacarpal neck just distal to the origin of the collateral ligaments with a saw or rongeur (Figure 25–8). A synovectomy is accomplished. The medullary canal of the metacarpal is hand reamed, taking care to not remove cortical bone. A trial implant is inserted to confirm fit and a level bone cut. The articular surface of the proximal phalanx is smoothed with a rongeur. The medullary canal is identified with an awl and reamed with a rasp or burr to create a rectangular

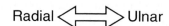

Radial ⟺ Ulnar

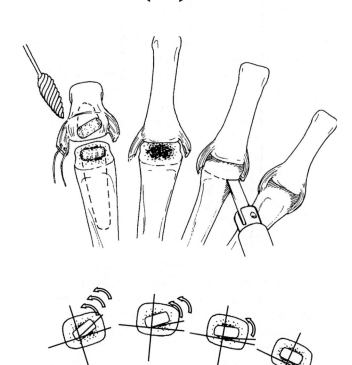

IF    MF    RF    SF

Figure 25–8:

**In the second stage of metacarpophalangeal (MCP) joint arthroplasty, the canal of the metacarpalis rearmed using a power burr. A power burr is also used to perforate the subchondral plate of the proximal phalanx. It is important to rearm the proximal phalanx of the index and middle finger with the digits in supination to prevent the pronated deformity that frequently occurs.**

opening that will accept the implant. The trial implant is again placed to confirm proper fit and stability. There should be no subluxation of the joint, and good canal fit should be seen both proximally and distally.

- With the implant selected and the bone prepared, the radial collateral ligament is reattached through drill holes placed prior to implantation. It is secured into place after implant insertion.

- *Implantation:* Because surface defects in these implants can lead to fracture, they are handled with a "no touch technique." The implant is held with smooth forceps and inserted first into the metacarpal and then into the proximal phalanx.

- *Closure:* The radial collateral ligament is repaired using the previously passed 4-0 suture. The radial sagittal band is imbricated to centralize the extensor tendon.

- *Immobilization:* Well-padded short arm resting pan splint positioning the MCP joints in extension and mild radial deviation.

- *Rehabilitation:* Follow-up at weeks 1, 2, 6, and 12.

- *Therapy:*
  - 3 days to 1 week: Wound and edema management. Fabrication of a static resting splint based on the forearm to include the fingers. The splint should include individual finger dividers encompassing radial influence and full extension for night wear. For day wear, a long dorsal outrigger (RA splint) is fabricated with alignment of rubber band traction at a 60-degree angle from the outrigger to the proximal phalanx. Both are made to limit stresses to the radial-sided repairs. Active and active-assisted range of motion exercises are initiated within the RA splint to include MP and IP flexion and extension.
  - 2 weeks: Wound, scar, and edema management. Splint adjustments for swelling reduction as needed. Assessment of range of motion. Radial walk and gentle passive exercises are initiated.
  - 6 weeks: Light prehensile activities out of the RA splint are encouraged. Assessment of alignment and range of motion.
  - 8 weeks: Discontinuation of RA splint. Dynamic flexion splinting initiated if passive MP flexion is less than 50 degrees. Dynamic flexion splinting can be initiated alone or compositely in cases of extrinsic extensor tautness. Gentle strengthening initiated.
  - 10–14 weeks: Dynamic flexion splinting discontinued. Functional assessment reevaluated.
  - 3–4 months: Static night splint discontinued.

### Resurfacing Arthroplasty

- The main difference in the design of these prostheses compared with silicone implants is that they resurface the articular surfaces, leave the collateral ligaments intact, and create a more secure bone–prosthesis interface. The interface is either cement or bone ingrowth.

- The techniques vary depending on the specific prosthesis. The technique manuals for each prosthesis should be studied prior to its use. The general differences in the technique include the following:
  - Preservation of the collateral ligament origins.
  - Bone cuts are made with the assistance of alignment guides.

# Proximal Interphalangeal Arthritis

## Clinically Relevant Anatomy

- The PIP joint is a simple diarthrodial joint with complex soft tissue balancing.

- The bicondylar proximal phalanx head has corresponding concavities in the base of the middle phalanx in both the sagittal and coronal planes. This conformity provides some joint stability.

- The static soft tissue stabilizers of the joint include the collateral ligaments, capsule, and volar plate. The collateral ligaments protect against radial and ulnar deviation and volar subluxation. The volar plate prevents dorsal subluxation and coronal instability.

- The dynamic restraints of the joint include the dorsal apparatus and the extrinsic flexor tendon. These stabilizers work not only on the PIP joint but along the chain of digit joints, including the DIP joint and MCP joint. Therefore, alteration of these stabilizers at any site has some effect on the adjacent joints.

- Dysfunction of these stabilizers is most commonly manifested as a swan-neck deformity or a boutonnière deformity. A swan-neck deformity is hyperextension of the PIP joint and flexion of the DIP joint. A boutonnière deformity is flexion at the PIP and hyperextension at the DIP. These deformities are further explained in Chapter 26.

- When a swan-neck or boutonnière deformity is associated with radiographic destruction of the PIP joint, surgical intervention with an arthrodesis or arthroplasty may be indicated.[16–18]

## Physical Examination

- A useful classification of RA swan-neck and boutonnière deformities was described by Nalebuff (Table 25–5). The four stages of swan-neck deformities and three stages of boutonnière deformi ties are defined by their physical examination and radiographic findings. This classification is useful to determine the appropriate surgical intervention.

- *Inspection:* The resting position of the hand and individual joints is observed. The status of the skin, presence of nodules, and synovial swelling should be assessed.

- *Manipulation:* Active and passive range of motion of the digit's joints should be measured.

| Table 25–5: | Nalebuff Classification of PIP Joint Deformities in RA |
|---|---|

**Swan-neck deformities**

| I. | Full flexibility of the PIP joint |
|---|---|
| II. | PIP joint flexion limited in certain positions (intrinsic tightness) |
| III. | Limited PIP joint flexion in all positions with normal articular surface |
| IV. | Limited PIP joint flexion with radiographic articular destruction |

**Boutonnière deformities**

| I. | Extensor lag 10–15 degrees |
|---|---|
| II. | Extensor lag 30–40 degrees with DIP and MCP compensation |
| III. | Flexion contracture of the PIP with radiographic articular destruction |

Millender LH, Nalebuff EA: Preventive Surgery—tenosynovectomy and synovectomy. *Orthop Clin North Am* 6:765–792, 1975.

- The Bunnell intrinsic tightness test is used in assessing swan-neck deformities. This test looks for a disparity in passive PIP joint flexion with the MCP joints extended and flexed. If intrinsic tightness is present, passive PIP joint flexion is greater when the MCP joint is flexed than when it is extended.
- The DIP joint must be assessed for mallet deformity, which may be the cause of reciprocal PIP hyperextension.
- An examination of the MCP joint as previously described is necessary to determine its effect on the PIP joint. MCP flexion contractures often are associated with swan-neck deformities. If the MCP joint is abnormal, arthroplasty of the PIP joint may be contraindicated as described in the section entitled Proximal Interphalangeal Arthritis: Operative Management.

## Radiographic Evaluation

- Biplanar radiographs of the affected PIP joints are useful to assess joint congruency, alignment, and status of the articular cartilage.
- Articular destruction of the PIP joint suggests the need for skeletal reconstruction, either arthrodesis or arthroplasty.

## Nonoperative Management

- Nonoperative management is based on medical management, hand therapy, injections, and splinting.
- Hand therapy has a comprehensive approach that includes education, exercise, activity modification, and splinting.
- Steroid injections may help symptomatic episodes.
- PIP joint extension blocking splints are used for swan-neck deformities. A figure-eight splint allows active PIP joint flexion and prevents hyperextension. It is well accepted by patients, helps decrease symptoms, and may assist in slowing progression of deformity.
- Boutonnière deformities can be treated with dynamic or nighttime static splints, which position the joint in full extension.

## Operative Management

- *Indications:* Skeletal reconstruction is indicated for patients with stage IV swan-neck deformities or stage III boutonnière deformities. Prior to the appearance of articular destruction on radiographs, soft tissue procedures are more indicated.[17]
- Surgical options include arthrodesis and arthroplasty. Arthrodesis is more commonly performed and is more reliable because of the frequent association with MCP joint disease. Concomitant arthroplasty of both PIP and MCP joints has performed poorly. In general, skeletal reconstruction in a single rheumatoid digit is most successful with arthrodesis of the PIP joint and arthroplasty of the MCP joint. In patients with PIP joint disease and unaffected MCP joints, most surgeons recommend arthrodesis of the index and middle fingers and arthroplasty of the ring and small fingers.
- PIP joint arthroplasty is indicated if the surrounding soft tissues, joints, and tendons are intact. Adequate bone stock to support the implant and intact flexor and extensor function to achieve postoperative motion must be available. Arthroplasty has not fared well with joint dislocation, contractures greater than 60 degrees, and fixed hyperextension.[18]
- Arthroplasty designs for the PIP joint are similar to those for the MCP joint. The most commonly used implant is the silicone hinged implant. Joint resurfacing implants are available with short-term follow-up.

### Arthrodesis Technique

- *Approach:* A dorsal longitudinal skin incision is made over the PIP joint. All dorsal veins and nerve branches should be preserved. The triangular ligament and central slip are incised longitudinally. The joint is exposed, and the collateral ligaments are released from their proximal phalangeal origins. Periarticular tissue is released circumferentially on both the proximal and middle phalanx.
- The articular surface is fashioned with a saw or rongeur. The base of the middle phalanx is denuded of articular cartilage down to cancellous bone while minimizing bone loss. The exposed cancellous bone edge should be cut perpendicular to the axis of the shaft. The proximal phalanx then can be cut to the desired angle of flexion. Flexion should increase from approximately 25 degrees at the index finger to 50 degrees at the small finger. The amount of flexion can be altered if there are fixed contractures of the adjacent MCP or DIP joints. Coaptation of the bone ends should be attempted to assess apposition and alignment.
- *Fixation:* Arthrodesis fixation can be achieved through many implants, which include Kirschner wires, interosseous wires, tension band wiring, and headless screws (Figure 25–9). We have found that the tension band technique is the most reliable. Fixation is achieved

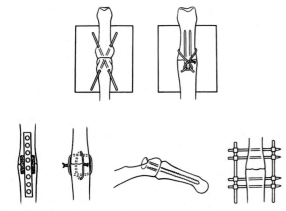

Figure 25–9:
**Methods of fixation used for proximal interphalangeal arthrodesis: crossed wires, tension band, plate and screws, intramedullary screw, and external fixation.**

by drilling a transverse 0.028-inch hole across the base of the middle phalanx to just beneath the dorsal cortex. A 26-gauge stainless steel wire is passed through this hole. Then two 0.028- or 0.035-inch Kirschner wires are placed from the dorsal aspect of the proximal phalanx across the arthrodesis site and into the intramedullary canal of the middle phalanx. These wires must be started proximal enough to prevent cutout into the arthrodesis site and should be parallel to each other. The stainless steel wire is crossed and looped around these pins proximally in a figure-eight fashion. Tensioning of the wire should be performed at the level of the arthrodesis so that the cut end can be buried into the arthrodesis site. The longitudinal wires are cut, bent, and impacted to hold the tension band wire in place (Figure 25–10).

* *Closure:* The dorsal apparatus is approximated with a 4-0 nonabsorbable suture.

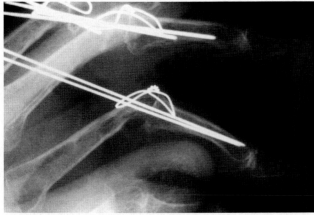

Figure 25–10:
**Lateral radiograph of multiple proximal interphalangeal arthrodeses with tension band fixation.**

* *Immobilization:* A short arm splint with extension past the PIP joints to maintain position.
* *Rehabilitation:* Follow-up at weeks 1, 3, and 6.
* *Therapy:*
  * 7–10 days: Wound and edema management. Fabrication of a digit gutter splint that provides lateral support to the PIP joint and holds the digit in full extension. If multiple digits are involved, a full extension resting pan splint is favored.
  * 2–3 weeks: Wound, scar, and edema management. Initiation of active DIP blocking exercises.
  * 10–12 weeks: Discontinuation of extension gutter splint if clinical and radiographic fusion has occurred.

## Arthroplasty Technique (Silicone Arthroplasty)

* *Dorsal approach:* A dorsal longitudinal skin incision is made over the PIP joint with exposure of the dorsal apparatus.
  * The joint is exposed between the central slip and the lateral band, taking care to preserve the central slip insertion.
  * The collateral ligaments are released from their proximal phalangeal origin. The proximal phalangeal head is resected through its neck with a saw cutting perpendicular to the axis of the shaft in the coronal and sagittal planes.
  * The medullary canals of the proximal and middle phalanges are prepared in a fashion similar to the MCP arthroplasty.
  * Medullary canals are sized with trial implants.
  * The permanent implant is inserted using the "no touch technique."
  * The split between the lateral band and central tendon is reapproximated with a 4-0 nonabsorbable suture.
* *Immobilization:* A short arm volar splint past the PIP joint with full extension.
* *Rehabilitation:* Follow-up at weeks 1, 2, 6, and 12.
* *Therapy:*
  * 3–5 days: Wound and edema management. Fabrication of a hand-based dynamic flexion block PIP splint limiting flexion to 40 degrees. A hand-based static extension gutter splint is used for night wear.
  * 2–3 weeks: Wound, scar, and edema management. Increase flexion block limit to 60 degrees. Gentle passive and active-assisted range of motion exercises to PIP and DIP.
  * 4–5 weeks: Emphasis placed on DIP exercises and MCP reverse extension blocking for PIP extension.
  * 6 weeks: Discontinue PIP flexion block splint. Gentle dynamic flexion splinting if needed. Gentle strengthening and functional activities encouraged.
  * 8–10 weeks: Discontinue night PIP extension splint if extensor lag is 25 degrees or less.
* *Volar approach:* A Bruner-type incision is centered over the PIP joint flexion crease. The neurovascular bundles

are visualized and protected. Exposure of the flexion tendons are obtained through a flap created from the A4 to A2 pulley. The flexor tendons are retracted to allow exposure of the volar plate. The volar plate is released from its proximal attachments. Collateral ligaments are resected from the head of the proximal phalanx. The PIP joint is hyperextended for joint exposure.

- Bony preparation for the implant is identical to the dorsal approach.
- The appropriate size implant is inserted.
- *Closure:* The volar plate is reattached to its proximal phalanx origin.
- *Immobilization:* A bulky volar short arm splint is applied, holding the digits in full extension.
- *Rehabilitation:* Follow-up at 1, 3, 6, and 12 weeks.
- *Therapy:* See dorsal approach.

## Conclusions

- Treatment of RA must always begin with medical management. With continuing advances in early detection and aggressive medical intervention, the need for surgical intervention in this disorder hopefully will decrease in the future.
- The decision to surgically intervene in RA in the wrist and hand should be based on relieving pain, restoring function, preventing further damage, and cosmesis.
- Although skeletal reconstruction can be successful at specific joints in the hand and wrist, perspective of the status and function of the entire upper extremity and patient as a whole must be maintained.

## References

1. Klippel JH: Rheumatoid arthritis. In Klippel JH, Weyand CM, Wortmann RL, editors: *Primer on the rheumatologic diseases,* ed 11. Atlanta, 1993, Arthritis Foundation.
   The authors review the latest understanding of rheumatoid arthritis etiology, pathogenesis, diagnosis, and medical management.

2. Harris ED: Clinical features of rheumatoid arthritis. In Kelley WN, Harris ED, Ruddy S, Sledge CB, editors: *Textbook of rheumatology,* ed 4. Philadelphia, 1993, WB Saunders.
   The author provides a complete overview of rheumatoid arthritis, covering the presentation, criteria for diagnosis, epidemiology, disease course, diagnosis, prognosis, and classification.

3. Lee DM, Weinblatt ME: Rheumatoid arthritis. *Lancet* 358: 903-911, 2001.
   The author reviews improvements in the understanding of the pathophysiology of rheumatoid arthritis, its medical management, especially DMARDs, and the changing rationale for medical intervention.

4. Gardner GC, Kadel NJ: Ordering and interpreting rheumatologic laboratory tests. *JAAOS* 11:60-67, 2003.
   The author reviews the standard rheumatology laboratory tests and a rationale for their use in confirming clinically suspected diagnoses.

5. Pisetsky DS, St. Clair EW: Progress in the treatment of rheumatoid arthritis. *JAMA* 286:278-290, 2001.
   This article reviews the current principles of medical treatment for rheumatoid arthritis and outlines the newer treatments.

6. Blank JE, Cassidy C: The distal radioulnar joint in rheumatoid arthritis. *Hand Clin* 12:499-513, 1996.
   The author provides an excellent review of the DRUJ anatomy, the regions affected by synovitis, deformity, radiographic assessment, and surgical reconstructions.

7. Clawson MC, Stern PJL: The distal radioulnar joint complex in rheumatoid arthritis: an overview. *Hand Clin* 7:373-381, 1991.
   The authors review the pathoanatomy of the DRUJ in rheumatoid arthritis, the nonoperative modalities, and operative options.

8. Dingman PV: Resection of the distal end of the ulna (Darrach operation); an end result study of twenty-four cases. *J Bone Joint Surg Am* 34A: 893–900, 1952.
   A review of twenty-four cases of the Darrach procedure. The author found no difference in the result of the procedure despite varying techniques in resection.

9. Shapiro JS: The wrist is rheumatoid arthritis. *Hand Clin* 12: 477-498, 1996.
   A review of the natural history of rheumatoid arthritis in the hand and wrist, patient examination, surgical decision making, and surgical treatment options.

10. Jebson PJ, Adams BD: Wrist arthrodesis: review of current techniques. *JAAOS* 9:53-60, 2001.
    The techniques of wrist arthrodesis including dorsal plating and intramedullary rod placement are discussed.

11. Carlson JR, Simmons BP: Total wrist arthroplasty. *JAAOS* 6:308-315, 1998.
    The authors review the indications, history, designs, technique, complications, and salvage procedures for total wrist arthroplasty.

12. Cobb TK, Beckenbaugh RD: Biaxial total wrist arthroplasty. *J Hand Surg* 21:1011-1021, 1996.
    Reports an 83% survivorship at 5 years in 64 implants.

13. Divelbiss BJ, Sollerman C, Adams BD: Early results of the universal total wrist arthroplasty in rheumatoid arthritis. *J Hand Surg* 27:195-204, 2002.
    The authors note encouraging results in 22 implants with 1- to 2-year follow-up but discourage use of this implant in patients with severe preoperative wrist laxity.

14. Abboud JA, Beredjiklian PK, Bozentka DJ: Metacarpophalangeal joint arthroplasty in rheumatoid arthritis. *JAAOS* 11:184-191, 2003.
    The authors provide a review of the anatomy, clinical assessment, indications, published outcomes, and surgical technique for silicone MCP prostheses in RA.

15. Stirrat CR: Metacarpophalangeal joints in rheumatoid arthritis of the hand. *Hand Clin* 12:515-529, 1996.

The author provides a review of the pathoanatomy of RA at the MCP joint, its clinical evaluation, decision making, and surgical technique and results of arthroplasty.

16. Rizio L, Belsky MR: Finger deformities in rheumatoid arthritis. *Hand Clin* 12:531-540, 1996.

The authors provide a review of the deformities that can affect the fingers in RA. They review the anatomy, classifications, clinical evaluation, and treatment options.

17. Kobayashi K, Terrono AL: Proximal interphalangeal joint arthroplasty of the hand. *JASSH* 3:219-226, 2003.

The authors review the indications and techniques for arthroplasty of the proximal interphalangeal joint.

18. Kiefhaber T, Strickland J: Soft tissue reconstruction for rheumatoid swan-neck and boutonnière deformities: long term results. *J Hand Surg* 18:984-989, 1993.

The authors review their results from soft tissue reconstruction for rheumatoid swan-neck and boutonnière deformities. Results deteriorated over time.

# CHAPTER 26

# Rheumatoid Arthritis—Hand and Wrist: Soft Tissue Reconstruction

## Peter J.L. Jebson

MD, Associate Professor, Chief Orthopaedic Hand Service, Department of Orthopaedic Surgery, University of Michigan Medical Center, Ann Arbor, MI

- Rheumatoid arthritis (RA) is a disease of unknown etiology that affects the synovium found in joints, tendon sheaths, and ligaments, resulting in deformity, weakness, and loss of function.
- There is a hereditary component to RA, with an increased incidence of expression of major histocompatibility grouping HLA-DR4 among involved individuals (70% incidence).
- The diagnosis of RA requires the presence of four of the seven diagnostic criteria (Box 26–1).
- Approximately 80% of patients have an elevated level of rheumatoid factor (RF), which is an immunoglobulin M antibody directed against host synovium. The 20% of patients who remain seronegative may have milder disease and fewer extraarticular manifestations.[1]
- Patients with RA frequently have an elevated erythrocyte sedimentation rate and C-reactive protein during the active phases of the disease.
- Biopsy of rheumatoid synovium or nodules demonstrates synovial inflammation with lymphocyte invasion and noncaseating granulomas.
- Management of the rheumatoid patient must involve a cooperative effort between the hand surgeon and rheumatologist, although differences of opinion exist between both specialties regarding the effectiveness of surgical intervention and the role of surgery in preventing disease progression.[2]
- The best outcomes following surgery can be found in patients who undergo surgery *before* the development of a fixed severe contracture, tendon rupture, joint subluxation, dislocation, or destruction.
- Not all patients with RA and a hand deformity require surgical treatment, because many patients adapt and have an acceptable functional level. It is important for the patient to understand that surgical treatment does not restore full function and actually may weaken the hand.
- In patients with bilateral hand problems requiring surgery, it is preferable to stage the procedures to allow the patient one useful extremity for functional activities during rehabilitation of the operated extremity.
- Preoperative evaluation of the rheumatoid patient with a hand/wrist deformity requiring surgical treatment must include an assessment of cervical spine stability and the status of the shoulder and elbow joints. If there is significant involvement with pain and limited function and mobility of the shoulder and/or elbow, proximal reconstruction usually is performed before any hand or wrist procedures so that rehabilitation of the hand is not impaired.

| Box 26–1 | American College of Rheumatology Diagnostic Criteria for Rheumatoid Arthritis |
|---|---|

- Morning stiffness located around joints for at least 1 hour lasting for at least 6 weeks
- Simultaneous arthritis with synovitis in three or more joints present for at least 6 weeks
- Arthritis of the hand joints (wrist, metacarpophalangeal or proximal interphalangeal) lasting at least 6 weeks
- Symmetric arthritis present for at least 6 weeks
- Presence of rheumatoid nodules
- Elevated rheumatoid factor titer
- Subchondral erosions or osteopenia adjacent to involved joints on radiographs

## Rheumatoid Nodules

- Occur in approximately 25% of patients.
- The nodules usually are located in the subcutaneous tissues, extensor surfaces, and are adjacent to the joints with which they communicate.
- The most common locations include the olecranon and dorsum of the hand.
- Their presence is associated with more aggressive joint disease.[3]
- Rheumatoid nodules can be painful and interfere with function, particularly if they are located on the volar surfaces of the fingers or thumb.
- Symptomatic nodules are injected with a corticosteroid, which may result in nodule regression; however, ulcerations can occur.
- Surgical excision is recommended for persistent, problematic nodules; however, recurrence and wound healing problems can occur.

## Extensor Tenosynovitis

- Can be the *first* presentation of RA and may precede intraarticular involvement by several months.
- Typically manifests as a nonpainful soft tissue mass on the dorsum of the wrist. If the patient complains of pain, joint involvement should be suspected.
- Extensor tenosynovitis usually is seen in combination with synovitis of the distal radioulnar joint (DRUJ), dorsal subluxation of the distal ulna, palmar subluxation of the distal radius and carpus with respect to the ulna, and supination of the carpus; this is referred to as *caput ulnae syndrome*.[4]
- Extensor tenosynovitis can be confined to an individual tendon or compartment, or it may involve multiple compartments. Initially the sheath appears distended. However, as the inflammation progresses the sheath fills with "rice bodies" and the synovium thickens, resulting

in tendon adhesions. Left untreated, the synovium proliferates and infiltrates the tendon, resulting in weakening and subsequent rupture.

- Although tendon rupture should be avoided, it is not possible to predict which patients with tenosynovitis will progress to tendon rupture. Tenosynovectomy has been shown to decrease the rate of tendon rupture.[5]
- The initial treatment for tenosynovitis involves a trial of medical therapy consisting of splinting, antirheumatologic medication, and judicious use of a local steroid injection.
- Surgical intervention is indicated in patients with persistent or progressive proliferative synovitis despite a 3–6 month course of maximal medical therapy, or if there is an actual or impending tendon rupture, significant functional limitation, or destructive joint changes.[6]

## Dorsal Tenosynovectomy Technique

- A straight longitudinal midline incision is used, with elevation of full-thickness skin flaps to expose the extensor retinaculum. The retinaculum is divided over the sixth compartment, and a transverse radially based flap is elevated to expose all diseased tendons. Exposure of the first compartment usually is unnecessary.
- A systematic, complete tenosynovectomy then is performed.
- After all hypertrophic synovial tissue has been removed, each tendon is inspected for fraying, attenuation, infiltration, or rupture (Figure 26–1).
- Frayed tendons are debrided with an assessment of the remaining tendon tissue for strength and quality, particularly with respect to the risk of rupture. If a rupture is considered imminent, the frayed area is resected and reconstruction (tendon transfer or grafting) is performed.
- Similarly, if a thin strand of tissue connecting normal tendon proximally and distally ("pseudotendon") is encountered, this tissue must be resected and tendon reconstruction (transfer vs. grafting) performed.
- The underlying wrist and distal radioulnar joints are inspected for proliferative synovitis and the presence of an irregular bony prominence that has developed as a consequence of bone invasion and destruction. Such a prominence attenuates the adjacent tendons, resulting in rupture, and should be removed. A joint synovectomy may decrease the symptoms of joint pain but has not been proven to change overall disease progression.
- The retinaculum is split transversely with the distal half placed beneath the tendons, whereas the proximal half is sutured back over the dorsal surface to prevent bowstringing. The extensor pollicis longus (EPL) tendon usually is transposed subcutaneously (Figure 26–2).

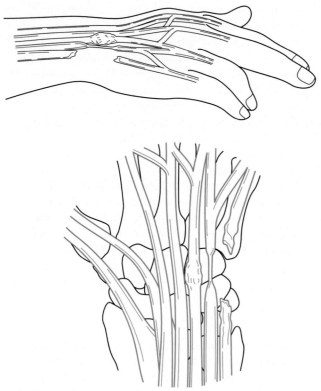

**Figure 26–1:**
**Tendon damage from rheumatoid disease can include tendon invasion with nodule formation, attenuation and pseudotendon formation, or tendon rupture.**

- Complications are rare following a tenosynovectomy but include dorsal skin slough, tendon adhesions, recurrence, and tendon rupture.
- *Rehabilitation:* Immediate active and passive range of motion. Dynamic splinting is used if an extensor lag develops.

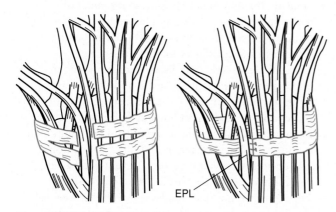

EPL

**Figure 26–2:**
**The retinaculum is split transversely, with half placed beneath the extensor tendons and the other half placed dorsally. Note the extensor pollicis longus (EPL) is transposed dorsally.**

# Extensor Tendon Rupture

- Tendon rupture may occur secondary to attritional wear, synovial infiltration, or ischemia. Thus the preoperative evaluation must include radiographs of the wrist to look for bony irregularities.
- The patient classically presents with the sudden loss of finger extension, occasionally following a trivial hand injury and usually after a delay in seeking medical attention.
- Other conditions that occur in the rheumatoid patient can mimic an extensor tendon rupture[7] (Box 26–2).
- The most frequent single extensor tendon rupture involves the extensor digiti minimi (EDM), which usually is an attritional rupture caused by a bony spike on the distal ulna. This is referred to as a *Vaughan-Jackson lesion.*[8]
- EDM rupture is a sign of impending additional extensor tendon ruptures and thus should be treated urgently.
- Rupture of the extensor digitorum communis (EDC) tendons also usually occurs at the wrist level, typically in association with an EDM rupture and caput ulnae syndrome.
- The EPL usually ruptures at the Lister tubercle on the distal radius.

| Box 26–2 | **Differential Diagnosis of the Inability to Extend the Digital Metacarpophalangeal Joints in the Rheumatoid Patient** |
|---|---|

1. Extensor tendon rupture
   - As the wrist is passively moved through a full flexion-extension arc, the MCP joints do not extend (loss of the tenodesis effect).
   - No palpable contraction of the tendons during attempted extension.
2. Extensor tendon dislocation at the MCP joint
   - Extensor tendons located ulnar to the MCP joint.
   - Fingers are in a flexed, ulnarly deviated position.
   - Tendons may be palpated along the hand.
   - When the fingers are brought into an extended position passively, the patient can maintain the extended position in contrast to ruptured tendons or a posterior interosseous nerve (PIN) palsy.
3. Dislocated MCP joints
   - The joints usually are positioned in flexion and ulnarly deviated.
   - The joints usually appear eroded and dislocated on radiographs.
4. PIN compression/palsy
   - Usually involves the inability to extend all four fingers and the thumb IP joint.
   - Occurs secondary to radiocapitellar joint synovitis.
   - No palpable contraction of the extensor tendons is noted when the patient is asked to extend the fingers.
   - The wrist radially deviates slightly on attempted extension because the ECU is paralyzed.
   - As the wrist is passively flexed, the MCP joints extend slightly secondary, indicating intact extensor tendons (tenodesis effect).

# Extensor Tendon Reconstruction

- Treatment of all extensor tendon ruptures involves a dorsal tenosynovectomy, removal of any bone spikes, excision with or without replacement of the ulnar head, and relocation of the retinaculum.
- The most common method for restoring tendon function following rupture of an extensor tendon is tendon transfer because end to end repair usually is not feasible due to loss of the substance of the tendon because of the erosive disease. Grafting also can be performed.[9]
- Tendon transfers can restore function if the patient has satisfactory motion of the metacarpophalangeal (MCP) joints. Rarely, the surgeon must replace the joints in combination with tendon reconstruction or as a staged procedure.
- EPL rupture is treated by transfer of the extensor indicis proprius (EIP), which is a reliable method for restoring thumb interphalangeal (IP) joint extension (Figure 26–3).
- EDM or small-finger EDC rupture is treated by side to side transfer of the distal tendon end to the ring finger EDC. Alternatively, an isolated EDM rupture can be treated with an EIP transfer to preserve independent small-finger extension.
- For an isolated EDC rupture involving the ring or long fingers, the distal end of the EDC is sutured to an adjacent EDC tendon.
- For ruptures involving two fingers (usually the EDM, EDC small, and EDC ring), the EIP is transferred to the small finger EDC and EDM, and the ring finger EDC is transferred side to side to the EDC of the long finger (Figure 26–4).
- When three or four tendons are ruptured, the aforementioned transfers can be used. Alternatively, the long- and ring-finger flexor digitorum superficialis (FDS) tendons can be transferred through the interosseous membrane or subcutaneously around the radius (Figure 26–5). Other options include intercalary free tendon grafts or, if an arthrodesis of the thumb MCP joint or wrist joint will be performed, the EPL or wrist extensors may be available for transfer.
- All transferred and grafted tendons should be sutured together using the Pulvertaft method, which consists of weaving one tendon end through the other at perpendicular angles to strengthen the repair.

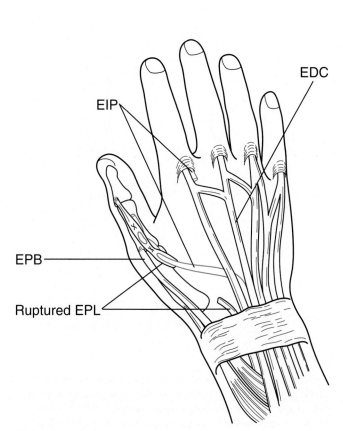

**Figure 26–3:**
Transfer of the extensor indicis proprius *(EIP)* for an extensor pollicis longus *(EPL)* rupture. *EDC,* Extensor digitorum communis; *EPB,* extensor pollicis brevis.

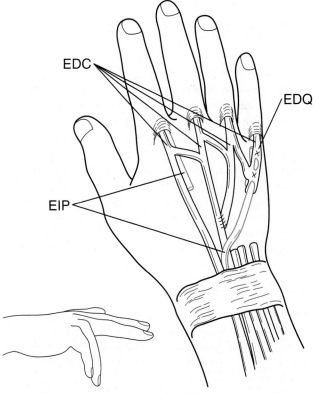

**Figure 26–4:**
Reconstruction of the ruptured small extensor digitorum communis *(EDC)* and extensor digiti quinti and ring EDC tendons can be accomplished with transfer of the extensor indicis proprius *(EIP)* to the small finger and side to side transfer of the ring EDC to the long finger EDC. EDQ, Extensor digiti quinti. (From Trumble TE, editor: *Principles of hand surgery and therapy.* Philadelphia, 2000, WB Sanders Company.)

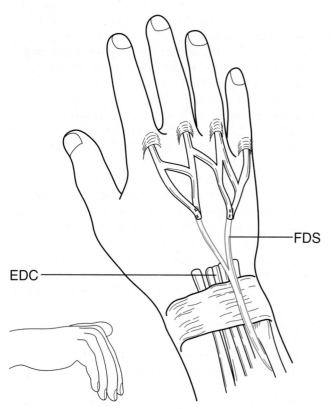

**Figure 26–5:**
**Transfer of the flexor digitorum superficialis *(FDS). EDC,* Extensor digitorum communis.**

- *Rehabilitation:* Following tendon transfer or grafting, the wrist is immobilized in 30 degrees extension, the MCP joints in slight flexion, and the IP joints are left free to move. One week later, dynamic extension splinting is started during the daytime, with splinting of the wrist and fingers in extension at night. Dynamic splinting permits active flexion and passive extension to simultaneously protect the transfer and allow tendon gliding to prevent adhesion formation. Dynamic splinting is discontinued at 4–6 weeks postoperatively and a range of motion program started. If an extensor lag is noted, dynamic splinting is used for an additional 3 weeks.

## Wrist Balancing

- Occasionally a patient presents with a wrist that is postured in radial deviation and extension. The deformity contributes to the characteristic ulnar deviation deformity of the fingers and is the result of ulnocarpal ligament destruction.
- If the wrist is not addressed when arthroplasties at the MCP joints are performed, early failure of the implants results.[10]
- If the wrist has good pain-free motion and a well-preserved joint surface and the radial deviation can be corrected passively, an extensor carpi radialis longus to

extensor carpi ulnaris (ECU) tendon transfer can be performed (Figure 26–6).
- *Rehabilitation:* Postoperatively the wrist is placed in a splint or a cast for 4 weeks to maintain the carpus and metacarpals in ulnar deviation with the MCP joints in radial deviation.

## Extensor Carpi Ulnaris Dislocation

- The ECU is an extrinsic stabilizer of the DRUJ. As proliferative synovitis occurs in the DRUJ, attenuation of the ECU subsheath, DRUJ ligaments and capsule, and ulnocarpal complex occurs, resulting in supination of the carpus, dorsal subluxation of the ulnar head, volar subluxation of the ECU, and loss of dynamic distal ulna stabilization.
- *Treatment:* Therapy involves repositioning the ECU and stabilizing it with a portion of the extensor retinaculum, which acts as a sling to maintain the ECU in the correct dorsal position.

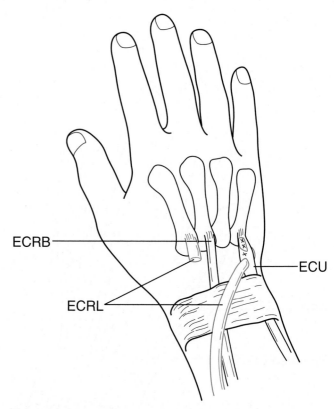

**Figure 26–6:**
**Patients with a severe radial deviation of the metacarpals develop an intercalated collapse of the hand with ulna deviation of the digits at the metacarpophalangeal (MCP) joints. Tendon transfer of the extensor carpi radialis longus (ECRL) to the extensor carpi ulnaris can be a useful adjunct coupled with MCP joint arthroplasty to prevent recurrent deformity.**

## Flexor Tenosynovitis

- Flexor tenosynovitis is common but not as clinically apparent as synovitis on the dorsum of the hand because the flexor tendons are located deep to the thick volar forearm fascia and transverse carpal ligament.
- Flexor tenosynovitis is suspected when morning stiffness and pain in the forearm and volar wrist are noted in the presence of relatively normal joints, and when passive flexion of the fingers exceeds active flexion.
- Clinical manifestations include loss of finger motion, locking or triggering of the fingers, carpal tunnel syndrome (23%–69% incidence), and flexor tendon rupture. In the palm and fingers, pain and swelling may be the initial complaint.
- Nonoperative treatment involves rest, splinting, and corticosteroid injection.
- Indications for surgical intervention include persistent or progressive proliferative synovitis despite maximal medical therapy, failed previous steroid injection, impending or actual tendon rupture, persistent or worsening carpal tunnel syndrome, or significant functional limitations.
- Surgical treatment consists of release of the transverse carpal ligament and flexor tenosynovectomy, including inspection of the carpal tunnel floor for erosion of the carpus and the subsequent development of bone spikes. If a trigger digit is present or flexor tenosynovitis is suspected, a separate incision is made at the proximal phalangeal level, which permits retraction and inspection of the flexor tendons both proximally and distally, thus facilitating a complete tenosynovectomy.
- If triggering is associated with proliferative tenosynovitis within the fibroosseous sheath, release of the A1 pulley should be avoided because it results in volar subluxation and a greater moment arm of the flexor tendons, which contributes to volar subluxation of the MCP joints and ulnar deviation deformities of the fingers.[11] Tenosynovectomy, sheath excision with preservation of the pulleys, and resection of the ulnar slip of the FDS to decompress the contents of the fibroosseous tunnel is recommended.
- Flexor tenosynovectomy combined with excision of the ulnar slip of the FDS is associated with reduced recurrence and reoperation rates.[12]
- Triggering may be caused by a nodular mass of tenosynovium impinging on the proximal edge of the transverse carpal ligament.[13]
- *Rehabilitation:* Active and passive range of motion exercises started several days postoperatively to prevent adhesion formation and a limitation of finger flexion.

## Flexor Tendon Rupture

- Flexor tendon rupture is not as common as rupture of the extensor tendons; however, they are more difficult to treat, and the clinical results are less favorable.

- Rupture most commonly occurs within the carpal tunnel and is caused by attrition or direct tenosynovial invasion. Synovitis and bone erosion result in the development of a bony spike that erodes through the volar wrist capsule, producing wear and abrasion of the adjacent flexor tendons. This phenomenon is known as the *Mannerfelt lesion* (Figure 26–7).[14]
- The most common location of the bone spike is the scaphoid, followed by the trapezium, distal ulna, hamate, lunate, and distal radius, in descending order of frequency.
- The flexor pollicis longus (FPL) is the most common flexor tendon to rupture, followed by the flexor digitorum profundus (FDP) of the index finger. This is because of the proximity of these tendons to the scaphoid.
- Although FPL or FDP ruptures may produce minimal functional disability, surgery is warranted to prevent further ruptures.

## Flexor Tendon Reconstruction

- Reconstruction of a flexor tendon rupture depends on the location of the rupture, the degree of arthritis in the joints moved by the tendon, and the functional loss.
- Treatment of a rupture at the level of the wrist or palm consists of debridement of involved synovium, carpal canal exploration, excision of any bony spikes, and coverage of the bone with a rotational flap of volar capsule. If a partial tendon rupture is encountered, a tenosynovectomy is performed and the tendon is left alone.
- Treatment of an FPL rupture is dependent on the status of the IP joint. If the joint is painless and has good motion, a free intercalary graft (most commonly the palmaris longus if available) is used when the distal stump can be brought into the palmar wound. If this is not possible, transfer of the ring- or long-finger FDS tendon is performed. If the IP joint is arthritic or unstable, arthrodesis is preferred.
- FDS ruptures usually do not require reconstruction if the FDP is intact. If the proximal interphalangeal (PIP) joint can be hyperextended, a tenodesis procedure may be necessary to prevent the development of a swan-neck deformity.

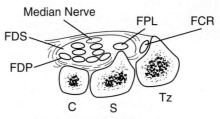

Figure 26–7:
**Proliferative synovitis results in a carpal erosion with attenuation of the adjacent flexor tendons. *C,* capitate; *FCR,* flexor carpi radialis; *FDP,* flexor digitorum profundus; *FDS,* flexor digitorum superficialis; *FPL,* flexor pollicis longus; *S,* scaphoid; *Tz,* trapezium.**

- FDP rupture at the level of the wrist or palm can be treated with side to side transfer to an adjacent intact FDP if the distal interphalangeal (DIP) joint is painless and supple. If the joint is arthritic or unstable, an arthrodesis is recommended. Reconstructive options for rupture of the FDP within the finger include free intercalary tendon grafting, staged reconstruction, or DIP arthrodesis. Less predictable outcomes have been associated with intercalary grafting and staged reconstruction.
- If the FDS and FDP tendons are ruptured within the carpal tunnel, transfer of an intact FDS to the FDP or intercalary grafting can be performed.
- If both the FDS and FDP tendons are ruptured in the finger, an arthrodesis of the PIP and DIP joints in a functional position is advocated because of the unsatisfactory outcomes associated with staged tendon reconstruction.
- Rehabilitation of flexor tendon grafting or transfer involves the initiation of active motion exercises on the third postoperative day to prevent adhesion formation.

# Rheumatoid Thumb

- Involvement of the thumb in rheumatoid arthritis often results in significant pain, deformity, and functional loss.
- Nalebuff[15] originally classified thumb deformities into three types; this has been subsequently revised to six types (Box 26–3).
- The specific pattern encountered is dependent on which joints are involved. Changes at one joint result in pathologic changes in adjacent joints. Extrinsic tendon involvement further contributes to the deformity. If the thumb remains untreated, it progresses from a passively correctable deformity to a fixed one.
- When evaluating the rheumatoid thumb, it is important to assess the degree of the deformity, active and passive motion in the individual thumb joints, tendon integrity, and the amount of joint destruction on plain radiographs.

- Type I is most common, followed by types III and IV. Types II and V are much less common.
- *Type I (Boutonnière deformity)* is characterized by MCP joint flexion and IP joint hyperextension. The deformity is most commonly caused by MCP joint synovitis, which attenuates the dorsal capsule, extensor pollicis brevis (EPB) insertion, and extensor mechanism, resulting in volar and ulnar subluxation of the EPL tendon. This results in MCP joint flexion and secondary hyperextension of the IP joint (Figure 26–8). Alternatively, EPB rupture at the wrist level, FPL rupture within the carpal tunnel, or IP joint volar plate attenuation can produce the same deformity.
- *Type II (boutonnière deformity with carpometacarpal [CMC] joint involvement)* is characterized by CMC subluxation or dislocation, MCP joint flexion, IP joint hyperextension, and first metacarpal adduction. The initial pathologic change occurs in the CMC joint, where synovitis attenuates the stabilizing structures and results in joint instability and adduction of the metacarpal.
- *Type III (swan-neck deformity)* is characterized by MCP joint hyperextension, IP joint flexion, and first metacarpal adduction (Figure 26–9). The deformity originates at the CMC joint, where synovitis results in dorsal and radial subluxation of the metacarpal base with secondary adduction. The resultant imbalance in extensor tendon forces, combined with volar plate laxity, results in MCP joint hyperextension and IP joint flexion.
- *Type IV (gamekeeper deformity)* is characterized by instability of the MCP joint. The ulnar collateral ligament attenuates because of chronic synovitis. The proximal phalanx radially deviates due to pressure from pinch activities, resulting in first metacarpal adduction and contraction of the first web space.
- *Type V (swan-neck without metacarpal adduction or CMC joint involvement)* is caused by MCP joint synovitis, which results in volar plate laxity with MCP joint hyperextension and secondary IP joint flexion.

| Box 26–3 | Nalebuff Classification of Rheumatoid Thumb Deformities | |
|---|---|---|
| Type | Description | |
| I | Boutonnière | |
| II | Boutonnière with CMC involvement | |
| III | Swan-neck | |
| IV | Gamekeeper deformity | |
| V | Swan-neck with no metacarpal adduction or CMC changes | |
| VI | Skeletal collapse with loss of bone substance (arthritis mutilans) | |

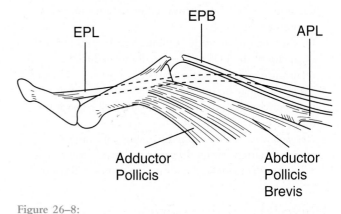

Figure 26–8:
**Boutonnière deformity of the thumb.** *APL,* Abductor pollicis longus; *EPB,* extensor pollicis brevis; *EPL,* extensor pollicis longus.

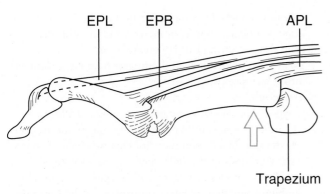

**Figure 26–9:**
Swan-neck deformity of the thumb. *APL,* Abductor pollicis longus; *EPB,* extensor pollicis brevis; *EPL,* extensor pollicis longus. (From Trumble TE, editor: *Principles of hand surgery and therapy.* Philadelphia, 2000, WB Saunders Company.)

Metacarpal adduction and CMC joint changes are not present.

- *Type VI (arthritis mutilans)* is characterized by marked skeletal collapse, loss of bone substance, and a very short, unstable thumb.

## Surgical Treatment of the Rheumatoid Thumb

- The goals of surgery are to provide pain relief, enhance function, prevent disease progression, and improve the cosmetic appearance.

### Type I

- If both the MCP and IP joints are passively correctable, MCP joint synovectomy combined with EPL transection and rerouting to the EPB insertion site and dorsal capsule is performed (Figure 26–10).

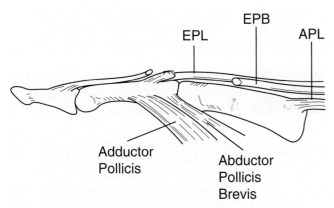

**Figure 26–10:**
Transfer of the extensor pollicis longus *(EPL)* for the flexible boutonnière deformity that passively corrects. *APL,* Abductor pollicis longus; *EPB,* extensor pollicis brevis. (From Trumble TE, editor: *Principles of hand surgery and therapy.* Philadelphia, 2000, WB Saunders Company.)

- If the MCP joint is rigid and the IP joint is passively correctable, an MCP joint arthrodesis in 30 to 45 degrees flexion with EPL rerouting is recommended.
- If both the MCP and IP joints are rigid, arthrodesis of both joints or MCP arthroplasty combined with an IP joint dorsal capsulotomy can be performed.

### Type II

- Treatment follows the principles for types I and III.

### Type III

- CMC resection arthroplasty with soft tissue interposition. If the MCP joint is passively correctable, a capsulodesis, flexor tenodesis, or sesamoidesis is performed. If the MCP hyperextension is fixed, MCP arthrodesis is performed. MCP implant arthroplasty is *not* recommended for a hyperextension deformity.

### Type IV

- Reconstruction of the ulnar collateral ligament with possibly a first web space contracture release. Advanced disease in the MCP joint usually requires an arthrodesis or arthroplasty.

### Type V

- Reconstruction involves MCP joint capsulodesis or sesamoidesis. Advanced disease requires an arthrodesis or arthroplasty.

### Type VI

- Treatment typically involves a combination of arthrodeses.

## Finger Deformities

- Finger deformities caused by rheumatoid arthritis impair hand function and are aesthetically displeasing.
- The three characteristic deformities are (1) MCP joint subluxation and ulnar drift, (2) boutonnière deformity, and (3) swan-neck deformity. Each deformity is caused by an imbalance of the normally delicate, complex extrinsic and intrinsic tendon system.[16,17]

## Metacarpophalangeal Joint Palmar Subluxation and Ulnar Deviation

- Proliferative synovitis attenuates the MCP joint capsule and ligamentous structures, resulting in a loss of stability. The strong pull of the flexor tendons and the weaker dorsal capsule results in palmar subluxation. The extensor tendons displace ulnarward from their normal position, contributing to ulnar deviation. Concomitant wrist pathology may contribute to "ulnar drift."
- Soft tissue reconstruction is indicated *before* significant articular disease is present. Any concomitant wrist and/or

PIP joint involvement should be addressed first for a satisfactory outcome following MCP joint soft tissue reconstruction.

- *Treatment:* Extensor tendon realignment with release of the ulnar sagittal fibers, relocation of the extensor tendon, and imbrication of the radial sagittal fibers. This usually is combined with transfer of a distally based ulnar slip of the extensor tendon through the capsule and back on to itself along the radial side (Figure 26–11). If ulnar drift is present, the ulnar intrinsic tendon is released. Release of the abductor digiti minimi (ADM) is necessary if ulnar deviation of the small finger is noted. Crossed intrinsic transfer has been advocated by some to prevent recurrent ulnar drift. This involves transfer of the ulnar intrinsic tendons of the index, long, and ring fingers to the adjacent finger radial intrinsic mechanism. Postoperatively the hand is splinted with the wrist in 20 degrees extension, the MCP joints in 30 degrees flexion and 10 degrees of radial deviation, and the IP joints in full extension.
- If severe joint destruction is present, MCP arthroplasties combined with soft tissue reconstruction is recommended.
- *Rehabilitation:* At 2 weeks, a dynamic outrigger splint is worn during the daytime for active flexion exercises. The splint is worn for 6 weeks, at which time active and active assisted exercises are initiated and light functional use is permitted. A static night splint is used to maintain the position of the fingers and wrist for 6 to 8 weeks.

## Swan-Neck Deformity

- Swan-neck deformity is characterized by PIP hyperextension and DIP flexion (see Figure 13–7).
- The deformity can be caused by attenuation of the PIP joint volar plate associated with proliferative synovitis within the joint or a rupture of the FDS tendon. The deformity also may occur following erosion and flexion of the DIP joint with attenuation of the terminal

extensor tendon. Proximal migration of the extensor hood secondarily results in increased tension on the central slip, creating PIP hyperextension.[16]
- Swan-neck deformities in the fingers have been classified into four types (Box 26–4).
- *Treatment*[18]:
  - *Type I:* Nonoperative treatment consists of PIP joint splinting to prevent hyperextension but permit flexion (extension block splinting). Surgical treatment involves an arthrodesis of the DIP joint combined with a sublimis tenodesis to correct PIP hyperextension. The sublimis tenodesis involves suturing a distally based slip of the FDS back to itself or the A2 pulley while the PIP joint is held in 20–30 degrees flexion.
  - *Type II:* Surgical treatment involves DIP arthrodesis combined with an ulnar intrinsic release, sublimis tenodesis with temporary pinning of the PIP joint in 20 degrees flexion for 3 weeks, and implant arthroplasty of the MCP joint.
  - *Type III:* If severe PIP joint articular disease is present, arthrodesis (index finger) or implant arthroplasty (long, ring, and small fingers) is performed. In the absence of significant joint disease, PIP joint manipulation under anesthesia with temporary pinning of the PIP joint in 20–30 degrees flexion for 3 weeks combined with MCP joint implant arthroplasty and mobilization of the dorsally migrated contracted lateral bands is performed. The flexor tendons are assessed and a concomitant tenosynovectomy performed if necessary.
  - *Type IV:* Surgical treatment involves PIP arthrodesis (index finger) or implant arthroplasty of the ulnar three fingers. If MCP joint implant arthroplasty is required, arthrodesis of the PIP joint is preferred.

## Technique for Distal Interphalangeal Joint Arthrodesis

- An H-shaped dorsal incision permits excellent exposure. The extensor tendon is divided transversely, and the collateral ligaments are released off the condyles of the

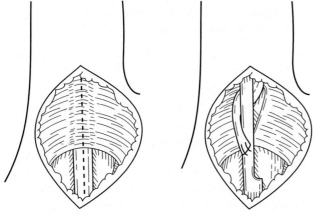

Figure 26–11:
**Realignment of the extensor tendon over the MCP joint.**

| Box 26–4 | Four Types of Swan-Neck Deformities in the Fingers |
|----------|----------------------------------------------------|
| **Type** | **Description** |
| I | Full flexibility of the PIP joint is present. The patient has difficulty of initiating PIP flexion. |
| II | PIP motion is limited and influenced by MCP joint position. PIP joint motion is limited when the MCP joint is passively extended (intrinsic tightness). |
| III | Little or no passive PIP flexion is present. PIP motion does not change with MCP joint position. |
| IV | Similar to type III but with radiographic features of severe articular destruction. |

middle phalanx. The joint surfaces are denuded and the joint stabilized with a longitudinal intramedullary screw (Figure 26–12) or K-wires with or without an interosseous wire. The screw can be inserted by drilling out the tip of the finger. The joint is reduced, and the screw hole is drilled across the DIP joint (Figure 26–13). The DIP joint is fused in 10–20 degrees of flexion with an increased amount of flexion required in the more ulnar digits. Local bone graft from the resected bone is inserted in the fusion site. The tendon is repaired and the skin closed with simple sutures.

## Technique of Sublimis Tenodesis

- A Brunner incision is centered over the volar aspect of the PIP joint. The C1 pulley is released to expose the flexor digitorum sublimis. The A2 pulley is preserved. The two slips of the FDS insertion are identified. The ulnar slip is sharply transected just proximal to the A1 pulley.

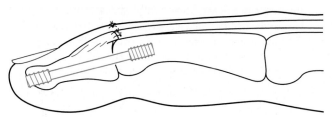

Figure 26–12:
**Arthrodesis of the distal interphalangeal joint with an intramedullary screw.** (From Trumble TE, editor: *Priniciples of hand surgery and therapy.* Philadelphia, 2000, WB Saunders Company.)

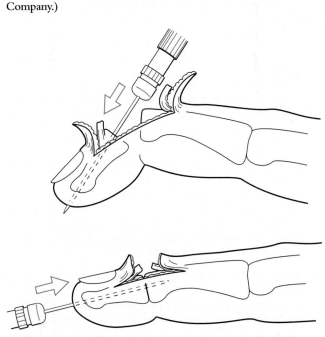

Figure 26–13:
**Arthrodesis of the distal interphalangeal joint with a K-wire technique.** (From Trumble TE, editor: *Principles of hand surgery and therapy.* Philadelphia, 2000, WB Saunders Company.)

The distally based slip is identified between the A1 and A2 pulleys. It is passed around the A2 pulley and with maximal tension is sutured to the A2 pulley or back upon itself distal to the A2 pulley as the PIP joint is held in 30 degrees flexion. The skin incision is closed, and a transarticular 0.035 K-wire is inserted to hold the joint in 30 degrees flexion for 3 weeks.

- *Rehabilitation:* The pin is removed at 3 weeks, at which time PIP joint flexion is permitted. A hand-based extension block splint maintaining the PIP joint in the flexed position is worn for an additional 3 weeks.

## Technique of Proximal Interphalangeal Joint Arthrodesis

- A gently curved longitudinal incision is used and the extensor tendon is split longitudinally. An oscillating saw is used to remove the distal end of the proximal phalanx at an angle necessary to achieve the desired amount of flexion. The index finger is fused in 30 degrees flexion, and an additional 5 degrees flexion is used for each finger in an ulnar direction. The volar plate and collateral ligaments may need to be released in order to mobilize the middle phalanx. After predrilling, a 24-gauge wire is passed through the base of the middle phalanx and the neck of the proximal phalanx with the aid of a 16-gauge needle. K-wires are drilled across the osteosynthesis site in a retrograde fashion, and the tension band wire is tightened (Figure 26–14).

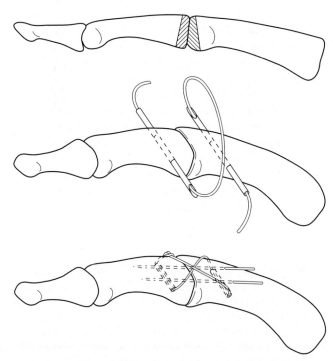

Figure 26–14:
**Proximal interphalangeal joint arthrodesis with a tension band wire technique.** (From Trumble TE, editor: *Principles of hand surgery and therapy.* Philadelphia, 2000, WB Saunders Company.)

# Boutonnière Deformity

- The deformity is caused by PIP joint synovitis that results in capsular distension, attenuation of the central slip, and PIP joint flexion. The lateral bands displace palmar to the joint axis further contributing to PIP flexion and DIP extension (see Figure 13–8).
- Nalebuff has classified the boutonnière deformity into three stages
  - *Stage I:* Consists of slight PIP joint flexion, but the joint is passively correctable. DIP flexion may or may not be present.
  - *Stage II:* The PIP joint flexion usually approaches 30 to 40 degrees. Early on, the deformity is passively correctable, but with time soft tissue contractures occur and passive motion is limited.
  - *Stage III:* The PIP joint is rigid and cannot be passively flexed or extended.
- *Treatment*[18]:
  - *Stage I:* Nonoperative treatment consists of nighttime splinting of the PIP joint in extension and a corticosteroid injection into the joint if significant synovitis is present. If more DIP joint flexion is desired, an extensor tenotomy (Fowler technique) distal to the triangular ligament (Fowler procedure) is recommended. Under local anesthesia, the tendon is divided transversely or obliquely over the middle phalanx.
  - *Stage II:* If the PIP joint is passively correctable, extensor mechanism reconstruction combined with extensor tenotomy to restore DIP joint flexion is preferred. Through a dorsal approach, the lateral bands are relocated dorsally after incision of the volar transverse retinacular ligament. The central slip is reefed by excising a segment. Extensor tenotomy is performed, and the PIP joint is pinned in extension for 3 to 4 weeks.
  - *Rehabilitation:* Immediate active motion of the DIP joint is performed. The PIP joint is splinted with a dynamic extension splint for an additional 3 weeks between exercises.
  - *Stage III:* If the patient complains of a loss of grip function, PIP joint arthrodesis using a tension band wiring technique is recommended.

# References

1. Bonagura VR, Wedgwood JF, Agostino N, et al: Seronegative rheumatoid arthritis, rheumatoid factor cross-reactive idiotype expression, and hidden rheumatoid factors. *Ann Rheum Dis* 48:488-495, 1989.
   The presence of RF is not diagnostic of RA. Approximately 80% of patients with rheumatoid arthritis have an elevated RF level. Seronegative patients (20%) tend to have milder disease.
2. Alderman AK, Chung KC, Kim HM et al: Effectiveness of rheumatoid hand surgery: contrasting perceptions of hand surgeons and rheumatologists. *J Hand Surg* 28A: 3–11, 2003.
   There is disagreement between hand surgeons and rheumatologists regarding the effectiveness of surgical reconstruction in patients with rheumatoid arthritis.
3. Duthie JJ, Brown PE, Truelove LH, et al: Course and prognosis in rheumatoid arthritis: a further report. *Ann Rheum Dis* 23:193, 1964.
   The subcutaneous nodules of rheumatoid arthritis usually are located on extensor surfaces. In general, their presence is associated with more aggressive joint disease.
4. Backdahl M: The caput ulna syndrome in rheumatoid arthritis: a study of the morphology, abnormal anatomy, and clinical picture. *Acta Rheum Scand* (suppl 5):1, 1963.
   A discussion of end-stage rheumatoid destruction of the DRUJ.
5. Ferlic DC, Clayton ML: Flexor tenosynovectomy in the rheumatoid finger. *J Hand Surg* 3:364-367, 1978.
   In treating the rheumatoid trigger finger, incision of the A1 pulley should be avoided because of persistent synovitis within the tendon sheath and the risk of digital ulnar drift. Rheumatoids should be treated by flexor tenosynovectomy combined with resection of one slip of the FDS.
6. Brown FE, Brown ML: Long-term results after tenosynovectomy to treat the rheumatoid hand. *J Hand Surg* 13:704-708, 1988.
   Tenosynovectomy is effective in preventing tendon ruptures and recurrent tenosynovitis. It is most effective when done before the development of significant tendon damage.
7. Wilson RL, DeVito MC: Extensor tendon problems in rheumatoid arthritis. *Hand Clin* 12:551-559, 1996.
   When 3 to 6 months of medical management fails to successfully treat extensor tenosynovitis, tenosynovectomy is indicated to prevent tendon rupture. Single tendon rupture should be treated promptly because further ruptures are likely. The differential diagnosis of loss of MCP joint extension is discussed.
8. Vaughan-Jackson OJ: Ruptures of tendons by attrition at the inferior radioulnar joint. Report of two cases. *J Bone Joint Surg Br* 30:528, 1948.
   DRUJ synovitis results in erosive changes of the ulnar head, leading to attritional rupture of the overlying extensor tendons. Tendon rupture usually proceeds in an ulnar to radial direction.
9. Mountney J, Blundell CM, McArthur P, Stanley D: Free tendon interposition grafting for the repair of ruptured extensor tendons in the rheumatoid hand: a clinical and biomechanical assessment. *J Hand Surg Br* 23:662-665, 1998.
   Reports satisfactory results for free tendon grafting for extensor tendon ruptures in patients with rheumatoid arthritis. They report that tendon grafting, rather than side to side tendon transfer, achieved greater force and more accurately reproduced the anatomic axis of tendon function.
10. Shapiro JS: The wrist in rheumatoid arthritis. *Hand Clin* 12:477-498, 1996.
    A discussion of rheumatoid wrist pathology and its influence on the MCP joints and the fingers. Wrist reconstructions are discussed.
11. deJager LT, Jaffe R, Learmonth ID, Heywood AW: The A1 pulley in rheumatoid flexor tenosynovectomy—to retain or divide? *J Hand Surg* 19B:202-204, 1994.

Division of the A1 pulley leads to increased volar subluxation of the MCP joint, bowstringing of the flexor tendons, and increased ulnar deviation of the fingers.

12. Wheen DJ, Tonkin MA, Green J, Bronkhorst M: Long-term results following digital flexor tenosynovitis in rheumatoid arthritis. *J Hand Surg* 20A:790-794, 1995.
An excellent or good result was noted in two thirds. Recurrence was noted in 31%, with a reoperation rate of 15%. Excising one slip of the FDS in conjunction with the tenosynovectomy was associated with a lower recurrence and reoperation rate.

13. Clayton ML: Surgical treatment of the wrist in rheumatoid arthritis. *J Bone Joint Surg* 47A:741, 1965.
Flexor tenosynovitis may result in locking or triggering of the flexor tendons at the level of the transverse carpal ligament. Hand pain may be the result of carpal tunnel syndrome.

14. Mannerfelt N, Norman O: Attrition ruptures of flexor tendons in rheumatoid arthritis caused by bony spurs in the carpal tunnel. *J Bone Joint Surg* 51B:270-277, 1969.
The two causes of flexor tendon rupture in RA are attrition and invasion of the tendon by tenosynovitis. Attritional ruptures are caused by tendon abrasion on prominent bony spicules in the floor of the carpal canal.

15. Nalebuff EA: Diagnosis, classification and management of rheumatoid thumb deformities. *Bull Hosp Joint Dis* 29:119-137, 1968.
A classification system is proposed in which rheumatoid thumb deformities are originally divided into three types. Treatment principles are reviewed for each deformity.

16. Littler JW: The finger extensor mechanism. *Surg Clin North Am* 47:415-432, 1967.
A classic article that provides a detailed description of digital extensor tendon anatomy and pathomechanics.

17. Rizio L, Belsky MR: Finger deformities in rheumatoid arthritis. *Hand Clin* 12:531-540, 1996.
The treatment approach for swan-neck and boutonnière deformities are reviewed, including potential complications.

18. Kiefhaber TR, Strickland JW: Soft tissue reconstruction for rheumatoid swan-neck and boutonnière deformities: long-term results. *J Hand Surg Am* 18:984-989, 1993.
Soft tissue reconstruction of rheumatoid swan-neck deformity led to initial improvement, but results deteriorated over time. The most predictable procedure for an advanced rheumatoid boutonnière deformity was an arthrodesis.

p

# CHAPTER 27

# Soft Tissue Neoplasms: Benign and Malignant

Peter M. Murray

MD, Associate Professor, Department of Orthopedic Surgery, Division of Hand and Microvascular Surgery, Mayo Clinic Graduate School of Medicine, Rochester, MN; Consultant, Department of Orthopaedic Surgery, Division of Hand and Microvascular Surgery, Mayo Clinic, Jacksonville, FL

## Introduction

- Neoplasms of the hand and wrist are not regarded with a high index of suspicion. The majority of soft tissue tumors of the hand and wrist are benign. Malignancy often is considered only as an afterthought.
- An estimated 6600 new cases of soft tissue sarcoma are diagnosed annually, with only 14% arising in the upper extremity.
- Soft tissue sarcomas of the hand and wrist, therefore, account for less than 0.5% of all cancer deaths per year.
- Most orthopedic surgeons will encounter only one or two undiagnosed soft tissue sarcomas in an entire career.
- Lesions that rapidly enlarge, ache, or exceed 5 cm in size should be considered potentially malignant. When lesions about the hand and wrist present in a worrisome fashion, a complete tumor workup is indicated.

## Basic Principles of the Tumor Workup

### Physical Examination

- The physical examination includes a careful inspection of the lesion, including measurements of lesion size, characterization of the texture of the mass (soft, mobile, firm, fixed), inspection of the skin overlying the mass, palpation for enlarged epitrochlear or axillary lymph nodes, and a comprehensive neurologic and vascular examination.
- Laboratory studies should include routine hematology, a chemistry panel, and baseline coagulation studies.
- The medical oncologist and the radiation oncologist are consulted and should follow the patient if malignancy is confirmed.

### Imaging Techniques

- Plain biplanar radiography is warranted whenever a hand or wrist mass seems suspicious. For lesions with familiar characteristics, however, radiographs do not alter the final treatment or outcome.
- Evaluation by magnetic resonance imaging (MRI) has become the gold standard for soft tissue masses. Image sequencing should include T1, fat-suppressed "turbo" T2, and short tau inversion recovery (STIR). T1 weighted images provide anatomic detail. Fat-suppressed, "turbo" T2 images highlight pus, subacute hematoma, and malignancy through image enhancement. An exception is fibrous tumors that typically are "dark" on T2. STIR images also suppress fat and help highlight abnormal lesions or fluid collections. Gadolinium contrast can provide spectacular enhancement of soft tissue tumors that otherwise show only intermediate intensity on T2 (Figure 27–1 A, B).
- The tumor workup for suspected malignancy includes standard chest radiography and total body scintigraphy

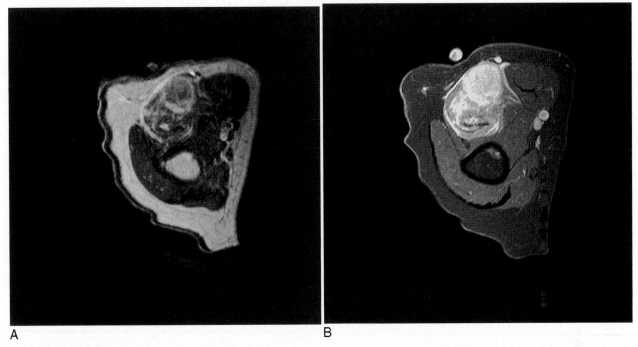

A          B

Figure 27–1:
**Marked enhancement of a soft tissue sarcoma on MRI using gadolinium: MRI without gadolinium (A). MRI following injection of gadolinium contrast material (B).**

(bone scan). Scintigraphy helps identify the presence of bone metastatic spread. Computerized tomography of the chest, abdomen, and pelvis should be included in the tumor workup.

## Biopsy

- If malignancy is highly likely, it is recommended that the biopsy be performed at the institution where all subsequent treatment and monitoring will be performed. Clinical studies have suggested that ultimate survival may be worse when the biopsy is performed at a different institution than the institution performing the definitive management.[1]
- For most lesions of the hand and wrist, an excisional biopsy is performed because of the small size of these lesions. Alternatives to open biopsy include fine needle aspiration and core needle biopsy. The open technique of biopsy has a higher accuracy rate and a higher diagnostic yield than the closed biopsy techniques. For the hand and wrist, open biopsy typically is preferred over a needle biopsy.
- Biopsy is best performed under tourniquet control, but the limb must be exsanguinated by elevation rather than by use of an elastic (Esmarch) bandage prior to tourniquet elevation.
- Because the resultant biopsy tract will be contaminated with tumor cells, subsequent removal of the tumor and biopsy tract en bloc will be necessary should the lesion prove malignant. Therefore, the biopsy incision must be

kept in line with the incision that ultimately would be required for reconstruction.
- Longitudinal incisions are preferred; transverse incisions are never used (Figure 27–2 A, B).
- Frozen sectioning may be helpful initially to ensure adequate tissue has been obtained for diagnosis, but final tumor treatment is based only on the reading of the permanent pathology preparation.

## Staging and Tumor Classification

- The American Joint Committee on Cancer (AJCC) has developed a classification system for the musculoskeletal tumors based the histologic grade, tumor depth, presence of nodes or metastasis, and size. Histology grade can be well differentiated ($G_1$), moderately well differentiated ($G_2$), poorly differentiated ($G_3$), or undifferentiated ($G_4$). The size of the tumor is characterized as less than 5 cm or greater than 5 cm. A tumor is considered deep if it is below the fascia (Table 27–1).
- Musculoskeletal tumors are excised according to one of four dissection methods: intralesional, marginal, wide, or radical (Table 27–2).

## Benign Tumors

### Desmoid

- The desmoid tumor is composed of muscle connective tissue or its overlying investments. Less than 5% of

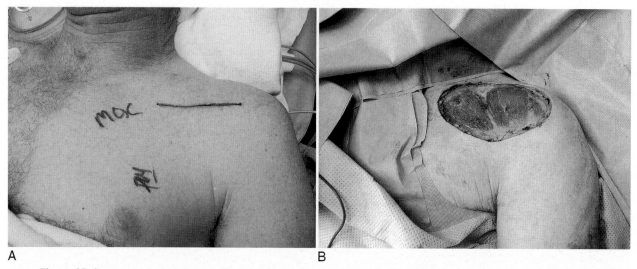

Figure 27–2:

**Original transverse biopsy incision of dermatofibroma protuberans (A) requiring subsequent large resection of contaminated tumor track (B).**

desmoid tumors occur in the hand and forearm region. Because of the intricate nature of the anatomy of the hand, wrist, and forearm and the infiltrative nature of this tumor, desmoid tumors can present challenging surgical problems in this region.

## Physical Examination

- The usual complaint is that of a painless, deep, firm, slowly growing mass. These findings are apparent on physical examination.
- Frequently the tumor, although histologically benign, behaves in an aggressive fashion. Desmoid tumors frequently are invasive.

## Operative Management

- Treatment is individualized, but wide excision is preferred when the tumor is in its early stages. Intralesional excision is inadequate and invariably leads to recurrence.

Obtaining wide margins in patients with desmoid tumor of the hand and wrist can be functionally devastating. In such instances, adjuvant low or median dose radiation therapy has been successful in several reports.

- Recurrence rates range from 24% to 65%. Recurrence is higher in children and adolescents.

## Nerve Tumors

### Neurolemmoma (Schwannoma)

- Most common benign nerve tumor of the upper extremity.

## Physical Examination

- Patients complain of a painless, well-circumscribed mass.
- A positive Tinel sign can generally be elicited over the lesion.
- Neurologic examination generally is normal.
- The cell of origin is the Schwann cell, which covers peripheral nerves, creating the outer myelinated layer of the nerve. Histologically, the tumor is composed of a cellular component (Antoni A region) and a matrix component (Antoni B region) (Box 27–1).

### Table 27–1: American Joint Committee on Cancer (AJCC) System for Staging Soft Tissue Sarcomas

| STAGE | SIZE | DEPTH | NODE | METASTASES | GRADE |
|---|---|---|---|---|---|
| I | Any | Any | None | None | $G_{1-2}$ (low) |
| II | <5 cm | Any | None | None | $G_{2-3}/G_{3-4}$ (high) |
| | >5 cm | Superficial | None | None | $G_{2-3}/G_{3-4}$ (high) |
| III | >5 cm | Deep | None | None | $G_{2-3}/G_{3-4}$ (high) |
| IV | Any | Any | Present | None | Any (high or low) |
| | Any | Any | None | Present | Any (high or low) |

$G_1$ = well differentiated; $G_2$ = moderately well differentiated; $G_3$ = poorly differentiated; $G_4$ = undifferentiated.
Adapted from Green FL, Page DL, Fleming ID, et al: *AJCC cancer staging handbook*, ed 6. New York, 2002, Springer-Verlag.

### Table 27–2: Musculoskeletal Tumor Dissection Method[34]

| | |
|---|---|
| Intralesional | Dissection plane is through tumor |
| Marginal | Dissection plane is through tumor "reactive zone" |
| Wide | Dissection plane well away from tumor in normal tissue but within the compartment |
| Radical | Dissection plane is extracompartmental |

### Box 27–1

- Histologically, the neurolemmoma is composed of a cellular region (Antoni A) and a matrix component (Antoni B).

## Operative Management

- Surgical excision only involves "shelling out" the tumor because it is confined to the outer layer or epineurium (Figure 27–3). In most instances this constitutes a marginal excision.
- Neurologic deficit following surgery is approximately 4%.[2]

## Neurofibroma

- In distinction to the neurilemoma, the neurofibroma arises in nerve fascicles, making excision without sacrificing normal nerve tissue difficult.

## Physical Examination

- Neurofibromas usually are encountered in patients with neurofibromatosis but can be found in any nerve. They typically are slow-growing, painless lesions. Any rapid increase in size should alert the surgeon to the possibility of malignant transformation. Most of the lesions occur in individuals 20 to 30 years old.
- Solitary neurofibromas are known to occur in the hand and wrist, causing enlargement of a single nerve.

## Operative Management

- Surgical removal often means sacrifice of the nerve. An intralesional or marginal resection is generally obtained.
- Nerve grafting may be necessary (Box 27–2).

## Tumor-Like Conditions

### Epidermal Inclusion Cyst

- Epidermal inclusion cysts are among the most common soft tissue lesions of the hand.

### Box 27–2

- The neurofibroma arises within nerve fascicles.

- The etiology of this tumor-like condition is the invagination of epithelium, typically from a puncture wound.

## Physical Examination

- The lesion usually is well circumscribed, firm, and painless. The most common location of epidermal inclusion cysts is the fingertip. However, other locations have been described (Figure 27–4).
- A history of injury is often not elicited.

## Operative Management

- Curative treatment is marginal surgical excision. Recurrence is not seen.

### Ganglion Cysts

- The ganglion cyst is the most common soft tissue lesion of the hand and wrist.
- The dorsal aspect of the wrist (originating from the scapholunate interosseous ligament) is the most common location (Figure 27–5). Other joints of origin include the scaphoid trapezium trapezoid joint of the wrist, the proximal interphalangeal (PIP) joints, and the distal interphalangeal (DIP) joints.
- Many have implicated a traumatic etiology for these lesions, with defects occurring in capsular structures. The lesion is formed by joint fluid material with the resultant "cyst" (perhaps a misnomer) lacking a true epithelial lining.
- Aspiration seems to be a reliable method of initial treatment for ganglions, especially because the retrieval of fluid allays patient fears.[3] Enhanced success rates may be

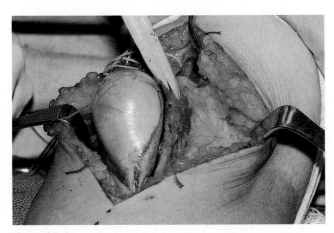

Figure 27–3:
**Large neurolemmoma in the upper arm.**

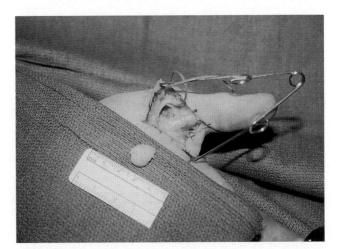

Figure 27–4:
**Epidermal inclusion cyst of the thumb.**

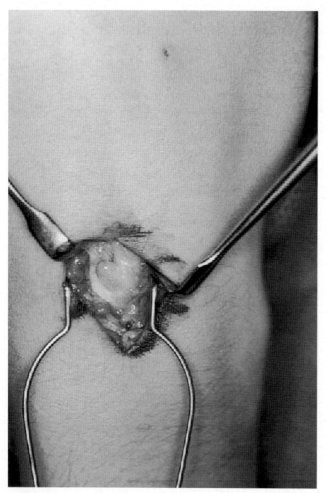

Figure 27–5:

**Dorsal wrist ganglion cyst arising from the scapholunate interosseous ligament.**

achieved with multiple aspirations. Reported success rates following ganglion aspiration range from 31% to 50%.
- Surgical indications include failure of conservative management as indicated by continued pain or dysfunction because of a persisting mass. In some instances, the diagnosis of ganglion cyst may be in doubt, prompting surgical extirpation of the mass before attempts at conservative management (Box 27–3).

### Physical Examination

- The mass is firm, nontender, and transilluminates on physical examination.
- One study found that MRI detected associated pathology in 30% of wrist ganglia imaged.[4] The exact pathogenesis of ganglion cysts, however, remains unclear.

---

**Box 27–3**

- Ganglion cyst removal is indicated when conservative management fails or the diagnosis is in question.

---

### Operative Management

- The most definitive treatment remains open surgical excision. The key to the procedure is the identification and removal of the ganglion stalk by tracing the stalk to the joint capsule. A cuff of capsule is excised with the stalk. The capsule is left open to prevent loss of motion. Recurrence rates with open surgical removal are as low as 5% (Box 27–4).
- Arthroscopic ganglion surgery for dorsal wrist ganglions is becoming increasing popular. At an average follow-up of 47.8 months, Rizzo et al.[5] reported successful treatment in 40 of 42 ganglion cysts using arthroscopic surgery.
- Whatever technique is used, it is important to consider the patient's perspective when treating the ganglion. In one study, 28% of patients sought medical attention for their ganglion over concern for malignancy. It is important to realize that many patients seek reassurance rather than treatment for ganglion cysts.[6]

## Giant Cell Tumor of Tendon Sheath

### Physical Examination

- This lesion is a commonly seen, slowly progressive, painless, firm, multilobular tumor predominating on the radial three digits of the hand (Figure 27–6).
- The histology is variable, but the tumors consistently contain multinucleated giant cells and xanthoma cells. Some lesions demonstrate increased cellularity and mitotic activity.

### Operative Management

- Treatment is marginal excision using standard digital incisions. It is important to assess adjacent joints for infiltration. MRI is helpful for evaluating the extent of the tumor because recurrence can be a problem. Recurrence is as high as 44% to 50% in series with extended follow-up. A study of 43 patients found that following surgical excision, the only lesions that recurred were lesions that originally had multiple discrete tumors. Tumors composed of single masses did not recur following surgical excision.[7]

## Vascular Tumors

### Glomus Tumor

- The normal glomus is an arteriovenous shunt that aids in thermal regulation and is most commonly found in the

---

**Box 27–4**

- The key to surgical removal of the ganglion cyst is removing the stalk and tracing it to the joint capsule.
- A cuff of capsule is removed with the stalk.

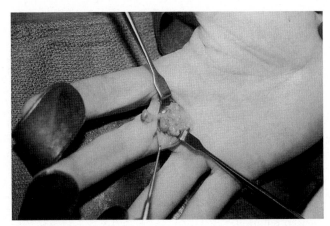

Figure 27–6:
**Multilobulated giant cell tumor of tendon sheath involving the long finger.**

subungual area of the digit but can occur elsewhere in the hand and forearm. The glomus tumor is a neoplasm of smooth muscle cells of this body. It is not composed of endothelial cells as once believed.

## Physical Examination

- Patients with glomus tumors complain of radiating pain, are generally very sensitive to temperature, and are point tender over the lesion. The tumor can become quite disabling for the patient reliant on the digits for occupational purposes (Box 27–5).
- MRI with gadolinium contrast enhancement is helpful for identifying the symptomatic glomus tumor.

## Operative Management

- The tumor is treated by marginal surgical excision. The recurrence rate varies from 0% to 10% in most reports.

## Hemangiomas

- Hemangiomas are benign vascular proliferations that can be superficial (capillary) or deep (cavernous). The deep hemangiomas often have high flow-characteristics.
- Hemangiomas generally appear during the first 4 weeks of life. Under normal circumstances, 70% of hemangiomas regress and ultimately involute by age 7 years (Box 27–6).
- Hemangiomas during the neonatal period and childhood are treated by observation only.

## Physical Examination

- Hemangiomas in the adult can be small, painless, discrete lesions, or they can be large and diffuse (Figure 27–7).

**Box 27–5**

- Patients with glomus tumors often have exquisite subungual tenderness over a relatively inconspicuous lesion.

**Box 27–6**

- Seventy percent of infantile hemangiomas regress and ultimately involute by age 7 years.

- Rapid growth during the first year of life can be alarming.
- MRI enhanced with gadolinium has the ability to differentiate these lesions from sarcomas and vascular malformations, eliminating the routine need for angiography.
- A rare complication of infantile hemangiomas is the Kasabach-Merritt syndrome, a potentially fatal coagulopathy that results from platelet trapping within the lesion.
- Maffucci's syndrome is a rare condition of both multiple hemangiomas and multiple enchondromas. The digits in Maffucci's syndrome are short and deviated. Deformity is common secondary to pathologic fractures. Chondrosarcomas or angiosarcomas may develop in as many as 20% of Maffucci patients.

## Operative Management

- Treatment of hemangiomas in adults is removal by marginal excision. More diffuse lesions are difficult to treat and are prone to recurrence (see Figure 27–7). Cryosurgery, laser ablation, and embolization are more recent successful treatment alternatives, but these modalities must be used with caution. Yakes, Rossi, and Odink[8] reported good results using embolization in otherwise inoperable hemangiomas of the upper limb. Embolization may be the only alternative in some patients with large, inaccessible lesions.

## Pyogenic Granuloma

- Pyogenic granuloma is a disorder of angiogenesis. The specific cause remains unknown. Infection and

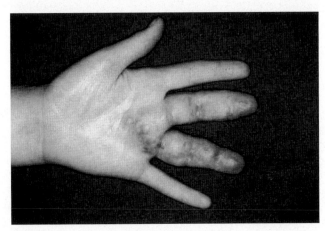

Figure 27–7:
**Diffuse hemangioma involving the long finger, ring finger, and palm in a 16-year-old boy.**

trauma are no longer believed to be the primary etiologic agents.

- In a report of 178 pediatric patients, 13% occurred in the upper extremity.

## Physical Examination

- These lesions usually are not painful. The lesions often break open and bleed following minimal trauma (Figure 27–8).

## Operative Management

- The most reliable treatment is marginal surgical excision while taking a small cuff of normal tissue. Recurrence following surgical excision is uncommon. Modalities such as simple shaving, silver nitrate application, or cautery are unreliable, making the lesions likely to recur.

# Tumors of Adipose Tissue

## Lipoma

- Generally painless, lipomas of the palm can reach substantial size (Figure 27–9). Neurologic symptoms can arise when the lipoma presents in the carpal tunnel or Guyon canal.

## Radiologic Examination

- MRI can be diagnostic because lipomas are of similar image intensity as surrounding fat on both T1- and T2-weighted images (Box 27–7). Additionally, lipomas differ little histologically from the surrounding fat. Lipomas are composed of mature lipocytes. They are considered more common in obese individuals.

## Operative Management

- Surgical excision with or without clear margins is curative, with recurrence unlikely.

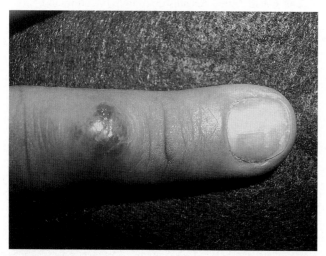

Figure 27–8:

**Pyogenic granuloma involving the dorsum of the long finger in a 20-year-old sailor.**

## Lipoblastoma

- Lipoblastomas are rare, rapidly enlarging benign tumors of embryonal fat. They are found in children usually during the first 3 years of life. Approximately 70% are found in the upper extremity as a painless mass.
- These tumors often are confused with malignancy. Histologically, lipoblastomas are composed of fibrous tissue separating groups of lipoblasts.

## Operative Management

- Marginal surgical excision is curative. Recurrence has not been reported.

# Malignant Tumors

## Clear Cell Sarcoma

- Clear cell sarcoma also is referred to as *malignant melanoma of soft parts*.
- Clear cell sarcoma accounts for 1% of all soft tissue sarcomas. Approximately 22% of all clear cell sarcomas involve the upper extremity.[9]

## Physical Examination

- The diagnosis of clear cell sarcoma should be considered when suspicious firm masses are found in proximity to tendons or aponeurotic junctions. Clear cell carcinomas typically are slow growing and may go undiagnosed for years.

## Radiographic Examination

- The standard tumor workup should include a careful assessment of the lymph nodes using computed tomography (CT) scan and sentinel node biopsy.
- Despite its name and its reference as a malignant melanoma of soft parts, this tumor can be distinguished from both melanoma and epidermal tissue. Histologically, the tumor can be distinguished from melanoma by round cells with clear cytoplasm.

## Operative Management

- Lymph node metastasis and local recurrence rates following treatment can be high.[9,10] With wide tumor resection and adjuvant radiation therapy, 5-year survival approaching 66% can be expected.[10,11] No particular benefit of chemotherapy for clear cell carcinoma has been found.[11]

## Dermatofibrosarcoma Protuberans

- Dermatofibrosarcoma protuberans (DFSP) is considered a low-grade sarcoma of the skin dermis (Box 27–8).

## Physical Examination

- DFSP may go undiagnosed for years because it often presents as a painless nodule in the forearm dermis.

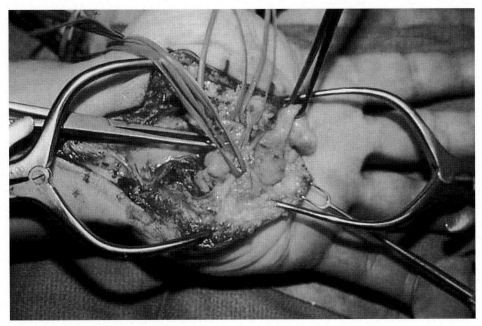

Figure 27–9:
**Large lipoma involving the palm.**

The lesion typically is characterized by overlying skin discoloration. It rarely occurs in the hand and wrist. In one series, the median age at diagnosis was 51 years.

- The tumor shares some histologic characteristics with fibrosarcoma, including slender spindle cells arranged in a storiform pattern.

## Operative Management

- With a surgical margin of 3 cm, including a deep fascial margin, high cure rates can be expected (see Figure 2, A, B).[2,12] Soft tissue coverage often is required following treatment of DFSP in the hand, wrist, and forearm. Inadequate margins lead to a high local recurrence rate with deeper tumor involvement.[2,12,13] Adjuvant radiation therapy may enhance control of the tumor.[14]

## Epithelioid Sarcoma

- Epithelioid sarcoma often is regarded as the most common soft tissue sarcoma of the hand and wrist.[2,15]

---

**Box 27–7**

- MRI can be diagnostic for lipomas because the lesions are of similar image intensity as surrounding fat.

---

**Box 27–8**

- DFSP is a low-grade sarcoma of the dermis with overlying skin pigmentation.
- The lesion may go undiagnosed for years.

---

## Physical Examination

- This tumor presents in a benign-appearing, slow-growing fashion. The tumor often is firm, typically affecting the digits, palm, or volar forearm. The median age in one study was 33 years, with an average delay in diagnosis of 18 months.[16]
- Histologically, epithelial cells are identified with a central region of necrosis.
- All too often these tumors are misdiagnosed or overlooked altogether. Epithelioid sarcoma ultimately may ulcerate and drain, leading to the misdiagnosis of infection. Epithelioid sarcomas also may be mistaken for palmar fibromas or Dupuytren contracture (Box 27–9).[2]
- Metastatic spread to regional lymph nodes is common.[15]

## Radiographic Examination

- MRI may reveal greater tumor involvement than originally thought, as spread along soft tissue planes is common.[2]

## Operative Management

- Treatment must include a wide or radical excision with sentinel lymph node sampling. In 55 patients reviewed retrospectively, a decreasing recurrence rate was seen with increasing aggressiveness of surgical resection.[17]

---

**Box 27–9**

- Epithelioid sarcomas often ulcerate and drain, leading to a misdiagnosis of infection.

Inadequate surgical margins, increasing tumor size, tumor necrosis of more than 30%, and vascular invasion may correlate with a high recurrence rate, a worse prognosis, or both.[15,17] External beam radiation or brachytherapy may be considered for local control of recurrent or larger lesions.[2] However, radiation does not compensate for inadequate surgical margins.

## Fibrosarcoma

### Physical Examination

- The clinical presentation of fibrosarcoma often can be obscure. This slow-growing, generally painless mass of the connective tissues may go undiagnosed for years (Figure 27–10). The average delay in diagnosis was 3 years in one study, and the average age at time of presentation was approximately 48 years.[18]
- The spindle cells arranged in a herringbone pattern with varying degrees of mitotic activity characterize the histology of the lesion (Box 27–10).

### Operative Management

- Wide or radical margins with adjuvant external beam radiation can be expected to yield low local recurrence rates and 5-year disease-free survival approaching 80%.[19,20] Limb salvage reconstructive surgery often is necessary. The most common site of metastatic involvement is the lung. Use of chemotherapy is generally recommended for locally extensive disease, high-grade tumors, or metastatic disease.

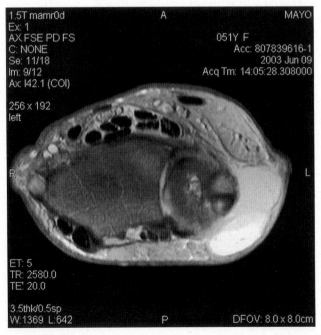

Figure 27–10:
**Fibrosarcoma of the ulnar border of the wrist in a 51-year-old schoolteacher.**

---

**Box 27–10**

- Fibrosarcoma is characterized histologically by spindle-shaped fibroblasts with varying degrees of mitotic activity, arranged in a herringbone pattern.

## Congenital Fibrosarcoma

- Congenital fibrosarcoma is a distinct clinical entity.[21,22] Approximately 90% of these tumors are present by the age of 3 months.[21] The hand, wrist, and forearm are common locations. These tumors may grow rapidly and can reach substantial size. Fortunately, a 5-year survival rate approaching 85% has been documented following treatment with wide excision.[21] The role of chemotherapy and radiation therapy is not clearly defined.

## Liposarcoma

- Liposarcoma can be divided into five different subtypes: well differentiated, myxoid, round cell, dedifferentiated, and pleomorphic.[2,23] The Air Force Institute of Pathology (AFIP) reported 10.6% of 1067 cases of liposarcoma arose in the upper extremity.[24]

### Physical Examination

- Patients typically present because of rapidly enlarging, painful masses of sizable proportions (Box 27–11). These tumors are seen most often during the sixth decade of life, with the exception of the myxoid and round cell varieties, which are tumors of younger adults. Considered together, the myxoid and round cell varieties compose more than half of all liposarcomas. Liposarcomas in infants are almost never seen.
- The myxoid liposarcoma is characterized histologically by a plexiform vascular latticework housing peripheral lipoblasts.
- Wide excision or amputation with adjuvant radiation therapy is the treatment of choice for liposarcomas in the adult. In high-grade lesions or lesions with associated metastatic spread, adjuvant chemotherapy should be considered. In one study of myxoid/round cell liposarcomas, 35% of patients developed metastasis and 31% ultimately died.[25] Patient age older than 45 years and presence of tumor necrosis were among the clinical features correlating with a poorer prognosis.[25]

## Malignant Fibrous Histiocytoma

- Considering all the extremities, malignant fibrous histiocytoma (MFH) is regarded as the most common soft

---

**Box 27–11**

- Liposarcomas typically present as rapidly enlarging, painful masses often reaching sizable proportions.

tissue sarcoma. MFH usually presents in the sixth to eighth decade of life,[23,26] but earlier presentation is well recognized. Although regarded by some as the most common sarcoma of the upper extremity, MFH has rarely been reported in the hand.[2,23]

### Physical Examination

- These tumors may present painlessly and go undiagnosed for months (Figure 27–11). The MFH may be first noticed following trauma, and rapid enlargement may occur. Often patients consider the mass to result from a coincident trauma and do not seek medical attention for months.
- Histologically MFH is composed of spindle-shaped fibroblasts arranged in a storiform pattern. Numerous atypical mitotic figures may be seen, along with multiple vascular channels, pleomorphism, and nuclear pyknosis (Box 27–12).

### Operative Management

- Resection with wide surgical margins and aggressive adjuvant therapies have lessened recurrence rates and improved survival. In one study, the local recurrence rate was 19%, metastatic rate 35%, and 5-year survival 65%.[27] The lung is the most common site of metastasis. Bone metastasis from soft tissue MFH is less common, and lymph nodal metastasis is unusual. Tumor size, depth, and histologic grade seem to correlate with metastatic rate and ultimate survival.[26,27]

## Rhabdomyosarcoma

- Rhabdomyosarcoma is the most common soft tissue sarcoma of children and young adults (Box 27–13).

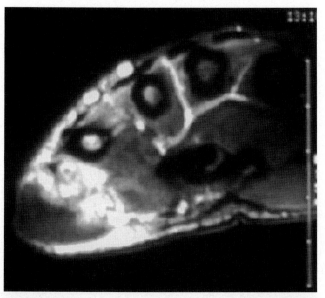

**Figure 27–11:**
**Malignant fibrous histiocytoma of the hypothenar aspect of the hand in 16-year-old patient diagnosed after a fall on an outstretched hand.**

---

> ### Box 27–12
>
> - MFH is characterized histologically by pleomorphic cells arranged in a storiform pattern.

The average age at diagnosis is 8 years.[24] Approximately 7% of rhabdomyosarcomas occur in the upper extremity. Hand involvement has been reported[2,24] but is extremely rare.

### Physical Examination

- These tumors can present as rapidly enlarging, painful masses. Much like liposarcoma in the adult, these tumors can achieve substantial size. The rhabdosarcoma is a tumor of skeletal muscle that is deep seated and hard. The diagnosis of rhabdomyosarcoma often is preceded by a history of trauma. Lesions involving the hand may be smaller in size and painless, with the most common location being the thenar eminence or the metacarpal interosseous spaces.
- Rhabdomyosarcomas can be divided histologically into four subtypes: embryonal, alveolar, botryoid, and pleomorphic. The alveolar variety is the most common subtype found in the upper extremity. The alveolar subtype is generally regarded as having the worst prognosis.
- The lung and lymph nodes are the most common metastatic locations. Sentinel node biopsy is helpful to rule out regional lymph node involvement. Unfortunately, metastatic involvement is present in approximately 20% of cases at presentation.[28]

### Operative Management

- Treatment is surgical excision with wide or radical margins, followed by limb salvage surgery if feasible. Survival from rhabdomyosarcoma is improving because of the use of chemotherapeutic agents such as vincristine, actinomycin-D, cyclophosphamide, and doxorubicin (Adriamycin) plus cisplatin, as well as high-dose methotrexate,[2,29] followed by hematopoietic cell rescue. External beam radiation has been shown to be effective in improving survival. Disease-free 5-year survival approaching 70% has been reported.[30]

## Synovial Cell Sarcoma

- Some authors regard synovial cell sarcoma, rather than epithelial sarcoma, the most common soft tissue sarcoma of the hand and wrist.[31]

---

> ### Box 27–13
>
> - Rhabdomyosarcoma is the most common soft tissue sarcoma of children and young adults.

## Physical Examination

- These tumors are slow-growing, painless, solid masses. They may be present for months to years before diagnosis is made. They arise in proximity to joints or bursae as opposed to within the joint as the name implies. In the hand and wrist, synovial cell sarcoma is most commonly found in proximity to the carpus (Box 27–14). Synovial cell sarcoma most often affects patients aged 15 to 40 years.
- Histologically, the tumor has a biphasic pattern composed of epithelial cells and spindle cells. The tumor is classified as biphasic type, monophasic fibrous type, monophasic epithelial type, or poorly differentiated.

## Operative Management

- Treatment is surgical with wide or radical margins, followed by adjuvant chemotherapy and external beam radiation therapy. Chemotherapeutic agents such as Adriamycin and ifosfamide have been successful. Five-year survival rates as high as 82% have been reported following surgical excision, but local recurrence is common.[32]

# Treatment and Outcome of Soft Tissue Sarcoma

- Limb-sparing tumor resection with adjuvant radiotherapy is preferred over amputation as the primary treatment for high-grade soft tissue sarcomas of the upper limb (Box 27–15). Because of the complex anatomy of the hand and wrist, a "radical" tumor resection in this region means an above-the-elbow amputation in most instances. Therefore, limb salvage considerations are important in the treatment of the upper extremity sarcoma. In general, the more distal the soft tissue sarcoma, the more likely amputation will be the more appropriate treatment (Box 27–16).

---

**Box 27–14**

- Synovial cell sarcomas arise in proximity to joints and bursae.
- In the hand and wrist it is most often found about the carpus.

---

**Box 27–15**

- Limb-sparing tumor resection surgery with adjuvant radiotherapy is preferred over amputation for high-grade soft tissue sarcoma of the upper limb.

---

**Box 27–16**

- Although limb salvage surgery is preferred, the more distal the location of the soft tissue sarcoma, the more likely amputation will be the more appropriate surgical treatment.

---

- In the case of soft tissue sarcomas affecting the distal digits, adequate surgical margins can be obtained under most circumstances by disarticulations at the DIP or PIP joints. For more proximal digital involvement, single or double ray amputations may be necessary. Microscopically negative surgical margins of at least 3 cm are preferred but cannot always be obtained. Forearm-level amputation may be necessary for lesions of the carpal tunnel. Use of "tumor barriers," such as the distal radius or the extensor retinaculum, may permit limb salvage when lesions are identified on the dorsum of the wrist. When needed, free tissue transfer options include contralateral radial forearm flap, contralateral lateral arm flap, and rectus abdominus flap. Local pedicled flaps must be considered carefully in the reconstruction following soft tissue sarcoma resection surgery because of concerns over tumor cross contamination.
- Well-controlled prospective trials have demonstrated equivalent 5-year survival among soft tissue sarcoma patients treated by amputation alone or limb salvage with external beam radiation (Box 27–17). The relative merits of preoperative irradiation versus postoperative external beam radiation for soft tissue sarcomas have been debated. Postoperative radiation therapy currently is favored in most situations if the tumor is radiosensitive. Preoperative radiation has the theoretical advantage of creating tumor necrosis and therefore decreasing tumor bulk. A tumor pseudocapsule is created, enhancing the possibility of limb salvage with negative surgical margins. Also, with preoperative radiation therapy, less radiation exposure typically is needed compared to postoperative radiation therapy.
- There is, however, a higher postoperative wound complication rate following neoadjuvant radiation therapy (Box 27–18). One soft tissue sarcoma study found quadruple the wound complication rate for patients receiving preoperative irradiation compared to patients receiving postoperative irradiation (31% vs. 8%).[20] Preoperative radiation therapy typically has been reserved for patients with a tumor located where standard wide resection techniques and limb salvage surgery are mutually prohibitive. An example is a

---

**Box 27–17**

- Studies have demonstrated equivalent 5-year survival between soft tissue sarcoma patients treated by amputation alone and patients treated by limb-sparing surgery and adjuvant external beam radiation.

---

**Box 27–18**

- A higher postoperative wound complication rate can be expected following the use of preoperative external beam radiation.

high-grade soft tissue sarcoma close to a major nerve or vessel.

- Recommended total postoperative radiation doses for soft tissue sarcomas are 50 to 70 Gy, with the first 45 Gy covering all possible fields of tumor spread. The upper end of this range is used in patients with microscopically positive surgical margins, with the lower end of this spread indicated in patients with microscopically negative margins. Preoperative irradiation doses typically are in the 45- to 50-Gy range given in fractions over 3 to 6 weeks. Following the conclusion of preoperative irradiation, surgery is delayed for at least 3 weeks to allow some recovery of the soft tissues. By limiting the field of radiation for soft tissue sarcomas of the hand and by initiating early, aggressive hand therapy, postradiation sequelae such as edema and stiffness can be minimized or even eliminated.

- Many believe that substantial sparing of surrounding normal tissues can be accomplished with brachytherapy. This technique uses multiple small catheters placed 1 cm apart throughout the wound (Figure 27–12). Commonly used isotopes include iridium 192 and iodine 125. These catheters can deliver specific quantities of the radioisotope directly to the tumor bed following surgical excision of the tumor. The catheters are placed at the time of surgery, but radiation is not delivered until 6 days postoperative to allow for wound healing. Decreased treatment time, diminished normal tissue irradiation, lower radiation doses, and less expense are theoretical advantages (Box 27–19).

- Adjuvant chemotherapy for treatment of soft tissue sarcomas remains controversial. More favorable results have been reported with neoadjuvant use of certain chemotherapeutic agents, particularly when used in combination with radiation therapy. Many of these

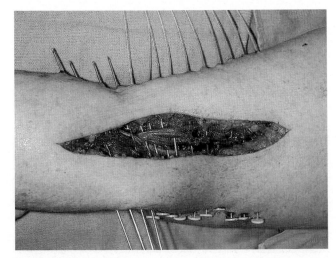

**Figure 27–12:**
**Brachytherapy tubes in place for delivery of radiation directly to the antecubital fossa.**

---

**Box 27–19**

- Theoretical advantages of brachytherapy include diminished normal tissue irradiation and lower doses.

---

chemotherapy protocols remain in the clinical trial phase and are subject to frequent modification.

- With limb salvage surgery techniques and adjuvant radiation therapy, 75% to 80% 5-year survival can be expected for many soft tissue sarcomas of the upper limb, with 85% to 95% of patients having sustained local control (Box 27–20).[20] These success rates can drop precipitously in the presence of positive surgical margins. Hand soft tissue sarcoma tumor size greater than 5 cm had a worse prognosis in one study.[33] Ultimate survival, however, is dependent on tumor grade, size, depth, and stage (Box 27–21).[19]

## Follow-Up Care for Patients with Soft Tissue Sarcoma

- Following definitive surgical management of soft tissue sarcoma, patients should be reevaluated at 4-month intervals for 3 years with chest CT, abdominal CT, and regional MRI examinations. Thereafter, if no recurrence has developed, the patient can be followed at 6-month intervals for 2 additional years with imaging studies. At the 5-year mark, the follow-up is individualized, with the majority having yearly follow-up with imaging studies.

## Tumors of Skin

- Skin cancers are the most common form of cancer in the United Stated, affecting one million people annually.

- As a group, skin cancers are the most common form of cancer in the hand and upper extremity.

- Host and environmental factors contribute to the risk of developing skin carcinomas and include sun exposure, fair skin, male gender, and advancing age.

- Cumulative lifetime ultraviolet (UV) light exposure and recent UV exposure are risks factors for nonmelanotic

---

**Box 27–20**

- With limb salvage surgery and adjuvant radiation therapy, 75% to 80% 5-year survival can be achieved for certain soft tissue sarcomas of the upper limb.

---

**Box 27–21**

- Ultimate survival from soft tissue sarcomas of the upper limb depends on tumor grade, size, depth, and stage.

skin carcinomas, whereas intermittent intense episodes of UV light are responsible for the development of malignant melanomas (Box 27–22).

## Actinic Keratosis

- Common premalignant skin lesion, caused by cumulative UV light exposure, also is known as *solar keratosis*.
- Most commonly seen in older, light-complexioned individuals.

### Physical Examination

- Multiple hyperkeratotic, scaly lesions are seen most commonly in atrophic, sun damaged skin.
- Actinic keratosis may be red or brown and rough in texture.

### Treatment

- Treatment is nonsurgical and includes 5-fluorouracil, chemical peel therapy, dermabrasion, electrodesiccation, or liquid nitrogen.
- Without treatment, an estimated 25% of actinic keratosis progress to invasive squamous cell carcinoma.

## Basal Cell Carcinoma

- Occurs mainly in middle-age to elderly, light-skinned individuals.
- Basal cell carcinomas arise from the basilar cell layer of the epithelium or from the hair follicle external root sheath.
- Up to 26 histologic subtypes of basal cell carcinomas exist, with the nodular and superficial types being the most common.

### Physical Examination

- Basal cell carcinomas present as slow-growing, irregular, often erosive or ulcerative tumors in areas of atrophic skin, frequently highlighted by red or brownish discoloration.

### Treatment

- Primary treatment of basal cell carcinoma of the hand and upper extremity is surgical, with 5-mm margins achieved and simple closure performed (Box 27–23).

- Mohs micrographic surgery can be considered for upper extremity basal cell carcinomas when more aggressive features are present. The advantage of Mohs surgery in these circumstances is the possibility of surrounding tissue conservation.
- Alternative surgical treatment techniques include electrodesiccation and curettage, cryosurgery, and laser phototherapy. These techniques are best indicated for superficial lesions or for patients who are poor surgical candidates given that pathologic tissue examination is not possible because of the destructive nature of these treatments.
- Reported cure rates for primary surgical excision, Mohs micrographic surgery, or the alternative surgical techniques range from 94% to 99%.
- Medical management for basal cell carcinoma includes intralesional interferon injection, chemotherapy, and radiotherapy. Cure rates with these therapies are generally considered less favorable.
- Incompletely excised basal cell carcinomas have a high recurrence rate.

## Squamous Cell Carcinoma

- Squamous cell carcinoma is the most common malignancy of the hand, with the dorsum of the hand the most common location. Approximately 16% of all squamous cell tumors arise in the upper extremity (Box 27–24).[34]
- These tumors are most commonly seen in elderly men.
- Squamous cell carcinoma is the most common malignancy of the nail bed, often misdiagnosed as trauma or infection.
- Squamous cell carcinomas typically arise in areas of premalignant conditions, such as sun-damaged skin, actinic keratosis, chronic ulcers, or draining sinuses.
- The primary risk factor is extensive solar radiation.

### Physical Examination

- Squamous cell carcinomas may present as small, scaly, discolored skin lesions or as large ulcerating masses.
- A careful lymph node examination of the upper extremity is mandatory because of the high metastatic potential of squamous cell carcinoma (Box 27–25).

---

**Box 27–22**

- Risk factors for skin cancers are sun exposure, fair skin, male gender, and advancing age.

**Box 27–23**

- Primary surgical treatment is preferred for basal cell carcinomas of the upper extremity, with acquisition of a 5-mm margin.

**Box 27–24**

- Squamous cell carcinoma is the most common malignancy of the hand.

**Box 27–25**

- A careful lymph node examination is critical in the examination of a patient with suspected skin cancer.

- Squamous cell carcinoma of the subungual region often presents with pain and discoloration. Secondary infections may be present at time of presentation.

### Treatment

- Squamous cell carcinomas are more aggressive than basal cell carcinomas and have a high metastatic potential. Therefore, squamous cell carcinoma is treated by either wide surgical excision or Mohs micrographic surgery.
- For lesions up to and including 3 cm, recommendations for surgical margins vary from 0.5 to 1 cm. For lesions larger than 3 cm, margins of 1 cm are recommended. More aggressive treatment is preferred for recurrent lesions or lesions showing evidence of ulceration or invasion.
- Superficial subungual lesions often can be managed by excision with a 1-cm margin and full-thickness skin grafting directly to the distal phalanx. More invasive or recurrent lesions are best managed by distal phalanx disarticulation (Box 27–26).

## Malignant Melanoma

- The incidence of malignant melanoma is increasing at an alarming rate, with the number of new diagnosed cases doubling every 10 years. The etiology of the condition is unknown, but intermittent, excessive sun exposure plays a role.
- The incidence of melanoma is greater in the more sun-exposed areas of the United States.
- The most common subtype of melanoma is the superficial spreading type. Acrolentigenous melanoma is more commonly found in the palm and subungual region.

### Physical Examination

- The diagnosis of melanoma usually can be made clinically, but any unusual or concerning skin lesion deserves a biopsy. A thorough examination of the epitrochlear and axillary lymph nodes must be performed.
- The physical examination findings of melanoma follow an ABCD rule:

  **A**symmetry of the lesion
  **B**order irregularity
  **C**olor dishomogeneity
  **D**iameters in excess of 6 mm

- CT scanning of the head, neck, chest, and abdomen generally are included in the workup, along with PET scanning and sentinel node biopsy.

- Frozen section is never relied upon to determine the presence or absence of melanoma because histologic diagnosis can be challenging. Tumor thickness is critically important as a prognostic factor for melanoma (Box 27–27).

### Treatment

- Treatment of melanoma is wide surgical resection. In general, 1 cm of negative resected skin margin is recommended for every 1-mm depth of melanoma. No more than a 3-cm margin is necessary, except in extraordinary circumstances.
- Lesions in the digits often are treated with ray amputation or proximal/distal interphalangeal joint disarticulation.[35] Treatment of metastatic melanoma is decidedly disappointing. Response to chemotherapy and radiation therapy is poor (Boxes 27–28 and 27–29).

## Summary

- Benign tumors are much more common than malignant tumors in the hand, wrist, and forearm. Soft tissue sarcomas occur only rarely. A delay in diagnosis is typical for soft tissue sarcomas of the upper extremity. Despite appropriate treatment, delays in diagnosis can lead to local recurrence, metastatic disease, and lessened ultimate survival.
- The current standard for imaging of suspicious soft tissue lesions is MRI. A full tumor workup should be obtained for any lesion that appears suspicious for malignancy. The most important step in any tumor workup is the biopsy. The biopsy should be performed through a longitudinal incision that can be incorporated in the definitive limb salvage exposure.
- Ganglion cysts, epidermal inclusion cysts, and giant cell tumors of tendon sheath are the more common benign lesions of the upper extremity. MFH is the most common

**Box 27–27**

- Frozen section is never relied upon for diagnosis of malignant melanoma.

**Box 27–28**

- Digital malignant melanoma lesions are often best treated with ray amputation or interphalangeal joint disarticulation.

**Box 27–26**

- Margins of 1 cm typically are recommended for surgical excision of squamous cell carcinoma.

**Box 27–29**

- Treatment of melanoma of the upper extremity is surgical, with acquisition of a 1- to 3-cm margin depending on lesion depth.

soft tissue sarcoma of the upper limb in general, whereas epithelioid sarcoma or synovial sarcoma is considered the most common soft tissue sarcoma of the hand and wrist.

- Benign soft tissue lesions of the upper extremity can, in most circumstances, be excised by marginal excision. The preferred treatment combination for high-grade soft tissue sarcomas of the upper extremity is wide resection, limb-sparing surgical reconstruction, and adjuvant radiation therapy. No survival benefit is obtained from preoperative radiation, and wound complications are significantly higher. Brachytherapy may provide equal or better local tumor control than external beam radiation therapy at less expense, while using less radiation and causing less collateral tissue damage. Overall survival from soft tissue sarcoma, however, is not improved with brachytherapy.

- The role of chemotherapy in the treatment of soft tissue sarcomas remains controversial. For many soft tissue sarcomas, 5-year survival rates following limb sparing surgery and adjuvant radiation therapy can approach 80%.

# References

1. Mankin HJ, Mankin CJ, Simon MA: The hazards of the biopsy, revisited. Members of the Musculoskeletal Tumor Society. *J Bone Joint Surg Am* 78:656-663, 1996.
   Among 597 musculoskeletal oncology patients treated at 21 different institutions, errors in diagnosis and changes in management were two to 12 times more likely to occur at the referring institution as opposed to the treating institution.

2. Athanasian EA: Bone and soft tissue tumors. In Green DP, Hotchkiss RN, Pederson WC editors: *Green's operative hand surgery,* ed 4. New York, 1999, Churchill Livingstone.
   This is a comprehensive review of the more commonly encountered bone and soft tissue tumors.

3. el-Noueam KI, Schweitzer ME, Blasbalg R, et al: Is a subset of wrist ganglia the sequela of internal derangements of the wrist joint? MR imaging findings. *Radiology* 212:537-540, 1999.
   Among MRI images of 625 patients with wrist ganglia, 28% of 97 radial-sided ganglia had associated ligament tears, suggesting that in certain circumstances ganglia may represent a secondary sign of wrist internal derangement.

4. Stephen AB, Lyons AR, Davis TR: A prospective study of two conservative treatments for ganglia of the wrist. *J Hand Surg [Br]* 24:104-105, 1999.
   One hundred nineteen patients with ganglions were treated with either aspiration or a multiple puncture technique, with aspiration leading to a slightly lower recurrence rate.

5. Rizzo M, Berger RA, Steinmann SP, Bishop AT: Arthroscopic resection in the management of dorsal wrist ganglions: results with a minimum 2-year follow-up period. *J Hand Surg [Am]* 29:59-62, 2004.
   Forty-two patients were followed-up at an average of 47.8 months following arthroscopic removal of symptomatic dorsal wrist ganglion cysts.

6. Thornburg LE: Ganglions of the hand and wrist. *J Am Acad Orthop Surg* 7:231-238, 1999.
   This review article covers the entire subject of diagnosis and treatment of ganglion cysts about the hand and wrist.

7. Al-Qattan MM: Giant cell tumours of tendon sheath: classification and recurrence rate. *J Hand Surg [Br]* 26:72-75, 2001.
   43 patients with giant cell tumor of tendon sheath were treated prospectively and followed for a mean of 4 years.

8. Yakes WF, Rossi P, Odink H: How I do it. Arteriovenous malformation management. *Cardiovasc Intervent Radiol* 19:65-71, 1996.
   Twenty patients with symptomatic arteriovenous malformations were embolized using absolute alcohol, with 19 of the 20 patients showing persistent occlusion at follow-up.

9. Kuiper DR, Hoekstra HJ, Veth RP, Wobbes T: The management of clear cell sarcoma. *Eur J Surg Oncol* 29:568-570, 2003.
   The surgical experience treating clear cell sarcoma at two university hospitals is presented.

10. Chung EB, Enzinger FM: Malignant melanoma of soft parts. A reassessment of clear cell sarcoma. *Am J Surg Pathol* 7:405-413, 1983.
    In this study of 141 patients with clear cell sarcoma, delay in diagnosis and recurrences were common.

11. Ferrari A, Casanova M, Bisogno G, et al: Clear cell sarcoma of tendons and aponeuroses in pediatric patients: a report from the Italian and German Soft Tissue Sarcoma Cooperative Group. *Cancer* 94:3269-3276, 2002.
    Twenty-eight pediatric patients with clear cell sarcoma were treated with multimodal therapeutic approach, with 5-year and event-free survival of 66.4% and 63.3% respectively.

12. Parker TL, Zitelli JA: Surgical margins for excision of dermatofibrosarcoma protuberans. *J Am Acad Dermatol* 32:233-236, 1995.
    Twenty patients with DFSP were studied to determine appropriate surgical margins. The authors found that a 2.5-cm margin cleared all tumors studied.

13. Khatri VP, Galante JM, Bold RJ, et al: Dermatofibrosarcoma protuberans: reappraisal of wide local excision and impact of inadequate initial treatment. *Ann Surg Oncol* 10:1118-1122, 2003.
    In a study of 35 patients with DFSP, the authors conclude that inadequate initial treatment results in larger recurrent lesions.

14. Suit H, Spiro I, Mankin HJ, et al: Radiation in management of patients with dermatofibrosarcoma protuberans. *J Clin Oncol* 14:2365-2369, 1996.
    The authors conclude that radiation alone is an effective alternative for treatment for patients with DFSP.

15. Steinberg BD, Gelberman RH, Mankin HJ, Rosenberg AE: Epithelioid sarcoma in the upper extremity. *J Bone Joint Surg Am* 74:28-35, 1992.
    Eighteen patients with epithelioid sarcoma of the upper extremity were treated with marginal or wide surgical excision, with disease-free survival markedly better following wide excision.

16. Ross HM, Lewis JJ, Woodruff JM, Brennan MF: Epithelioid sarcoma: clinical behavior and prognostic factors of survival. *Ann Surg Oncol* 4:491-495, 1997.
    Sixteen patients with epithelioid sarcoma were prospectively followed.

17. Halling AC, Wollan PC, Pritchard DJ, et al: Epithelioid sarcoma: a clinicopathologic review of 55 cases. *Mayo Clin Proc* 71:636-642, 1996.
    In a review of 55 cases of epithelioid sarcoma, the authors found that the recurrence rate decreased with increased aggressiveness of tumor resection.

18. Pritchard DJ, Sim FH, Ivins JC, et al: Fibrosarcoma of bone and soft tissue of the trunk and extremities. *Orthop Clin North Am* 8:869-881, 1977.
    The authors reviewed 199 patients with soft tissue fibrosarcomas and recommend wide ablative surgery for adults with soft tissue fibrosarcoma.

19. Gibbs CP, Peabody TD, Mundt AJ, et al: Oncological outcomes of operative treatment of subcutaneous soft-tissue sarcomas of the extremities. *J Bone Joint Surg Am* 79:888-897, 1997.
    Sixty-two patients with subcutaneous soft tissue sarcomas were evaluated following treatment with wide surgical margins.

20. Cheng EY, Dusenbery KE, Winters MR, Thompson RC: Soft tissue sarcomas: preoperative versus postoperative radiotherapy. *J Surg Oncol* 61:90-99, 1996.
    One hundred twelve patients with nonmetastatic soft tissue sarcomas were treated with limb-sparing surgery and either preoperative or postoperative radiotherapy.

21. Chung EB, Enzinger FM: Infantile fibrosarcoma. *Cancer* 38:729-739, 1976.
    In a review of 53 cases of infantile fibrosarcomas, the authors recommend wide local excision as the treatment of choice.

22. Soule EH, Pritchard DJ: Fibrosarcoma in infants and children: a review of 110 cases. *Cancer* 40:1711-1721, 1977.
    In a review of 110 children with fibrosarcoma, the authors recommend local excision of the tumor in patients younger than 5 years.

23. Murray PM: Soft tissue neoplasms: Benign and malignant. In Trumble T, editor: *Hand surgery update: a guide to the hand, elbow and shoulder.* Rosemont, IL, 2003, American Society for Surgery of the Hand.
    An update of the current treatment recommendations for the more common benign and malignant tumors of the upper extremity

24. Lattes R, Stout AP, Armed Forces Institute of Pathology (U.S.), et al. Tumors of the soft tissues. In: *Atlas of tumor pathology, 2nd ser., fasc. 1, Rev.* Washington, DC, 1982, Armed Forces Institute of Pathology under the auspices of Universities Associated for Research and Education in Pathology.
    A comprehensive review text of tumors of the soft tissues.

25. Kilpatrick SE, Doyon J, Choong PF, et al: The clinicopathologic spectrum of myxoid and round cell liposarcoma. A study of 95 cases. *Cancer* 77:1450-1458, 1996.
    Ninety-five patients with myxoid or round cell liposarcoma were reviewed between 1970 and 1992.

26. Enzinger FM, Weiss SW: Malignant fibrohistocytic tumors. In Weiss SW, Goldblum JR, Enzinger FM, editors: *Enzinger and Weiss's soft tissue tumors,* ed 4. St. Louis, 2001, Mosby.
    This comprehensive chapter reviews the clinical behavior, histologic characteristics, and treatment alternatives of malignant fibrohistocytic tumors of the extremities.

27. Salo JC, Lewis JJ, Woodruff JM, et al: Malignant fibrous histiocytoma of the extremity. *Cancer* 85:1765-1772, 1999.
    Among 239 patients undergoing surgical excision of malignant fibrous histiocytoma, 5- and 10-year disease-free survival rates were 65% and 59%, with age older than 50 years, local recurrence, and tumors greater than 5 cm associated with an unfavorable outcome.

28. Lawrence W Jr, Gehan EA, Hays DM, et al: Prognostic significance of staging factors of the UICC staging system in childhood rhabdomyosarcoma: a report from the Intergroup Rhabdomyosarcoma Study (IRS-II). *J Clin Oncol* 5:46-54, 1987.
    Five hundred five patients were enrolled in the intergroup rhabdomyosarcoma study group and were retrospectively reviewed.

29. Pappo AS, Bowman LC, Furman WL, et al: A phase II trial of high-dose methotrexate in previously untreated children and adolescents with high-risk unresectable or metastatic rhabdomyosarcoma. *J Pediatr Hematol Oncol* 19:438-442, 1997.
    Fifteen patients with unresectable rhabdomyosarcoma received high-dose methotrexate along with multiagent chemotherapy and local agent chemotherapy.

30. Pappo AS, Shapiro DN, Crist WM: Rhabdomyosarcoma. Biology and treatment. *Pediatr Clin North Am* 44:953-972, 1997.
    Rhabdomyosarcoma is the most common soft tissue sarcoma of childhood. Cure rates with multimodal therapy approach 70%.

31. Brien EW, Terek RM, Geer RJ, et al: Treatment of soft-tissue sarcomas of the hand. *J Bone Joint Surg Am* 77:564-571, 1995.
    Twenty-three patients treated for soft tissue sarcoma of the hand were followed retrospectively at 49 months.

32. Varela-Duran J, Enzinger FM: Calcifying synovial sarcoma. *Cancer* 50:345-352, 1982.
    Thirty-two patients with calcifying synovial sarcoma showed a more favorable prognosis than synovial cell sarcoma without calcification.

33. Gustafson P, Arner M: Soft tissue sarcoma of the upper extremity: descriptive data and outcome in a population-based series of 108 adult patients. *J Hand Surg [Am]* 24:668-674, 1999.
    In a review of 108 patients, the authors conclude that soft tissue tumors of the upper extremity are smaller at diagnosis and carry a more favorable prognosis than similar lesions of the trunk and lower extremity.

34. Chakrabarti I, Watson JD, Dorrance H: Skin tumours of the hand. A 10-year review. *J Hand Surg [Br]* 18:484-486, 1993.
    Among 98 skin lesions in 85 patients studied over a 10-year period, the most common tumor was squamous cell carcinoma.

35. Park KG, Blessing K, Kernohan NM: Surgical aspects of subungual malignant melanomas. The Scottish Melanoma Group. *Ann Surg* 216:692-695, 1992.
    Among 100 cases of subungual melanoma, the overall 5-year survival was only 41% regardless of level of amputation.

# 28

# Bone Tumors: Benign and Malignant

David P. Moss[*] and Keith B. Raskin[†]

[*]MD, BA, Senior Resident, Department of Orthopaedic Surgery, New York University School of Medicine, Hospital for Joint Diseases, New York, NY
[†]Clinical Associate Professor of Orthopaedic Surgery, New York University School of Medicine; Former Chief of Hand Surgery, New York University Medical Center, New York, NY

## Introduction

- Primary bone tumors can be classified into three categories[1]:
  - Benign bone tumors
  - Malignant bone tumors or sarcomas (malignant neoplasms of mesenchymal origin)
  - Lesions that imitate bone tumors, such as cystic lesions and Brown tumor
- Lesions that present in bone but are not of mesenchymal origin include metastatic bone disease, myeloma, and lymphoma (Table 28–1).

## History

- Patients with bone tumors often complain of deep, dull pain. Pain may be intermittent, constant, occur at night, or associated with certain activities.
- It is important to ask of factors that relieve the pain. The pain related to osteoid osteoma, for example, is classically relieved with nonsteroidal antiinflammatory drugs (NSAIDs). Patients with more aggressive lesions usually present with a shorter duration of pain, whereas patients with benign lesions may describe a longer history of pain.
- Prior history of cancer or a family history of cancer should be obtained, paying particular attention to lesions that frequently metastasize to bone, including prostate, breast, renal, thyroid, and lung carcinoma.

### Table 28–1: Common Benign and Malignant Bone Lesions of the Upper Extremity

| BENIGN | MALIGNANT |
|---|---|
| Enchondroma | Chondrosarcoma |
| Unicameral bone cyst | Osteogenic sarcoma |
| Aneurysmal bone cyst | Angiosarcoma |
| Osteochondroma | Ewing sarcoma |
| Osteoid osteoma | Lymphoma of bone |
| Osteoblastoma | Myeloma |
| Giant cell tumor of bone | Metastases |
| Fibrous dysplasia | |
| Chondroblastoma | |

- The patient's age is extremely important in making a diagnosis.
  - Most primary bone tumors occur in younger patient populations.
  - Metastases are more common in those older than 50 years.
- Males have a slightly higher incidence than females of primary bone tumors, with the exception of giant cell tumors, which are slightly more common in females.[2]

## Physical Examination

- Examine the area of concern for an extraosseous or soft tissue component and overlying skin changes. Adenopathy is rare in musculoskeletal neoplasms.
- With metastatic disease, the appropriate organ system should be evaluated.
- All masses in the hand should be evaluated for the presence of a pulse, because arterial aneurysms are relatively common. Cystic masses may transilluminate (Tables 28–2 and 28–3).

| Table 28–2: | Differential Diagnosis of an Upper Extremity Mass |
| --- | --- |
| Tumor/neoplasm | |
| Infection | |
| Inflammatory process | |
| Metabolic disorder | |
| Vascular malformation | |
| Trauma | |

| Table 28–3: | Common Ages of Presentation and Most Common Locations in the Upper Extremity of Select Tumors | |
| --- | --- | --- |
| **TUMOR** | **AGE (Yr)** | **LOCATION** |
| Enchondroma | 10–30 | Hand, proximal humerus |
| Unicameral bone cyst | 5–10 | Proximal humerus |
| Aneurysmal bone cyst | 5–20 | Humerus |
| Osteochondroma | 10–35 | Hand |
| Osteoid osteoma | 10–35 | Carpus, proximal phalanges |
| Osteoblastoma | 5–25 | Proximal humerus |
| Giant cell tumor of bone | 20–40 | Distal radius |
| Fibrous dysplasia | 2–30 | Phalanges, metacarpals |
| Chondroblastoma | 2–20 | Proximal humerus |
| Chondrosarcoma | >60 | Shoulder girdle, hand |
| Osteogenic sarcoma | 5–15 | Hand |
| Angiosarcoma | 20–40 | Metacarpals, phalanges |
| Ewing sarcoma | 5–30 | Clavicle, proximal humerus |
| Lymphoma of bone | 30–60 | Shoulder girdle |
| Myeloma | >50 | Proximal humerus |
| Metastatic bone disease | >40 | Proximal humerus, hand |

## Imaging

- *Plain radiographs* of the entire affected bone in at least two planes and of the joints proximal and distal to the lesion should be obtained.
- A geographic pattern of bone destruction suggests a benign lesion, whereas moth-eaten or permeative patterns of bone destruction suggest a malignant process.
- The anatomic location of the lesion in both the long axis of the bone (diaphyseal, metaphyseal, or epiphyseal) and the transverse axis (central or eccentric) can aid in diagnosis. Giant cell tumors commonly begin in the metaphysis and extend to the epiphysis, whereas Ewing sarcomas are more common in the diaphysis.
- The presence of a periosteal reaction and/or soft tissue component should be noted.
- Cartilage-derived lesions can be differentiated from osteoid-derived lesions by the radiographic features of the matrix. Cartilage-derived matrix shows arcs and rings, whereas osteoid-derived matrix usually is cloud-like and fluffy.
- *Bone scan* can be used to identify the presence of other lesions or metastases.
- *Computed tomography* (CT) is the preferred imaging modality for evaluating the extent of bony involvement. *Magnetic resonance imaging* (MRI) is preferred for evaluation of soft tissue involvement.
- *Arteriography* may be indicated to determine vascular anatomy and pathology.
- *Ultrasonography* can be used to differentiate cystic from solid lesions.
- If malignancy is suspected, a chest x-ray film and/or chest CT scan should be obtained at the very least.

## Laboratory Tests

- An elevated erythrocyte sedimentation rate (ESR) is common in patients with round cell tumors.
- Metastases, metabolic bone disease, and Paget disease can elevate serum calcium. The clinical and radiographic appearance of metabolic bone disease can mimic neoplasms (Table 28–4).

## Staging

- Separate staging systems exist for benign and malignant lesions.
- Malignant tumors are divided into low-grade and high-grade lesions (Table 28–5).[2]
  - Low-grade ($G_1$)
    - Slow growth
    - Recognizable, mature stem cell
    - Few mitotic figures

| Table 28–4: | Indicated Laboratory Tests, Depending upon the Patient's Age and Gender | |
| --- | --- | --- |
| **AGE 5–40 YR** | **AGE 40–80 YR** | |
| CBC with differential | CBC with differential | |
| Peripheral blood smear | ESR | |
| ESR | Calcium and phosphate | |
| | Serum and urine protein electrophoresis | |
| | Urinalysis | |
| | Prostate specific antigen | |

CBC, Complete blood count; ESR, erythrocyte sedimentation rate.

| Table 28–5: | Staging of Malignant Tumors | |
| --- | --- | --- |
| **STAGE** | **GRADE** | **SITE** |
| IA | Low (G$_1$) | Intracompartmental (T$_1$) |
| IB | Low (G$_1$) | Extracompartmental (T$_2$) |
| IIA | High (G$_2$) | Intracompartmental (T$_1$) |
| IIB | High (G$_2$) | Extracompartmental (T$_2$) |

- High-grade (G$_2$)
  - Rapid growth
  - Primitive cells
  - High degree of cellularity
  - More mitotic figures

## Biopsy

- Minimizing the number of compartments violated is important to prevent possible tumor seeding of other compartments.
- Extensile incisions are used in open biopsies.
- Use of an Esmarch bandage to exsanguinate the limb should be avoided. Instead, the limb can be exsanguinated by 3 minutes of elevation while maintaining manual compression of the brachial artery and then inflating the tourniquet.
- Meticulous hemostasis is used to prevent hematoma formation.

## Benign Bone Tumors

### Enchondroma

#### Basics

- Enchondroma is a benign cartilage tumor of bone.
- *Prevalence:* Enchondroma is the most common benign tumor of bone[2] and the most common osseous tumor in the hand.[3]

- *Age:* Lesions usually appear in the skeletally mature in the second to fourth decades of life.
- *Presentation:* Most enchondromas are asymptomatic and are discovered incidentally. Patients may present after pathologic fracture, often associated with minimal trauma.
- *Location:* In the hand, the metacarpals and proximal and middle phalanges are most commonly involved. The proximal humerus also is commonly affected. Growth usually begins in the metaphysis, extending to the diaphysis. Involvement of the epiphysis is rare.
- Associated conditions:
  - Ollier disease is the presence of multiple enchondromas, also known as *multiple enchondromatosis*. There is a 30% risk of malignant transformation to chondrosarcoma.
  - Maffucci disease is multiple enchondromas and hemangiomas. The risk of malignant transformation to chondrosarcoma is 100%.[1]

### Imaging

- Radiographs can show symmetric fusiform expansion of the bone with endosteal scalloping and calcifications within the lesion (Figure 28–1).

### Histology

- Microscopically, benign cartilage is seen. High cellularity may be present in enchondromas of the hand, but no mitotic figures are seen. Lesions in the humerus usually are hypocellular (Figure 28–2).
- The pathologist should be informed of the specimen's source. A similar specimen from the pelvis may behave in a malignant manner.

### Treatment

- If the lesion is asymptomatic, particularly in the proximal humerus, it may be followed with serial radiographs to ensure a benign course.
- Recommended treatment is excision with curettage and bone grafting of the defect. In the hand, excision followed by internal fixation and bone cementing has shown good results at 2-year follow-up.[4]
- Histologically, acute and healing pathologic fracture callus in an enchondroma may be confused with low-grade chondrosarcoma. If the patient presents with a pathologic fracture, the fracture should be immobilized and healed before curettage and bone grafting is performed. In addition, immediate operative fixation has been shown to increase complication rates, including fracture angulation and loss of reduction.[5]
- An attempt should be made to treat unstable or malaligned fractures with closed reduction and protective cast or splint immobilization. Only if a significant rotational or angulational deformity persists would a corrective osteotomy be needed at the time of curettage

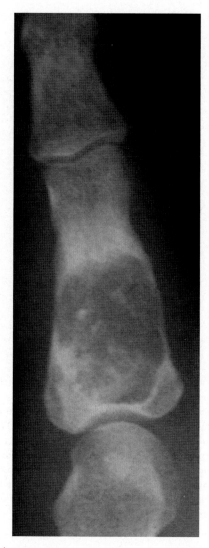

Figure 28–1:
Enchondroma presents with a lytic lesion of bone involving the region of the metaphysis and expanding toward the epiphysis of the original bone. There usually is a scalped appearance as the tumor slowly expands the bone compared with the destructive pattern of a malignant tumor. Wispy calcifications usually are seen within the lytic region from the calcified cartilage. (From Trumble TE, Berg D, Bruckner J, McCallister WV: Benign and malignant neoplasms of the upper extremity. In Trumble TE, editor: *Principles of hand surgery and therapy.* Philadelphia, 2000, WB Saunders.)

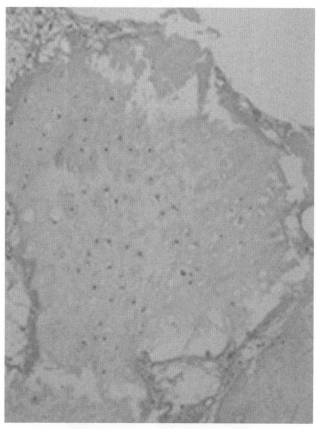

Figure 28–2:
Histologically, the enchondroma demonstrates the appearance of poorly organized but normal-appearing cartilage within the marrow space of bone. The cartilage appears to be slowly encroaching on the cortical margins without gross destruction or permeation of the cortical margins. (From Trumble TE, Berg D, Bruckner J, McCallister WV: Benign and malignant neoplasms of the upper extremity. In Trumble TE, editor: *Principles of hand surgery and therapy.* Philadelphia, 2000, WB Saunders.)

and bone grafting. Open fractures or grossly unstable or irreducible fractures may undergo provisional minimally invasive operative fixation with curettage and grafting, if necessary. In this situation, the surgical pathologist should be made aware of the suspected clinical diagnosis, history, radiographs, and MRI results to assist in histologic examination of the biopsy specimen.

## Unicameral Bone Cysts

### Basics

- *Age:* Unicameral bone cysts (UBC) are most common in skeletally immature patients 5 to 10 years old.
- *Presentation:* Patients usually present with pathologic fracture after activities such as throwing a baseball.
- *Location:* The proximal humerus is the most common site, but it is seen rarely in the metacarpals and phalanges. UBC growth begins in the metaphysis and extends toward the physis.

### Imaging

- Radiographs show a cystic, expansile lesion with symmetrically thinned cortices that may be trabeculated (Figure 28–3). A cyst in contact with the physis is called *active,* whereas a cyst away from the physis is termed *latent.*

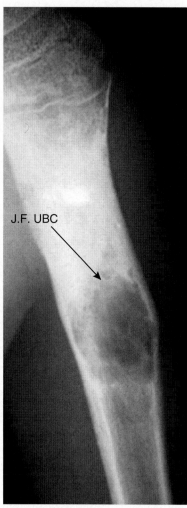

Figure 28–3:
The unicameral bone cyst has a propensity for the humerus. The cyst often appears as a lucent defect on plain radiographs with septations within the lesion. (From Trumble TE, Berg D, Bruckner J, McCallister WV: Benign and malignant neoplasms of the upper extremity. In Trumble TE, editor: *Principles of hand surgery and therapy*. Philadelphia, 2000, WB Saunders.)

## Histology

- The cyst has a thin fibrous lining consisting of fibrous tissue, giant cells, hemosiderin pigment, and inflammatory cells (Figure 28–4).[1]

## Treatment

- Spontaneous involution of symptomatic UBC lesions is reported in less than 10% of cases.[6]
- Excision and curettage has a high rate of recurrence, as well as pathologic fracture.
- The cyst can be aspirated and then injected with methylprednisolone acetate.[7] This technique may need to be repeated.

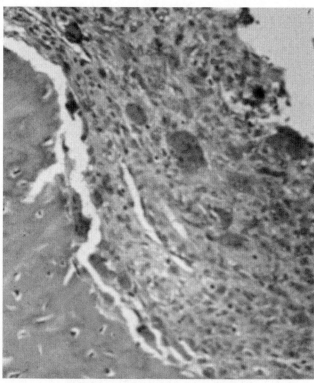

Figure 28–4:
The unicameral bone cyst is filled with fluid. There is a thin fibrous lining covering the bony walls of the cyst. This lining consists of benign fibrous tissue plus granulation-type tissue containing giant cells and macrophages. (From Trumble TE, Berg D, Bruckner J, McCallister WV: Benign and malignant neoplasms of the upper extremity. In Trumble TE, editor: *Principles of hand surgery and therapy*. Philadelphia, 2000, WB Saunders.)

- Techniques substituting demineralized bone matrix for methylprednisolone acetate are described.
- Bone grafting usually is reserved for cysts in the lower extremities.

## Aneurysmal Bone Cysts

### Basics

- Aneurysmal bone cyst (ABC) is a nonneoplastic condition that can be associated with severe bone destruction.
- *Age:* ABCs are most common in skeletally immature patients younger than 20 years.
- *Presentation:* Patients typically present with pain and swelling in the involved extremity.
- *Location:* ABCs may be seen in the humerus but are rare in the forearm and hand.
- ABCs differ from UBCs in that radiographically ABCs usually are eccentrically located and histologically ABCs are blood filled.

## Imaging

- On radiographs ABCs characteristically show eccentric, lytic, expansile lesions in the metaphysis.

## Histology

- ABC is a blood-filled cyst without an endothelial lining. Thin strands of bone may be present. Benign giant cells can be seen, much like in UBC.

## Treatment

- Curettage and bone grafting is the preferred treatment, with a high incidence of local recurrence. Use of cryosurgery in addition to curettage and bone grafting has shown a lower incidence of recurrence.[8]

# Osteochondroma

## Basics

- Osteochondromas are benign surface masses thought to be related to an aberrant physis producing a second epiphysis. Grossly, they appear as an osseous outgrowth with a cartilaginous cap.
- *Age:* Usual age of presentation is 10 to 35 years.
- *Presentation:* Lesions usually are found incidentally but they can be painful, particularly when they occur near a tendon origin or insertion.
- *Location:* These lesions are common throughout the body but are rarely seen in the hand, except in association with multiple hereditary exostosis. When osteochondroma does occur in the hand, the distal aspect of the proximal phalanx is most commonly involved.[9]
- Risk of malignant transformation to chondrosarcoma is well known but has never been described for lesions in the hand. Pain in the absence of mechanical factors should alert the physician of possible malignant change.

## Imaging

- On plain radiographs, the stalk may appear sessile or pedunculated (Figure 28–5). The cortex of the stalk is confluent with the cortex of the bone from which it originated.

## Histology

- Microscopically normal-appearing cartilage and bone are seen, with a distinct cartilaginous cap that may be several millimeters thick on the end of the stalk. In a child, the cartilaginous cap may be up to 2 to 3 cm thick.

## Treatment

- Symptomatic lesions should be excised.
- Local recurrences can be seen, particularly in children.

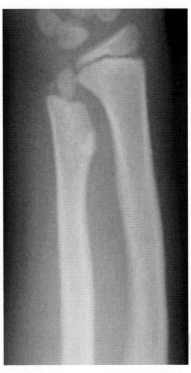

**Figure 28–5:**
The bulge on the radial aspect of the ulna is the site of the osteochondroma that is causing tethering and shortening of the ulna. The hallmark of the osteochondroma is the cartilage cap with stalk, which can be either broad based or narrow. The stalk demonstrates a marrow space that is in continuity with the marrow of the involved bone. (From Trumble TE, Berg D, Bruckner J, McCallister WV: Benign and malignant neoplasms of the upper extremity. In Trumble TE, editor: *Principles of hand surgery and therapy.* Philadelphia, 2000, WB Saunders.)

# Osteoid Osteoma

## Basics

- Osteoid osteoma is a benign lytic lesion of bone that usually causes pain.
- *Age:* Patients between 10 and 35 years old are most commonly affected.
- *Presentation:* Pain, often occurring at night, is the typical presentation. The pain usually resolves with aspirin or NSAIDs. These medicines may be less effective for lesions in the distal phalanges.[1] In the hand, osteoid osteoma may present simply as swelling without pain.
- *Location:* Lesions can occur anywhere in the body but usually are seen in the diaphysis of long bones and the pedicles of the spine. In the hand and wrist, osteoid osteoma is most common in the carpus and proximal phalanx.

## Imaging

- Radiographs show a radiolucent nidus surrounded by a well-defined area of reactive sclerosis (Figure 28–6). By definition, the lesion must be less than 1.0 cm.
- CT can be helpful in further characterizing the lesion. On bone scan the lesion shows an intense area of uptake.

## Histology

- Microscopically the nidus is vascular, with benign osteoblasts forming osteoid strands (Figure 28–7). The nidus is surrounded by a sclerotic rim.

## Treatment

- Definitive treatment requires complete and thorough excision of the nidus. Incomplete nidus excision is associated with recurrence.
- CT-guided radiofrequency (RF) ablation has been shown to be a safe and effective treatment, although no published data report on the use of RF for osteoid osteoma in the hand.[10]

## Osteoblastoma

- Osteoblastoma has many of the same clinical and radiographic features as osteoid osteoma.
- By definition, osteoblastoma lesions are greater than 1 cm in diameter, whereas osteoid osteomas are less than 1 cm in diameter.

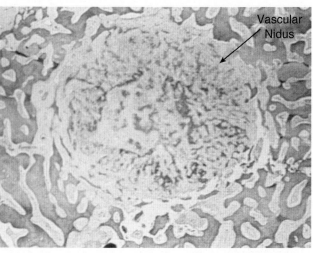

Figure 28–7:
Histologically, the osteoid osteoma demonstrates a small vascular nidus within the center of the lesion that contains osteoid and benign osteocytes. The vascular nidus is surrounded by a wall of dense reactive bone. (From Trumble TE, Berg D, Bruckner J, McCallister WV: Benign and malignant neoplasms of the upper extremity. In Trumble TE, editor: *Principles of hand surgery and therapy.* Philadelphia, 2000, WB Saunders.)

- *Location:* Osteoblastoma occurs more commonly in the spinal pedicles and pelvis. Lesions in the proximal humerus are common.
- Treatment consists of excision.

# Giant Cell Tumor of Bone

## Basics

- Giant cell tumors (GCTs) are benign but locally aggressive lesions of the metaphysis that can behave in a malignant fashion. GCTs can metastasize and can even cause death.
- GCTS are more common in women than men.
- *Age:* The age range usually is the third or fourth decade of life.
- *Presentation:* Progressive swelling and pain are characteristic for GCT presentation. Pathologic fracture can be seen.
- *Location:* GCT usually arises in the metaphysis, extending to the epiphysis, of tubular bones, but this presentation is less common in the hand. The distal radius is the third most common site in the body for GCT (Figure 28–8).[9]

## Imaging

- An eccentric lytic lesion, lacking internal matrix, appears in the metaphysis and epiphysis approaching or involving the articular surface.
- Expansion or destruction of the cortex and a soft tissue mass may be seen.

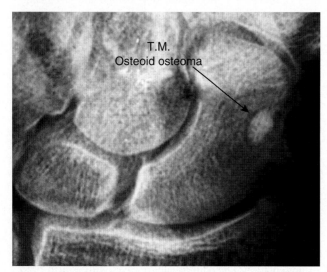

Figure 28–6:
The osteoid osteoma occurs as a sclerotic nidus within the diaphysis of a bone. Although it appears most frequently in long bones, this osteoid osteoma occurred in the carpal scaphoid. By definition, the osteoid osteoma is less than 1.0 cm in diameter. (From Trumble TE, Berg D, Bruckner J, McCallister WV: Benign and malignant neoplasms of the upper extremity. In Trumble TE, editor: *Principles of hand surgery and therapy.* Philadelphia, 2000, WB Saunders.)

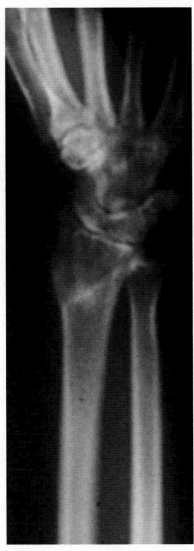

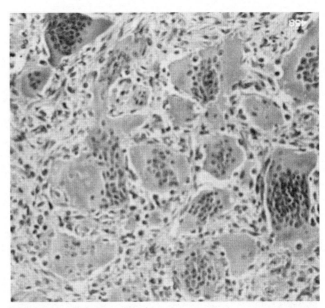

Figure 28–9:
On high-power microscopy, this giant cell tumor of bone demonstrates a field of multinucleated giant cells. The nuclei within the giant cells appear to be confluent with the nuclei of the stroma. (From Trumble TE, Berg D, Bruckner J, McCallister WV: Benign and malignant neoplasms of the upper extremity. In Trumble TE, editor: *Principles of hand surgery and therapy*. Philadelphia, 2000, WB Saunders.)

Figure 28–8:
Giant cell tumors of the distal radius occur in the area of the old epiphysis. (From Trumble TE, Berg D, Bruckner J, McCallister WV: Benign and malignant neoplasms of the upper extremity. In Trumble TE, editor: *Principles of hand surgery and therapy*. Philadelphia, 2000, WB Saunders.)

- CT and MRI can assist in evaluating bony destruction and soft tissue masses, respectively.

## Histology

- A dense, even distribution of multinucleated giant cells is seen (Figure 28–9).

## Treatment

- Wide excision, while preserving the joint, is the preferred treatment.
- Local recurrence rates reportedly are as high as 30%. Success has been reported using curettage, cryotherapy, and packing with polymethylmethacrylate.

- If resection of the distal radius is required, autograft using vascularized fibula graft or allograft can be used to reconstruct the defect.

## Fibrous Dysplasia

### Basics

- Fibrous dysplasia is an abnormality that can affect a single bone or multiple bones.
- An error in the expression of collagen genes is responsible, resulting in malformed, weakened bone.
- *Age:* Fibrous dysplasia most commonly occurs up to age 30 years.
- *Presentation:* Deformity and pathologic fracture may result. Consequences can be devastating for lesions in weight-bearing bones, such as the proximal femur.
- When associated with neurofibromatosis, café au lait spots may be observed. Association with endocrine abnormalities, such as early menarche, is termed *Albright syndrome*.
- *Location:* In the upper extremity, the phalanges and metacarpals may be affected but rarely require treatment.[2]

### Imaging

- Radiographs show a lytic, "ground glass" appearance, usually with a defined sclerotic margin. The metacarpals may develop a rectangular appearance (Figure 28–10).

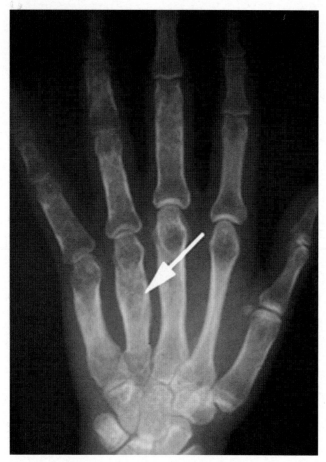

Figure 28–10:
The ring finger metacarpal *(arrow)* appears to be the most significantly involved bone in the hand of this patient with polyostotic fibrous dysplasia. (From Trumble TE, Berg D, Bruckner J, McCallister WV: Benign and malignant neoplasms of the upper extremity. In Trumble TE, editor: *Principles of hand surgery and therapy*. Philadelphia, 2000, WB Saunders.)

- Bone scans are helpful for determining the extent of skeletal involvement.

## Histology

- The intramedullary canal consists of poorly formed osteoid. Fibroblasts produce a dense collagen matrix, often containing trabeculae of osteoid, called *Chinese characters* (Figure 28–11).[1]

## Treatment

- Treatment is aimed at relieving symptoms or stabilizing weight-bearing bones.
- Polyostic fibrous dysplasia has a small risk of malignant transformation, and patients with the condition should be followed. Almost all malignant conversions occur during adulthood and frequently are symptomatic.

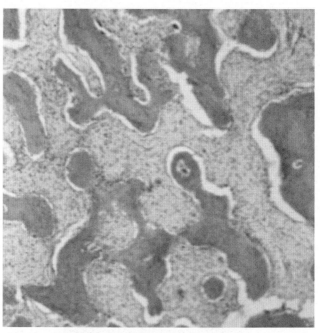

Figure 28–11:
Histologically, the fibrous dysplasia demonstrates a marrow canal filled with nonossified osteoid that displaces the normal marrow. (From Trumble TE, Berg D, Bruckner J, McCallister WV: Benign and malignant neoplasms of the upper extremity. In Trumble TE, editor: *Principles of hand surgery and therapy*. Philadelphia, 2000, WB Saunders.)

## Chondroblastoma

### Basics

- These are benign cartilage lesions of the epiphysis of long bones, usually in patients with open physes.
- *Age:* Lesions present by the second decade of life.
- *Presentation:* Pain of the involved joint is the most frequent complaint in presentation.
- *Location:* The most common locations for chondroblastoma are about the knee and in the proximal humerus. The epiphysis is commonly affected, but the apophysis also may be involved.

### Imaging

- Radiographs show a lucent area with a distinct sclerotic border. Mineralization may be present (Figure 28–12).

### Histology

- Chondroblastoma consists of numerous chondroblasts, with giant cells dispersed throughout, and zones of chondroid and lace-like calcifications. This pattern has been termed a *cobblestone* appearance (Figure 28–13).

### Treatment

- Chondroblastomas are treated by curettage and bone grafting.

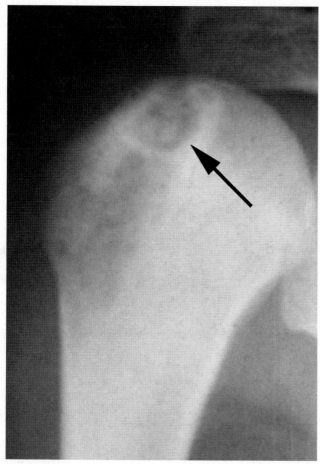

Figure 28–12:
The chondroblastoma presents as a lytic lesion *(arrow)* within the epiphyseal region of a long bone in an adult. This uncommon tumor has a predilection for the proximal humerus. (From Trumble TE, Berg D, Bruckner J, McCallister WV: Benign and malignant neoplasms of the upper extremity. In Trumble TE, editor: *Principles of hand surgery and therapy.* Philadelphia, 2000, WB Saunders.)

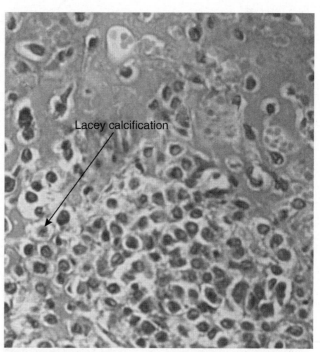

Figure 28–13:
The tissue contains ovoid cells that resemble chondrocytes. There is an intracellular matrix with lace-like calcifications producing a "cobblestone" appearance. (From Trumble TE, Berg D, Bruckner J, McCallister WV: Benign and malignant neoplasms of the upper extremity. In Trumble TE, editor: *Principles of hand surgery and therapy.* Philadelphia, 2000, WB Saunders.)

# Malignant Bone Tumors

## Chondrosarcoma

### Basics

- Chondrosarcoma is the most common primary malignant bone tumor of the hand.[9] Chondrosarcoma may arise as a primary lesion or from a preexisting enchondroma.
- *Age:* This lesion is most common in patients older than 60 years.
- *Presentation:* Patients usually present with pain or a mass.
- *Location:* The shoulder girdle, pelvic girdle, knee, and spine are most frequently affected. When chondrosarcoma occurs in the hand, the metacarpals and proximal phalanges usually are involved.[9]

### Imaging

- Radiographs show a matrix of stippled calcifications in rings and arcs. Areas of lucency may be present, and the border is poorly defined (Figure 28–14). Cortical expansion or erosion and soft tissue extension may be present.
- Chest CT should be obtained because metastasis to the lungs is common.

### Histology

- Under the microscope, cartilage cells have increased mitotic figures, plump nuclei, and hypercellularity (Figure 28–15).
- Histologic evaluation in the presence of clinical data and radiographs are suggested because of the difficulty of this diagnosis.

### Treatment

- Excision with wide margins is required to prevent recurrence (Figure 28–16).
- Chemotherapy and radiation therapy have no role in treatment of chondrosarcoma of the hand.

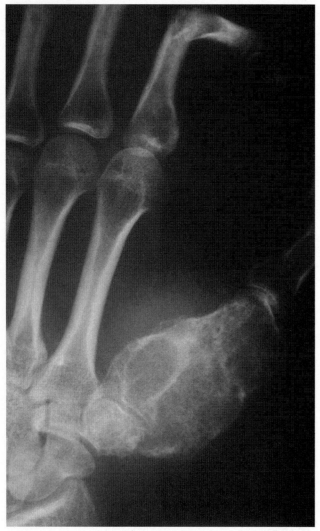

**Figure 28–14:**
Radiograph of the hand demonstrates expansion of the cortices of the metacarpal with alternating areas of benign scalloping of the cortex and destructive changes consistent with the presence of the benign enchondroma and the malignant chondrosarcoma, respectively. (From Trumble TE, Berg D, Bruckner J, McCallister WV: Benign and malignant neoplasms of the upper extremity. In Trumble TE, editor: *Principles of hand surgery and therapy.* Philadelphia, 2000, WB Saunders.)

## Osteogenic Sarcoma

### Basics

- Osteogenic sarcoma rarely presents in the upper extremity.
- Males are affected more than females.
- *Age:* Usually, osteogenic sarcoma presents in the first or second decade of life. In the hand, presentation can occur at a more advanced age.[9]
- *Presentation:* Patients present with a rapidly enlarging, firm, painful mass.

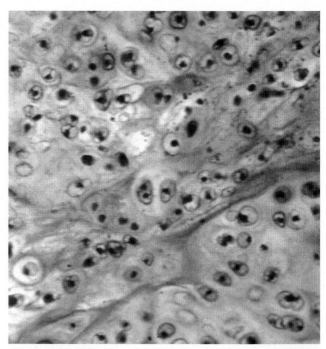

**Figure 28–15:**
Microscopically, the tissue from the chondrosarcoma demonstrates bizarrely shaped chondrocytes containing anaplastic nuclei. (From Trumble TE, Berg D, Bruckner J, McCallister WV: Benign and malignant neoplasms of the upper extremity. In Trumble TE, editor: *Principles of hand surgery and therapy.* Philadelphia, 2000, WB Saunders.)

- *Location:* The most common area affected is about the knee. Upper extremity involvement is uncommon. When the hand is involved, the metacarpals and phalanges usually are involved.

### Imaging

- Radiographs show an expansile lesion that may be lytic, blastic, or both (Figure 28–17).
- Soft tissue involvement is common and may be seen best on MRI (Figure 28–18).

### Histology

- Malignant osteoblasts with high nucleus to cytoplasm ratio, bizarre nuclei, and increased mitotic figures are seen on microscopic section (Figure 28–19).

### Treatment

- Neoadjuvant chemotherapy is used to decrease the size of the lesion and is followed by wide resection and adjuvant chemotherapy.
- Long-term prognosis is better for osteogenic sarcoma of the hand than for lesions elsewhere in the skeleton.

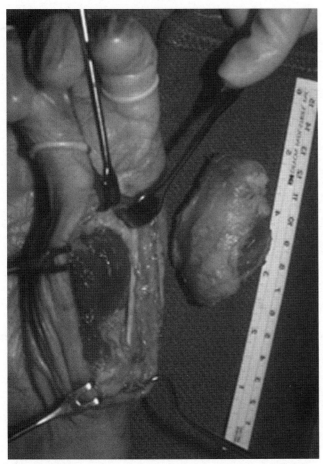

Figure 28–16:
A wide resection required en bloc excision of the entire thumb metacarpal. (From Trumble TE, Berg D, Bruckner J, McCallister WV: Benign and malignant neoplasms of the upper extremity. In Trumble TE, editor: *Principles of hand surgery and therapy.* Philadelphia, 2000, WB Saunders.)

## Angiosarcoma

### Basics

- *Age:* Diagnosis usually is made in the third and fourth decades of life.
- *Location:* Angiosarcoma most commonly affects the metacarpals and phalanges in the hand.

### Imaging

- Plain radiographs show sclerosis and deformity of the bone trabeculae (Figure 28–20).[2]
- MRI shows signal change in affected bone and soft tissue (Figure 28–21).

### Histology

- Mitotic figures in angiosarcoma differentiate it from hemangioendothelioma (Figure 28–22). Abnormal endothelial cells containing red blood cells are seen microscopically.

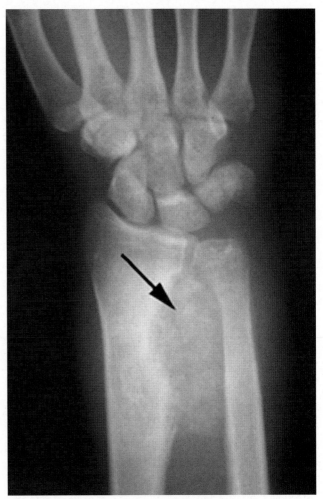

Figure 28–17:
Anteroposterior radiograph demonstrates destruction of the ulnar cortex of the distal radius and extraosseous bone formation between the radius and the ulna in a patient with osteogenic sarcoma *(arrow).* (From Trumble TE, Berg D, Bruckner J, McCallister WV: Benign and malignant neoplasms of the upper extremity. In Trumble TE, editor: *Principles of hand surgery and therapy.* Philadelphia, 2000, WB Saunders.)

### Treatment

- Wide surgical resection is advised. Angiosarcoma is unresponsive to chemotherapy and radiation therapy.

## Ewing Sarcoma

### Basics

- *Age:* Usual presentation is in children older than 5 years.
- *Presentation:* Children present with a rapidly expanding painful mass and may have fever and chills. The white blood cell count and ESR may be elevated.
- *Location:* The pelvis and long bones (usually the diaphyses) are most frequently affected. Clavicle and proximal humerus involvement are common. In the hand, the metacarpals and phalanges are commonly affected.

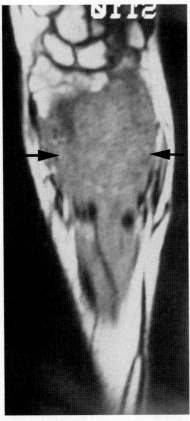

**Figure 28–18:**
Magnetic resonance image in a patient with an osteogenic sarcoma demonstrates the extent of soft tissue involvement that extends far beyond the original cortical margins of the bone as indicated by the *black arrows*. (From Trumble TE, Berg D, Bruckner J, McCallister WV: Benign and malignant neoplasms of the upper extremity. In Trumble TE, editor: *Principles of hand surgery and therapy*. Philadelphia, 2000, WB Saunders.)

## Imaging

- X-ray films demonstrate a lytic lesion with or without a soft tissue component. Periosteal reaction of the Codman triangle, "sunburst" pattern (Figure 28–23), or "onion skin" may be present.
- MRI is the best modality to evaluate soft tissue involvement.

## Histology

- Biopsy sample shows densely packed small, round blue cells (Figure 28–24).

## Treatment

- Ewing sarcoma is responsive to chemotherapy, making limb salvage surgery more feasible. Neoadjuvant chemotherapy and then wide resection followed by adjuvant chemotherapy and/or radiation therapy is recommended.
- In some reports, recurrence was highly associated with fatality.[11]

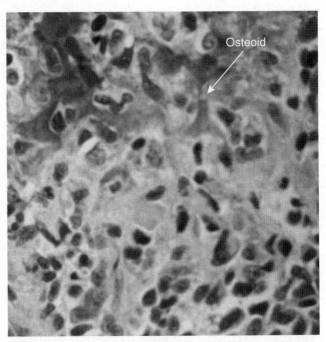

Osteoid

**Figure 28–19:**
On a high-power field, the diagnosis of an osteosarcoma can be confirmed based on the anaplastic nuclei of the malignant osteocytes surrounded by immature osteoid. (From Trumble TE, Berg D, Bruckner J, McCallister WV: Benign and malignant neoplasms of the upper extremity. In Trumble TE, editor: *Principles of hand surgery and therapy*. Philadelphia, 2000, WB Saunders.)

## Lymphoma of Bone

### Basics

- *Age:* Lymphoma usually occurs in adults in the fourth to sixth decades of life.
- *Presentation:* Pain and soft tissue mass are the most common presenting complaints.
- *Location:* The major long bones, in the diaphysis, usually are involved. The shoulder girdle is most commonly affected among upper extremity sites.

### Imaging

- Radiographs have a moth-eaten appearance, lacking a periosteal reaction.
- MRI can reveal a substantial soft tissue mass.

### Histology

- A high concentration of small, round cells is seen on microscopy.

### Treatment

- The mainstays of treatment are radiation therapy and chemotherapy. Surgery can be used to achieve local control or for palliative measures.

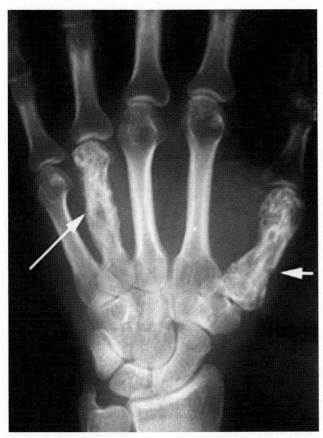

Figure 28–20:
The alternating pattern of sclerotic and lyric changes is particularly evident in the thumb metacarpal and ring finger metacarpal in this patient with angiosarcoma. (From Trumble TE, Berg D, Bruckner J, McCallister WV: Benign and malignant neoplasms of the upper extremity. In Trumble TE, editor: *Principles of hand surgery and therapy*. Philadelphia, 2000, WB Saunders.)

## Myeloma

### Basics

- *Age:* Myeloma occurs in the adult population, usually in patients older than 50 years.
- *Presentation:*
  - Bone pain, fatigue associated with anemia, and pathologic fracture may be seen on presentation. Renal symptoms may be present.
  - Laboratory values may include elevated λ chain on protein electrophoresis, anemia, hypercalcemia, and elevated creatinine.[2]
- *Location:* Myeloma frequently occurs in bone with great hematopoietic potential, such as the pelvis, spine, sternum, proximal femur, and humerus.

### Imaging

- X-ray films may show the classic "punched out" appearance or may simply show osteopenia.

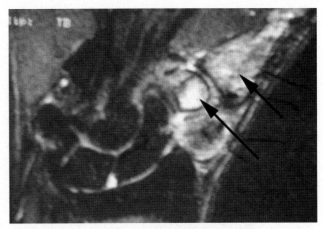

Figure 28–21:
Magnetic resonance imaging is helpful in this patient with an angiosarcoma, because it demonstrates extension of the tumor from the thumb metacarpal *(upper arrow)* into the trapezium *(lower arrow).* (From Trumble TE, Berg D, Bruckner J, McCallister WV: Benign and malignant neoplasms of the upper extremity. In Trumble TE, editor: *Principles of hand surgery and therapy*. Philadelphia, 2000, WB Saunders.)

- Bone scan is negative. Instead, a skeletal survey is used to scan for bony involvement.

### Histology

- Densely packed plasma cells with eccentric, "clock face" nuclei are seen.
- A perinuclear clear zone represents the Golgi apparatus (Figure 28–25).[1]

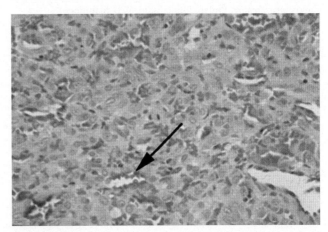

Figure 28–22:
Histologically, the angiosarcoma demonstrates poorly formed lumen *(arrow),* some of which contain red blood cells. The cuboidal, endothelial-like cells lining the lumen demonstrate mitotic figures and other abnormalities of the nuclei. (From Trumble TE, Berg D, Bruckner J, McCallister WV: Benign and malignant neoplasms of the upper extremity. In Trumble TE, editor: *Principles of hand surgery and therapy*. Philadelphia, 2000, WB Saunders.)

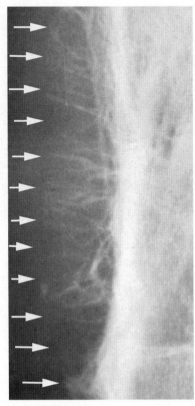

**Figure 28–23:**
Ewing sarcoma on radiographs demonstrates a permeative destructive pattern often associated with a periosteal reaction that produces striations of bone formation, as in this figure, or an "onion skin" pattern as the rapidly displaced periosteum tries to respond to tumor growth. (From Trumble TE, Berg D, Bruckner J, McCallister WV: Benign and malignant neoplasms of the upper extremity. In Trumble TE, editor: *Principles of hand surgery and therapy.* Philadelphia, 2000, WB Saunders.)

## Treatment

- Radiation therapy decreases bone pain.
- Surgical intervention is predominantly palliative, aimed at stabilizing pathologic or impending fractures and relieving pain.
- Chemotherapy lengthens short-term survival but does not significantly affect the 5-year survival rate.[2] Overall survival is approximately 2 years.[1]

## Metastatic Bone Lesions

### Basics

- Primary tumors include renal, lung, breast, colon, prostate, thyroid, and bone malignancies. Lung tumor is the most common source, followed by breast and kidney.[12]
- *Age:* Metastases should be part of the differential diagnosis for all persons older than 40 years with a destructive bone lesion.

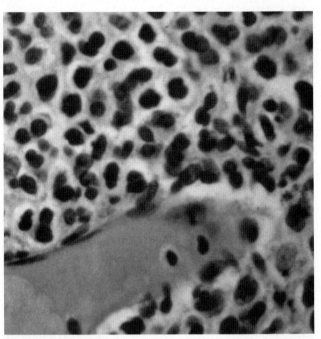

**Figure 28–24:**
Biopsy sample from a patient with Ewing sarcoma demonstrates densely packed round cells and destruction of bone trabeculae with minimal bone reaction from the host. (From Trumble TE, Berg D, Bruckner J, McCallister WV: Benign and malignant neoplasms of the upper extremity. In Trumble TE, editor: *Principles of hand surgery and therapy.* Philadelphia, 2000, WB Saunders.)

- *Presentation:* Patients with metastases often present with bone pain or pathologic fracture. Swelling and erythema may be present, particularly in the hand.
- *Location:* Most metastases are to the spine, pelvis, and proximal long bones. Metastases to the hands are rare but, when they occur, the metacarpals and phalanges usually are involved.[9]

### Imaging

- Radiographs show a lytic lesion, except for prostate metastases, which can be blastic.
- Bone scan is used to survey for other lesions.

### Treatment

- Treatment is palliative, aimed at relieving pain and preserving function. Survival expectancy should be considered in all treatment plans.

## Conclusion

- Tumors of the upper extremity are relatively common entities. Initially, a broad differential diagnosis should be considered, including neoplasm, infection, metabolic disorder, and trauma, at the very least. In the upper extremity, bone tumors can be broadly classified as

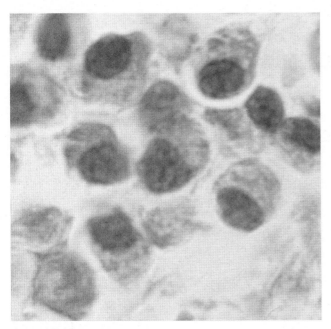

**Figure 28–25:**
Biopsy sample of the marrow from a patient with myeloma demonstrates densely packed plasma cells. These cells have darkly staining nuclear material that often has a cartwheel pattern. (From Trumble TE, Berg D, Bruckner J, McCallister WV: Benign and malignant neoplasms of the upper extremity. In Trumble TE, editor: *Principles of hand surgery and therapy.* Philadelphia, 2000, WB Saunders.)

benign, malignant, or tumor-like. Benign masses are significantly more common than malignancies.

- When confronted with a mass, it is important to obtain a detailed history (focusing on the nature and duration of pain) and a medical history and to perform a complete physical examination. When appropriate, other organ systems should be evaluated.
- The patient's age may be the single most important factor in forming an initial differential diagnosis.
- Imaging studies, including radiography, CT, MRI, and bone scan, can be valuable tools for delineating a lesion and possible metastases. Results of laboratory studies may be abnormal and should be obtained when appropriate.
- Many bone tumors in the upper extremity can be appropriately treated by a knowledgeable hand surgeon. If concern exists over treatment or in the case of metastases, oncology consultation or referral can be obtained.

## References

1. Miller MD: *Review of orthopaedics,* ed 3. Philadelphia, 2000, WB Saunders.

2. Trumble TE: *Principles of hand surgery and therapy.* Philadelphia, 20002, WB Saunders.

3. Sekiya I, Matsui N, Otsuka T, et al: The treatment of enchondromas in the hand by endoscopic curettage without bone grafting. *J Hand Surg [Br]* 22B:230-234, 1997.
   Nine patients with enchondroma were treated successfully by endoscopic curettage of the lesions without bone grafting.

4. Bickels J, Wittig JC, Kollender Y, et al: Enchondromas of the hand: treatment with curettage and cemented internal fixation. *J Hand Surg [Am]* 27:870-875, 2002.
   Thirteen patients with enchondroma underwent successful excision of the tumor, followed by reconstruction of the defect with bone cement and intramedullary hardware.

5. Ablove RH, Moy OJ, Wheeler DR: Early versus delayed treatment of enchondroma. *Am J Orthop* 29:771-772, 2000.
   Among 16 patients presenting with pathologic fracture through enchondroma, a higher complication rate was found for those enchondromas treated prior to fracture healing.

6. Ahn JI, Park JS: Pathologic fractures secondary to unicameral bone cysts. *Int Orthop* 18:20-22, 1994.
   In a retrospective review of 75 children with UBC, the cyst recurred and sometimes enlarged without showing acceleration of healing post fracture.

7. Scaglietti O, Narchetti PG, Bartolozzi P: The effects of methylprednisolone acetate in the treatment of bone cysts. Results from three years follow-up. *J Bone Joint Surg Br* 61B: 200-204, 1979.
   Sixty-nine of 72 patients with bone cysts treated by injection of methylprednisolone acetate had positive results with healing and varying degrees of bone repair.

8. Marcove RC, Sheth DS, Takemoto S, Healey JH: The treatment of aneurysmal bone cyst. *Clin Orthop* 311:157-163, 1995.
   Thirty-four primary ABCs and 17 secondary ABCs were treated by excision and application of liquid nitrogen with an overall cure rate of 82%.

9. Green DP, Hotchkiss RN, Pederson WC: *Green's operative hand surgery,* ed. 4. Philadelphia, 1999, Churchill Livingstone.

10. Rosenthal DI, Hornicek FJ, Torriani M, et al: Osteoid osteoma: percutaneous treatment with radiofrequency energy. *Radiology* 229:171-175, 2003.
    Radiofrequency ablation of suspected osteoid osteoma was performed in 126 patients with complete relief of symptoms in 112 patients (89%).

11. Gasparini M, Lonbardi F, Ballerini E: Long-term outcome of patients with monostotic Ewing's sarcoma treated with combined modality. *Med Pediatr Oncol* 23:406-412, 1994.
    Patients with Ewing sarcoma were treated with radiotherapy, resection and radiotherapy, or radical surgery. All patients received chemotherapy. The progression-free survival rate reached at plateau at 46% after the seventh year from diagnosis, but relapses were observed as late as 14 years from diagnosis.

12. Kerin R: The hand in metastatic disease. *J Hand Surg [Am]* 12:77-83, 1987.
    A meta-analysis of the literature was performed, analyzing 163 cases of metastatic hand tumors for location and primary source of metastasis.

# CHAPTER 29

# Pediatric Hand Trauma

### Roger Cornwall* and Peter M. Waters†

*MD, Pediatric Hand and Upper Extremity Surgeon, The Children's Hospital of Philadelphia; Assistant Professor of Orthopaedic Surgery, University of Pennsylvania School of Medicine, Philadelphia, PA
†MD, Associate Professor, Department of Orthopaedic Surgery, Harvard Medical School; Associate Chief, Department of Orthopaedic Surgery, Children's Hospital; Director, Hand and Upper Extremity Surgery, Children's Hospital, Boston, MA

## Introduction

- The hand is the second most common site of fractures in children.[1] The hands of children are vulnerable to injury. Children use their hands as tools of exploration and are constantly placing them in precarious places such as door jambs. Young children are curious and lack good motor control in their exploration of their environment, making them more prone to injury. The increasing participation of young children in organized sports places their hands at risk for significant injuries.[2]
- The child's hands are important for proper social interaction and development, so significant injuries can have profound ramifications.
- This chapter discusses the principles of management of hand injuries in children and describes in more detail those injuries that are unique to children or that have special considerations in children. Fractures and injuries proximal to the carpus in children are not discussed here, as they are covered in detail in the book *Pediatric Orthopaedics,* from the Core Knowledge in Orthopaedics series.

## Principles of Management

- Children's hand injuries differ from those in adults in several meaningful ways.
  - The mechanical properties of immature bone allow buckle and greenstick fractures and plastic deformation

because of the higher collagen to mineral ratio than in adult bone.
- The speed and reliability of bony healing can be both advantageous and disadvantageous. Whereas simple fractures heal reliably and quickly, displaced fractures progress to a malunion in a short time if not diagnosed and treated promptly.
- The dynamic nature of the child's skeleton enables remodeling of malunited fractures but also adds a layer of complexity to the assessment and treatment of injuries involving the physes.
- The ability of a child to prevent or overcome stiffness in the hand and fingers allows for use of forms of immobilization that are not appropriate in the adult population.
- A child's compliance with activity restrictions cannot be assured, making immobilization important in the treatment of injuries for which activity modification suffices in an adult.
- Examining the child's hand can be challenging, especially when the hand is injured and painful. Young children may not elucidate specific complaints or follow specific commands. The fatty nature of young hands can mask swelling from a fracture and allow underestimation of angular deformities. The close proximity of various structures in a small hand makes precise localization of tenderness difficult. Therefore, evaluation of the child's injured hand relies heavily on observation and passive clinical tests.

- Earn the child's trust. Do not palpate for tenderness at the injury site as the first step of the examination: you will lose all hope of interacting in a calm and fruitful way with the child. Perhaps examine the opposite, uninjured extremity first, even if not clinically warranted, just to "break the ice." Save potentially painful portions of the examination until the very end.
- Watch the child play or move. You can get a good sense of the nature and severity of an injury based on the child's voluntary use of the hand. Much information can be gained by simple observation. If possible, engage the child with interesting toys or objects.
- Enlist the parents in the examination. A child might follow a parent's command more readily than an examiner's. Children usually are more comfortable and cooperative with examinations when they are close to their parents, such as on their lap.
- Examine the resting posture of the hand. Tendon injuries can be detected simply by observing the finger flexion cascade, without requiring the child to follow commands to bend the fingers (Figure 29–1).
- Always check for rotational deformities in finger or hand injuries. Benign-appearing two-dimensional radiographs may mask a three-dimensional rotational deformity. If the child will not voluntarily flex a finger, passively extend the wrist with a thumb in the palm.

The resulting tenodesis flexion suffices to detect many rotational deformities (Figure 29–2).

- Parents play important roles on both sides of the therapeutic relationship. They are important members of the evaluation and management team, but they can be as challenging to "treat" as the child. For example, many children's hand injuries result from accidents in which the parents were involved, such as the finger slammed in a car door, bringing parental guilt and denial into the picture. Education of parents or caregivers often is as critical to the success and safety of treatments as the actual interventions performed on the child.
- Most hand injuries in children can be treated successfully by nonoperative means. However, a subset of hand fractures and dislocations can cause significant complications and disability if not treated aggressively.[3] It is imperative to recognize such injuries and treat them appropriately.

# Wrist Fractures and Dislocations

## Carpal Fractures

- Carpal fractures are uncommon in children.[4] The most commonly fractured carpal bone in children is the scaphoid, with a peak incidence around age 15 years.

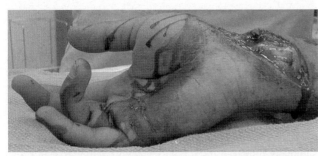

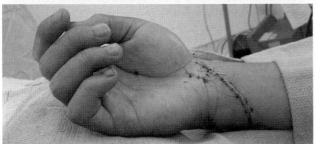

Figure 29–1:
**A,** A 14-year-old boy punched a window and sustained a large laceration to his volar wrist. In this position of wrist extension, the extended position of all fingers except the ring finger demonstrates several flexor tendon lacerations. Upon exploration, all flexor tendons except the ring finger flexor digitorum profundus were transected. **B,** After repair, the normal cascade is returned.

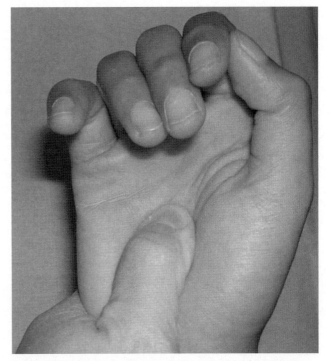

Figure 29–2:
Passive flexion of the wrist produces enough tenodesis finger flexion to detect a rotational malalignment of the small finger, in this case produced by a displaced proximal phalangeal neck fracture.

Scaphoid fractures in children younger than 10 years are uncommon. Fractures of the other carpal bones are rare in children.

- The immature carpus can be difficult to evaluate when injured because of its largely cartilaginous nature. The capitate and hamate are the first carpal bones to ossify (6–8 months), followed by the triquetrum (2–3 years), lunate (4 years), scaphoid (4–5 years), trapezium and trapezoid (5–6 years), and pisiform (10 years).
  - An easy way to remember this order is to imagine a posteroanterior view of the right carpus as a clock with the capitate in the 12 o'clock position. Ossification starts at 12 o'clock and progresses clockwise around the carpus: hamate, triquetrum, lunate, etc., until being punctuated by the pisiform. If you forget the direction of the clock, remember that, after the capitate, the hamate is next (capitate–hamate, or CH, short for "CHILD").
- A high index of suspicion is required to detect a scaphoid fracture because radiographs may be normal initially,[5] and examination of the child's wrist may not allow precise localization of tenderness. Use of magnetic resonance imaging (MRI) and computed tomography (CT) has allowed better and earlier detection of carpal fractures in children, and it is possible that scaphoid fractures occur more frequently than previously thought.[6] Scaphoid fractures can occur in conjunction with other fractures about the wrist, further complicating the evaluation.
- The most common type of scaphoid fracture in children previously was the distal pole fracture (Figure 29–3).[5] Such fractures usually are nondisplaced and can be treated successfully with 6 to 8 weeks in a thumb spica cast. Insufficient data exist to determine the necessity of above-the-elbow immobilization for such fractures in children, and the decision should be left up to the treating physician.
- Scaphoid waist fractures now occur more commonly and should be treated with a long arm thumb spica cast if nondisplaced or with open reduction and internal fixation if displaced more than 2 mm. CT scans may be necessary to determine the degree of displacement.
- Scaphoid nonunions usually follow waist fractures that were not recognized initially[6] or were treated nonoperatively when displaced. These nonunions, like adult injuries, can be treated with open reduction, internal fixation, and bone grafting.[7]
- Fractures of the other carpal bones usually follow direct trauma to the wrist or other high-energy trauma. Most are nondisplaced and can be treated by closed immobilization. Significantly displaced fractures may require operative reduction and fixation. The rare capitate waist fracture requires careful evaluation, as the proximal pole can rotate 180 degrees.

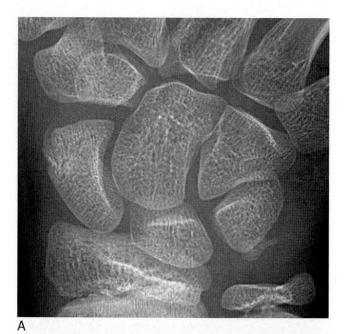

A

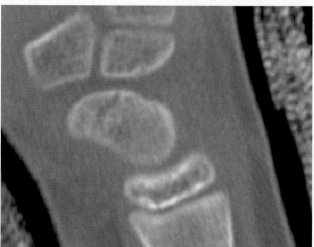

B

Figure 29–3:
**Minimally displaced distal pole scaphoid fracture as seen on a posteroanterior radiograph (A) and sagittal CT scan reconstruction (B).**

## Wrist Ligament Injuries

- Wrist ligament injuries, like carpal fractures, are uncommon in children. Evaluation of the alignment of the immature carpal bones is difficult, given that few data defining normal radiographic relationships are available.[8]
- Perilunate dislocations can occur in adolescents and are treated like those injuries in adults.
- Triangular fibrocartilage complex (TFCC) tears occur in children and adolescents and usually are traumatic avulsions from the ulna (Palmer class 1B).[9] Persistent ulnar-sided wrist pain following wrist trauma should raise the suspicion of a TFCC tear. MRI may be helpful in the

assessment, but arthroscopy remains the best diagnostic tool. Most TFCC tears in children and adolescents can be successfully repaired, as long as all other concomitant injuries are addressed.

# Hand Fractures and Dislocations

- Metacarpal fractures are common in children and adolescents, and their treatment does not vary in most cases from that in adults. However, the presence of growth plates complicates the assessment and treatment while allowing remodeling with growth. An important consideration is the location of the physes: proximal in the thumb metacarpal and distal in the rest!

## Metacarpal Base Fractures

- Metacarpal base fractures are common in the thumb. These fractures can be either Salter II fractures of the physis or metaphyseal fractures (Figure 29–4). The potential for growth arrest is low with a physeal fracture. Conversely, the remodeling potential is excellent because of the multiplanar motion of the adjacent trapeziometacarpal joint and the proximity of the fracture to the physis. Closed reduction and cast immobilization typically is sufficient. Salter III or IV fractures at the base

of the thumb (pediatric Bennett fracture), however, often require closed or open reduction and pin fixation if there is displacement at the joint surface or the physis.

- Fractures of the finger metacarpal bases are not physeal fractures but may be intraarticular. Such fractures can be associated with dislocation of the adjacent carpometacarpal joints. As long as the fracture is extraarticular and the joint is anatomic, the fracture can be treated closed (Figure 29–5). Closed or open reduction and pin fixation are required for displaced intraarticular or subluxed fractures. CT scans may be necessary to determine articular alignment.

## Metacarpal Shaft Fractures

- Metacarpal shaft fractures are not uncommon in children, especially adolescents. The mechanisms of injury, evaluation, and treatment are similar to that in adults.

- Most fractures can be treated closed if nondisplaced. However, rotated, angulated, or shortened fractures should be reduced and stabilized with percutaneous or internal fixation (Figure 29–6). It is imperative to check for malrotation on clinical examination regardless of the radiographic appearance of the fracture.

- Shaft fractures are slower to heal than metaphyseal or base fractures, even in children and adolescents. Close follow-up is required to ensure maintained alignment during healing and to prevent refracture with early activity.

## Metacarpal Neck Fractures

- Metacarpal neck fractures are common in children and adolescents. The mechanism of injury is an axial load to a flexed metacarpophalangeal (MP) joint, usually during a punch or fall on a clenched fist. Depending on the position

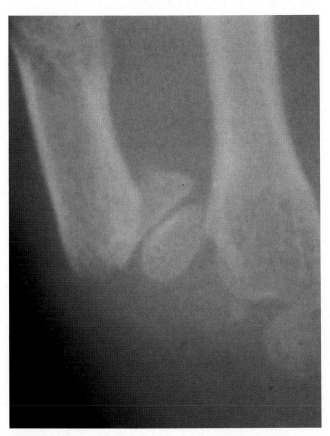

Figure 29–4:
**Metaphyseal fracture at the base of the thumb metacarpal.**

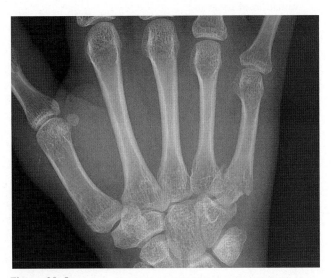

Figure 29–5:
**Minimally displaced, extraarticular small finger metacarpal base fracture that was treated closed.**

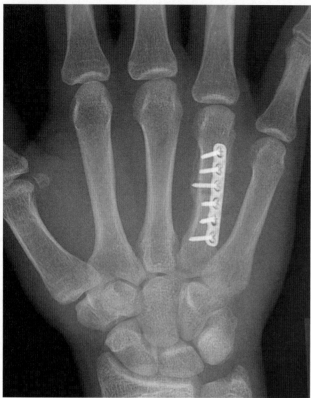

Figure 29–6:
Displaced, rotated metacarpal shaft fracture in a 16-year-old boy treated with open reduction and internal fixation 18 days after the injury.

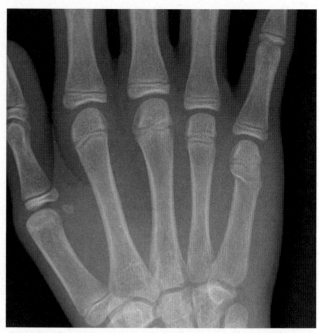

Figure 29–7:
Buckle fracture of the small finger metacarpal neck. A common pediatric equivalent of the adult boxer's fracture.

of the hand with the trauma, any metacarpal can bear the load and fracture. A variety of fracture patterns are seen, most commonly a metaphyseal fracture (Figure 29–7).

• Assessment of metacarpal neck fractures must include evaluation of rotation.

• Most fractures can be treated with closed reduction and cast immobilization. In children, the MP joints can be immobilized in extension without major concern for collateral ligament tightening and stiffness. Immobilization with the MP joint extended allows better three-point molding at the fracture site and therefore better maintenance of reduction. The age at which stiffness becomes an issue has not been established, although we treat adolescents successfully in this manner. Surgical fixation is rarely needed. Minimally angulated fractures need not be reduced. The exact criteria for acceptable angulation have not been elucidated in children, but it is generally accepted that the ulnar rays tolerate more flexion deformity than the radial rays.

• These fractures are juxtaphyseal and have significant remodeling potential. Remodeling occurs in the planes of joint motion. Risk of growth arrest is low. Malaligned fractures at skeletal maturity are rare but can be treated with corrective osteotomy if problematic.

## Metacarpal Head Fractures

• Metacarpal head fractures are uncommon but potentially serious injuries. Metacarpal head fractures can be open, usually a result of a punch to the mouth, or closed, also from axial load to a flexed MP joint.

• Any metacarpal head fracture with an overlying laceration should be considered an open fracture with a contaminated joint until proven otherwise. Such metacarpal head fractures often are simple indentations of the articular cartilage and subchondral bone and can be difficult to see radiographically. The treatment centers upon thorough irrigation and debridement of the joint, repair of the extensor mechanism if torn, and reduction and fixation of the fracture if displaced.

• Displaced metacarpal head fractures should be reduced anatomically, which usually requires open reduction. Sutures and pins can be used for fixation (Figure 29–8).

## Metacarpophalangeal Joint Dislocations

• Metacarpophalangeal joint dislocations are more common in children than adults but do not differ substantially from those in adults. Most are dorsal dislocations. The most important feature to remember is that the misguided use of longitudinal traction to reduce the dislocation can result in a complex dislocation with entrapment of the volar plate. Simple dislocations should be reduced by exaggerating the hyperextension deformity and applying volarly directed force on the base of the proximal phalanx.

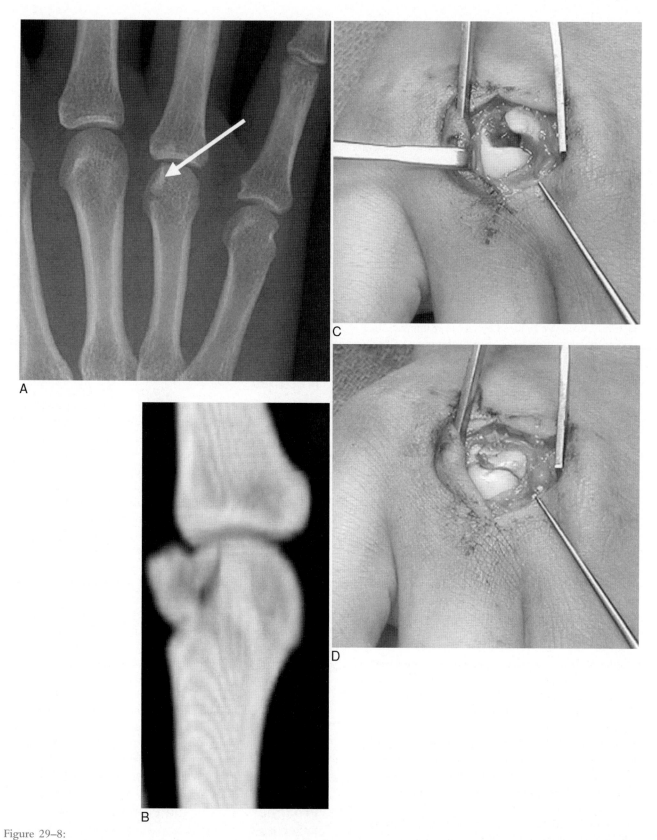

Figure 29–8:
Fracture of the ring finger metacarpal head in a 15-year-old girl seems innocuous on the plain radiograph (A) but is widely displaced on a CT scan (B). Open reduction confirmed the articular displacement (C). Fixation was achieved with absorbable sutures and a Kirschner wire (D).

Complex (irreducible) dislocations are treated by incising the volar plate longitudinally through a dorsal incision or by reducing the dislocated metacarpal head through a volar incision. Care must be taken to prevent injury to the neurovascular bundle with volar exposure. At times, reduction can be performed by flushing the volar plate out of the joint with an intraarticular injection of saline or lidocaine (Figure 29–9).

# Finger Fractures and Dislocations

## Proximal Phalanx Base Fractures

- Fractures at the base of the proximal phalanges are common. Most phalangeal base fractures occur in the small finger and are termed the *extra-octave* fracture because of the typical abduction deformity (Figure 29–10). These typically are Salter II fractures. Such fractures usually are reduced by closed manipulation, as long as the patient presents prior to the onset of healing. Cast immobilization including adjacent digit(s) usually is sufficient. Rarely, open reduction is required for substantially displaced fractures with interposed soft tissue. Percutaneous pinning can be used in unstable fractures (Figure 29–11). Because of the proximity to the physis and the multiplanar motion of the finger MP joints, substantial remodeling can occur. Growth arrest is uncommon.

- Salter III fractures of the thumb proximal phalanx represent a more serious injury. These are intraarticular fractures that destabilize the MP joint because of avulsion of the ulnar collateral ligament insertion at the base of the proximal phalanx. As such, they bear the eponym "pediatric skier thumb." If displaced, these fractures should be treated with open reduction and internal fixation (Figure 29–12). Suture anchors can be used for fixation as long as injury to an open physis is avoided.

## Middle Phalanx Base Fractures

- Middle phalanx base fractures come in several varieties. Metaphyseal or Salter II fractures resemble those in the proximal phalanx (Figure 29–13) and can be treated closed in most cases. Remodeling occurs in the flexion-extension plane, but radial or ulnar deviation and rotation must be corrected. Surgical fixation is rarely needed.

- Epiphyseal fractures can represent avulsions of the volar plate, central slip, or collateral ligaments. Volar plate avulsion fractures (Figure 29–14) are common and result from hyperextension injuries. They should be treated with early mobilization after a brief period (up to 1 week) of splinting. It is important to stress to the child and parents that perfect motion is not guaranteed, and that swelling and stiffness can persist for a long time. Avulsion fractures of the collateral ligaments or central slip are distinctly

uncommon but can be treated with protected mobilization most of the time. It is rarely necessary to rigidly fix a displaced fracture.

## Proximal and Middle Phalanx Shaft Fractures

- Fractures of the shafts of the proximal and middle phalanges are similar to those seen in adults. If nondisplaced, the fractures heal reliably and quickly because of ample intact periosteum. If displaced, closed reduction and cast immobilization often are successful. In young children, up to 20 to 30 degrees of angulation in the flexion-extension plane is well tolerated and can remodel. All malrotated fractures should be reduced, as should those angulated in the radial-ulnar plane. If reduction cannot be maintained in a cast, fixation with pins or screws should be used.

- Crush fractures can be seen in young children, with significant comminution of the phalangeal shaft. Such fractures are generally minimally displaced, with an intact periosteum, and heal reliably with closed immobilization.

## Proximal and Middle Phalanx Neck Fractures

- Fractures of the phalangeal neck occur almost exclusively in children and are relatively common.[10] These are problem fractures. Most fractures are displaced, with dorsal translation and extension angulation (Figure 29–15). The adjacent interphalangeal joint is left in hyperextension, and the subcondylar fossa is obliterated by the volar spike on the proximal fragment. This situation leads to a block of flexion. Angulation in radial or ulnar deviation also occurs, as does malrotation.

- All displaced fractures should be reduced. Cast immobilization is sometimes successful, but most need percutaneous pinning for secure fixation (Figure 29–16). Open reduction sometimes is required but is associated with a risk for avascular necrosis of the condyles from excessive soft tissue stripping. Risk of this disastrous complication can be lessened by performing a percutaneous reduction, using a K-wire as a joystick in the fracture site. Pins used for fixation are left in place for 4 weeks, which usually is sufficient for complete healing. Stiffness is common after fracture healing, and formal therapy sometimes is required to overcome it.

- Remodeling of phalangeal neck malunion can occur in the flexion-extension plane,[11] but a substantial block to flexion also can be addressed using a subcondylar fossa reconstruction.[12]

## Proximal and Middle Phalanx Condyle Fractures

- Fractures of the phalangeal condyles are intraarticular fractures that can involve one or both condyles (Figure 29–17). Most are displaced. An anatomic reduction is

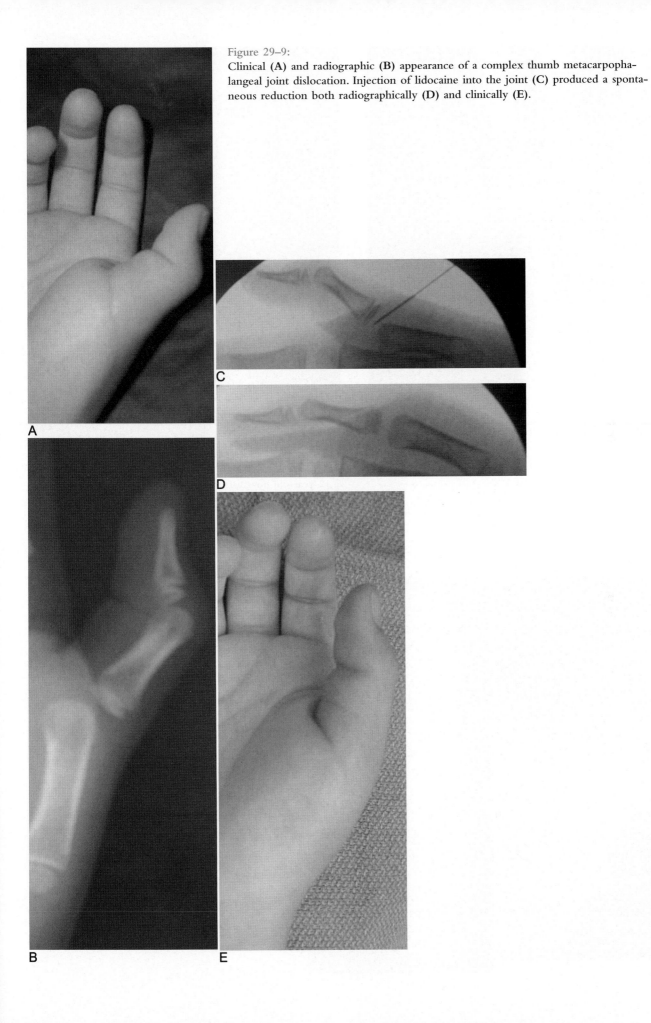

Figure 29–9:
Clinical **(A)** and radiographic **(B)** appearance of a complex thumb metacarpophalangeal joint dislocation. Injection of lidocaine into the joint **(C)** produced a spontaneous reduction both radiographically **(D)** and clinically **(E)**.

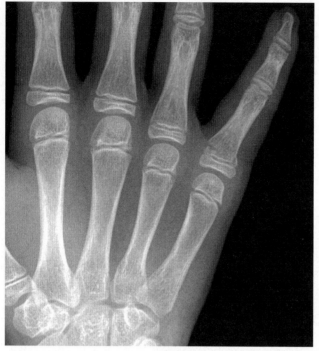

Figure 29–10:
"Extra-octave" fracture at the base of the small finger proximal phalanx treated with closed reduction and cast immobilization.

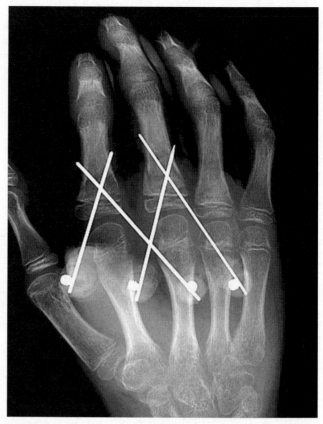

Figure 29–11:
A 12-year-old boy sustained a crush injury to his right hand, with bayonetted metaphyseal fractures of his index and middle finger proximal phalanges. Both fractures required open reduction because of interposed periosteum and required pin fixation because of instability.

Figure 29–12:
Displaced avulsion fracture of the thumb metacarpophalangeal joint ulnar collateral ligament treated with open reduction and pin fixation.

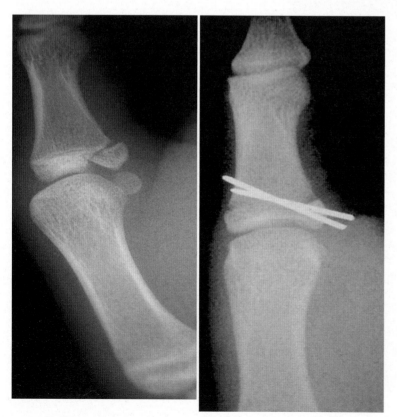

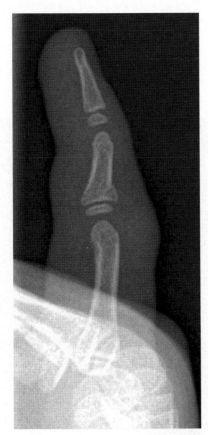

Figure 29–13:
Buckle fracture at the base of the middle phalanx. Angulation in the plane of flexion-extension remodels reliably.

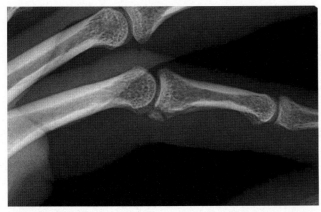

Figure 29–14:
Volar plate avulsion fracture at the proximal interphalangeal joint. After assuring joint stability clinically, allow early protected motion to prevent stiffness.

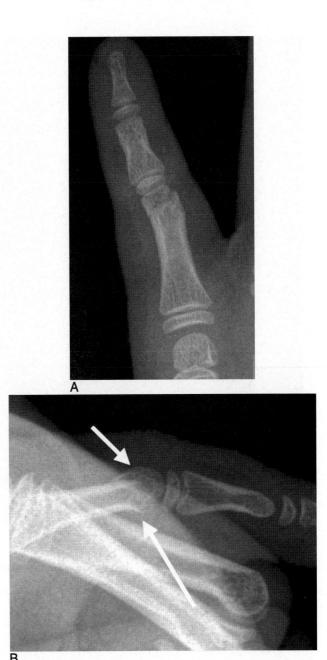

Figure 29–15:
**A,** Posteroanterior radiograph of a displaced phalangeal neck fracture. **B,** On the lateral view, note the extended distal fragment *(short arrow)* and the volar spike on the proximal fragment protruding into the subcondylar fossa *(long arrow)*.

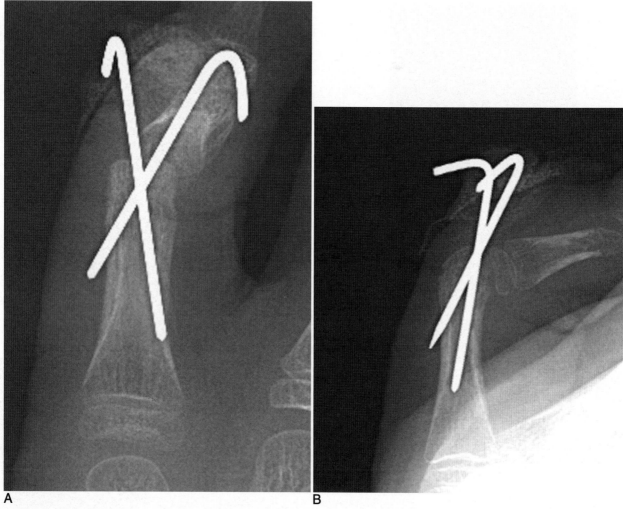

Figure 29–16:
**Posteroanterior (A) and lateral (B) radiographs of a displaced phalangeal neck fracture treated with closed reduction and percutaneous pin fixation.**

required to restore proper joint alignment, and such a reduction often requires an open approach. Fixation is obtained using miniscrews or pins. Remodeling does not occur, and clinical deformity can result from a malunion. Osteotomy of a malunion carries a high risk of avascular necrosis.

## Distal Phalanx Fractures

- The "Seymour fracture" is a problem fracture that can lead to significant complications if missed. The Seymour fracture is a Salter I or II fracture of the distal phalanx physis, with avulsion of the proximal edge of the nail from the eponychial fold (Figure 29–18). Because the nail is avulsed and the germinal matrix is torn, the fracture is an open fracture. The proximal edge of the torn nail matrix often is incarcerated in the opened physis, blocking reduction. If the injury is not recognized and treated properly, osteomyelitis, nail deformity or absence, and impaired bone growth can result.

- Hallmarks on clinical examination include a mallet posture of the finger, with an exposed proximal nail plate. Although the nail bed laceration typically is not visible, the proximal edge of the nail sits atop the eponychial fold, and the length of the visible nail is too long.

- Radiographs must be carefully inspected for signs of physeal injury. Widening of the dorsal physis is common, as is flexion of the distal segment. When in doubt, nail removal displays the open physis (Figure 29–19).

- Treatment consists of removal of the nail plate, thorough irrigation and debridement of the fracture, gentle removal of the incarcerated nail bed from the fracture, reduction of the fracture (with or without pinning depending on the stability), repair of the nail bed if a substantial proximal flap can be isolated, replacement of the nail under the eponychial fold, and splinting or casting. Adequate visualization of the nail bed injury and the fracture site may require incising

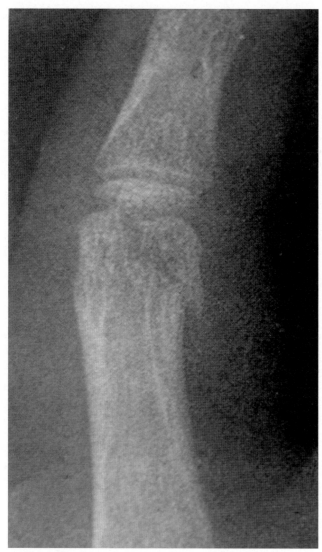

Figure 29–17:
**Displaced phalangeal condyle fracture.**

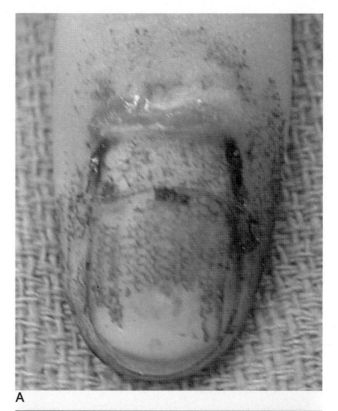

A

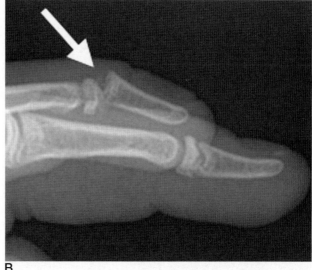

B

Figure 29–18:
**Seymour fracture. A,** In the clinical appearance, note the elongated fingernail with exposure of the proximal end atop the eponychial fold. **B,** Lateral radiograph demonstrating widening of the physis dorsally *(arrow)* and the typical flexion angulation.

and reflecting the eponychial fold (Figure 29–20). Antibiotics should be given postoperatively.

- Salter III fractures of the distal phalanx represent avulsion of the terminal extensor tendon, the "pediatric mallet finger." Such fractures are generally amenable to closed reduction and splinting.
- Fractures of the distal phalanx shaft and tuft generally result from crush injuries and often have associated nail bed injuries. The nail bed injury should dictate the type of treatment. Nail bed lacerations are common in children, and the resident should be able to repair injuries with proficiency. Repairs are discussed in detail in other chapters, so only features with particular relevance to children are discussed here:
  - Because of the very small size of children's fingertips, loupe magnification is helpful.

- In infants, a digital block usually is sufficient. The child typically is exhausted from the pain and from waiting in the emergency room, so the child usually sleeps soundly as soon as the pain is relieved by a digital block. Sedation, although helpful for the administration of the digital block, may disinhibit the child and cause

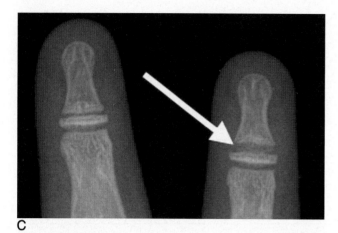

**C**

**Figure 29–18: cont'd**
**C, Posteroanterior radiograph demonstrating subtle widening of the physis** *(arrow)* **compared with adjacent physes.**

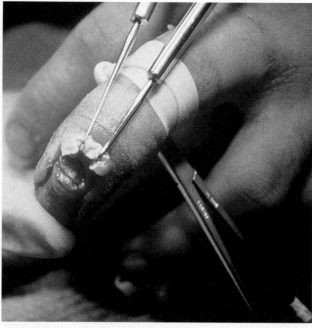

**Figure 29–20:**
**Exposure of the proximal end of the nail bed by incising and reflecting the eponychial fold.**

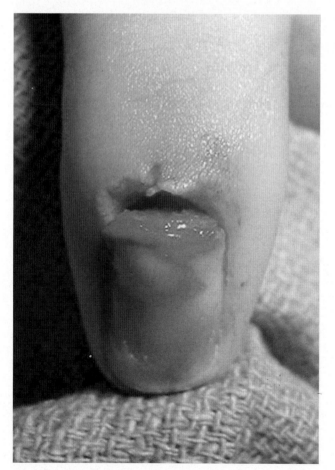

**Figure 29–19:**
**Seymour fracture after nail removal. Note the torn nail bed and widely open physis.**

squirming during the repair. The momentary pain of the digital block is not outweighed by the risks of the sedation. Older children, however, typically need sedation. Adolescents may be able to cooperate with local anesthesia.

- Prep and drape the entire hand and wrist. Attempting to drape only one tiny finger causes great frustration and frequent breaks in sterility.
- Never use nonabsorbable sutures. Suture removal from the fingertip of a previously traumatized child often requires general anesthesia, posing an entirely unnecessary risk to the child's health.
- Use the smallest needle possible so as to minimize additional trauma to the nail bed during the repair. Ophthalmic needles with a 6-0 chromic suture work well.
- A long arm mitten cast covering all fingers should be used in infants and small children. Finger splints and short arm casts tend to quickly fall off small hands.
- In the absence of nail bed injury, tuft fractures can be treated symptomatically, and distal phalanx shaft fractures can be treated with closed splinting until union (Figure 29–21). Symptomatic nonunion is rare but can be treated with bone grafting.
- Children usually but do not always "bounce back" from significant fingertip injuries. Fear of reinjury may prevent the child from initially reincorporating the injured finger into daily activities even after complete clinical healing.

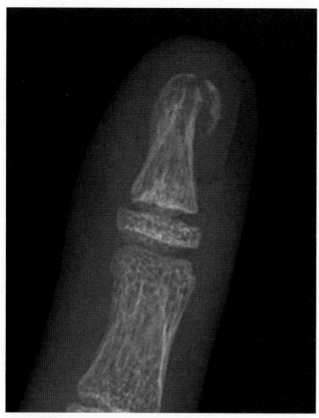

Figure 29–21:

**Tuft fracture of the distal phalanx. Most such fractures, when isolated, can be treated symptomatically.**

Brief occupational therapy may be necessary in these young children.

## Interphalangeal Joint Dislocations

- Interphalangeal joint dislocations are less common in children than in adults (Figure 29–22). Treatment does not differ substantially from that in adults. Closed reduction is the treatment of choice with early, protected mobility to prevent permanent stiffness, especially at the proximal interphalangeal joint. The surgeon should have a high index of suspicion and emergency surgery to properly debride, evacuate, and treat a small hand may be the better part of valor.

## Soft Tissue Injuries

- Soft tissue injuries in children are largely treated as they are in adults. Some features differ substantially enough to deserve specific mention here.

## Flexor Tendon Injuries

- Flexor tendon injuries are not as common in children as they are in adults. The diagnosis of a flexor tendon injury may be difficult. Penetrating trauma on the volar aspect of the hand and/or fingers should raise suspicion. As described in the section on principles of management,

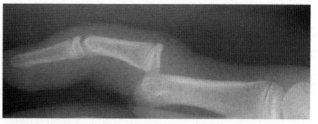

Figure 29–22:

**Dorsal proximal interphalangeal dislocation treated with closed reduction and extension block splinting.**

passive signs are of key importance. Signs of flexor tendon disruption include disruption of the cascade of finger flexion or lack of tenodesis finger flexion with wrist extension. When a complex wound exists and passive signs are equivocal, operative exploration may be warranted.

- Flexor tendons are repaired in children as they are in adults, although multistrand repairs often are not feasible in very small tendons. Suture diameter chosen for repair is dependent on the size of the child and tendon.

- Postoperative care of the child with a repaired flexor tendon in zone II depends on the age and cooperative ability of the child. Generally, children younger than 9 or 10 years cannot cooperate reliably with strict early motion protocols. Rather, cast immobilization is used for 4 weeks, with good protection against rerupture and no substantially increased risk of stiffness.[13,14] The cast is fashioned with the wrist and finger flexed and without a hard surface at the volar aspect of the fingers. This design prevents the child from exerting isometric force though the repaired tendon.

- Overall, the results of flexor tendon repairs do not differ substantially from those in adults. Tenolysis, if necessary, is generally performed after age 10 years, as results of tenolyses performed at younger ages are poor.

## Digital Nerve Injuries

- Digital nerve injuries are difficult to diagnose in young children. Young children may not understand "numbness" or "feeling," and even if they do, will not always answer consistently. An appropriately placed laceration should raise suspicion. Acutely, the "wrinkle" test can be used. The phenomenon of skin wrinkling following immersion in warm water depends on intact digital nerves. If a digital nerve is cut, the area of the fingertip supplied by that nerve usually does not wrinkle after immersion in lukewarm water for more than 5 minutes. In the days to weeks following an injury, dryness of the skin at the fingertip can indicate nerve dysfunction. Two-point discrimination is reliable in children older than 5 to 7 years.

- The decision to explore and repair a suspected digital nerve laceration is complex. Important variables include patient age, location of the injury, and nature of the injury. In young children, replantations and microvascular toe transfers without nerve suture lead to excellent sensation, suggesting that spontaneous reinnervation of finger skin is possible in children.[15] Such a phenomenon argues against exploration for nerve repair in young children with distal injuries. However, the definitions of "young" and "distal" are far from clear. A workable algorithm could include the following:

- In a child younger than 2 years with a laceration distal to the distal interphalangeal (DIP) joint, do not explore the nerve(s).
- In a child older than 2 years with a complex laceration over a neurovascular bundle proximal to the DIP joint, explore the nerve at the time of skin suture. If the skin has already been sutured, evaluate the possibility of nerve injury clinically using the wrinkle test and other signs. If nerve injury is likely, explore. If nerve injury is clinically unlikely, do not explore.
- In a child of any age with a large, complex laceration proximal to the DIP joint that requires volar soft tissue coverage procedures, explore the nerve to assess the need for nerve grafting.
- The results of nerve repair in children are superior to those in adults.[16,17] A high rate of normal sensation can be expected.

## Conclusions

- Most hand injuries in children require simple treatments and heal reliably, leading to excellent outcomes. Several types of injuries exist, however, that require aggressive treatment. Prompt recognition of these injuries is crucial to a good outcome.
- Skill in the clinical examination of the child's hand is important, because subtle radiographic abnormalities may belie the severity of the injury.
- Children are not small adults. Treatments must respect the dynamic nature of the skeleton, the rapid healing potential, and the cooperative ability of the child and parents.

## References

1. Worlock PH, Stower MJ: The incidence and pattern of hand fractures in children. *J Hand Surg [Br]* 11:198-200, 1986.
   The authors present a population-based epidemiologic analysis of hand fractures in children.

2. Taylor BL, Attia MW: Sports-related injuries in children. *Acad Emerg Med* 7:1376-1382, 2000.
   Of 611 pediatric sports-related injuries, 28% occurred in the hand and wrist, with basketball and football being the leading culprit sports.

3. Hastings H 2nd, Simmons BP: Hand fractures in children. A statistical analysis. *Clin Orthop* 188:120-130, 1984.
   The authors retrospectively reviewed 354 pediatric hand fractures and highlighted several fractures that cause problems: dis-

placed intraarticular fractures, Salter I distal phalanx fractures, displaced subcondylar fractures, and open fractures.

4. Light TR: Carpal injuries in children. *Hand Clin* 16:513-522, 2000.
   The author reviews carpal injuries in children, reporting a high rate of missed or delayed diagnosis because of lack of suspicion.

5. Christodoulou AG, Colton CL: Scaphoid fractures in children. *J Pediatr Orthop* 6:37-39, 1986.
   The authors review 64 pediatric scaphoid fractures, most of which were nondisplaced and in the distal pole, and for most of which cast immobilization led to union.

6. Toh S, Miura H, Arai K et al: Scaphoid fractures in children: problems and treatment. *J Pediatr Orthop* 23:216-221, 2003.
   The authors review 64 pediatric scaphoid fractures, 46 of which were nonunions at diagnosis.

7. Mintzer CM, Waters PM: Surgical treatment of pediatric scaphoid fracture nonunions. *J Pediatr Orthop* 19:236-239, 1999.
   The authors treated 13 pediatric scaphoid nonunions with either Matti-Russe bone grafting or bone grafting plus Herbert screw fixation with good results in all cases.

8. Kaawach W, Ecklund K, Di Canzio J et al: Normal ranges of scapholunate distance in children 6 to 14 years old. *J Pediatr Orthop* 21:464-467, 2001.
   The authors measured scapholunate distances on bone age radiographs in 85 children, establishing age-based norms.

9. Terry CL, Waters PM: Triangular fibrocartilage injuries in pediatric and adolescent patients. *J Hand Surg [Am]* 23:626-634, 1998.
   Of 29 skeletally immature patients with arthroscopically documented TFCC tears, 79% had Palmer class 1B tears that typically did well with surgical treatment.

10. Al-Qattan MM: Phalangeal neck fractures in children: classification and outcome in 66 cases. *J Hand Surg [Br]* 26:112-121, 2001.
    The author reviews 67 pediatric phalangeal neck fractures and proposes a classification scheme.

11. Cornwall R, Waters PM: Remodeling of phalangeal neck fracture malunions in children: case report. *J Hand Surg [Am]* 29:458-461, 2004.
    A case is presented of a 5-year-old boy whose 60-degree extension malunion of a phalangeal neck fracture remodeled completely over 2 years.

12. Simmons BP, Peters TT: Subcondylar fossa reconstruction for malunion of fractures of the proximal phalanx in children. *J Hand Surg [Am]* 12:1079-1082, 1987.
    The authors describe a technique of subcondylar fossa reconstruction for dorsally displaced malunions of phalangeal neck fractures that cause a block to adjacent interphalangeal joint flexion.

13. O'Connell SJ, Moore MM, Strickland JW et al: Results of zone I and zone II flexor tendon repairs in children. *J Hand Surg [Am]* 19:48-52, 1994.
    The authors reviewed the results of 78 children younger than 16 years with 95 zone 1 or 2 flexor tendon repairs, reporting

that immobilization for 3 to 4 weeks did not adversely affect outcome of zone 2 repairs.

14. Kato H, Minami A, Suenaga N et al: Long-term results after primary repairs of zone 2 flexor tendon lacerations in children younger than age 6 years. *J Pediatr Orthop* 22:732-735, 2002.
The authors report good results of 12 children younger than 6 years with zone 2 flexor tendon repairs immobilized in a cast postoperatively.

15. Faivre S, Lim A, Dautel G et al: Adjacent and spontaneous neurotization after distal digital replantation in children. *Plast Reconstr Surg* 111:159-165, 2003; discussion 111:166, 2003.
Normal sensory results were obtained in eight children (mean age 9 years) who underwent distal finger replantations without nerve suture.

16. Efstathopoulos D, Gerostathopoulos N, Misitzis D et al: Clinical assessment of primary digital nerve repair. *Acta Orthop Scand Suppl* 264:45-47, 1995.
Among 64 primary digital nerve repairs in 50 patients, only children achieved a high rate of normal sensation.

17. Weinzweig N, Chin G, Mead M et al: Recovery of sensibility after digital neurorrhaphy: a clinical investigation of prognostic factors. *Ann Plast Surg* 44:610-617, 2000.
In a multicenter retrospective review of 172 digital nerve repairs in patients aged 5 to 64 years, the authors found age correlated strongly with results, with patients younger than 40 years having better results.

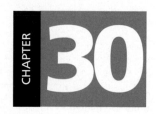
# Congenital Anomalies of the Upper Extremity

## Roger Cornwall* and Scott H. Kozin†

*MD, Pediatric Hand and Upper Extremity Surgeon, The Children's
Hospital of Philadelphia; Assistant Professor of Orthopaedic Surgery, University of
Pennsylvania School of Medicine, Philadelphia, PA
†MD, Associate Professor, Department of Orthopaedic Surgery, Temple University School of
Medicine; Hand and Upper Extremity Surgeon, Shriner's Hospital for Children,
Philadelphia, PA

- Congenital anomalies affect 1% to 2% of newborns, and approximately 10% of these children have upper extremity abnormalities. Congenital anomalies of the limb are second only to congenital heart disease in the incidence of birth malformations.[1]
- Most anomalies are either spontaneous occurrences or inheritable. Only a small subset of anomalies is attributed to teratogens.
- During the period of embryogenesis, many organ systems are developing concurrently. Any aberration during limb formation can disturb formation of these other systems. Certain upper limb anomalies, such as radial deficiency, are associated with concomitant systemic disorders. Other limb anomalies, such as ulnar deficiency, occur in isolation or are combined with other musculoskeletal problems. The discrimination between the various types of anomalies is crucial, because many of the systemic conditions are more important than the limb anomaly and require accurate evaluation to prevent life-threatening consequences.
- This chapter reviews many congenital conditions that manifest in the upper extremity. The intention is to familiarize the resident with common problems and the principles governing their evaluation and management.

## Approaching the Child with a Congenital Difference

- All parents hope for a perfect child, and the awareness that their newborn baby may have a "birth defect" can be an earth-shattering event in the family. Awareness of this impact is of paramount importance to the treating physicians. Parents may notice what may seem a trivial problem, such as a child who just holds her thumb in her palm, but the actuality may be much worse, such as a hypoplastic thumb associated with a radial ray deficiency and profound extraskeletal abnormalities.
- Parents, especially those with their first child, can be frightened by any abnormality and will have many questions about the possible outcome once an abnormality is diagnosed. Therefore, before the diagnosis of a congenital malformation is made, the physician needs a working knowledge of the prognosis of the condition, the possible associated anomalies, and the likelihood and nature of corrective treatments and surgeries. In conditions that may be associated with extraskeletal abnormalities, having a genetic counseling team or various subspecialists at ready disposal ensures a thorough

evaluation and provides the parents with a sense that their child is being well cared for. Parents generally do not take kindly to prolonged waits for further evaluations.

- Parents, especially mothers, may have a sense of guilt if a congenital condition carries with it a poor prognosis or a need for major reconstruction. Conversely, for milder conditions, especially those shared by the child and a parent, parents can look to their own outcomes as reassurance regarding the child's expected outcome.

- Regardless of the anomaly, educating parents about the priorities for treatment is most important. For example, in the case of an unreconstructable hypoplastic thumb, three fingers and a functional thumb (pollicization) is better than four fingers and a nonfunctional thumb. In general, function should not be sacrificed for cosmetic appearance.

- Children typically learn to cope well with deformities. Although this occurrence maximizes potential function, major surgical corrections (e.g., pollicization) should be performed before the child has firmly established compensatory coping strategies that would be disrupted by the correction.

- Corrections for cosmetic gains can be performed before the child reaches school age to avoid teasing from peers or later when the child is old enough to express his/her own displeasure with the appearance.

- Whereas parents and doctors typically focus on children's *abnormalities*, young children focus on their *normalities*. It pays to reorient ourselves and parents to this optimistic point of view periodically.

## Embryology

- The limb bud is first visualized 26 days after fertilization. At that time, the joints form by condensation of the chondrogen to form dense plates between juxtaarticular bones. Proper joint development requires motion for final modeling of the articular surface. Eight weeks after fertilization, embryogenesis is complete and all limb structures are present.[2]

- Most upper extremity congenital anomalies occur during embryogenesis, which is a precarious period of rapid limb development. The three axes of limb development are proximodistal, anteroposterior, and dorsoventral. Three signaling centers control these different aspects of limb development: apical ectodermal ridge (AER), zone of polarizing activity formation (ZPA), and Wnt (wingless-

type) signaling center (Table 30–1).[2] These pathways are interconnected such that limb patterning and growth partly depend on their coordinated effort.

- The limb bud develops in a proximal to distal direction, controlled by the AER, a thickened layer of ectoderm that forms at the apex between the dorsal and ventral ectoderm and centralizes over the limb bud. The cells from the somatic mesoderm form the muscle, nerve, and vascular elements of the limb bud. The cells from the lateral plate become bone, cartilage, and tendon.

- The limb also develops in an anteroposterior (i.e., radioulnar or preaxial-postaxial) direction under the guidance of the ZPA and the sonic hedgehog compound signaling molecule. Transplantation of the ZPA or sonic hedgehog protein causes mirror duplication of the ulnar aspect of the limb.

- Dorsoventral limb development is not well understood but involves the Wnt signaling pathway, which induces dorsal characteristics unless inhibited by the ventralizing Engrailed-1 gene.

## Molecular Defects in Hand Abnormalities

- The number of limb anomalies that have been mapped to specific chromosomal segments and defined at the molecular level is small but is growing each year. Several reputable web sites provide a mechanism for keeping informed of this growing body of information. The National Institutes of Health web site (available at www.ncbi.nlm.nih.gov) allows Internet access to Online Mendelian Inheritance in Man and valuable updated information regarding genes and disease. This source is readily available, frequently updated, and invaluable when evaluating children with congenital anomalies.

- A more detailed discussion of associations between congenital upper limb anomalies and specific genetic defects is beyond the scope of this chapter but has been reviewed.[3]

## Classification of Limb Anomalies

- Numerous classification systems exist for upper extremity limb anomalies based on embryology, teratologic sequencing, and/or anatomy. Each proposal has merit at the time of its inception, although many systems become

| Table 30–1:  Signaling Pathways During Embryogenesis | | |
|---|---|---|
| **SIGNALING CENTER** | **RESPONSIBLE SUBSTANCE** | **ACTION** |
| Apical ectodermal ridge | Fibroblast growth factors | Proximal to distal limb development, interdigital necrosis |
| Zone of polarizing activity | Sonic hedgehog protein | Radioulnar limb formation |
| Wingless-type (Wnt) pathway | Lmx-1 | Dorsalization of the limb |

outdated as our understanding of embryogenesis and genetics expands.

- The most widely accepted classification of congenital limb anomalies is based on embryonic failure during development and relies on clinical diagnosis for categorization. Each limb malformation is classified according to the most predominant anomaly and placed into one of seven categories (Table 30–2). Different clinical presentations within similar categories are explained by variable degrees of damage. This classification scheme represents a valiant attempt to comprehensively classify congenital anomalies.

- However, valid criticisms of this system have arisen concerning the difficulty with classifying the

| Table 30–2: Embryologic Classification of Congenital Anomalies | | | |
|---|---|---|---|
| **CLASSIFICATION** | **SUBHEADING** | **SUBGROUP** | **CATEGORY** |
| I. Failure of formation | A. Transverse arrest | 1. Shoulder | |
| | | 2. Arm | |
| | | 3. Elbow | |
| | | 4. Forearm | |
| | | 5. Wrist | |
| | | 6. Carpal | |
| | | 7. Metacarpal | |
| | | 8. Phalanx | |
| | B. Longitudinal arrest | 1. Radial deficiency | |
| | | 2. Ulnar deficiency | |
| | | 3. Central deficiency | |
| | | 4. Intersegmental | Phocomelia |
| II. Failure of differentiation | A. Soft tissue | 1. Disseminated | a. Arthrogryposis |
| | | 2. Shoulder | |
| | | 3. Elbow and forearm | |
| | | 4. Wrist and hand | a. Cutaneous syndactyly |
| | | | b. Camptodactyly |
| | | | c. Thumb-in-palm |
| | | | d. Deviated/deformed digits |
| | B. Skeletal | 1. Shoulder | |
| | | 2. Elbow | Synostosis |
| | | 3. Forearm | a. Proximal |
| | | | b. Distal |
| | | 4. Wrist and hand | a. Osseous syndactyly |
| | | | b. Carpal bone synostosis |
| | | | c. Symphalangia |
| | | | d. Clinodactyly |
| | C. Tumorous conditions | 1. Hemangiotic | |
| | | 2. Lymphatic | |
| | | 3. Neurogenic | |
| | | 4. Connective tissue | |
| | | 5. Skeletal | |
| III. Duplication | A. Whole limb | | |
| | B. Humeral | | |
| | C. Radial | | |
| | D. Ulnar | 1. Mirror hand | |
| | E. Digit | 1. Polydactyly | a. Radial (preaxial) |
| | | | b. Central |
| | | | c. Ulnar (postaxial) |
| IV. Overgrowth | A. Whole limb | | |
| | B. Partial limb | | |
| | C. Digit | 1. Macrodactyly | |
| V. Undergrowth | A. Whole limb | | |
| | B. Whole hand | | |
| | C. Metacarpal | | |
| | D. Digit | 1. Brachysyndactyly | |
| | | 2. Brachydactyly | |
| VI. Constriction band syndrome | | | |
| VII. Generalized skeletal abnormalities | | | |

"predominant" deformity and the inability to categorize peculiar anomalies. Also, several authors have noted numerous similarities and differences between various congenital anomalies, creating conflict within this embryologic failure classification scheme.[4–6]

# Radial Deficiency ("Radial Club Hand" and Thumb Hypoplasia)

## Definition

• Radial deficiency is a complex congenital anomaly that involves deficiencies in any or all parts of the preaxial border of the limb.[7] The term *radial club hand* refers to the radial deviation posturing that resembles a clubfoot (Figure 30–1). The underlying pathoanatomy is very different, however, as radial ray deficiency relates to hypoplasia of the radius and radial carpal structures but clubfoot does not involve tibial hypoplasia.

## Epidemiology

• Radial deficiency is bilateral in 50% of cases and slightly more common in males than females (3:2). Most cases are sporadic without any definable cause; however, exposure to teratogens (e.g., thalidomide and radiation) can yield radial deficiencies. The incidence of radial deficiency within the same family is small, ranging from 5% to 10% of reported cases.

• Radial deficiency is the classic anomaly associated with systemic conditions.[7] Irrespective of the degree of expression, all forms warrant systemic evaluation. The prominent syndromes are Holt-Oram; thrombocytopenia with absent radius (TAR); vertebral, anal, cardiac, tracheal, esophageal, renal, and limb (VACTERL); and Fanconi anemia. The principal organ systems involved in these syndromes are the cardiac, renal, and hematology cell lines (Table 30–3). Children with VACTERL syndrome also can have vertebral, tracheoesophageal, and anal problems.

• The most devastating associated condition is Fanconi anemia, an aplastic anemia that affects all hematopoietic cell lines and can cause death during childhood. Children with Fanconi anemia do not have signs of bone marrow failure at birth; therefore, the diagnosis is not initially apparent. Most children experience signs of aplastic anemia between the ages of 3 and 12 years (median age 7 years). A chromosomal challenge test currently is available that allows detection of the disease prior to the onset of bone marrow failure. Because bone marrow transplant is the only cure for Fanconi anemia, this prefatory diagnosis is crucial for the child and affected family. Early diagnosis provides ample time to search for a suitable bone marrow donor or to consider preimplantation genetic diagnosis to conceive an unaffected and human leukocyte antigen-matched sibling for cord blood donation.

• Children with VACTERL syndrome warrant additional evaluation for spinal abnormalities, such as congenital scoliosis, and require x-ray films of the spinal column. Children with VACTERL syndrome often appear similar to children with Fanconi anemia: both have small stature,

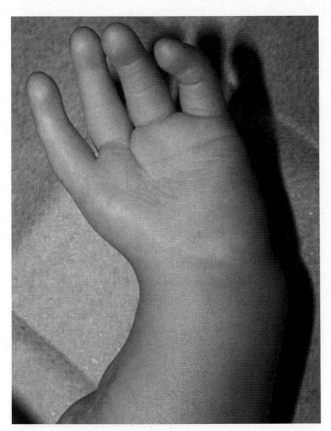

Figure 30–1:
**Radial club hand with thumb aplasia. (From Trumble TE, editor:** *Principles of hand surgery and therapy.* **Philadelphia, 2000, WB Saunders.)**

| Table 30–3: | Syndromes Associated with Radial Deficiency | |
|---|---|
| **SYNDROME** | **CHARACTERISTICS** |
| Holt-Oram | Heart defects, most commonly cardiac septal defects |
| TAR | Thrombocytopenia absent radius syndrome; thrombocytopenia present at birth but improves over time |
| VACTERL | Vertebral abnormalities, anal atresia, cardiac abnormalities, tracheoesophageal fistula, esophageal atresia, renal defects, radial dysplasia, lower limb abnormalities |
| Fanconi anemia | Aplastic anemia not present at birth, develops at approximately age 6 years; fatal without bone marrow transplant; chromosomal challenge test now available for early diagnosis |

feeding difficulties, and similar musculoskeletal anomalies. Therefore, a chromosomal challenge test is warranted in a child with a presumed diagnosis of VACTERL syndrome.
- Children with TAR syndrome can be differentiated from those with Fanconi anemia by the presence of a thumb. Children with TAR have present thumbs even when the radius is completely absent, whereas children with Fanconi anemia and complete radial absence lack thumbs (Figure 30–2).

## Classification

- The degree of preaxial deficiency can range from mild thumb hypoplasia to complete absence of the radius and thumb.[6]
- The severity of radial deficiency is graded from one to four based on x-ray interpretation (Table 30–4). The user must be aware that ossification of the radius is delayed in radial deficiency, and the differentiation between total and partial absence (types III and IV) cannot be established until approximately age 3 years.

- The severity of thumb hypoplasia is graded from one to five based mostly on clinical examination (Table 30–5). The severities of radial deficiency and thumb hypoplasia do not always coincide.

## Evaluation

- Radial ray deficiencies typically are noticed at birth, although milder forms may be missed until later in infancy. Complete absence of the radius is the most common variant, and the primary manifestations occur in the forearm segment and radial side of the carpus and hand. The forearm is always decreased in length because the ulna is approximately 60% of normal length at birth.[7] Forearm rotation is absent in partial or complete aplasia of the radius, although considerable intercarpal supination and pronation are present. The index and long fingers often are stiff and slender, with decreased motion at the metacarpophalangeal (MP) and interphalangeal joints. The ring and small fingers are less affected. Elbow motion may not be normal, and an extension contracture may exist.

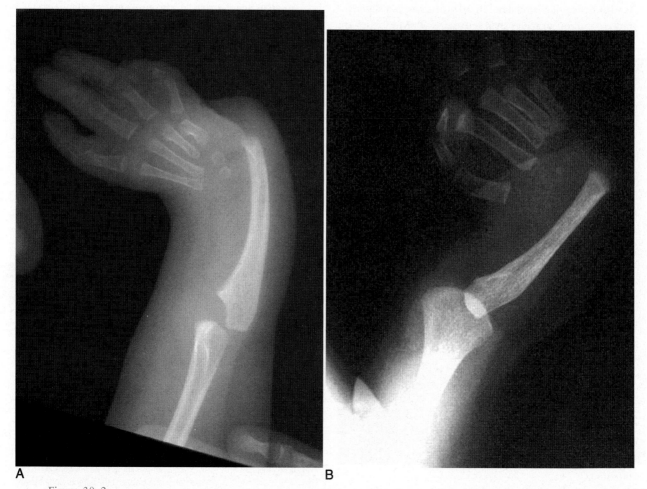

**A**                                                      **B**

Figure 30–2:
Radial club hands in Fanconi anemia and thrombocytopenia with absent radius (TAR) syndrome. The absent radius in Fanconi anemia is accompanied by thumb absence (A), whereas the TAR hand has a thumb despite an absent radius (B).

### Table 30–4:   Radial Deficiency Classification

| TYPE | X-RAY FINDINGS | CLINICAL FEATURES |
|---|---|---|
| I.  Short radius | Distal radial epiphysis delayed in appearance<br>Normal proximal radial epiphysis<br>Mild shortening of radius without bowing | Minor radial deviation of the hand<br>Thumb hypoplasia is the prominent clinical feature requiring treatment |
| II.  Hypoplastic | Distal and proximal epiphysis present<br>Abnormal growth in both epiphyses<br>Ulna thickened, shortened, and bowed | Miniature radius<br>Moderate radial deviation of the hand |
| III.  Partial absence | Partial absence (distal, middle, proximal) of radius<br>Distal one third to two thirds absence most common<br>Ulna thickened, shortened, and bowed | Severe radial deviation of the hand |
| IV.  Total absence | No radius present<br>Ulna thickened, shortened, and bowed | Most common type<br>Severe radial deviation of the hand |

Because ossification of the radius is delayed in radial club hand, the differentiation between total and partial absence (types III and IV) cannot be established until approximately age 3 years. Centralization is required for types II, III, and IV.

- Radiographs demonstrate the aforementioned radial anomalies. In addition, the ulna is thickened and frequently bowed toward the absent radius with an apex posterior curve.
- The appropriate workup for associated conditions necessitates referral to pediatric subspecialists. The heart is evaluated by auscultation and echocardiography, the kidneys are examined by ultrasound, and platelet status is assessed by blood count and peripheral blood smear.

## Management

- The basic goals of treatment in radial deficiency are the following:
  - Correct the radial deviation of the wrist.
  - Balance the wrist on the forearm.
  - Maintain wrist and finger motion.
  - Promote growth of the forearm.
- Nonoperative management of the wrist deformity begins shortly after birth. Passive stretching of the taut radial structures is instructed at the initial visit and performed at each diaper change and at bedtime. Splint fabrication is difficult in the newborn with a shortened forearm and usually is delayed until the forearm is long enough to accommodate a splint. Type I deficiencies often can be managed successfully with splinting intermittently throughout growth without requiring surgical correction.
- Surgical correction of the wrist deformity is generally indicated for type II, III, and IV radial deficiencies. Contraindications for surgical intervention are children with a very limited life expectancy, mild deformity with adequate support for the hand (type I), an elbow extension contracture that prevents the hand from reaching the mouth in a centralized position (child must use the radial deviation deformity to reach the mouth), and adults who have adjusted to their deformity.
- Centralization remains the principal procedure for realigning the carpus onto the distal ulna (Figure 30–3).
- Numerous technical modifications and advancements have been proposed to sustain a well-aligned wrist position, including correction of the ulnar bow, radialization or overcorrection of the carpus, tendon transfer, capsular plication, and prolonged pin fixation.[7–9] Unfortunately, no method reliably and permanently corrects the radial deviation, balances the wrist, and allows continued growth of the forearm.[6,9] Currently, maintenance of the carpus on the end of the ulna without sacrificing wrist mobility or stunting forearm growth remains a daunting task. Recurrence is the most common source of failure after centralization, and the cause appears multifactorial. Operative causes include the inability to obtain complete correction at surgery, inadequate radial soft tissue release, and failure to balance the radial force. Postoperative reasons consist of early pin removal, poor postoperative splint use, and the natural tendency for the shortened forearm and hand to deviate in a radial direction for hand-to-mouth use.
- Adequate centralization results in a shortened forearm segment secondary to altered growth of the ulna. The short forearm is both a cosmetic and functional problem

### Table 30–5:   Thumb Deficiency Classification

| TYPE | FINDINGS | TREATMENT |
|---|---|---|
| I | Minor generalized hypoplasia | Augmentation |
| II | Absence of intrinsic thenar muscles<br>First web space narrowing<br>Ulnar collateral ligament (UCL) insufficiency | Opponensplasty<br>First-web release<br>UCL reconstruction |
| III | Similar findings as type II plus:<br>   Extrinsic muscle and tendon abnormalities<br>   Skeletal deficiency<br>A:  Stable carpometacarpal joint<br>B:  Unstable carpometacarpal joint | A:  Reconstruction<br>B:  Pollicization |
| IV | Pouce flottant or floating thumb | Pollicization |
| V | Absence | Pollicization |

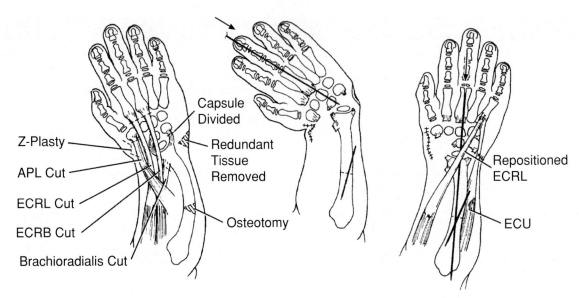

Figure 30–3:
**Centralization procedure for radial club hand.** (From Trumble TE, editor: *Principles of hand surgery and therapy.* Philadelphia, 2000, WB Saunders.)

for the teenager with radial deficiency.[6] Lengthening of the ulna can be accomplished using distraction osteogenesis. Uniplanar and multiplanar devices have been used, depending on the deformity, forearm size, and surgeon preference. Successful lengthening results in functional improvement because of the increased volume of space available for the hand, although complications are common.[10] The appropriate indications, age for surgery, and amount of length obtainable remain questions.

- The basic goals of treatment in thumb hypoplasia are the following:
  - Ensure stability at the thumb carpometacarpal (CMC) and MP joints.
  - Improve intrinsic and extrinsic tendon function.
  - Provide a sufficient web space.
  - Improve the cosmetic appearance of the hand.
- Nonoperative management of thumb hypoplasia consists of splinting and stretching for a tight web space. However, the ulnar collateral ligament of the MP joint often is insufficient, and splinting can worsen joint instability without improving the web space. Type I hypoplastic thumbs generally do not need treatment, because function is good.
- Surgical correction of the hypoplastic thumb depends on the severity of hypoplasia, specifically the stability of the CMC joint. Thumbs with a stable CMC joint can be reconstructed, whereas thumbs without basal stability usually require ablation of the hypoplastic thumb and pollicization of the index finger (Figure 30–4). The clinical differentiation between types IIIA and IIIB can be difficult. The child often helps discriminate between a type IIIA and IIIB deficiency during the development of pinch and grasp. A stable IIIB thumb is incorporated into routine use, whereas an unstable thumb is ignored as prehension

develops between the index and long digits. The index finger repositions itself by pronation and rotation out of the palm. In equivocal cases, the decision may be further complicated by delayed ossification of the trapezium and trapezoid, which normally ossify between age 4 and 6 years. Radiographs may demonstrate absence of the proximal half of the metacarpal at birth in type IIIB thumbs.

- Thumb reconstruction in types II and IIIA requires addressing all elements of the hypoplasia. The adducted posture of the thumb is corrected with web space deepening and reconstruction by Z-plasty or dorsal transposition flap. The MP joint instability is rectified by ulnar collateral ligament reconstruction. Transfer of the

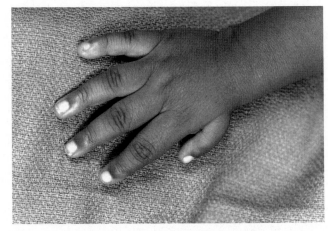

Figure 30–4:
**Type IIIB hypoplastic thumb devoid of a carpometacarpal joint that was treated by pollicization.** (From Trumble T, editor: *Hand surgery update 3.* Rosemont, IL, 2003, American Society for Surgery of the Hand.)

abductor digiti quinti or a flexor digitorum superficialis tendon for opposition augments the thenar hypoplasia. A type IIIA thumb may also require transfers to overcome the extrinsic musculotendinous abnormalities of the extensor pollicis longus and/or flexor pollicis longus tendons.

- Pollicization is the procedure of choice for types IIIB, IV and V hypoplasia (Figure 30–5). This procedure involves neurovascular transposition of the index digit to the thumb position with reconstruction of the intrinsic muscles of the thumb. The index digit must be rotated at least 120 degrees to attain proper orientation of the new thumb. The index is shortened by removing the diaphysis of the metacarpal, and a metacarpal epiphysiodesis should be performed to prevent excessive length of the thumb. The neurovascular bundles are carefully protected throughout the procedure. The proper digital artery to the radial side of the long digit is ligated to allow index finger transposition. Joint and tendon reorganization is necessary for optimal pollicization.[6] Attempts at microsurgical joint transfer to restore the CMC joint in types IIIB and IV have been reported. Currently, the results appear mediocre compared to index finger pollicization and involve considerable microsurgical expertise.[11]

- The results after pollicization are directly related to the status of the transposed index digit and surrounding musculature.[6,12,13] A mobile index finger transferred to the thumb position provides stability for grasp and mobility for pinch. In contrast, a stiff index finger provides a stable thumb for gross grasp but does not participate in pinch. Therefore, pollicization of the index finger provides good functional and cosmetic results in patients with isolated thumb hypoplasia but is less reliable in patients with radial forearm deficiencies. Early good results have persisted into adulthood.[13]

- Timing of radial deficiency reconstruction should be tailored to the severity of deformities and number of procedures needed. If surgery is required for both wrists and both thumbs, the first procedure can be performed at age 6 months so that all procedures can be completed before age 18 months with adequate spacing between the procedures (6 weeks–3 months).

# Ulnar Deficiency ("Ulnar Club Hand")

## Definition

- *Ulnar longitudinal deficiency* refers to a range of abnormalities involving hypoplasia or absence of any or all structures on the postaxial border of the limb, although preaxial abnormalities may also exist.

## Epidemiology

- Ulnar longitudinal deficiency is less common than radial longitudinal deficiency and less often associated with

syndromes and extraskeletal abnormalities.[14] Deficiencies are bilateral in approximately one fourth of cases.

## Classification

- Ulnar deficiency has been classified according to the extent of forearm and elbow involvement (Table 30–6).
- Since the late 1990s, ulnar deficiency has been indexed according to the anatomy of the first web space.[15] This scheme emphasizes surgical indications for ulnar deficiency, which primarily involve the thumb and first-web abnormalities. Interestingly, the progressive deficiency of the first web space and thumb does not correlate with severity of forearm and elbow anomalies.

## Evaluation

- Ulnar deviation is noted at birth; however, unlike radial club hands, the deviation usually is mild.
- Hand abnormalities are much more prevalent and varied. As many as 85% of cases have missing fingers, usually entire ulnar rays. Approximately one third have syndactyly, and one third have radial-sided hand defects.
- The elbow frequently is affected, with abnormalities ranging from radial head dislocation to radiohumeral synostosis.

## Management

- Despite the range of abnormalities present in this condition, function can be good. Passive stretching and splinting should be used early in life to correct deviation deformities at the wrist.
- Surgical corrections in ulnar deficiency depend on the specific deformities present and can be organized into procedures for the hand, wrist, forearm, and elbow. Procedures in the hand most often consist of syndactyly releases and thumb web space deepening. Reconstruction of the wrist deviation is similar to that for radial club hands, although such correction often is unnecessary. The forearm can be addressed in many ways, including creation of a one-bone forearm, fusing the proximal ulna (if present) to the distal radius. At the elbow, radial head resection can be performed in adolescents for symptomatic radial head dislocations with an intact proximal ulna. No good procedure exists for obtaining elbow motion from a radiohumeral synostosis.

# Transverse Deficiencies

## Definition

- Transverse deficiencies are also called *congenital amputations* and are defined according to the last remaining bone segment.

## Epidemiology

- Transverse deficiencies usually are unilateral and occur sporadically. A vascular insult to the AER and subsequent

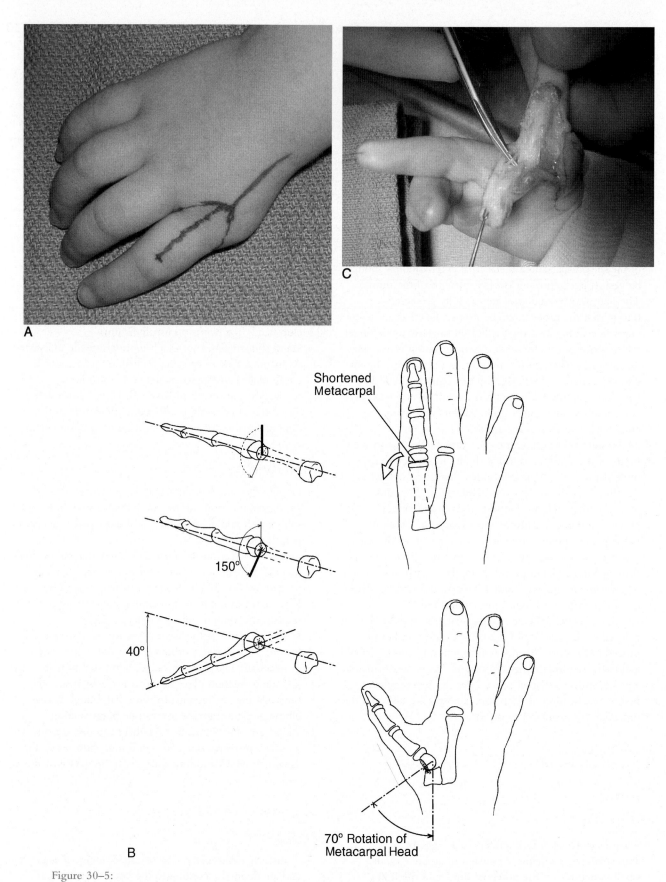

Figure 30–5:

Pollicization of the index finger for absent thumb. **A,** Preoperative planning of skin flaps. **B,** Schematic of reconstruction. (From Trumble TE, editor: *Principles of hand surgery and therapy.* Philadelphia, 2000, WB Saunders). **C,** Mobilization of the index digit.

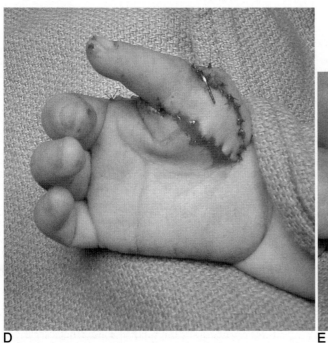

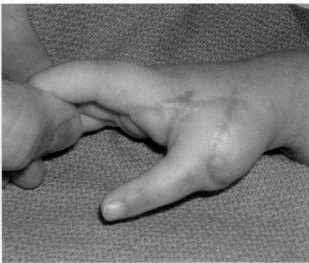

D                                                                 E

Figure 30–5: cont'd
**D, Postoperative appearance. E, Final result.**

limb truncation during limb development is the most
prevalent explanation for these deficiencies.

## Evaluation

- An amputation through the proximal third of forearm
  (i.e., short below the elbow) is the most common
  transverse deficiency of the upper extremity. The end of
  the residual limb usually is cushioned and may possess
  rudimentary nubbins or mild dimpling (Figure 30–6).

## Management

- Management of congenital amputations consists of
  protheses and/or reconstructions.
  - For a forearm amputation, initial prosthetic fitting is
    done when independent sitting is achieved (usually age
    6–9 months) and consists of a passive terminal device.
    Early fitting before age 2 years increases the acceptance
    rate of upper limb prosthetics. Family acceptance and

support are the other crucial variables affecting prosthetic
wear. Between age 15 months and 2 years, the child is
transitioned to some form of body-powered prosthesis. A
supracondylar socket, figure-of-nine harness, and
voluntary opening terminal device is often the prosthesis
of choice. Myoelectric devices usually are introduced
later (age 3–5 years) to ensure acceptance of a prostheses
and to encourage use of both a conventional and a
myoelectric device. The conventional prosthesis is more
durable and often is the preferred prosthesis for certain
activities in adolescent and adult life.

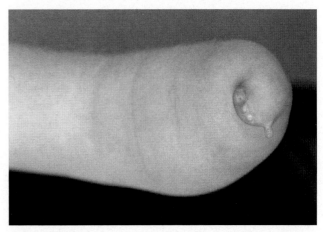

Figure 30–6:
**Short-below-the-elbow amputation with rudimentary nubbins
along the end of the residual limb.** (From Trumble T, editor:
*Hand surgery update 3.* Rosemont, IL, 2003, American Society
for Surgery of the Hand.)

| TYPE | GRADE | CHARACTERISTICS |
|------|-------|-----------------|
| I | Hypoplasia | Hypoplasia of the ulna with presence of distal and proximal ulnar epiphysis, minimal shortening |
| II | Partial aplasia | Partial aplasia with absence of the distal or middle third of the ulna |
| III | Complete aplasia | Total agenesis of the ulna |
| IV | Synostosis | Fusion of the radius to the humerus |

**Table 30–6: Classification of Ulnar Deficiencies**

- Surgery usually is not indicated in short-below-the-elbow transverse deficiencies. The stump often is well padded and can support a prosthesis without skin irritation or breakdown. Occasionally, a small bone spicule or rudimentary nubbins irritates the residual stump, and excision of the bone or removal of the nubbins can alleviate this problem. Use of limb lengthening for transverse deficiencies is controversial. At this level of amputation, an increase in limb length would not eliminate the use of a prosthesis, and the expected gains do not outweigh the risks.
- A less common level of transverse deficiency is through the hand or metacarpals. This deficiency creates considerable unilateral impairment that can be lessened by prosthetic fitting and/or advanced surgical procedures. The long residual limb length, however, dissuades the child from accepting a prosthesis and promotes use of this limb as a sensate helper. The ultimate goal is restoration of prehension to allow independent usage. Advances in pediatric microsurgery have offered optimism for this lofty goal. Single and multiple toe-to-hand transfers are being applied to congenital and traumatic amputations at this level. The procedure requires considerable expertise and careful postoperative monitoring. Successful toe-to-hand transfer(s) has achieved some form of prehensile activity and augmented function.[16]

# Cleft Hand

## Definition

- The typical cleft hand is a central deficiency with varying degrees of absence about the long ray. The term *lobster claw hand* refers to this condition but is not the preferred name.

## Epidemiology

- Cleft hand is rare, with an incidence of less than one per 10,000 live births. The malformation can be sporadic or inherited. The condition of split hand/split foot, with central deficiencies of both hands and both feet, has been localized to chromosome 7.[17] Many associated anomalies have been described, both skeletal and extraskeletal.

## Evaluation

- A range of abnormalities can be detected. Total absence of the long finger ray leaves a cleft to the midpalm. Syndactyly of the remaining border digits can occur. Greater degrees of absence can lead to a two-digit hand, whereas concomitant central polydactyly and syndactyly in combination with central deficiencies can create complex malformations. The clinical appearance may belie the underlying skeletal disorganization.

## Management

- In general, the cleft hand is a "functional triumph, yet social disaster,"[18] meaning the function of the cleft hand is good despite significant cosmetic deformity (Figure 30–7).
- Surgical correction is not routinely required, depending on the functionality of the hand. Surgery is recommended in infancy for thumb-index syndactyly causing angulation of the index finger. Otherwise, delaying surgery until later childhood makes the reconstructions technically easier. Surgical correction should never jeopardize function for the sake of appearance.
- Closure of the cleft with dermodesis and intermetacarpal ligament reconstruction can improve the cosmetic appearance, although a cleft hand missing only the central rays is a functional triumph. An abnormal transverse bone can exist in the cleft and must be excised to close the cleft (Figure 30–8). Reconstruction of the transverse intermetacarpal ligament can lead to scissoring during flexion and may require derotational osteotomy for correction.[19]
- The functional triumph of the cleft hand requires an adequate first web space and thumb. Syndactyly and central deficiency can occur jointly in the same hand,[5] with the syndactyly affecting the ring-small and/or thumb-index web space. Ring-small web space syndactyly usually is purely soft tissue (simple) and is treated by conventional release and skin grafting. The extent of thumb-index syndactyly is variable and requires individualized treatment. Progressive syndactyly is associated with malrotation of the thumb into the plane of the other digits, intrinsic muscle anomalies (primarily opposition), and extrinsic tendon dysfunction. Mild thumb-index syndactyly can be managed by web

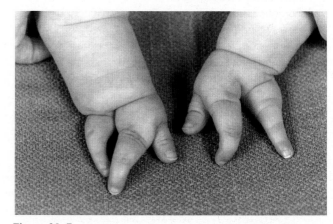

Figure 30–7:
Bilateral typical cleft hand, which often is hereditary, affects both hands, involves the feet, and usually includes the long digit. (From Trumble T, editor: *Hand surgery update 3*. Rosemont, IL, 2003, American Society for Surgery of the Hand.)

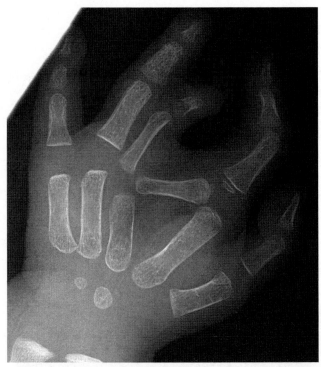

Figure 30–8:
**Abnormal cross bone in the cleft of a cleft hand. Removal of the bone allows closure of the cleft.**

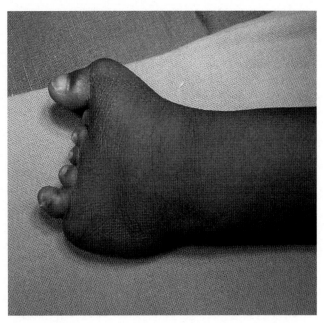

Figure 30–9:
**Symbrachydactyly. Note relative preservation of the thumb.**

deepening and local flap coverage. A four-flap Z-plasty deepens the web and provides a more rounded contour than a two-flap configuration. Moderate involvement requires a local dorsal rotation flap for adequate deepening. Severe thumb-index narrowing can be treated at the time of cleft closure using an ingenious flap harvested from the cleft and transposed into the thumb-index commissure.[19] This Snow-Littler technique results in restoration of the first web space with improved function and appearance.

# Symbrachydactyly

## Definition

- Symbrachydactyly consists of shortened, coalesced digits, often with nubbins resembling fingertips protruding from a shortened hand (Figure 30–9). Symbrachydactyly had been called *atypical cleft hand,* but the term is no longer used.

## Epidemiology

- Symbrachydactyly typically is a sporadic anomaly, although several associated syndromes exist. Unilateral involvement is common.

## Evaluation

- Symbrachydactyly can manifest anywhere along a spectrum from simple shortening of the middle phalanges to absence

of all digits. In intermediate forms, a thumb and small finger are the only digits present, leading to confusion with typical cleft hand. When the digits are just nubbins, soft tissue pouches often replace the absent phalanges.

## Management

- Surgical management depends on the nature of the deformity. Slightly short fingers may not need correction.
- For absent phalanges with good soft tissue envelopes distal to the metacarpals, nonvascularized transfer of a toe proximal phalanx is a viable option. Inclusion of the periosteum and collateral ligaments appears to limit graft resorption; however, a patent physis does not translate into continued longitudinal growth. In growth plates that remain active, variable amounts of activity have been reported.[20,21] An additional concern following nonvascularized toe transfers is the capability of obtaining enough length to truly enhance function.
- Digital lengthening is an alternative to toe phalanx transfer. Use of a one-stage intercalary graft has been replaced by distraction lengthening. Gradual distraction is able to achieve greater length (30%–100% of the bone) and prevents the morbidity associated with bone graft harvest. Digital lengthening devices are more applicable to the border digits as central digit fixation traverses the palm. However, distraction lengthening is not without complications, which are related to adjacent joint stiffness, pin tract infection, and problems with the regenerate bone.[22] The principal limitation of distraction lengthening is

that the procedure does not provide new joints, only length.

- Web space deepening between short, syndactylized digits can create functional and cosmetic lengthening and is technically easier than other reconstructive options.
- Other joint structures and length can be added using vascularized toe transfers. Microsurgical reconstruction provides a sensate digit with exceptional growth potential. The success of this procedure is dictated by the experience of the surgeon and the ability to locate recipient vessels, nerves, and tendons.[16,23,24] The results after vascularized toe transfers have shown some stiffness in the transferred digit but enhanced function in daily activities (Figure 30–10).[16,24] These results represent a considerable addition to the adactylous and/or monodactylous hand.

# Polydactyly

## Definition

- *Polydactyly* refers simply to duplication of digits in part or completely. Polydactyly may be an isolated anomaly or exist as a feature of more complex hand deformities.

## Epidemiology

- Postaxial or ulnar polydactyly often demonstrates familial propagation and racial preference.[25] The duplication is transmitted via an autosomal dominant pattern and occurs more commonly in black individuals. Preaxial duplication or radial polydactyly also demonstrates racial predilection toward white children but usually is unilateral and sporadic.

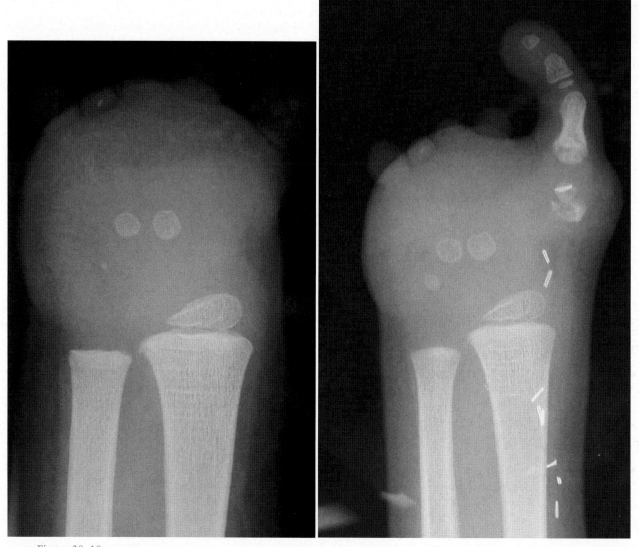

Figure 30–10:

**A–C,** Sequential toe-to-hand transfers in a child with symbrachydactyly. **D,** Tenolysis for stiffness following second transfer.

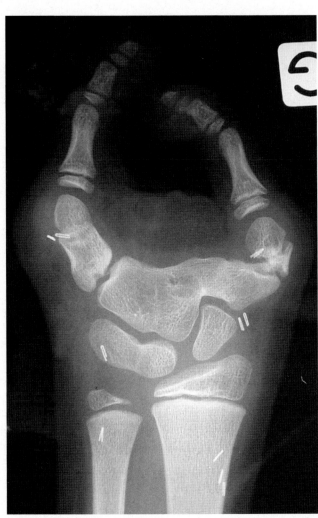

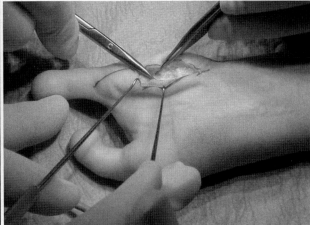

Figure 30–10:  cont'd

## Evaluation

- Polydactyly, when isolated, is easily detected at birth. Family history often reveals parents and siblings with similar findings. When part of a more complex problem, the polydactylism may be underappreciated until radiographs are taken (Figure 30–11).

## Classification

- Postaxial polydactyly or duplication of the small finger is categorized as type A (extra digit is well developed) or type B (extra digit is rudimentary and pedunculated) (Figure 30–12).
- Preaxial polydactyly, or thumb duplication, is categorized according to Wassel[26] (Figure 30–13). The Wassel classification is easy to remember: count the abnormal bones. For example, two distal phalanges plus a V-shaped proximal phalanx equals three abnormal bones (Wassel 3); two distal phalanges plus two proximal phalanges equals four abnormal bones (Wassel 4); and so on. The Wassel type 4 is the most common form of thumb duplication.

## Management

- Surgical correction of polydactyly centers on ablation of extra digits while preserving function of adjacent structures. Although untreated polydactyly may not present a functional problem, injury to the extra digits, which may protrude and have poor or no control, is common.
- In postaxial polydactyly, type A duplication is treated by formal surgical removal. Postaxial polydactyly can occur on both hands and both feet, and all four extremities can be operated on at the same time without causing undue stress on the baby or parents (although it causes undue stress on the anesthesiologist without access to any extremities intraoperatively!)
- Type B postaxial polydactyly frequently is suture ligated in the nursery. Tying the type B duplication has been shown to be safe and effective. The most common residual is a small bump at the base in 40% of children.[25] This bump, which occurs if the suture is not tied at exactly the base of the stalk, can be cosmetically

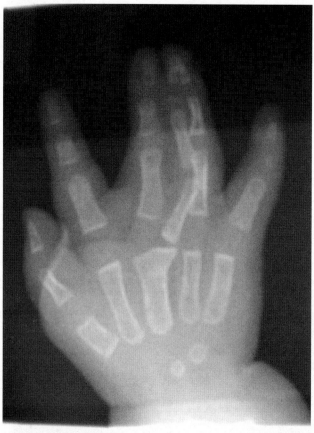

Figure 30–11:

**Central synpolydactyly. The polydactylous nature may be underappreciated based on the clinical appearance resembling typical syndactyly.**

displeasing. Therefore, some prefer formal surgical excision of type B digits, which leaves a well-hidden linear scar at the glabrous/nonglabrous junction.

- Thumb or preaxial polydactyly represents a split rather than a true duplication; therefore, the contents of both digits should be combined to create a single thumb (Figure 30–14). Selection of a dominant thumb and ablation of the lesser counterpart is the standard of treatment. The soft tissues from the ablated thumb are used to augment the retained thumb ("spare parts surgery"). The collateral ligament is retained with an osteoperiosteal sleeve from the deleted thumb and transferred to the preserved thumb. Articular surface modification and tendon realignment are necessary to optimize thumb function. Osteotomy or articular surface recontouring may be necessary to correctly align the thumb and prevent progressive angulatory deformity. The thenar intrinsic muscles may require transfer from the deleted thumb to the retained thumb. The ultimate goal is to create a functional thumb that is well aligned and has an acceptable appearance.[27]

## Syndactyly

### Definition

- Syndactyly describes the partial or total fusion of adjacent digits, including soft tissue alone or soft tissue and bone together.

### Epidemiology

- Inheritable, spontaneous, and syndromic forms of syndactyly have been identified with various similarities

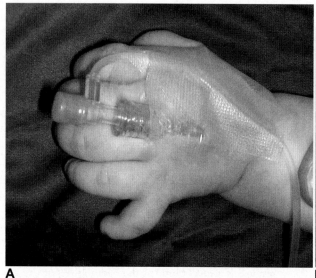

**A**

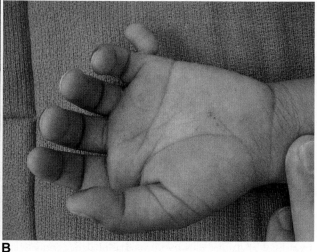

**B**

Figure 30–12:

**Postaxial polydactyly type A (A) and type B (B).**

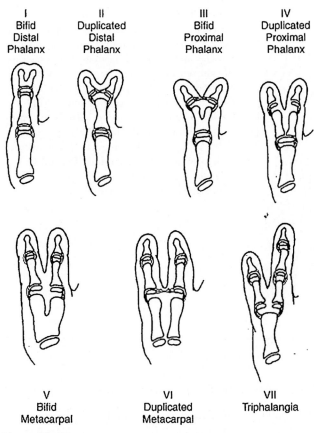

**Figure 30–13:**
Wassel classification of thumb duplication. (From Trumble TE, editor: *Principles of hand surgery and therapy.* Philadelphia, 2000, WB Saunders.)

and dissimilarities. Inheritable syndactylism is associated with genetic defects involving particular candidate regions on the second chromosome (2q34-q36).[28] The mode of inheritable syndactyly transmission is considered autosomal dominant with variable expressivity and incomplete penetrance. This terminology signifies familial propagation, although the syndactyly may skip a generation (incomplete penetrance) and may not be present in full form (variable phenotype). Inheritable syndactyly is associated with syndactyly of the second and third toes. Syndactyly is more prevalent in male offspring, which may indicate a decreased penetrance in females.

## Classification

- Syndactyly can be described as complete, extending to the tips of the fused fingers, or incomplete, involving only part of the length of the finger. Further classification includes simple, which involves soft tissue only, and complex, which involves bone fusions. *Acrosyndactyly* refers to fusion of only the distal segments of digits, with a patent web space proximal to the fusion. Acrosyndactyly is typical of constriction band syndrome.

## Evaluation

- Simple syndactyly is easily evaluated with physical examination and radiographs. The location of the syndactyly is important, as border syndactyly (thumb-index, ring-small) can cause deviation of the longer digit toward the shorter digit during growth. Attention should be paid to whether the fingernails are fused, because this condition can require a toe skin graft for reconstruction of the missing lateral nail fold(s).

## Management

- Mild incomplete syndactyly that does not interfere with function does not require treatment. In contrast, simple syndactyly of any considerable degree warrants surgical reconstruction of the web space for improved function and appearance.
  - The timing of release and the technique of separation are controversial but abide by certain guidelines. Border digits (thumb-index and ring-small web spaces) or digits with marked differences in their respective lengths should be separated within the first few months of life. Separation prevents tethering of the longer digit, which results in a flexion contracture and rotational deformity. In contrast, digits of relatively equal lengths (e.g., long-ring syndactyly) negate the development of a flexion contracture and separation can be delayed, which facilitates surgical reconstruction. This wait is valuable, because surgery performed after age 18 months has a lower incidence of complications and unsatisfactory results (e.g, web creep). Separation can be performed even in adults (Figure 30–15).
- Surgical reconstruction should include only one side of an affected digit at a time to prevent vascular compromise of the skin flaps or digit. Therefore, complete separation of three connected adjacent fingers requires staged surgical procedures.
- Complete syndactyly almost always requires supplemental skin graft. Full-thickness grafts provide better skin quality than split-thickness grafts. A technique to decrease digital volume by extensive defatting the full length of the fingers and the interdigital space can achieve complete closure with minimal tension.[29] Because the circumference of two digits separated is 22% greater than those digits conjoined, use of this technique requires further study.[28] Irrespective of flap design, supple skin (not graft) must be placed within the commissure to prevent interdigital contracture and motion-limiting scar.
- Complex syndactyly adjoins the soft tissue and bone along a portion or the entire length of the adjacent digits. This form of syndactyly is less common than simple syndactyly and more challenging to treat, especially as the quantity of bony union increases.

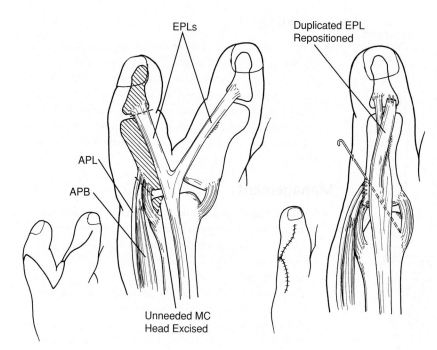

EPLs

Duplicated EPL
Repositioned

APL

APB

Unneeded MC
Head Excised

Figure 30–14:
Schematic of reconstructive procedure for Wassel type 4 thumb duplication. The intrinsic muscles and collateral ligament that attach to the ablated thumb must be preserved and reattached to the thumb being preserved. Crossing the extensor pollicis longus (EPL) tendon may be necessary to balance the coronal plane forces at the interphalangeal joint. *APB*, Abductor pollicis brevis, *APL*, abductor pollicis longus. (From Trumble TE, editor: *Principles of hand surgery and therapy.* Philadelphia, 2000, WB Saunders.)

Determining the correct plane of cleavage, realigning the joints, and managing the soft tissue are the difficult issues. Identifying the proximal and distal extents of the bony connection and probing for an interconnecting ridge or axilla can guide division. Actual separation of the bone into individual components can be accomplished using a knife blade. Soft tissue coverage is more difficult and neurovascular anomalies are more frequent, which complicate surgical reconstruction.

## Syndactyly in Other Syndromes

- Complicated syndactyly is a broad category that encompasses many difficult forms of abnormal web space connection and bony abnormalities. Many of these cases are associated with a syndrome, most notably Poland syndrome, constriction bands, or acrocephalosyndactyly. The treatment algorithm is more involved, and a meticulous physical examination and parental discussion

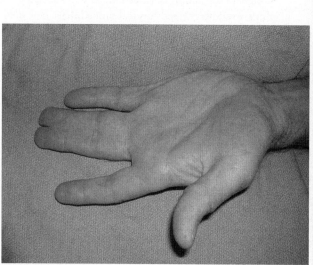

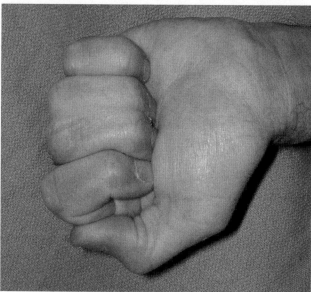

Figure 30–15:
Long-ring syndactyly may not pose a functional problem. A 54-year-old man elected operative correction of his left long-ring syndactyly prior to getting married so that he could wear a wedding ring.

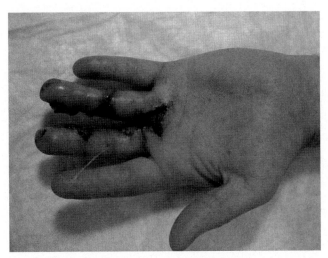

Figure 30–15: cont'd

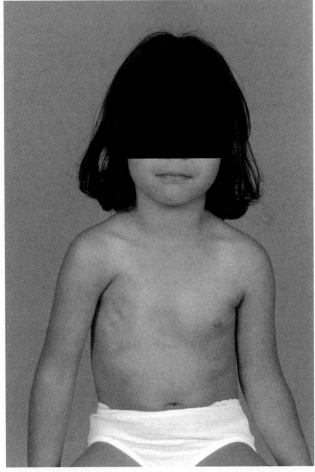

Figure 30–16:
Poland syndrome. Note absent nipple and underdeveloped chest wall musculature. (From Trumble T, editor: *Hand surgery update 3*. Rosemont, IL, 2003, American Society for Surgery of the Hand.)

are essential components during formulation of a treatment strategy.

- *Poland syndrome* is an ipsilateral anomaly of the hand and chest wall. The most common form is described as a small hand with incomplete simple syndactyly and an absence of the sternocostal portion of the pectoralis major muscle. The brachydactyly component characteristically involves the middle phalanx. More severe forms involve progressive bony reduction beginning in the central digits and resembling a symbrachydactyly.[30] The proximal muscle deficiencies and breast underdevelopment can progress to a shallow chest wall deformity with complete absence of the breast (Figure 30–16).

- Syndactyly associated with *constriction bands* is not hereditary and often is called *pseudosyndactyly* or *acrosyndactyly* (distal connection of digits). The cause remains controversial, with intrinsic and extrinsic theories.[31] The extrinsic postulate reasons that either the amniotic membrane traps the developing hand or an amniotic band encircles the affected part, leading to a variable amount of injury. Mild digital damage initiates an embryonic repair process and yields variable amounts of circumferential stricture. This inflammatory response can merge adjacent digits distal to the rudimentary web. Complete vascular ischemia results in truncation of the digits and syndactyly of the affected parts at the site of amputation. Irrespective of the magnitude of constriction, a web space or sinus cleft remains present between the volar and dorsal aspects of the digits (Figure 30–17). Surgical reconstruction follows the principles established for syndactyly release, although modifications are necessary to accommodate the peculiar anatomy. Unfortunately, any available web space often is located too distal, and formal commissure reconstruction is required.

- *Apert syndrome* or acrocephalosyndactyly is rare and represents a constellation of congenital anomalies that necessitates a multidisciplinary approach to management. The hand anomalies are consistent and include a shortened thumb with radial deviation, complex syndactyly of the index, long, and ring digits with symphalangism, and simple syndactyly of the ring-small web space (Figure 30–18).[32] These children often suffer from severe craniofacial deformities that are life threatening. The presence of MP joints provides markers for commissure reconstruction. Considerable neurovascular anomalies are present, especially within the central conglomeration of digits. Distal bifurcation of the common digital arteries and median nerve is frequent, which complicates separation of the complex central syndactyly. Extrinsic flexor and

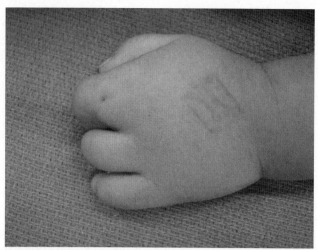

**Figure 30–17:**
**Constriction band syndrome with amputations and syndactyly. Note the dimple indicating a sinus cleft at the base of the conjoined digits.**

extensor tendon abnormalities are widespread, and peculiar intrinsic muscle anatomy is prevalent. Syndactyly correction in these cases is a formidable task that requires multiple procedures to obtain digital independence. Similar to simple syndactyly, priority is given to separation of border syndactyly to allow prehensile function and unimpeded growth without additional deformity. The thumb-index and ring-small web spaces can be created at the same time. The index finger is released approximately 6 months after

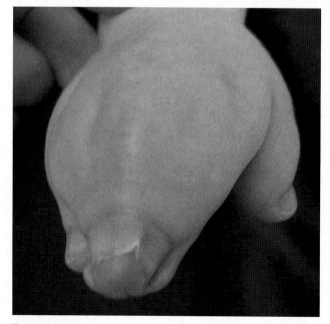

**Figure 30–18:**
**Apert syndrome. Note the conjoined fingernails and the radially deviated thumb.**

separation of the border digits. Following segregation of the thumb, index, and small digits, the long-ring finger syndactyly is assessed for possible release. Complex interconnections and marked skin deficiency must be considered when planning separation. Options include leaving the digits conjoined, amputation of the long digit at the MCP joint (i.e., creation of a three-fingered hand), and syndactyly release with pedicle groin flap coverage.[32] The specific reconstruction varies with the patient (intellect, compliance, motivation), mobility of the digits, and surgeon preference.

# Miscellaneous Finger Anomalies

- Various congenital finger anomalies exist. A comprehensive discussion is beyond the scope of this text, but the following section describes three deformities that should be easily recognizable.

## Camptodactyly

### Definition

- Camptodactyly is a nontraumatic flexion deformity of the proximal interphalangeal (PIP) joint.

### Epidemiology

- Camptodactyly may occur in as many as 1% of the population. Cases may be sporadic or inherited in an autosomal dominant pattern.[33]

### Classification

- Two forms of camptodactyly appear to exist. One form is present at birth and is distributed evenly between males and females. Progressive contractures develop within the first few years of life. The second form develops during adolescence, mostly in females, and progressively worsens until skeletal maturity.

### Evaluation

- The small finger is most often involved, although multiple fingers can be involved. A careful history should rule out trauma to the PIP joint, especially in the adolescent form. A central slip injury generally leads to a boutonnière deformity, whereas camptodactyly does not cause secondary distal interphalangeal (DIP) hyperextension. Radiographs typically are normal in camptodactyly.

### Management

- The contracture of camptodactyly typically progresses, especially during growth spurts. Splinting may be beneficial in some cases, although indications, techniques, and results are highly varied. Surgical releases of tight volar structures, with or without tendon transfers to augment the extensor apparatus, are complex procedures with mixed results. Fortunately, mild flexion contractures of the small finger PIP joint are well tolerated, functionally and cosmetically.

## Clinodactyly

### Definition

- Clinodactyly is an angular deformity of the finger in a coronal (radioulnar) plane. Clinodactyly is a physical finding rather than a specific disease or condition.

### Epidemiology

- Curvature of the small finger in the coronal plane is common, and the threshold between normal and abnormal is difficult to define. Clinodactyly can be inherited as an autosomal dominant trait, associated with various chromosomal disorders, or result from physical or thermal injury to the finger with subsequent asymmetric growth plate disturbance.

### Evaluation

- The small finger is most often involved, with curvature toward the ring finger. Radiographs may reveal a shortened/angulated middle phalanx (Figure 30–19). In cases associated with other congenital abnormalities, any ray can be involved, and radiographs may reveal an abnormal phalanx known as a *delta phalanx*. A delta phalanx is an angulated bone with proximal *and* distal physes connected on the shorter side of the shaft. A history of trauma should be obtained to rule out posttraumatic growth disturbance.

### Management

- Correction of clinodactyly is necessary only if the curvature causes a functional disturbance, usually when the deformity is greater than 30 to 40 degrees.[34] Splinting does not correct the angulation. A closing wedge osteotomy can be performed through the angulated middle phalanx, although disagreement exists as to whether this procedure should be performed before or after skeletal maturity. When a delta phalanx exists, the deformity can be corrected by surgically removing the continuity between the proximal and distal physes, by closing wedge osteotomy, or by using combinations of surgical procedures.

## Kirner Deformity

### Definition

- Kirner deformity is a flexion and radial deviation deformity of the distal phalanx of the small finger. The deformity exists in the bone, not at the DIP joint (Figure 30–20).

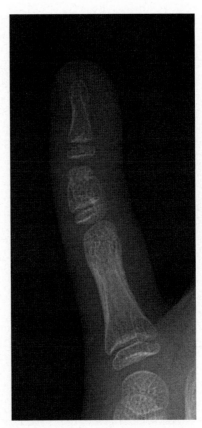

Figure 30–19:
**Clinodactyly with a shortened, angulated middle phalanx (brachymesophalangia).**

### Epidemiology

- The exact prevalence of this deformity is unknown. It may be more common in girls.[35]

### Evaluation

- Physical examination reveals a mildly curved small fingertip with a beak-shaped nail in some cases. Finger motion typically is normal. Radiographs reveal a characteristic abnormality of the diaphysis with a relatively normal metaphysis.

### Management

- Most patients do not require treatment. Splinting is not typically effective at correcting the deformity. Multiple volar opening-wedge osteotomies can be performed after skeletal maturity.

## Congenital Synostoses

- Synostosis, or bony fusion, can occur as a congenital abnormality at many levels in the upper extremity. This section describes synostoses at the elbow, forearm, wrist, and hand. Finger synostoses are discussed in the section on syndactyly.

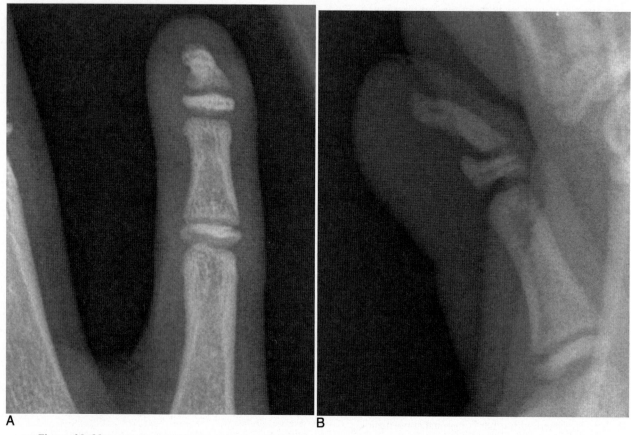

**Figure 30–20:**
Kirner deformity on posteroanterior **(A)** and lateral **(B)** radiographs. The angulation originates in the distal phalanx, not at the distal interphalangeal joint or middle phalanx.

## Humeroradial and Humeroulnar Synostoses

- Humeroradial synostosis is much more common than humeroulnar synostosis and can be divided into two types. Type I involves ulnar hypoplasia, usually is sporadic, and has an elbow usually fixed in extension. Type II is less common, usually is familial, is not associated with ulnar hypoplasia, and usually is fused in flexion.[36] Both types can be associated with genetic syndromes, and extraskeletal abnormalities are present in numerous cases. Referral to a geneticist or to subspecialists is warranted.

- Treatment of elbow synostoses depends on the position of the elbow and forearm. No procedure has successfully created and maintained a flexible elbow. These synostoses usually are unilateral and are well compensated by a normal contralateral hand. If the hand is positioned in front of the body with moderate elbow flexion and forearm pronation, surgical correction is not indicated. However, in patients in whom the elbow is positioned in such hyperextension that the hand is behind the body,

corrective osteotomies through the fusion mass are recommended.

## Radioulnar Synostosis

- Proximal radioulnar synostosis is the most common upper extremity synostosis. Most cases are bilateral. This synostosis can occur sporadically but often is transmitted as a dominant trait with variable penetrance. Several classification systems exist, although they are of limited use in deciding treatment. The radial head often is dislocated (Figure 30–21). The diagnosis often is missed until the child is in school, as compensatory wrist rotation can exceed 100 degrees and be enough to permit nearly normal function in young children.[37] In the physical examination, the examiner must not be fooled by wrist rotation: always measure forearm rotation by palpating motion of the distal radius, not the hand.

- Treatment depends on the position of the fused forearm(s). The forearm can be fused in any position, but most often both forearms are positioned in slight pronation. In such a position, function can be excellent without surgery. Shoulder

Figure 30–21:
**Bilateral congenital radioulnar synostoses with posterior dislocation of the radial heads. The child presented at age 4 years when his mother noticed that he could not throw a ball like his friends could.**

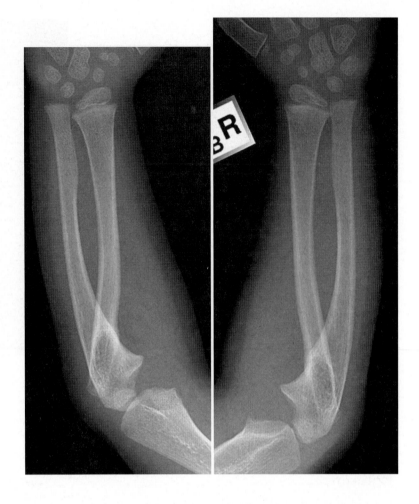

motion is used in addition to wrist rotation to compensate for the fusion. The indications for surgical correction are controversial. Takedown of the fusion mass historically has failed as the synostosis invariably recurs, although vascularized fat grafting may prove useful.[38] Derotational osteotomy of a malpositioned forearm is recommended for forearms in nonfunctional positions; however, the optimal target position in bilateral cases is controversial.[39,40] Some recommend placing the dominant forearm in slight pronation for writing and the nondominant forearm in slight supination for perineal hygiene. However, modern times require two pronated hands for computer keyboard use, and given the excellent functional outcomes of untreated patients with bilateral mild pronation fusions, this position may be the best goal of derotational osteotomies.

## Carpal Coalition

- Carpal coalitions are synostoses between carpal bones. Most coalitions are lunotriquetral or capitohamate,

although all possible combinations have been reported. Carpal coalitions can be associated with tarsal coalitions or many other syndromes, or they can occur sporadically. Unlike tarsal coalitions, carpal coalitions typically do not cause pain or wrist dysfunction, and treatment generally is not needed.

## Metacarpal Synostoses

- Fusion between adjacent metacarpals can appear as an isolated abnormality or as part of more complex hand deformities. As an isolated abnormality, bilateral fusion of the ring and small finger metacarpals is the most common metacarpal synostosis (Figure 30–22). In severe cases, the small finger is abducted because the small finger metacarpal head is nestled against the ring finger metacarpal neck. Surgical correction is aimed at widening the intermetacarpal space to allow small finger adduction. Lengthening the short metacarpal can be obtained achieved by various osteotomies.

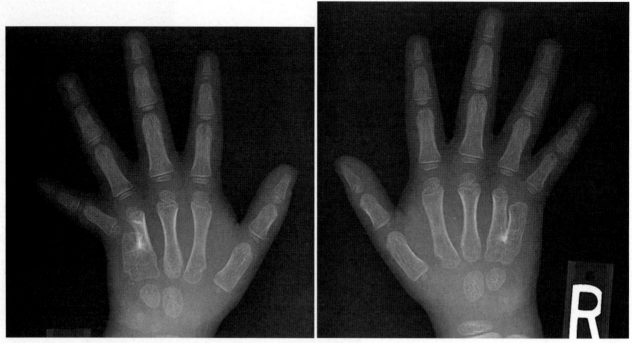

Figure 30–22:
**Bilateral congenital synostosis of the small and ring metacarpals. Note abduction of the small finger because of the proximity of the metacarpals.**

# References

1. Bamshad M, Watkins WS, Dixon ME, et al: Reconstructing the history of human limb development: lessons from birth defects. *Pediatr Res* 45:291-299, 1999.
   This article reviews the embryogenesis and developmental programs used to modify the architecture of the hominoid limb. The signaling pathways and their crucial role in limb axes formation are discussed.

2. Riddle RD, Tabin CJ: How limbs develop. *Sci Am* 280:74-79, 1999.
   A concise review of limb embryogenesis including axis development in normal and abnormal limbs.

3. Daluiski A, Yi SE, Lyons KM: The molecular control of upper extremity development: implications for congenital hand anomalies. *J Hand Surg* 26A:8-22, 2001.
   A general review of the various signaling pathways and molecular tracks that control limb development, with an update of syndromes attributed to defined molecular abnormalities.

4. Miura T, Nakamura R, Horii E: The position of symbrachydactyly in the classification of congenital hand anomalies. *J Hand Surg* 19B:350-354, 1994.
   Clinical features of 53 cases of intercalated hypoplasia and 113 cases of distal aplasia are compared with each other and with 129 cases of syndactyly, with discussion of implications for classification.

5. Ogino T: Congenital anomalies of the hand. The Asian perspective. *Clin Orthop* 323:12-21, 1996.
   Clinical scenarios of congenital differences were reviewed and compared to deformities created experimentally in rat fetuses in an effort to identify common underlying pathogeneses.

6. McCarroll HR: Congenital anomalies: a 25-year overview. *J Hand Surg* 25A:1007-1037, 2000.
   An overview of the major advances in the treatment of congenital hand anomalies over 25 years.

7. Lourie GM, Lins RE: Radial longitudinal deficiency. A review and update. *Hand Clin* 14:85-99, 1998.
   A review of radial deficiency that covers the gamut, including pathoanatomy, demographics, diagnosis, and treatment.

8. Buck-Gramcko D: Radialization as new treatment for radial clubhand. *J Hand Surg* 10A:964-968, 1985.
   This article describes the technique of "radialization" for treatment of radial deficiency.

9. Damore E, Kozin SH, Thoder JJ, Porter S: The recurrence of deformity after surgical centralization for radial clubhand. *J Hand Surg* 25A:745-751, 2000.
   Fourteen children (19 cases of radial deficiency) were reviewed retrospectively following centralization and found to have high rates of deformity recurrence despite excellent initial correction.

10. Hülsbergen-Krüger S, Preisser P, Partecke B-D: Ilizarov distraction-lengthening in congenital anomalies of the upper limb. *J Hand Surg* 23B:192-195, 1998.
    Distraction lengthening was applied to the congenitally short limb in nine patients. Five radial deficient limbs obtained an

average of 5.8-cm increase in length. In two patients with sym-brachydactyly, pinch grip between a radial and an ulnar digit was obtained by lengthening of the short ray. A patient with monodactyly underwent unsuccessful lengthening of the three transplanted proximal toe phalanges.

11. Foucher G, Medina J, Navarro R: Microsurgical reconstruction of the hypoplastic thumb, type IIIB. *J Reconstr Microsurg* 17:9-15, 2001.
Five cases of type IIIB thumb reconstruction using a free vascularized metatarsophalangeal joint combined with standard tendon transfers had persistent cosmetic deformity and limited function.

12. Kozin SH, Weiss AA, Webber JB, et al: Index finger pollicization for congenital aplasia or hypoplasia of the thumb. *J Hand Surg* 17A:880-884, 1992.
Fourteen hands (10 patients) evaluated after index finger pollicization had an average of 70% of the dexterity expected for normal hands.

13. Clark DI, Chell J, Davis TR: Pollicisation of the index finger. A 27-year follow-up study. *J Bone Joint Surg* 80-B:631-635, 1998.
Long-term follow-up of 11 patients treated by pollicization of the index finger after 20 to 38 years found lasting good-to-excellent function in most patients.

14. Lovett RJ: The treatment of longitudinal ulnar deficiency. *Prosthet Orthot Int* 15:104-105, 1991.
The author provides a thorough review of literature to date, including epidemiology, classifications, treatments, and functional outcomes.

15. Cole RJ, Manske PR: Classification of ulnar deficiency according to the thumb and first web. *J Hand Surg* 22A:479-488, 1997.
Fifty-five upper extremities with ulnar deficiency were reviewed, with particular focus on the hand abnormalities.

16. Vilkki SK: Advances in microsurgical reconstruction of the congenitally adactylous hand. *Clin Orthop* 314:45-58, 1995.
Microsurgical toe transfers were performed for adactylous hands, with the ability to pinch restored successfully in 14 of 17 hands.

17. Buss PW: Cleft hand/foot: clinical and developmental aspects. *J Med Genet* 31:726-730, 1994.
The author provides a review of the epidemiology, genetic basis, and functionality of patients with isolated central defects.

18. Flatt AE: Cleft hand and central defects. In Flatt AE, editor: *The care of congenital hand anomalies,* ed 2. St Louis, 1994, Quality Medical Publishing.
A classic single-author textbook on congenital hand anomalies in which the chapter on cleft hand delineates the functional triumph of the hand missing part or all of the long ray.

19. Rider MA, Grindel SI, Tonkin MA, Wood VE: An experience of the Snow-Littler procedure. *J Hand Surg* 25B:376-381, 2000.
The authors review results of the Snow-Littler procedure in 12 hands with classic central longitudinal deficiency and in one hand with symbrachydactyly.

20. Radocha RF, Netscher D, Kleinert HE: Toe phalangeal grafts in congenital hand anomalies. *J Hand Surg* 18A:833-841, 1993.
In a review of 73 toe phalangeal grafts, physeal growth in the transferred phalanx was found to decline with age at time of procedure, with the best results in patients operated before age 1 year.

21. Buck-Gramcko D: The role of nonvascularized toe phalanx transplantation. *Hand Clin* 6:643-659, 1990.
Ninety-seven toe phalanx transplantations were performed in 57 children, with 100% graft take but variable functional results when joint reconstruction was attempted.

22. Dhalla R, Strecker W, Manske PR: A comparison of two techniques for digital distraction lengthening in skeletally immature patients. *J Hand Surg* 26A:603-610, 2001.
Twenty metacarpals and seven phalanges were lengthened in 16 skeletally immature patients, with average lengthening of 12 to 13 mm but high complication rates.

23. Van Holder C, Giele H, Gilbert A: Double second toe transfer in congenital hand anomalies. *J Hand Surg* 24B:471-475, 1999.
Fourteen patients with congenital hand anomalies received staged double second toe transfers for functional restoration.

24. Kay SP, Wiberg M: Toe to hand transfer in children. Part 1: technical aspects. *J Hand Surg* 21B:723-734, 1996.
Forty children with either congenital or acquired hand deformities underwent microvascular transplantation of one or more toes with 100% survival of the digits, but secondary procedures were required in 75%.

25. Watson BT, Hennrikus WL: Postaxial type-B polydactyly. Prevalence and treatment. *J Bone Joint Surg* 79A:65-68, 1997.
A prospective screening program of 11,161 newborns delineated the incidence of postaxial polydactyly type B and described the results of 20 cases of suture ligation in the nursery.

26. Wassel HD: The results of surgery for polydactyly of the thumb. A review. *Clin Orthop* 64:175-193, 1969.
A classic article in which Wassel puts forth his classification of thumb duplication and his surgical correction techniques and results.

27. Ogino T, Ishii S, Takahata S, Kato H: Long-term results of surgical treatment of thumb polydactyly. *J Hand Surg* 21A:478-486, 1996.
One hundred thirteen hands with thumb polydactyly were treated and outcome assessed at an average of 49 months.

28. Kozin SH: Syndactyly. *J Am Soc Surg Hand* 1:1-13, 2001.
A review of syndactyly, including inheritable, spontaneous, and syndromic forms.

29. Greuse M, Coessens BC: Congenital syndactyly: defatting facilitates closure without skin graft. *J Hand Surg* 26A:589-594, 2001.
Syndactyly was corrected without skin grafts in 16 consecutive patients (24 syndactylies).

30. Al-Qattan MM: Classification of hand anomalies in Poland's syndrome. *Br J Plast Surg* 54:132-136, 2001.
Twenty cases of Poland syndrome are reviewed, and a classification of the hand anomalies is presented.

31. Wiedrich TA: Congenital constriction band syndrome. *Hand Clin* 14:29-38, 1998.
An overview of constriction band syndrome with a discussion of proposed etiologies. Various clinical presentations are addressed, and potential treatment options are reviewed.

32. Van Heest AE, House JH, Reckling WC: Two-stage reconstruction of Apert acrosyndactyly. *J Hand Surg* 22A:315-322, 1997.

Twenty-eight hands (14 children) with Apert acrosyndactyly were evaluated to develop a classification system that guides the type and staging of hand reconstruction.

33. Engber WD, Flatt AE: Camptodactyly: an analysis of sixty-six patients and twenty-four operations. *J Hand Surg [Am]* 2:216-224, 1977.
    The authors review a series of 66 patients with camptodactyly and highlight the futility of surgical procedures.

34. Burke F, Flatt A: Clinodactyly. A review of a series of cases. *Hand* 11:269-280, 1979.
    A series of 50 patients is reviewed, and the authors recommend early surgery only if a delta phalanx is present.

35. Freiberg A, Forrest C: Kirner's deformity: a review of the literature and case presentation. *J Hand Surg [Am]* 11:28-32, 1986.
    A review of the literature pertaining to Kirner deformity is presented.

36. McIntyre JD, Benson MK: An aetiological classification for developmental synostoses at the elbow. *J Pediatr Orthop B* 11:313-319, 2002.
    The authors review reported cases of humeroulnar, humeroradial, and humeroradioulnar synostoses, proposing a classification scheme to account for mode of occurrence and association with other upper extremity malformations.

37. Ogino T, Hikino K: Congenital radio-ulnar synostosis: compensatory rotation around the wrist and rotation osteotomy. *J Hand Surg [Br]* 12:173-178, 1987. Erratum in: *J Hand Surg [Br]* 12:402, 1987.
    The authors review 40 cases of congenital radioulnar synostosis in which compensatory rotation through the carpus was found to exceed 100 degrees and the most functional position was found to be approximately 20 degrees pronation.

38. Kanaya F, Ibaraki K: Mobilization of a congenital proximal radioulnar synostosis with use of a free vascularized fascio-fat graft. *J Bone Joint Surg Am* 80:1186-1192, 1998.
    The authors describe a novel technique of excising a congenital radioulnar synostosis and interposing a free vascularized fat graft from the upper arm with modest functional gains.

39. Green WT, Mital MA: Congenital radio-ulnar synostosis: surgical treatment. *J Bone Joint Surg Am* 61:738-743, 1979.
    The authors review the results of 13 patients who underwent rotational osteotomy for congenital radioulnar synostosis and conclude that the optimal positions for bilateral synostoses are 30 to 45 degrees pronation for the dominant arm and 20 to 35 degrees supination for the nondominant arm.

40. Simmons BP, Southmayd WW, Riseborough EJ: Congenital radioulnar synostosis. *J Hand Surg [Am]* 8:829-838, 1983.
    The authors review the results of 33 patients who underwent rotational osteotomy for congenital radioulnar synostosis and conclude that the optimal positions for bilateral synostoses are 10 to 15 degrees pronation for the dominant arm and neutral rotation for the nondominant arm.

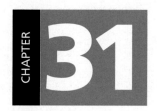

# Management of the Upper Extremity in Cerebral Palsy and Following Brain Injury in Adults

## Michael R. Hausman[*] and James M. Savundra[†]

[*]MD, Department of Orthopaedics, Mount Sinai School of Medicine, New York, NY
[†]MBBS, FRACS, Consultant Plastic Surgeon, Royal Perth Hospital, Perth, Australia; Consultant Plastic Surgeon, Fremantle Hospital, Fremantle, Australia

- Insult to the brain during the period of brain plasticity and adult brain injury are distinct disorders but share many common symptoms and physical findings.
- The causes of brain injury in this adult population include cerebrovascular accident, brain trauma, brain parenchymal disorders, and injury following brain surgical procedures.
- The causes of cerebral palsy are far more ill defined. They include intrauterine, perinatal, and postnatal insults to the brain that are nonprogressive.
- Although the early priorities following brain injury may be preservation of life and maintenance of critical organ function, the management of the musculoskeletal problems should commence early after the irreversible brain injury is diagnosed.
- The patient often benefits from involvement of specialists in upper extremity management, including hand therapists and hand surgeons.
- The long-term sequelae of brain injury often include major upper limb dysfunction. In some patients, surgical and nonsurgical interventions may help a range of problems in the upper limb.

- Spasticity is the key problem that reconstructive surgeons deal with because weakness, which is the other major consequence of an upper motor neuron lesion, is rarely treatable.

## Etiology

- Strokes (cerebrovascular accidents) tend to present with classic patterns of motor dysfunction, whereas cerebral palsy, brain injury from trauma or surgery, and other neurologic disorders cause motor dysfunction with variable patterns.
- The number of limbs affected often is included in the description of the condition: monoplegia (single limb), diplegia (bilateral limbs, either upper or lower), hemiplegia (both limbs on one side of the body), and tetraplegia (all four limbs).

### Cerebral Palsy

- Cerebral palsy results from a nonprogressive lesion in the developing brain, which causes a permanent musculoskeletal dysfunction that may change as the child physically matures.[1]

- With an incidence of 2.0 to 2.5 per 1000 live births, cerebral palsy is the most common cause of physical disability affecting children in developed countries.[2]
- In addition to the motor dysfunction, the other features of cerebral palsy include epilepsy, learning difficulties, behavioral challenges, and sensory impairments.[3]
- As with most insults that occur during very early childhood and infancy, the patient learns to cope and manage with the deficits present, but the condition may affect musculoskeletal development.

## Cerebrovascular Accident

- Cerebrovascular accidents or strokes affect one in 1000 individuals each year. They cause 200,000 deaths per year and the majority of hemiplegia in the United States. If patients survive the initial 6 months, they usually live for 6 years or more.[4–6]
- The middle cerebral artery is the most commonly involved vessel in stroke; therefore, the sensory and motor strips usually are affected, often producing a pattern of hemiplegia.[7]

## Trauma Causing Brain Injury

- Motor vehicle accident, assaults, and falls can cause irreversible brain injury. These incidents are the most common cause of neurologic deficit leading to spasticity in the limbs occurring in late childhood and early adulthood. As opposed to cerebrovascular accident, this group of patients have a heterogeneous group of dysfunction in the upper limb that may lead to atypical patterns of spasticity.

## Surgery and Surgical Pathology Causing Brain Injury

- Many brain surgical procedures performed through craniotomy and minimal exposure techniques can cause motor disorders (including spasticity), and, like trauma, the resultant spasticity may not fall into classic predictable patterns.

## Acquired Brain Disorders

- Conditions such as multiple sclerosis, meningitis, and encephalitis all can lead to spasticity affecting the upper limb.

## Spasticity

### Definition

- Spasticity is an increase in muscle tone resulting from a velocity-dependent increase in tonic spinal stretch reflexes that have lost their normal inhibitory cortical control.

- Spasticity is part of an upper motor neuron syndrome having positive features (e.g., spasticity) and negative features (e.g., weakness).[8]

## Pathophysiology Key

- Abnormal processing of proprioceptive input in the spinal cord.[8]
- Mediated by the afferent nerves (Ia) in the muscle spindle (neuronal end-organ that senses tension in a skeletal muscle).
- Results from loss of inhibition of the spinal stretch reflexes, which normally are controlled by the upper motor neuron pathways.
- During normal purposeful motion, the muscle that is being intentionally activated causes stretch in its antagonist muscle. This passive stretch of the antagonist sends signals from its muscle spindle to the lower motor neuron that would activate its contraction, except that this activation normally is inhibited by upper motor neurons. This inhibition allows relaxation of the antagonistic muscle during purposeful movement (Figure 31–1).
- An upper motor neuron syndrome may cause involuntary cocontraction because of loss of the upper motor neuron pathways that normally inhibit the antagonist muscle during voluntary motion. This simultaneous cocontraction of the agonist and its antagonist makes movement ineffectual. When the attempt at voluntary movement is discontinued, both muscle groups relax.
- Immediately after an irreversible injury to upper motor neurons, flaccidity occurs. The spasticity of the upper motor neuron syndrome occurs only after a period of several days to weeks.
- Flexor spasms (clonus) are different than spasticity (abnormal proprioceptive reflexes) because they result from disinhibited normal flexor withdrawal reflexes (e.g., standing barefoot on a pin).[8]
- Figure 31–2 shows the relationship of positive and negative features of upper motor neuron syndrome to limb dysfunction.

## Assessment

- Assessment can be performed in conjunction with a multidisciplinary team and can be especially useful in children with cerebral palsy. Often review of more than one occasion is a necessary part of the clinical assessment.
- The upper limb should be completely exposed and compared throughout the clinical assessment to the other side.
- The resting posture should be noted, including the integrity of the skin, subcutaneous tissues, and joints.
- All the positive and negative features of the upper motor neuron syndrome should be sought and noted.
- Joint contracture should be noted. Absolute shortening of the musculotendinous unit should be separated from joint contracture.

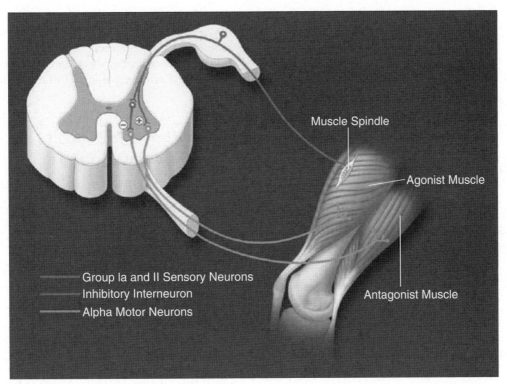

Figure 31–1:
**Stretch reflex arc.**[13] (**From Satkunam LE:** *Can Med Assoc J* 169:1173, 2003.)

## Deformities

- Abnormal function and deformity may present several months to years after the insult in cerebral palsy. The first presentation may be failure to reach learning and motor milestones.
- Following brain injury, flaccid paralysis occurs prior to any spasticity. Spasticity may take several days to weeks to develop.
- Complex regional pain syndrome (reflex sympathetic dystrophy) may occur early in any limb affected by neurologic injury. Swelling, stiffness, and pain are common sequelae.
- The spasticity that develops in the upper limb tends to fall into a classic pattern, but the clinician must be prepared for variations in this pattern.
- Box 31–1 lists the classic patterns of spasticity in the upper limb.

## Early Intervention

### Splinting, Positioning, and Mobilization

- Early management of the upper limbs and lower limbs following a neurologic insult follows the principles used for any lower or upper motor neuron injury.

- Early splinting is important when flaccid paralysis or any degree of paresis is present. Also, when the conscious state is diminished, the limbs must be kept in "safe" positions.
- Positioning of patient and limbs is important to prevent early sequelae of brain injury, such as decubitus ulcers, deep venous thrombosis, and pneumonia.
- Passive mobilization is commonly practiced and, although safe, probably has not proved to be beneficial to long-term outcome.
- The main aim of these measures is to prevent joint contracture and musculotendinous unit shortening.

### Pain Management and Associated Procedures (Blocks)

- Complex regional pain syndromes can affect the patient with brain injury and tend to present in the first few weeks following the injury. The early involvement of pain specialists and physical and occupational therapists is crucial.
- Once an upper motor neuron syndrome is established, pain can be a debilitating symptom. Each of the positive and negative features carries specific patterns of pain.[9]
- Sympathetic blockade can be beneficial in some of these patients.

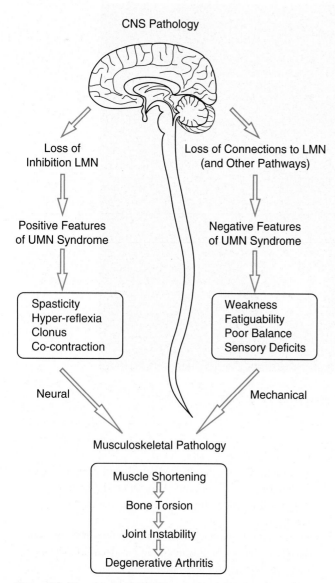

CNS Pathology

Loss of Inhibition LMN

Loss of Connections to LMN (and Other Pathways)

Positive Features of UMN Syndrome

Negative Features of UMN Syndrome

Spasticity
Hyper-reflexia
Clonus
Co-contraction

Weakness
Fatiguability
Poor Balance
Sensory Deficits

Neural

Mechanical

Musculoskeletal Pathology

Muscle Shortening

Bone Torsion

Joint Instability

Degenerative Arthritis

Figure 31–2:
Upper motor neuron syndrome.[1] *CNS*, central nervous system; *LMN*, lower motor neuron; *UMN*, upper motor neuron. (From Graham H, Selber P: *J Bone Joint Surg Br* 85B:157, 2003.)

| Box 31–1 | Patterns of Spasticity in the Upper Limb |
| --- | --- |
| Shoulder | Internal rotation, adduction |
| Elbow | Flexion |
| Forearm | Pronation |
| Wrist | Flexion, ulnar deviation |
| Thumb | Adduction, flexion |
| Fingers | Variable, extension of interphalangeal joints; flexion of MCP joints, swan-neck deformity |

- Shoulder subluxation is a common cause of pain in the upper limb and can be treated with simple measures such as splinting. Other procedures, such as shoulder arthrodesis and functional electrical stimulation, can be used for the primary purpose of treating pain.

## Nonsurgical Techniques and Neurologic Procedures

### Therapy and Functional Appliances

- Therapists play an important role in the long-term care of patients with upper limb dysfunction following brain injury. Their intervention with aids for walking and activities of daily living is important.
- Use of therapy, such as mobilization techniques, muscle lengthening and strengthening, motor relearning, and splinting, to prevent long-term sequelae is less proven but probably has a role.[10]

### Medical Treatment

- The general goal of medical management is to decrease spinal reflex excitability by reducing the release of excitatory neurotransmitters or by potentiating the activity of inhibitory circuits.[11]
- Long-acting benzodiazepines such as diazepam can help produce generalized relaxation.
- Baclofen, which is a drug that stimulates γ-aminobutyric acid (GABA)-B receptors, can be given systemically or intrathecally to specifically affect the activity of the spinal reflex pathways. Baclofen can be delivered intrathecally by a continuous pump.
- Other medications, such as tizanidine ($\alpha_2$-agonist) and dantrolene (affects intracellular calcium release), are used in some situations.

### Botulinum Toxin A

- Since botulinum toxin became available in the United States, its uses have increased to include conditions with debilitating spasticity and muscle overactivity.
- Botulinum toxin A works at the neuromuscular junction by irreversibly blocking release of acetylcholine.
- The toxin is easier to use than nerve blockade techniques because the injections need only be given within the affected muscles rather than precisely located at the nerve. A sound knowledge of the upper limb anatomy is important.
- The effect of botulinum toxin A lasts between 3 and 6 months. Therefore, it can be used not only to counter long-term spasticity but also for diagnostic purposes so that voluntary function of agonist and antagonist muscles can be assessed without spasticity clouding the assessment.

## Nerve and Neurosurgical Procedures

- As with botulinum toxin, motor nerves can be blocked for therapeutic and diagnostic purposes. Local anesthetic agents can be used for short-term diagnostic purposes. Phenol can be injected for an effect that lasts approximately 5 months. Phenol can be toxic, and percutaneous delivery may be hazardous to surrounding structures. Open nerve approaches can be used to decrease the collateral damage associated with phenol blockade.
- More long-term benefit may be gained by formal open sectioning of peripheral motor nerves. Nerves have the propensity to regrow, so removing a section of nerve may be important. Intraoperative, intraneural assessment can be made using a nerve stimulator so that sectioning can be fascicle specific if needed.
- Dorsal rhizotomy is a surgical interruption of afferent pain and muscle proprioceptive fibers as they enter the spinal cord. This procedure selectively disrupts the influence of pain and proprioception on the spinal cord reflexes, thereby decreasing their overactivity. The newer techniques aim for greater precision and are termed *dorsal root entry zone-otomy* (DREZotomy). For the upper limb, the spinal cord is approached through a laminectomy between levels C4 and C7, which allows access to all the cord levels affecting upper limb function.[12]

## Surgery

### Indications

- Upper limb surgery for patients with brain injury has limited but specific benefits. The aims of surgery can be grouped into three main areas: hygiene reasons, improved function, and aesthetic (social) reasons.
- Issues of hygiene are an important indication for surgery. The skin of contracted joints is difficult to clean. Normal skin integrity and physiology requires regular toileting. When the affected person or his/her caretaker cannot clean the skin, breakdown can result.
- Functional improvement is less predictable but aims to neutralize the forces causing deformity (e.g., spasticity) and therefore improve the ability of the functioning motors to drive the part of the limb affected. Improved control of the limb may be gained by simply releasing the musculotendinous units causing contracture and possibly also releasing joint capsular contracture. Occasionally, tendon transfer improves function, but this is less likely with adult brain injury than in the cerebral palsy group.
- Box 31–1 describes the pathologic postures that may afflict the limb after brain injury. A limb carried in this manner has significant connotations for the sufferer and those with whom they interact in the community. Improving the position of a limb for socialization is an important service that can be provided by relatively simple surgery.

### Planning

- The multidisciplinary model works well in the management of the upper limb affected by brain injury and is a critical part of planning for surgical intervention.
- When presented with the spastic, seemingly useless upper limb, the surgeon must assess each muscle to determine whether the muscle is spastic or has some voluntary control. An assessment as to the degree of spasticity and the degree of voluntary control may be difficult.
- Use of nerve blockade (local anesthetic or phenol) and botulinum toxin A may inhibit function of spastic muscles to allow further assessment of voluntary control or spasticity within the remaining muscles. The advantage of the longer-acting agents is that patients can return to their activities of daily living and determine whether they are better off without the overfunctioning muscles. Surgical results then can be more predictable.
- A little spasticity can improve function in specific situations, as in the finger intrinsics. Finger intrinsic spasticity can leave the finger in an intrinsic plus position that is a more functional position, as opposed to long finger flexor spasticity that tends to leave the fingers in an intrinsic minus position.
- Dynamic surface electromyography has been used to predict functioning muscles in lower limb spasticity. It may have some use in planning surgical intervention in the upper limb but at this stage has not been widely used.

### Releases

- Multiple surgical procedures performed at different times in this group of patients are not preferred. Most releases, fusions, and transfers can be performed at multiple levels in the upper limb during a single operation.

#### Anterior Shoulder Release

- The patient is placed with a bolster behind the scapula. A standard deltopectoral approach is used.
- The tendon of pectoralis major is divided near its insertion on the humerus. The subscapularis muscle is carefully separated from the anterior glenohumeral capsule and divided.
- If adequate release has not been achieved by this stage, the teres major and latissimus dorsi muscles can be divided near their humeral insertions.
- The wound is closed, and formal abduction splinting usually is not necessary.

#### Elbow Release

- The elbow flexors are exposed through a lateral incision in the distal arm, which curves medially at the antecubital crease.

- The brachioradialis muscle and biceps tendon are completely released. The brachialis is lengthened at the musculotendinous junction by dividing the tendinous portion within the muscle substance.
- The elbow is splinted in a straighter position for 2 to 3 weeks.

### Pronator Release

- The pronator teres is approached over the volar midforearm between the mobile wad and the flexor carpi radialis.
- The tendon is identified near the muscle belly and divided within the myotendinous junction to allow fractional lengthening.
- The pronator quadratus is approached more distally in the forearm through a longitudinal volar incision.
- The finger flexor tendons are retracted radially, and the pronator quadratus is completely divided.
- The wounds are closed. The patient is placed in an above elbow splint in slight supination for 2 weeks, and then full mobilization is allowed.

### Volar Wrist Release

- A longitudinal midline forearm incision is made to access all the volar tendons.
- The flexor carpi radialis and flexor carpi ulnaris tendons are divided, taking care to preserve the ulnar and median nerves. Tendon lengthening can be performed if needed at either the musculotendinous junction or within the substance of the tendon.
- This procedure is often associated with long finger flexor tendon lengthening.

### Thumb Adductor Release

- A four-flap Z-plasty is created in the first web space to allow wide exposure of the adductor pollicis and the thenar muscles and soft tissue lengthening of the contracted web space (Figure 31–3).
- As much adductor pollicis muscle belly is divided as necessary to allow release of the first web space, starting with the transverse muscle fibers and then the oblique fibers if necessary.
- The skin is closed to allow the points of the Z-plasty to be placed where they allow maximum lengthening. A splint is applied for 3 weeks.

### Finger Flexor Lengthening

- This procedure often is combined with a wrist flexor release and can be performed through the same incision. The aim is to have all the tendons lengthened proximal to the carpal tunnel.
- A step cut is placed in each of the tendons to be lengthened and then resutured in the elongated position (Figure 31–4).
- Postoperative splint protection is needed for at least 4 weeks to allow the tendons to heal. Early active

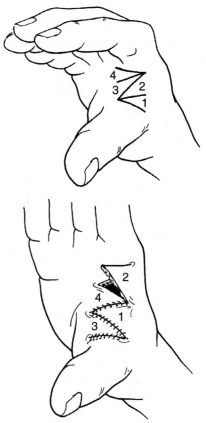

**Figure 31–3:**
**Four-flap Z-plasty provides an excellent means of improving the thumb index web space when there is concomitant contracture of the skin as well as the adductor pollicis muscle.** (From Trumble T: *Principles of hand surgery and therapy.* Philadelphia, 2000, WB Saunders Company.)

mobilization therapy regimens are less likely to work in this patient population and probably are less necessary in zone 4 tendon repairs.

### Transfers

- Tendon transfers can be beneficial in specific cases where multiple muscles within a compartment are under voluntary control. These patients must be assessed for their individual donor musculotendinous units using the techniques described in the section on Planning.
- Tendon transfers tend to be less useful in the adult brain injury population compared to the cerebral palsy and spinal injury groups.

### Flexor Carpi Ulnaris to Extensor Carpi Radialis Brevis Transfer

- The patient must have a functioning flexor carpi radialis for this transfer to be performed. In addition, little spasticity of both wrist flexors is preferable.
- The flexor carpi ulnaris is approached through a generous longitudinal incision. The tendon is divided at the insertion into the pisiform and raised proximally

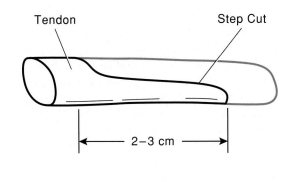

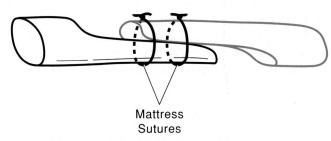

**Figure 31–4:**
Step-cut lengthening of tendons.

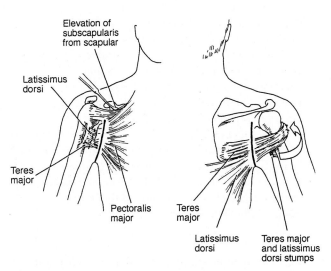

**Figure 31–5:**
The L'Episcopo procedure is performed to regain external rotation following an upper trunk injury. The latissimus dorsi muscle is detached from the humerus, usually through an incision along the interior axillary fold that borders the anterior margin of the latissimus dorsi muscle. A posterior approach is then used to redirect the latissiumus dorsi muscle and insert this into the lateral aspect of the humerus in line with the fibers of the infraspinatus to provide external rotation. The teres major muscle runs parallel to the latissimus dorsi and its tendon is transfered as well. (From Trumble T: *Principles of hand surgery and therapy.* Philadelphia, 2000, WB Saunders Company.)

as far as possible. Care must be taken not to injure the ulnar neurovascular bundle.

- Another incision is made in the distal dorsal forearm, and the extensor carpi radialis brevis tendon is localized.
- The flexor is tunneled subcutaneously around the ulnar border of the forearm. A weave is performed into the divided end of the extensor tendon at the appropriate tension to give 10 to 20 degrees wrist extension with the forearm in neutral position.
- The patient is splinted in an above elbow splint with the wrist in extension and the forearm in neutral position.

## L'Episcopo Transfer (Latissimus Dorsi/Teres Major Rerouting)

- The standard deltopectoral approach is used along with release of the pectoralis major and subscapularis as described in the section entitled Anterior Shoulder Release.
- The tendon of the latissimus dorsi is divided 1 cm from its insertion. A tunnel is bluntly dissected around the lateral and posterior surfaces of the upper humerus, and the latissimus tendon is brought posteriorly around to be reattached to the original tendon stump (Figure 31–5).
- The same procedure is performed for the teres major.

## STP Transfer (Flexor Superficialis to Flexor Profundus Transfer)

- This transfer is used for the clenched fist deformity where tendon lengthening will not provide adequate finger opening for hand toileting. As a general rule, if the pulp-palm distance is less than 6 cm with the wrist

in neutral position, then tendon lengthening probably will not provide enough improvement in digital position.

- STP transfer is preferable to long flexor tenotomy because simple tenotomy may have the undesirable aesthetic effect of a functionless open hand.
- The superficialis is commonly spastic. The STP transfer is rarely active but may provide some function in conjunction with normal extensors and the tenodesis effect.
- Release of the clenched fist deformity often uncovers significant finger intrinsic spasticity, which can be treated by neurectomy of the motor branch of the ulnar nerve in the hand or intrinsic release. Neurectomy usually provides enough improvement in intrinsic spasticity. However, if significant MCP joint contracture greater than 10 to 20 degrees with the wrist in neutral position is present, intrinsic release should be considered.
- Through the same longitudinal volar forearm incision used in multiple other procedures, the flexor digitorum superficialis tendons are sutured together proximal to the carpal tunnel and divided distal to the suture.
- The flexor digitorum profundus tendons are sutured together near their musculotendinous junctions and then divided just proximal to this suture.

- The proximal superficialis tendons are sutured to the distal profundus tendons at the desired tension so that passive wrist extension causes a degree of finger flexion and passive wrist flexion causes finger extension. For severe contractures, the flexor digitorum profundus (FDP) can be transferred to the flexor digitorum superficialis (Figure 31–6).
- This procedure usually is performed for more severe deformities and can be performed in conjunction with a wrist fusion so that no tenodesis effect is possible. In that case, the fingers should be in a comfortable position that allows easy cleaning of the hand but they should not be in full extension.

## Joint Fusions

- Most joints can be effectively fused in the upper limb. The shoulder and wrist fusions are the most commonly fused in the spastic upper limb to improve position and function.

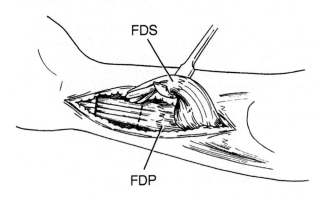

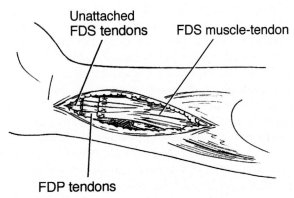

Figure 31–6:
The superficialis-to-profundus transfer is performed by transecting the flexor digitorum profundus (FDP) tendons proximally and the flexor digitorum superficialis (FDS) tendons distally. The superficialis tendons are then attached to their respective profundus tendon after the tendons have been lengthened sufficiently to allow full extension of the digits with the wrist in neutral position. (From Trumble T: *Principles of hand surgery and therapy.* Philadelphia, 2000, WB Saunders Company.)

- The wrist fusion usually is associated with flexor tendon release. The standard technique of a wrist fusion plate and cancellous iliac bone graft is reliable in this group of patients. Carpectomy, either proximal row or total, may be required if significant wrist flexor contracture occurs after flexor tendon release.
- Small joint fusion, as in the thumb interphalangeal joint, can be useful for improving function. This fusion can be achieved using a headless compression screw technique.

## Conclusion

- Brain injury and cerebral palsy may cause deforming and disabling spasticity because of loss of central inhibition of spinal reflex arcs.
- Treatment can be directed at multiple levels to minimize or release deforming forces, thus preventing or releasing contractures (Figure 31–7).
- Restoration of limited voluntary control may be possible in selected cases if deforming forces can be eliminated or controlled.

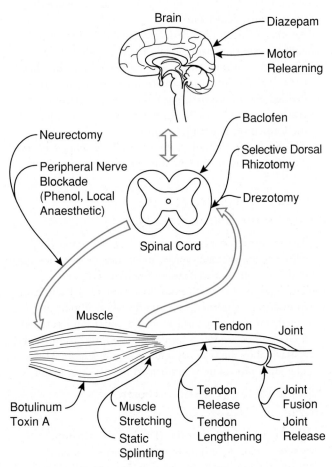

Figure 31–7:
Interventions for spasticity.

- When surgical intervention is indicated, the whole upper limb should be treated for maximal benefit to the patient.
- In the group of patients with brain injury after the period of brain plasticity, transfers are of less value than in the cerebral palsy group; however, both groups benefit from correctly indicated releases.

# References

1. Graham H, Selber P: Musculoskeletal aspects of cerebral palsy. *J Bone Joint Surg Br* 85B:157, 2003.
   Important information on the epidemiology of cerebral palsy that often is quoted by authors on this topic. Discusses etiologic considerations.

2. Standley F, Blair E, Alberman E: Cerebral palsies: epidemiology and causal pathways. *Clin Dev Med* :151, 2000.
   A review of the musculoskeletal aspects of cerebral palsy. Presents data and a good overview of the principles of nonsurgical and surgical management.

3. Rosenbaum P: Cerebral palsy: what parents and doctors want to know. *Br Med J* 326:970, 2003.
   A thorough overview of cerebral palsy, which also is useful to patients with cerebral palsy and their parents. Not much detail on specific treatments.

4. Fuchs Z, Blumstein T, Novikov I, et al: Morbidity, comorbidity, and their association with disability among community-dwelling oldest-old in Israel. *J Gerontol A Biol Sci Med Sci* 53:M447, 1998.
   An often quoted epidemiologic study of medical conditions affecting the elderly.

5. Lackland DT, Bachman DL, Carten TD, et al: The geographic variation in stroke incidence in two areas of the southeastern stroke belt: the Anderson and Pee Dee Stroke Study. *Stroke* 29:2061, 1998.
   An often quoted study of the epidemiology of strokes in two North American populations.

6. Sacco RL, Boden-Albala B, Gan R, et al: Stroke incidence among white, black and Hispanic residents of an urban community: the Northern Manhattan Stroke Study. *Am J Epidemiol* 147:259-268, 1998.
   An important study on the epidemiology of stroke in a North American population.

7. Trumble TE, Van Heest A: Stroke, traumatic brain injury, and cerebral palsy. In Trumble T, editor: *Principles of hand surgery and therapy*. Philadelphia, 2000, WB Saunders.
   Brief chapter that mainly discusses clinical assessment and surgical treatment.

8. Sheean G: The pathophysiology of spasticity. *Eur J Neurol* 9:3, 2002.
   Overview of the pathophysiology of spasticity, critical to the understanding of the deformities and treatment options.

9. Ward AB, Kadies M: The management of pain in spasticity. *Disabil Rehabil* 24:443, 2002.
   Overview of the management of pain in patients with spasticity. Brings together the use of many treatments with the aim of improving pain but not necessarily motion.

10. Richardson D: Physical therapy in spasticity. *Eur J Neurol* 9:17, 2002.
    Review of physical therapy techniques used in patients with spasticity.

11. Abbruzzese G: The medical management of spasticity. *Eur J Neurol* 9:30, 2002.
    Good overview of medications used for treatment of spasticity, featuring diazepam, dantrolene, and baclofen. However, botulinum toxin is not discussed.

12. Lazorthes Y, Sol JC, Sallerin B, Verdie JC: The surgical management of spasticity. *Eur J Neurol* 9:35, 2002.
    Describes neurosurgical techniques of the central and peripheral nervous systems. Discusses indications, expected outcomes, and briefly describes techniques.

13. Satkunam LE: Rehabilitation medicine: 3. Management of adult spasticity. *Can Med Assoc J* 169:1173, 2003.
    Overview of spasticity in adults, including assessment and treatment. Written from the point of view of a rehabilitation physician. Brief with regard to surgical intervention.

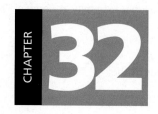

# Tetraplegia

## Michael W. Keith

MD, Professor of Orthopedics and BioMedical Engineering, Case Western Reserve University; Chief, Hand Service, Metrohealth Medical Center, Cleveland, OH

- This chapter is written for the hand surgical resident who is consulting to the spinal cord injury (SCI) service or assists senior faculty in the care of persons with tetraplegia.

## Spinal Cord Injuries

- Approximately 10,000 new cases of SCI occur in the United States every year. The prevalence now is approximately 250,000 persons. Among tetraplegics, about half have injuries in the middle of the cervical spine with American Spinal Injury Association (ASIA) class C5 or C6 injuries.
- Today in western nations with access to good continuing medical and surgical care, persons with SCI have a normal life expectancy and are entitled to complete social participation. The level of medical and social support a person receives is dependent on his/her preinjury work history and benefits, geographic location within the country, and social status rather than the type of injury sustained or its consequences. Initially all injured persons receive uniform acute care support through commercial hospitalization insurance or Medicaid coverage.
- Two years after injury, patients are entitled to receive more limited Medicare benefits. In some states with no-fault insurance for motor vehicle accidents, they are entitled to excellent life-long care and attendant support. Military service injured beneficiaries receive broad and life-long support through the Veteran's Affairs Medical Centers. Constant reference to these entitlements is needed to optimize treatment.
- Data from the National Institute on Disability and Rehabilitation Research (NIDRR) Spinal Cord Injury Model Centers reveal that, for a survivor, trauma causation is seasonal. It occurs more often in the summer, is most often a disease of young men, and is linked to interpersonal and vehicular violence and in some cases negligent behavior. SCI patients often are the victims rather than the cause of injury.
- A high-energy form of injury differs from injury resulting from tumors, vascular accidents, and infections, as does the prognosis. We differentiate potentially recurrent spinal cord diseases such as tumors from isolated injuries.
- Mechanically the spinal cord is damaged when the spinal column ligaments or vertebral bodies of the vertebrae fail when loaded. Frequently the mechanism of injury is head and spine flexion and axial compression during diving accidents; flexion and distraction during motor vehicle accidents; and direct injury from gunshot and stabbing incidents.
- The resulting translation of the bony fragment posteriorly produces varied forces on the spinal cord and begins a cascade of structural and cellular events, including *apoptosis* (a remarkable programmed cellular death of neurons), which disrupts the anatomy and functionality of the complex nervous interconnections. It is not a simple bony compression, although we discuss

"decompressing" the cord. It is not a vascular insufficiency, although we discuss improving circulation by alignment. The spinal cord responds to trauma by edema and cell death, central formation of a hematomyelia (blood and necrotic nerve), and eventually resorption. Subsequent intrinsic and extrinsic scar, syrinx formation (a central fluid cavity that may enlarge), and local bony instability all contribute to the persistence of paralysis. There is no known reliable intervention—surgical, pharmacologic, or other method—for reversing these processes.

- Natural recovery can occur but usually to a limited degree, such as a spinal root level in ASIA "complete" injuries. We expect the root level muscles below the voluntary level to improve through reversal of neurapraxia of the peripheral nerves, axonal regeneration from some intact motor neurons, and some cord plasticity of the cord neuron pool.
- The damaged level of the cord as viewed by magnetic resonance imaging represents irreparable disorganization and a block to descending control and ascending responsiveness.
- We can expect patients examined during the first week and classified by the ASIA scales to improve at least one muscle level to the next lowest root level, but the improvement varies among cases. Consultants as a group should present a single, cautiously advised opinion to the patient and family to avoid false hope, conflict, or confusion.

## Consultation

- The consultation should make a diagnosis, recommend intervention at the proper time, define the expectations for improvement, and define and reinforce the life-long process of adaptation and rehabilitation.

## Diagnosis

- A high degree of suspicion of head and neck injury is required upon initial examination of all persons with a high-velocity or high-energy injury. Routinely, first-responder emergency personnel place injured persons in a splint for cervical spine injury at the scene of accidents and perform a preliminary screen for paralysis.
- Removal of neck collars and subsequent examination, x-ray films, and secondary examination by knowledgeable and responsible physicians are required.
- Medical clearance for head and neck movement is highly formalized and documented. With this greater attention to prevention of reinjury or propagation of initial injury, the incidence of partial SCI and survival is increasing.
- Remember that children often have a higher-level spine injury[1] or can have cord injury without a bony injury, that is, spinal cord injury without radiographic abnormality (SCIWORA).[10] Repeat neurologic

examination is valuable for charting progression, thus affecting the timing of intervention, or for documenting stability.

## Examination and Classifications

- Classification of patients into groups based on preservation of distal motor function may help identify the patients with better prognoses. We have assembled the relevant classifications and innervation and root level information in a single worksheet (Figure 32–1).
- Classically, a differentiation was made between patients with and patients without sensation in the thumb. Those with 10 mm or less of two-point discrimination in the thumb were referred to as *cutaneous,* which was considered the minimum sensibility required to control grip and pinch. Those with greater than 10 mm of two-point discrimination were referred to as *ocular,* indicating they would have to rely on vision for afferent information and grip control. Patients with ocular designations had reconstruction of only one hand because only one hand could be watched at a time. Although sensation still is considered important, it is not decisive in surgical planning, and both hands still may benefit from reconstruction even in patients with decreased sensation. Therefore, the "cutaneous/ocular" designation may no longer be of critical importance.
- ASIA classifies patients according to grade 3 muscle strength. When discussing cases with rehabilitationists, the ASIA scale is most appropriate. This scale refers to preserved muscles, not spine bony injury level.[7]
- Upper extremity surgeons use the World Health Organization (WHO) International Classification of Function based on grade 4 motor strength of a progressive series of muscles to initially plan reconstruction. Surgical procedures improve function based on increasing movements beyond the preserved voluntary level.

## Earlier Intervention: Spinal Stabilization and Upper Limb Reconstruction

- Where recumbent and body cast treatment for spinal column instability once were common, internal fixation and stabilization now are the rule. With earlier mobilization of the patient, protection against spinal displacement, and removal of fragments from the bony canal, acute spinal cord care has improved.
- By developing specialized units for SCI care and rehabilitation, management of the complications of SCI, such as pressure sores and respiratory and genitourinary infection, and psychological adjustment are optimized. Shorter lengths of acute stay and transfers to long-term

## International Classification for Surgery of the Hand in Tetraplegia

| GROUP | MOTOR CHARACTERISTICS | FUNCTION | DEFICIT |
|---|---|---|---|
| 0 | No muscle below elbow | Flexion of elbow, supination of forearm | Complete, no hand function |
| 1 | Brachioradialis | Flexion of elbow, supination of forearm | Complete, no hand function |
| 2 | Extensor carpi radialis longus | Extension of wrist with radial deviation | Lack pronation wrist flexion, finger and thumb flexion/extension and intrinsic function |
| 3 | Extensor carpi radialis brevis | Strong extension of the wrist | Same as above |
| 4 | Pronator teres | Wrist extension, forearm pronation | Same as above except pronation |
| 5 | Flexor carpi radialis | Flexion of the wrist | Lack finger and thumb flexion/extension and intrinsic function |
| 6 | Finger extensors | Extrinsic extension of the finger | Lack finger and thumb flexion, thumb extension, and intrinsic function |
| 7 | Thumb extensors | Extrinsic extension of the thumb and intrinsic function | Lack finger and thumb flexion and intrinsic function |
| 8 | Partial digital flexors | Extrinsic flexion of the fingers (weak) | Lack thumb flexion and intrinsic function |
| 9 | Lack only intrinsics | Lack only intrinsics | Lack intrinsics |

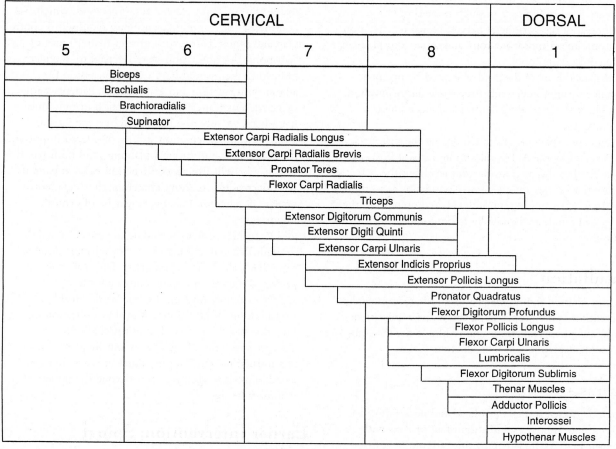

Figure 32–1:
The segmental innervation of the muscles of the upper extremity is demonstrated with the corresponding cervical spine level. (From Zancolli, E. A.: Structure and Dynamice Basis of Hand Surgery. Philadelphia, J.B. Lippincott, 1979.)

care facilities for rehabilitation also are mandated by third party payers.

- Intervention for upper extremity reconstruction may occur as early or late as the patient, caregivers, and supporters can visualize and understand the recovery possible for the injured patient.
- We recommend preventing joint and muscle contractures, early functional use of the hand to maintain supple fingers and wrist, training toward tenodesis

movements, and strengthening all muscle groups until neurologic function reaches a plateau.

## Patient Selection

- We delay or reconsider surgery after consultation with those persons who have a history of recurrent infection, rigidity and severe contractures, immune deficiency, emotional instability, excessive spasticity uncontrolled by medication, expectations of cure or return to normal hand function, substance abuse and dependency, long distance to travel for treatment, uncertain access to medical care, therapy, or medication received during the postoperative period.

- The decisions often are dependent upon socioeconomic issues, prior medical history, and future support analysis rather than simply physical condition. Past success in nonoperative management, such as use of splints, attendance at therapy, and clarity of planning for the patient's future, is an incentive to surgical reconstruction.

## Surgical Reconstruction Planning

- Table 32–1 provides an overview of current recommendations for surgical procedures. See the referenced book chapters for descriptions of the procedures and alternatives.[2-4] Single-tendon transfers are abbreviated with the letters of the muscles and the destination of the transfer. The left column shows the function created.
- As the elbow positions and stabilizes the hand in space, it must be addressed first, before the hand. Dysfunctional positions (usually of flexion and supination) must be treated. Triceps function should be restored simultaneous with hand reconstruction. Elbow extension strengthens wrist extension by tensioning the extensor carpi radialis longus and the brachioradialis, which often are transferred to motor reconstructions of the hand.
- The biceps to triceps transfer predictably restores elbow extension (Figure 32–2). Although some supination power may be sacrificed, the supinator usually is innervated and intact. This can be determined by palpating the supinator during resisted supination with the elbow extended.
- The first functional goal of tetraplegic hand reconstruction is key pinch (Figure 32–3).
- For patients with only a brachioradialis functioning, a modified Moberg transfer is performed (Figure 32–4). A split flexor pollicis longus (FPL) transfer (New Zealand Y) is performed to prevent overflexion of the interphalangeal joint, which would impede pulp pinch (Figure 32–5).
- Two-stage reconstruction is performed to ensure that the more easily stretched extensor transfers have time to become anchored before the mechanically stronger and forceful muscles are transferred. In the first stage, the extensor digitorum communis and extensor pollicis longus are tenodesed by anchoring them to the radius (Figure 32–6).
- The House intrinsic reconstruction[5] uses the extensor digiti quinti as a free tendon graft split in half longitudinally into two thin, long tendon slips. One free end of a tendon graft is woven into the index finger's lumbrical hood. It is passed through the index finger's radial lumbrical canal, volar to the intermetacarpal ligament and metacarpal neck, and passed through the radial lumbrical canal of the middle finger. Its other free end is woven into the middle finger's lumbrical hood. This passive tenodesis increases extension at the proximal interphalangeal (PIP) joint. The other free tendon slip is similarly used to reconstruct the intrinsics to the ring and small fingers (Figure 32–7).

- After 6 weeks, the second stage is performed. A wrist extensor is transferred to the flexor digitorum profundus of the index and middle fingers and the flexor digitorum superficialis (FDS) of the ring and small fingers. The FDS of the ulnar digits is chosen to prevent excessive flexion posturing of those digits, which may inhibit grasp. If those digits are already contracted in a flexed position, then their flexor tendons are not motored. The brachioradialis is transferred to the FPL for pinch (Figure 32–8).
- Thumb posture may be positioned by arthrodesis of the carpometacarpal (CMC) joint (Figure 32–9).
- Intrinsic reconstruction by the Lasso procedure involves cutting the FDS tendon just distal to the A2 pulley, wrapping it around the A1 pulley and the proximal 20% of the A2 pulley, and suturing it to itself. This procedure turns it from a flexor of the PIP joint into a flexor of the MCP joint, allowing it to preflex the metacarpophalangeal joint and prevent clawing (see Figure 18–13).
- For tendon transfers to the thumb, the term *adductor-opponensplasty* is used to denote the fact that the vector of the tendon transfer is between that of adduction and an opponensplasty. Adductor-opponensplasty uses the pronator teres as the motor and extends its length with a bipolar (double-sided) FDS transfer, which is attached distally to both the tendinous insertion of the abductor pollicis brevis and the extensor hood of the thumb (Figure 32–10 and Boxes 32–1, 32–2, 32–3, and 32–4).

## Therapy

- Postoperative and continuing hand therapy consultation is recommended to provide adaptive equipment, functional bracing, and training on adaptation to disability (see the case studies for details).

## Outcomes Determination

- Surgical restoration that overcomes a physical impairment does not always translate into additional measured function, and people with disabilities may develop adaptive movements that achieve functional objectives.
- Outcomes instruments that capture both results are important. The results of SCI management are measured by the patient's performance on standardized tests of

## Table 32–1: International Classification

| | GROUP: 0 | GROUP: 1 | GROUP: 2 | GROUP: 3 | GROUP: 4 | GROUP: 5 | GROUP: 6 | GROUP: 7 | GROUP: 8 | GROUP: 9 |
|---|---|---|---|---|---|---|---|---|---|---|
| **Intact Motor Grade 4** | None | BR | ECRL | ECRB | PT | FCR | EDC | EPL | FDP | Intrinsic (−) |
| **Retained Function** | Elbow flexion | Forearm supination | Wrist extension | | Forearm pronation | Wrist flexion extension | Partial or full finger | Thumb extension | Partial finger flexion | Full finger flexion |
| **GOALS FOR RECONSTRUCTION** | | | | | | | RECONSTRUCTION RECOMMENDED | | | |
| Elbow Extension | Posterior deltoid or biceps to triceps transfer | | | | | | | Intact | | |
| Wrist Extension | | BR→ECRB or ECRL | | | Intact | | | | | |
| Thumb Key Pinch | | | One stage key pinch BR→FPL | | | | | | | |
| Grasp/Release | | | | ECRL→FDP | Two stage extensor/ flexor reconstruction | | EPL+EDC single flexor phase | | | |
| Intrinsic Function Fingers | | | | | | FDS lasso or intrinsic tenodesis | | | FDS lasso | |
| Thumb | CMC arthrodesis key pinch | | | | | Adductor-opponensplasty or CMC arthrodesis | | BR→FPL | | |

Surgical procedures for tetraplegia are determined by the level of voluntary function in the limb. The International Classification groups are indicated on the top line. The achievable additional hand function is indicated in the first column. The surgical procedures indicated for each level and the anticipated function are listed.

Adapted from Trumble T, editor: *Hand surgery update 3.* Rosemont, IL, 2003, American Society for Surgery of the Hand.

Front          Back

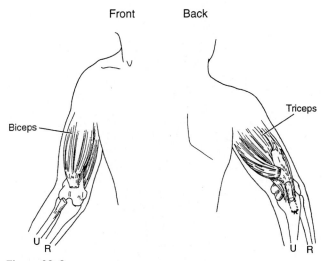

Figure 32–2:
The biceps-to-triceps is performed using an S-shaped incision over the antecubital fossa. The biceps tendon is detached after releasing the lacertus fibrosis. The biceps is rerouted around the medial aspect of the arm in a subcutaneous plane superficial to the ulnar nerve. A posterior incision is used to expose the insertion of the triceps onto the olecranon. The biceps tendon is woven through the tendon of the triceps and then through drill holes of the olecranon for a secure fixation.

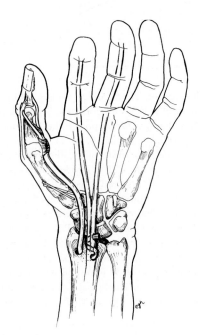

Figure 32–4:
Modification of the Moberg simple key pinch procedure. (1) Transfer of the brachioradialis (BR) into the extensor carpi radialis brevis (ECRB) for wrist extension. The BR is mobilized proximally to improve its excursion. Its distal tendon is detached and interwoven into the ECRB. The tension of the transfer is set later while other transfers are adjusted. (2) Thumb carpometacarpal (CMC) arthrodesis in 20 to 30 degrees extension, 30 to 40 degrees abduction, and 10 to 15 degrees pronation. (3) Flexor pollicis longus (FPL) split tenodesis through a single radial midaxial incision. (4) FPL is tenodesed to the distal radius. The proximal free end is woven in and out of the volar distal radius through 4.5-mm drill holes, 1.5 cm apart. (5) As the FPL emerges from the radius, it is interwoven to the index and long finger flexor profundi. The tension of the tenodesis is adjusted to create a reverse cascade with slightly more flexion in the index finger. (6) The extensor pollicis longus is tenodesed to the distal radius by weaving it through the retinaculum over its fibroosseous tunnel. (7) Extensor digitorum communis synchronization and tenodesis. The seven surgical steps are part of a single-stage reconstruction. The flexor pulleys of the thumb are left undisturbed. Arthrodesis of the CMC joint of the thumb is an important early step. Tension of tenodeses around the thumb and wrist can be adjusted properly until the desired "release" is accomplished with the wrist in 20 degrees flexion. With the wrist in 20 to 30 degrees extension, lateral key pinch should be restored. The extremity is immobilized with the elbow in 90 degrees flexion and the wrist and fingers in a position of "function." (Reprinted from The Spinal Cord Injury Patient, Second Edition, New York: Demos Medical Publishing, 2001.)

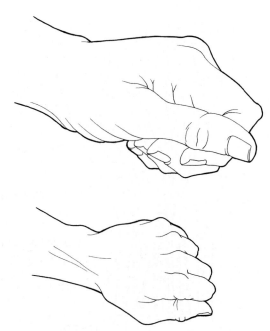

Figure 32–3:
Typical lateral key pinch after reconstruction. (Reprinted from The Spinal Cord Injury Patient, Second Edition, New York: Demos Medical Publishing, 2001.)

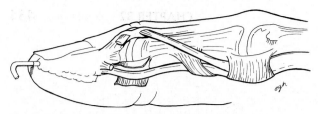

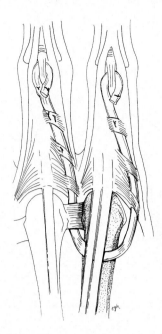

Figure 32–5:

Modified split transfer, flexor pollicis longus (FPL) to extensor pollicis longus (EPL). 1) We perform the procedure with a single midlateral, radial incision, exposing the A2 pulley, which is volar to the interphalangeal (IP) joint. 2) The A2 pulley is released, leaving the volar plate of the IP joint intact. The more radial fascicle of the FPL is divided at its insertion on the distal phalanx and dissected proximally, preserving the oblique pulley of the thumb. 3) The detached FPL slip is rerouted, in a direct line of pull, to the EPL and woven into it. Tension is adjusted by tensioning the FPL at the wrist level, stabilizing the IP joint in neutral. The Pulvertaft weave is sutured with 4-0 nonabsorbable braided suture. A 0.062 K-wire is placed across the IP joint and removed at 4 to 6 weeks. (Reprinted from The Spinal Cord Injury Patient, Second Edition, New York: Demos Medical Publishing, 2001.)

Figure 32–7:

House intrinsic reconstruction. A free tendon graft such as the extensor digiti quinti is harvested. One free end of the graft is woven and sutured into the radial lateral band about the index finger MCP joint. The other free end is passed under the extrinsic extensors of the index and into the lumbrical canal of the long finger, passing deep to the transverse intermetacarpal ligament. It is woven into the radial lateral band of the long finger. A second graft is used around the dorsum of the fourth metacarpal neck for intrinsic tenodesis of the ring and small digits. (Adapted from House et al. *J Hand Surg* 1(2): 152–159,1976.) (Reprinted from The Spinal Cord Injury Patient, Second Edition, New York: Demos Medical Publishing, 2001.)

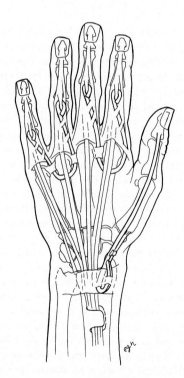

Figure 32–6:

Extensor tenodesis. The extensor pollicis longus (EPL), abductor pollicis longus (APL), and extensor digitorum communis (EDC) are tenodesed into the distal radius. The APL is rerouted through the third extensor compartment and, together with the EPL, is tenodesed into a boney window in the distal radius or into the extensor retinaculum. The floor of the fourth extensor compartment is exposed, and a 2- × 2-cm ulnar-sided periosteal flap is developed. A high-speed burr is used to create a cortical grove in the shape of a U. The EDC tendons are sutured together to synchronize finger extension and then are tucked under the U bone clip without dividing them proximally. The House intrinsic reconstruction is shown distally. (Reprinted from The Spinal Cord Injury Patient, Second Edition, New York: Demos Medical Publishing, 2001.)

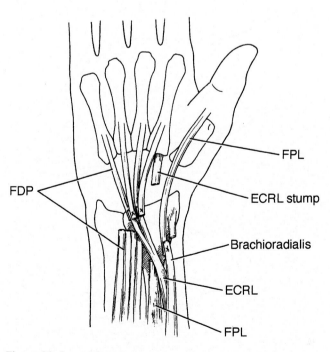

Figure 32–8:

Thumb and finger flexion is restored by transferring the extensor carpi radialis longus (ECRL) to the flexor digitorum profundus (FDP) and the brachioradials to the flexor pollicis longus (FPL).

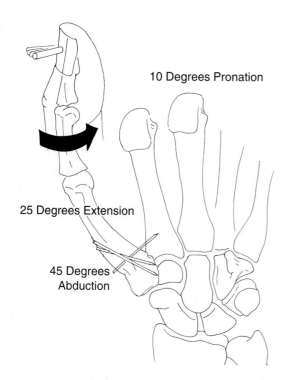

10 Degrees Pronation

25 Degrees Extension

45 Degrees Abduction

Figure 32–9:
Carpometacarpal (CMC) arthrodesis of the thumb significantly improves the posture of the thumb for pinch and release. The position for CMC arthrodesis is 45 degrees abduction, 25 degrees extension, and 10 degrees pronation. The precise position for arthrodesis ultimately is determined intraoperatively. Excessive abduction places the thumb too anterior to the flexed digits, missing them altogether while attempting pinch. Adding pronation at the fusion site has two important advantages: (1) thumb pulp opposition is better, and (2) abduction is better tolerated because the plane of thumb interphalangeal joint flexion is made to coincide with the platform made by the flexed digits. Abduction at the thumb metacarpal improves first web space opening during the release phase, which translates into the ability to grasp larger objects. In addition, with a more abducted thumb, the plane for lateral key pinch is shifted into pronation such that patients with limited forearm pronation can more easily grab objects from a horizontal table top. Patients are able to substitute for the lack of pronation with shoulder abduction and internal rotation. Patients with weaker triceps function will have difficulty with this substitution maneuver when they try to reach an object because extending the elbow with the arm abducted and internally rotated requires an active elbow extensor working against gravity. (Reprinted from The Spinal Cord Injury Patient, Second Edition, New York: Demos Medical Publishing, 2001.)

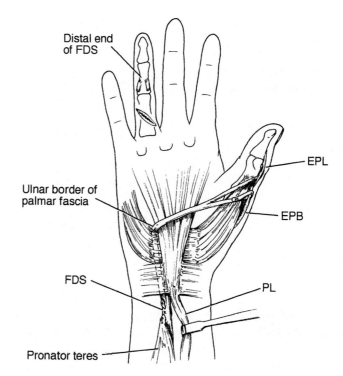

Distal end of FDS

Ulnar border of palmar fascia

EPL

EPB

FDS

PL

Pronator teres

Figure 32–10:
A tendon transfer to provide thumb adduction-opposition can be performed using the pronator teres as a motor (BR as an alternate); the ring finger FDS tendon as an in-situ graft; the ulnar border of the plamar fascia as a pulley in the palm; and the EPB and EPL as an insertion.

## Box 32–1  Case Example 1

- ASIA C6, group 3 tetraplegia
  - Elbow extension obtained by posterior deltoid transfer to triceps.
  - Similar results are obtained from biceps transfer to triceps.
  - Postoperatively, posterior splint is used for 4 weeks, then active assisted range of motion and progressive resistive exercises with a brace permitting 15 additional degrees of flexion per week.

## Box 32–2  Case Example 2

- ASIA C6, group 3 tetraplegia
  - Hand reconstructed by one-stage key grip and release.
  - Procedures included CMC arthrodesis, EPL tenodesis, brachioradialis to FPL transfer, and EDC tenodesis.
  - Arthrodesis is protected for 6 to 8 weeks in a short arm cast. Transfers are protected for 4 weeks and then mobilized.

| Box 32–3 | Case Example 3 |
|---|---|

- ASIA C7, group 5 tetraplegia
  - Reconstructed in two stages for grasp and release.
  - Stage 1 consists of EDC and EPL tenodesis and intrinsic tenodesis.
  - Stage 2 is performed 2 to 3 months later, after stabilization of the tenodeses, consisting of brachioradialis to FPL tendon transfer and ECRB to FDP transfer via interosseous membrane.
  - Postoperative range of motion is permitted with tenodesis grasp exercises for 6 weeks. Task-oriented resistive exercises are permitted at 8 weeks.
  - Weight-bearing is permitted after 3 months.

| Box 32–4 | Case Example 4 |
|---|---|

- ASIA C6, group 3 tetraplegia
  - Severe elbow flexion-supination contractures managed by staged elbow and biceps release and fractional lengthening, and then tendon transfer of posterior deltoid to triceps and forearm radius osteotomy for pronation.
  - The second stage is performed after the anterior elbow wound reaches stability. Serial cast correction of the elbow flexion deformity is used after the release, and adjustable splints are maintained after the extensor-plasty and allow 15 degrees of additional flexion per week.
  - Weight-bearing for transfers and weight shifts is permitted at 3 months.

impairment, activities of daily living, and societal participation within the context of the World Health Organization International Classification of Function.[6] Only *valid* and *reliable* surveys and outcomes instruments should be used rather than subjective grading scales. Some examples include the Functional Independence Measure (FIM)[9] and the Canadian Occupational Performance Measure (COPM).[8] It is important to determine the patient's perception of his/her progress as a result of interventions and to compare that perception to those of other patients with the disability.
- Surveys of patient satisfaction with hand surgery show high satisfaction and improved hand use, quality of life, and appearance.[11]

# References

1. Betz RR, Mulcahey MJ, editors: *The child with a spinal cord injury.* American Academy of Orthopaedic Surgery. 1996.
   Complete synopsis of the management of a child with a spinal cord injury.

2. Keith M, Gonzalez E: Surgical management of the upper limb in tetraplegia. In Lee B, Ostrander L, editors: *The spinal cord injured patient.* New York, 2001, Demos Medical Publishing.
   Discusses most surgical methods and neuroprostheses and provides procedure drawings.

3. Hentz VR, LeClercq C: *Surgical rehabilitation of the upper limb in tetraplegia.* London, New York, W.B. Saunders, 2002.
   New and current textbook of tetraplegia featuring surgical procedures commonly used.

4. Hand Clinics: The tetraplegic upper limb. LeClercq C, ed, 18(3): xiii, 2002.
   Recent and comprehensive international synopsis of current thinking of a wide variety of authors on reconstruction of the upper extremity in tetraplegia.

5. Van Heest A: Tetraplegia. In Green D, editor: *Green's operative hand surgery.* New York, 1998, Churchill Livingstone.
   This is the classic resource from among the field's most experienced writers and surgeons, now in its fourth edition with excellent illustrations.

6. World Health Organization International Classification of Functioning, Disability and Health. Available at *http://www3.who.int/icf/icftemplate.cfm*.

7. American Spinal Injury Association. Available at *http://www.asia-spinalinjury.org/home/index.html*.

8. Canadian Occupational Performance Measure (COPM). Available at *http://www.caot.ca/copm/description.html*.

9. Functional Independence Measure. Available at *http://www.udsmr.org/*.

10. Cirak B, Ziegfeld S, Knight VM, et al: Spinal injuries in children. *J Pediatr Surg* 39:607-612, 2004.

11. Wuolle KS, Bryden AM, Peckham PH, et al: Satisfaction with upper-extremity surgery in individuals with tetraplegia. *Arch Phys Med Rehabil* 84:1145-1149, 2003.

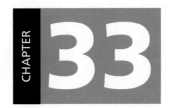

# Forearm Anatomy and Forearm Fractures

David Ring

MD, Instructor of Orthopaedics, Harvard Medical School; Director of Research, Department of Orthopaedic Surgery, Hand and Upper Extremity Unit, Massachusetts General Hospital, Boston, MA

- The rotary movements (pronation/supination) provided by the unique two-bone, dual intraarticulation structure of the forearm greatly expand the variety of ways in which objects can be positioned and manipulated by the hand.
- Loss of this motion as a result of malunion, prolonged immobilization, and/or proximal or distal radioulnar joint incongruity following trauma to the adult forearm can be disabling.
- The gradual improvement in functional outcomes and decrease in the rate of complications associated with the management of forearm fractures during this century parallels the history of the development of sound, stable techniques of internal skeletal fixation that permit mobility while assuring maintenance of skeletal alignment during fracture union.
- Forearm fractures often are the sequelae of high-energy injury, and a relatively large percentage are open fractures.
- Injury and treatment-related complications include compartment syndrome, neurovascular injury, soft tissue loss, bone loss, refracture after plate removal, and posttraumatic radioulnar synostosis. Infection is unusual, even in the case of an open fracture, partly because of the relative ease of wound debridement and the well-perfused forearm musculature.

## Evolutionary Anatomy

- The pattern of evolution at both the elbow and the wrist reflects a transition from stability to mobility.[1,2]
- The development of bipedalism freed the upper extremity for enhanced manipulative function.
- In conjunction with the increase in brain size and the development of the prehensile thumb, the acquisition of forearm rotation is considered one of the three most important aspects differentiating the most highly developed hominids, as these factors are important in determining the ability to manipulate one's environment, particularly for tool use.[1,3]

## Skeletal Anatomy

### Ulna

- There is a slight apex posterior bow along the entire length of the ulna as seen on a lateral radiograph.
- In the anteroposterior plane the ulna has a slight double curvature, apex lateral in the proximal half and apex medial distally.[4,5]
- The ulna is triangular in cross section through the majority of its midportion and becomes cylindrical distally. The laterally directed apex of the triangle

corresponds with the insertion of the interosseous ligament. The posterior apex remains essentially subcutaneous as it divides the flexor and extensor musculature on the ulnar border of the forearm and is palpable along the entire length of the bone.

## Radius

- The radius has a double curvature in both the anteroposterior and lateral planes.[6] The bicipital tuberosity, representing the insertion of the biceps brachii tendon, is at the apex of the smaller, proximal, convex medial curve, whereas the large, distal, convex lateral curve has at its apex the insertion of the pronator teres. This circumstance provides these powerful muscles with longer lever arms through which to produce rotatory torque of the radius. According to Sage's measurements, the proximal curvature of the radius averages approximately 13 degrees apex medial in the coronal and 13 degrees apex anterior in the sagittal anatomic planes.[6,7] The distal curvature averages approximately 9.3 degrees apex lateral in the coronal and 6.4 degrees apex posterior in the sagittal plane.
- The large ulnar concavity of the distal curvature of the radius allows for overriding of the ulna without restriction of pronation.[8] The limit of forearm pronation is reached as the flexor musculature is compressed between the forearm bones.[8] Loss of this "radial bow" was shown by Schemitch and Richards to be associated with limitation in both forearm rotation and grip strength.[9,10]
- Numerous studies have demonstrated a direct relationship between the degree of forearm bone angular and rotational malalignment and restriction of rotational motion.[6,10–16]

- The biceps inserts onto the roughened posterior aspect of the bicipital tuberosity. The orientation of the tuberosity can provide an indication of the rotation of the proximal radius, which may prove useful in the treatment of forearm fractures.[12] Its apex is directed roughly opposite to that of the distal radial styloid. It points directly medial or ulnar in full supination and directly lateral in full pronation and is not visible when the proximal radius is in the neutral position.[11,12]

## Radioulnar Articulation

- The radius rotates about the relatively stationary ulna along an axis that passes roughly through the center of the radial head proximally and the fovea of the ulnar head distally (Figure 33–1).
- Rotation of the radius occurs via axial rotation of the radial head at the proximal radioulnar joint, whereas distally, the motion is a combination of axial rotation and translation of the radius relative to the ulna.[8,17–23]
- The association of the radius and ulna is maintained by ligamentous structures at the proximal and distal radioulnar joints and by the interosseous ligament, a ligamentous sheet interconnecting the two bones along their midportion.
- The proximal radioulnar joint is stabilized by the annular and quadrate ligaments proximally and by the interosseous ligament.[24,25]
- The quadrate ligament is described as a thin ligamentous structure that covers the capsule at the inferior margin of the annular ligament and attaches to the ulna.[8,26] Its existence as a discrete entity and its contributions to

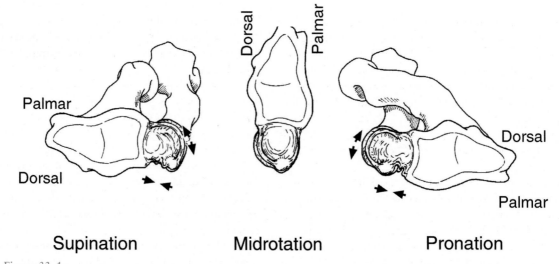

**Figure 33–1:**
In supination the palmar ligament supports the triangular fibrocartilage complex (TFCC) and distal radioulnar joint (DRUJ), becoming taunt whereas in pronation the dorsal ligaments bordering the TFCC become taunt to support the DRUJ

the stability of the proximal radioulnar joint has been disputed by some authors.[24]

- The distal radioulnar articulation is stabilized by the triangular fibrocartilage complex. The complex represents a combination of structures that are inseparable in anatomic dissections including the articular disc, the dorsal and volar radioulnar ligaments, and the sheath of the extensor carpi ulnaris.[27]

## Muscle-Tendon Units

- Four muscles produce active forearm rotation, two that originate and insert in the forearm and two that cross the elbow joint. Both the supinator and biceps insert on the proximal radial shaft and produce supination. The pronator teres and pronator quadratus insert on the midshaft and distal radius, respectively, and produce pronation.

- Contraction of the brachioradialis encourages neutral forearm rotation.

- The power of supination exceeds that of pronation by approximately 15%.[28]

- Malunion of the radius can decrease the mechanical efficiency of the muscles, producing forearm rotation by shortening the lever arms.[8]

- The forearm musculature is commonly considered as three separate compartments based on fascial divisions and nerve supply: the volar or flexor compartment innervated by the median and ulnar nerves; the dorsal or extensor compartment innervated by the posterior interosseous nerve; and the mobile wad of Henry (brachioradialis and the extensor carpi radialis longus and brevis) innervated by the radial nerve. The divisions between the compartments delineate commonly used and relatively safe intervals for operative exposure.

- Anatomic studies suggest that the fascial divisions between these compartments are sufficiently pliant that fascial release of one compartment usually decompresses the remaining two.[29,30] As a result, in the treatment of compartment syndrome of the forearm, pressures in the dorsal and mobile wad compartments rarely, but occasionally, remain elevated following release of the volar forearm musculature.[29,30]

- Muscle tissue becomes sparse in the distal forearm where the transition from muscle to tendon is completed.

- On the extensor surface of the distal radius and ulna, the tendons organize and are confined within compartments defined by the attachment of the extensor retinaculum to the dorsal radial and ulnar periosteum. Commonly referred to by number counting radial to ulnar, the first dorsal compartment contains the abductor pollicis longus and the extensor pollicis brevis; the second contains the radial wrist extensors, the extensor carpi radialis brevis and longus; the third contains the extensor pollicis longus as it angles about the fulcrum provided by Lister's

tubercle; the fourth contains the extensor digitorum communis and extensor indicis tendons; the fifth contains the extensor digiti quinti tendon; and the sixth compartment the extensor carpi ulnaris, lying in a groove in the ulnar head, just dorsoradial to the ulnar styloid.

## Neurovascular Anatomy

- Three large nerves enter the forearm at the elbow: the ulnar, radial and median nerves.

- For the ulnar nerve, the forearm is primarily a conduit to the hand. It passes from the extensor compartment of the arm to the flexor compartment of the forearm under the medial epicondyle of the distal humerus. It then dives below the flexor carpi ulnaris, under the fascial band formed by the connection between its humeral and ulnar heads, innervating this muscle and the ulnar half of the flexor digitorum profundus. The ulnar nerve is incorporated into the epimysium of the flexor digitorum profundus, lying between the flexor carpi ulnaris and the flexor digitorum superficialis muscles. The ulnar nerve lies just lateral to the tendon of the flexor carpi ulnaris at the wrist.

- The remainder of the flexor musculature of the hand and wrist is innervated by the median nerve. The median nerve is found medial to the brachial artery, overlying the brachialis muscle at the elbow. After entering the forearm in the cubital fossa, it passes between the humeral and ulnar heads of the pronator teres and then disappears under the superior margin of the flexor digitorum superficialis between its radial and ulnar origins. It lies between the superficial and deep digital flexor musculature, often incorporated into the epimysium of the flexor digitorum superficialis, until it reaches the wrist at which point the nerve emerges in a relatively superficial position between the flexor carpi radialis and flexor digitorum superficialis tendons.

- The anterior interosseous branch of the median nerve arises as a separate fascicle well proximal to the elbow and is a distinct branch at the level of the superior margin of the flexor digitorum superficialis muscle. This branch supplies the flexor pollicis longus and the radial half of the flexor digitorum profundus muscle and the pronator quadratus.

- The radial nerve bifurcates just proximal to the elbow. Its deep branch, the posterior interosseous nerve, courses over the radial head and dives between the two heads of the supinator muscle at the arcade of Frohse, a fibrous thickening of the fascial margin of the superficial head of the supinator. The posterior interosseous nerve typically is separated from the radial shaft by the deep head of the supinator muscle, but occasionally it lies in direct contact with the periosteum of the radial neck, making it particularly susceptible to damage when internal fixation devices are implanted in this region.[31] The posterior interosseous nerve terminates in an articular branch that lies in the floor of the fourth compartment of the extensor retinaculum.

- The superficial branch of the radial nerve runs along the undersurface of the brachioradialis with the radial artery and provides sensory branches to the dorsoradial aspect of the wrist and hand.

- The skin of the forearm is supplied primarily by three nerves: the medial, lateral, and posterior antebrachial cutaneous nerves.

- The lateral antebrachial cutaneous nerve is the continuation of the musculocutaneous nerve, which emerges from between the biceps brachii and the brachialis muscles on the lateral aspect of the distal arm. This nerve innervates the skin of the lateral half of the anterior aspect of the forearm and the direct lateral aspect of the forearm.

- The medial antebrachial cutaneous nerve is a branch from the medial cord of the brachial plexus, which runs down the arm with the brachial artery. It emerges in the middle of the arm and divides into an anterior and a posterior branch. These large branches supply the majority of the anteromedial and posteromedial skin surface of the forearm.

- The posterior antebrachial cutaneous nerve of the forearm supplies the posterolateral aspect of the forearm integument.

- The arterial supply to the upper extremity is characterized by extensive longitudinal collateralization. The brachial artery, which enters the forearm superficial to the brachialis muscle, lateral and adjacent to the median nerve, represents the primary blood supply of the forearm. However, distal branches such as the radial, ulnar and interosseous arteries also are supplied by large collaterals: the radial recurrent, anterior and posterior ulnar recurrent, and interosseous recurrent arteries, respectively. The radial recurrent artery represents the continuation of the radial collateral branch of the profunda brachii artery and travels with the radial nerve onto the anterior aspect of the elbow. The middle collateral branch of the profunda brachii becomes the interosseous recurrent artery on the posterolateral aspect of the elbow. The anterior and posterior ulnar recurrent arteries are named for their position relative to the elbow joint. They begin as the inferior and superior ulnar collateral arteries, respectively, in the arm.

- Bifurcation of the brachial artery into the radial and ulnar arteries occurs at the level of the radial neck.

- The ulnar artery is crossed by the median nerve as it courses under the pronator teres and flexor digitorum superficialis. It eventually meets the ulnar nerve with which it continues through the forearm lying between the flexor digitorum superficialis and the flexor carpi ulnaris and overlying the flexor digitorum profundus.

- The radial artery passes medial to the biceps tendon and lies on the surface of the supinator muscle, meeting the superficial radial nerve, with which it courses toward the wrist on the undersurface of the brachioradialis muscle.

- The radial artery lies radial to the flexor carpi radialis tendon, and the ulnar artery lies radial to the flexor carpi ulnar tendon and ulnar nerve. As in most parts of the body, the nerves that course near arteries (superficial radial sensory nerve, ulnar nerve) are more peripheral and more superficial and thus more vulnerable to injury than the deeper and more central arteries.

- The common interosseous artery arises just below the bicipital tuberosity and almost immediately branches into anterior and posterior interosseous arteries at the superior margin of the interosseous ligament. These arteries, which are associated with their corresponding nerves, run along the anterior and posterior surfaces of the interosseous ligament, anastomosing in the distal forearm.

## Kinesiology

- It is difficult to separate the forearm and carpal contributions to the total pronation and supination of the hand.[32,33] Some studies found that when carpal rotation is included, total forearm rotation approaches 260 degrees, whereas isolated distal radioulnar (or forearm) motion is closer to 190 degrees.[33]

- Pronation is limited by compression of the flexor musculature between the radius and ulna, whereas supination is limited proximally by the restraint of the annular ligament (as reinforced by the anterior fibers of the lateral and medial collateral ligament complexes of the elbow), the quadrate ligament, the tone of the pronator quadratus, and impingement of the ulnar styloid process on the posterior margin of the sigmoid notch of the distal radius.[8]

- Using simple goniometric measurements, pronation averages between 71 and 80 degrees and supination between 80 and 84 degrees.[34–37] More sophisticated techniques demonstrate a total arc of forearm rotation less than 160 degrees, with supination (75–88 degrees) greater than pronation (70–71 degrees).[38–42]

- Most simple activities of daily living can be performed within an arc of approximately 50 degrees each of pronation and supination.[39,43] On the other hand, many activities such as supporting a tray or accepting objects into the hand require near full supination, whereas many other activities such as pressing downward, leaning upon an object, and dribbling a basketball become restricted even with relatively small decreases in pronation.[8]

- As a result of the translational contribution to forearm rotation at the distal radioulnar joint, the axis of rotation is not constant. The so-called instant center of rotation, or the center of rotation at any given position of forearm rotation, translates a few millimeters about the center of the radial and ulnar heads as the forearm courses through a full arc of rotation.[17,33,44–47] Distally, the average center of rotation usually is found near the fovea of the ulnar head.[33,44,45]

- Ulnar variance increases between 1 and 2 mm with pronation or grasp.[3,27,48-53] A corresponding increase in radiocapitellar contact and force transmission has been measured during pronation.[54] Tightening of the soft tissues with forearm rotation, particularly the interosseous ligament, has been offered as an explanation for these observations.[54]

- Studies differ with regard to the relative proximal migration of the radius with respect to the ulna following radial head resection and serial sectioning of the soft tissue stabilizing structures. One study found little (0.4 mm) whereas another study found substantial (7 mm) relative shortening with radial head excision alone.[55,56] Both investigations demonstrated that loss of both the triangular fibrocartilage complex and the interosseous ligament was required for marked (>10 mm) proximal migration to occur. Sectioning of only one of these structures resulted in shortening between 4 and 10 mm under axial load.[55,56] A similar study of Galeazzi fractures reported similar results.[57]

- Hotchkiss et al.[58] measured stiffness rather than displacement of the forearm under axial load after radial head excision and serial sectioning of the soft tissue structures. They found that sectioning of the triangular fibrocartilage complex decreased the axial stiffness by only 8%, whereas isolated sectioning of the central band of the interosseous ligament decreased axial stiffness by 71%.[58]

- In the clinical setting, provided the normal curvatures of the radius and ulna are maintained, the integrity of the interosseous ligament usually is sufficient to maintain proximal radioulnar joint congruity despite rupture of the annular and quadrate ligaments, as occurs in Monteggia type fracture-dislocations of the forearm.[26] Similarly, provided the interosseous ligament remains intact, substantial proximal migration of the radius following radial head fracture or excision is unusual.[59] Complete dislocation of the distal radioulnar joint cannot occur with disruption of the triangular fibrocartilage complex alone. The interosseous ligament must also be at least significantly disrupted.[60] Radioulnar diastasis also indicates damage to the interosseous ligament.[52,60]

## Operative Exposures
### Skin Incision

- The skin of the upper extremity is well vascularized because of the large number of distinct angiosomes (collections of tissue with a distinct arterial supply) and the excellent collateralization.[61] As a result, large flaps can be raised with little risk to skin of adequate quality.
- The skin over the extensor surfaces of the hand, wrist, and elbow is sufficiently lax and elastic that the relaxed

skin tension lines can be crossed without causing scar contracture or hypertrophy. On the other hand, incisions should cross the flexor creases of the wrist or elbow obliquely.[62]

- It is preferable to not incise the skin directly over neurovascular structures or tendons in the setting of acute trauma. If excessive swelling prevents closure of the wound, these structures will remain exposed. For forearm compartment release, we incise the skin on the ulnar aspect of the wrist, creating a radially based flap to ensure coverage of the median nerve. Preservation of subcutaneous venous structures should help limit edema formation.

### Ulna

- The posterior apex of the ulnar shaft defines the plane between the extensor forearm musculature innervated by the radial nerve and the flexor musculature innervated by the ulnar nerve (Figure 33–2). Incise the skin in line with the ulna. You can start with a 10-cm incision and

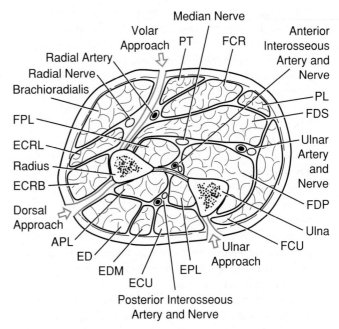

Figure 33–2:

Cross-sectional anatomy of the forearm. The subcutaneous apex of the ulna defines the interval between the flexor carpi ulnaris *(FCU)* and extensor carpi ulnaris *(ECU)*. The flexor side of the ulna is further from the interosseous membrane. The median nerve and the ulnar nerve and artery lie between the superficial and deep digital flexor musculature. The Henry exposure uses the interval between the median and radial nerves. The Thompson exposure uses the interval between the radial nerve and the posterior interosseous nerve. *APL,* Abductor pollicis longus; *ECRB,* extensor carpi radialis brevis; *ECRL,* extensor carpi radialis longus; *ED,* extensor digitorum communis: *EDM,* extensor digiti minimi; *EPL,* extensor pollicis longus; *FCR,* flexor carpi radialis; *FDP,* flexor digitorum profundus; *FDS,* flexor digitorum superficialis; *FPL,* flexor pollicis longus; *PL,* palmaris longus; *PT,* pronator teres.

lengthen it as needed after the fracture site is localized and the plate length is selected.

- In the midforearm, it is preferable to expose the volar (flexor or medial) surface rather than the dorsal (extensor or posterior) surface of the ulna to avoid violating the interosseous ligament, which can contribute to the formation of a radioulnar synostosis. Elevate the muscle extraperiosteally from only one side of the bone. Extraperiosteal means that you leave the periosteum on the bone and only elevate the muscle.
- The ulnar nerve and artery lie underneath the flexor carpi ulnaris on top of the flexor digitorum profundus. They are easily avoided provided elevation of the flexor carpi ulnaris is performed close to the bone and does not stray into its substance.

## Radius

### Dorsal or Thompson Exposure

- The dorsal (or Thompson) approach has waned in popularity because of the potential for injury to the posterior interosseous nerve, which must be dissected from the substance of the supinator and protected, and the narrow skin bridge, which remains between the incision used for exposure of the radius and that used to expose the ulna when both bones require exposure.[9]
- A straight longitudinal skin incision is made along the line connecting the lateral epicondyle at the elbow with Lister's tubercle at the wrist while the elbow is in 90 degrees flexion and the forearm is in neutral rotation.
- The internervous interval between the extensor digitorum communis (supplied by the posterior interosseous nerve) and the extensor carpi radialis brevis (supplied by the radial nerve) is most easily identified by locating the point at which the abductor pollicis longus and extensor pollicis brevis emerge from between the mobile wad and the dorsal compartment musculature in the distal half of the forearm.
- The deep fascia is incised directly adjacent to this interval, and the muscles are separated in a distal to proximal direction until their common aponeurosis is encountered. The supinator muscle covering the proximal radius is thereby exposed.
- Use of the proximal portion of the dorsal surface of the radius for plate fixation requires identification and mobilization of the posterior interosseous nerve, because this nerve may lie almost directly adjacent to the bone at this level and potentially could be trapped beneath a plate.[31] The posterior interosseous nerve emerges from between the superficial and deep heads of the supinator muscle approximately 1 cm proximal to the distal limit of this muscle. It can be identified at this point and then dissected free from the muscle, being careful to preserve its muscular branches (Figure 33–3). Following sufficiently proximal mobilization of the nerve, exposure

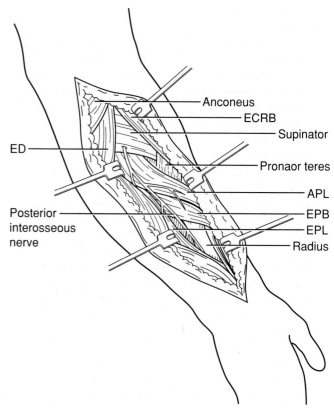

Figure 33–3:

**The dorsal Thompson exposure of the radius has waned in popularity because of frequent problems with the posterior interosseous nerve. *APL,* Abductor pollicis longus; *ECRB,* extensor carpi radialis brevis; *ED,* extensor digitorum communis: *EPB,* extensor pollicis brevis; *EPL,* extensor pollicis longus.**

of the radial shaft can be performed by rotating the radius into full supination and detaching the insertion of the supinator from the anterior aspect of the radius.

- Exposure of the midportion of the bone is facilitated by mobilizing and retracting the crossing abductor pollicis longus and extensor pollicis brevis muscles. Exposure of the radius distal to the extensor pollicis brevis is performed in the interval between the radial wrist extensors (extensor carpi radialis brevis and longus muscles) and the extensor pollicis longus muscle, which ultimately produce the tendons occupying the third and second dorsal extensor compartments, respectively.

### Anterior or Henry Exposure

- Exposure of the anterior surface of the radius is safer and more extensile than a dorsal exposure (Figure 33–4).[63]
- A straight longitudinal incision along a line between the lateral margin of the biceps tendon at the elbow and the radial styloid process at the wrist affords access to the plane between the mobile wad and the flexor musculature of the forearm.

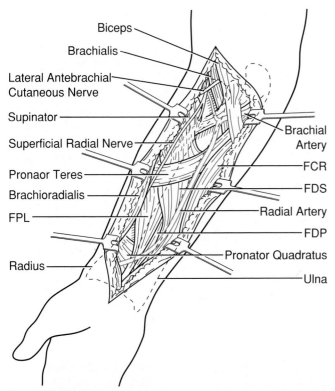

**Figure 33–4:**
**Henry's extensile exposure to the anterior surface of the radius provides easy access to the entire bone.** *FCR,* flexor carpi radialis; *FDP,* flexor digitorum profundus; *FDS,* flexor digitorum superficialis; *FPL,* flexor pollicis longus.

- The deep fascia is incised adjacent to the medial border of the brachioradialis, and a plane is developed between this radial nerve-innervated muscle and the median nerve-innervated flexor carpi radialis and pronator teres muscles. Dissection is initiated distally and proceeds proximally following the course of the radial artery.
- Arterial branches to the brachioradialis and the recurrent radial artery arising near the elbow are ligated, and the radial artery is mobilized and retracted medially with the flexor carpi radialis muscle.
- The superficial radial nerve is encountered on the undersurface of the brachioradialis and remains lateral with this muscle.
- Deep dissection is initiated proximally where the biceps tendon is followed toward its insertion on the bicipital tuberosity of the radius. Full supination of the forearm displaces the posterior interosseous nerve laterally and brings the insertion of the supinator muscle anterior. The insertion of the supinator muscle is identified by deepening the muscular plane along the lateral aspect of the biceps tendon. Here you may encounter a bursa between the biceps tendon and the supinator, which further facilitates this dissection.
- The posterior interosseous nerve remains well protected within the substance of the supinator muscle during

elevation of its insertion from the radius, provided excessive lateral traction is not applied.
- The insertion of the pronator teres can be detached or the plate can be placed directly on top of the insertion. The body of the flexor digitorum superficialis must be elevated to expose the midportion of the radius.
- In the distal portion of the wound, the pronator quadratus and the flexor pollicis longus are elevated from the bone, usually extraperiosteally.

## Forearm Compartment Release

- Fascial release for compartment syndrome can be performed through the standard volar Henry-type exposure in the setting of a forearm fracture or through a straight ulnar McConnell-type incision when exposure of the bones is not required (Figure 33–5).[63,64]
- This ulnar incision provides a flap for median nerve coverage at the wrist and allows exposure of the median and ulnar nerves under the superficial flexor muscles when required. Access to the deep flexor musculature is obtained without dissection through the superficial flexors.

## Treatment

- Despite numerous descriptions of the relevant anatomy and proper methods of reducing forearm fractures that appeared early in the twentieth century,[12,65–73] these fractures remained "problem" fractures and attracted a variety of early attempts at operative treatment.
- Early attempts at internal fixation, although sufficient to hold open reductions, did not preclude the need for external immobilization, resulting in comparably poor functional outcomes in fractures treated by open or closed methods.[70,74]

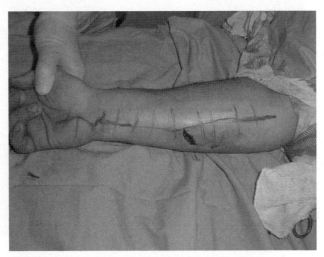

**Figure 33–5:**
**Approach for compartment release.**

- The development of larger, corrosion-resistant compression plates led to a dramatic decrease in the rate of fracture nonunion while providing sufficient stability for confident early mobilization of the forearm.[75–78] The dynamic compression plates and the emphasis on immediate mobilization of the limb developed by the AO/ASIF (Arbeitsgemeinschaft für Osteosynthesefragen/Association for the Study of Internal Fixation) in particular made open reduction and internal fixation a predictable treatment for diaphyseal forearm fractures with a rate of nonunion less than 5% and excellent functional results.

- Intramedullary implants are reintroduced periodically but they have inherent weaknesses, including difficulty maintaining rotational alignment, difficulty restoring the anatomic radial bow, the need for supplemental immobilization, a high nonunion rate, and the technical difficulty of device insertion with frequent splitting of the cortex and protrusion of the nail through the cortex or into a joint.[6,7,79,80]

- The results of intramedullary nailing of forearm fractures have improved modestly following the introduction of nails of square and triangular cross section intended to better control rotation, improved nail design and insertion techniques intended to restore the anatomic radial bow, and closed nailing under fluoroscopic guidance.[6,80,81] However, despite these improvements, intramedullary nailing continues to lack the predictability and stability of modern plate and screw fixation that have essentially solved the "problem" of forearm fractures and made plate fixation the treatment of choice.

- Isolated fractures of the ulna without associated radioulnar instability *(nightstick fracture)* usually heal with nonoperative treatment. Operative treatment is considered when there is greater than 50% translation or greater than 10° angulation of the fracture fragments.

- Isolated fractures of the radius are more common than previously recognized, as pointed out by Rettig and Raskin[82] (Figure 33–6). These fractures benefit from plate fixation unless they are nondisplaced. The distal

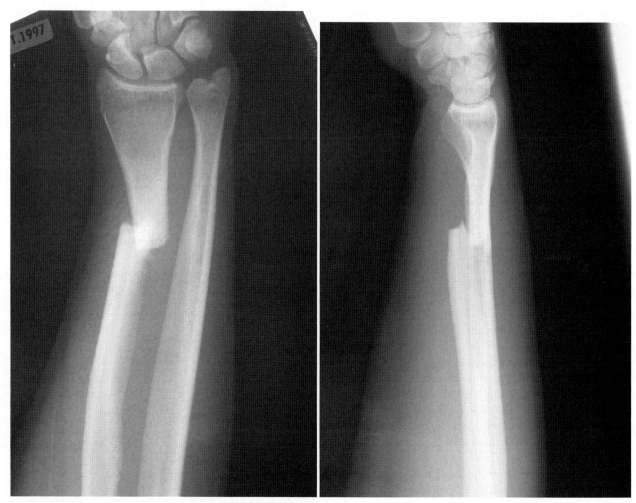

Figure 33–6:

Not all isolated radius fractures are Galeazzi injuries. This displaced fracture of the radius shows no displacement of the distal radioulnar joint in either the anteroposterior or lateral plane.

radioulnar joint should be carefully evaluated after the radius is stabilized.

## Open Fractures

- Immediate plate fixation of all but the most complex and contaminated forearm fractures is associated with an acceptably low rate of infection in open forearm fractures treated by immediate plate and screw fixation (0%–3%) when perioperative antibiotics are given and thorough wound debridement and delayed primary closure of the traumatic wounds are performed.[77,83–86]
- When infection occurs, its eradication is not necessarily dependent upon implant removal. As long as all bone fragments and soft tissues are well vascularized, stable internal fixation will facilitate wound care and help maintain length and alignment, range of motion, and overall function, without hindering treatment of the infection.

## Fracture-Dislocations of The Forearm (Galeazzi, Monteggia, and Essex-Lopresti Lesions and Their Variants)

- The Galeazzi fracture is a fracture of the radial diaphysis (often the distal third) in association with dislocation of the distal radioulnar joint (Figure 33–7).[82]
- The Monteggia fracture and its variants represent a fracture of the proximal ulna associated with proximal radioulnar joint disruption (Figure 33–8).[87]
- The Essex-Lopresti lesion is a fracture of the radial head with rupture of the interosseous ligament of the forearm (Figure 33–9).[88]
- Bipolar forearm fracture-dislocation or radioulnar dissociation represents a more complex injury with associated disruption of the interosseous ligament.[89]
- Clinical and anatomic investigations have determined a number of clues indicating distal radioulnar joint disruption that can be detected on radiographs: (1) fracture of the ulnar styloid at its base, (2) widening of the distal radioulnar joint space, (3) dislocation of the radius relative to the ulna seen on a true lateral radiograph, and (4) shortening of the radius beyond 5 mm relative to the distal ulna under a constant applied load (see Figure 33–9).[57,90]
- Proximally, the radio-humeroulnar joint is dislocated if a line through the radial shaft and head does not bisect the capitellum in all positions of flexion/extension.[91,92]
- Galeazzi fracture-dislocations are treated with anatomic reduction and plate and screw fixation.[93,94] If the ulnar

styloid is fractured at its base, it should be repaired. The distal radioulnar joint usually is stable, and the forearm can be mobilized immediately postoperatively.[93] If the distal radioulnar joint remains unstable, the forearm can be immobilized in midsupination for 4 weeks, occasionally with transfixion of the distal ulna to the radius with one or two stout smooth Kirschner wires that often results in the loss of forearm rotation.[95]
- Anterior and lateral Monteggia fractures (Bado[96] types 1, 3, and 4 [which is a fracture of both bones with anterior or lateral dislocation of the radial head from the proximal radioulnar joint]) usually are treated with anatomic reduction and internal fixation of the ulna and early mobilization. Instability or incomplete reduction of the radial head most commonly results from ulnar malalignment. The annular ligament should rarely require exploration or repair.[97] Posterior Monteggia lesions (Bado type 2) are more complex and best considered along with elbow fracture-dislocations (Figure 33–10 and Table 33–1).
- With Essex-Lopresti and bipolar fracture-dislocations, the treatment principles include stable anatomic reduction of all fractures,[98,99] preservation of radiocapitellar contact with operative fixation or prosthetic replacement, and addressing the soft tissue injury with either direct repair or immobilization in a reduced position (with or without cross pinning).

## Compartment Syndrome

- Prompt diagnosis of compartment syndrome is dependent upon clinical suspicion and frequent, careful examination focusing on pain out of proportion to injury, pain with passive stretch of the fingers, and compartment palpation.
- Gelberman et al.[29] found a change in two-point discrimination was associated with compartment syndrome. Even better would be detecting a change in threshold (or light-touch sensation), which can be achieved in an objective manner with Semmes-Weinstein monofilaments. Loss of discriminatory sensation (two-point) and weakness usually are late findings.
- A reliable examination is dependent upon patient understanding and cooperation. In a patient with altered mental status (because of associated traumatic injury, intoxication, or narcotic medication), in the presence of associated neurologic deficit, or in any case in which the physician is not confident of his/her examination, serial measurement of intracompartmental forearm pressures is useful.[100]
- Elevated or rising pressures indicate the need for fasciotomy. The absolute pressure at which fasciotomy is indicated is debated. Pressures above 30 mm Hg are of concern. Forearm fascial release should be strongly considered at pressures above 45 mm Hg.
- Gun shot fractures of the forearm are particularly prone to compartment syndrome. Moed and Fakhouri[101]

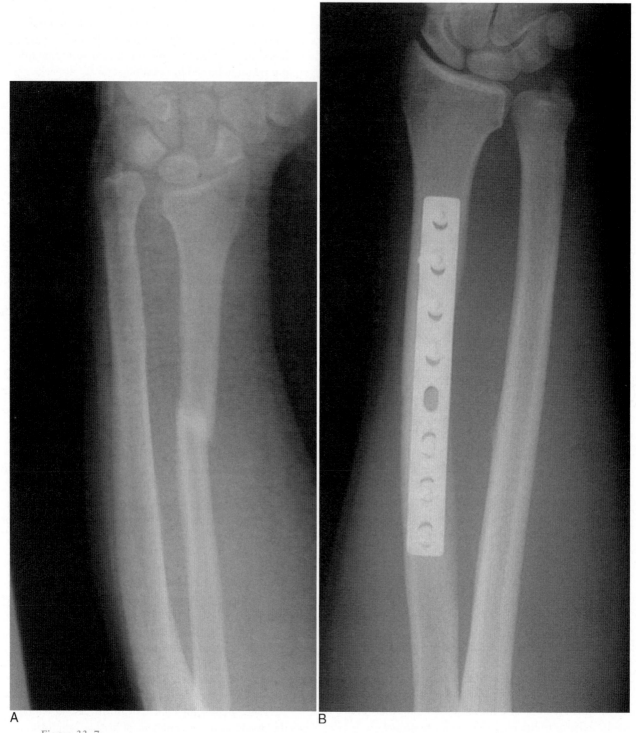

A                                                                                    B

Figure 33–7:
Isolated radius fractures may be associated with dislocation of the distal radioulnar joint. **A,** The distance of the fracture from the radiocarpal joint is not always predictive of radioulnar instability. This midshaft fractures has a widened and shorted distal radioulnar joint indicating injury to the triangular fibrocartilage complex and interosseous membrane. **B,** Following plate fixation, the distal radioulnar joint was stable, allowing immediate active motion.

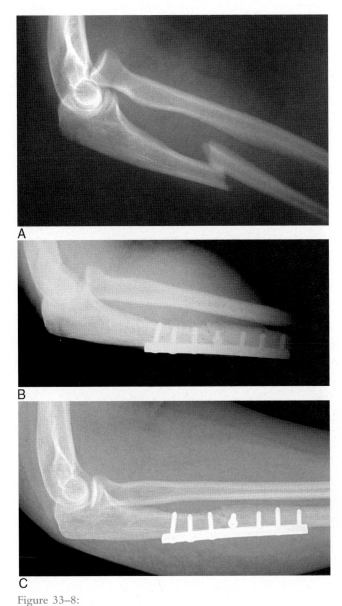

Figure 33–8:
Anterior (Bado type I) Monteggia fracture. **A,** The anterior
Monteggia fracture (fracture of the ulnar diaphysis with anterior dislocation of the proximal radioulnar joint) is uncommon
in adult patients and usually reflects high-energy injury. **B,**
Persistent subluxation of the proximal radioulnar (and radiocapitellar) joints nearly always reflects residual malalignment of
the ulna. **C,** Revision of the ulnar fixation achieved better
alignment and function of the forearm.

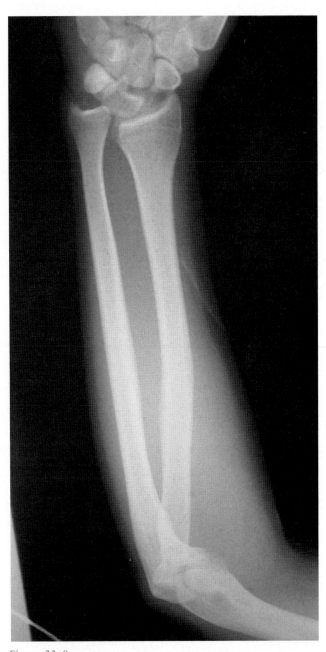

Figure 33–9:
Essex-Lopresti lesion is a fracture of the radial head associated
with injury to the triangular fibrocartilage complex and the
interosseous ligament. This patient also has a transscaphoid
perilunate fracture dislocation.

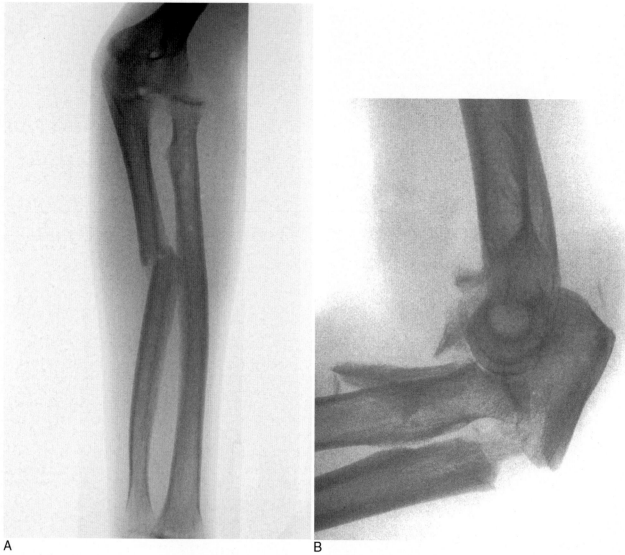

A

B

Figure 33–10:
**Monteggia fractures, Bado types. A, Type 3. B, Type 2.**

recorded a 15% overall incidence among 60 gunshot fractures of the forearm. Comminuted, severely displaced, and proximal third fractures were more commonly associated with compartment syndrome.

- Compartment release usually is achieved by exposing the radius and ulna for plate fixation.

## Nonunion

- The current rate of nonunion is less than 5% when proper technique is used in compliant patients.[77]
- Nonunions most often are related to technical errors, such as use of plates of inadequate size (e.g., semitubular plates) or length, inadequate reduction, and failure to bone graft comminuted and open fractures.[77,102–105]
- The majority of nonunions, including most nonunions with segmental bone defects, can be treated successfully with plate and screw fixation and autogenous cancellous bone grafting.
- The key elements of nonunion treatment are realignment (mobilization can be done with osteoperiosteal and/or soft tissue stripping), removal of synovial and fibrous tissues, opening of sclerotic bone ends, autogenous cancellous bone graft (except for hypertrophic nonunions, which do not need bone graft), and stable internal fixation.

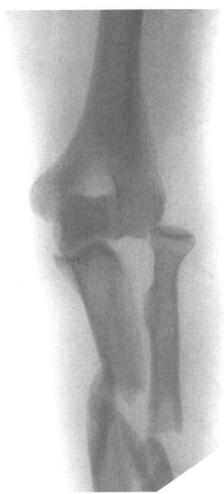

**C**

Figure 33–10: cont'd
**C, Type 4.**

• The majority of forearm diaphyseal nonunions are atrophic and associated with a segmental bony defect. Because one bone often is intact, the bone cannot be shortened. Therefore, in the majority of forearm nonunions, a plate is applied, bridging the defect with autogenous cancellous bone graft placed in the defect. Some surgeons use structural (corticocancellous) bone grafts, but we have not found this to be necessary.

## Refracture

• Initially the AO/ASIF recommended removal of all implants following fracture healing. However, because removal of forearm plates has been associated with the risk of refracture (either through the old fracture site or a screw hole) and the risks of a second operation (injury to the posterior interosseous nerve in particular), most surgeons no longer remove the plates unless they are causing definable problems.[67,106–110] This applies to athletes as well.

• The risk of refracture following plate removal is believed to result from a combination of incomplete healing and the osteoporosis that occurs under a plate because of some combination of disruption of the vascular supply to the bone and stress shielding. Risk factors for refracture following plate removal include fracture comminution or the inability to gain compression of fracture fragments,[106,110] implant size (Chapman Gordon, and Zissimos[77] noted that refracture was less likely following removal of 3.5-mm than 4.5-mm plates), implant removal earlier than 1 year after injury,[107,110] radiolucency beneath the plate,[106] and inadequate protection following plate removal.[107,110]

## References

1. Almquist EE: Evolution of the distal radioulnar joint. *Clin Orthop* 275:5-13, 1992.

2. Larson SG: Phylogeny. In Morrey BF, editor: *The elbow and its disorders.* Philadelphia, 1993, WB Saunders.

3. Linscheid RL: Biomechanics of the distal radioulnar joint. *Clin Orthop* 275:46-55, 1992.

4. Goss CM: Anatomy of the human body. In Goss CM, editor: *29th American edition of Gray's anatomy.* Philadelphia, 1973, Lea & Febiger.

5. Williams PI, Warwik R: *Gray's anatomy, 36th British edition,* ed 36. Philadelphia, 1980, WB Saunders.

6. Sage FP: Medullary fixation of fractures of the forearm. A study of the medullary canal of the radius and a report of fifty fractures of the radius treated with a prebent triangular nail. *J Bone Joint Surg* 64A:857-863, 1982.

| Table 33–1: | Monteggia Fractures: Bado Types |
| --- | --- |
| **BADO TYPE** | **DEFINITION** |
| H1, 3 (Figure 33–9A) | • Diaphyseal fracture of the ulna<br>• Anterior (type 1), lateral (type 3), or anterolateral dislocation of the radius from the proximal radioulnar and radiocapitellar joints<br>• High-energy injury in children or young adult |
| 2 (Figure 33–9B) | • Ulna fracture more often metaphyseal or intraarticular than diaphyseal<br>• Posterior dislocation of the radius with respect to the capitellum, with relative sparing of the proximal radioulnar relationship often relatively spared<br>• More often older, osteoporotic patients |
| 4 (Figure 33–9C) | • Both bones fracture of the forearm with proximal radioulnar joint dislocation<br>• Very high energy |

The results of intramedullary nails to treat diaphyseal forearm fractures have not been able to match those achieved with plate and screw fixation.

7. Sage FP, Smith H: Medullary fixation of forearm fractures. *J Bone Joint Surg Am* 39A:91-98, 1957.

8. Kapandji IA: *The physiology of the joints,* ed 5. Edinburgh, 1982, Churchill Livingstone.

9. Richards RR: Chronic disorders of the forearm. *J Bone Joint Surg Am* 78:916-930, 1996.

10. Schemitsch EH, Richards RR: The effect of malunion on functional outcome after plate fixation of fractures of both bones of the forearm in adults. *J Bone Joint Surg Am* 74:1068-1078, 1992.
    This study demonstrated an association between failure to restore the anatomic bow of the radius and diminished forearm rotation.

11. Evans EM: Fractures of the radius and ulna. *J Bone Joint Surg* 33B:548-561, 1951.
    This cadaveric study demonstrated diminished forearm rotation with relatively small angular deformities in the forearm.

12. Evans EM: Rotational deformities in the treatment of fractures of both bones of the forearm. *J Bone Joint Surg* 27:373-379, 1945.

13. Matthews LS, Kaufer H, Garver DF, Sonstegard DA: The effect on supination-pronation of angular malalignment of fractures of both bones of the forearm. *J Bone Joint Surg Am* 64:14-17, 1945.

14. Patrick J: A study of supination and pronation, with special reference to the treatment of forearm fractures. *J Bone Joint Surg* 28B:737-748, 1946.

15. Sarmiento A, Ebramzadeh E, Brys D, Tarr R: Angular deformities and forearm function. *J Orthop Res* 10:121-133, 1992.

16. Tarr RR, Garfinkel AI, Sarmiento A: The effects of angular and rotational deformities of both bones of the forearm. An in vitro study. *J Bone Joint Surg Am* 66:65-70, 1984.

17. Cone RO, Szabo R, Resnick D et al: Computed tomography of the normal radioulnar joints. *Invest Radiol* 18:541-545, 1983.

18. af Ekenstam F, Hagert CG: Anatomical studies on the geometry and stability of the distal radio ulnar joint. *Scand J Plast Reconstr Surg* 19:17-25, 1985.

19. Gemmill F: On the movement of the lower end of the radius in pronation and supination, and on the interosseous membrane. *J Anat Physiol* 35:101-109, 1900.

20. Hagert CG: The distal radioulnar joint in relation to the whole forearm. *Clin Orthop* 275:56-64, 1992.

21. Kapandji IA: The inferior radioulnar joint and pronosupination. In Tubiana R, editor: *The hand*. Philadelphia, 1981, WB Saunders.

22. Olerud C, Kongsholm J, Thuomas KA: The congruence of the distal radioulnar joint. A magnetic resonance imaging study. *Acta Orthop Scand* 59:183-185, 1988.

23. Schuind F, An KN, Berglund L et al: The distal radioulnar ligaments: a biomechanical study. *J Hand Surg [Am]* 16:1106-1114, 1991.

24. Martin BF: The annular ligament of the superior radial ulnar joint. *J Anat* 52:473-481, 1958.

25. Spinner M, Kaplan EB: Extensor carpi ulnaris. Its relationship to the stability of the distal radio-ulnar joint. *Clin Orthop* 68:124-129, 1970.

26. Spinner M, Kaplan EB: The quadrate ligament of the elbow: its relationship to the stability of the proximal radio-ulnar joint. *Acta Orthop Scand* 41:632-647, 1970.

27. Palmer AK, Werner FW: The triangular fibrocartilage complex of the wrist: anatomy and function. *J Hand Surg [Am]* 6:153-162, 1981.

28. Askew LJ, An KN, Morrey BF, Chao EY: Isometric elbow strength in normal individuals. *Clin Orthop* 222:261-266, 1987.

29. Gelberman RH, Garfin SR, Hergenroeder PT et al: Compartment syndromes of the forearm: diagnosis and treatment. *Clin Orthop* 161:252-261, 1981.

30. Gelberman RH, Zakaib GS, Mubarak SJ et al: Decompression of forearm compartment syndromes. *Clin Orthop* 134:225-229, 1978.
    The forearm is not like the lower leg; release of one compartment usually releases all of the compartments.

31. Davies F: The supinator muscle and the deep radial (posterior interosseous) nerve. *Anat Rec* 101:234-250, 1948.

32. Cyriaz EF: On the rotatory movements of the wrist. *J Anat* 60:199-201, 1926.

33. King GJ, McMurtry RY, Rubenstein JD, Gertzbein SD: Kinematics of the distal radioulnar joint. *J Hand Surg [Am]* 11:798-804, 1986.

34. Boone DC, Azen SP: Normal range of motion of joints in male subjects. *J Bone Joint Surg Am* 61:756-759, 1979.

35. Dorrison SM, Wagner ML: An exact technique for clinically measuring and recording joint motion. *Arch Phys Med Rehab* 29:468-475, 1948.

36. Glanville AD, Kreezer G: The missed Monteggia fracture. *Radiology* 10:45-47, 1974.

37. Silver D: Measurement of the range of motion in joints. *J Bone Joint Surg* 5:569-578, 1923.

38. Darcus HD, Salter N: The amplitude of pronation and supination with the elbow flexed to a right angle. *J Anat* 87:169-184, 1953.

39. Morrey BF, Askew LJ, Chao EY: A biomechanical study of normal functional elbow motion. *J Bone Joint Surg Am* 63:872-877, 1981.
    At least 50 degrees each of supination and pronation was required to perform 12 daily functional tasks.

40. Salter N, Darcus HD: The amplitude of forearm and of humeral rotation. *J Anat* 87:407-418, 1953.

41. Wagner C: Determination of the rotatory flexibility of the elbow joint. *J Appl Physiol* 37:47-59, 1977.

42. Youm Y, Dryer RF, Thambyrajah K et al: Biomechanical analyses of forearm pronation-supination and elbow flexion-extension. *J Biomech* 12:245-255, 1979.

43. Chao EY, An KN, Askew LJ, Morrey BF: Electrogoniometer for the measurement of human elbow joint rotation. *J Biomech Eng* 102:301-310, 1980.

44. Adams BD: Effects of radial deformity on distal radioulnar joint mechanics. *J Hand Surg [Am]* 18:492-498, 1993.

45. Adams BD: Partial excision of the triangular fibrocartilage complex articular disk: a biomechanical study. *J Hand Surg [Am]* 18:334-340, 1993.

46. Carret JP, Fischer LP, Gonon GP, Dimnet J: [Cinematic study of prosupination at the level of the radiocubital (radioulnar) articulations]. *Bull Assoc Anat (Nancy)* 60:279-295, 1976.

47. Robbin ML, An KN, Linscheid RL, Ritman EL: Anatomic and kinematic analysis of the human forearm using high-speed computed tomography. *Med Biol Eng Comput* 24:164-168, 1986.

48. Epner RA, Bowers WH, Guilford WB: Ulnar variance: the effect of wrist positioning and roentgen filming technique. *J Hand Surg [Am]* 7:298-305, 1982.

49. Friedman SL, Palmer AK, Short WH et al: The change in ulnar variance with grip. *J Hand Surg [Am]* 18:713-716, 1993.

50. Palmer AK, Glisson RR, Werner FW: Relationship between ulnar variance and triangular fibrocartilage complex thickness. *J Hand Surg [Am]* 9:681-682, 1984.

51. Palmer AK, Glisson RR, Werner FW: Ulnar variance determination. *J Hand Surg [Am]* 7:376-379, 1982.

52. Palmer AK, Werner FW: Biomechanics of the distal radioulnar joint. *Clin Orthop* 187:26-35, 1984.

53. Schuind FA, Linscheid RL, An KN, Chao EY: Changes in wrist and forearm configuration with grasp and isometric contraction of elbow flexors. *J Hand Surg [Am]* 17:698-703, 1992.

54. Morrey BF, An KN, Stormont TJ: Force transmission through the radial head. *J Bone Joint Surg Am* 70:250-256, 1988.

55. Rabinowitz RS, Light TR, Havey RM et al: The role of the interosseous membrane and triangular fibrocartilage complex in forearm stability. *J Hand Surg [Am]* 19:385-393, 1994.
The forearm is only markedly destabilized when both the triangular fibrocartilage complex and the interosseous ligament are disrupted.

56. Reardon JP, Lafferty M, Kamaric E et al: Structures influencing axial stability to the forearm: the role of the radial head, interosseous membrane, and distal radio-ulnar joint. *Orthop Trans* 15:436-437, 1991.

57. Moore TM, Lester DK, Sarmiento A: The stabilizing effect of soft-tissue constraints in artificial Galeazzi fractures. *Clin Orthop* 194:189-194, 1985.

58. Hotchkiss RN, An KN, Sowa DT et al: An anatomic and mechanical study of the interosseous membrane of the forearm: pathomechanics of proximal migration of the radius. *J Hand Surg [Am]* 14(2 pt 1):256-261, 1989.

59. Morrey BF, Chao EY, Hui FC: Biomechanical study of the elbow following excision of the radial head. *J Bone Joint Surg Am* 61:63-68, 1979.

60. King GJ, McMurtry RY, Rubenstein JD, Ogston NG: Computerized tomography of the distal radioulnar joint: correlation with ligamentous pathology in a cadaveric model. *J Hand Surg [Am]* 11:711-717, 1986.

61. Taylor GI, Palmer JH, McManamny D: The vascular territories of the body (angiosomes) and their clinical applications. In McCarthy JG, editor: *Plastic surgery*. Philadelphia, 1990, WB Saunders.

62. Kraissl CJ: The selection of appropriate lines for elective surgical incisions. *Plast Reconstr Surg* 8:1-28, 1951.

63. Henry AK: *Extensile exposure,* ed 2. Edinburgh, 1973, Churchill Livingstone.
Classic text describing some of the most commonly used exposures in detail.

64. McConnell AA: Approach to the median nerve in the forearm. *Med Sci* 149:90-92, 1920.

65. Bagley CH: Fracture of both bones of the forearm. *Surg Gynecol Obstet* 42:95-102, 1926.

66. Bolton H, Quinlan AG: The conservative treatment of fractures of the shaft of the radius and ulna in adults. *Lancet* 2:700-705, 1952.

67. Bednar DA, Grandwilewski W: Complications of forearm-plate removal. *Can J Surg* 35:428-431, 1992.

68. Buxton JD: Treatment of closed fractures of the radius and ulna. *BMJ* 2:795-799, 1939.

69. Carrell WB: Fractures of both bones of the forearm excluding those at the elbow joint and wrist joint. *Surg Gynecol Obstet* 66:506-511, 1938.

70. Compare EL: The treatment of fractures of both bones of the forearm. *Surg Clin North Am* 25:48-58, 1948.

71. Eliason EL, Brown RB, Kaplan L: Fractures of the forearm; except Colles'. *Am J Surg* 38:511-525, 1937.

72. Magnuson PB: Mechanics of treatment of fractures of the forearm. *JAMA* 78:789-794, 1922.

73. Whipple AO: A study of one hundred consecutive fractures of the shafts of both bones of the forearm with the end-results in ninety-five. *Surg Gynecol Obstet* 25:77-91, 1917.

74. Knight RA: Fractures of both bones of the forearm in adults. *J Bone Joint Surg* 31A:755-764, 1949.
Demonstrated the disadvantages of nonoperative and limited operative techniques, including intramedullary nailing.

75. Anderson LD, Sisk D, Tooms RE, Park WI III: Compression-plate fixation in acute diaphyseal fractures of the radius and ulna. *J Bone Joint Surg Am* 57:287-297, 1975.

Documented the effectiveness of the relatively new AO 4.5-mm plates. The results were far better than any previously reported and have only been slightly improved upon since.

76. Burwell HN, Charnley AD: Treatment of forearm fractures in adults with particular reference to plate fixation. *J Bone Joint Surg* 46B:404-424, 1964.
    Documented that longer plates achieve better results. As plates became larger and stronger, internal fixation was more effective.

77. Chapman MW, Gordon JE, Zissimos AG: Compression-plate fixation of acute fractures of the diaphyses of the radius and ulna. *J Bone Joint Surg Am* 71:159-169, 1989.
    The first paper to report an extensive experience with the newer AO 3.5-mm plates. Reported nearly 100% union with relatively few problems.

78. Grace TG, Eversmann WW Jr: Forearm fractures: treatment by rigid fixation with early motion. *J Bone Joint Surg Am* 62:433-438, 1980.

79. Caden JG: Internal fixation of fractures of the forearm. *J Bone Joint Surg* 43:1115-1121, 1961.

80. Street DM: Intramedullary forearm nailing. *Clin Orthop* 212:219-230, 1986.

81. Marek FM: Axial fixation of forearm fractures. *J Bone Joint Surg* 43A:1099-1114, 1961.

82. Rettig M, Raskin K: Galeazzi fracture-dislocation: a new treatment-oriented classification. *J Hand Surg [Am]* 26:228-235, 2001.

83. Duncan R, Geissler W, Freeland AE, Savoie FH: Immediate internal fixation of open fractures of the diaphysis of the forearm. *J Orthop Trauma* 6:25-31, 1992.

84. Jones JA: Immediate internal fixation of high-energy open forearm fractures. *J Orthop Trauma* 5:272-279, 1991.

85. Lenihan MR, Brien WW, Gellman H et al: Fractures of the forearm resulting from low-velocity gunshot wounds. *J Orthop Trauma* 6:32-35, 1992.

86. Moed BR, Kellam JF, Foster RJ et al: Immediate internal fixation of open fractures of the diaphysis of the forearm. *J Bone Joint Surg Am* 68:1008-1017, 1986.
    The upper extremity is so well vascularized that all but the most complex and severely comminuted fractures can be treated with immediate plate fixation.

87. Ring D, Jupiter JB, Simpson NS: Monteggia fractures in adults. *J Bone Joint Surg* 80A:1733-1744, 1998.
    The majority of adult Monteggia fractures are posterior in direction. These fractures can compromise both elbow and forearm function and often need secondary procedures.

88. Essex-Lopresti P: Fractures of the radial head with distal radioulnar dislocation. *J Bone Joint Surg* 33B:244-247, 1951.
    The classic description of longitudinal forearm instability.

89. Odena IC: Bipolar fracture-dislocation of the forearm. *J Bone Joint Surg* 34:968-976, 1952.

90. Schneiderman G, Meldrum RD, Bloebaum RD et al: The interosseous membrane of the forearm: structure and its role in Galeazzi fractures. *J Trauma* 35:879-885, 1993.

91. Giustra PE, Killoran PJ, Furman RS, Root JA: The missed Monteggia fracture. *Radiology* 110:45-47, 1974.

92. Mclaughlin HL: *Trauma.* Philadelphia, 1959, WB Saunders.

93. Kraus B, Horne G: Galeazzi fractures. *J Trauma* 25:1093-1095, 1985.

94. Moore TM, Klein JP, Patzakis MJ, Harvey JP Jr: Results of compression-plating of closed Galeazzi fractures. *J Bone Joint Surg Am* 67:1015-1021, 1985.

95. Mikic ZD. Galeazzi fracture-dislocations. *J Bone Joint Surg Am* 57:1071-1080, 1975.
    The largest paper on Galeazzi fractures demonstrates the importance of anatomic reduction and stable internal fixation.

96. Bado JL: The Monteggia lesion. *Clin Orthop* 50:71-76, 1967.
    Although Monteggia lesions had long been described in terms of the direction of radial head displacement, Bado's numeric classification has become widely used.

97. Boyd HB, Boals JC: The Monteggia lesion. A review of 159 cases. *Clin Orthop* 66:94-100, 1969.

98. Eglseder WA, Hay M: Combined Essex-Lopresti and radial shaft fractures: case report. *J Trauma* 34:310-312, 1993.

99. Jupiter JB, Kour AK, Richards RR et al: The floating radius in bipolar fracture-dislocation of the forearm. *J Orthop Trauma* 8:99-106, 1994.
    Description of complex longitudinal forearm instability.

100. Mubarak SJ, Owen CA, Hargens AR et al: Acute compartment syndromes: diagnosis and treatment with the aid of the wick catheter. *J Bone Joint Surg Am* 60:1091-1095, 1978.

101. Moed BR, Fakhouri AJ: Compartment syndrome after low-velocity gunshot wounds to the forearm. *J Orthop Trauma* 5:134-137, 1991.

102. Hadden WA, Reschauer R, Seggl W: Results of AO plate fixation of forearm shaft fractures in adults. *Injury* 15:44-52, 1983.

103. Langkamer VG, Ackroyd CE: Internal fixation of forearm fractures in the 1980s: lessons to be learnt. *Injury* 22:97-102, 1991.

104. Ross ER, Gourevitch D, Hastings GW et al: Retrospective analysis of plate fixation of diaphyseal fractures of the forearm bones. *Injury* 20:211-214, 1989.

105. Stern PJ, Drury WJ: Complications of plate fixation of forearm fractures. *Clin Orthop* 175:25-29, 1983.
    The majority of complications are associated with complex injuries and technical errors.

106. Deluca PA, Lindsey RW, Ruwe PA: Refracture of bones of the forearm after the removal of compression plates. *J Bone Joint Surg Am* 70:1372-1376, 1988.

107. Hidaka S, Gustilo RB: Refracture of bones of the forearm after plate removal. *J Bone Joint Surg Am* 66:1241-1243, 1984.

108. Labosky DA, Cermak MB, Waggy CA: Forearm fracture plates: to remove or not to remove. *J Hand Surg [Am]* 15:294-301, 1990.

109. Mih AD, Cooney WP, Idler RS, Lewallen DG: Long-term follow-up of forearm bone diaphyseal plating. *Clin Orthop* 299:256-258, 1994.

110. Rumball K, Finnegan M: Refractures after forearm plate removal. *J Orthop Trauma* 4:124-129, 1990.

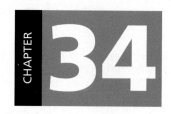

# Elbow Anatomy and Physical Examination

Christopher J. Veneziano,* Matthew J. Nofziger,† and Robert P. Nirschl‡

*MD, Orthopaedic Sports Medicine Fellow, Georgetown University Medical Center, Washington, DC; Orthopaedic Sports Medicine Fellow, Nirschl Orthopaedic Center for Sports Medicine and Joint Reconstruction, Virginia Hospital Center, Arlington, VA
†MD, Orthopaedic Surgeon, Southwestern Vermont Medical Center, Taconic Orthopaedics, Bennington, VT
‡MD, MS, Associate Clinical Professor, Department of Orthopedic Surgery, Georgetown University Medical Center, Washington, DC; Director, Orthopaedic Sports Medicine Fellowship Program, Nirschl Orthopaedic Center for Sports Medicine and Joint Reconstruction, Virginia Hospital Center, Arlington, VA

## Anatomy

- The elbow is a complex joint consisting of three separate articulations: the ulnohumeral, radiocapitellar, and proximal radioulnar joints. Its primary function is to assist the shoulder and wrist in positioning the hand in space. Although not technically a weight-bearing joint, the elbow is subjected to significant loads, especially in laborers and athletes participating in throwing and racquet sports. In order to diagnose and treat elbow injuries, it is essential to understand the anatomy and physiology of the elbow joint.
  - The normal range of elbow flexion/extension is approximately 0 to 150 degrees and normal forearm pronation/supination is 80 to 80 degrees. Functional range of motion (ROM) is 30 to 130 degrees of flexion/extension and 50 to 50 degrees of pronation/supination.

### Osteology

- The distal humerus terminates at the elbow in medial and lateral columns, epicondyles and condyles. The condyles articulate at the elbow joint as the trochlea medially and the capitellum laterally. The articular surface is angled approximately 30 degrees anterior to the axis of the humeral shaft (Figures 34–1, 34–2, and 34–3).[1]
- The medial ridge of the trochlea is larger than the lateral ridge and the capitellum. This gives the articular surface a slight valgus position, approximately 6 degrees, compared to the epicondylar axis.
- The coronoid fossa and olecranon fossa, just proximal to the articular surface, accommodate the coronoid process and olecranon process of the ulna in the extremes of flexion and extension, respectively. They are separated by a thin section of bone or, at times, a fibrous membrane. A smaller, radial fossa accepts the contour of the radial head when the elbow is fully flexed.
- The medial epicondyle is the prominent terminus of the medial supracondylar ridge. It is the point of origin for the flexor/pronator musculature. The distal portion of the medial epicondyle is the origin of the medial (ulnar) collateral ligament complex. The ulnar nerve runs along the smooth posterior portion of the medial epicondyle.
- The lateral epicondyle is the terminus of the lateral supracondylar ridge. It is less prominent than the medial epicondyle and is the point of origin of the extensor musculature and the radial collateral ligament (RCL).

Figure 34–1:
**Anterior aspect of distal humerus.**

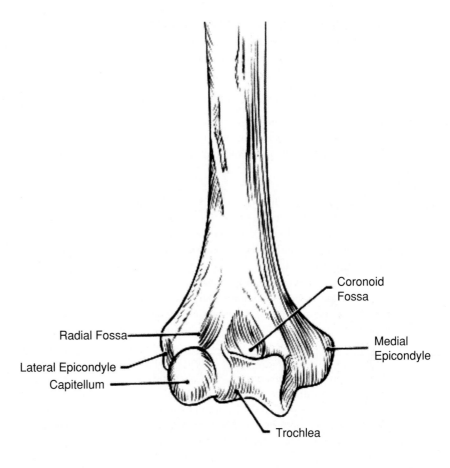

Coronoid
Fossa

Radial Fossa

Lateral Epicondyle

Capitellum

Medial
Epicondyle

Trochlea

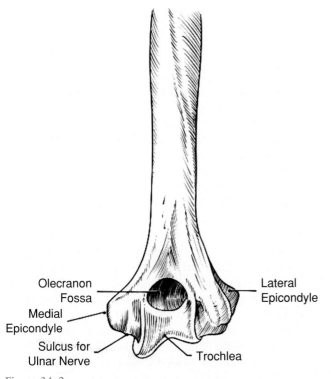

Olecranon
Fossa

Medial
Epicondyle

Sulcus for
Ulnar Nerve

Lateral
Epicondyle

Trochlea

Figure 34–2:
**Posterior aspect of distal humerus.**

- The olecranon and coronoid process coalesce to form the greater sigmoid notch, the articulating portion of the proximal ulna. It commonly is not completely covered with articular cartilage centrally.
- The coronoid process, on its lateral aspect, contains the lesser sigmoid (radial) notch (articulates with the radial head), the supinator crest (ulnar origin of the supinator muscle), and the crista supinatoris (insertion of the accessory lateral collateral ligament [LCL]). The medial side of the coronoid provides the insertion site (sublime tubercle) for the anterior bundle of the medial collateral ligament (MCL).
- The radial head articulates with the capitellum. Both the head and neck are considered intraarticular structures. Distal to the neck is the radial (bicipital)

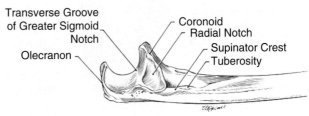

Transverse Groove
of Greater Sigmoid
Notch

Olecranon

Coronoid
Radial Notch
Supinator Crest
Tuberosity

Figure 34–3:
**Lateral aspect of proximal ulna.**

tuberosity, which is extraarticular. The radial head is covered with articular cartilage on its surface and along its periphery, which allows it to articulate smoothly in the lesser sigmoid (radial) notch.

## Capsuloligamentous Structures

- Stability of the elbow results from a combination of its bone structure, the articular congruence of the ulnohumeral joint, and its capsuloligamentous structures.
  - The medial collateral ligament complex originates on the distal portion of the medial epicondyle and consists of three bundles: anterior (inserts on the sublime tubercle on the medial surface of the coronoid), posterior (inserts on the medial olecranon), and transverse (Figure 34–4).[1]
  - Tension in the ligamentous complex varies throughout elbow ROM because its humeral origin lies posterior to the axis of rotation in flexion/extension.[2] Fibers of the anterior bundle sequentially tighten throughout the ROM from 20 to 120 degrees. The anterior bundle is the primary restraint to valgus stress within this ROM.[3] The radiocapitellar articulation provides a secondary restraint to valgus stress.
  - From 0 to 20 degrees flexion (i.e., in full extension), the MCL, capsule, and joint congruity contribute equally to stability.[3] The anterior MCL provides the majority of resistance to valgus stress in flexion. The posterior bundle of the MCL provides minimal stability to valgus stress but contributes somewhat in full flexion and provides constraint to hyperflexion.[4]
  - The LCL complex consists of the annular ligament, the RCL, the accessory collateral ligament, and the lateral ulnar collateral ligament (LUCL) (Figure 34–5).[1] There is tension in the LCL throughout motion because of its isometric position.[2] The RCL originates from the

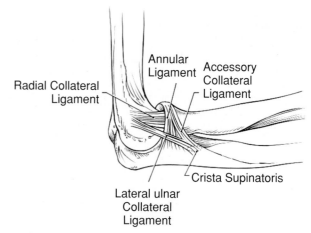

Figure 34–5:
**Lateral collateral ligament complex.**

lateral epicondyle and inserts along the course of the annular ligament. Because of its isometric position, it is taut throughout flexion. The LUCL is a separate, posterior portion of the RCL, which attaches to the crista supinatoris on the ulna. It is taut only in flexion beyond 110 degrees. It becomes lax in the presence of load or valgus stress. With varus load, the LUCL is taut throughout the ROM.[5] LUCL insufficiency leads to posterolateral rotatory instability (PLRI) of the elbow.[6]

- The annular ligament stabilizes the proximal radioulnar joint. It also plays a role in providing stability to varus stress (Figure 34–6).[7] The accessory collateral ligament is formed from a band of the annular ligament. It also attaches on the crista supinatoris.[1]

## Musculature

- The muscles on the anterior and posterior aspects of the elbow facilitate flexion and extension. The muscles on the medial side function to flex the wrist and fingers and to pronate the forearm, whereas the muscles on the lateral side extend the wrist and fingers and supinate the forearm (Figure 34–7).[1]
- The triceps is composed of three heads: long (origin at infraglenoid tubercle), lateral (origin from the posterior humerus), and medial or deep (origin from the posterior humerus). It crosses the posterior elbow and inserts broadly on to the posterior olecranon. Laterally, a band courses over the anconeus and attaches to the dorsal fascia of the forearm; this can provide weak elbow extension with essentially complete triceps rupture in some cases. The triceps is innervated by the radial nerve.
- The medial and lateral intermuscular septa separate the triceps (posterior compartment) from the anterior compartment in the distal two thirds of the arm.
- The brachialis and biceps are the muscles overlying the anterior elbow. The brachialis originates from the anterior

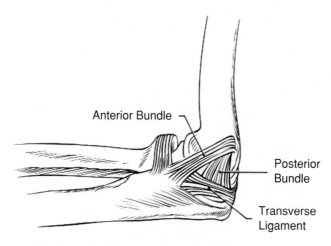

Figure 34–4:
**Medial collateral ligament complex.**

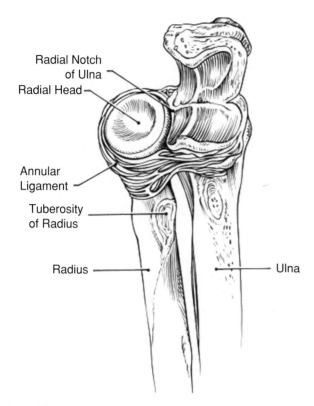

Radial Notch of Ulna

Radial Head

Annular Ligament

Tuberosity of Radius

Radius

Ulna

Figure 34–6:
**Proximal radioulnar joint.**

surface of the humerus and inserts on to the proximal ulna, just distal to the tip of the coronoid and on the ulnar tuberosity. It is innervated primarily by the musculocutaneous nerve; the lateral portion receives some supply from the radial nerve.

• The biceps originates as two heads, short (from the coracoid process) and long (from the superior glenoid), and blends into a single tendon distally, which inserts on to the radial (bicipital) tuberosity. It also inserts through the bicipital aponeurosis (lacertus fibrosis) broadly over the common flexor origin and proximal forearm. It is innervated by the musculocutaneous nerve.

• Medially, the flexor/pronator muscles originate from the medial epicondyle and course distally. They fan out laterally to medially as the pronator teres (PT), flexor carpi radialis (FCR), palmaris longus (PL), and flexor carpi ulnaris (FCU) superficially and the flexor digitorum sublimis (FDS) deeply.

• The PT originates as two heads, the superficial (humeral) head from the medial epicondyle and the deep (ulnar) head, and inserts on to the lateral aspect of the middle third of the radius. It functions to pronate the forearm and provides some elbow flexion. It is innervated by the median nerve, which passes between the two heads.

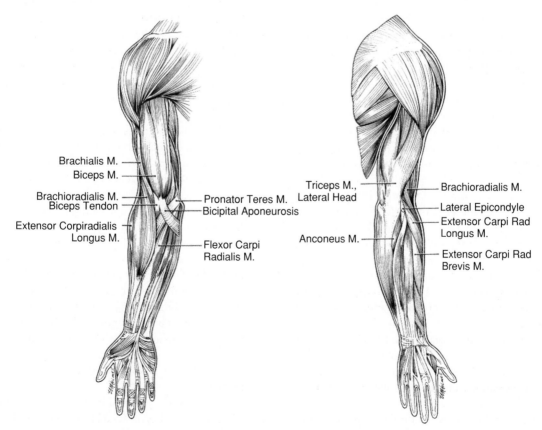

Brachialis M.
Biceps M.

Brachioradialis M.
Biceps Tendon

Extensor Corpiradialis Longus M.

Pronator Teres M.
Bicipital Aponeurosis

Flexor Carpi Radialis M.

Triceps M., Lateral Head

Anconeus M.

Brachioradialis M.

Lateral Epicondyle

Extensor Carpi Rad Longus M.

Extensor Carpi Rad Brevis M.

Figure 34–7:
**Superficial musculature of the upper extremity (anterior on *left,* posterior on *right).***

- The FCR originates from the medial epicondyle and inserts on to the volar base of the second metacarpal. It functions to flex the wrist and is innervated by the median nerve.
- The PL originates from the medial epicondyle and inserts into the palmar fascia. It functions as a weak wrist flexor and is innervated by the median nerve. It is absent in approximately 10% of patients.
- The FCU originates from the medial epicondyle and the posterior ulna and inserts onto the pisiform. It functions to flex the wrist powerfully and is innervated by the ulnar nerve.
- The flexor digitorum superficialis (FDS) is considered to be located in the middle layer of the forearm. It originates from the medial epicondyle and the anterior radius and inserts on the middle phalanges. It functions to flex the proximal interphalangeal (PIP) joints of the hand. It is innervated by the median nerve.
- Laterally, the mobile wad (brachioradialis [BR], extensor carpi radialis longus [ECRL], extensor carpi radialis brevis [ECRB]), the finger extensors (extensor digitorum communis [EDC]), and the anconeus cross the elbow.
- The BR, the most anterior muscle of the mobile wad, originates from the lateral supracondylar ridge of the humerus and inserts on the lateral aspect of the distal radius. Its primary function is elbow flexion. As a result of its insertion on the lateral border of the radius, it produces a rotational pull on the forearm that encourages a position of neutral rotation. It is, therefore, both a pronator and a supinator, depending on the starting position of the forearm. Innervation is supplied by the radial nerve.
- The ECRL is adjacent to the BR, originating just distally on the lateral supracondylar ridge of the humerus. It inserts on to the base of the second metacarpal. It functions to extend the wrist and produces slight radial deviation. Innervation is supplied by the radial nerve.
- The ECRB, the final muscle of the mobile wad, originates just distal and deep to the ECRL on the lateral epicondyle of the humerus and to some degree on the anteromedial edge of the extensor aponeurosis. It inserts on to the base of the third metacarpal and functions to extend the wrist. Because of the more central position of the third metacarpal base, the ECRB produces less radial deviation than does the ECRL. Innervation is supplied by the radial nerve.
- The EDC originates just distal to the ECRL and ECRB on the tip of the lateral epicondyle, and inserts into the extensor mechanism of the dorsal hand and fingers. It functions to extend the fingers. It is innervated by the posterior interosseous nerve (PIN).
- The anconeus originates distally on the more posterior aspect of the lateral epicondyle and inserts on to the proximal, dorsal ulna. It functions to extend the elbow and is innervated by the radial nerve.
- The extensor digiti minimi originates from the common extensor tendon, just distal to the elbow and inserts into the small finger extensor mechanism. It functions to assist extension of the small finger and is innervated by the PIN.
- The supinator originates from two heads. The superficial head originates from the lateral epicondyle, the LCL, and the supinator crest of the ulna. The deep head originates from the supinator crest. Together they insert onto the anterior aspect of the radius. It functions to supinate the forearm and is innervated by the PIN.

## Neurovascular

- The musculocutaneous nerve is derived from the lateral cord of the brachial plexus. It pierces the coracobrachialis muscle 5 to 8 cm distal to the coracoid process and runs distally between the brachialis and biceps. It emerges as the lateral antebrachial cutaneous nerve of the forearm just above the elbow. It innervates the coracobrachialis, brachialis, and biceps.
- The radial nerve is derived from the posterior cord of the brachial plexus. It courses around the posterior humerus in the spiral groove then travels anteriorly between the brachialis and BR. It crosses the elbow between them and divides in the cubital fossa anterior to the radiocapitellar joint into the PIN and the superficial radial nerve. The PIN enters the body of the supinator and continues distally on the dorsal aspect of the forearm, whereas the superficial radial nerve continues on the deep surface of BR. The radial nerve innervates the triceps, anconeus, BR, ECRL, and ECRB. The PIN supplies the supinator and the remainder of the finger extensors.
- The median nerve is derived from the medial and lateral cords of the brachial plexus. It runs with the brachial artery in the arm, starting on its lateral side. It then passes anterior to the brachial artery to its medial side before reaching the elbow. It crosses the medial side of the elbow, where it lies superficial to brachialis, just deep to the bicipital aponeurosis. It then passes distally between the two heads of the PT into the forearm between the FDS and flexor digitorum profundus (FDP). It innervates the PT, FCR, PL, FDS, and, in most cases (though some variation exists), the FDP-3. Distally, it supplies the index and middle finger lumbricals, the abductor pollicis brevis, opponens pollicis, and (though variations exist) flexor pollicis brevis. The anterior interosseous nerve branches off and supplies the FDP-2 (sometimes also the FDP-3), flexor pollicis longus, and pronator quadratus.
- The ulnar nerve is derived from the medial cord of the brachial plexus. It runs medial to the brachial artery in the arm before passing posteriorly through the medial

intermuscular septum and posterior to the medial epicondyle. It continues distally into the anterior compartment of the forearm between the two heads of the FCU, distal to the medial epicondyle, where it lies on the anterior surface of the FDP. It supplies the FCU and the ulnar half of the FDP.

- The brachial artery enters the cubital fossa on the anterior surface of the brachialis, lateral to the median nerve. Both then pass under the bicipital aponeurosis. In the cubital fossa the artery divides into the radial and ulnar arteries. The radial artery lies medial to the biceps tendon and immediately sends the radial recurrent artery laterally. It then continues distally superficial to the supinator and the PT, deep to the BR (running with the superficial radial nerve). The ulnar artery quickly branches into the anterior and posterior interosseous arteries and the ulnar recurrent artery (which runs proximally with the ulnar nerve). The ulnar artery exits the cubital fossa passing deep to the deep head of the PT and continues distally beneath the FCU and FDS, on the surface of the FDP (with the ulnar nerve as they course along the forearm).

# Physical Examination of the Elbow

## Keys to Effective Examination

- Taking a thorough history can provide a working differential diagnosis to guide the subsequent physical examination. Important when taking a history is to inquire about the location and severity of pain, exacerbating activities, and mechanism of injury. Also ask about such mechanical complaints as loss of motion, catching, locking, crepitus, and instability.[8]

## Initial Examination

- Before examining the elbow, evaluate the neck and shoulder to rule out radiculopathy, referred pain, or shoulder weakness. Next, evaluate elbow strength and perform a full distal neurovascular examination. Look for visual clues such as ecchymosis, swelling, gross deformity, altered carrying angle, and muscle spasm or atrophy. Continue with palpation, ROM, and tests for instability to help arrive at a differential diagnosis. Provocative tests (tests that place specific structures under stress) can be used to confirm the diagnosis.[8,9]

## History

### Introduction

- Although the elbow is not a "weight-bearing" joint, large forces are transmitted across it. During heavy lifting, the elbow's joint reaction forces reach two to three times body weight.[8] Overuse injuries can result from a number of popular sports, such as tennis, golf, baseball, and weight lifting, as well as activities of daily living.

### Patient Interview

- A thorough history is crucial in assessing an elbow injury and can provide a working differential diagnosis to guide the subsequent physical examination. The examiner should obtain the following information from the patient:
- *What is the character of the pain?* Pain is the most common complaint. Define its location and severity, exacerbating activities, and the mechanism of injury. Is the pain radiating or worse at night? The physician may consider referral of pain from the cervical spine or possibly a double crush neurologic injury. Does the pain involve several joints, possibly suggesting joint diseases (e.g., rheumatoid arthritis or osteoarthritis)?[8,10]
- *Where is the pain?* This question probably determines the most important characteristic from a diagnostic standpoint. Common causes of lateral pain include tennis elbow, radiocapitellar injury, and radial tunnel syndrome. Medial pain usually results from injury to the flexor-pronator origin, the MCL, ulnar nerve compression or subluxation, or rarely, from a snapping triceps tendon. Posterior pain may be associated with triceps tendinopathy or posterior impingement of the olecranon in its fossa from hypertrophic spurs. Anterior pain often represents distal biceps pathology, anterior capsular strain, median nerve entrapment, or osteoarthritis. Localizing the pain can allow further questions that focus on structures in that anatomic region.[8]
- *Are there any exacerbating activities?* Specific motions or activities stress specific structures, resulting in pain or injury. Medial elbow pain that occurs during the late cocking or acceleration phases of throwing, when valgus forces are maximized, often results from injury to the MCL. In acute injuries there may be an associated pop and sharp pain with an inability to continue throwing. Other times there is a gradual onset with progressively increasing pain during or after heavy throwing. There may be associated complaints of ulnar nerve paresthesias, caused by inflammation about the MCL, thus irritating the nerve as it passes through the cubital tunnel, or by valgus laxity, which causes traction on the nerve. These paresthesias are characterized mainly by medial elbow pain radiating to the ring and little finger. They also may produce a heavy or clumsy feeling in the hand after throwing.
  - Symptoms of ulnar nerve irritation can be associated with repetitive or prolonged elbow flexion, valgus force, forceful triceps activity (i.e., weight lifting), or direct pressure, with pain often worst at night or upon awakening.[8,11–13] Repetitive forearm rotation, wrist motion, gripping, or lifting stresses the tendons

of the extensor and flexor-pronator muscle masses. These actions are commonly seen in occupations such as carpentry, plumbing, and textile production, and in sports such as golf, throwing and racket sports.

○ Valgus forces in throwing can cause repetitive microtrauma, usually affecting the capitellum (osteochondritis dissecans) and, in adolescents, cause stress fractures of the medial epicondyle (Little Leaguer's elbow). Usually asymptomatic, a snapping medial head of the triceps can cause symptoms with repetitive elbow motion, as can a snapping synovial plica over the radial head.[8,13]

○ Postactivity ache or pain at rest typically results from joint effusion and synovitis but may be associated with nerve compression.[8]

○ Systemic inflammatory disorders, tumors, or infections may cause pain not related to activity.[8]

○ Elbow pain may be caused by tendinopathies, peripheral nerve entrapment, or cervical radiculopathy.[8]

○ Coldness or swelling of the hand may indicate a vascular injury or obstruction (i.e., brachial artery or vein obstruction).[8]

- *What is the severity and duration of symptoms?* How long has the patient had the problem? Does the severity of symptoms fluctuate? These questions can give an indication of the seriousness of the condition or to the amount of functional compromise for the patient.[8,10]

- *What was the mechanism of injury?* Was there an acute episode of pain, swelling, or ecchymosis associated with a specific traumatic event? Was it direct or indirect trauma, that is, a fall directly on the elbow or outstretched hand, or is there a history of repetitive microtrauma or recent change or increase in activity level?[8,10]

- *Are there mechanical complaints?* There may be loss of motion, locking, catching, instability, or recurrent effusions.

○ *Loss of motion, locking, and catching.* Elbow motion and forearm rotation may be limited by intraarticular and extraarticular pathologies affecting many articulations: the ulnohumeral, radiohumeral, proximal radioulnar, forearm, or distal radioulnar articulations. Loss of motion may not be functionally limiting (functional range 30–130 degrees extension-flexion, 50–50 degrees pronation-supination) but may suggest past or present injury. Loose bodies commonly arising from osteochondritis dissecans, or osteophytes from posterior impingement may produce symptoms of catching or locking, whereas osteoarthritis often produces crepitus.[8,10]

○ *Instability.* Instability may occur with injuries to the major stabilizing ligaments, that is, the MCL and LCL complexes. Instability also may occur with severe arthritis secondary to bone loss. The alteration in

elbow biomechanics may cause pain, synovitis, and osteophyte formation. Chronic MCL laxity, commonly seen in pitchers, allows the medial olecranon to impinge on the olecranon fossa during terminal extension or the follow-through phase of overhand throwing, causing elbow pain and swelling. Injury to the LCL, whether occurring acutely in an elbow dislocation or "sprain" or iatrogenically induced as a complication of lateral elbow surgery, can cause PLRI. Symptoms may include feelings of elbow instability, locking, catching, or snapping when the elbow is extended with the forearm supinated, or with elbow flexion from an extended position coupled with pronation, manifested as an uncomfortable "clunk" as the joint relocates from a subluxed position.[8,10,13]

## Initial Physical Examination

### Observation

- The patient must be suitably undressed to allow full examination of the trunk and neck down to the hand and full comparison of both upper limbs. Note any focal ecchymosis, swelling, atrophy, asymmetry, or gross deformity. Full body posture should be observed for possible referral of symptoms, especially in patients with a history of insidious onset of elbow pain.[10]

  - The carrying angle (the angle formed by the long axis of the humerus and the long axis of the ulna) is best viewed when the elbow is straight and the forearm is fully supinated (Figure 34–8). The normal valgus carrying angle in males is 5 to 10 degrees and in females is 10 to 15 degrees. A carrying angle less than 5–10 degrees is called *cubitus varus* and an angle greater than 10–15 degrees is called *cubitus valgus*. The normal carrying angle changes linearly depending on the degree of extension or flexion, ultimately reaching varus in full flexion. Discrepancy in carrying angles may indicate former trauma (i.e., a fracture), growth disturbance (i.e., epiphyseal injury to the distal humerus), or chronic valgus overload leading to valgus deformity secondary to bony remodeling. Chronic valgus overload is seen in baseball pitchers who started throwing competitively before they reached skeletal maturity. In general, carrying angle differences are of cosmetic rather than functional significance.[8,10,12]

- Ecchymosis may indicate an area of direct trauma, signifying contusion or tendon injury. However, ligaments on the opposite side of the impact also may be injured secondary to tension overload.[8]

- The anconeus soft spot (lateral infracondylar recess) is the most sensitive area to detect a joint effusion, whether secondary to hemarthrosis, synovitis, infection, dislocation, or fracture. This is the triangular area

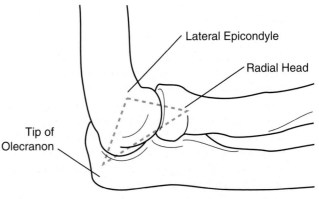

Figure 34–9:
Anconeus soft spot (lateral infracondylar recess) is the most sensitive area to detect a joint effusion. This triangular area located on the lateral aspect of the elbow is outlined by the radial head, tip of the olecranon, and lateral epicondyle.

ulna and the medial and lateral epicondyles of the humerus at 90 degrees flexion (Figure 34–10). With the elbow fully extended, these points should form a straight line. This relationship can be altered by intraarticular pathology, including fracture, malunion, or an unreduced elbow dislocation.[8,10]

- Discrepancy in muscle girth when comparing contralateral limbs may be a sign of disuse atrophy secondary to injury, or a sign of hypertrophy as often seen in athletes, such as pitchers or throwers who have a greater forearm muscle mass on the dominant side.[8,14]

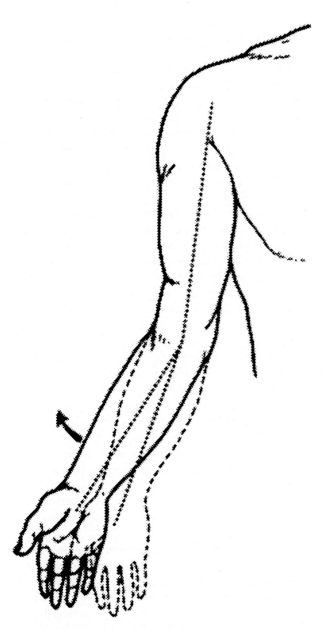

Figure 34–8:
Normal carrying angle of the elbow *(dotted outline)*. Cubitus valgus *(solid outline)* may occur secondary to former trauma, growth disturbance, or chronic valgus overload. (From Magee DJ: *Orthopaedic physical assessment,* ed 3. Philadelphia, 1997, WB Saunders.)

outlined by the radial head, tip of the olecranon, and lateral epicondyle (Figure 34–9). This is also an ideal location for joint aspiration or injection of the elbow joint. The anatomic position that allows for maximum joint capacity, as seen with a tense effusion, is with the elbow held at approximately 70 to 80 degrees flexion. More discrete swelling over the olecranon process usually results from olecranon bursitis.[8,10]

- The normal osseous landmarks of the elbow form an isosceles triangle between the olecranon process of the

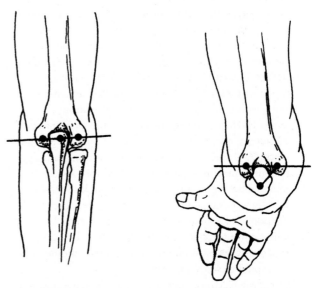

Figure 34–10:
The normal osseous landmarks of the elbow form an isosceles triangle between the olecranon process of the ulna and the medial and lateral epicondyles of the humerus at 90 degrees flexion. In full extension, these points should form a straight line. (From Magee DJ: *Orthopaedic physical assessment,* ed 3. Philadelphia, 1997, WB Saunders.)

## Examination

- It is essential to start the physical examination with the neck and shoulder to rule out radiculopathy, referred pain, or shoulder weakness, especially if the history indicates elbow symptoms of insidious onset.
  - *Range of motion.* Perform both active and passive ROM, remembering to do active movements first and painful movements last. Normal active elbow flexion is approximately 140 to 150 degrees flexion, with movement usually stopped by contact between the soft tissues of the forearm and the arm.
  - Full active extension may range from 0 to 10 degrees hyperextension, depending on the patient's degree of ligamentous laxity. Hyperextension is more common in women and is considered normal if it is symmetric with the contralateral elbow and the patient has no history of trauma. Pain with hyperextension of the elbow may be a sign of posterior impingement between osteophytes on the olecranon and the walls of the olecranon fossa. This phenomenon is most common in patients exposed to repetitive hyperextension overload, such as gymnasts and throwing athletes.
  - Full extension often is the first parameter lost after injury and may be a sensitive indicator of intraarticular pathology. However, terminal extension is not required for many daily activities, and loss of flexion often is believed to be more disabling. The functional range of flexion-extension motion, necessary for most activities of daily living (hand to mouth, hand to buttocks) is within the range from 30 to 130 degrees.
  - Active supination and pronation should approach 80 degrees in both directions, measured with the arm at the side to prevent the patient from using shoulder motion (adduction or abduction) to compensate for any deficiencies of forearm rotation. However, the functional ROM needed for most daily activities is only 50 degrees of supination and pronation.
  - Wrist ROM should be included in the examination because of the shared musculature between wrist and elbow. Any specific movements or positions causing patient complaint recorded in the history should be included in the examination. Mechanical blocks to motion may suggest an osseous blockage (abrupt endpoint) or soft tissue interposition or capsular contraction (rubbery endpoint).[10,13,15]
  - If active ROM is limited, passive motion should be attempted to test endpoints.[10]
- *Motor strength.* Motor strength is tested through resisted isometric movements of the muscles of the elbow complex. Elbow flexion power is greatest at 90 to 110 degrees flexion and in supination or neutral forearm rotation. In normal subjects, flexion strength is 30% greater than extension strength, and pronation strength approximately 75% that of supination strength,

with the dominant arm commonly 5% to 10% stronger than the nondominant side. Weak and pain-free isometric contraction may signify a myotendinous injury, but without a history of trauma suggests a neurologic origin.[8,10,12]

- *Palpation.* Palpation is a key part of the examination of the elbow in forming a differential diagnosis. In palpating the elbow, the examiner tries to elicit point tenderness or searches for abnormalities, including changes in temperature or texture, or any suspicious masses. The painful regions are palpated last and always compared to the uninjured side.[10,15]
  - The anterior elbow, or antecubital fossa, bounded laterally by the BR and medially by the PT, contains many important structures. Both the median and lateral antebrachial cutaneous nerves course within the fossa but are not palpable. Rarely, entrapment of the median nerve deep to the lacertus fibrosis (bicipital aponeurosis) occurs, and then a Tinel sign may be elicited. The biceps tendon can be easily palpated within the fossa, especially as it is placed under tension with resisted elbow flexion and supination. Pain to palpation can be a sign of strain or tendinosis. The coronoid process of the ulna and radial head can be palpated for potential abnormality. The anterior capsule can be strained in a hyperextension injury and produce tenderness to palpation along its origin on the distal humerus. Palpation of a strained brachialis muscle, especially through resisted elbow flexion in pronation, can produce pain.
  - The pulse of the brachial artery can be palpated as it crosses the elbow joint just medial to the biceps tendon.
  - Important structures that take origin from the medial epicondyle include the wrist flexor-pronator muscle mass and the MCL. The anterior band of the MCL can be palpated from its origin on the humerus to its insertion on the ulna at the base of the coronoid (sublime tubercle) with the elbow positioned in 30 to 60 degrees flexion.
  - Tenderness to palpation of the flexor-pronator mass just distal and anterior to the medial epicondyle usually signifies a tendinopathy of the PT and/or the FCR, also called golfer's elbow or medial tennis elbow.
  - The ulnar nerve, located just posterior to the medial epicondyle, runs in the cubital tunnel, deep to a fascial covering or retinaculum, before passing between the two heads of the FCU. Pathologic thickening of this retinaculum may cause sites of nerve compression, which can be diagnosed with a positive Tinel's sign and elbow flexion test. Flexing and extending the elbow during palpation helps detect any nerve subluxation at or just proximal to the epicondyle, which may predispose a patient to ulnar neuritis.[10,15–17]

○ "Tennis elbow," or degenerative tendinosis of the ECRB, is the most common cause of lateral elbow pain. Point tenderness over the ECRB origin, just anterior and distal to the tip of the lateral epicondyle, is diagnostic. When palpating the elbow, it is important to remember that the ECRL originates above the epicondyle along the epicondylar ridge. If the EDC is involved (in 30% of patients with lateral tennis elbow), tenderness also will be present just posterior and distal to the tip of the lateral epicondyle.

○ Included in the differential diagnosis of lateral elbow pain is radial tunnel syndrome, caused by compression of the PIN as it passes between the two heads of the supinator muscle under the arcade of Frohse. This commonly leads to pain and tenderness within the extensor mass. Tenderness to palpation can be localized to the area just distal to the radial head along the proximal edge of the supinator. Provocative tests, described later, are useful in differentiating lateral tennis elbow from radial tunnel syndrome.

○ The anconeus soft spot, described earlier, not only is a sensitive area to detect joint effusions or hemarthrosis but also can be used to palpate the capitellum, which may become tender from osteochondral injury. Supination and pronation of the forearm aids in palpation of both the radial head and the annular ligament. Crepitus and/or pain to palpation during rotation may represent a radial head fracture, radiocapitellar arthritis, chondromalacia, plica, osteochondritis dissecans, or a loose body.[10,15,18–20]

○ The triceps muscle, olecranon fossa, olecranon process, and its bursa can be palpated at the posterior aspect of the elbow. Flexing the elbow to approximately 30 degrees relaxes the triceps muscle and allows access to the olecranon process as it is delivered from the olecranon fossa. This allows palpation of any olecranon exostosis or loose bodies as are seen with chronic hyperextension overload, especially in throwing athletes. The olecranon bursa overlying the olecranon process may feel thickened, warm, tender, or distended with fluid and may contain "rice bodies," fragments of fibrous tissue that can act as further irritants to the bursa. Tenderness along the triceps tendon may represent tendinosis or "posterior tennis elbow" as a result from repetitive overload, whereas a defect or gap in the substance suggests rupture.[10,13,15,21]

## Instability and Provocative Tests

• The patient history should help direct the examiner to perform any special tests relevant to confirming a diagnosis. When elbow instability is suspected, stress tests can be performed to evaluate for ligamentous injury.[10]

• The anterior band of the MCL is the primary stabilizer during valgus stress in flexion, whereas the osseous architecture and the anterior joint capsule provides a large degree of elbow stability in extension. Valgus instability can be detected by applying a valgus force to the patient's elbow with the humerus stabilized in external rotation, and the elbow flexed 25 to 30 degrees (Figure 34–11). One hand can be used to stabilize the elbow while the other hand is used to palpate the ligament and joint line to detect tenderness or gapping (Figure 34–12). Placing the patient in the supine position offers easier control for maximum external rotation of the humerus, while in the seated or standing position the examiner uses his/her torso to stabilize the patient's arm, thus freeing up both hands to further stabilize and palpate the medial joint line.[10,14]

• Four important variables to determine during stress testing are degree of laxity, endpoint quality, pain elicited, and focal tenderness. MCL sprains can be graded on the degree of laxity, starting with minor sprains (grade 1) presenting with pain and no laxity, partial tears (grade 2)

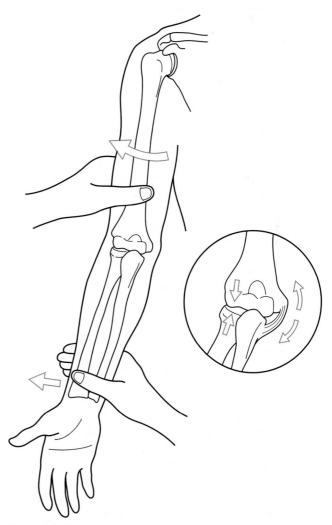

Figure 34–11:
**Testing for valgus instability.**

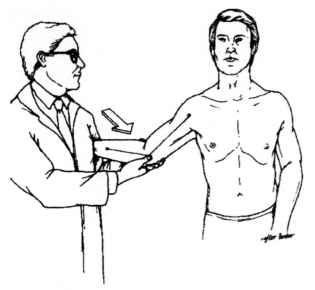

Figure 34–12:
For elbow valgus stress testing, the patient's upper extremity can be stabilized by holding the humerus in full external rotation and placing the patients forearm within the examiner's axilla, allowing both the examiner's hands to be free to palpate the joint line and medial collateral ligament. (From Morrey BF: *J Am Acad Orthop Surg* 4:117, 1996.)

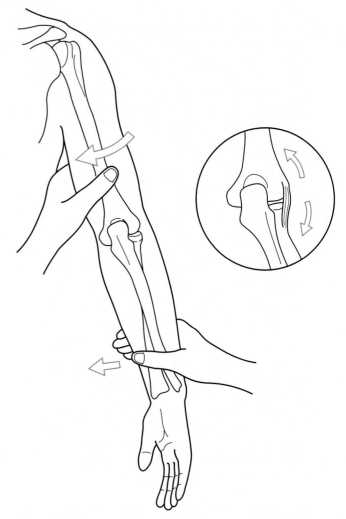

Figure 34–13:
**Varus laxity is tested similar to valgus stress testing, except with the humerus held in internal rotation and the forearm in supination, while adduction force is applied to the elbow.**

allowing some laxity but maintaining a solid endpoint, and complete tears (grade 3) demonstrating gross valgus laxity without a firm endpoint.[13,15]

- True instability of the anterior MCL is present during both pronation and supination of the forearm. When valgus instability in supination resolves in pronation, PLRI should be suspected.[12,15]

- Attenuation of the LCL complex with true varus laxity, a much less common injury, is tested similar to the valgus stress test, except with the humerus stabilized in internal rotation, and the forearm supinated, while adduction stress is applied to the elbow (Figure 34–13).[10,15]

- PLRI, caused by insufficiency of the LUCL, is a rotatory subluxation. When valgus stress is applied with the forearm in supination and the elbow near full extension, the radius and ulna rotate together as a unit away from the humerus. There is subluxation of the ulna from the trochlea and posterior subluxation of the radius off the capitellum. Pronation of the forearm and flexion of the elbow reduces PLRI. Pure varus laxity occurs only rarely, most likely because of the restraint from the LCL in combination with the osseous architecture of the ulnohumeral articulation.[6,15,21]

## Provocative Tests

- *Provocative tests,* which place specific structures under stress, help to determine which structure in an anatomic region is symptomatic.[9] A presumed diagnosis of lateral tennis elbow is tested by stressing the ECRB through resisted wrist extension. First, the patient holds the elbow in extension and is asked to make a fist, pronate the forearm, and extend the wrist while the examiner resists the motion (Figure 34–14).[9,10] A positive sign is pain at the origin of the ECRB. Coonrad described a positive "coffee cup test," or pain with picking up a cup of liquid, as pathognomonic for lateral tennis elbow.[9]

- EDC involvement can be tested, using the same position of elbow extension and forearm pronation but with the wrist now at neutral, by resisting extension of the middle finger. Pain at the origin of the EDC is suggestive of a tendinosis.[9,10] This maneuver may also increase compression on the radial nerve, possibly exacerbating symptoms of radial tunnel syndrome. However, in contradistinction to tennis elbow, the pain of radial tunnel syndrome is localized more distally.[9]

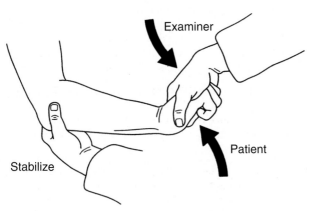

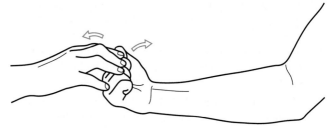

**Figure 34–15:**
**Resisted wrist flexion test is specific for flexor carpi radialis involvement.**

**Figure 34–14:**
**Test for lateral tennis elbow with the patient's arm held in extension, forearm pronated, and wrist radially deviated while resisting wrist extension. A positive sign is pain at the extensor carpi radialis brevis origin.** (From Magee DJ: *Orthopaedic physical assessment,* ed 3. Philadelphia, 1997, WB Saunders.)

- Provocative testing of the supinator may be more helpful in differentiating lateral tennis elbow from radial tunnel syndrome. This test is carried out through resisted supination from a fully pronated position with the elbow held in extension (to eliminate the supination effects of biceps). Symptoms are reproduced if there is PIN compression at the arcade of Frohse.[9,10]
- The differential diagnosis of lateral elbow pain includes radiocapitellar arthritis, synovitis, and a symptomatic radiocapitellar plica. All of these conditions typically lead to a more diffuse pain that can be reproduced through passive rotation of the forearm with axial compression. It is important to be aware of coexistent pathologic conditions (<5% in our experience) that may be present along with lateral tennis elbow, including intraarticular injury, synovitis, plica, or posterolateral chondromalacia.[9]
- Tendinosis of the flexor-pronator muscle mass, or medial tennis elbow, usually affects the PT and FCR. Symptoms can be reproduced through the resisted wrist flexion test and resisted pronation test.[9,10] The resisted wrist flexion test is more specific for FCR involvement and involves resisted wrist flexion with the elbow slightly flexed and forearm supinated (Figure 34–15). Provoked pain is localized to the origin of the FCR. When the PT is involved, resisted pronation with the elbow extended and forearm in neutral rotation produces pain at the origin of this tendon. Paresthesias in the median nerve distribution that occur with resisted forearm pronation suggest entrapment of the median nerve as it passes through the two heads of the PT (pronator syndrome).
- Cubital tunnel syndrome may occur as an isolated entity or may coexist with other medial elbow pathology, such as MCL insufficiency, which leads to traction on the

ulnar nerve, medial tennis elbow, or medial and/or posterior compartment osteophytes causing friction or compression on the nerve.[9] While the patient with cubital tunnel syndrome flexes and extends the elbow, the examiner palpates the medial epicondyle to test for ulnar nerve subluxation. The nerve can be palpated as it dislocates from the cubital tunnel anteriorly with elbow flexion.[9] The elbow flexion test is a provocative test for cubital tunnel syndrome. It is performed by having the patient fully flex and supinate the elbow. The pressure of a digit over the cubital tunnel can be added to increase sensitivity. A positive result is reproduction of paresthesias to the ulnar digits within 30 seconds.[9,10]
- Diagnostic injections of anesthetic can help validate a diagnosis from intraarticular pathology to tendinosis to nerve compression syndromes. Injections to specific pathoanatomic locations with pain relief often is confirmatory.[9]

## References

1. Nicholas JA, Hershman EB: *The upper extremity in sports medicine,* pp 273-283. St. Louis, 1990, Mosby.
   This chapter provides a review of elbow anatomy, both soft tissue and osseous.

2. Morrey BF, An Kai-Nan: Functional anatomy of the ligaments of the elbow. *Clin Orthop* 201:84, 1985.
   This article reviews the ligaments about the elbow and their three-dimensional anatomy throughout the range of motion.

3. Tullos HS, Bryan WJ: Functional anatomy of the elbow. In Zarins B, Andrews JR, Carson WD Jr, editors: *Injuries to the throwing arm.* Philadelphia, 1985, WB Saunders.
   This chapter provides a review of the function and contributions of the bony and capsuloligamentous structures of the elbow to stability throughout the arc of motion.

4. Fuss FK: The ulnar collateral ligament of the human elbow joint. *J Anat* 175:203-212, 1991.
   This article evaluates the ulnar (medial) collateral ligament complex of the elbow, assessing the contributions of the individual components of the complex.

5. Regan WD, Korinek SL, Morrey BF, et al: Biomechanical study of the ligaments around the elbow joint. *Clin Orthop* 271:170-179, 1991.

   This article evaluates the ligamentous contribution to elbow joint stability throughout the range of motion. The anterior portion of the MCL was the strongest and stiffest.

6. O'Driscoll SW, Bell DF, Morrey BF: Posterolateral rotatory instability of the elbow. *J Bone Joint Surg* 73A:440-446, 1991.

   Description of posterolateral rotatory instability of the elbow, its cause, and its physical examination.

7. Sojbjerg JO, Overssen J, Nielsen S: Experimental elbow instability after transection of the medial collateral ligament. *Clin Orthop* 218:186-190, 1987.

   The stability of the elbow is independent of the MCL at less than 20 degrees and greater than 120 degrees flexion. Maximum instability occurred between 60 and 70 degrees flexion.

8. Budoff JE, Nirschl RP: Elbow complaints: keys to effective examination. *Consultant* 2:509-516, 2001.

   Part one of three review articles. A review of appropriate history taking to help guide the physical examination in evaluating elbow complaints.

9. Budoff JE, Nirschl RP: Office examination of the elbow: how provocative tests can help clinch the diagnosis. *Consultant* 2:1004-1013, 2001.

   Part three of three review articles. A review of provocative tests used to help distinguish the cause of most common elbow disorders.

10. Magee DJ: *Orthopedic physical assessment*, ed 2. Philadelphia, 1997, WB Saunders.

    Textbook of physical diagnosis as pertaining to orthopedics.

11. Jobe FW, Kvitne RS. The elbow. *Instr Course Lect* 40:17, 1991.

    Review article of elbow injuries, especially as pertaining to the athlete.

12. Morrey BF, editor: *The elbow and its disorders*, ed 2. Philadelphia, 1993, WB Saunders.

    Textbook with a thorough description of the anatomy, pathology, diagnosis, and treatment of elbow disorders.

13. Jobe FW, Nuber G: Throwing injuries of the elbow. *Clin Sports Med* 5:621-636, 1986.

    A thorough history and physical examination combined with a firm understanding of biomechanics helps the physician make the proper diagnosis and initiate successful treatment.

14. Morrey BF: Acute and chronic instability of the elbow. *J Am Acad Orthop Surg* 4:117-128, 1996.

    Review article describing how to recognize and treat acute and chronic instability of the elbow. Both osseous and soft tissue reconstructive options are described.

15. Budoff JE, Nirschl RP: *Office examination of the elbow: palpation and instability tests. Consultant* 2:878-887, 2001.

    Part two of three review articles. Describes the physical examination of the elbow with respect to palpation and instability testing.

16. Schwab GH, Bennett JB, Woods G, et al: Biomechanics of elbow stability: role of the medial collateral ligament. *Clin Orthop Rel Res* 146:42, 1980.

    The anterior MCL is a major stabilizer. Fractures of the medial epicondyle must be anatomically reduced and fixed because lengthening may result in chronic elbow instability.

17. Nirschl RP: Medial tennis elbow, surgical treatment. *Orthop Trans Am Acad Orthop Surg* 7:298, 1980.

    Review of the diagnosis and treatment of medial tennis elbow, that is, "golfer's elbow."

18. Nirschl RP: Elbow tendinosis/tennis elbow. Tendinitis, II: clinical considerations. *Clin Sports Med* 11:851-870, 1992.

    The histology of tennis elbow demonstrates noninflammatory tissue, named angiofibroblastic hyperplasia. Nonoperative treatment consists of rehabilitative exercise. Surgical treatment involves excision of the pathologic tissue with repair of the tendon.

19. Nirschl RP: Tennis elbow. *Orthop Clin North Am* 4:787, 1973.

    Review of tennis elbow, including anatomy, pathology, diagnosis, and treatment.

20. Eversman WW Jr. Entrapment and compression neuropathies. In Green DP, editor. *Operative hand surgery*. New York, 1993, Churchill Livingstone.

    Discusses nerve entrapment and compression syndromes in the upper extremity. Anatomy and clinical signs and symptoms are described.

21. Andrews JR, Wilk KE, Satterwhite YE, Tedder JL: Physical examination of the throwers elbow. *J Orthop Sports Phys Ther* 17:296-304, 1993.

    Review of the evaluation of thrower's elbow.

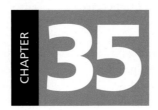
# Tendon Injuries and Tendinopathies About the Elbow

Jeffrey E. Budoff

MD, Assistant Professor, Hand and Upper Extremity Institute, Department of Orthopaedic Surgery, Baylor College of Medicine; Houston Veterans Affairs Medical Center, Houston, TX

## Tennis Elbow

- Tendinopathies usually are the result of overuse from repetitive tensile overload. Overuse injuries occur when the stress applied to a tissue exceeds its stress tolerance, which is a function of strength, flexibility, and endurance. When the tissue's stress tolerance is exceeded, tissue damage may occur. When repetitive tissue damage occurs at a rate exceeding the body's ability to heal it, tissue degeneration and subsequent symptoms of pain and disability may occur.[1]

- Approximately 50% of tennis players may get tennis elbow at some point, but the term *tennis elbow* probably is a misnomer because 95% of cases occur in non-tennis players.[2] The condition now is more commonly an industrial injury.[1] Specific predisposing tasks involve repetitive forearm rotation, overuse of the wrist or finger extensors, lifting with the forearm pronated, and athletic activities including racket sports, throwing, and swimming.[3] Throwing athletes tend to develop medial epicondylitis tennis elbow because of the valgus stresses experienced. Golfers tend to develop medial tennis elbow of the dominant arm and lateral tennis elbow of the nondominant arm. Posterior tennis elbow is seen with repetitive sudden elbow extension, as occurs during pitching, football line play, shot put, javelin throw,

bowling, and heavy weight lifting. Lateral tennis elbow is three to seven times as frequent as medial tennis elbow.[4] Posterior tennis elbow is uncommon, accounting for only approximately 2% of cases,[1] and usually occurs in combination with other pathology, such as posterior impingement.[1,5]

- The term *tendonitis* has been used to describe the theoretical chronic inflammatory changes in the overused tendon. However, histologic examination has found that acute inflammatory cells are invariably absent. Chronic inflammatory cells, if present, are those of traumatic repair, such as the cells found in granulation tissue and scar.[3,5] Therefore, the term *tendonitis* also is a misnomer and should be replaced by the term *tendinosis*. Tendinosis more accurately defines the histopathology of the degenerative process. The characteristic appearance of this tissue consists of invasion of immature fibroblasts and disorganized, nonfunctional vascular elements. This granulation-like tissue has been termed *angiofibroblastic hyperplasia* by Nirschl.[6]

- Angiofibroblastic hyperplasia is theorized to result from an aborted healing response to microtears. Healing may fail because of disruption of the repair response by continuing injury, the poor vascularity of the tendon origin, or the possibility that the degenerative tendinosis itself deters the process of repair.[6] The angiofibroblastic hyperplasia/tendinosis tissue appears to be the primary source of pain, and its amount appears to correlate with the duration of symptoms and the intensity of the pain.[3,5] However, what makes this tissue intrinsically painful is not fully clear. The pain may result from tissue ischemia, as electron microscopy has demonstrated that the vascular elements do not possess lumen and therefore have no oxygen transporting capability.[7]

## History and Physical Examination

- The onset of symptoms usually is gradual, often appearing after vigorous activity. Less commonly, acute onset is associated with an extreme effort or direct trauma.[3] In many instances no predisposing activity can be determined.[2]
- Lateral tennis elbow is degenerative tendinosis of the origin of the extensor carpi radialis brevis (ECRB). In addition, the anterior origin of the extensor digitorum communis (EDC) is involved in 30% of cases. Both of these tendons take origin from the lateral epicondyle. The extensor carpi radialis longus (ECRL) and the extensor carpi ulnaris are rarely involved.[3] Lateral tennis elbow presents with pain over the origin of the ECRB, and often the EDC. It often is associated with weakness of the wrist extensors. The pain often is described as "burning," and may radiate down the forearm, occasionally to the dorsal hand. Radiating pain does not necessarily imply a neurogenic origin.[1] As noted by Coonrad,[2] pain at the origin of the ECRB while picking up a full cup of coffee (or any other fluid) is almost pathognomonic for lateral tennis elbow.
- Medial tennis elbow is degenerative tendinosis of the conjoined tendon interface of the pronator teres (PT) and the flexor carpi radialis (FCR), but it also has been noted in the origin of the flexor carpi ulnaris and rarely on the underside of the flexor digitorum superficialis origin.[3,5,8] All of these tendons originate from the medial epicondyle. Medial tennis elbow typically presents with pain over the flexor-pronator mass. Ulnar nerve irritation, medial collateral ligament injury, and olecranon osteophytes may be associated with medial tennis elbow because they also are induced by repetitive valgus stress and overuse.[5]
- Posterior tennis elbow is degenerative tendinosis of the triceps insertion and presents with pain there.

## Point of Maximum Tenderness

- Lateral tennis elbow causes tenderness over the origin of the ECRB, just anterior and slightly distal to the tip of the lateral epicondyle. If the EDC also is involved, it will be tender just posterior and distal to the tip of the lateral epicondyle. Associated bony exostosis of the lateral epicondyle can result in tenderness over the lateral epicondyle itself.
  - *Pearl:* The point of maximum tenderness is invariably within 1 to 2 cm of the lateral epicondyle. If the point

of maximum tenderness is distal to the level of the radial head, other diagnoses, such as radial tunnel syndrome, should be suspected.[1]
- The point of maximum tenderness for radial tunnel syndrome is on the lateral side of the proximal forearm, in the soft spot just posterior to the mobile wad of Henry, approximately 4 to 5 cm distal to the lateral epicondyle. The lateral epicondyle, the radial head, and the radial tunnel lie in a line equidistant from each other.[1,4] Tenderness here should be compared to the other side because this region often is a little tender to deep pressure.
  - *The differential diagnosis* of lateral elbow pain includes radial tunnel syndrome, radiocapitellar disorder, (arthritis, fracture, avascular necrosis, osteochondral lesion) and cervical radiculopathy. Pain also may radiate from the shoulder, especially from the rotator cuff, to the lateral elbow.
- Medial tennis elbow causes tenderness over the origin of the flexor-pronator mass, just distal to the medial epicondyle. In addition, the PT has an origin proximal to the medial epicondyle, which may also be tender.
  - *Pearl:* In medial tennis elbow, the point of maximum tenderness should be within 1 to 2 cm of the medial epicondyle. If the tenderness is more distal, other diagnoses should be considered.[2]
  - *The differential diagnosis* of medial elbow pain includes injury to the medial collateral ligament (MCL), ulnar neuritis/cubital tunnel syndrome, ulnotrochlear arthritis or fracture, and a snapping medial triceps tendon.
- Posterior tennis elbow leads to tenderness at the insertion of the triceps tendon.
  - *The differential diagnosis* of posterior elbow pain includes posterior impingement (from chronic hyperextension or valgus extension overload), olecranon stress fracture, olecranon periostitis, olecranon bursitis, or ulnotrochlear arthritis.

## Provocative Tests for Lateral Tennis Elbow

- Loading the injured musculotendinous unit(s) should reproduce the patient's symptoms. The ECRB (a wrist extensor) is tested by having the patient hold the elbow extended and the forearm pronated while he/she makes a fist and extends the wrist. The patient should hold this position while the examiner applies resistance, ie., attempts to forcibly flex the wrist. Pain at the origin of the ECRB is diagnostic of lateral tennis elbow. The test should be repeated with the elbow flexed 90 degrees. As the ECRB crosses the elbow anterior to its axis of rotation, it is tensioned by elbow extension and relaxed by elbow flexion. Provoked pain often is increased by elbow extension and lessened by elbow flexion. Pain that is not lessened by elbow flexion implies a greater extent of tendon degeneration and a poorer prognosis for successful nonoperative management.

- The EDC should also be tested. With the wrist in neutral, the forearm pronated, and the elbow extended, all of the fingers should be extended. The patient attempts to maintain this position as the examiner applies a downward (flexing) force to the metacarpophalangeal joint of the long digit or of all digits simultaneously. Pain at the origin of the EDC (as opposed to over the radial tunnel) is suggestive of EDC tendinosis. The finger extension test previously has been described as provocative for radial tunnel syndrome, where it is theorized to provoke pain by driving the medial edge of the ECRB, or its fascial extension, against the posterior interosseous nerve (PIN).[9] However, pain with resisted long digit extension probably more commonly represents degenerative tendinosis of the EDC origin.[1] It is important to note the location of the provoked pain. Provocative testing in cases of PIN entrapment should refer pain to the radial tunnel, *not* the lateral epicondyle. Pain referred to or about the lateral epicondyle is consistent with lateral tennis elbow. The finger extension test may not reliably distinguish between these two pathologic entities.[1]

## Provocative Tests for Medial and Posterior Tennis Elbow

- Symptoms of medial tennis elbow may be reproduced by resisted wrist flexion and pronation. With the elbow slightly flexed and the forearm supinated, the patient makes a fist and flexes the wrist. The patient maintains that position as the examiner attempts to forcibly extend the wrist. If resisted wrist flexion elicits pain at the flexor-pronator origin, the FCR tendon is involved. With the elbow extended and the forearm in neutral rotation, the patient should "shake hands" with the examiner. The patient should then try to forcefully pronate the forearm, which the examiner resists. If resisted pronation causes pain at the flexor-pronator origin, the PT is involved.
  - *Pearl:* Symptoms caused by entrapment of the median nerve between the two heads of the PT (the pronator syndrome) may be reproduced by resisted forearm pronation with the elbow extended. However, in the pronator syndrome, resisted pronation leads to paresthesias of the radial digits, not medial elbow pain. In addition, resisted pronation with the elbow flexed should not reproduce symptoms caused by the pronator syndrome because only the ulnar head of the PT is tense in this position, and therefore the median nerve should not be compressed.
- Symptoms of posterior tennis elbow may be reproduced by resisted elbow extension.

## Radiography

- Standard radiographs should be evaluated for the presence of fracture, dislocation, subluxation, avascular necrosis, and degenerative changes. Radiographic exostosis of the lateral epicondyle occurs in 7% to 20% of patients with lateral tennis elbow.[5,10] Although of questionable prognostic significance, consideration can be given to exostosis removal at the time of surgery, especially if they are tender. Medial tennis elbow is usually not associated with radiographic changes.
- Magnetic resonance imaging (MRI) of the elbow is not routinely necessary in patients with tennis elbow. Physical examination is the gold standard for diagnosis of the condition, with advanced radiologic studies adding little with regard to staging, prognosis, or the determination of treatment.[1]

## Diagnostic Injection

- In cases of diagnostic dilemma, a diagnostic injection often can be helpful in determining the cause of the patient's symptoms. Lidocaine injected deep to the origin of the ECRB over the anterior aspect of the lateral epicondyle should relieve pain caused by lateral tennis elbow. Injections just deep to the flexor-pronator mass for medial tennis elbow achieve the same result. Intratendinous injections should be avoided because they may further damage an already injured tendon. Subdermal injection of steroid superficial to the tendon may lead to subcutaneous fat atrophy, leaving a permanent dimple, thinner skin, and a poorly padded, tender epicondyle.
- Injection of lidocaine into the radial tunnel should relieve the pain of radial tunnel syndrome. The ECRB should be injected first because forceful wrist extension will not be possible after the injection.
  - *Author's technique:* Use a 22-gauge, 1.5-inch needle and 10 ml lidocaine (and 1 ml steroid if desired). The elbow should be flexed and pronated. Penetrate the skin over the radial tunnel, aiming somewhat posteriorly, for the radial neck. After contacting the radial neck, pull back 1 to 2 mm and inject all 10 ml. A PIN palsy should occur within a few minutes, confirming appropriate placement of the injection.
- An intraarticular injection of lidocaine, most often through the anconeus soft spot, should relieve pain resulting from intraarticular pathology.

## Treatment

- The aim of nonoperative management of tendinopathies is twofold: decreasing the stress applied to the injured tendon and increasing the tendon's stress tolerance (i.e., strength). Approximately 75% to 95% of patients improve with nonoperative management.[1,11]
  - *Pearl:* It is critical to distinguish between comfort and cure. Therapeutic modalities (rest, nonsteroidal antiinflammatory drugs, and steroid injections) may temporarily relieve pain, but the pain relief does not necessarily imply healing or improvement of tissue quality. These interventions have no long-term curative

efficacy, and reliance upon them may result in further deconditioning and delay of the rehabilitative process. Therefore, these measures must be used only in the perspective of a larger treatment plan.

- If pain prevents the patient from performing the prescribed exercise program, an injection of corticosteroid is appropriate. However, the efficacy of steroid injections is questionable, as a randomized prospective trial found no difference in symptoms between patients injected with steroid and lidocaine and those injected with only saline at 3 and 12 months.[12] Repetitive injections are inappropriate because they may cause cellular death, further tissue weakness, and actually slow the healing process.[1,3,12]

- Rest should be relative. The patient should refrain from symptom-aggravating or abusive activities, not all activities. Work or play can be continued if the injured tissue can be protected through a reduction in stress.[1] Faulty athletic or workplace techniques that place unnecessarily high stresses on the tendon origins should be identified and corrected. The patient's tennis swing, throwing motion, or other sport-specific task should be evaluated by an athletic trainer, coach, or professional. In cases of work-induced lateral tennis elbow, grasping or lifting with the forearm pronated (palm down) should be avoided,[2] and the patient should be instructed to lift with the forearm supinated.[1,4]

- Counterforce bracing reduces the transmission of externally applied forces to the tendon origins and decreases symptoms of tennis elbow.[6] This brace should be worn during rehabilitative exercise, stressful daily activities, and upon return to work or sport. The brace usually is not necessary at rest or during light activities of daily living. Counterforce bracing also may function by preventing full muscular expansion, thereby not allowing maximal contraction, which further decreases force at the muscle's tendinous origin.[12] In addition, the brace probably reminds the patient to exercise due caution. Wrist splints can be used to decrease stress during a specific activity. Continuous splint use or casting may relieve pain but at the price of atrophy, stiffness, and further deconditioning, and is not recommended.[3]

- Although stress minimization is important, the mainstay of treatment is improvement of tissue quality through rehabilitative exercise, to allow the myotendinous unit to safely absorb the imposed forces. Activity modification to eliminate the motions causing pain may be necessary for three months. The term, "no pain, no gain," does not apply to elbow tendinosis. The six key forearm exercises are wrist extension, wrist flexion, forearm pronation, forearm supination, finger extension, and the ball squeeze (Figures 35–1, 35–2, and 35–3). The patient should be instructed *not* to work through pain. If pain occurs, the resistance, number of repetitions, or arc of motion should be decreased.

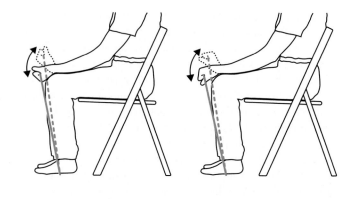

Wrist Flexion          Wrist Extension

Figure 35–1:
**Wrist flexion/extension.**

- The elbow should be flexed 90 degrees and the forearm supported on the thigh or a table to minimize tension at the tendon origins. More is not better and may exacerbate symptoms. Repetitions should be increased every few days as pain allows, until the patient is comfortably performing one to three sets of 10 repetitions per day. Athletes may work up to three sets per day, whereas some deconditioned workers' compensation patients may do better performing only one set per day. The elastic resistance or weight may then be slowly increased. Remember that the goal is to relieve the patient's symptoms, not to have him/her exercise with an ever-increasing amount of resistance.

- If program advancement is desired (as in athletes), once 5 lb of resistance is reached, the elbow is gradually straightened from 90 degrees, with the forearm still supported. To avoid overloading the tendons, the resistance should be decreased and reprogressed.

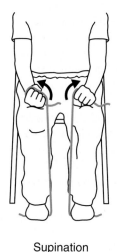
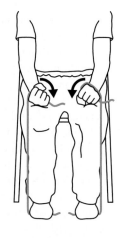

Supination          Pronation

Figure 35–2:
**Wrist supination/pronation.**

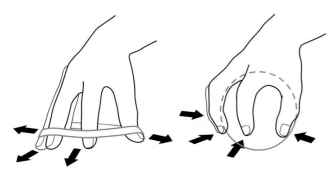

Figure 35–3:
**Finger extension and ball squeeze.**

- The final stage involves performing the exercises with the elbow extended and the forearm unsupported. Depending upon symptoms, the resistance should be decreased and reprogressed. It is important to continue the strengthening program as return to work or sport occurs; otherwise the patient risks reinjury or the return of symptoms.[1]
- The ECRB is stretched by wrist flexion with the forearm pronated and the elbow extended. This maneuver may be best performed in a hot shower.
- Nonoperative management may require 2 to 3 months to decrease symptoms. Work-related tendinopathies often are more resistant to nonoperative management, probably because athletes can often reduce participation in the aggravating activity, whereas those with work-related tendinosis often do not have that option.[4]
- The efficacy of extracorporeal shock wave therapy for treatment of lateral tennis elbow is controversial.[13–16]

## Operative Management

- Following at least 3 months of appropriate nonoperative management with no improvement (not necessarily complete symptom resolution),[12] the patient has the choice of either accepting the pain and disability, lowering his/her activity level to the point where the pain is tolerable, or seeking a surgical solution.
- The key to successful tendinopathy surgery is identifying and excising the pathologic tendinosis while minimizing iatrogenic injury to normal tissue. This option is preferable to tendon releases or slides, which fail to remove the pathology and weaken the force generators, leading to less predictable results with a greater incidence of persistent pain and weakness.[3]

### Lateral Tennis Elbow

- The Nirschl technique of lateral tennis elbow excision has reported consistently good results: 85% of patients reported complete pain relief, full strength, and full return to all prior activities without pain. Twelve percent reported significant but not complete pain relief and

return of strength. Only 3% failed to improve. No patient had increased symptoms postoperatively. Complications have been minimal: 1% superficial infection and 1% mild (<5 degrees) loss of extension.[3,5]

### Modified Nirschl Technique[17]

- *Pearl:* The key to this surgery is realizing that the ECRB is hidden under the ECRL, which merges with the EDC at a thickening called the *extensor aponeurosis.* The ECRL must be mobilized and retracted to expose the ECRB.
1. A longitudinal incision is made just anterior to the tip of the lateral epicondyle, centered over it proximodistally (Figure 35–4). The tendinous layer is exposed (Figure 35–5).
2. The ECRL muscle is red. It merges posteriorly with the EDC at a palpably firm white structure called the *extensor aponeurosis.* This aponeurosis is incised 3 mm posterior to the ECRL, paralleling it, to leave a tendinous cuff for firm repair (Figure 35–6).
3. This layer is incised to a depth of only 2 to 3 mm.
   - *Pitfall:* Incising too deeply distorts the origin of the ECRB, which lies beneath the ECRL.
4. The ECRL (red) is sharply dissected off the underlying ECRB tendon origin (white-gray). The ECRL is dissected medially until the entire triangular origin of the ECRB is exposed (Figure 35–7).
5. The entire ECRB proximal origin is excised down to bone. Often it is easiest to cut down to bone proximally on two sides of the triangle and then lift the origin off the bone from proximally to distally to the level of the radiocapitellar joint (Figure 35–8). Only rarely is tendinosis found distal to the radiocapitellar joint. The ECRB origin is excised to this level. The lateral joint capsule is just deep to the ECRB and is optimally spared. However, it often is inadvertently incised, which leads to no negative consequences, even if it is not repaired. The

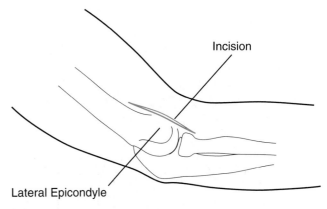

Figure 35–4:
**Lateral tennis elbow excision: incision.**

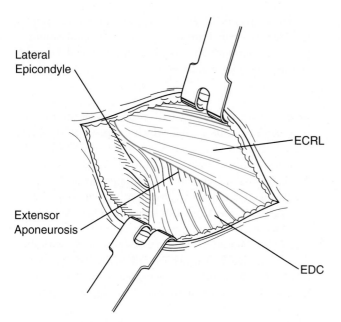

Figure 35–5:
Lateral tennis elbow excision: fascial exposure. *ECRL,*
Extensor carpi radialis longus; *EDC,* extensor digitorum communis.

elbow joint can be inspected if intraarticular pathology is suspected, but this is not routinely performed.

6. Tendinosis tissue appears grayer than the normal white tendon and more edematous. The more steroid injections a patient has had, the more pronounced the tendinosis. In mild to moderate cases the superficial tendon may be relatively normal, with most of the pathology in the

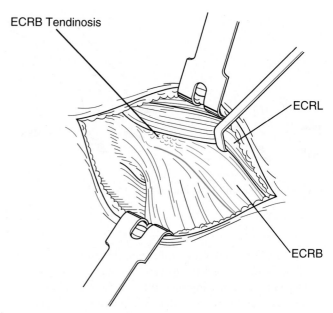

Figure 35–7:
Lateral tennis elbow excision: exposure of extensor carpi radialis brevis *(ECRB)* tendinosis. *ECRL,* Extensor carpi radialis longus.

deep tendon. The *Nirschl scratch test* is used to remove all tendinosis while leaving normal tendon behind. Using a fresh blade in a scraping fashion (as opposed to a cutting or stabbing fashion) will not injure normal tendon. Tendinosis is more friable and will be scraped off. In 30% of cases the anterior EDC also is involved (Figure 35–9).

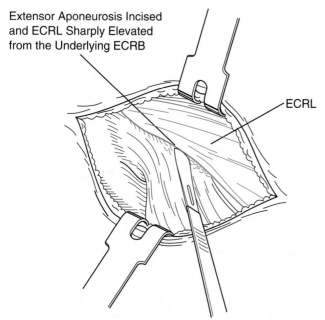

Figure 35–6:
Lateral tennis elbow excision: fascial incision. *ECRL,* Extensor carpi radialis longus.

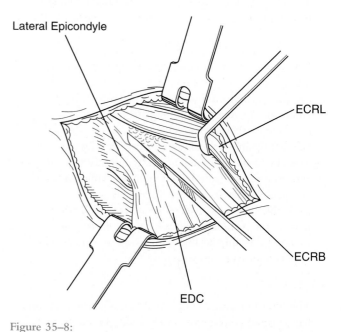

Figure 35–8:
Lateral tennis elbow excision: extensor carpi radialis brevis (ECRB) origin excision. *ECRL,* Extensor carpi radialis longus; *EDC,* extensor digitorum communis.

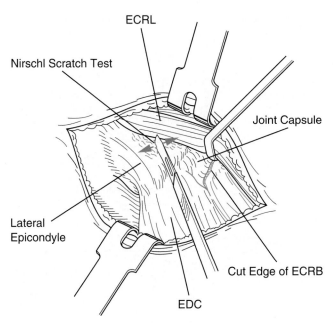

**Figure 35–9:**
Lateral tennis elbow excision: Nirschl scratch test. *ECRL,* Extensor carpi radialis longus; *EDC,* extensor digitorum communis.

7. *Pearl:* No bone is removed, drilled, or altered. Tender excrescences present on the tip of the lateral epicondyle may be removed, but any bony work significantly increases postoperative pain and morbidity and delays return to full activity.

8. The ECRL muscle and tendinous cuff are repaired back to the EDC with a running no. 1 Vicryl stitch (Figure 35–10). The knot is anchored in the middle

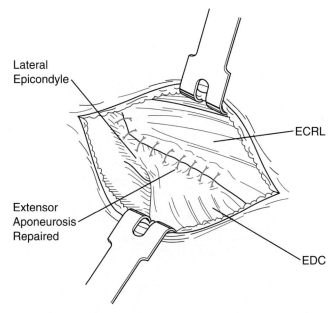

**Figure 35–10:**
Lateral tennis elbow excision: fascial closure. *ECRL,* Extensor carpi radialis longus; *EDC,* extensor digitorum communis.

(proximodistally), where the tendon is strongest. It is run proximally and then distally, where it is tied buried deep to the fascia. The fascia becomes weaker proximally and may not provide as secure a closure if tied there. A firm closure of this layer is important to prevent synovial cyst formation secondary to fluid leakage from the elbow. The skin is closed in subcuticular fashion.

- *Postoperative:* Early motion is started within a few days. Strengthening is started as tolerated by the patient, usually within 3 to 4 weeks. Soreness may persist for 3 to 6 months, but relief from the most severe pain often is fairly rapid.[1,17,18]

  - *Pearl:* Because of the extensive origin of the ECRB from the annular ligament, the undersurface of the extensor aponeurosis, the undersurface of the ECRL, and the lateral epicondyle, the ECRB tendon does not retract even when the majority of its origin is excised. Therefore, it is not necessary to reattach the tendon to bone. Doing so only risks creating a flexion contracture.[17]

## Revision Surgery

- The three most common reasons for failure of lateral tennis elbow surgery are (1) failure to identify and completely remove all tendinosis (most common), (2) iatrogenic trauma to the lateral collateral ligament or other structures, and (3) misdiagnosis.

- Tendinosis excision works well following failed lateral tennis elbow surgery, leading to 83% good or excellent results at average 64-month follow-up, and is my preferred revision procedure.[19]

- Postoperative synovial cysts are caused by an iatrogenic defect in the extensor layer. Failing nonoperative management, an anconeus flap can be used to cover this defect or to provide more padding over the lateral epicondyle in cases of severe fat atrophy from multiple steroid injections.[20] Normal tendon should not be transected or debrided in order to rotate this flap.

## Medial Tennis Elbow

- The results of surgery for medial tennis elbow excision are less predictable than those for lateral tennis elbow. In a study of 50 cases, all patients reported partial or complete pain relief, with increased strength. However, 26% were not able to return to their same level of sporting activity. No major complications occurred.[3,8]

### Modified Nirschl Technique[1,8]

1. A curvilinear incision is made over the cubital tunnel. Dissection is carried down to the ulnar nerve, taking care to dissect out and preserve branches of the medial antebrachial cutaneous nerve (Figure 35–11).

2. An in situ release of the ulnar nerve is performed from the level of the epicondyle distally to prevent postoperative swelling from inducing an iatrogenic

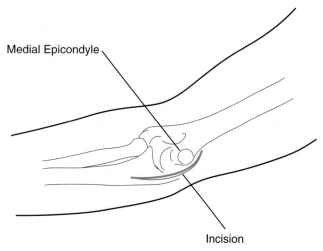

**Figure 35–11:**
**Medial tennis elbow excision: incision.**

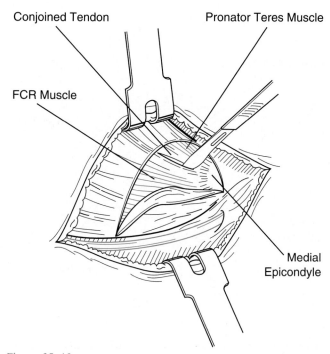

**Figure 35–13:**
**Medial tennis elbow excision: excision of conjoined tendon.**
*FCR,* Flexor carpi radialis.

neuropathy. To prevent subluxation, the nerve is not released proximal to the epicondyle. If symptomatic cubital tunnel syndrome is present, the nerve may be transposed subcutaneously.

3. The conjoined tendon of the PT and FCR can be exposed by raising a medially based semicircular fascial flap, as for a subcutaneous transposition (Figure 35–12). This procedure exposes the white conjoined tendon, which is excised (Figures 35–13 and 35–14). Care is taken to avoid disrupting the MCL, which is deep to this tendon. The ligament is part of the joint capsule and appears smooth compared to the rougher tendon fibers. The Nirschl scratch test is used to excise all tendinosis while

leaving normal tendon, as for lateral tennis elbow (Figure 35–15).
• *Pearl:* Please note that the bone is not altered. No epicondylectomy, drilling, or abrasion is performed.

4. The fascial sling is repaired and the skin routinely closed (Figure 35–16).
• *Postoperative:* As for lateral tennis elbow.

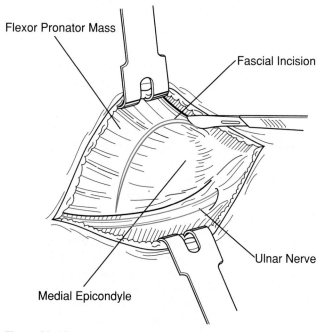

**Figure 35–12:**
**Medial tennis elbow excision: fascial incision.**

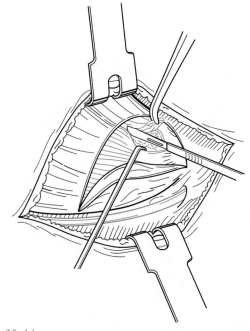

**Figure 35–14:**
**Medial tennis elbow excision: excision of conjoined tendon.**

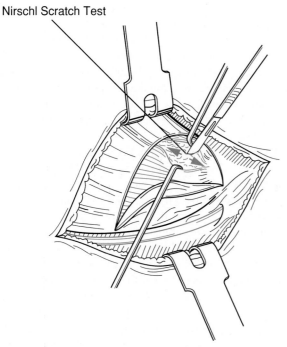

Nirschl Scratch Test

Figure 35–15:
**Medial tennis elbow excision: Nirschl scratch test.**

## Posterior Tennis Elbow

- This procedure is essentially the same as that used to treat Achilles tendinosis or patellar tendinosis.
  1. The triceps tendon is exposed through a posterior incision (Figure 35–17). The tendon is incised in the line of its fibers (Figure 35–18).

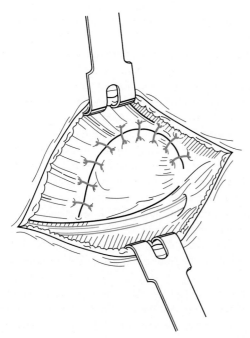

Figure 35–16:
**Medial tennis elbow excision: fascial repair.**

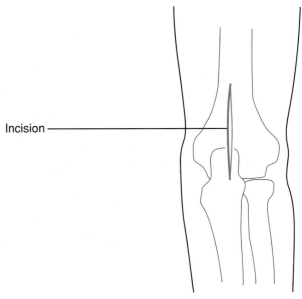

Incision

Figure 35–17:
**Posterior tennis elbow excision: incision.**

  2. The Nirschl scratch test is used to remove pathologic tendinosis, while leaving normal tendon behind (Figure 35–19). Consideration should be given to not excising more than 50% of the triceps insertion, although the amount removed is usually significantly less.
  3. The remaining tendon is closed side to side (Figure 35–20). The skin is routinely closed.
- *Postoperative:* As for lateral tennis elbow.

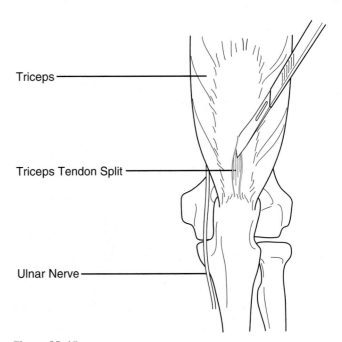

Triceps

Triceps Tendon Split

Ulnar Nerve

Figure 35–18:
**Posterior tennis elbow excision: tendon incision.**

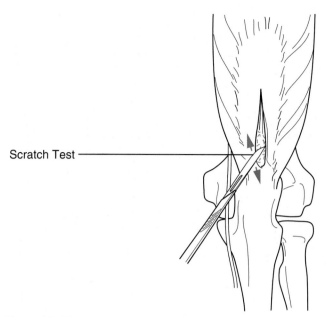

**Figure 35–19:**
**Posterior tennis elbow excision: Nirschl scratch test.**

# Distal Biceps Rupture

## History and Physical Examination

- Tendon degeneration in the hypovascular zone close to its radial tuberosity insertion predisposes to distal biceps rupture. Smoking leads to a 7.5 times greater risk of rupture, probably by further decreasing tendon oxygenation in this hypovascular zone.[21] Use of anabolic steroids is a risk factor. Mechanical irritation has been

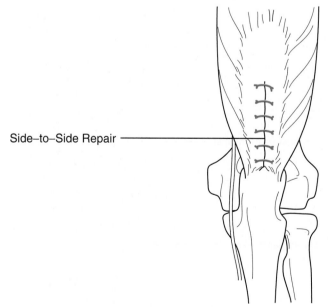

**Figure 35–20:**
**Posterior tennis elbow excision: tendon repair.**

theorized to play a role because of a 50% decrease in the interosseous space during pronation.[22]

- Rupture occurs most commonly in the dominant arm of men 40 to 60 years old who engage in manual labor, athletics, or weight lifting. Rupture usually is associated with a painful pop following an episode of eccentric tensile overload, when the arm is forced from a flexed position, as occurs when lifting or moving heavy objects.
- Physical examination often reveals antecubital tenderness, swelling, and ecchymosis. The biceps muscle is retracted proximally, and the normal proximal-distal tracking of the biceps muscle belly with passive forearm rotation is lost. Flexion power is mildly reduced, supination power is markedly reduced, and resisted flexion and supination is painful.
  - *Pitfall:* Do not mistake the intact lacertus fibrosus (bicipital aponeurosis) for the ruptured biceps tendon. Compare the affected elbow to the contralateral side, and note that the bicipital aponeurosis does not move significantly with forearm rotation.
- MRI is not routinely necessary to diagnose a complete tear but can be helpful in unclear cases or in the workup of a partial tear.

## Treatment

- Nonoperative management leads to a 30% loss of flexion strength and a 40% decrease in supination strength and endurance.[23,24]
- Surgical reattachment to the radial tuberosity is indicated for active individuals with complete ruptures. This procedure is best done within the first 2 to 3 weeks, before scarring and retraction make dissection difficult and obliterate the tunnel the tendon follows to the tuberosity.[22]
- Either a single-incision technique using two to three suture anchors or a two-incision technique using a bone trough may be used. Both techniques lead to excellent results in acute injuries, with good return of supination and flexion power and endurance in most cases and predictably excellent functional results and patient satisfaction.[23,24] However, in one comparison, the two-incision technique showed fewer complications and more rapid recovery of flexion strength.[25] Repair of the nondominant arm does not lead to as good results as repair of the dominant arm, with less than full recovery of strength and endurance.[26]
- For chronic tears, the biceps tendon may not easily reach the tuberosity because of retraction and scarring. An autograft or allograft may be necessary to prolong the tendon. It may first be attached to the radial tuberosity as for an acute tear, and then secured to the remaining distal biceps tendon at the appropriate length and tension using a Pulvertaft weave. Results of chronic tear repair are not as good as those following acute repair. Although strength

is improved, it does not return to the preinjury level, and the biceps muscle contour frequently is only partially corrected.[22,26]

- Partial-thickness tears often present with atraumatic onset of pain at the insertion of the distal biceps tendon. These tears initially may be treated nonoperatively with splinting and decreased activity level. Failing this, operative intervention involves completion of the tear, debridement of the symptomatic tendinosis, and reinsertion.

## Two-Incision Technique

1. A transverse incision is made in the antecubital crease (Figure 35–21). Dissection is carried down to the distal biceps tendon, which is milked into the wound. Care is taken to avoid injuring the lateral antebrachial cutaneous nerve. Degenerative tendinosis is debrided off the tendon end sharply and/or using the Nirschl scratch test. The tendon end is rounded off. Two no. 2 fiber-wire stitches of different colors are woven into the tendon in either Bunnell or running locked fashion (Figure 35–22).

   - *Pearl:* The biceps tendon sheath may still be intact, giving the false impression of continuity to the radial tuberosity. This sheath is opened to identify the free tendon end.

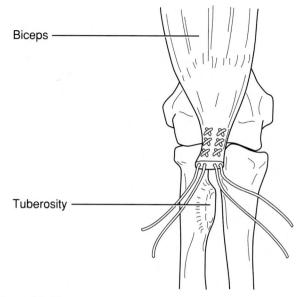

Figure 35–22:
**Distal biceps repair: suture placement.**

2. With the forearm supinated (to avoid the PIN), a tonsil forceps is placed through the biceps tendon tunnel, hugging the radial tuberosity (staying away from the ulna), and is punched through the interosseous space to tent the skin posteriorly (Figure 35–23). The interosseus tunnel is bluntly enlarged to allow easy passage of the biceps tendon.

3. A longitudinal posterior incision is centered over the tonsil's tip (see Figure 35–23). The common extensor and supinator muscles are split, staying away from the ulna, until the radial tuberosity is visualized. Pronation improves visualization of the tuberosity and protects the PIN. The entire tuberosity is cleaned of residual soft tissue with a

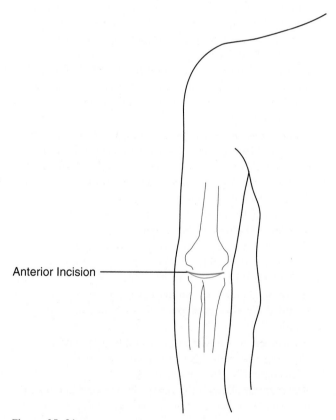

Figure 35–21:
**Distal biceps repair: incision.**

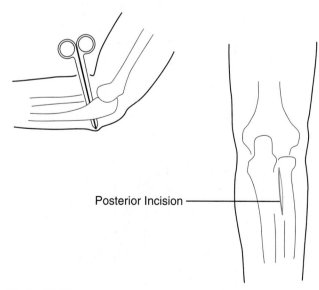

Figure 35–23:
**Distal biceps repair: posterior incision.**

rongeur, curette, and/or elevator, and its limits are defined. A 5-mm burr is used to make a trough as medial as possible (toward the free end of the tuberosity) while leaving the cortical wall intact. The trough is approximately 6 mm wide and 12 mm long (Figure 35–24).

4. A 3-mm drill is used to make a hole from the radial shaft into the trough, one proximal and one distal, with a large bone bridge between. All bone dust is thoroughly irrigated out of the wound.

5. The biceps tendon's lead sutures are passed through the interosseous space into the posterior wound. One free end of each stitch is passed through each of the two drill holes using a Hewson suture passer.

6. The forearm is rotated to neutral and the sutures are tensioned to pull the tendon into the bone trough. A freer elevator is used to help "shoe-horn" it into position. Each suture is firmly tied (Figure 35–25).

7. To determine postoperative restrictions, supinate the forearm and note the amount of elbow extension that occurs before the tendon repair becomes tensioned. Routine closure is performed.

- *Postoperative:* The elbow is splinted at 90 degrees flexion and full supination for 1 week before noncomposite elbow motion is begun. After 1 week, supervised elbow extension is allowed with the forearm supinated to the degree determined intraoperatively. No active flexion is allowed. Full forearm rotation is allowed with the elbow flexed 90 degrees. Full active and gentle passive motion is

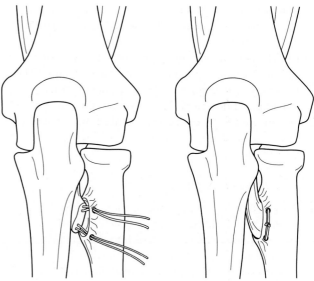

Figure 35–25:
**Distal biceps repair: tendon reduction and fixation.**

allowed after 4 weeks. Progressive strengthening is allowed at 3 months, heavy lifting at 4 months, and contact sports at 6 months.

# Triceps Tendon Ruptures

- Rupture of the triceps tendon is the rarest of all tendon ruptures. Predisposing factors include renal insufficiency with secondary hyperparathyroidism, use of systemic steroids, and steroid injections. Triceps rupture occurs by a similar mechanism to olecranon fractures: either a sudden forceful flexion of the extended elbow, as occurs during a fall on the outstretched hand, or a direct blow to the olecranon area.[22]

- The most common site of rupture is the tendo-osseous junction. Avulsion often occurs with a small fleck of bone, which may be visible on radiography. Examination usually reveals swelling and a palpable gap in the tendon proximal to the olecranon.

- A modified Thompson test for the triceps has been described: The upper arm is supported, allowing the elbow to flex 90 degrees with the elbow relaxed, such as a prone position with the forearm hanging over the end of the table. The triceps muscle belly is squeezed. If elbow extension is produced, the triceps is not completely ruptured. Absence of elbow extension suggests a complete rupture.[22]

- A complete tear results in the inability to extend the elbow against even slight resistance. Operative reattachment is recommended.

- A partial tear allows some active elbow extension. It can be treated nonoperatively in a splint at 30 degrees flexion for 4 weeks. However, some active elbow extension may be present even in cases of near-complete

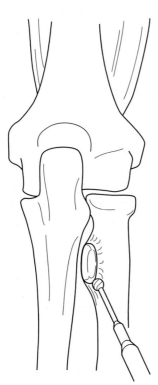

Figure 35–24:
**Distal biceps repair: trough preparation.**

tears from the lateral triceps expansion onto the forearm fascia. In this case, elbow extension can be maintained with the elbow straight but not attained from greater than 90 degrees flexion. Whether nonoperative treatment of both large and small partial tears will produce a good functional outcome is unknown. Therefore, if a large tear of greater than 50% of the triceps is noted on MRI and is associated with a significant loss of triceps power, operative repair should be considered, especially in athletic individuals.[22]

- MRI can assist in differentiating partial from complete ruptures.
- As for distal biceps ruptures, surgical repair is easiest performed within the first 2 to 3 weeks. Results of surgical repair generally are excellent, with no pain, normal strength, and full motion.[22]

## Technique of Triceps Repair

1. Make a longitudinal posterior incision, just medial to the olecranon (Figure 35–26). The triceps tendon is retrieved and its end debrided of tendinosis (Figure 35–27). Two no. 2 or no. 5 fiber wire sutures of different colors are placed in Bunnell or running locked fashion (Figure 35–28).

2. Identify and protect the ulnar nerve. Clean soft tissue off the superficial olecranon. Use a 5- to 6-mm burr to make a unicortical hole in the superficial/posterior portion of the proximal olecranon, where the triceps naturally inserts. Do not violate the posterior cortex. When this trough has been partially drilled, place a freer inside of it and move the elbow to ensure the hole is extraarticular. Place two distal 3-mm drill holes through posterior

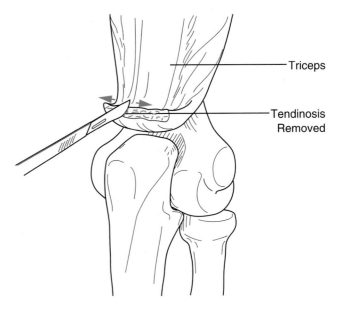

Figure 35–27:
**Distal triceps repair: excision of tendinosis.**

cortex into the trough, with a large bone bridge between (see Figure 35–28).

3. Bring one of each suture's free end through each drill hole with a Hewson tendon passer. Extend the elbow and firmly tie these stitches (Figure 35–29). A tendon turndown flap can be used as needed to reinforce the repair or to prolong a retracted tendon.[17]

- *Postoperative:* The elbow is immobilized at 30 degrees flexion for 4 weeks, followed by progressive motion. Full use is restricted for 4 months.

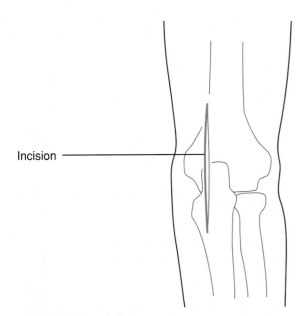

Figure 35–26:
**Distal triceps repair: incision.**

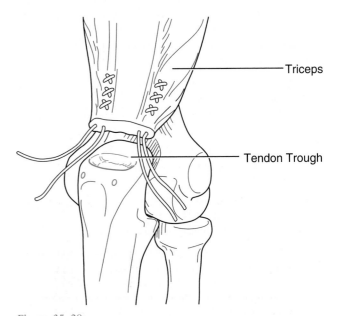

Figure 35–28:
**Distal triceps repair: suture placement, trough preparation and drill holes.**

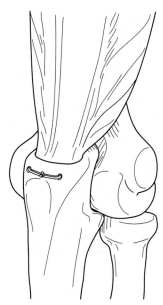

Figure 35–29:
**Distal triceps repair: tendon-bone fixation.**

# References

1. Budoff JE, Nirschl RP: Tendinopathies about the elbow. In Garrett WE, Speer KP, Kirkendall, editors: *Principles and practice of orthopaedic sports medicine.* Philadelphia, 2000, Lippincott Williams & Wilkins.
   In-depth review of lateral and medial tennis elbow.

2. Coonrad RW. Tennis elbow. *Instr Course Lect* 35:94, 1986.
   Presents the epidemiology of tennis elbow.

3. Nirschl RP: Sports and overuse injuries to the elbow. In Morrey BF, editor: *The elbow and its disorders,* ed 2. Philadelphia, 1993, WB Saunders.
   Classic work on the pathology and treatment of lateral and medial tennis elbow.

4. Gellman H: Tennis elbow (lateral epicondylitis). *Orthop Clin North Am* 23:75-82, 1992.
   Includes a discussion of tennis elbow as an industrial injury.

5. Nirschl RP: Elbow tendinosis/tennis elbow. Tendinitis II: clinical considerations. *Clin Sports Med* 11:851-870, 1992.
   Covers the pathology, diagnosis, phases, and treatment of lateral and medial tennis elbow.

6. Nirschl RP: The etiology and treatment of tennis elbow. *Am J Sports Med* 2:308-319, 1974.
   Early paper on the pathology of tennis elbow.

7. Kraushaar BS, Nirschl RP: Tendinosis of the elbow. Clinical features and findings of histological, immunohistochemical and electron microscopy studies. *J Bone Joint Surg* 81A:259-278, 1999.
   Excellent paper on the pathology of tennis elbow, complete with photographs.

8. Olliviere CO, Nirschl RP, Pettrone FA: Resection and repair for medial tennis elbow. *Am J Sports Med* 23:214-221, 1995.
   Fifty of 50 patients noted improvement following resection of tendinosis for medial tennis elbow at 37 months.

9. Lister G: *The hand,* ed 3. New York, 1993, Churchill Livingstone.
   Described the "finger extension test" as suggesting radial tunnel syndrome; however, this test may also cause pain in patients with lateral tennis elbow.

10. Pomerance J: Radiographic analysis of lateral epicondylitis. *J Shoulder Elbow Surg* 11:156-157, 2002.
    Documents the prevalence of lateral calcifications associated with tennis elbow.

11. Bowen RE, Dorey FJ, Shapiro MS: Efficacy of nonoperative treatment for lateral epicondylitis. *Am J Orthop* 30:642-646, 2001.
    Reported nonoperative management to be successful in 75% of cases of lateral tennis elbow.

12. Wolf BR, Altchek DW: Elbow problems in elite tennis players. *Tech Shoulder Elbow Surg* 4:55-68, 2003.
    Notes that steroid injections may not be efficacious and may potentially be harmful.

13. Speed CA, Richards C, Nichols D, et al: Extracorporeal shock-wave therapy for tendonitis of the rotator cuff. A double-blind, randomized, controlled trial. *J Bone Joint Surg Br* 84:509-512, 2002.
    Reported that extracorporeal shock wave therapy did not lead to improved results over sham treatment. There seemed to be a significant placebo effect in both groups.

14. Haake M, Konig IR, Decker T, Riedel C, Buch M, Muller HH: Extracorporeal shock wave therapy in the treatment of lateral epicondylitis: a randomized multicenter trial. *J Bone Joint Surg Am* 84A:1982-1991, 2002.
    Found extracorporeal shock wave therapy was ineffective in treatment of lateral tennis elbow.

15. Wang CJ, Chen HS: Shock wave therapy for patients with lateral epicondylitis of the elbow: a one- to two-year follow-up study. *Am J Sports Med* 30:422-425, 2002.
    Reported 91% success at 1- to 2-year follow-up of extracorporeal shock wave therapy.

16. Ko JY, Chen HS, Chen LM: Treatment of lateral epicondylitis of the elbow with shock waves. *Clin Orthop* 387:60-67, 2001.
    Reported 73% good or excellent results at 6 months following extracorporeal shock wave therapy.

17. Budoff JE, Nirschl RP: Resection and repair of lateral tennis elbow. *Oper Tech Sports Med* 9:211-216, 2001.
    Detailed the technique of resection and repair (excision) of lateral tennis elbow.

18. Khashaba A: Nirschl tennis elbow release with or without drilling. *Br J Sports Med* 35:200-201, 2001.
    Showed superior results for tennis elbow excision if bony work was not performed.

19. Organ SW, Nirschl RP, Kraushaar BS, Guidi EJ: Salvage surgery for lateral tennis elbow. *Am J Sports Med* 25:746-750, 1997.

Reports 83% success for resection of lateral tennis elbow on patients who did not respond to prior surgical intervention.

20. Almquist EE, Necking L, Bach AW: Epicondylar resection with anconeus muscle transfer for chronic lateral epicondylitis. *J Hand Surg [Am]* 23:723-731, 1998.
    Reported 94% patient satisfaction at a mean of 48 months following anconeus muscle transfer for lateral tennis elbow.

21. Safran MR, Graham SM: Distal biceps tendon ruptures: incidence, demographics, and the effect of smoking. *Clin Orthop Relat Res* 404:275-283, 2002.
    Reports that smoking is associated with a 7.5x greater risk of distal biceps tendon rupture.

22. Strauch RJ: Biceps and triceps injuries of the elbow. *Orthop Clin North Am* 30:95-107, 1999.
    The common biceps and triceps injuries about the elbow are reviewed. The relevant anatomy, presenting signs, symptoms, and treatment of these injuries are discussed.

23. Baker BE, Bierwagen D: Rupture of the distal tendon of the biceps brachii. Operative versus non-operative treatment. *J Bone Joint Surg Am* 67:414-417, 1985.
    Ten patients showed a return to normal elbow flexion and supination strength and endurance following surgical repair of a distal biceps rupture.

24. Morrey BF, Askew LJ, An KN, Dobyns JH: Rupture of the distal tendon of the biceps brachii. A biomechanical study. *J Bone Joint Surg Am* 67:418-421, 1985.
    Nonoperative management of distal biceps ruptures led to a mean loss of 40% of supination strength and a mean loss of 30% of elbow flexion strength.

25. El-Hawary R, Macdermid JC, Faber KJ, Patterson SD, King GJ: Distal biceps tendon repair: comparison of surgical techniques. *J Hand Surg [Am]* 28:496-502, 2003.
    This comparison of outcomes for distal biceps repair through either one or two incisions showed minor differences between these techniques, with the two-incision technique showing a slightly more rapid recovery of flexion strength and fewer complications.

26. Morrison KD, Hunt TR 3rd: Comparing and contrasting methods for tenodesis of the ruptured distal biceps tendon. *Hand Clin* 18:169-178, 2002.
    Notes that repair of the biceps tendon in the nondominant arm does not lead to results as good as repair in the dominant arm, with less than full recovery of strength and endurance.

# 36

# Elbow Instability and Arthroscopy

David S. Ruch* and Anastasios Papadonikolakis†

*MD, Professor, Department of Orthopaedic Surgery, Wake Forest University School of Medicine, Winston-Salem, NC
†MD, Resident, Department of Orthopaedic Surgery, Wake Forest University School of Medicine, Winston-Salem, NC

## Introduction

- Elbow instability following ligamentous and bony trauma remains complex.
- Outcome studies demonstrate that injuries resulting in significant ligamentous disruption have worse results than fractures in isolation.[1,2]
- Key determinants of stability are the coronoid process, medial collateral ligament (MCL) complex, and the lateral/posterolateral ligament complex.

## Anatomy

### Medial Collateral Ligament Complex

- The MCL originates posterior to the axis of rotation and inserts onto the medial aspect of the coronoid process (Figure 36-1).[3]
- The MCL complex is composed of the anterior bundle, posterior bundle, and transverse ligament. Some authors refer to the MCL as the *ulnar collateral ligament complex* (Box 36-1).

### Lateral Collateral Ligament

- Originates at the lateral humeral epicondyle and inserts into the supinator crest of the ulna (Figure 36-2).
- This broad, flat ligament remains taut throughout the range of elbow flexion and extension, with little change throughout the range of motion in the distance between its origin and insertion points.[6]

- It can be divided into lateral, medial, and anterior bundles.[7] The relative contribution of each bundle to stabilizing the elbow remains controversial; however, it is accepted that disruption of the posterior lateral ligamentous complex results in loss of the "sling" effect on the radial head, which suspends the radial head to the capitellum, maintaining articular congruity.
- Without this effect, the radial head rotates away from the capitellum, resulting in subluxation or dislocation of the radiocapitellar joint, and subsequently the ulnohumeral articulation.[7]

## Secondary Stabilizers

### Bony Structures

- The articulation between the capitellum and radial head is an important secondary stabilizer to valgus stress. Cadaveric studies indicate that following division of the anterior bundle of the MCL, the radial head is the primary stabilizer preventing valgus instability.[8]
- The coronoid process also is key and acts as a direct buttress and an insertion point for critical ligaments.[9] Cadaveric studies indicate that if more than 50% of the coronoid height is lost, a statistically significant increase in posterior translation in the elbow may occur in response to axial load.[9]

### Muscular Structures

- Cadaveric studies indicate that the common extensor origin with the interdigitating fascial bands and

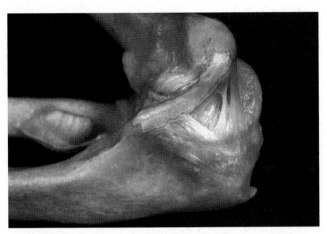

Figure 36–1:
Anatomic specimen of the medial side of the elbow showing the components of the medial collateral ligament. The anterior bundle is outlined to demonstrate its origin on the undersurface of the epicondyle and its insertion at the base of the coronoid.

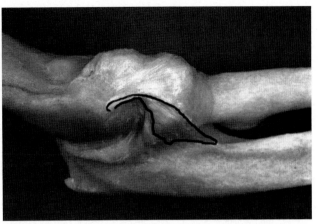

Figure 36–2:
Anatomic specimen demonstrating the origin and the insertion of the medial bundle of the lateral collateral ligament.

intramuscular septate stabilize the lateral aspect of the elbow.[10]

- On the medial aspect of the elbow, the flexor carpi ulnaris muscle, positioned directly over the MCL, works with the common digital flexors to provide medial support in the case of ligamentous laxity.[11] Despite anatomic positioning, electromyographic studies do not demonstrate increased electrical activity in flexor carpi ulnaris and common digital flexors when assessing a group of baseball pitchers with MCL insufficiency. This finding suggests that the muscles on the medial side of the elbow do not augment the role of the MCL during a baseball pitch.[12]

- The brachialis, brachioradialis, and triceps brachii function as direct buttresses to prevent anteroposterior subluxation and may also dynamically stabilize the elbow. The brachialis muscle with its broad insertion across the coronoid provides a direct buttress to posterior

subluxation. In addition, the compressive loads by biceps and triceps during forced coupling may compress the articular surface, thus maximizing joint surface contact and subsequently diminishing instability (Box 36–2).

## Acute Injury

### Presentation and Diagnosis

- Acute instability is commonly seen following dislocation of the elbow.
- Avulsion of the flexor pronator origin from the medial side of the elbow is frequently seen.
- The diagnosis of valgus instability may be readily apparent. Examination reveals hemorrhage along the medial epicondyle and gross instability to valgus stress (Boxes 36–3 and 36–4).

## Chronic Instability

- Chronic instability commonly results from repetitive microtrauma caused by chronic overload during overhead throwing (Box 36–5).

### Imaging

- Plain radiographs should be made with the elbow in flexion and under significant valgus stress.[17] These dynamic radiographs may reveal widening of the joint space in up to 80% of patients, but many patients do not "open up" until they are under anesthesia.

---

### Box 36–1 | Anatomy of the MCL Complex

1. The anterior bundle is divided into anterior and posterior segments. The anterior segment provides the majority of stability.[4]
2. The anterior bundle has an isometric point where some fibers are taut in extension and others are taut in elbow flexion.[3]
3. The transverse ligament originates at the central two thirds of the anteroinferior undersurface of the medial epicondyle.[5] It does not have a defined function; however, it deepens the greater sigmoid notch.
4. The posterior bundle has fibers that become taut during both maximum elbow extension and maximum elbow flexion.[4] It lies posterior to the axis of rotation. Because of the cam effect of the MCL, the posterior bundle may require partial release to achieve full elbow flexion in patients with long-standing stiffness.

---

### Box 36–2 | Patterns of Valgus Instability

- Valgus instability may be seen either acutely following trauma or chronically following attenuation of repetitive injury. The primary stabilizer to valgus load is the anterior bundle of the MCL. Cadaveric studies indicate that 100% of the anterior bundle of the MCL must be sectioned before demonstrating significant valgus or intrarotatory elbow instability.[13,14]

| **Box 36–3** | **Treatment of Acute Injuries** |
|---|---|

- A reduction should be performed and an assessment of range of motion initiated.
  - With loss of stability in elbow extension, the elbow should be placed in pronation and flexed to 90 degrees.
  - Range of motion should be initiated with an extension block at the point at which the elbow becomes unstable.
  - The elbow should be extended approximately 30% per week such that the elbow is in full extension by the end of 3 weeks.
  - Surgical exploration is indicated if the patient is unable to maintain reduction in pronation at 45 to 60 degrees flexion.
  - Possible causes:
    1. Entrapment of the medial epicondyle
    2. Loose body
    3. Unrecognized coronoidal/radial head/capitellum trauma

- Computerized tomography with arthrography and magnetic resonance imaging (MRI) with or without arthrography are of higher sensitivity than ultrasound, and are best at demonstrating abnormalities of the MCL.[18]
- A computerized tomography arthrogram allows best visualization of partial undersurface tears of the MCL.[19]
- Arthroscopy can confirm the diagnosis, but visualization of the MCL is incomplete and the diagnosis more likely is made by excessive laxity when the arthroscope is passed through the ulnohumeral articulation. Arthroscopy is more useful for assessing secondary changes. Cadaveric studies indicate that 100% of the anterior bundle of the MCL must be cut before 1 to 2 mm of joint space opening is present and visible arthroscopically (Figure 36–3 and Box 36–6).[14]

| **Box 36–4** | **Acute Instability Operative Treatment** |
|---|---|

- Acute instability can be treated with direct repair of the avulsed MCL using drill holes or suture anchors. MCL almost always fails at its humeral origin. Suture anchors usually are not strong enough for repair. In such cases, drill holes through the medial epicondyle should be used.
- Care should be taken to reattach the ligament to the undersurface of the medial epicondyle at the anatomic origin.
- Following repair, tension in the anterior bundle of the ligament should be demonstrated in both flexion and extension. *Only the middle bundle of the anterior portion of the ligament demonstrates isometry.*
- If the elbow subluxes or dislocates as the elbow is brought down into extension, the forearm should be placed in pronation at 90 degrees elbow flexion.
- If stability is restored, then a hinge brace or cast brace can be applied.
- The elbow should be brought down out of flexion over a 3-week period such that, at the end of 3 weeks, full arc of motion is permitted.

| **Box 36–5** | **Critical Points in the Evaluation of MCL Insufficiency** |
|---|---|

- Patients complain of increasing pain after repetitive throwing, particularly during the early and middle phases of the throwing motion. Approximately 25% present with ulnar sensory symptoms.
- Typically patients demonstrate pain and tenderness posteroinferior to the medial epicondyle at the ulnar attachment of the ligament.
- Insufficiency is most evident with the elbow flexed from 70 to 90 degrees.[15]
- During the cocking phase of throwing, the elbow is subjected to tremendous valgus stress. As the laxity progresses, increased loading of the capitellum leads to cartilage wear. Abutment of the olecranon against the posterior medial aspect of the humerus also occurs, resulting in osteophyte formation.[16] Intraarticular trauma and increased capitellar loading can occur, leading to cartilage wear and loose body formation. Traction on the ulnar nerve may result as instability increases, leading to neuritis in 30% of cases.

## Treatment of Chronic Injuries

- Nonoperative treatment involves rest and physical therapy. Pain-free motion is necessary prior to gradual resumption of competition level play.
- Forty-two percent of athletes treated nonoperatively can return to their previous level of competition at an average of 24.5 weeks following diagnosis.

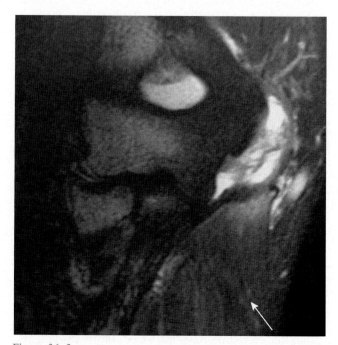

Figure 36–3:
Avulsion of the proximal portion of the medial collateral ligament with fluid extravasation medially.

- In a series of 72 baseball pitchers who underwent arthroscopic or open elbow surgery, postmedial olecranon osteophytes occurred in 65%, ulnar collateral ligament (MCL) injuries in 25%, and ulnar nerve neuritis in 15%. The authors noted that in the presence of posterior medial olecranon osteophytes, attenuation of the medial collateral ligament can be considered the cause of the osteophyte formation.[6]

| Box 36–7 | Modifications of Reconstruction Technique for Chronic Valgus Instability Repair |

- Cadaveric studies indicate single-strand repair results in stability equal to a two-stranded repair through drill holes in the humerus.[21]
- No significant acute difference in reconstruction strength using bone anchors or a bone tunnel has been observed.[22]
- The potential benefit of using bone anchors is reduced exposure of the olecranon, which allows for a muscle-splitting approach. Because the flexor pronator is not detached, routine transposition of the ulnar nerve is not necessary. Results following this procedure are uniformly excellent, with 90% of athletes returning to their previous level of competition. In one series of 36 patients, 92% exceeded their previous level of competition.[23]

- No particular findings demonstrate whether or not a patient will be successful with nonoperative management.
- If nonoperative management is unsuccessful, ligament reconstruction is indicated. Attempts at direct ligament repair are less reliable than reconstruction using tendon graft (Figure 36–4, Boxes 36–7 and 36–8).[20]

## Postoperative Management

- The elbow is splinted at 40 degrees flexion for 10 to 14 days. Active motion in a hinged elbow brace with a

20-degree extension stop is performed for 4 more weeks. The elbow brace can be unlocked at 6 weeks. Light activity should be resumed at 3 months. Full restoration of activity is expected at 1 year.

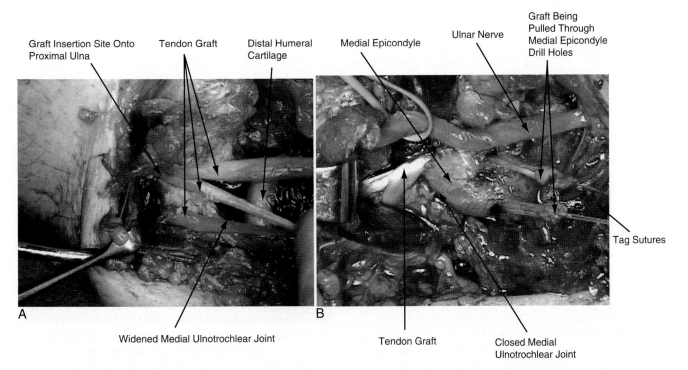

Figure 36–4:

A, Location of the drill holes in the sublime tubercle of the ulna. Distal is to the *left,* proximal is to the *right,* anterior is *up,* and posterior is *down.* Note widening of the medial ulnotrochlear joint because of valgus instability. The gloved digit is holding the tensioned graft over the medial epicondyle. The ulnar nerve is visualized just anterior to the graft. B, Location of graft placement through drill holes in the medial epicondyle. The graft can be sutured directly to itself at this level. Any extra length can be turned distally and sutured back over the middle of the graft to reinforce it. Note the medial ulnotrochlear joint now is held closed.

| Box 36–8 | Authors' Preferred Technique for MCL Reconstruction |
|---|---|

- The procedure is performed with the patient in supine position under tourniquet control. Prior to starting the procedure, I prefer to document insufficiency with fluoroscopic images performed with the elbow flexed to approximately 45 degrees compared to the contralateral side. After documentation of insufficiency, I make a longitudinal incision slightly posterior to the medial epicondyle in line with the ulnar nerve. The ulnar nerve is identified proximally and dissected from proximal to distal, with release of the arcade of Struthers, excision of the intermuscular septum and release of Osborne's fascia. Once the nerve has been decompressed, a muscle-splitting approach is used and the flexor pronator muscle mass is gently retracted. The origin of the MCL on the epicondyle is identified. The ligament is isolated. The insertion on the olecranon is identified through the muscle-splitting approach and retractors are placed. At this point, the anterior bundle of the MCL can be identified. There usually is an elliptical region of insufficient tissue in this area that may or may not be frankly disrupted but permits significant gapping of the humeral ulnar articulation with valgus stress. If there is a frank tear, it may be incorporated into the approach. If there is no tear, then a longitudinal incision is made in the MCL in line with its fibers through the most attenuated portion of the ligament. Again, tension is placed on the origin of the MCL at the inner two thirds of the epicondyle. A drill bit (3.2-mm in females, 4.5-mm in males) is used to create divergent drill holes in the medial epicondyle. A single hole is used to create one tunnel going cephalad and one tunnel going medial. The tunnels are connected again using the drill.
- Convergent drill holes are created in the ulna at the level of the tubercle on the medial aspect of the coronoid process. The sublime tubercle can be palpated; it usually is the hardest bone on the medial aspect of the coronoid. Care should be taken to avoid penetrating the articular surface.
- At this point, the palmaris graft is harvested from the ipsilateral upper extremity. If this is unavailable, either the contralateral palmaris or a toe extensor is used, harvested from a skin incision at the wrist crease and a separate incision at the muscular tendonous junction. The median nerve with its palmar cutaneous branch must be identified prior to harvesting the tendon to avoid iatrogenic injury to these structures.
- I prefer to harvest some of the muscle as well in order to obtain the maximum graft length possible. A suture passer is used to pass the tendon through the tunnels. Ideally, two strands of the palmaris are placed into the entry site at the medial epicondyle. These strands can be either tied in a half-hitch over the epicondyle if the graft is long enough or sutured to each other using nonabsorbable suture. Prior to suturing the graft, the elbow is placed at 45 degrees flexion. I usually apply a slight varus load and have not experienced problems with a tight graft.
- The elbow is brought to full range of motion, and care is taken to smooth any rough edges that might abrade the graft.
- The remaining limbs of the MCL can be used to reinforce the graft with a 3-0 Vicryl suture.
- The ulnar nerve is often transposed. I prefer to make a Z-plasty in the flexor pronator fascia and suture the limbs loosely over the transposed nerve.
- In patients with no evidence of preoperative ulnar nerve palsy, the nerve can be left in situ. A formal transposition is not performed.
- Postoperatively, the patient is placed in a long arm splint with the elbow flexed 90 degrees and the forearm in neutral rotation. At 10 days to 2 weeks, range of motion of the shoulder, wrist, and elbow in neutral forearm rotation is performed. Supination is started at 4 weeks, and strengthening is added at 6 weeks.

## Patterns of Instability

### Posterolateral Instability

- Chronic subluxation or dislocation of the radial head in a posterolateral direction has been associated with attenuation of the posterior lateral corner of the lateral collateral ligament. O'Driscoll[7] referred to the posterior region of the lateral collateral ligament complex as the *lateral ulnar collateral ligament* (LUCL). The significance of the LUCL is reflected in its role in securing the ulna to the humerus and preventing posterolateral rotatory instability. They documented the kinematics of elbow subluxation and dislocation in which the forearm rotates away from the humerus in valgus and external rotation during flexion from the extended position. Despite an intact MCL, the radial head can rotate away from the capitellum, and the ulna essentially "pivots" on the MCL and rotates off the lateral trochlea (Boxes 36–9 and 36–10).

### Imaging

- Confirming a chronic tear of the lateral ulnar collateral ligament with MRI can be difficult, but it may demonstrate thinning.

## Treatment of Posterolateral Instability

- Treatment of acute posterolateral rotatory instability may require repair or reconstruction of the radial head so that the intact ligament has an osseous structure to support.
- The ligament may be disrupted either at its origin or (rarely) at its insertion.
- Acute injuries may be treated with immediate repair of the ligament back to bone.

| Box 36–9 | Presentation and Diagnosis of Posterolateral Rotatory Instability |
|---|---|

- Diagnosis can be made historically based upon presentation of painful, recurrent clicking, snapping, or locking of elbow with pain located posterior to the proximal radio-ulnar joint as the elbow moves into supination and extension.
- Lateral pivot-shift test: Radial head is subluxed with a combination of full supination, axial compression, and valgus load as the elbow is placed in 40 degrees flexion. Because of patient apprehension and pain, this test is best done under anesthesia.

- Cohen and Hastings[10] and Imatani et al.[24] documented that the LUCL itself is a relatively slender structure and may not contribute significantly to stability. Subsequent sequential sectioning studies documented that both the ulnar bundle of the LUCL and either the anterior bundle or the annular ligament must be disrupted in order to result in reproducible subluxation of the ulnar humeral joint.[25] It appears critical for the radial head to have a posterior lateral sling, which allows rotation of the radial head without permitting it to sublux away from the distal humerus.

- Chronic injuries require reconstruction of the ligament using a free tendon graft.[7]
- In a cadaveric study, reconstruction of the LUCL restored elbow stability to that of the intact state (Box 36–11).[6]

## Instability Associated with Fracture-Dislocations

- Successful restoration of elbow stability following fracture-dislocation is dependent on the following factors:
- Restoration of the anatomy of the ulna, including the coronoid

- Restoration of the radial buttress, either by repair or by reconstruction of the radial head
- Direct or indirect repair of the medial and lateral ulnar collateral ligaments, either by direct repair to bone or by maintaining the elbow in the reduced position and allowing these ligaments to heal in an anatomic position.

### Treatment

- In a retrospective series of 56 patients with fracture-dislocations of the elbow, 13 patients had a posterior dislocation of the elbow associated with both a fracture of the radial head and the coronoid process. Ten of the 13 elbows remained unstable following operative treatment, with early arthritis seen in all 10 patients. The authors found that recurrent instability was noted in type 2 and 3 coronoid fractures. In addition, 90% of the patients who had removal of a fractured radial head had an unsatisfactory outcome, whereas only one third of patients in whom the radial head was fixed had an unsatisfactory result.[26]
- The injury of a posterior dislocation of the elbow with associated fracture of the radial head and a greater than 50% fracture (type 2 or 3) of the coronoid process of the elbow has been referred to as a *terrible triad*. Based on these results, the surgeons recommend the following[27]:

| Box 36–11 | Authors' Preferred Technique: Lateral Collateral Ligament Reconstruction |
|---|---|

- Under general anesthesia, a posterior lateral rotatory instability assessment is performed with the patient supine. The elbow is supinated, and a valgus load is applied. The elbow subluxates in full extension and then reduces as the elbow is brought back into flexion. This situation can be confirmed with simultaneous fluoroscopy, which demonstrates that the radial head subluxates off the capitellum. We prefer that with additional stress and valgus load, the ulnohumeral articulation also truly dislocate.
- Reconstruction is performed under tourniquet control. The preferred graft is the palmaris longus from the ipsilateral upper extremity; however, if none is available, a toe extensor can be taken.
- A 10-cm Kocher incision is made over the extensor carpi ulnaris–anconeus interval. The common wrist extensors are peeled off the humerus anteriorly, and the lateral epicondyle and supinator crest of the ulna are visualized.
- Typically, in acute trauma, this procedure reveals an avulsion of the majority of the soft tissue off the lateral epicondyle in one soft tissue sleeve. In chronic situations, the avulsion may have already healed back to the epicondyle and require dissection. Two connecting drill holes are made in the ulna. The most proximal drill hole is made on the supinator crest at the level of the middle-distal annular ligament insertion; the other is placed 10 to 12 mm distally.
- The most distal wall of the humeral tunnel should be at the 3:00 o'clock position on the lateral epicondyle. After placing the drill holes, it often is useful to place a suture through the drill holes in the same path that the graft will take and use this suture to determine the isometric point on the distal humerus. Although, based on cadaver studies there is no true isometric point for this ligament because of multiple bundles, there is an obvious point at which the graft must originate in order to prevent posterolateral subluxation with elbow extension. A graft that is placed too posteriorly on the lateral aspect of the humerus may permit too much posterolateral subluxation with elbow extension; therefore care must be taken to ensure that the graft is sufficiently anterior to prevent recurrent instability. After determining the isometric point, two additional converging holes are made in the distal humerus.
- The palmaris graft can be woven through the holes in the humerus and ulna and then pulled taut prior to being sutured to itself. While the graft is pulled taut, the elbow is brought down into supination and extension with a valgus stress. Make note that there is no further subluxation of the radial head posterolaterally. The graft is then tensioned and sutured with the forearm fully pronated and the elbow flexed 40 degrees.
- The graft can be sutured into position. If the graft appears to be insufficient, it can be augmented using a large (no. 2 or 5) Ethibond suture.
- Postoperatively, the patient is placed in a cast in full pronation for approximately 3 weeks. I then permit full range of motion, with the elbow maintained in neutral rotation and prevented from terminal extension for an additional 3 weeks. At 3 weeks, full range of motion from 0 to 150 degrees is permitted, with restoration of full supination with the elbow maintained at 90 degrees. Patients then can be started on gentle strengthening, with emphasis on avoiding simultaneous full supination and full extension.

1. Operative stabilization of type 2 and 3 coronoid fractures
2. Repair and reconstruction of the radial head with either stable internal fixation or an implant
3. Repair of the lateral ulnar-collateral ligament

- Even with operative treatment in a review of 11 patients at a minimum 2-year follow up, 3 of the 11 patients were considered failures. In the remaining 8 patients the results were rated as "excellent" in 2, "good" in 2, "fair" in 3, and "poor" in 1. Overall, the results were rated as unsatisfactory for 7 of 11 patients (Box 36–12).

## Longitudinal Instability

### Anatomy

- Longitudinal stability of the forearm is provided by three major anatomic constraints:
  1. Palmar and dorsal radioulnar ligaments
  2. Central band of the interosseous membrane (IOM)
  3. Radial head
- The individual contribution of the distal radioulnar joint (DRUJ) ligaments and the central band of the IOM remains somewhat controversial.
- The central band of ligamentous IOM tissue, approximately twice the thickness of the membrane on either side, is responsible for the majority of longitudinal stiffness of the IOM after radial head excision. This central band has properties similar to those of the patellar tendon. The ligament has a modulus of elasticity of 120% of the patellar tendon and an ultimate tensile strength of 84% of the patellar tendon.[30]
- Disruption of the longitudinal stiffness of the forearm permits shortening of the radius relative to the intact ulna. Resection of the radial head results in late proximal migration of the radius, which leads to distal ulnar impaction syndrome and DRUJ incongruity.
- When axial loading of the distal radius results in sufficient displacement of the radius relative to the ulna, disruption of the IOM and triangular fibrocartilage complex (TFCC) may occur. Resection of the fractured radial head alone without repair or reconstruction may result in DRUJ incongruity with ulnar impaction syndrome and pain (Essex-Lopresti fracture-dislocation).
- One author documented a fibrous tract from the distal dorsal corner of the sigmoid notch, which extends to the IOM of the forearm.[31] These fibers may contribute

to dorsal stability of the DRUJ and to longitudinal stability.
- Complications are more common and prognosis is worse for displaced fractures such as the Essex-Lopresti fracture-dislocation.

### Imaging

- Results of late reconstruction of the IOM continue to be problematic. To avoid resection of the radial head in the face of IOM injury, several cadaveric studies examined the role of imaging modalities.
- MRI using axial T2-weighted fast-spin echo images with fat suppression in the middle third of the forearm may provide accurate information.[32]
- Dynamic ultrasound, which permits visualization of the IOM over the length from its radial and ulnar insertions, may be useful.[33]

### Diagnosis

- MRI or ultrasound for diagnosis of IOM rupture?
  - No statistically significant difference in accuracy between MRI and ultrasound has been observed.[34]
  - Diagnosis can be made intraoperatively prior to replacing the radial head. Longitudinal traction on the radial neck can be combined with fluoroscopic evaluation of the DRUJ. If proximal migration greater than 6 mm occurs, gross longitudinal instability is present with disruption of both the IOM and the DRUJ ligaments. In this case, reconstruction or direct repair of the ligament may be indicated.[35]

### Treatment

#### Acute

- If the IOM injury is recognized acutely, one article has documented the feasibility of a direct primary repair of the torn IOM through an open approach.[36] In this article, successful repair of an acute IOM disruption with evidence of healing at follow-up was documented. This technique can be combined with repair or reconstruction of the radial head.

#### Chronic

- Following proximal migration, ulnar shortening osteotomy can be combined with reconstruction of the IOM and possibly TFCC.
- Reconstruction of the IOM can may performed with patellar tendon graft, allograft, or pronator teres rerouting.[37]
- Reconstruction of the radial head with either prostheses or allograft can be performed.[31,38]
- When forearm rotation is severely limited and pain relief is the primary operative indication, creation of a one-bone forearm has been performed. The results were rated as excellent and good in 37% and 32%, respectively.[38]

---

| **Box 36–12** | **Role of Hinged External Fixation** |
| --- | --- |

- Hinged external fixation has been investigated for management of complex elbow fracture-dislocations, with some success.[2,28,29] In all cases, hinged external fixation was used to treat fractures that had previously failed operative treatment or had a late presentation. Although the technique is demanding, results are satisfactory.[29]

- No comparative studies have been performed on reconstructive options, but poor outcome has been associated with infection, severe nerve injury, and multiple previous surgical procedures.

# Other Causes of Mechanical Elbow Pain Treatable by Arthroscopy

- In a review of 414 cases of elbow arthroscopy, the most common final diagnoses were osteoarthritis in 150 cases, loose bodies in 112 cases, and rheumatoid disease in 75 cases. The most common procedures include synovectomy (134), debridement of joint surfaces (180), excision of osteophytes (164), diagnostic arthroscopy (154), and loose body removal (144).

## Plicae

- Antuna and O'Driscoll[39] described the snapping plica syndrome in which a band of tissue snaps over the radial head between 90 and 110 degrees elbow flexion and pronation.
- Subsequent snapping may mimic either loose body formation or instability in some cases.
- Subsequent histologic studies demonstrated that this tissue is highly vascularized and innervated.
- *Treatment:* Arthroscopic excision of this band of tissue relieves symptoms.

## Osteoarthritis

- With the exception of throwing athletes, patients tend to be older men. Classic findings include osteophytes from the coronoid and olecranon, loose bodies, and bony hypertrophy of the distal humerus. A flexion contracture is a common finding secondary to posterior mechanical impingement. Bony changes produce mechanical symptoms.
- Retrospective reviews of the treatment of osteoarthritis of the elbow indicate that the degree of improvement is dependent upon intrinsic degenerative changes in the elbow. In a series of 70 patients, 73% benefitted in some way from arthroscopic procedures to the elbow. Overall, diagnostic arthroscopy was beneficial in 64% of elbows, whereas operative arthroscopy was of therapeutic value in 70% of elbows. However, the degree to which the procedure was deemed beneficial was in diagnosing discrete articular lesions or loose bodies.[40]
- In another series of 22 patients treated arthroscopically for loose bodies and osteochondrotic lesions, 12 rated the results as good or excellent, four had slight improvement, and six were not satisfied. The patients who remained dissatisfied with the procedures were those in whom marked degenerative changes were encountered during arthroscopy.[41]

## Rheumatoid Arthritis

- Arthroscopic synovectomy appears to be an excellent option. In a series of 29 elbows with rheumatoid arthritis followed for a minimum of 42 months, short-term results appear to be good, with clinical recurrence of synovitis in five of 21 elbows. Overall, only patients with early or moderate (Larsen grade I or II arthritis) appeared to have favorable long-term results (Box 36–13).[42,43]

## Osteochondritis Dissecans

- *Presentation:* The condition is most commonly seen in patients between 10 and 17 years old. The patients usually participate in sport activities in which the elbow functions as a weight-bearing joint.
- *Diagnosis:* Symptoms are pain with activity, dull aching at rest, catching, and locking. Swelling, tenderness over the

| Box 36–13 | Larsen Classification[44] | |
|---|---|---|
| **Grade** | **Characteristics** | |
| 0 | • Normal conditions<br>• Abnormalities not related to arthritis, such as marginal bone deposition, may be present | |
| I | • Slight abnormality<br>• Periarticular soft tissue swelling, or osteoporosis and slight joint space narrowing | |
| II | • Definite early abnormality<br>• Erosion and joint space narrowing corresponding to the standards | |
| III | • Medium destructive abnormality<br>• Erosion and joint space narrowing corresponding to the standards | |
| IV | • Severe destructive abnormality<br>• Erosion and joint space narrowing corresponding to the standards | |
| V | • Mutilating abnormality<br>• Original articular surfaces have disappeared<br>• Dislocation and bony ankylosis, which are late and secondary, should not be considered in the grading; if present, the grading should be made according to the concomitant bone destruction or deformation | |

radiocapitellar joint, and limitations in elbow motion (flexion-extension) usually are the objective findings.

- *Treatment:* Arthroscopic management of osteochondritis dissecans of the humeral capitellum has been successful.
- The goal of surgery is resection of the osteochondritic lesion and removal of loose bodies with limited synovectomy.
- Success rates at 2- to 5-year follow-up are approximately 90%.[45-48]
- The more advanced the lesion and the older the patient, the worse the result.
- *Postoperative management:* A postoperative course of continuous passive motion and early active range of motion using a bivalve extension cast helps prevent flexion contraction.

## Arthrofibrosis

- *Presentation and diagnosis:* The resulting loss of motion may cause significant morbidity. Flexion contracture, that is, loss of elbow extension, can have several causes, such as fractures, dislocations, osteoarthritis, burns, or increased spasticity.
- *Treatment:* When arthrofibrosis is associated with lesions of the radial head and capitellum, debridement may yield excellent results. However, when degenerative changes are noted in the trochlea or olecranon, patients appear to have a more protracted recovery, according to the degree of articular cartilage degeneration.
- Arthroscopic capsulectomy is a procedure that requires the highest level of experience. Among nonexperienced surgeons, the risk of causing injury to a major nerve is very high. However, capsular release does not appear to be as effective as capsulectomy or capsulotomy (Box 36–14).[49-51]
- *Postoperative management:* Passive motion is started in the recovery room. Active therapy should be initiated the day after surgery. The goal is to achieve full active motion. Splinting can be used at night for at least 3 weeks after surgery.

## Valgus Extension Overload

- *Presentation and diagnosis:* Commonly seen in athletes who throw overhead. Valgus extension overload typically presents as a bony block to full extension secondary to osteophytes on the olecranon process.

---

| Box 36–14 | Pearls and Pitfalls |
|---|---|

- *Pitfall:* Possibility of iatrogenic radial nerve injury is a concern during arthroscopic anterior capsule release.
- In a stiff elbow, capsular tissue expansion capacity is approximately 6 to 7 mm compared to a normal of 14 mm. Consequently, the safe zone is decreased, and tethering of the radial nerve and direct injury from shaving may result.[52]

---

- *Treatment:* Arthroscopy is effective for removal of loose bodies and debridement of posterior osteophytes (Figure 36–5).[53]
- *Treatment limitations:* Any degree of medial collateral insufficiency associated with valgus extension overload will not be corrected by arthroscopy.
- *Postoperative management:* Passive motion is started in the recovery room. Active therapy should be initiated the day after surgery. The goal is to achieve full active motion. Splinting can be used at night for at least 3 weeks after surgery.

## Lateral Epicondylitis

- *Presentation and diagnosis:* Presents as pain on the lateral epicondyle or 1 to 2 cm forward of it on the tendon. It usually is worse with strong gripping with the elbow in an extended position. It usually is seen in tennis players, but this disease can occur in those who participate in golf and other sports or after repetitive use of tools.
- *Treatment:* Before surgery is considered, a trial of appropriate non-operative management is indicated, with a maximum of three cortisone injections in 1 year.
- Arthroscopic management of lateral epicondylitis may have some clinical utility. The degenerative changes in the common extensor origin are debrided from inside the joint from the anterolateral portal and the cortex may be abraded. Tendon repair is not performed.[54]
- In one series of 42 releases with follow-up of 2.8 years, patients demonstrated a high satisfaction rate and returned to work at an average of 2.2 weeks.[54]

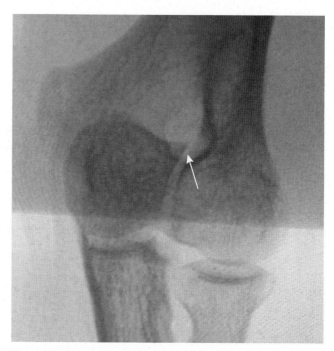

Figure 36–5:
**Characteristic osteophyte on olecranon process in a baseball player with chronic medial collateral insufficiency.**

- Arthroscopic evaluation also allows identification of intraarticular pathology, which has been noted in approximately 20% of cases, including synovitis, osteophytes, plicae, and loose bodies.[55]
- Arthroscopy allows adequate debridement of the common extensor origin without instability, provided care is taken to avoid resection posterior to the midaxis of the radial head. Arthroscopy also facilitates identification of intraarticular pathology.[55]
- *Postoperative management:* Some patients are relatively pain-free with simple movements at the initial follow-up visit. Resistance exercises usually are not permitted for 3 to 4 weeks after surgery. Unrestricted use of the elbow usually is allowed at 12 weeks.

# References

1. Ring D, Jupiter JB, Zilberfarb J: Posterior dislocation of the elbow with fractures of the radial head and coronoid. *J Bone Joint Surg* 84A:547-551, 2002.
   Discussion of elbow dislocations with a fracture of the coronoid process and radial head.

2. McKee MD, Bowden SH, King GJ et al: Management of recurrent, complex instability of the elbow with a hinged external fixator. *J Bone Joint Surg* 80B:1031-1036, 1998.
   Discusses use of the fixator in the management of recurrent complex elbow instability after failure of conventional treatment.

3. Morrey BF, An KN: Functional anatomy of the ligaments of the elbow. *Clin Orthop Relat Res* 201:84-90, 1985.
   Discusses the anatomy of the lateral and medial collateral ligaments based on 10 cadaveric dissections.

4. Floris S, Olsen BS, Dalstra M et al: The medial collateral ligament of the elbow joint: anatomy and kinematics. *J Shoulder Elbow Surg* 7:345-351, 1998.
   This study defines the anterior band as the primary constraint to valgus forces.

5. O'Driscoll SW, Jaloszynski R, Morrey BF, An KN: Origin of the medial ulnar collateral ligament. *J Hand Surg* 17A:164-168, 1992.
   The anterior medial collateral ligament originates exclusively from the anteroinferior surface of medial epicondyle, and only 20% of the width of the medial epicondyle in the coronal plane can be removed without violating a portion of its origin.

6. King GJ, Dunning CE, Zarzour ZD et al: Single-strand reconstruction of the lateral ulnar collateral ligament restores varus and posterolateral rotatory stability of the elbow. *J Shoulder Elbow Surg* 11:60-64, 2002.
   This study demonstrates that both single- and double-strand lateral ulnar collateral ligament reconstructions restore varus and posterolateral elbow stability.

7. O'Driscoll SW: Elbow instability. *Hand Clin* 10:405-415, 1994.
   Classification of the spectrum of elbow instability, from subluxation to dislocation, is presented.

8. Morrey BF, Tanaka S, An KN: Valgus stability of the elbow. A definition of primary and secondary constraints. *Clin Orthop Relat Res* 265:187-195, 1991.
   This study defines the MCL as the primary constraint of the elbow joint to valgus stress and the radial head as a secondary constraint. Comminuted radial head fracture uncomplicated by MCL insufficiency can be treated by excision without replacement.

9. Closkey RF, Goode JR, Kirschenbaum D, Cody RP: The role of the coronoid process in elbow stability. A biomechanical analysis of axial loading. *J Bone Joint Surg* 82A:1749-1753, 2000.
   Elbows with a fracture involving more than 50% of the coronoid process displace more readily than elbows with a fracture involving 50% or less.

10. Cohen MS, Hastings H: Rotatory instability of the elbow. The anatomy and role of the lateral stabilizers. *J Bone Joint Surg* 79A:225-233, 1997.
    Forty fresh cadavers were studied to define the ligamentous anatomy of the lateral aspect of the elbow as it relates to rotatory instability.

11. Davidson PA, Pink M, Perry J, Jobe FW: Functional anatomy of the flexor pronator muscle group in relation to the medial collateral ligament of the elbow. *Am J Sports Med* 23:245-250, 1995.
    The flexor carpi ulnaris and the flexor digitorum superficialis muscles are the muscles best positioned to support the MCL.

12. Hamilton CD, Glousman RE, Jobe FW et al: Dynamic stability of the elbow: electromyographic analysis of the flexor pronator group and the extensor group in pitchers with valgus instability. *J Shoulder Elbow Surg* 5:347-354, 1996.
    This study suggests that the muscles on the medial side of the elbow cannot supplant the role of the medial collateral ligament during the fastball pitch.

13. Kenter K, Behr CT, Warren RF et al: Acute elbow injuries in the National Football League. *J Shoulder Elbow Surg* 9:1-5, 2000.
    This retrospective review found that professional football players with medial collateral ligament injuries and valgus instability were able to function without operative reconstruction, and no evidence of valgus instability remained at average 3.4-year follow-up. This is in contrast to baseball players, in whom the mechanics and demands may differ.

14. Field LD, Altchek DW: Evaluation of the arthroscopic valgus instability test of the elbow. *Am J Sports Med* 24:177-181, 1996.
    The authors found that the entire anterior bundle must be sectioned before measurable and reproducible arthroscopic evidence of valgus instability is seen.

15. Eygendaal D, Olsen BS, Jensen SL et al: Kinematics of partial and total ruptures of the medial collateral ligament of the elbow. *J Shoulder Elbow Surg* 8:612-616, 1999.
    This study indicates that valgus instability should be evaluated at 70 to 90 degrees flexion. Detection of partial ruptures in the anterior bundle of the medial collateral ligament based on medial joint opening and increased valgus movement is impossible.

16. Azar FM, Andrews JR, Wilk KE, Groh D: Operative treatment of ulnar collateral ligament injuries of the elbow in athletes. *Am J Sports Med* 28:16-23, 2000.
    Reconstruction of the ulnar collateral ligament was effective in correcting valgus elbow instability and allowed most athletes to return to sport in less than 1 year.

17. Lee GA, Katz SD, Lazarus MD: Elbow valgus stress radiography in an uninjured population. *Am J Sports Med* 26:425-427, 1998.
Uninjured elbows have significant medial ulnohumeral gapping on valgus stress radiography but should be compared to the contralateral elbow.

18. Sasaki J, Takahara M, Ogino T et al: Ultrasonographic assessment of the ulnar collateral ligament and medial elbow laxity in college baseball players. *J Bone Joint Surg* 84A:525-531, 2002.
Valgus laxity of the dominant elbow was increased in baseball players compared with nonplayers.

19. Timmerman LA, Schwartz ML, Andrews JR: Preoperative evaluation of the ulnar collateral ligament by magnetic resonance imaging and computed tomography arthrography. Evaluation in 25 baseball players with surgical confirmation. *Am J Sports Med* 22:26-31, 1994.
Both computed tomography(CT) arthrograms and MRIs were accurate in diagnosing a complete tear of the ulnar collateral ligament, with CT arthrograms advantageous in evaluating partial undersurface tears.

20. Conway JE, Jobe FW, Glousman RE, Pink M: Medial instability of the elbow in throwing athletes. Treatment by repair or reconstruction of the ulnar collateral ligament. *J Bone Joint Surg* 74A:67-83, 1992.
Good or excellent results are reported in 10 of 14 patients following MCL repair (seven returned to sport) and in 45 of 56 (80%) following reconstruction; 38 (68%) returned to sport. Follow-up averaged 6.3 years.

21. Armstrong AD, Dunning CE, Faber KJ et al: Single-strand ligament reconstruction of the medial collateral ligament restores valgus elbow stability. *J Shoulder Elbow Surg* 11:65-71, 2002.
The central portion of the anterior bundle of the MCL is an important valgus stabilizer of the elbow, whose injury can be reliably treated with a simplified single-strand reconstruction.

22. Hechtman KS, Tjin ATE, Zvijac JE et al: Biomechanics of a less invasive procedure for reconstruction of the ulnar collateral ligament of the elbow. *Am J Sports Med* 26:620-624, 1998.
MCL reconstruction using bone anchors reproduced normal anatomy and mechanical function more closely than bone tunnel reconstruction, but with no significant difference in reconstruction strength.

23. Rohrbough JT, Altchek DW, Hyman J et al: Medial collateral ligament reconstruction of the elbow using the docking technique. *Am J Sports Med* 30:541-548, 2002.
Describes the docking technique for MCL reconstruction.

24. Imatani J, Ogura T, Morito Y et al: Anatomic and histologic studies of lateral collateral ligament complex of the elbow joint. *J Shoulder Elbow Surg* 8:625-627, 1999.
This cadaveric study suggests that the lateral ulnar collateral ligament contributes to posterolateral rotatory stability as part of the lateral collateral ligament complex but is not the major constraint.

25. Hannouche D, Begue T: Functional anatomy of the lateral collateral ligament complex of the elbow. *Surg Radiol Anat* 21:187-191, 1999.
A new technique of ligamentoplasty using the fascia of the extensor carpi ulnaris muscle is reported.

26. O'Driscoll SW, Jupiter JB, King GJ et al: The unstable elbow. *Instr Course Lect* 50:89-102, 2001.

27. Ring D, Jupiter JB: Reconstruction of posttraumatic elbow instability. *Clin Orthop Relat Res* 370:44-56, 2000.
Describes the necessities of successful reconstruction for post-traumatic elbow instability.

28. Fox RJ, Varitimidis SE, Plakseychuk A et al: The Compass Elbow Hinge: indications and initial results. *J Hand Surg* 25B:568-572, 2000.
Describes use of the compass elbow hinge in 11 patients with degenerative disease, contracture, or instability.

29. Jupiter JB, Ring D: Treatment of unreduced elbow dislocations with hinged external fixation. *J Bone Joint Surg* 84A:1630-1635, 2002.
Describes successful treatment of unreduced elbow dislocations with open reduction and hinged external fixation as much as 30 weeks postinjury.

30. Pfaeffle HJ, Tomaino MM, Grewal R et al: Tensile properties of the interosseous membrane of the human forearm. *J Orthop Res* 14:842-845, 1996.
Determined that the interosseous membrane is stiff and capable of bearing high loads, especially its central band.

31. Szabo RM, Hotchkiss RN, Slater RR Jr: The use of frozen-allograft radial head replacement for treatment of established symptomatic proximal translation of the radius: preliminary experience in five cases. *J Hand Surg* 22A:269-278, 1997.
Describes forearm reconstruction with radial head allograft implantation for proximal translation of the radius following radial head excision (Essex-Lopresti lesion).

32. Starch DW, Dabezies EJ: Magnetic resonance imaging of the interosseous membrane of the forearm. *J Bone Joint Surg* 83A:235-238, 2001.
The intact and disrupted interosseous membrane can be evaluated using magnetic resonance imaging.

33. Jaakkola JI, Riggans DH, Lourie GM et al: Ultrasonography for the evaluation of forearm interosseous membrane disruption in a cadaver model. *J Hand Surg* 26A:1053-1057, 2001.
Noted ultrasonography was 96% accurate in detecting interosseous membrane injuries.

34. Fester EW, Murray PM, Sanders TG et al: The efficacy of magnetic resonance imaging and ultrasound in detecting disruptions of the forearm interosseous membrane: a cadaver study. *J Hand Surg* 27A:418-424, 2002.
Noted that MRI and ultrasonographic imaging should both be considered when forearm interosseous membrane integrity is in question.

35. Smith AM, Urbanosky LR, Castle JA et al: Radius pull test: predictor of longitudinal forearm instability. *J Bone Joint Surg* 84A:1970-1976, 2002.
Following radial head resection, 3 mm of proximal radial migration with longitudinal traction indicates disruption of the interosseous membrane; 6 mm or more implies disruption of all ligamentous structures of the forearm.

36. North ER, Meyers S: Wrist injuries: correlation of clinical and arthroscopic findings. *J Hand Surg* 15A:915-920, 1990.

37. Ruch DS, Chang DS, Koman LA: Reconstruction of longitudinal stability of the forearm after disruption of interosseous

ligament and radial head excision (Essex-Lopresti lesion). *J South Orthop Assoc* 8:47-52, 1999.
Technique for reconstruction of the central band of the interosseous membrane in conjunction with surgical repair of the DRUJ and radial head prosthesis is presented.

38. Peterson CA, Maki S, Wood MB: Clinical results of the one-bone forearm. *J Hand Surg* 20:609-618, 1995.
Reports less predictable results for one-bone forearm construction than previously reported.

39. Antuna SA, O'Driscoll SW: Snapping plicae associated with radiocapitellar chondromalacia. *Arthroscopy* 17:491-495, 2001.
Reports 14 patients who were treated arthroscopically for snapping elbow caused by hypertrophic synovial folds associated with radiocapitellar chondromalacia.

40. O'Driscoll SW, Morrey BF: Arthroscopy of the elbow. Diagnostic and therapeutic benefits and hazards. *J Bone Joint Surg* 74A:84-94, 1992.
Analysis of the results and complications of 71 elbow arthroscopies.

41. Rupp S, Tempelhof S: Arthroscopic surgery of the elbow. Therapeutic benefits and hazards. *Clin Orthop Relat Res* 313:140-145, 1995.
Twelve of 22 patients who underwent arthroscopic surgery of the elbow mainly for loose bodies or osteochondrotic lesions rated the result as good or excellent. Patients without severe damage of the articular cartilage benefitted most.

42. Lee BP, Morrey BF: Arthroscopic synovectomy of the elbow for rheumatoid arthritis. A prospective study. *J Bone Joint Surg* 79B:770-772, 1997.
Recognition of the short-term gain and the potential for serious nerve injury should be considered when offering arthroscopic synovectomy.

43. Horiuchi K, Momohara S, Tomatsu T et al: Arthroscopic synovectomy of the elbow in rheumatoid arthritis. *J Bone Joint Surg* 84A:342-347, 2002.
Arthroscopic synovectomy in an elbow affected by rheumatoid arthritis is a reliable procedure that can alleviate pain.

44. Larsen A, Dale K, Eek M: Radiographic evaluation of rheumatoid arthritis and related conditions by standard reference films. *Acta Radiol Diagn (Stockh)* 18:481-491, 1977.
Review of radiographic evaluation of rheumatoid arthritis is given.

45. Jackson DW, Silvino N, Reiman P: Osteochondritis in the female gymnast's elbow. *Arthroscopy* 5:129-136, 1989.
Once bony changes are detected from capitellar osteochondritis dissecans in high-performance teenage female gymnasts, symptoms may be improved by surgery, but persistent pain makes return to high-level competitive gymnastics unlikely.

46. Baumgarten TE, Andrews JR, Satterwhite YE: The arthroscopic classification and treatment of osteochondritis dissecans of the capitellum. *Am J Sports Med* 26:520-523, 1998.
Arthroscopic abrasion chondroplasty and treatment of any accompanying pathologic lesions provided good results in most patients in a young population with capitellar osteochondritis dissecans at short-term follow-up.

47. Ruch DS, Cory JW, Poehling GG: The arthroscopic management of osteochondritis dissecans of the adolescent elbow. *Arthroscopy* 14:797-803, 1998.
Reports that 11 of 12 pediatric patients were highly satisfied following arthroscopic debridement for capitellar avascular necrosis at a mean 3.2 years of follow-up.

48. Baker CL Jr, Jones GL: Arthroscopy of the elbow. *Am Sports Med* 27:251-264, 1999.

49. Kim SJ, Kim HK, Lee JW: Arthroscopy for limitation of motion of the elbow. *Arthroscopy* 11:680-683, 1995.
Notes that elbow arthroscopy is an effective diagnostic and therapeutic procedure for limited motion caused by intra-articular pathology.

50. Phillips BB, Strasburger S: Arthroscopic treatment of arthrofibrosis of the elbow joint. *Arthroscopy* 14:38-44, 1998.
Arthroscopic treatment of stiff elbow joints appears to result in improvement equal to that obtained by open techniques, with less morbidity and earlier rehabilitation.

51. Savoie FH III, Nunley PD, Field LD: Arthroscopic management of the arthritic elbow: indications, technique, and results. *J Shoulder Elbow Surg* 8:214-219, 1999.
Describes the arthroscopic modification of the Outerbridge-Kashiwagi procedure.

52. Jones GS, Savoie FH III: Arthroscopic capsular release of flexion contractures (arthrofibrosis) of the elbow. *Arthroscopy* 9:277-283, 1993.
Describes treatment of elbow flexion contractures by arthroscopic capsular release and debridement of the olecranon fossa.

53. Ogilvie-Harris DJ, Weisleder L: Fluid pump systems for arthroscopy: a comparison of pressure control versus pressure and flow control. *Arthroscopy* 11:591-595, 1995.
Arthroscopic pumps that separately control pressure and flow are significantly better than pumps that control pressure alone.

54. Baker CL Jr, Murphy KP, Gottlob CA, Curd DT: Arthroscopic classification and treatment of lateral epicondylitis: two-year clinical results. *J Shoulder Elbow Surg* 9:475-482, 2000.
Arthroscopic tennis elbow release is a reliable treatment.

55. Owens BD, Murphy KP, Kuklo TR: Arthroscopic release for lateral epicondylitis. *Arthroscopy* 17:582-587, 2001.
Arthroscopic release effectively treats lateral epicondylitis while also affording visualization of the joint space to address associated intraarticular pathology.

# Fractures of the Elbow

Ajay K. Seth* and Mark E. Baratz†

*MD, Spectrum Orthopedics, Canton, OH
†MD, Professor of Orthopedics, Drexel University School of Medicine, Philadelphia, PA;
Vice Chairman, Department of Orthopaedic Surgery, Director, Division of Hand and
Upper Extremities, Allegheny General Hospital, Pittsburgh, PA

## Introduction

- Elbow fractures can be subdivided into distal humerus fractures, radial head fractures, and olecranon fractures.
- Types of elbow fractures depend primarily on the position of the elbow and the axis of the force from the trauma.

## Distal Humerus Fractures

- Treatment depends on anatomic reduction of fracture fragments, rigid fixation, preservation of the soft tissue envelope, and early motion.

### Anatomy

- The distal humerus consists of two columns: medial and lateral (Figure 37–1).
- The medial column consists of the medial flare of the metaphysis, the medial epicondyle, and the medial condyle including the trochlea.
- The lateral column consists of the lateral metaphyseal flare, the lateral epicondyle, and the lateral condyle including the capitellum.
- Between the two columns is the coronoid fossa anteriorly and the olecranon fossa posteriorly.

### Mechanism of Injury

- Supracondylar fractures generally result from a fall from a standing height.

- Intraarticular fractures result from high-energy injuries in young individuals and lower-energy injuries to osteopenic bone in elderly individuals.

## Evaluation

- Assess the elbow for skin lacerations, nerve function, and pulses in the upper extremity. Note the potential for ulnar nerve compromise in T-condylar distal humerus fractures and radial nerve and anterior interosseous nerve palsy in pediatric supracondylar fractures.
  - Anterior interosseous nerve the palsy causes deficit in the flexor pollicis longus, the flexor digitorum profundus to the index finger, and the pronator quadratus.
  - Radial nerve palsy presents with deficits in extension of the wrist, thumb and fingers.
  - Check the arm, forearm, and hand for compartment syndrome. Signs of compartment syndrome are
    - Pain with passive range of motion
    - Pain out of proportion to the injury
    - Paresthesias
    - Poikilothermia (coolness of extremity)
    - Loss of pulse (often the last sign)
- Examine the shoulder and wrist for associated injuries.
- Radiographic examination should include anteroposterior (AP) and lateral radiographs of the elbow. (Radiographs should also include the shoulder and wrist.)
- Oblique views should be ordered to diagnose subtle fractures. For example, the radial head oblique view is

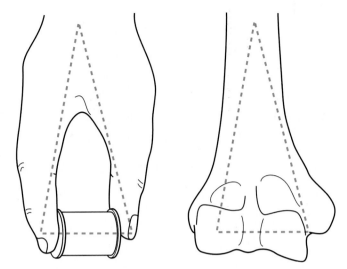

Figure 37–1:
**Distal humerus consists of two columns: medial and lateral columns.**

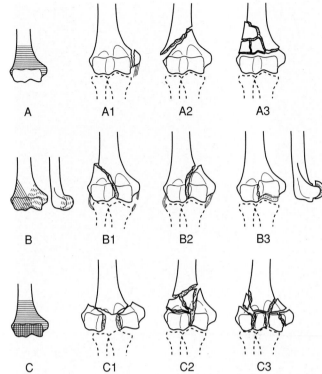

Figure 37–2:
**AO classification.**

shot 30 degrees cephalad to a true lateral view to diagnose occult radial head fractures.
- Radiographs should be inspected for dislocations, positive posterior or anterior fat pad signs, fractures, and subluxations.
- Computed tomography (CT) can be used for finer bony detail of intraarticular fractures.

## Classification

- Divided into supracondylar, transcondylar, and intercondylar fractures.
  - Supracondylar fracture: above the olecranon fossa
  - Transcondylar fracture: through the olecranon fossa
  - Intercondylar fracture: between the condyles of the distal humerus
- AO classification (Figure 37–2) divides fractures into
  - Type A: extraarticular
  - Type B: extension into the articular surface
  - Type C: complete separation of the articular surface from the shaft
  - Numerical attachments are used, depending on the degree of comminution (1–3, with 3 being highly comminuted)
- Intercondylar fractures divided by the Riseborough and Radin types (all types include a supracondylar component)
  - Type I: nondisplaced fracture between the capitellum and trochlea
  - Type II: displaced, nonrotated fracture between the condyles
  - Type III: displaced and rotated fracture between the condyles
  - Type IV: severe comminution of the articular surface of one or both condyles (Figure 37–3)

- Capitellar fractures: shear injury to the distal humerus
  - Type I: fracture of the entire capitellum and lateral trochlear ridge (Hahn-Steinthal fracture) (Figure 37–4)
  - Type II: involves only the articular surface of capitellum with subchondral bone (Kocher-Lorenz fracture)
  - Type III: comminuted fractures of capitellum (Figure 37–5)

## Treatment

### Nonoperative

- Limited role for nonoperative treatment of distal humerus fractures.
- Goal of treatment is early motion to prevent stiffness.
- Elderly patients with multiple medical problems can be treated with the "bag of bones" method: splint in 60 degrees flexion for 2 to 3 weeks, followed by gentle motion.

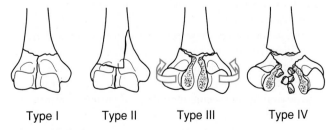

Type I        Type II        Type III        Type IV

Figure 37–3:
**Riseborough and Radin classification.**

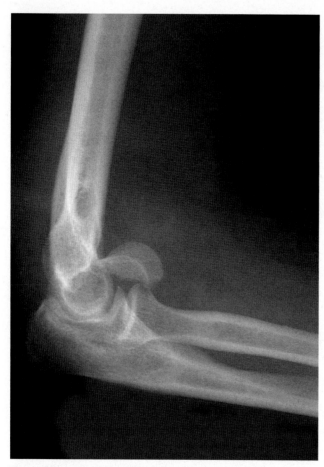

Figure 37–4:
**Type I capitellar fracture.**

## Operative

- Goals of treatment are a pain-free joint with functional motion (30 degrees extension, 130 degrees flexion, 50 degrees supination and pronation).
- Stable fixation allows elbow motion as soon as the skin is sealed.
- Plate fixation consists of double plating the distal humerus: medial and posterolateral, or medial and lateral.

## Surgical Procedure

- Patient placed in the lateral decubitus position with the affected arm over a padded post.
- Identify and mobilize the ulnar nerve.
- Extensile posterior approach: olecranon osteotomy or triceps retraction
  - Olecranon osteotomy: excellent exposure, particularly when the articular surface is comminuted. However, nonunions may occur at the osteotomy site. Note nonunion rates are decreased with use of a chevron osteotomy and secure tension band wiring or plate fixation.
  - Retraction of the triceps can be used when there are three major fragments and no articular comminution.

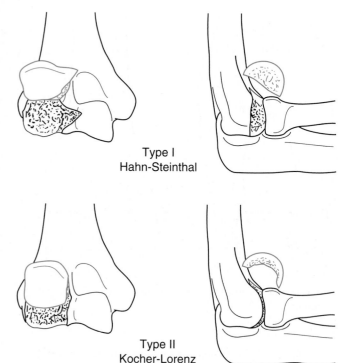

Type I
Hahn-Steinthal

Type II
Kocher-Lorenz

Figure 37–5:
**Classification of capitellar fracture.**

- The view of the trochlea can be improved by removing approximately 1 cm of the tip of the olecranon process.
- Studies have shown that plates can be aligned in orthogonal planes or parallel. Allow the fracture pattern to dictate the placement of plates.[1-4]
- The articular surface is assembled and then attached to the shaft.
- Provisional fixation with pins can be used first, then a 3.5-mm DC plate can be contoured to the posterior surface of the lateral column and a 3.5-mm reconstruction plate contoured to fit the medial column (new precontoured plates may simplify this process) (Figure 37-6).
- Take care not to compress the articular segment from medial to lateral, by using a fully threaded, cortical screw.
- Metaphyseal–diaphyseal contact is important to avoid nonunions.
- Use a structural graft. Use corticocancellous iliac crest graft when there is a break in cortical continuity of the triangle: medial column, joint surface, lateral column. Use cancellous graft when the triangle is intact and there is loss of metaphyseal bone.
- Key points to remember in fixation:
  - Place as many screws as possible into the distal fragments.
  - Screws from the medial and lateral plates should be placed into as many comminuted fragments as possible.
  - Plates can be placed on the medial and lateral surfaces.[5,6]

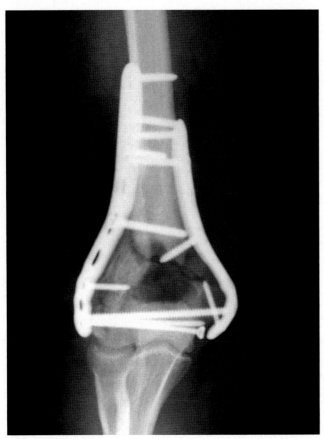

Figure 37–6:
**Fracture fixation of the elbow.**

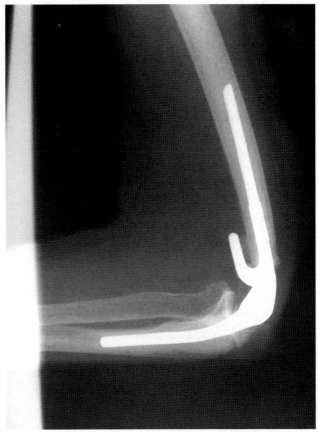

Figure 37–7:
**Example of post fracture total elbow arthroplasty.**

## Alternative Treatment: Total Elbow Arthroplasty

- Considered for patients with severe comminution and osteoporosis[7,8]
- In low-demand patients, total elbow arthroplasty (TEA) can restore motion and hand function.
- Technique similar to TEA for degenerative conditions.
  1. Long-stemmed components should be available in case of proximal fracture extension.
  2. *Operative Pearls:*
- Use a posterior approach. Similar steps taken to open reduction internal fixation (ORIF) humerus.
- Transpose the ulnar nerve anteriorly.
- Work on both sides of the triceps to remove condylar pieces. *(Key: Do not take down/off the triceps from the olecranon during approach.)*
- You can remove the entire distal humerus to the olecranon fossa without a problem because it is replaced by the prosthesis. Removal of an additional 1 to 2 cm does not lead to any significant sequelae.
- After removing the condyles, use the triceps muscle to gauge proper tension of the humeral prosthesis.

- Remove the proximal tip of the olecranon to allow better access for implanting the ulnar component (Figure 37–7).

## Postoperative Care

- The elbow is immobilized in a posterior splint for 3 to 5 days.
- The splint is removed, and the patient is started on active-assisted motion as long as the skin is sealed. Wait longer after a TEA to ensure the skin has healed. (May leave elbow in an extension splint for 2 weeks to help obtain better extension.
- A removable splint is fashioned to protect the limb while allowing frequent removal for range of motion excercises.
- Active motion is started when healing is eminent, usually at 6 to 8 weeks.
- Passive stretch is started when the fracture is fully healed.

## Articular Shear Fractures of the Distal Humerus

- Fractures of the capitellum and trochlea often result from shear forces.
- Oblique views or CT scans may be needed to identify fracture fragments.

- Nondisplaced fracture fragments are treated with a brief period of immobilization.
- X-ray films of the fracture are needed weekly for 2 to 3 weeks to check the maintenance of reduction.

### Displaced Fractures

- Type I: capitellar fractures
  - Treat with ORIF.
  - Lateral approach allows best access to the fracture fragment.
  - Headless compression screws are placed anterior to posterior.
  - Short threaded malleolar screws are placed posterior to anterior (Figure 37–8).
- Types II and III
  - Fixation is difficult.
  - Best to perform excision of the fracture fragments.
  - Check valgus stability to rule out associated medial collateral ligament injury.
  - Begin early motion.
- An isolated displaced trochlea fracture is addressed with ORIF.
  - An olecranon osteotomy or extended lateral approach is required to inspect and reduce articular fragments.[10]

### Complications of Distal Humerus Fractures

- Complications of distal humerus fractures include loss of motion, nonunion, malunion, heterotopic ossification,

infection, nerve injury, extensor tendon dysfunction, and symptomatic hardware.

## Fractures of the Radial Head

- Result from axial load applied through a flexed elbow.
- Radial head fractures that occur with elbow dislocation often have associated disruptions of the medial and lateral collateral ligaments, anterior joint capsule, and coronoid process.
- High-energy axial load to the forearm can lead to an Essex-Lopresti lesion, which consists of:
  - A comminuted fracture of the radial head
  - Rupture of the interosseous membrane
  - Injury to the triangular fibrocartilage complex (TFCC)

### Classification of Radial Head Fractures

- Hotchkiss modification of Mason-Johnston:
  - Type I: nondisplaced or minimally displaced fracture of the head or neck; no block to pronation or supination
  - Type II: displaced (>2 mm) fractures of the head or neck; may have incongruity at the neck or fracture site causing a block to motion
  - Type III: comminuted fracture (Figure 37–9)

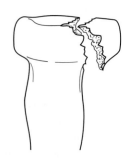

Type I

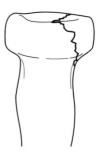

Type II

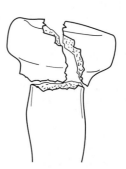

Type III

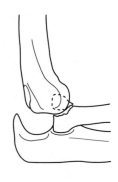

Type IV

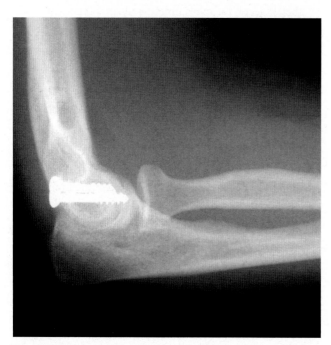

Figure 37–8:
**Postoperative image of a type I capitellar fracture.**

Figure 37–9:
**Radial head classification.**

## Evaluation

- Appropriate treatment of radial head fractures is guided by the following four factors:
  1. Forearm rotation
  2. Elbow stability
  3. Wrist pain
  4. Imaging
- The patient with a suspected fracture has tenderness over the radial head and an elbow effusion.
- May have limited forearm pronation or supination.
- The limitations in rotation should improve with aspiration of the elbow and injection of anesthetic.
- The limitation may improve with 1 week of rest and gentle immobilization.
- A block to forearm rotation is an indication for operative intervention.
- Tenderness over the medial collateral ligament with elbow laxity during a valgus stress confirms associated elbow instability.
- Wrist pain and tenderness in the region of the distal radioulnar joint may indicate a concurrent rupture of the TFCC and interosseous membrane.

## Radiographs

- AP and lateral projections of the elbow.
- Oblique projection: 30 degrees anterior to a true lateral; may help identify impacted fractures.
- Wrist radiographs of both the injured and uninjured arms should be obtained when a patient has a radial head fracture and wrist pain suggesting the possibility of an Essex-Lopresti lesion.

## Treatment

- The most common problem is elbow stiffness.
- The goal should be to design a treatment option that permits early motion.

### Type I

- Rarely associated with injury to the elbow's collateral ligaments or interosseous membrane.
- If the elbow is stable and the wrist is not tender, place in a sling for comfort and have the patient work on elbow motion and forearm rotation.

### Type II

- May be associated with an elbow dislocation and have associated medial or lateral collateral ligament injuries.
- The marginal fracture of the radial head may create a block to forearm rotation.
- The medial fracture fragment may impinge on the sigmoid notch of the proximal ulna, limiting rotation. This is best visualized on an oblique radiograph.

- Operative treatment is highly successful for type II fractures. If a block to motion exists, surgical intervention is the treatment of choice.
- A lateral approach to the elbow is used.
- Large fragments of the radial head are treated with ORIF.
- The safe zone for screw placement is formed by a 110-degree arc from a line perpendicular to the radial styloid and one perpendicular to Lister's tubercle. The safe zone is centered laterally with the forearm in neutral rotation, and extends 65 degrees anteriorly and 45 degrees posteriorly. This is the portion of the radial head that does not articulate with the proximal radioulnar joint.
- Fixation is accomplished with headless screws, lag screws, or plates.

### Type III

- Highly comminuted fractures reflect a high-energy injury with the possibility of associated damage to the collateral ligaments, coronoid process, and interosseous membrane.
- During the lateral approach, care must be taken to inspect for injury to the lateral complex.
- If the ligament complex has been stripped from the lateral epicondyle, it should be repaired using sutures passed through bone tunnels at the completion of surgery. (Suture anchors are often not adequate for this repair.)
- Three or fewer head fragments may allow an internal fixation to be performed.[9,10]
- More than three fragments may necessitate either radial head replacement or excision of the radial head.[10–12]
- If the radial head cannot be repaired, the surgeon must assess the status of the:
  - Medial collateral ligament with valgus stress testing using intraoperative imaging
  - Integrity of the interosseous membrane with the "pull test"
    - A posteroanterior image of the wrist is obtained before and after applying traction to the fractured end of the proximal radius.
    - Translation of 6 mm or more suggests disruption of the interosseous membrane and the TFCC.
- If there is no valgus laxity or longitudinal instability (distal migration of the radius), the radial head can be excised, which is the exception. However, if there is any other ligamentous or osseous injury to the elbow, a radial head prosthesis should be used.
- The remaining metaphyseal bone should be trimmed distal to the sigmoid notch to avoid neck-notch impingement.
- If there is evidence of valgus or axial laxity, then a metallic radial head prosthesis is inserted.
- The head diameter is estimated by assembling the fractured head fragments.

- Images should be obtained intraoperatively to evaluate for (Figure 37–10):
  - Match of the radial head with the capitellum
  - Match of the radial head with the sigmoid notch
  - Alignment of the prosthesis in the shaft
  - The medial joint space
- If the elbow remains stable at 30 degrees of flexion, the wounds are closed.
- If the elbow dislocates at 30 degrees, consideration is given to repairing the medial collateral ligament through a separate incision.

## Postoperative Care

- Patients are placed in a posterior splint for approximately 5 days to allow the swelling to subside and the incision to heal.
- Patients then begin active-assisted motion.

# Olecranon Fractures

- Fractures result from a direct blow to the dorsal surface of the proximal ulna.
- The humeral articular surface often functions as a wedge to fracture the proximal ulna.

## Evaluation

- Evaluate the soft tissues for disruption, including the presence of an open fracture.
- Nerve dysfunction and vascular status must be evaluated (particularly the ulnar nerve).
- Palpate and check range of motion of the shoulder and wrist to identify any associated injuries.
- AP and lateral x-ray films should be obtained. The lateral radiograph of the elbow helps determine fracture displacement, comminution, and joint congruity.

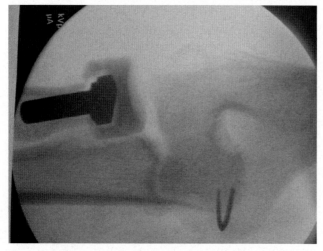

Figure 37–10:
**Intraoperative image of a radial head implant performed for a type III fracture of the radial head.**

- Oblique views of the AP projection help assess medial and lateral wall reduction and comminution.
- CT can help define the size and location of articular fragments.

## Classification

- Fractures are divided into three types using the Mayo classification system (Figure 37–11):
  - Type I: nondisplaced fractures
  - Type II: displaced fractures but the elbow is stable
  - Type III: fractures are displaced and the elbow is unstable (either from rupture of the medial collateral ligament or fracture comminution that extends to and disrupts the insertion of the medial collateral ligament) (Figure 37–12)

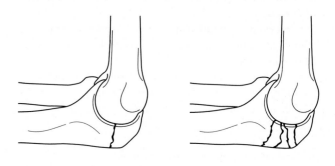

Type I Undisplaced

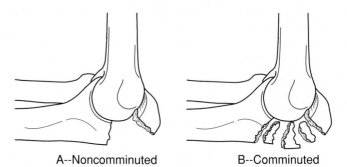

A--Noncomminuted          B--Comminuted

Type II Displaced-Stable

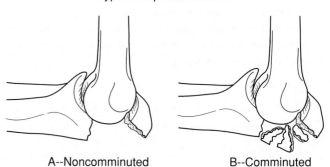

A--Noncomminuted          B--Comminuted

Type III Unstable

Figure 37–11:
**Mayo classification for olecranon fractures.**

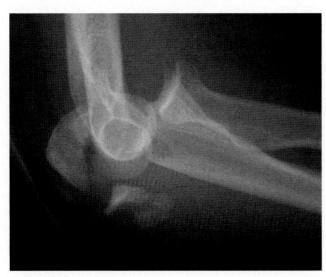

**Figure 37–12:**
**Displaced olecranon fracture with instability.**

## Treatment

- Management depends on displacement, comminution, and elbow stability.

### Nondisplaced Fractures

- Nondisplaced fractures can be immobilized in a long arm cast or splint in 30 degrees of flexion.
- Repeat radiographs are obtained in 1 week to evaluate fracture displacement.
- Immobilization is discontinued within 2 weeks, and active motion without resistance is initiated (use a similar protocol for comminuted fractures in elderly, debilitated patients).

### Displaced Fractures

- Displaced fractures are treated according to fracture pattern.
- The patient is placed in the lateral decubitus position.
- Use a posterior approach with the incision curving medial to the olecranon.
- Options for treatment include tension band wiring, plate fixation, and primary excision.

### Tension Band Wiring[13,14]

- Recommended for transverse fractures with minimal comminution.
- A large bone tenaculum is used to help reduce and compress the fracture fragments.
- Two 0.062-inch Kirschner wires are inserted into the tip of the olecranon and advanced across the fracture and into the anterior cortex of the ulna. (We do not use screws, because they are not as forgiving when trying to compress the fracture with a tension band wire.)

- Using an angiocatheter placed anterior to the triceps tendon, an 18-gauge wire is passed so that it rests on the olecranon. The angiocatheter is placed from medial to lateral to avoid injuring the ulnar nerve.
- A 2.0-mm drill hole is created in the posterior cortex approximately 2 cm distal to the fracture site.
- The wire is passed through the tunnel to create a figure-eight pattern. The wire is pulled and twisted taut.
- The pins are bent and cut at 180 degrees and impacted into the olecranon tip.
- Check to ensure that full motion has been preserved (Figure 37–13).

### Plate Fixation[15,16]

- Plate fixation is indicated in comminuted fractures, fractures distal to the coronoid process, oblique fractures distal to the midpoint of the trochlear notch, and Monteggia fracture-dislocations of the elbow.
- Plates can be placed posteriorly or medially. There is no difference except that the posterior position minimizes malreduction in the sagittal plane (Figure 37–14).
- Can use a posterior plate to help with fracture reduction. Place screws peripherally to allow placement of an intramedullary screw.
- Severely comminuted fractures often require dual plating to achieve stability.

### Resection of the Proximal Fragment[17]

- Option for managing severely comminuted olecranon fractures.
- Often used for elderly patients in whom the fracture fragments constitute less than 70% of the articular surface and are too comminuted for fixation.
- Extent of the resection is dictated by the insertion of the medial collateral ligament.
- The triceps tendon is reattached using nonabsorbable suture passed through drill holes toward the proximal edge of the articular surface. This method creates a sling

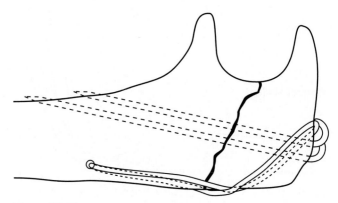

**Figure 37–13:**
**Fracture treated with tension band wiring.**

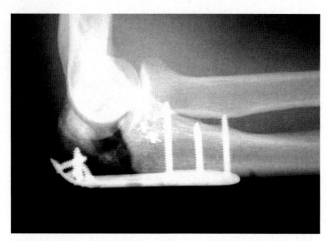

Figure 37–14:

**Postoperative fixation for olecranon fracture with repair of the collateral ligaments.**

and a smooth surface for articulation with the distal humerus; however, it may decrease extensor strength secondary to a shortened tricep's moment arm (Figure 37–15).

- The remaining olecranon should be cut transversely.

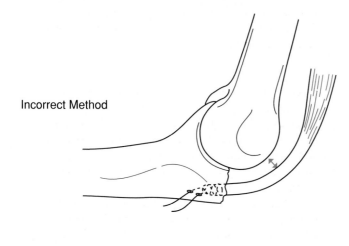

Incorrect Method

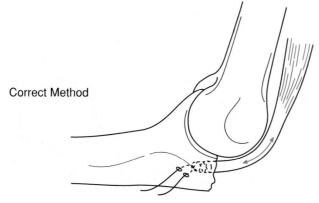

Correct Method

Figure 37–15:

**Resection of an olecranon fracture.**

## Postoperative Care for Resection or Plate Fixation

- The elbow is splinted in approximately 60 degrees of flexion.
- Reevaluate the patient in 5 to 7 days. If the skin is sealed, initiate active-assisted motion.
- Between exercises, the elbow is protected in a posterior splint.
- The splint is discontinued at 2 weeks and active motion is started.
- Passive and resisted exercises are started when the fracture has healed, usually around 8 weeks. If the fracture fragment was excised with triceps advancement, resistive exercises begin after week 12.

## Complications

- Complications of tension band wire include loss of fixation, nonunion, skin breakdown, infection, and prominent hardware.
- Complications of plate fixation include metal prominence, loss of reduction, malreduction, and nonunion (<10%).

## References

1. Pajarinen J, Bjorkenheim JM: Operative treatment of type C intercondylar fractures of the distal humerus: results after a mean follow-up of 2 years in a series of 18 patients. *J Shoulder Elbow Surg* 11:48-52, 2002.
   A good or excellent result was obtained in 56% of patients, including all patients younger than 40 years but only two of 10 patients older than 50 years. Stiffness was seen more frequently in men, those immobilized for more than 3 weeks, and with the triceps-splitting approach.

2. O'Driscoll SW, Sanchez-Sotelo J, Torchia ME: Management of the smashed distal humerus. *Orthop Clin North Am* 33:19-33, 2002.
   An excellent review of the technique of operative fixation of comminuted distal humerus fractures.

3. Gofton WT, MacDermid JC, Patterson SD, et al: Functional outcome of AO Type C distal humeral fractures. *J Hand Surg [Am]* 28:294-308, 2003.
   Reported 93% satisfactory results in 23 patients at mean 45-month follow-up but significantly poorer results in those with high levels of articular comminution.

4. McKee MD, Wilson TL, Winston L, et al: Functional outcome following surgical treatment of intra-articular distal humeral fractures through a posterior approach. *J Bone Joint Surg Am* 82:1701-1707, 2000.
   DASH and SF-36 scores revealed minor but significant impairment consistent with the loss of motion and weakness noted in these patients.

5. Ring D, Jupiter JB, Gulotta L: Articular fractures of the distal part of the humerus. *J Bone Joint Surg Am* 85:232-238, 2003.

This study evaluated 21 patients with capitellar or trochlear fractures fixed with implants buried beneath the articular cartilage. Motion averaged 96 degrees.

6. Helfet DL, Kloen P, Anand N, Rosen HS: Open reduction and internal fixation of delayed unions and nonunions of fractures of the distal part of the humerus. *J Bone Joint Surg Am* 85:34-40, 2003.
   The authors recommended extensive exposure, rigid fixation, bone grafting, judicious soft tissue release, and immediate mobilization for successful treatment of these complicated cases.

7. Gambirasio R, Riand N, Stern R, Hoffmeyer P: Total elbow replacement for complex fractures of the distal humerus. *J Bone Joint Surg Br* 83:974-978, 2001.
   The authors conclude that total elbow replacement is the treatment of choice for elderly patients with comminuted distal humerus fractures.

8. Garcia JA, Mykula R, Stanley D: Complex fractures of the distal humerus in the elderly: the role of total replacement as primary treatment. *J Bone Joint Surg Br* 84:812-816, 2002.
   This study supports the use of elbow replacement as a primary treatment of comminuted distal humerus fractures in elderly patients.

9. Ring D, Quintero J, Jupiter JB: Open reduction and internal fixation of fractures of the radial head. *J Bone Joint Surg Am* 84:1811-1815, 2002.
   Comminuted Mason type 3 fractures with more than three articular fragments have a high percentage of unsatisfactory results following ORIF, whereas those split into two to three fragments have a better prognosis.

10. Caputo AE, Mazzocca AD, Santoro VM: The nonarticulating portion of the radial head: anatomic and clinical correlations for internal fixation. *J Hand Surg [Am]* 23:1082-1090, 1998.
    The nonarticulating portion of the radial head subtends an average arc of 113 degrees and is the "safe zone" for hardware placement. It can be localized as the arc between the radial styloid and Lister's tubercle.

11. Harrington IJ, Sekyi-Otu A, Barrington TW, et al: The functional outcome with metallic radial head implants in the treatment of unstable elbow fractures: a long-term review. *J Trauma* 50:46-52, 2001.
    The radial head prosthesis restored elbow stability in the setting of a comminuted radial head fracture with a dislocated elbow, ruptured medial collateral ligament, fractured proximal ulna, or fracture of the coronoid process.

12. Fuchs S, Chylarecki C: Do functional deficits result from radial head resection? *J Shoulder Elbow Surg* 8:247-251, 1999.
    Clinical and isokinetic tests were superior for patients undergoing primary resection compared with those undergoing secondary resection.

13. Karlsson MK, Hasserius R, Karlsson C, et al: Fractures of the olecranon: a 15- to 25-year follow-up of 73 patients. *Clin Orthop* 403:205-212, 2002.
    Ninety-six percent of patients had an excellent or good outcome.

14. Karlsson MK, Hasserius R, Besjakov J, et al: Comparison of tension-band and figure-of-eight wiring techniques for treatment of olecranon fractures. *J Shoulder Elbow Surg* 11:377-382, 2002.
    No differences were found when the two techniques were compared, except for an 81% rate of hardware removal with tension band wiring compared to 43% with figure-of-eight wiring.

15. Bailey CS, MacDermid J, Patterson SD, King GJ: Outcome of plate fixation of olecranon fractures. *J Orthop Trauma* 15:542-548, 2001.
    Twenty-five patients underwent plate fixation for displaced olecranon fractures. The mean DASH score was consistent with almost normal upper extremity function.

16. Ring D, Jupiter JB, Sanders RW, et al: Transolecranon fracture-dislocation of the elbow. *J Orthop Trauma* 11:545-550, 1997.
    Large coronoid fragments and extensive comminution of the trochlear notch do not preclude a good result provided stable anatomic fixation is achieved.

17. Gartsman GM, Sculco TP, Otis JC: Operative treatment of olecranon fracture. Excision or open reduction with internal fixation. *J Bone Joint Surg* 63:718-721, 1981.
    No difference was noted with regard to pain, functional range of motion, elbow stability, degenerative changes, or biomechanical testing. The open reduction group had 13 local complications, and the excision group had only two.

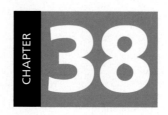

# Elbow Arthritis

## Steven H. Goldberg*, Mark S. Cohen†, and Leonid I. Katolik‡

*MD, Chief Resident, Department of Orthopaedic Surgery, Rush University Medical Center, Chicago, IL

†MD, Professor, Department of Orthopaedic Surgery; Director, Hand and Elbow Section; Director, Orthopaedic Education, Department of Orthopaedic Surgery, Rush University Medical Center, Chicago, IL

‡MD, Assistant Professor, Department of Orthopaedic Surgery, University of Washington, Seattle, WA

## Introduction

- Three primary patterns of arthritis affect the elbow: rheumatoid (inflammatory), posttraumatic, and primary osteoarthritis. Each occurs in different patient populations and with different presentations.
- The elbow has two main functions:
  1. Position the hand in space
  2. Stabilize the upper extremity for power and fine motor activities
- Clinical consequences of progressive arthritis (Box 38–1):
  - Pain that can result in further morbidity from disuse, exacerbating stiffness
  - Functional difficulty using the hand for activities of daily living. A 100-degree flexion/extension arc of motion from 30 to 130 degrees typically is quoted for normal activities. However, flexion is much more important than extension, as loss of extension can be compensated for by moving closer to an object. Functional forearm rotation is quoted as 100 degrees, with 50 degrees pronation and 50 degrees supination. However, supination is more important than pronation, which can be compensated for by shoulder abduction.[1]

## Rheumatoid Arthritis (Figure 38–1)

- Most frequent type
- Majority of cases are bilateral
- Immunologically mediated inflammatory disorder of synovial joints
- Elbow arthritis affects 20% to 50% patients with rheumatoid disease
- Women are affected three times more commonly than men
- Prolonged inflammation and synovitis can lead to secondary changes
  - Fixed joint contracture
  - Ligamentous attenuation
    - Ulnar collateral ligament incompetence can lead to valgus ulnohumeral instability and ulnar nerve dysfunction
    - Lateral collateral ligament incompetence can lead to posterolateral rotatory instability

---

### Box 38–1 Symptoms of Elbow Arthritis

- Pain with range of motion (flexion-extension or rotation)
- Stiffness with loss of flexion-extension and/or rotation
- Swelling or effusion, more common with inflammatory arthritis
- Neurologic symptoms or deficits, most commonly involving ulnar nerve
- Instability, more common with end-stage inflammatory arthritis

---

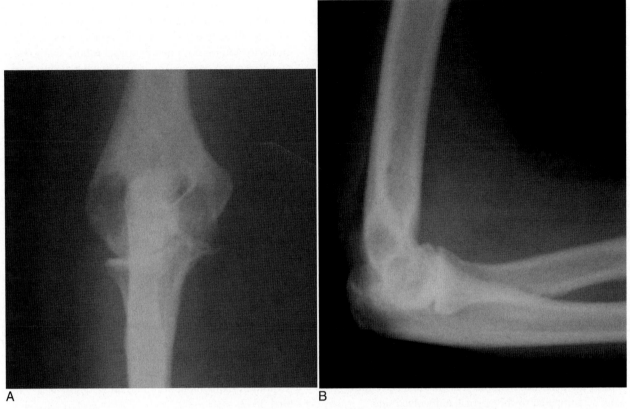

Figure 38–1:

**A,** Anteroposterior radiograph of an elbow with rheumatoid arthritis. Note the symmetric ulnohumeral and radiocapitellar complete loss of joint space, a large subchondral cyst in the lateral epicondyle, periarticular osteopenia, and absence of osteophytes. **B,** Lateral radiograph showing loss of ulnohumeral and radiocapitellar joint spaces with intussusception of the distal humerus into the greater sigmoid notch of the ulna because of bone loss of the coronoid and greater sigmoid notch. Note the olecranon osteopenia, normal radial head-capitellar alignment, and absence of osteophytes.

- ○ Annular ligament incompetence can lead to radial head subluxation
- ○ Combined ligamentous injury with bone loss leads to greater instability
- Cyst formation
  - ○ Results from proliferation of synovium (pannus)
  - ○ Predisposes to subarticular fracture
  - ○ Can cause compression of the ulnar and/or radial nerves

## Posttraumatic Arthritis

- The second most prevalent type of arthritis
- May affect any age group but more common in young and middle-aged individuals
- The elbow is one of the joints in the body most intolerant to trauma, with a high propensity for stiffness and arthritis following injury
- Prolonged immobilization following trauma may predispose to stiffness
- The primary complaint often is restricted motion

## Primary Osteoarthritis

- Least common and represents only 1% to 2% of patients presenting with degenerative arthritis[2]
- Most commonly seen in middle-aged and older patients
- Predilection for males
- More common in individuals exposed to repetitive manual labor
- Osteophyte formation at the tip of coronoid and the olecranon tip
- Radiocapitellar narrowing common and may be the "wear generator"
- Typically presents with pain at the end range of motion, mechanical block to flexion and extension, pain carrying an object with the arm in extension, often with mechanical symptoms of clicking and catching from loose bodies[2]

## Physical Examination

- It is important to perform a thorough evaluation of the cervical spine, shoulder, elbow, and wrist to determine if the patient's complaints are limited to the elbow or are more diffuse in nature. For example, isolated elbow involvement in rheumatoid arthritis is rare.[3] Associated wrist (distal radioulnar joint) pathology can contribute to loss of forearm rotation and affect axial radial stability if radial head excision is being considered. Limited shoulder abduction can prevent the ability to compensate for loss of pronation.

- Inspect the elbow for evidence of prior incisions, ecchymosis, or gross deformity.
- Effusion can be best appreciated by palpation of a "soft spot" at the center of an equilateral triangle formed by the olecranon, radial head, and lateral epicondyle.
- Radial head identification is facilitated by palpation during forearm rotation.
- Synovial thickening can be palpated medially and laterally as a boggy fullness along the joint line.
- Test active and passive range of motion with a goniometer. Normal elbow motion is 0 to 140 degrees, with 0 degrees defined as full elbow extension. Pronation and supination are measured with the arm at the side at 90 degrees elbow flexion. Normal is approximately 75 degrees pronation and 85 degrees supination. Some rotation can take place through the wrist. Placement of pens in the hand can help measure rotation. All values must be compared to the normal, uninvolved side.
- Careful neurologic assessment of sensory (normal static two-point discrimination is 5 mm or less) and motor function of the radial, posterior interosseous, ulnar, median, and anterior interosseous nerves should be performed.
- Provocative testing can elicit symptoms of ulnar neuropathy (Tinel percussion along the ulnar nerve at the elbow, the elbow flexion test with simultaneous manual ulnar nerve compression), radial tunnel syndrome (manual pressure directly over the mobile wad to compress the posterior interosseous nerve), carpal tunnel syndrome (median nerve compression test, Tinel percussion over the median nerve in the volar palm, Phalen maneuver), and tests for medial collateral and lateral collateral instability.

## Radiographic Assessment

- Anteroposterior, lateral, and oblique radiographs should be obtained at the initial evaluation. When full extension is not possible, the beam should not be centered on the antecubital crease. For distal humerus pathology, the beam is centered perpendicular to the distal humerus. For proximal forearm pathology, the beam is centered perpendicular to the radial head. The lateral view should be shot in 90 degrees flexion with the forearm in neutral rotation. A medial oblique view improves visualization of the trochlea, olecranon fossa, and coronoid tip. A lateral oblique view provides visualization of the radiocapitellar joint, medial epicondyle, radioulnar joint, and coronoid tubercle.
- Common radiographic findings are given in Box 38–2.
- Rheumatoid arthritis has a specific radiographic classification system (Table 38–1 and see Figure 38–1).
- Ultrasound and magnetic resonance imaging typically are unnecessary in the diagnosis and treatment of elbow arthritis.
- Computed tomography occasionally is needed in preoperative planning.

---

### Box 38–2   Common Radiographic Findings

1. Soft tissue swelling
   - Can indicate inflammation and subcutaneous rheumatoid nodules.
2. Visualization of fat pad
   - Signifies an effusion causing the fat pad to lift away from the bone. An anterior fat pad can be normally seen, but the presence of a posterior fat pad is abnormal because it normally sits deep in olecranon fossa.
3. Osteophytes
   - Often present on the coronoid and olecranon (best seen on lateral views) or the radial head.
4. Loose bodies
   - Often best seen on lateral view. Opacification of the fossa above the trochlea on anteroposterior view can suggest bony overgrowth or loose bodies.
5. Joint line narrowing
   - Assess the ulnohumeral and radiocapitellar joints. Asymmetry or gapping at the medial ulnohumeral joint can suggest medial collateral ligament incompetence.
6. Radial head position
   - Ensure the center of the radial head lines up with the capitellum on all views. Disruption of this relationship indicates radial head subluxation or, more commonly, posterolateral joint subluxation.
7. Bone quality
   - Note the presence of periarticular osteopenia, which is more common in rheumatoid arthritis.

| GRADE | DESCRIPTION |
|---|---|
| I | Periarticular osteopenia and soft tissue swelling associated with mild synovitis |
| II | Mild-to-moderate joint space narrowing without architectural distortion, usually associated with synovitis refractory to isolated NSAIDs |
| III | More advanced joint space narrowing with or without cyst formation, associated with architectural changes such as olecranon thinning or trochlear destruction<br>Synovitis may be present or burnt out |
| IV | Extensive articular damage with loss of subchondral bone and subluxation or ankylosis of joint |

**Table 38–1:   Mayo Clinic Classification of Disease Severity[21]**

## Nonsurgical Treatment (Box 38–3)

- Activity modification: Limit activities that exacerbate symptoms
- Nonsteroidal antiinflammatory drugs (NSAIDs)
  - Decrease synovial reactivity and alleviate pain and swelling in milder cases
  - Represents first-line treatment of all types of arthritis
- Immunosuppressive agents, such as gold salts, methotrexate, and antimalarial agents, are used for recalcitrant inflammatory arthritis. Serious side effects, including thrombocytopenia, hepatic or renal insufficiency, and pulmonary toxicity, complicate their use. Newer immunosuppressive agents, such as leflunomide and infliximab, are effective but may impair the patient's ability to mount a response to infection.
- Oral and intraarticular corticosteroid injections can be effective for acute episodes of painful synovitis and "flares" about the elbow. Elbow arthrocentesis or injection should be performed through the lateral soft spot described in the physical examination section.

### Box 38–3 | Treatment Options

**Nonoperative Treatment**
- Activity modification
- NSAIDs
- Disease-modifying agents in inflammatory arthritis (methotrexate, gold, leflunomide, infliximab)
- Steroids (oral vs. intraarticular)
- Splinting
- Ice/heat

**Operative Treatment**
- Ulnohumeral debridement
  - Open vs. arthroscopic
- Synovectomy
  - Open vs. arthroscopic
  - With/without radial head excision (inflammatory arthritis)
- Ulnohumeral interposition arthroplasty
- Total elbow arthroplasty
  - Semiconstrained
  - Unconstrained

- Static nighttime splinting can improve the range of motion early in the disease process.[4] Turnbuckle braces or, more commonly, patient-adjusted, static progressive splints can be used to improve range of motion.[5]
- Intermittent heat can loosen up muscles prior to exercise, with cold therapy used to limit swelling after exercise or during acute exacerbations.

## Surgical Treatment

- *Indications:* Failed response to appropriate nonsurgical management with functional limitations because of pain or loss of motion and patients who will be compliant with postoperative rehabilitation.
- The following surgical procedures represent a spectrum, from joint debridement and soft tissue release to elbow replacement (see Box 38–3).

### Ulnohumeral Debridement

- *Indications*[6,7]: Most commonly used for osteoarthritis and posttraumatic arthritis with soft tissue contracture, impingement in flexion and/or extension, and mechanical symptoms. A normal central ulnohumeral joint is required. The goal is to remove any soft tissue or bony constraints to flexion, extension, or rotation (Figures 38–2 and 38–3).

### Open Technique

- Open options include either lateral and/or medial column approaches.[7,8]
- Anesthesia with axillary block is preferred.
- Positioning supine with arm table.
- Midline posterior incision allows access to both medial and lateral arthrotomies and exposure of ulnar nerve if transposition is necessary.
- Alternatively, medial and lateral approaches can be used.

### Lateral Column Procedure (Lateral Collateral Ligament Complex Preserved)[7]

- Can use midline posterior or lateral incision.
- Fasciocutaneous flaps are elevated.
- Starting proximally, the lateral supracondylar ridge is palpated.

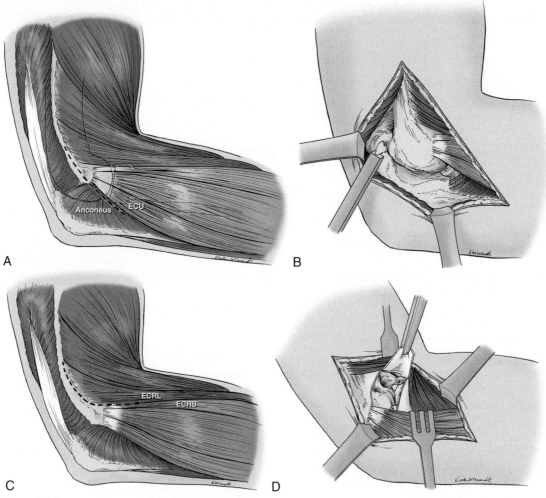

Figure 38–2:

Lateral view of the elbow. **A,** *Dotted line* shows incision from supracondylar ridge proximally to the anconeus–extensor carpi ulnaris (ECU) interval. **B,** Retraction of anconeus posteriorly and ECU anteriorly allows visualization of the posterior ulnohumeral joint. The olecranon tip is removed with an osteotome. **C,** *Dotted line* shows incision extending from supracondylar ridge proximally to the interval between extensor carpi radialis longus (ECRL) and extensor carpi radialis brevis (ECRB) distally. **D,** Retraction of ECRL anteriorly and ECRB posteriorly allows exposure of the anterior ulnohumeral and radiocapitellar joints.

- The triceps and anconeus are elevated and reflected posteriorly, exposing the posterior ulnohumeral joint (see Figure 38–2, *A).*
- Triceps tenolysis is performed, the olecranon fossa cleaned, and spurs and loose bodies removed (see Figure 38–2, *B).*
- The anterior joint is exposed by first sliding along the lateral humeral supracondylar ridge above the epicondyle and splitting distally between the extensor carpi radialis longus (ECRL) muscle anteriorly and the remaining extensor origin covered by fascia posteriorly. The deep dissection is between the ECRL and the extensor carpi radialis brevis, which is tendinous and lies deep to the ECRL (see Figure 38–2, *C).*

- The joint capsule is exposed by elevating the brachialis (blunt Metzenbaum scissors are helpful to avoid entering the joint prior to isolating the entire capsule).
- The capsule is excised, the anterior coronoid and radial fossae cleaned, and spurs and loose bodies removed (see Figures 38–2, *D* and 38–3, *A).*
- The Y-shaped split in the lateral fascia is repaired with no violation of the lateral ligament complex.

## Medial Column Approach (Medial Collateral Ligament Preserved)[8]

- Find and protect the medial antebrachial cutaneous nerves.

Figure 38–3:
Ulnohumeral debridement. Loss of motion can occur secondary to soft tissue contracture or bony impingement. **A,** Improved extension is obtained by anterior capsulectomy, brachialis tenolysis, removal of soft tissue and bony overgrowth in the olecranon fossa. and excision of olecranon tip osteophytes. **B,** Improved flexion is obtained by posterior capsular release, triceps tenolysis, removal of soft tissue and bony overgrowth within the coronoid and radial head fossae, and debridement of coronoid or radial head osteophytes.

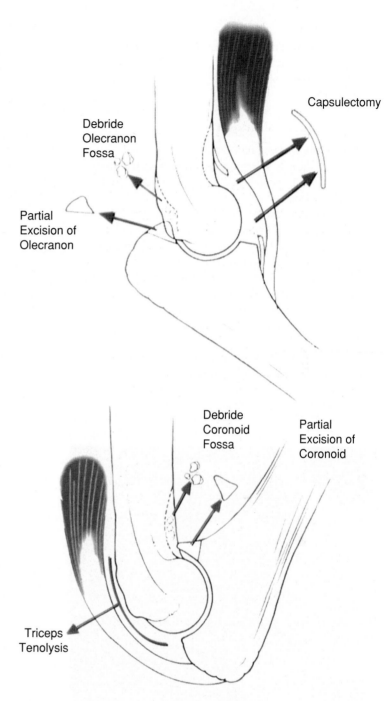

- Mobilize the ulnar nerve and free it proximally and distally.
- Expose the medial intermuscular septum and origin of the flexor-pronator muscle mass.
- The intermuscular septum is used to help reflect the triceps posteriorly.
- The posterior ulnohumeral joint is debrided of soft tissue and any olecranon tip and fossa osteophytes are removed.
- From the intramuscular septum, slide along the anterior humerus, reflecting the brachialis anteriorly. Distally, the flexor-pronator is split and elevated anteriorly, exposing the anterior joint capsule. The medial collateral ligament is protected beneath the posterior flexor-pronator muscle.
- The brachialis is retracted anteriorly and the joint capsule excised.
- Soft tissue is debrided from the coronoid and radial head fossae and osteophytes are removed.
- Reattach the flexor-pronator tendinous origin.
- The ulnar nerve is transposed anteriorly into a subcutaneous position.

## Open Outcome

- Good to excellent pain relief up to 36 months after open procedures[7,9]
- Range of motion averages 8 to 137 degrees after open release[7]

## Arthroscopic Technique

- Much more challenging
- Usually indicated in less severe contractures because risk of neural injury is increased secondary to decreased capsular volume
- Patient position can be:
  - Supine: requires overhead traction, which can limit elbow manipulation, or an assistant to hold the arm; has limited access to the posterior joint.
  - Prone: improved access to the posterior joint, easier to manipulate elbow, no traction needed.
  - Lateral decubitus: easier to position, improved airway access for anesthesia (Figure 38–4).
- Equipment:
  - 4-mm, 30-degree arthroscope (2.7-mm arthroscope may be needed in small contracted joints)
  - Coban to wrap hand and forearm to limit fluid extravasation and swelling

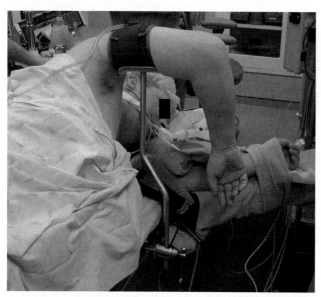

Figure 38–4:

**Arthroscopy positioning with patient in the lateral decubitus position. A bean bag is placed beneath the sheets to help maintain the patient's position. A tourniquet is placed on the arm, and the arm is placed over a bolster. Note the bolster is proximally located on the arm, leaving the distal brachium without any anterior pressure or contact. This position prevents compression of the anterior soft tissues against the humerus, facilitating portal placement and minimizing neural injury. The anesthesiologist has improved access to the airway compared with the prone position.**

- 18-gauge spinal needle to insufflate joint with 15 to 25 ml saline, cannulas with no side fenestrations to prevent soft tissue extravasation, mechanical shaver and radiofrequency ablation device for soft tissue debridement, power burr for bony debridement, retractors to improve visualization, switching sticks to facilitate changing portals
- Portals (Figure 38–5):
  - Scalpel used to incise through skin only, followed by blunt dissection with a hemostat to the capsule, then blunt trocars used to enter the joint
  - Proximal medial
    - 2 cm proximal to the medial epicondyle just anterior to the medial intermuscular septum; ulnar nerve the located posterior to septum
    - Can visualize the entire anterior joint
    - Contraindication to this portal is prior anterior transposition of ulnar nerve
    - Posterior branch of the medial antebrachial cutaneous nerve is at highest risk for injury
  - Proximal lateral (proximal anterolateral)
    - 2 cm proximal and 1 cm anterior to the lateral epicondyle
    - Can visualize the entire anterior joint
    - Posterior branch of the lateral antebrachial cutaneous nerve is at highest risk for injury
  - Anterolateral
    - Several locations described
    - Preferred location is between the radial head and capitellum 1 cm anterior and 1 cm distal to the lateral epicondyle
    - Radial nerve at risk
  - Direct lateral
    - "Soft spot" at center of triangle formed by olecranon, lateral epicondyle, and radial head
    - Can visualize the inferior radial head, capitellum, and radioulnar joint
    - At the beginning of the procedure, insufflate the joint with saline through this portal and remove the needle. If this portal is needed for visualization or work, use it at the end of the procedure because of an increased incidence of fluid extravasation.
  - Anteromedial
    - 2 cm distal and 2 cm anterior to the medial epicondyle
    - Medial antebrachial cutaneous nerve at risk
    - Consider using inside-out technique to create portal
  - Posterolateral
    - 3 cm proximal to olecranon tip and lateral to the edge of the triceps tendon
    - Make portal with elbow in 45 degrees flexion to relax posterior capsule and triceps
    - Can visualize the tip of the olecranon, olecranon fossa, and medial and lateral gutters

- Straight posterior
  - 3 cm proximal to the olecranon tip through the triceps in center of tendon
- Radial nerve at risk during anterior capsulectomy near anterolateral portal
- Ulnar nerve at risk during posteromedial debridement
- Methods to decrease injury:
  - Flex elbow to 90 degrees during anterior portal placement to release tension on the anterior capsule and nerves.

- Distend joint with 15 to 25 ml saline injected through lateral soft spot to displace the capsule and nerves during portal placement.
- Using retractors during debridement can maintain capsule and nerve displacement.
- Debride synovium, osteophytes, and loose bodies first and remove capsule last to decrease risk of fluid extravasation and swelling.
- Arthroscopic outcome (Figure 38–6):

Figure 38–5:
**Commonly used elbow arthroscopy portals. A,** Medial portals. **B,** Lateral portals.

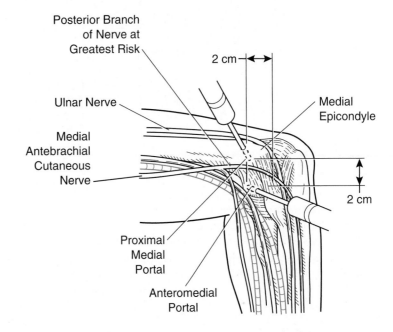

A

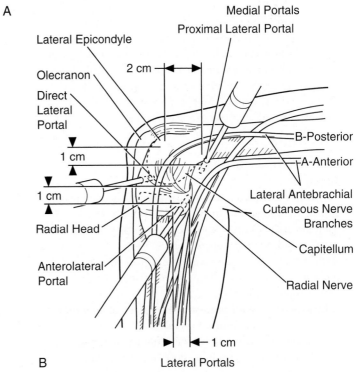

B

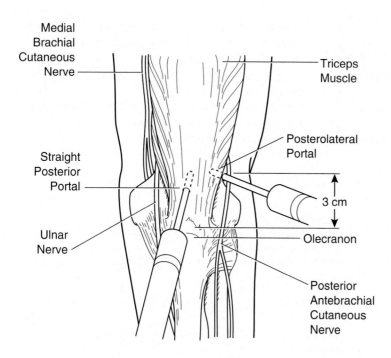

Medial Brachial Cutaneous Nerve

Triceps Muscle

Posterolateral Portal

Straight Posterior Portal

3 cm

Ulnar Nerve

Olecranon

Posterior Antebrachial Cutaneous Nerve

C          Posterior Portals

Figure 38–5: cont'd
**C, Posterior portals.**

- 80% regain functional arc of motion; 10% are within 5 to 10 degrees of full motion.[10]
- The ulnar nerve must be evaluated prior to open or arthroscopic procedures. In the presence of limited flexion (extension contracture), ulnar nerve symptoms, or sensitivity to percussion, decompression and transposition are recommended.

### Rehabilitation

- Restoration of motion typically is excellent but requires an extensive rehabilitation program, including continuous passive motion starting immediately postoperatively in the recovery room and continued at home for several weeks. Formal therapy begins on postoperative day 1 and includes edema control, weighted wrist stretches, and patient-adjusted, static progressive bracing.

### Complications

- Wounds (hematoma, seroma, ischemia)
- Infection
- Neuritis is minimized if the ulnar nerve is decompressed and/or transposed in patients with less than approximately 90 to 115 degrees flexion or with any nerve tension signs preoperatively.
- Arthroscopy is associated with a higher incidence of multiple nerve injuries during portal placement.
- Heterotopic ossification:
  - Increased risk with open surgery, history of heterotopic bone, or multiple surgical insults.
  - Consider several weeks of oral indomethacin (Indocin) sustained release or a single dose of radiation on

postoperative day 1 if heterotopic bone formation is of concern.

## Synovectomy

### Indications

- As a palliative procedure to reduce pain in inflammatory arthritis in early disease (Mayo I or II) with preservation of articular surfaces and subchondral bone.
- Some studies suggest efficacy in more radiographically advanced stages.[11,12]

### Open

- The open technique is the gold standard for synovectomy.
- Can approach joint through medial or lateral column approaches described in the ulnohumeral debridement section.
- *Possible disadvantage:* increased potential for wound problems.
- Outcomes:
  - Up to 90% excellent pain relief in the first 2 to 5 years after surgery.
  - Late results demonstrate deterioration over time, with success rates falling to 60% at 5 to 10 years.[11–13]
  - No significant change in range of motion.
  - Largest study reviewed 171 rheumatoid elbows with synovectomy and radial head excision.[11] Failure was defined by the need for revision surgery or significant pain. The study reported a 1-year survival rate of 81%, 6.5-year survival rate of 45%, and deterioration rate of

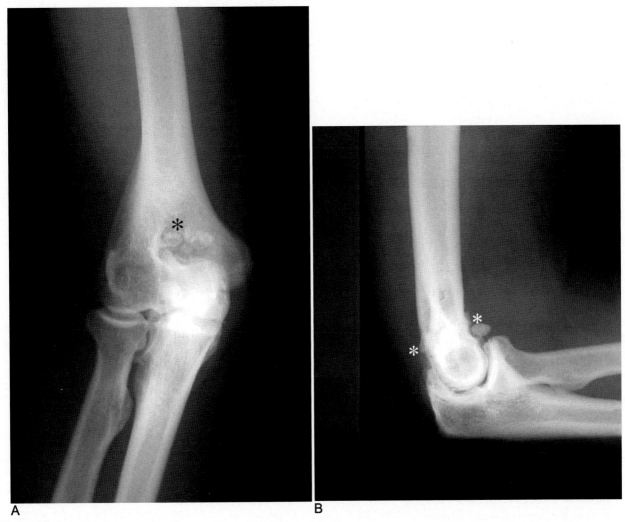

**Figure 38–6:**
**A,** Anteroposterior radiograph showing osteoarthritis with mild ulnohumeral joint space narrowing and presence of loose bodies *(asterisk)* in either the coronoid or olecranon fossa. **B,** Lateral radiograph showing radiocapitellar joint space narrowing and presence of loose bodies *(asterisks)* in both the coronoid and olecranon fossae.

3% per year. The strongest predictor of success was greater than 50% limitation of forearm rotation preoperatively. There was no association between radiographic severity and outcome. Failure correlated with recurrent synovitis (43%), instability, limitation of flexion-extension less than 60 degrees, prolonged preoperative symptoms, ulnar neuritis, and poor upper extremity function.

## Arthroscopic Synovectomy

- Equipment, positioning, portals as described in the section on ulnohumeral debridement.
- Offers potential for decreased morbidity and faster rehabilitation.[6]
- *Disadvantages:* With disease progression, alteration of bony and soft tissue landmarks makes spatial orientation during arthroscopy difficult. Capsular contracture leads to decreased working space and more limited visualization. Increased risk to neurovascular structures.[2]

- *Outcomes:* Greater than 76% to 90% good and excellent pain relief for 3 to 4 years, after which pain and recurrent synovitis can recur with no improvement in range of motion.[14,15]

## Concomitant Radial Head Excision

- Can be performed open or arthroscopically but is controversial, with trend toward radial head preservation unless pain with forearm rotation is a major symptom.
- *Advantages:* Elimination of a painful contact area between the head and humeral capitellum. May improve forearm rotation.
- *Disadvantages:* The radial head is an important secondary stabilizer to valgus load.[16] Resection can lead to valgus instability of the elbow and accelerate ulnohumeral arthritis if the medial collateral ligament is attenuated.[17]
- *Rehabilitation:* Typically less intensive therapy is required than after complete ulnohumeral debridement, but all modalities described in the section on ulnohumeral

debridement can be used as necessary. Begin early active and passive motion and edema control. Continuous passive motion typically is not necessary.

## Interposition Arthroplasty

- Involves debridement and "resurfacing" of the joint articulation with a layer of soft tissue.
- *Indications:*
  - Ideal candidate is a young, active patient with severe posttraumatic arthritis associated with severe pain and limited motion.
  - Patient is too young or active for total joint arthroplasty.[18]
- *Contraindications:*
  - Significant joint destruction with gross loss of architecture
  - Active infection
  - Gross joint instability
  - Need for elbow to assist in transfers/weight bearing, because excessive loading leads to destabilization[18]
  - Inflammatory arthritis resulting from progressive disease
- Resurfacing materials include autologous fascia lata from the thigh, autologous skin, and more commonly allograft soft tissue. Preferred allograft is the Achilles tendon because of its availability, size, and the ability to use part of it for concomitant ligament reconstruction.[18]
- Surgical technique[18]:
  - Supine position.
  - Posterior midline skin incision to expose the ulnar nerve.
  - Lateral extensile Kocher approach through the anconeus–extensor carpi ulnaris interval.
  - Release the lateral collateral ligament.
  - Excise the anterior and posterior capsule.
  - Preserve the radial head if possible.
  - Remove a small amount of bone from the greater sigmoid notch, trochlea, and capitellum to accommodate the tendon graft and create concentric, fluid joint motion.
  - Place drills holes from posterior to anterior in the distal humerus to pass sutures that will secure the graft to bone.
  - The achilles tendon graft is contoured to the size of the distal humerus and then draped over the trochlea and capitellum, and sutures placed through the bone to secure the graft.
  - Excess graft can be used to reconstruct lateral collateral and ulnar collateral ligaments through bone tunnels.
  - The tourniquet is released and hemostasis achieved.
  - A hinged external fixator is applied.
  - The triceps is reattached through drill holes in the olecranon.
  - Kocher's interval is closed.
- *Rehabilitation:* Motion is started early, with possible use of continuous passive motion. The fixator is removed under

anesthesia with examination to determine motion and stability. Gentle manipulation is performed as needed. Progressive static splinting is applied for residual stiffness.
- *Outcome:* 35 rheumatoid elbows with an average follow-up of 6 years. Outcome was rated fair for joint mobility and joint stability but good for pain relief. Radiographic destruction progressed in half of all elbows, with bone loss making reoperation difficult or impossible. The authors recommend total elbow replacement as the first choice in the surgical treatment of advanced rheumatoid arthritis.[19]
- *Complications:*
  - Bone resorption
  - Continued pain, stiffness, instability
  - Heterotopic bone formation
  - Triceps rupture
  - Infection
  - Deterioration in results over time

## Total Elbow Arthroplasty

- *Indications:* rheumatoid, posttraumatic, or primary arthritis with advanced symptoms and radiographic destruction after failed medical or less aggressive surgical treatment. The patient must agree to postoperative limitations of no lifting more than approximately 5 to 10 lb and no repetitive lifting of any object more than 2 to 3 lb to limit the risk of early failure.
- *Contraindications:*
  - Sepsis
  - Need for soft tissue coverage
  - Severe muscle weakness or paralysis
  - Noncompliant patient
- *Types:*
  - Constrained (historical)
    - Linked prosthesis with high incidence of loosening of 24% at 4 years because of excessive load transfer to the bone–cement interface[20]
  - Semiconstrained (Figure 38–7)
    - "Sloppy" hinged prosthesis with metal and polyethylene articulation that allows limited rotational and varus/valgus motion between humeral and ulnar components to decrease the bone–cement interface loading. However, stress concentration at the hinge can lead to polyethylene wear, debris, osteolysis, and component loosening. Newer designs have been developed in an effort to decrease stress transfer at the joint articulation and diminish these problems. Clinical results are pending.
    - *Outcome:*
      - Variable because of different indications, multiple different prostheses, and multiple generations within individual prostheses.
      - Significant pain relief reported in 76% to 92%.[3,20]
      - Improved final arc of flexion-extension of 29 to 131 degrees.[20]

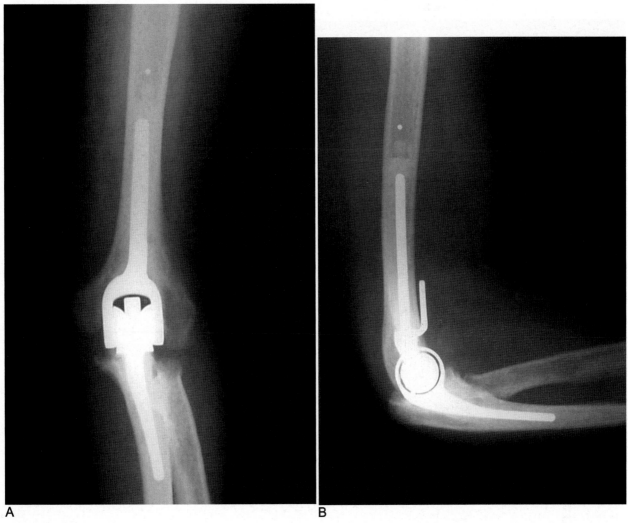

Figure 38–7:
**Anteroposterior (A) and lateral (B) radiographs of a semiconstrained total elbow arthroplasty.**

- Results of total elbow replacement in 45 elbows of 38 patients with rheumatoid arthritis compared with results of radial head excision with synovectomy in 45 age-matched patients showed better pain reduction and higher complications after replacement, with no differences in motion.
  - *Complications:*
    - Radiographic loosening up to 8%[3]
    - Revision for loosening 3% to 15%[20,21]
    - Postoperative neuropathy 14%[20]
    - Overall minor and major complication rate up to 55%[20]
- Unconstrained (Figure 38–8)
  - No linkage between the humeral and ulnar components with a metal on polyethylene articulation. Relies on ligaments and muscles for joint stability. Theoretically decreases loosening at the bone–cement

interface with greater longevity (not proven). Carries a greater risk for instability, especially in the rheumatoid population. Newer designs have the ability to be inserted semiconstrained or unlinked. Clinical data are pending.
  - *Outcome:*
    - Variability because of different indications, multiple different prostheses, and multiple modifications within individual prostheses
    - Significant pain relief reported in 79% to 94%[22,23]
    - Improved final arc of flexion-extension of 32 to 136 degrees[24]
  - *Complications:*
    - Radiographic loosening 0% to 70%[25,26]
    - Instability 2% to 29%[23,26,27]
    - Revision for loosening or instability 0% to 11%[25,26]
    - Complication rate up to 80%[3]

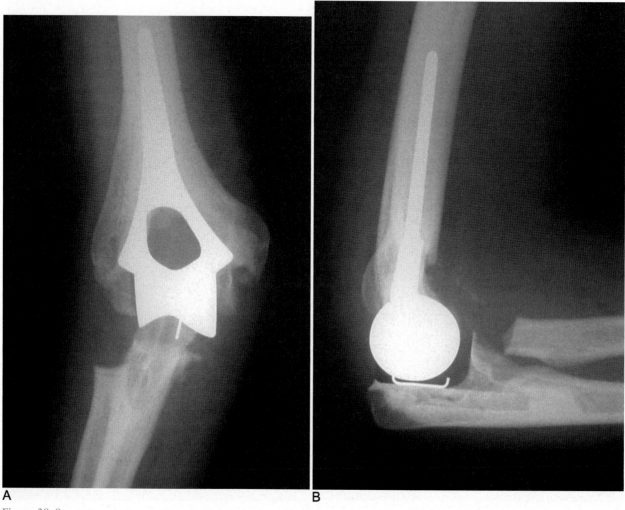

Figure 38–8:

**Anteroposterior (A) and lateral (B) radiographs of an unconstrained total elbow arthroplasty.**

- Surgical technique:
  - Lateral decubitus position with body supported by bean bag and bony prominences padded
  - Posterior midline incision
  - Ulnar nerve mobilized and transposed and protected throughout procedure
  - Triceps reflecting approach from medial to lateral most commonly used to expose the joint
  - Alternatives are the triceps midline split and the triceps preserving approach, which involves release of the entire flexor-pronator and extensor origins, allowing the humerus to be delivered medial and lateral to the triceps insertion on the ulna
  - The tip of the olecranon is resected and the elbow is hyperflexed to expose the trochlea
  - The radial head is resected if required
  - The humeral and ulnar canals are entered with a burr and enlarged with rasps
  - Trial prostheses are placed and motion and stability checked, then the trials are removed

- The canals are irrigated with pulsatile lavage and then dried to remove marrow contents
  - Cement plugs are placed in the humeral and ulnar canals to limit cement within the canal, allow pressurization, and improve the cement mantle
  - The polymethylmethacrylate is often mixed with antibiotics and the canals are filled in retrograde fashion with long, flexible tubing attached to the injection gun
  - The components are placed and the cement allowed to harden
  - The triceps is meticulously repaired
- *Rehabilitation:*
  - Short-term immobilization in a posterior long arm splint to protect the skin closure
  - No lifting over 10 lb as a single event or 2 lb repeatedly
  - Usually minimal formal therapy needed
  - A night elbow extension splint in maximum extension can be helpful in limiting flexion contracture

# References

1. Morrey BF, Askew LJ, Chao EY: A biomechanical study of normal functional elbow motion. *J Bone Joint Surg Am* 63:872-877, 1981.
   Most activities of daily living can be accomplished with 100 degrees elbow flexion (from 30–130 degrees) and 100 degrees forearm rotation (50 degrees pronation and 50 degrees supination).

2. Norberg FB, Savoie FH 3rd, Field LD: Arthroscopic treatment of arthritis of the elbow. *Instr Course Lect* 49:247-253, 2000.
   A review of arthroscopy and elbow arthritis.

3. Kauffman JI, Chen AL, Stuchin S, Di Cesare PE: Surgical management of the rheumatoid elbow. *J Am Acad Orthop Surg* 11:100-108, 2003.
   Review article discussing primarily synovectomy and total elbow arthroplasty.

4. Bonutti PM, Windau JE, Ables BA, Miller BG: Static progressive stretch to reestablish elbow range of motion. *Clin Orthop* 303:128-134, 1994.
   Patient-controlled static progressive stretch using a new orthosis led to a mean 31-degree increase in motion, with all patients expressing satisfaction.

5. Green DP, McCoy H: Turnbuckle orthotic correction of elbow-flexion contractures after acute injuries. *J Bone Joint Surg Am* 61:1092-1095, 1979.
   Fifteen patients with flexion contractures were treated with a turnbuckle splint. The average improvement in motion was 43 degrees after 20 weeks.

6. Ramsey ML: Elbow arthroscopy: basic setup and treatment of arthritis. *Instr Course Lect* 51:69-72, 2002.
   This article summaries arthroscopy setup, portal placement, and the treatment of arthritis.

7. Cohen MS, Hastings H 2nd: Operative release for elbow contracture: the lateral collateral ligament sparing technique. *Orthop Clin North Am* 30:133-139, 1999.
   This technique of elbow release and debridement uses a lateral approach designed to spare the lateral collateral ligament complex and extensor tendon origins of the elbow.

8. Mansat P, Morrey BF, Hotchkiss RN: Extrinsic contracture: "the column procedure": lateral and medial capsular releases. In Morrey BF, editor: *The elbow and its disorders*. ed 3. Philadelphia, 2000, WB Saunders.

9. Ogilvie-Harris DJ, Gordon R, MacKay M: Arthroscopic treatment for posterior impingement in degenerative arthritis of the elbow. *Arthroscopy* 11:437-443, 1995.
   Reports 100% good or excellent results for arthroscopic treatment of posterior impingement associated with degenerative elbow arthritis at 35 month follow-up.

10. O'Driscoll SW: Elbow reconstruction. In Kasser JR, editor: *Orthopaedic knowledge update 5: home study syllabus*. Rosemont, 1996, American Academy of Orthopaedic Surgeons.

11. Gendi NS, Axon JM, Carr AJ, et al: Synovectomy of the elbow and radial head excision in rheumatoid arthritis. Predictive factors and long-term outcome. *J Bone Joint Surg Br* 79:918-923, 1997.
    Survival analysis of elbow synovectomy and radial head excision performed on 171 rheumatoid elbows was 81% at 1 year, which decreased by an average of 3% per year.

12. Tulp NJ, Winia WP: Synovectomy of the elbow in rheumatoid arthritis. Long-term results. *J Bone Joint Surg Br* 71:664-666, 1989.
    At a mean follow-up of 6.5 years, 70% of elbow synovectomies were satisfactory, with no significant difference in the results based on preoperative radiological destruction.

13. Maenpaa HM, Kuusela PP, Kaarela K, et al: Reoperation rate after elbow synovectomy in rheumatoid arthritis. *J Shoulder Elbow Surg* 12:480-483, 2003.
    Reports complete pain relief in 44%, with excellent or good outcomes in 72% following synovectomy for Juvenile rheumatoid arthritis. The cumulative survival rate was 84% at 5 years. There was no significant improvement in functional ability or range of motion.

14. Horiuchi K, Momohara S, Tomatsu T et al: Arthroscopic synovectomy of the elbow in rheumatoid arthritis. *J Bone Joint Surg Am* 84A:342-347, 2002.
    Concludes that arthroscopic synovectomy is a reliable procedure that can alleviate pain, particularly in patients with mild preoperative radiographic changes.

15. Lee BP, Morrey BF: Arthroscopic synovectomy of the elbow for rheumatoid arthritis. A prospective study. *J Bone Joint Surg Br* 79:770-772, 1997.
    Although 93% had short-term good or excellent results, at 42 months only 57% maintained these results, which deteriorated more rapidly than following open synovectomy.

16. Morrey BF, Chao EY, Hui FC: Biomechanical study of the elbow following excision of the radial head. *J Bone Joint Surg Am* 61:63-68, 1979.
    Radial head excision for fracture led to 1.9 mm of proximal migration of the radius. Overall, the patients did well, and no deterioration of results occurred with time.

17. Rymaszewski LA, Mackay I, Amis AA, Miller JH: Long-term effects of excision of the radial head in rheumatoid arthritis. *J Bone Joint Surg Br* 66:109-113, 1984.
    Notes a common pattern of deterioration from what was often a satisfactory initial result, and recommends retention or replacement of the radial head.

18. Morrey BF: Nonreplacement reconstruction of the elbow joint. *Instr Course Lect* 51:63-67, 1984.
    Review of interposition arthroplasty.

19. Ljung P, Jonsson K, Larsson K, Rydholm U: Interposition arthroplasty of the elbow with rheumatoid arthritis. *J Shoulder Elbow Surg* 5:81-85, 1996.
    At 6-year follow-up, pain relief was good, but joint mobility and stability were only fair. Radiographic elbow destruction progressed in half. The authors recommend TEA instead.

20. Morrey BF, Bryan RS, Dobyns JH, Linscheid RL: Total elbow arthroplasty. A five-year experience at the Mayo Clinic. *J Bone Joint Surg Am* 63:1050-1063, 1981.
    Reports 60% good, 16% fair, and 24% poor results. Pain relief was excellent, and both flexion-extension and supination-

pronation improved. Revisions were performed in 24 percent, mainly because of loosening or deep infection.

21. Morrey BF, Adams RA: Semiconstrained arthroplasty for the treatment of rheumatoid arthritis of the elbow. *J Bone Joint Surg Am* 74:479-490, 1992.
    At 3.8-year follow-up, there was little or no pain in 53 of 58. Motion was improved. They noted no loosening, but a 22% rate of complications was reported.

22. Sjoden GO, Lundberg A, Blomgren GA: Late results of the Souter-Strathclyde total elbow prosthesis in rheumatoid arthritis. 6/19 implants loose after 5 years. *Acta Orthop Scand* 66:391-394, 1995.
    Although pain relief was initially achieved in all patients, at 5-year follow-up six prostheses had radiographic loosening and two patients had symptomatic loosening.

23. Weiland AJ, Weiss AP, Wills RP, Moore JR: Capitellocondylar total elbow replacement. A long-term follow-up study. *J Bone Joint Surg Am* 71:217-222, 1989.
    Pronation, supination, and flexion improved considerably, but improvement in extension was limited. Malarticulation or dislocation occurred in 25%. 25% had asymptomatic radiolucent lines.

24. Trancik T, Wilde AH, Borden LS: Capitellocondylar total elbow arthroplasty. Two- to eight-year experience. *Clin Orthop* 223:175-180, 1987.
    Reported pain relief in 34 of 35 at 5.6-year follow-up. Range of motion increased in all planes except extension. There was a 57% complication rate but no unstable elbows.

25. Davis RF, Weiland AJ, Hungerford DS et al: Nonconstrained total elbow arthroplasty. *Clin Orthop* 171:156-160, 1982.
    Report improved pain and range of motion for 30 capitellocondylar arthroplasties at 39.9-month follow-up. Deep wound infections occurred in 6.6%. Subluxation, which responded to treatment with long-arm casting, occurred in 13.2%.

26. Kudo H, Iwano K: Total elbow arthroplasty with a non-constrained surface-replacement prosthesis in patients who have rheumatoid arthritis. A long-term follow-up study. *J Bone Joint Surg Am* 72:355-362, 1990.
    Report 29 good, 1 fair, and 7 poor results at 9.5-year follow-up. Poor results most commonly were caused by posterior displacement of the humeral component, which subsided in 70%. Ulnar component loosening occurred in 5%. A humeral component with an intramedullary stem was recommended.

27. Trail IA, Nuttall D, Stanley JK: Survivorship and radiological analysis of the standard Souter-Strathclyde total elbow arthroplasty. *J Bone Joint Surg Br* 81:80-84, 1999.
    Twelve-year survivorship was 87% with revision as the endpoint. If the endpoint was revision or a 1-mm circumferential lucency, survivorship fell to 80%.

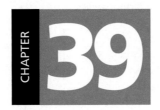

CHAPTER

# 39

# Humeral Shaft Fractures

Lisa A. Taitsman* and David P. Barei†

*MD, MPH, Assistant Professor, Department of Orthopaedics and Sports Medicine, University of Washington; Attending Surgeon, Department of Orthopaedics, Harborview Medical Center, Seattle, WA
†MD, FRCSC, Assistant Professor, Department of Orthopaedics and Sports Medicine, University of Washington, Harborview Medical Center, Seattle, WA

## Introduction

- Humeral shaft fractures compose approximately 3% to 5% of all fractures.
- Humeral shaft fractures can be isolated injuries or one of many fractures in a polytraumatized patient.
- Most humeral shaft fractures do not require operative intervention.

## Anatomy

- The humeral diaphysis is the segment of the humerus extending from the proximal aspect of the pectoralis major insertion to the supracondylar ridge.
- Functionally there are two compartments in the arm: anterior and posterior. The biceps, coracobrachialis, brachioradialis, and brachialis are the muscles of the anterior compartment. The triceps is the sole muscle of the posterior compartment. It is composed of a long head, lateral head, and medial head. The lateral and medial heads take origin from the posterior humeral shaft proximal and distal to the spiral groove, respectively.
- The median, ulnar, and musculocutaneous nerves are located in the anterior compartment. Unlike the radial nerve, they are rarely injured by nonpenetrating trauma.
- The radial nerve is located in the posterior compartment and courses immediately adjacent to the posterior aspect of the humerus in the spiral groove. As it travels diagonally across the humerus, it courses 20 cm proximal

to the medial epicondyle and 14 cm proximal to the lateral epicondyle.[1] The nerve remains along the posterior humerus and pierces the intermuscular septum approximately 10 cm proximal to the distal humeral articular surface.[1,2,3]

- The incidence of radial nerve palsy associated with humeral shaft fractures reportedly is 15% to 20%,[4,5,6] with midshaft fractures accounting for the majority.[4,5,7]
- The brachial artery provides the predominant arterial supply for the arm. The first major branch is the profunda brachii artery. Distally the brachial artery splits to form the radial and ulnar arteries. The anterior humeral circumflex artery is a branch of the axillary artery and provides the majority of the blood supply to the humeral head. The posterior humeral circumflex artery travels with the axillary nerve under the deltoid through the quadrangular space.
- Fracture displacement is partly dependent upon the location of the fracture relative to the origin and insertion of the major muscle groups about the humeral shaft. The pectoralis major and deltoid muscles are the major deforming forces that involve the proximal half of the humerus. The pull of the biceps and triceps may result in additional angulation and fracture shortening.

## Physical Examination

- Circumferential inspection of the skin identifies abrasions, contusions, and open wounds.

- Detailed neurologic examination of the arm is essential. Motor and sensory evaluation of the median, ulnar, axillary, and radial nerves should be performed and documented. Particular care should be directed toward identifying and documenting any injury to the radial nerve, given the frequent coexistence of radial nerve injuries and humeral shaft fractures.
- Arterial injuries are not common but they do occur. Pulses must be palpated. Excessive swelling must be critically assessed for occult arterial injury.

## Radiographic Examination

- Orthogonal radiographs (anteroposterior and lateral) are obtained. Both the shoulder and elbow joints should be imaged to rule out associated fractures.
- Occasionally traction views are useful, particularly for evaluating comminuted fractures in the supracondylar region.
- Angiography may be indicated if vascular injury is suspected.
- Computed tomographic scanning or magnetic resonance imaging are rarely indicated in the initial evaluation of these injuries.

## Classification

- No universally accepted classification system is used to describe humeral shaft fractures. In the AO classification scheme, type A fractures are simple fractures with spiral, oblique, or transverse characteristics; type B fractures have an associated "wedge" fragment; and type C fractures are significantly comminuted/segmental (Figure 39–1).
- More commonly, however, humeral shaft fractures are classified in descriptive terms, such as fracture location and characteristics.
- Holstein and Lewis identified a unique spiral fracture pattern of the distal third of the humerus, commonly referred to as a *Holstein-Lewis fracture*. In their case series, the authors demonstrated a high incidence of radial nerve palsies associated with these fractures.[8] However, others have demonstrated that the most common region associated with radial nerve palsy remains the mid-diaphysis.[5]

## Treatment

- The vast majority of isolated humeral shaft fractures are amenable to nonoperative management (Figure 39–2).

### Nonoperative Treatment

- Initially, patients are placed in a coaptation splint and collar-and-cuff immobilization.[9] Oddly enough, the most challenging patients can be the ones with a simple transverse fracture with distraction. A high percentage of

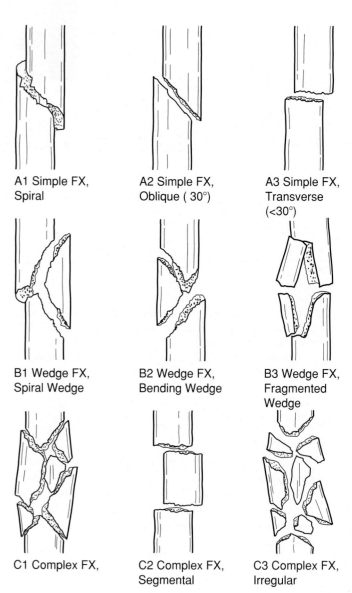

A1 Simple FX, Spiral

A2 Simple FX, Oblique ( 30°)

A3 Simple FX, Transverse (<30°)

B1 Wedge FX, Spiral Wedge

B2 Wedge FX, Bending Wedge

B3 Wedge FX, Fragmented Wedge

C1 Complex FX,

C2 Complex FX, Segmental

C3 Complex FX, Irregular

**Figure 39–1:**

**AO classification of humeral shaft fractures.**

these patients go into delayed union or nonunion without internal fixation. To improve alignment, the patient can be placed in a semi-sitting or full upright position, using gravity to improve alignment. The coaptation splint is placed from the axilla medially, around the elbow distally, and ends about the superior aspect of the acromioclavicular joint. Prior to plaster setting, the splint can be gently molded to reduce the major displacements. Anteroposterior and lateral radiographs are obtained to assess fracture position. The neurologic examination, particularly of the radial nerve, is then repeated. Patients should understand that they will be transitioned into several splints/braces while awaiting union.

- Patients are placed into a prefabricated functional brace (Sarmiento brace) within 1 to 2 weeks after injury. The patient is instructed on how to tighten the straps to

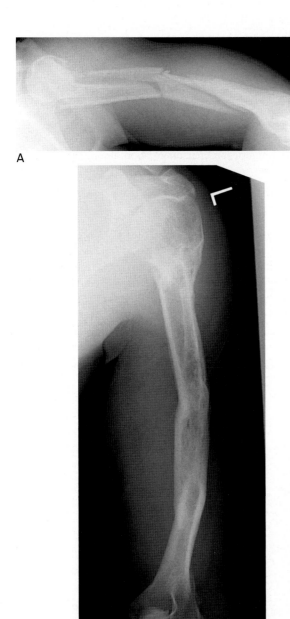

A

B

Figure 39–2:

**A,** A 45-year-old man with a comminuted isolated humeral shaft fracture. He was treated with a Sarmiento brace. **B,** At 1-year follow-up, the patient has full range of motion of his shoulder and elbow.

maintain a snug fit, as fracture reduction is obtained and maintained by the hydrostatic pressure within the soft tissue envelope created by the brace. After brace application, immediate orthogonal radiographs are obtained. Adjustments can be made to neutralize specific deformities. For example, a small abduction pillow at the patient's waist can be used to eliminate a varus deformity, and pads can be placed in the axilla to eliminate a valgus deformity. [10–13]

- Patients are encouraged to begin active range of motion exercises of the fingers, wrist, elbow, and shoulder as tolerated.
- Radiographs are obtained weekly for the first 3 to 4 weeks to ensure satisfactory maintenance of reduction and initiation of range of motion exercises. Radiographic and clinical healing usually becomes apparent at the 6- to 8-week mark. Weaning of the brace can begin at this time.
- Shoulder and elbow stretching and strengthening exercises are subsequently encouraged.
- Hanging casts, rather than coaptation splints, occasionally are used acutely, provided the top of the cast ends at least 2 cm above the fracture. They are mainly indicated in oblique or spiral fractures with shortening. Patients are transitioned into a functional brace. The main concern with hanging casts is the potential for overdistraction of the fracture and subsequent nonunion.
- With all of these techniques, significant hand and forearm edema may develop. The edema usually is a benign occurrence secondary to dependency. Encouraging active finger, wrist, and elbow range of motion and ensuring there are no constrictions in the region of the antecubital fossa often improve the situation.
- Acceptable alignment:
  - 20 degrees anterior or posterior angulation
  - 30 degrees varus or valgus angulation
  - Up to 2 cm of shortening

## Operative Treatment

### Indications

- Most of the indications for operative management of humeral shaft fractures are relative.
- Failure of nonoperative management is an indication for operative fixation. Inability to maintain acceptable alignment is a relative indication for surgical stabilization. Patients with a large body habitus are more prone to unacceptable reductions with varus deformities.
- The presence of multiple injuries is a relative indication for operative management. The rationale is to facilitate mobilization, nursing care, personal hygiene, and early weight bearing on the arm. [14]
- Associated vascular injuries requiring repair invariably require fracture stabilization to maintain the integrity of the vascular supply.
- Associated brachial plexus injuries often result in flaccid paralysis of the musculature of the upper extremity. Fracture distraction is particularly difficult to manage with closed methods and frequently leads to delayed or nonunion. [15]
- Pathologic fractures should be treated operatively. In these cases, humeral nails have superior biomechanical properties compared to plates, and are the usual implant of choice. [16]

- Open fractures requiring surgical debridement and irrigation often are stabilized to promote soft tissue healing, minimize dead space, and facilitate wound care. Injuries without significant soft tissue injury and with favorable fracture patterns can, however, be managed with functional bracing after operative debridement.
- Associated ipsilateral upper extremity fractures, such the "floating elbow," are relative indications for operative fixation.
- Segmental humeral fractures are a relative indication for surgical management because they may be difficult to manage with functional bracing. However, successful treatment can be obtained with nonoperative means.
- Intraarticular extension, either proximal or distal, is a relative indication for shaft fixation.
- Radial nerve palsy following closed reduction is a relative indication for operative intervention. Although controversial, evidence supports observation, provided alignment of the humeral shaft remains satisfactory and no other relative indications for surgical treatment are present.[7,17–19]

## Plate Osteosynthesis

- Plate stabilization has demonstrated satisfactory union rates with low complications and remains the gold standard for the majority of humeral shaft fractures[20–24] (Figure 39–3).
- The choice of surgical approach is dependent upon associated injuries and fracture location, among other factors.

## Surgical Approaches

### Posterior: Triceps Splitting

- The patient is positioned in the lateral or prone position.
- A longitudinal posterior skin incision is made. Distally, the incision is curved around the tip of the olecranon. The deep investing muscular fascia is incised. The interval between the long head and lateral heads of the triceps is identified and developed.
- The radial nerve (with the accompanying profunda brachii artery) is located, mobilized, and protected as it crosses from medial to lateral along the posterior aspect of

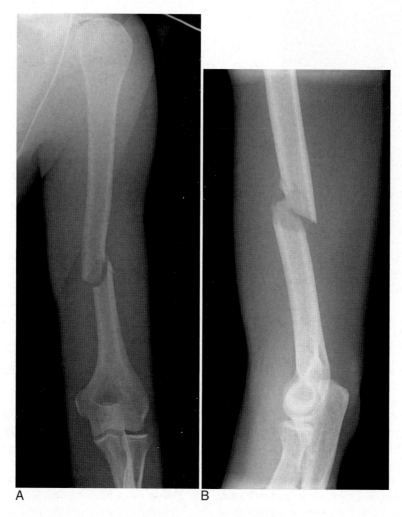

A                                    B

Figure 39–3:
A 25-year-old man with multiple injuries, including tibial shaft and pelvic ring fractures. **A, B,** Injury radiographs.

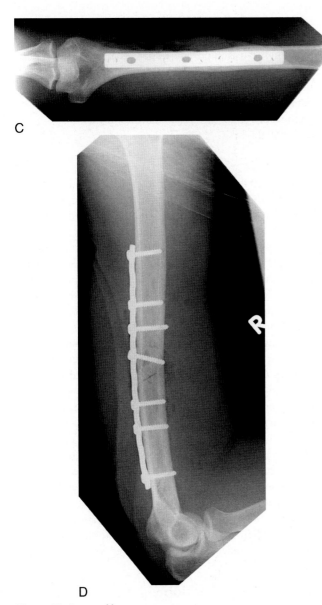

C

D

Figure 39–3: cont'd
**C, D,** The patient was treated with open reduction internal fixation via the modified extensile posterior approach.

the humerus in the spiral grove. The medial head of the triceps originates from the posterior aspect of the humerus distal to the spiral groove. The medial head is incised and elevated in a subperiosteal manner (Figure 39–4). This approach allows access to the posterior aspect of the humerus for plating. With mobilization of the radial nerve, this approach allows for exposure of approximately 75% of the humeral shaft.[1]

## Posterior: Modified Extensile

- The patient is positioned in the lateral or prone position.
- A midline longitudinal posterior skin incision is performed.

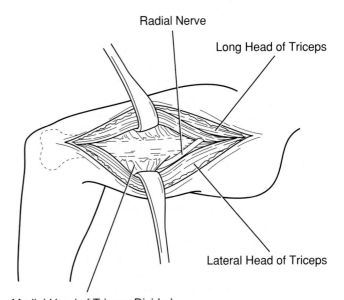

Figure 39–4:
**Triceps splitting posterior approach.**

- The lower lateral brachial cutaneous branch of the radial nerve is identified on the posterior aspect of the lateral intermuscular septum and followed proximally to identify the radial nerve proper along the posterior aspect of the humerus (Figure 39–5).
- At the lateral border of the humerus, the radial nerve trifurcates into three branches: the lower lateral brachial cutaneous nerve, a branch to the medial head of the triceps, and the continuation of the radial nerve into the distal aspect of the upper arm and forearm. Once the

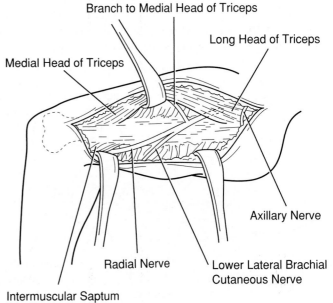

Figure 39–5:
**Modified extensile posterior approach to the humerus.**

radial nerve is identified, it is followed distally to the lateral intermuscular septum. The lateral intermuscular septum is incised proximally and distally, allowing for mobilization of the radial nerve.

- The triceps is elevated from lateral to medial (see Figure 39–5). This exposure is more extensile than the triceps splitting approach with visualization of approximately 94% of the humeral diaphysis.[1] It is limited proximally by the course of the axillary nerve and the posterior humeral circumflex artery.

### Lateral

- The patient is positioned in the supine position.
- The incision is made on the lateral aspect of the arm from the deltoid insertion to the lateral epicondyle.
- Identification of the radial nerve is performed as described in the extensile posterior approach.
- This approach should be considered for surgical stabilization of humeral shaft fractures in the multiply injured patient.[25]

### Anterior

- The patient is positioned in the supine position. Proximally, this exposure is extensile via the deltopectoral interval.
- The incision is made along the lateral border of biceps and ends proximal to elbow crease. Proximally, the interval is between the deltoid (lateral) and the pectoralis major (medial) muscles.
- The biceps muscle is retracted medially, exposing the brachialis muscle, which covers the anterior aspect of the humerus. The musculocutaneous nerve is identified between the biceps and the brachialis.
- The brachialis muscle is incised longitudinally, exposing the anterior aspect of the humerus (Figure 39–6).
- Distally the radial nerve lies between the brachialis (medial) and the brachioradialis (lateral). Controversy

exists regarding the need to expose the radial nerve in this approach. Although it is not necessary to expose the radial nerve, it is important to be certain of the intervals used and the lack of the radial nerve in the wound or under the plate.

- This exposure should be considered when managing fractures involving the proximal third of the humeral diaphysis.

### Fixation Strategies

- Most humeral shaft fractures can be managed using 4.5-mm limited contact dynamic compression plates. Traditional teaching advocated the use of broad 4.5-mm implants for fractures of the humeral shaft; however, current practice suggests most fractures can be adequately managed with narrow 4.5-mm implants. This later finding likely results from improved handling of comminuted fracture fragments and their soft tissue attachments and understanding the superior mechanical benefits afforded with longer plates and fewer screws.
- Lag screws applied through the plate substantially improve the construct strength and should be used whenever possible. Compression plating techniques are advocated for transverse or short oblique fractures.
- Highly comminuted fractures usually require bridging rather than compressing techniques.
- Double plating, with plates placed orthogonal to each other, may be needed for fixation of distal fractures.
- Acute bone grafting is rarely necessary, provided good soft tissue technique is used during reduction and stabilization.
- At the conclusion of posterior plate applications, the location where the nerve crosses the plate should be noted and included in the operative report, in case future surgery is required.

### Intramedullary Fixation

- Intramedullary nailing of humeral shaft fractures has not been as successful as in the lower extremity and remains controversial.
- The main concerns with humeral nailing are
  - Shoulder pain and decreased range of motion (thought to be secondary to rotator cuff injury at the time of antegrade nailing)
  - Radial nerve injury (during closed nailings)
  - Nonunion (particularly if the fracture is left distracted)
  - Iatrogenic fracture in the supracondylar region (retrograde nailing)
- Two randomized trials failed to demonstrate any superiority of humeral nailing over compression plate techniques.[4,14]
- Despite this finding, intramedullary nailing of humeral shaft fractures remains an important device in the armamentarium of the orthopaedic trauma surgeon and should be used in the appropriate situation.[26,27]

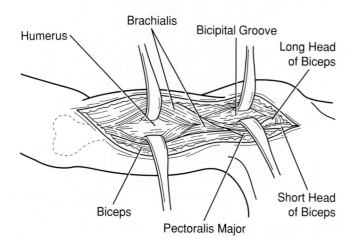

Figure 39–6:
**Anterior approach to the humerus.**

Humerus
Brachialis
Bicipital Groove
Long Head of Biceps
Biceps
Pectoralis Major
Short Head of Biceps

- The majority of humeral nailings performed in North America use an antegrade statically locked nail with a minimally reamed technique.
- Multiple nail designs are available. Standard antegrade nails are placed just medial to the greater tuberosity and require the rotator cuff to be incised and retracted to allow nail passage. Newer nails are available that allow antegrade nailing yet do not require violation of the rotator cuff (Figure 39–7). Hopefully these devices can

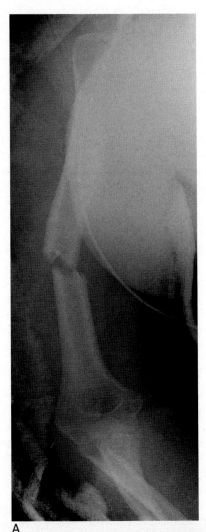

**A**

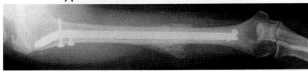

**B**

Figure 39–7:
**A 24-year-old woman was polytraumatized in a motor vehicle collision. A,** The patient sustained a closed humerus fracture. **B,** The radial nerve function was unknown at the time of treatment. A small incision was made to ensure the nerve was not entrapped in fracture. Reduction was achieved, and a humeral nail was inserted.

decrease the shoulder morbidity identified with standard antegrade nailing technique, but data supporting this hypothesis are lacking. Other devices allow multiple screws to be placed within the humeral head and are useful for humeral shaft fractures with associated fractures in the region of the surgical neck.

- Retrograde nailing avoids breaching the rotator cuff but requires the creation of an entrance hole in the supracondylar region of the humerus that is associated with iatrogenic fracture.
- Unlocked flexible nails, such as elastic nails or Enders nails, are infrequently used for management of these fractures. Despite reports of their successful use, they have poor rotational control and are suboptimal for comminuted fractures. Although their use is acceptable, other treatments are commonly preferred.

## Radial Nerve Management During Intramedullary Nailing of the Humerus

- Radial nerve injury during closed humeral nailing is the biggest detractor from the technique.
- Two established techniques to prevent this complication are as follows:
  1. Direct operative visualization of the fracture ends during reduction and nail passage to ensure that the nerve is not trapped within the fracture. Using this technique, the nerve does not need to be explored, but it must be verified to be out of harm's way.
  2. Utilization of somatosensory evoked potentials during closed nailings.[28]
- Fractures can be nailed without using the aforementioned techniques in the following situations:
  - Fractures that are well proximal or distal to the region of the spiral groove
  - Near anatomic fracture reduction that can be obtained without undue manipulation or force
  - Patients who can be examined preoperatively and postoperatively
- We have a low threshold for proceeding with open visualization of the radial nerve during humeral nailing.

## Antegrade Technique

- The patient is placed supine or in the beach chair position. This position allows the injured extremity to be elevated and rotated "away" from the surgeon.
- Fluoroscopy equipment is located on the contralateral side of the operating table. Combined with the rotation of the patient, the C-arm can traverse a near 90-degree arc without the patient's torso obscuring the image.
- A small longitudinal incision is made from the lateral aspect of the acromion distally. Blunt dissection is performed down to the rotator cuff. The rotator cuff is incised in line with its fibers and retracted.
- The starting point is confirmed radiographically.

- Neurovascular structures, including the radial, median, and musculocutaneous nerves and the brachial artery, are at risk with distal interlocking.

## Retrograde Technique

- The patient is placed in the lateral or prone position.
- Fluoroscopy equipment is generally located at the patient's head.
- The distal portion of a triceps splitting approach is performed.
- The staring point is in the midline approximately 2.5 cm proximal to the proximal extent of the olecranon fossa.
- When placing the proximally locking screws, the axillary nerve is at risk, so blunt dissection to bone is important.
- Great care must be taken when creating the entry portal, because the most common complication of retrograde nailing is fracture in this region.[29–31]

## External Fixation

- Rarely indicated.
- When used, the pins should be placed with direct visualization of bone when neurovascular structures are at risk.
- Consider this technique for high-energy open injuries.
- Successful outcomes in properly selected cases have been demonstrated.[32]

## Rehabilitation

- Immediate active finger, wrist, elbow, and shoulder range of motion is encouraged.
- Early weight bearing should be considered, particularly in the polytraumatized patient if the extremity is needed for mobilization.[14]
- Strengthening is emphasized at approximately 6 to 8 weeks.
- Radiographs typically are obtained at 6, 12, and 24 weeks.

# Complications

## Nerve Injury

- The radial nerve is the nerve injury most frequently associated with humeral shaft fractures. The majority of these injuries (90%) are neuropraxias, and spontaneously recovery is the rule.
- Open humeral shaft fractures have a higher incidence of radial nerve lacerations. These injuries should be explored initially and repaired (or grafted) at a secondary surgery, once the wound is stable and clean and the level of nerve injury is clearly demarcated.
- Closed humeral shaft fractures with radial nerve injuries are managed with observation, as the prognosis for nerve recovery is excellent. During the time of paralysis, passive range of motion of the fingers and wrist is imperative. Use of a "cock-up" wrist brace facilitates function.

- Use of electromyography for monitoring nerve recovery is controversial. Changes in electromyographic (EMG) recordings typically occur only 1 month prior to clinical signs of recovery and limit their usefulness. Some patients may not demonstrate spontaneous recovery for up to 6 months after injury, but the majority begin recovery within 4 months.[33]
- Nerve regeneration typically occurs at the rate of 1 mm/day and follows a reproducible pattern of muscle reinnervation.
- A progressive clinical sequence of recovery begins with radially deviated wrist extension (extensor carpi radialis longus), followed rapidly by wrist extension in a neutral plane (extensor carpi radialis brevis). Finger extension (extensor digitorum communis) occurs subsequently, with extension of the thumb interphalangeal joint (extensor pollicis longus) recovering later. The extensor indicis proprius is the last muscle to recover.
- The two treatment strategies for management of a nonrecovering radial nerve palsy are exploration and nerve grafting versus tendon transfers. Nerve grafting is a long, uncertain process that offers the chance at independent finger extension. Tendon transfers are more predictable but are limited in that the patient will not have fine independent finger extension.
- Iatrogenic nerve injuries are not uncommon. The radial nerve is at risk with most open reduction internal fixation procedures. With humeral nailing, the axillary nerve is vulnerable with proximal interlocking, whereas the radial, median, and musculocutaneous nerves all are at risk with distal locking. Injuries to the brachial artery have been described.

## Nonunion

- Nonunion rates are slightly higher in series of patients treated operatively for humeral shaft fractures compared to nonoperatively managed groups. Up to 29% nonunion rates have been reported.[34] More commonly, nonunion rates of 5% to 10% are presented. Overall, union rates may be higher in patients treated with plate osteosynthesis compared to humeral nailing.
- Compression plating with or without bone grafting has been the treatment of choice for humeral nonunions. Several small series have supported humeral nailing for treatment of nonunion.[10,31,35–37]

## Shoulder Pain

- Shoulder pain more commonly is experienced following antegrade humeral nailing. Theoretically it is less of a problem with antegrade humeral nails with entry sites distal to the rotator cuff. The reported rates of shoulder dysfunction or pain range from nearly none to nearly all patients.[34] Some patients treated by all methods, even closed management, report shoulder pain and functional loss.[13]

## Elbow Pain

- Elbow pain has been described following retrograde nailing of the humerus and following open reduction internal fixation and antegrade humeral nailing.
- Measurable elbow stiffness has been identified with plating fractures of the distal third of the humeral shaft.[20]

# References

1. Gerwin M, Hotchkiss RN, Weiland AJ: Alternative operative exposures of the posterior aspect of the humeral diaphysis. *J Bone Joint Surg Am* 78A:1690-1695, 1996.
   Description of three posterior approaches to the humerus, the location of the radial nerve, and the exposure of the humerus possible with each approach.

2. Uhl RL, Larosa JM, Sibeni T, Martino LJ: Posterior approaches to the humerus: when should you worry about the radial nerve. *J Orthop Trauma* 10:338-340, 1996.
   Describes the path of the radial nerve, particularly where it pierces the intramuscular septum and travels in the spiral groove.

3. Fleming P, Lenehan B, Sankar R et al: One-third, two-thirds: relationship of the radial nerve to the lateral intermuscular septum in the arm. *Clin Anat* 17:26-29, 2004.
   Describes the location of the radial nerve, with special attention to where it penetrates the intramuscular septum and enters the anterior compartment.

4. Hartsock LA: Humeral shaft fractures. In Kellam JF, Fischer TJ, Tornetta P III, Bosse MJ, Harris MB, editors: *Orthopaedic knowledge update trauma 2.* Rosemont, 2000, American Academy of Orthopaedic Surgeons.

5. Kettlekamp DB, Alexander H: Clinical review of radial nerve injury. *J Trauma* 7:424-432, 1967.
   Thirty-three patients with humeral shaft fractures are discussed. The demographics, treatments, and outcomes are reviewed.

6. Mast JW, Spiegel PG, Harvey JP Jr, Harrison C: Fractures of the humeral shaft: a retrospective study of 240 adult fractures. *Clin Orthop* 112:254-262, 1975.
   The epidemiology, treatment, and outcomes of humeral shaft fractures are discussed.

7. Shaw JL, Sakellarides H: Radial-nerve paralysis associated with fractures of the humerus. A review of forty-five cases. *J Bone Joint Surg* 49A:899-902, 1967.

8. Holstein A, Lewis GB: Fractures of the humerus with radial nerve paralysis. *J Bone Joint Surg Am* 45A:1382-1388, 1963.
   Reports a less than 2% rate of radial nerve palsies with humeral shaft fractures. Seven of eight patients with palsies had spiral fractures of the distal third of the humerus. The authors advocate open reduction internal fixation and nerve exploration for these fractures.

9. Spak I: Humeral shaft fractures. Treatment with a simple hand sling. *Acta Orthop Scand* 49:234-239, 1978.
   Outcomes of humeral shaft fractures treated with a simple sling are discussed.

10. Sarmiento A, Kinman PB, Galvin EG et al: Functional bracing of fractures of the shaft of the humerus. *J Bone Joint Surg* 59A:596-601, 1977.
    Reports a nonunion rate of less than 2% in closed fractures and 6% in open injuries. Eighty-seven percent had less than 16 degrees of varus/valgus angulation and 81% had less than 16 degrees flexion or extension deformity.

11. Sarmiento A, Latta LL: Functional fracture bracing. *J Am Acad Orthop Surg* 7:66-75, 1999.
    Functional bracing for treatment of multiple fractures is described. The nonunion rate in closed and type I open humeral shaft fractures was approximately 3%.

12. Sarmiento A, Horowitch A, Aboulafia A, Vangsness CT Jr: Functional bracing for comminuted extra-articular fractures of the distal third of the humerus. *J Bone Joint Surg* 72B:283-287, 1990.
    Reports a 96% union rate for distal third humeral shaft fractures managed with functional bracing. Varus deformity averaging 9 degrees in 81%, but motion and functional results were good.

13. Sharma VK, Jain AK, Gupta RK et al: Non-operative treatment of fractures of the humeral shaft: a comparative study. *J Indian Med Assoc* 89:157-160, 1991.
    Review of humeral shaft fractures treated by nonoperative means. Functional bracing had better results than U braces.

14. Tingstad EM, Wolinsky PR, Shyr Y, Johnson KD: Effect of immediate weightbearing on plated fractures of the humeral shaft. *J Trauma* 49:278-280, 2000.
    Weight bearing had no effect on union or malunion rates.

15. Brien WW, Gellman H, Becker V et al: Management of fractures of the humerus in patients who have an injury of the ipsilateral brachial plexus. *J Bone Joint Surg* 72A:1208-1210, 1990.
    Discusses the results of various treatment techniques for these fractures. Plating was the most consistently successful in a small number of patients.

16. Damron TA, Rock MG, Choudhury SN et al: Biomechanical analysis of prophylactic fixation for middle third humeral impending pathologic fractures. *Clin Orthop* 363:240-248, 1999.
    Locked intramedullary nails provided stronger fixation of simulated impending pathologic midhumerus fractures compared to compression plating and Rush rods.

17. Bostman O, Bakalim G, Vainionpaa S et al: Immediate radial nerve palsy complicating fracture of the shaft of the humerus: when is early exploration justified? *Injury* 16:499-502, 1985.
    Distal third humeral shaft fractures were more commonly associated with radial nerve laceration or entrapment compared to midshaft fractures. Nearly 80% had significant nerve recovery.

18. Pollock FH, Drake D, Bovill EG et al: Treatment of radial neuropathy associated with fractures of the humerus. *J Bone Joint Surg* 63A:239-243, 1981.
    The authors recommended initial observation with exploration at 3 to 4 months if there is no evidence of recovery.

19. Shah JJ, Bhatti NA: Radial nerve paralysis associated with fractures of the humerus. A review of 62 cases. *Clin Orthop* 172:171-176, 1983.

Ninety-five percent had full or near-full recovery. EMG studies are recommended at 4 to 6 months, with tendon transfers deferred for at least 6 months and preferably for 1 year.

20. Chapman JR, Henley MB, Agel J, Benca PJ: Randomized prospective study of humeral shaft fracture fixation: intramedullary nails versus plates. *J Orthop Trauma* 14:162-166, 2000.
    Both intramedullary nailing and compression plating provided predictable healing with comparable union rates.

21. McCormack RG, Brien D, Buckley RE et al: Fixation of fractures of the shaft of the humerus by dynamic compression plate or intramedullary nail. A prospective, randomized trial. *J Bone Joint Surg* 82B:336-339, 2000.
    The authors advocate the use of plate osteosynthesis for humeral shaft fractures requiring fixation, reserving nail stabilization for special situations. They noted no significant differences in shoulder or elbow function for plates or nails, but the overall complication rate was higher in the nailed group.

22. Niall DM, O'Mahony J, McElwain JP: Plating of humeral shaft fractures—has the pendulum swung back? *Injury* 35:580-586, 2004.
    Forty-seven of 49 humeral shaft fractures treated with plate osteosynthesis healed uneventfully. All patients regained full shoulder and elbow motion.

23. McKee MD, Pedlow FX, Cheney PJ, Schemitsch EH: Fractures below the end of locking humeral nails: a report of three cases. *J Orthop Trauma* 10:500-504, 1996.
    Three cases of fracture following antegrade humeral nailing at the distal interlocking site are described. All patients were treated with secondary surgeries.

24. Modabber MR, Jupiter JB: Operative management of diaphyseal fractures of the humerus. *Clin Orthop* 347:93-104, 1998.
    Reviews surgical stabilization humeral shaft fractures. Plate fixation is preferred to intramedullary nailing to allow visualization of the radial nerve.

25. Mills WJ, Hanel DP, Smith DG: Lateral approach to the humeral shaft: an alternative approach for fracture treatment. *J Orthop Trauma* 10:81-86, 1996.
    Describes a lateral, limited muscle splitting exposure for treatment of humeral shaft fractures that can be performed with the patient in the supine position.

26. Lin J: Treatment of humeral shaft fractures with humeral locked nail and comparison with plate fixation. *J Trauma* 44:859-864, 1998.
    Reports shorter operative times, comparable union rates, and decreased complications for locked nails compared to compression plating.

27. Stannard JP, Harris HW, McGwin G Jr et al: Intramedullary nailing of humeral shaft fractures with a locking flexible nail. *J Bone Joint Surg Am* 85A:2103-2110, 2003.
    Discusses antegrade and retrograde nailing for humeral shaft fractures.

28. Mills WJ, Chapman JR, Robinson LR, Slimp JC: Somatosensory evoked potential monitoring during closed humeral nailing: a preliminary report. *J Orthop Trauma* 14:167-170, 2000.
    Somatosensory evoked potential monitoring reliably reflected the radial nerve status in 13 patients undergoing closed intramedullary nailing of humeral shaft fractures.

29. Blum J, Janzing H, Gahr R et al: Clinical performance of a new medullary humeral nail: Antegrade versus retrograde insertion. *J Orthop Trauma* 15:342-349, 2001.
    Retrograde nailing of the humerus is more technically demanding, with higher intraoperative complication rates than antegrade nailing.

30. Rommens PM, Verbruggen J, Broos PL: Retrograde locked nailing of humeral shaft fractures. A review of 39 patients. *J Bone Joint Surg* 77B:84-89, 1995.
    Overall shoulder function was excellent in greater than 90%, elbow function was excellent in 87%, and end-result function was excellent in 85%. Complications are described.

31. Rommens PM, Blum J, Runkel M: Retrograde nailing of humeral shaft fractures. *Clin Orthop* 350:26-39, 1998.
    Reports a 7% nonunion rate and a 4% radial nerve palsy rate with complete recovery in all cases. Entry site fractures occurred in 4%. Shoulder and elbow function was excellent in almost 90%.

32. Mostafavi HR, Tornetta P 3rd: Open fractures of the humerus treated with external fixation. *Clin Orthop* 337:187-197, 1997.
    Discusses results and complications of open humeral shaft fractures treated with immediate external fixation.

33. Ring D, Chin K, Jupiter JB: Radial nerve palsy associated with high-energy humeral shaft fractures. *J Hand Surg* 29:144-147, 2004.
    The majority of radial nerves recovered, except for the transected nerves. The average time to full nerve recovery was 6 months.

34. Farragos AF, Schemitsch EH, McKee MD: Complications of intramedullary nailing for fractures of the humeral shaft: a review. *J Orthop Trauma* 13:258-267, 1999.
    Complications following nailing of humeral shaft fractures are described and compared to studies of plate fixation, for which lower complication rates are seen.

35. McKee MD, Miranda MA, Riemer BL et al: Management of humeral nonunion after the failure of locking intramedullary nails. *J Orthop Trauma* 10:492-499, 1996.
    Twenty-one humeral nonunions following intramedullary nailing are described. Repair with open reduction internal fixation with plate fixation had higher success rates than exchange nailing.

36. Volgas DA, Stannard JP, Alonso JE: Nonunions of the humerus. *Clin Orthop* 419:46-50, 2004.
    Review of the etiology and treatment strategies for humeral nonunions.

37. Sarmiento A, Waddell JP, Latta LL: Diaphyseal humeral fractures: treatment options. *Instr Course Lect* 51:257-269, 2002.
    Comprehensive review of management strategies and outcomes of humeral shaft fractures.

# CHAPTER 40

# Examination of the Shoulder

Jeffrey E. Budoff

MD, Assistant Professor, Hand and Upper Extremity Institute, Department of Orthopaedic Surgery, Baylor College of Medicine; Houston Veterans Affairs Medical Center, Houston, TX

## Introduction

- The majority of shoulder disorders can be diagnosed based on a thorough history and physical examination. Overreliance on diagnostic imaging is discouraged because the sensitivity of magnetic resonance imaging (MRI) and other studies used to detect common shoulder disorders still is suboptimal. Conversely, imaging studies may detect many asymptomatic abnormalities that do not require intervention.
- Physical examination can be relatively straightforward. The physician determines the location of the patient's pain by history, localizes the area(s) of tenderness and then applies his/her knowledge of anatomy to determine "what lives there." This process generates a differential diagnosis of potentially injured structures. The physician then stresses those individual structures to determine which reproduces the patient's pain. That structure most probably is the source of the patient's symptoms. If an anesthetic agent can be reliably injected into a localized area, the clinical impression can be confirmed with diagnostic injections. Although no test is perfect, if an injection decreases the patient's pain, the anesthetized structure probably is contributing to the patient's symptoms.

## Anatomy and Biomechanics

- The shoulder consists of three synovial joints (glenohumeral, acromioclavicular [AC], and sternoclavicular) and two articulations (scapulothoracic,

and acromiohumeral). The glenohumeral joint is the most mobile joint in the body. Unlike the hip, the glenoid socket is not intrinsically stable; it relies on static and dynamic soft tissue stabilizers to remain centered. Because of its lack of osseous stabilizers, it is the most commonly dislocated large joint in the body (Figure 40–1).

### Static Stabilizers: Glenohumeral Joint Capsule

- The joint capsule originates on the glenoid neck and inserts along the proximal humerus (Figure 40–2). Important capsular thickenings include the superior glenohumeral ligament (SGHL), the middle glenohumeral ligament (MGHL) and the inferior glenohumeral ligament (IGHL). The IGHL is a complex structure composed of an anterior bundle (aIGHL) and a posterior bundle (pIGHL), with the axillary pouch spanning the interval between them (Figure 40–3). This setup has been compared to a hammock that supports the humeral head during arm elevation.[1] Although clinically, individual ligaments are not tightened in isolation, they are differentially tensioned according to the degree of elevation.
  - With the shoulder adducted at rest, the SGHL and negative intraarticular pressure stabilize against inferior subluxation.[2]
  - At 45 degrees elevation, all capsuloligamentous components are at their loosest, with the MGHL, aIGHL, and subscapularis being the main restraint to anteroinferior translation.[3,4]

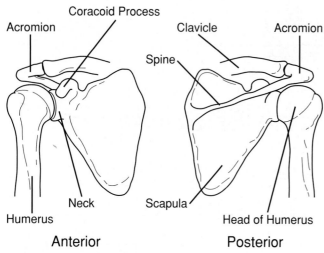

Figure 40–1:
Shoulder anatomy: osteology.

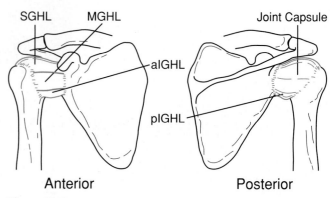

Figure 40–2:
Shoulder anatomy: glenohumeral capsule. *aIGHL,* Anterior bundle of inferior glenohumeral ligament; *MGHL,* middle glenohumeral ligament; *pIGHL,* posterior bundle of inferior glenohumeral ligament; *SGHL,* superior glenohumeral ligament.

- The IGHL complex is the prime stabilizer preventing anterior instability at higher degrees of abduction.[2,3]
- The capsuloligamentous restraints function as checkreins, maintaining stability at the end range of motion when they tighten. The anterior ligaments oppose anterior humeral translation in external rotation, and the posterior ligaments oppose posterior humeral translation in internal rotation. In the midrange of motion, where most activities of daily living occur, the capsuloligamentous structures are lax; therefore, their contribution to stability is limited. Stability is maintained by dynamic means.

## Dynamic Stabilizers

- The dynamic stabilizers include all musculature around the shoulder, with the rotator cuff playing a major role

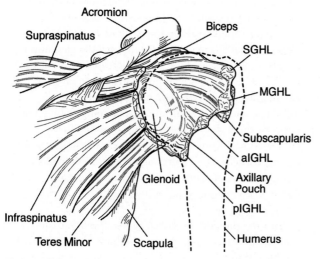

Figure 40–3:
Glenohumeral capsular ligaments. *aIGHL,* Anterior bundle of inferior glenohumeral ligament; *MGHL,* middle glenohumeral ligament; *pIGHL,* posterior bundle of inferior glenohumeral ligament; *SGHL,* superior glenohumeral ligament.

(Figures 40–4 and 40–5). The rotator cuff is composed of four tendons: the supraspinatus, infraspinatus, teres minor, and subscapularis. All rotator cuff muscles originate from the scapula and insert onto the greater tuberosity (supraspinatus, infraspinatus, teres minor) or lesser tuberosity (subscapularis). The subscapularis functions as an internal rotator; the infraspinatus and teres minor function as external rotators of the glenohumeral joint.

## Mechanisms of Dynamic Stabilization[3]

- Concavity-Compression
  - In the absence of rotator cuff function, deltoid activation approximates its insertion on the humerus to its origin on the acromion, leading to superior humeral migration and ineffective elevation. To prevent this occurrence, the rotator cuff compresses the convexity of the humeral head into the concavity of the glenoid, like a golf ball into a tee (Figures 40–6 and 40–7, *A*). With the humeral head stabilized within the glenoid, deltoid

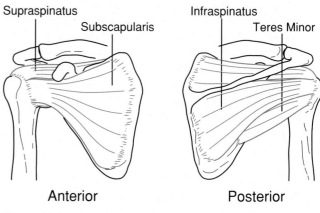

Figure 40–4:
Shoulder anatomy: rotator cuff.

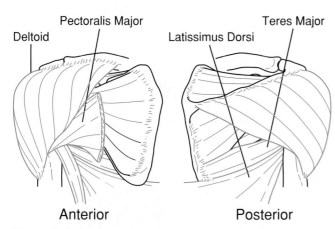

Figure 40–5:
**Shoulder anatomy: superficial muscles.**

activation then can effectively elevate the arm. Lippitt et al.[5] showed that this mechanism resists the superior shearing moment of the deltoid with a high efficiency approaching 60%.

- The long head of the biceps originates from the superior glenoid labrum and the supraglenoid tubercle and exits the shoulder in the intertubercular/bicipital groove. In abduction-external rotation, the biceps tendon runs almost perpendicular to the glenoid surface and may help increase compression of the humeral head into the glenoid, especially in cases of rotator cuff deficiency or shoulder instability.[6,7]

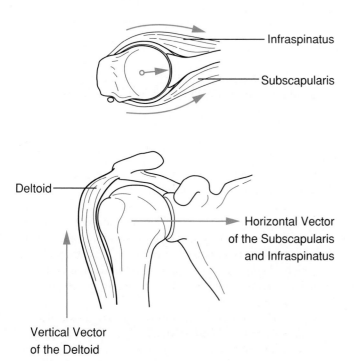

Figure 40–6:
**Concavity-compression.**

- Muscle contraction actively centers the humeral head on the glenoid.
- *Passive barrier effect:* The subscapularis muscle is an important barrier resisting anteroinferior humeral head displacement. The supraspinatus, infraspinatus, and teres minor are important barriers to posterior subluxation.

## Scapulothoracic Motion

- The scapula provides the stable base from which glenohumeral mobility occurs. The scapula is the origin for the rotator cuff and deltoid, so its stability is required for optimal function of these muscles. The scapulothoracic muscles position the glenoid in synchrony with glenohumeral motion in order to optimize concavity-compression. This synchronous motion has been likened to a "ball balanced on the tip of a seal's nose" to illustrate the glenoid's active response that keeps the humeral head centered during motion. This coordination of motion is especially important during midrange motion, where the capsuloligamentous constraints are lax. Important scapulothoracic stabilizers include the serratus anterior, the rhomboids, and the trapezius.[8]
- Scapulothoracic weakness, fatigue, or dysfunction increases stresses on the rotator cuff and static stabilizers, especially during high-demand activities such as overhead athletics (see Figure 40–7, *B*).[8] Conversely, the scapular stabilizers are inhibited by painful shoulder conditions, leading to scapulothoracic dysfunction in up to 68% of rotator cuff disorders and 100% of glenohumeral instabilities.[9]

## Rotator Cuff Cable and Crescent[10,11]
(Figures 40–8 and 40–9)

- The rotator cuff has a cable-like thickening that runs from the anterior supraspinatus to the inferior infraspinatus. This cable is consistently located at the margin of the avascular zone. The cable itself rarely degenerates.
- The rotator cuff crescent consists of the insertions of the supraspinatus and infraspinatus tendons, lateral to the cable. The vast majority of tendon degeneration and tearing occurs within the rotator cuff crescent, where the blood supply is poor.[12]
- The anatomic cable corresponds well to the functional "anteroposterior force couple" of the rotator cuff. This force couple consists of the subscapularis anteriorly, balanced against the inferior infraspinatus and teres minor posteriorly. Both sides of this force couple must be intact in order for the rotator cuff to function. Torn rotator cuffs can function biomechanically as long as the cable/force couple is intact. If a rotator cuff tear extends outside the cable and involves either the subscapularis or the most inferior infraspinatus and teres minor, the

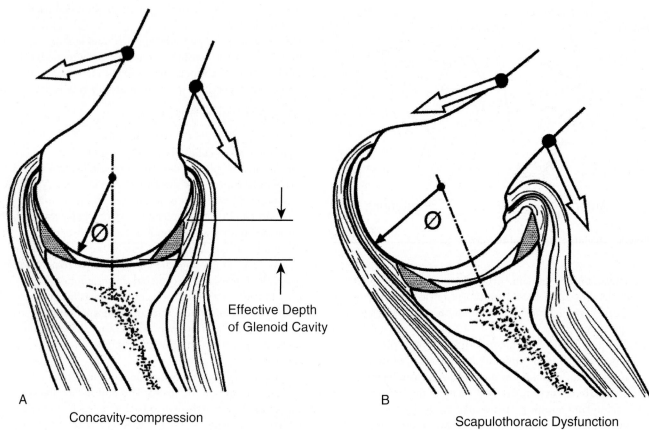

Effective Depth
of Glenoid Cavity

A

Concavity-compression

B

Scapulothoracic Dysfunction

Figure 40–7:

**A,** Concavity-compression actively stabilizes the glenohumeral joint. The rotator cuff compresses the humeral head into the glenoid-labral concavity. **B,** Scapulothoracic dysfunction alters kinematics, causing the net joint reaction force to fall outside of the glenoid concavity, stressing the dynamic and soft tissue static stabilizers. (Modified from Lippitt S, Matsen F: *Clin Orthop* 291:20-38, 1993.)

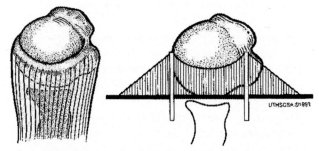

Figure 40–8:

Rotator cuff cable, with analogy to a suspension bridge model. The cable is located at the free margin of the tear, with the anterior and posterior attachments of the tear corresponding to the supports at each end of the cable's span. Loss of continuity not involving the cable allows continued load transmission through the cable. (From Burkhart SS: *Orthop Clin North Am* 24:111-123, 1993.)

shoulder becomes dysfunctional, and active elevation is compromised.

## History

- Chief complaints include pain, stiffness, weakness, instability, and mechanical issues, such as painful snapping or catching.
- *History of present illness:* Note the pain's location, symptom duration, exacerbating activities, the presence of nocturnal pain, any history of trauma, overuse, or neck disorders, whether symptoms are improving or worsening, and any treatments attempted (operative or otherwise) and their effectiveness.
- Pain of rotator cuff origin usually is located laterally, anterolaterally, or posterolaterally. Scapulothoracic pain is located posteromedially, or over the trapezius, medial to pain of rotator cuff origin. Biceps pain is universally anterior.

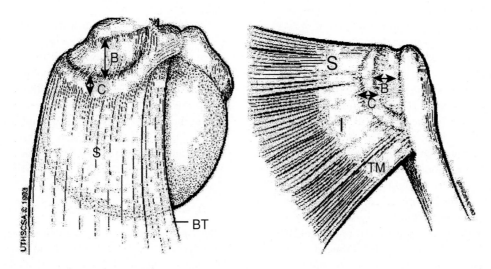

Figure 40–9:
Superior and posterior projections of the rotator cuff cable and crescent. The rotator cuff cable extends from the anterior margin of the supraspinatus to the inferior margin of the infraspinatus, spanning the supraspinatus and infraspinatus insertions. *B,* Mediolateral diameter of rotator crescent; *BT,* biceps tendon; *C,* width of rotator cuff cable; *I,* infraspinatus; *S,* supraspinatus; *TM,* teres minor. (From Burkhart SS: *Arthroscopy* 10:4-19, 1994.)

- Rotator cuff symptoms often are exacerbated by arm elevation, internal rotation, lifting, sudden motions, overhead athletics, and other strenuous activities. Pain frequently worsens at night and may wake the patient from sleep. Pain of rotator cuff origin may radiate as far distally as the lateral elbow. This radiation need not imply neurogenic origin.
- *Instability:* Note provocative positions, whether the initial onset was traumatic or atraumatic, whether frank dislocation or only subluxation has occurred, the number of instability events, and the direction of dislocation. Also note any residual symptoms between instability episodes, which often are referable to the rotator cuff, posttraumatic synovitis, and/or arthritis.
- *Past medical history:* Note any history of rheumatoid or inflammatory arthritis, crystal deposition disease, diabetes mellitus, or hypothyroidism.
- *Differential diagnosis:*
  - Lateral pain (including anterolateral or posterolateral pain): rotator cuff injury
  - Anterior pain: rotator cuff injury (including subscapularis injury), bicipital tendinosis, arthritis
  - Superior pain: trapezial strain (usually secondary to rotator cuff dysfunction), AC joint pain, os acromiale (rare)
  - Posterior pain: rotator cuff injury, strain of the scapulothoracic stabilizers, suprascapular nerve compression
  - Generalized pain: Rotator cuff injury, arthritis
  - Painful snapping: glenohumeral instability, biceps tendon instability, SLAP lesions, arthritis, scapulothoracic "bursitis"

- Feelings of instability: glenohumeral instability, biceps tendon instability, loose body, SLAP lesion
- Note that pain can radiate to the shoulder from the cervical region, intraabdominal and intrathoracic viscera, or Pancoast tumors. Although uncommon, one should always be aware of these potential sources of shoulder pain.
- Rotator cuff injury nearly always is in the differential diagnosis of shoulder disorders and is the most common source of symptoms referable to the shoulder. However, it is important to ensure that any rotator cuff involvement is not secondary to another primary disorder, such as instability or scapulothoracic dysfunction.

## Physical Examination

- The single most important diagnostic procedure performed on the shoulder.
- *Observation at rest:* Note atrophy of the supraspinatus or infraspinatus and any scapular protraction (anterolateral migration of the scapula from the midline).
- *Observation with (attempted) elevation:*
  - Scapulothoracic asymmetry: Results from scapulothoracic weakness and often is more pronounced in descent. It commonly presents as a hitch or jump in the normally smooth motion of the scapula and in subtle cases may require a few repetitions to become evident.[8]
  - Scapular shrug: The patient elevates the scapula to substitute trapezius function for that of a painful rotator cuff. This overuse may lead to trapezial pain.

- Uncontrolled anterosuperior instability: Inability to elevate the arm, associated with the fullness of the humeral head appearing under the anterior subcutaneous tissues, following surgical resection of the coracoacromial arch.
- *Observation during wall push-ups:* Winging of the scapula is a sign of significant serratus anterior dysfunction.
- *Neck:* Note tenderness of the paraspinals, sternocleidomastoid, or trapezius. Note range of motion and any radicular pain with motion or compression. C5 radiculopathy occasionally refers pain to the shoulder.
- *Active and passive shoulder motion:* External and internal rotation are most accurately measured with the arm abducted 90 degrees, not behind the back. With one hand on the acromion the humerus is rotated until scapular motion is noted. This defines true glenohumeral motion. As noted by Kibler et al.,[13] measurements of shoulder rotation based upon the vertebrae to which the thumb reaches are less reliable because they are affected by factors other than pure glenohumeral motion. These factors include scapulothoracic motion, elbow motion, forearm rotation, wrist radioulnar deviation, thumb motion and alignment, and imprecise location of the spinous processes.[13]
  - Loss of passive range of motion indicates adhesive capsulitis, guarding, arthritis, or a congenital or posttraumatic deformity.
  - Loss of active motion with passive motion retained (an "elevation lag") indicates dysfunction of the deltoid and/or rotator cuff caused by pain, neurologic injury, muscle weakness, or loss of tendon continuity.

- *Palpation:*
  - The rotator cuff can be palpated just anterior to the acromion with the shoulder extended. Rotation of the arm may allow palpation of full-thickness rotator cuff tears. According to Wolf and Agrawal,[14] in skilled hands palpation may be as accurate as MRI for assessment of full-thickness rotator cuff tears.
  - The rhomboids, levator scapulae, and trapezius should be palpated. The coracoid may be tender at the pectoralis minor insertion. In addition, the long head of the biceps and the AC and sternoclavicular joints should be palpated.

## Provocative Examinations

- *Scapulothoracic stress test:* The patient actively retracts the scapulae. Burning pain that occurs in less than 15 to 20 seconds indicates scapulothoracic weakness and/or dysfunction.
- *Lateral scapular slide test:* Measure the distance between the thoracic spinal processes and the inferomedial angle of the scapulae in three positions: (1) with the arms adducted at the side, (2) with hands on hips (thumbs posterior), and (3) with the arms elevated in the scapular plane in internal rotation (thumbs down/empty can position). A distance 1.5 cm greater than the contralateral side in any position suggests scapulothoracic weakness with secondary scapulothoracic protraction (Figure 40–10).[8]
- *Scapular assistance test:* This test is performed if the patient has rotator cuff symptoms elicited by active forward flexion. Retract the scapula and stabilize it against the thorax by pulling back on the acromion and pushing

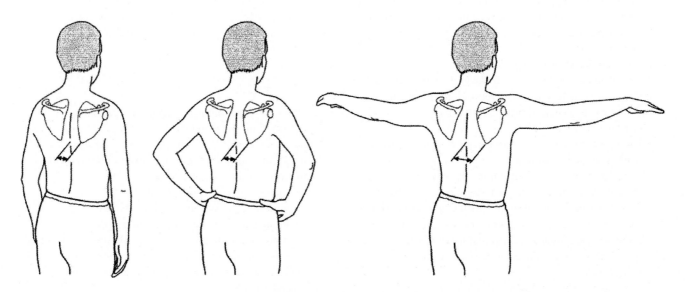

Lateral Scapular Slide Test

Figure 40–10:
**Lateral scapular slide test.**

down on the inferomedial scapular angle. Have the patient repeat active shoulder flexion. Diminution of pain suggests that the rotator cuff is being impinged secondary to inappropriate scapular protraction, which allows the acromion to fall forward onto the rotator cuff during arm elevation. Decreasing their pain by this maneuver can motivate patients to perform scapulothoracic strengthening to be better able to control their scapula and reduce their symptoms (Figure 40–11).[8]

- *Provocative tests: Rotator cuff*
  - Neer test: Stabilize the acromion and flex the internally rotated shoulder (Figure 40–12).[15]
  - Hawkins test: Flex the shoulder 90 degrees and flex the elbow 90 degrees, then internally rotate the arm (Figure 40–13).[16]
  - "Thumb down" or "empty can test": Elevate the shoulder to 90 degrees in the scapular plane with the elbow straight and the shoulder internally rotated, while the patient resists a downward force (Figure 40–14).[17]
  - "Thumb up" or "full can test": This test is performed in similar fashion to the "thumb down" or "empty can test," except that the arm is externally rotated (see Figure 40–14).[17]

- Whipple test: Elevate the arm to 90 degrees and adduct it so that the hand is in front of the opposite shoulder, with the elbow straight and the palm down. Have the patient resist a downward force. The Whipple test is sensitive for anterior supraspinatus pathology (Figure 40–15).[18]
- External rotation strength may be tested with the arm adducted against the side to assess infraspinatus function (Figure 40–16). Pain and/or weakness may indicate pathology of that tendon.[10]
- *Napoleon test:* Inability to bring the elbow anteriorly with the hand pressed against the belly is specific for subscapularis dysfunction (Figure 40–17).[19]
- *Lift-off test:* Inability to lift the hand off the lower lumbar region without extending the elbow is specific for subscapularis deficiency. This position may be difficult for patients to assume because of pain or restricted motion (Figure 40–18).[11]
- *Speed test:* Provokes the pain of bicipital tendinosis. It is performed by having the patient resist forward flexion of the shoulder with it flexed 90 degrees, the elbow extended, and the forearm supinated. A positive test reproduces pain at the bicipital groove. Pain reproduced

Figure 40–11:
**Scapular assistance test.**

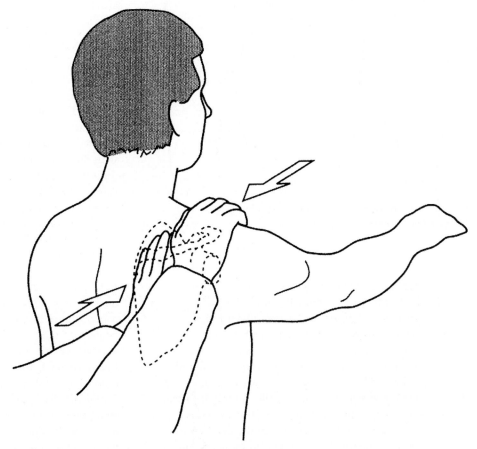

Scapular Assistance Test

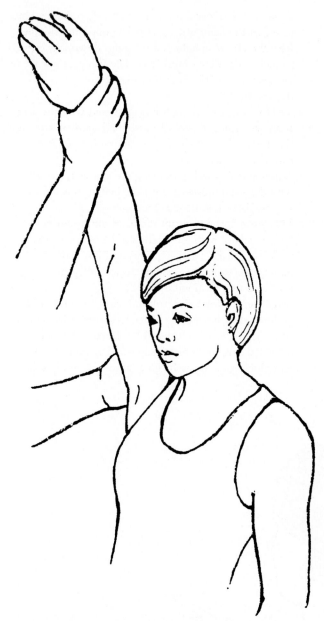

Figure 40–12:
**Neer test.** (From Valadie AI III, Jobe CM, Pink MM et al: *J Shoulder Elbow Surg* 9:36-46, 2000.)

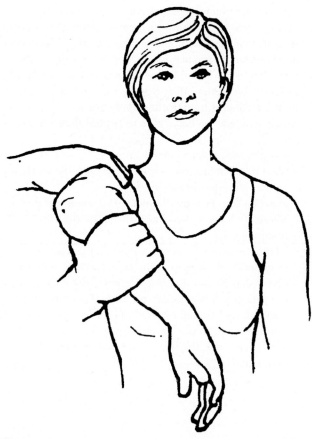

Figure 40–13:
**Hawkins test.** (From Valadie AI III, Jobe CM, Pink MM et al: *J Shoulder Elbow Surg* 9:36-46, 2000.)

in other areas may be related to a variety of other shoulder pathologies (Figure 40–19).[20]

- *O'Brien active compression test:* The shoulder is flexed 90 degrees and adducted 10 to 15 degrees to the sagittal plane of the body. The elbow is fully extended and the shoulder internally rotated so that the thumb points down. The patient resists a downward force. The test is repeated with the forearm fully supinated so that the palm points upward (Figure 40–20). The test is considered positive if pain elicited in the first position is relieved in the second position. Pain localized "on top" of the shoulder suggests an AC joint abnormality,

whereas pain located "inside" of the shoulder suggests a SLAP lesion.[21]

- *Biceps load test II:* The arm of the supine patient is elevated 120 degrees and maximally externally rotated with the elbow at 90 degrees flexion and the forearm supinated. The patient is asked to flex the elbow while it is resisted by the examiner. Reproduction of pain or an increase in pain with elbow flexion is a positive test. No pain or no change in preexisting pain with elbow flexion is a negative test (Figure 40–21).
  - Reported by Kim et al.[22] to be 89.7% sensitive and 96.9% specific.
- *Instability testing:* Especially important in patients younger than 40 years. This testing may be difficult because of patient apprehension, and definitive examination may not be possible in the awake patient.
- *Glenohumeral translation versus glenohumeral instability:* Instability refers to excessive, pathologic, symptom-producing translation. Not all increased translation is pathologic. For example, throwers may develop increased asymptomatic anterior glenohumeral translation in their dominant shoulder.
- Examine the contralateral, presumably normal, shoulder first to assess physiologic translation for the patient and to

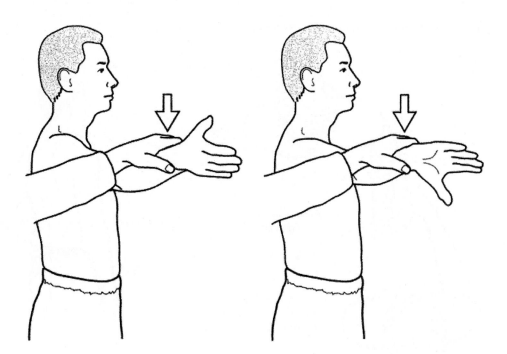

Figure 40–14:
Thumb up and thumb down tests.

Thumb Up-Thumb Down Tests

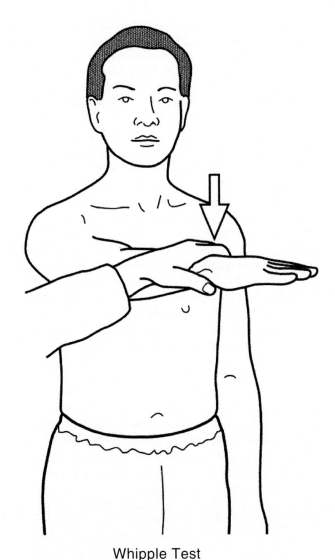

Whipple Test

Figure 40–15:
Whipple test.

reassure the patient that the examination will not hurt, possibly decreasing guarding.

- *Author's preferred technique for office examination of the awake patient:* This is similar to Andrews and Dugas' "Lachman test" for instability[23] and Cofield and Irving's examination under anesthesia.[24] Stand in the supine patient's axilla. Grasp the superior shoulder with the hand closer to the patient. The ulnar digits secure the scapula, and the thumb and index finger grasp the humeral head so that any motion that is noted is glenohumeral in origin. The examiner's other hand grasps the patient's wrist. The shoulder is held in neutral rotation; abduction can be varied between 45 and 90 degrees. Anterior translation is produced by gently lowering the arm as the index finger pushes the humeral head anteriorly. Posterior translation is produced by gently raising the arm as the thumb pushes the humeral head posteriorly (Figure 40–22). After the amount of glenohumeral translation in neutral rotation is noted, the arm is externally rotated. At maximal external rotation, no anterior glenohumeral translation should be possible; there should be a firm endpoint because of capsuloligamentous tensioning. The presence of continued anterior translation is indicative of instability, similar to the Lachman test for the knee. Posterior instability is similarly evaluated by assessing posterior translation with the shoulder held in maximal internal rotation.
- *Glenohumeral translation[25]:*
  - 1+: Increased translation compared to the contralateral, presumably normal side, without distinct subluxation of the humeral head over the glenoid rim. 1+ anterior translation can be normal in the dominant extremity, especially in overhead athletes.

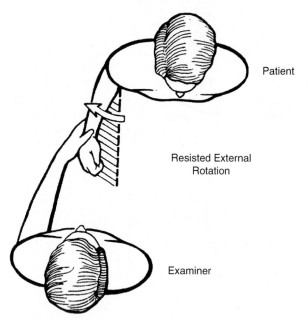

Figure 40–16:
Testing external rotation strength of the adducted shoulder.
(From Burkhart SS: *Orthop Clin North Am* 24:111-123, 1993.)

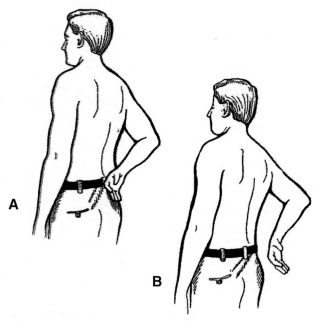

Figure 40–18:
Lift-off test: **A,** Starting position with the shoulder internally rotated and the elbow flexed so that the back of the hand rests on the lower lumbar area. **B,** The patient actively lifts the hand away from the lower back without extending the elbow. (From Burkhart SS: *Orthop Clin North Am* 24:111-123, 1993.)

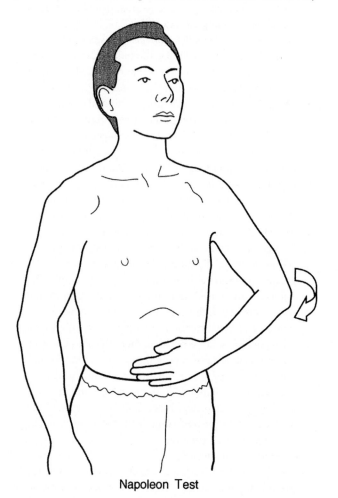

Napoleon Test

Figure 40–17:
**Napoleon test.**

- 2+: Humeral head is subluxable to the rim of the glenoid but does not lock in frank dislocation. 2+ anterior translation is pathologic, whereas this degree of translation can be normal in the posterior direction.
- 3+: Humeral head can be dislocated and locked over the glenoid rim. 3+ translation always is abnormal.
- *Jobe anterior apprehension/posterior relocation test:* Abduct, extend, and maximally externally rotate the shoulder of the supine patient. Apprehension that the arm may dislocate, which is relieved by a posteriorly directed force applied to the proximal humerus, is highly sensitive and specific for instability (Figures 40–23 and 40–24). Pain alone is not a positive test, because pain can be caused by rotator cuff pathology in the absence of instability.[26]
  - An alternative way to perform this test is the reverse posterior relocation test. A posteriorly directed force is placed against the patient's proximal humerus before and during placement of the arm into abduction-external rotation. This often elicits less discomfort. After the patient has been placed in this position, the posterior force is slowly decreased. Apprehension concerning impending instability strongly suggests anterior glenohumeral instability.
- *Posterior stress test:* Flex the supine patient's shoulder to 90 degrees, then internally rotate and adduct it. The elbow also is flexed 90 degrees. A posterior directed force is applied. Painful posterior subluxation or apprehension suggests posterior instability. Symptoms should diminish

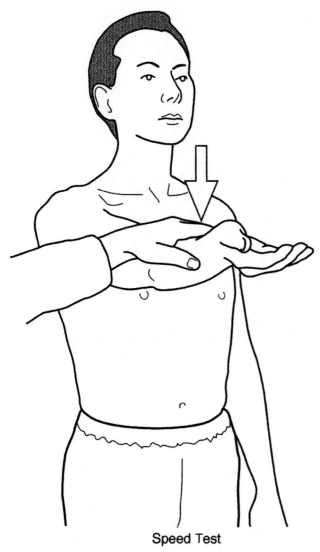

**Speed Test**

Figure 40–19:
**Speed test.**

with abduction/extension. If scapular malpositioning is contributing to the instability, the patient's assistance may be needed to recreate the symptoms (Figure 40–25).[27]

- *Sulcus sign:* Pull inferiorly on the relaxed patient's adducted arm. Significantly increased space, especially more than 2 to 3 cm, observed/palpated beneath the lateral acromion suggests inferior glenohumeral hyperlaxity. Failure of the sulcus to diminish with external rotation suggests a tear of the rotator interval. As for the other instability tests, comparison should be made to the opposite shoulder (Figure 40–26).[25]

- *Diagnostic injections:* Helpful in determining the source of pain in closely related anatomic regions. For example, a decrease in superior shoulder pain and a cross-arm adduction test made negative by an AC joint injection are strongly suggestive of symptomatic pathology at this location. Steroid placed in the injection has the

potential to provide at least temporary symptomatic relief.

- *Pearl:* Probably the least painful way of injecting the subacromial space is to insert a 22-gauge 1.5-inch needle through the Neviaser portal, medial to the acromion, anterior to the scapular spine, and posterior to the clavicle. Aim anterolaterally toward the greater tuberosity. Make sure to start medial enough that you do not hit the inferior acromion, which may cause significant pain (Figure 40–27).

- Another common method of injection is to start just inferior to the posterolateral corner of the acromion and aim anteriorly and slightly medially.
    - *Pearls:*
        ○ Most symptomatic rotator cuff pathology begins on the articular side. Therefore, although the subacromial injection may relieve the often considerable pain of secondary impingement, it may not completely eliminate the patient's pain.
        ○ Look at the patient's anteroposterior radiograph before injecting the AC joint to determine its slope, which varies. Following this slope often makes entering the AC joint easier. The AC joint often is easier to enter in its posterior half. The inside of the joint often feels gritty because of the intraarticular disc. Once the joint is full, there is often a back-pressure on the syringe's plunger. If you go through the AC joint, your needle will be in the subacromial space. For this reason, when trying to differentiate between sources of pain, it is often preferable to inject the subacromial space before injecting the AC joint.

## Diagnostic Imaging

- *Plain radiographs:* Shoulder radiographs should include an anteroposterior radiograph in the plane of the scapula with the humerus externally rotated, a transscapular lateral ("Y") view, and an axillary lateral.

- The axillary radiograph most clearly demonstrates glenohumeral dislocation or subtle arthritis.
    - *Emergency Room Pearls:*
        ○ Always get an axillary radiograph.
        ○ In cases of acute trauma precluding comfortable shoulder abduction, a Velpeau axillary view may easily be substituted. In this view, the arm remains in a sling and the standing patient leans backwards into the XR beam, which is positioned vertically. Alternatively, the patient may be supine (Figure 40–28).[28]
        ○ Never accept suboptimal radiographs. Many emergency room technicians are not highly experienced in taking good shoulder radiographs. Decisions often are made, and diagnoses ruled out, based on those radiographs. If you are unsure, repeat the radiographs. You may have to assist with patient

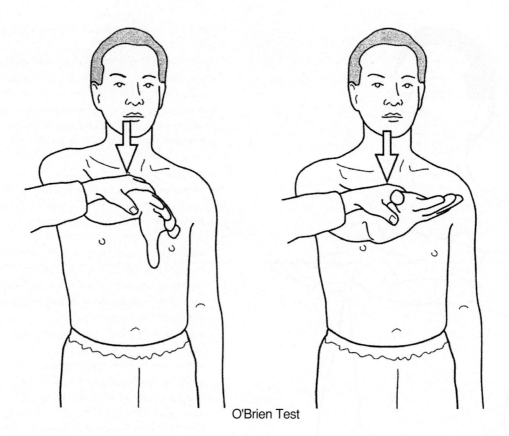

O'Brien Test

Figure 40–20:
O'Brien test.

positioning in order to obtain the radiographs you require.

- *Ultrasound:* Although isolated reports show efficacy in diagnosing full-thickness rotator cuff tears, results are operator dependent, and ultrasound currently is not commonly used.
- *Magnetic resonance imaging:* Provides excellent soft tissue detail. Especially good at diagnosing avascular necrosis, tumors, cysts, osteomyelitis, and rotator cuff muscle atrophy.

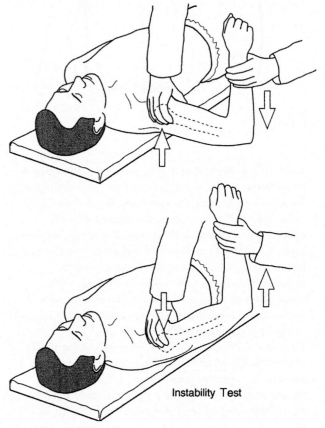

Instability Test

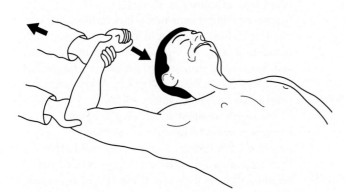

Figure 40–21:
Biceps load II test.

Figure 40–22:
Instability test.

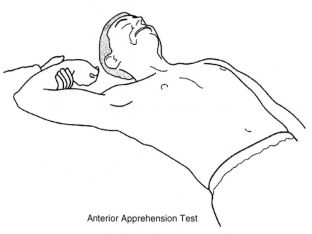

Anterior Apprehension Test

Figure 40–23:
Anterior apprehension test.

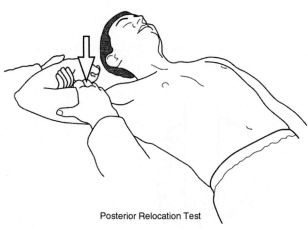

Posterior Relocation Test

Figure 40–24:
Posterior relocation test.

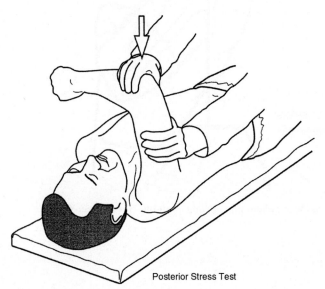

Posterior Stress Test

Figure 40–25:
Posterior stress test.

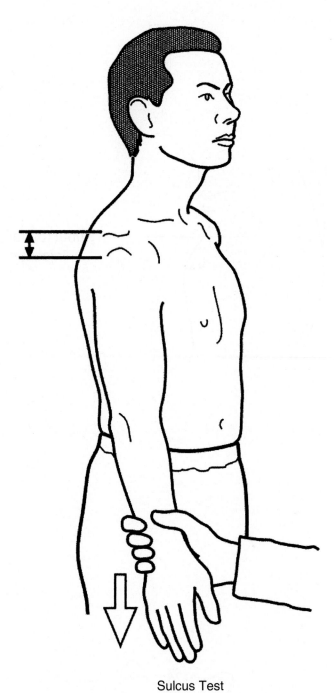

Sulcus Test

Figure 40–26:
Sulcus test.

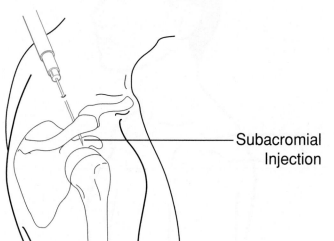

Figure 40–27:
Subacromial injection via Neviaser portal.

Subacromial
Injection

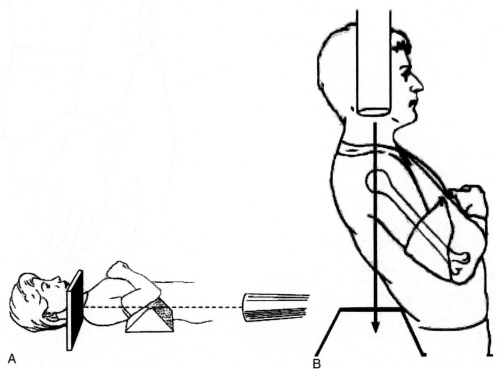

Figure 40–28:
**A,** Velpeau axillary radiograph, supine position. **B,** Velpeau axillary radiograph, upright position. (From Neer CS II: *J Shoulder Elbow Surg* 11:389-400, 2002.)

# References

1. O'Brien SJ, Neves MC, Arnoczky SP et al: The anatomy and histology of the inferior glenohumeral ligament complex of the shoulder. *Am J Sports Med* 18:449-456, 1990.
   Describes the anatomy of the inferior glenohumeral ligament complex and compares it to a hammock that supports the humeral head during arm elevation.

2. Warner JJ, Deng XH, Warren RF, Torzilli PA: Static capsuloligamentous restraints to superior-inferior translation of the glenohumeral joint. *Am J Sports Med* 20:675-685, 1992.
   Discusses ligament tensioning in multiples positions of abduction and rotation.

3. Itoi E, Hsu HS, An KN: Biomechanical investigation of the glenohumeral joint. *J Shoulder Elbow Surg* 5:407-424, 1996.
   The roles of the static and dynamic glenohumeral stabilizers are discussed.

4. Turkel SJ, Panio MW, Marshall JL, Girgis FG: Stabilizing mechanisms preventing anterior dislocation of the glenohumeral joint. *J Bone Joint Surg* 63A:1208-1217, 1981.
   Discusses the role of the static glenohumeral stabilizers at different degrees of abduction.

5. Lippitt SB, Vanderhooft JE, Harris SL et al: Glenohumeral stability from concavity-compression: a quantitative analysis. *J Shoulder Elbow Surg* 2:27-35, 1993.
   Concavity-compression is reported to have an efficiency of 60% in resisting tangential shear forces. This is decreased by labral resection.

6. Kido T, Itoi E, Konno N et al: The depressor function of biceps on the head of the humerus in shoulders with tears of the rotator cuff. *J Bone Joint Surg Br* 82:416-419, 2000.
   The biceps is an active depressor of the head of the humerus in shoulders with lesions of the rotator cuff.

7. Itoi E, Newman SR, Kuechle DK et al: Dynamic anterior stabilisers of the shoulder with the arm in abduction. *J Bone Joint Surg* 76B:834-836, 1994.
   The biceps becomes a more important stabilizer than the rotator cuff muscles as stability from the capsuloligamentous structures decrease.

8. Kibler WB: The role of the scapula in athletic shoulder function. *Am J Sports Med* 26:325-337, 1998.
   Physical examination of the scapula is reviewed, including the scapular stress test and the scapular slide test.

9. Warner JJ, Micheli LJ, Arslanian LE et al: Scapulothoracic motion in normal shoulders and shoulders with glenohumeral instability and impingement syndrome: a study using Moire topographic analysis. *Clin Orthop* 285:191-199, 1992.
   Scapulothoracic dysfunction occurs in up to 68% of rotator cuff disorders and 100% of glenohumeral instabilities.

10. Burkhart SS: Arthroscopic debridement and decompression for selected rotator cuff tears. Clinical results, pathomechanics, and patient selection based on biomechanical parameters. *Orthop Clin North Am* 24:111-123, 1993.
    The force couples of the shoulder and the biomechanics of the rotator cuff cable are discussed.

11. Burkhart SS: Reconciling the paradox of rotator cuff repair versus debridement: a unified biomechanical rationale for the treatment of rotator cuff tears. *Arthroscopy* 10:4-19, 1994.
    Discussion of functional and nonfunctional rotator cuff tears, the force couples of the shoulder, and the cable and its suspension bridge analogy.

12. Budoff JE, Nirschl RP, Guidi EJ: Debridement of partial-thickness tears of the rotator cuff without acromioplasty. Long-term follow-up and review of the literature. *J Bone Joint Surg Am* 80:733-748, 1998.
    Notes that the vast majority of rotator cuff tendon degeneration and tearing occurs within the rotator cuff crescent, lateral to the cable, where the blood supply is poor.

13. Kibler WB, Chandler TJ, Livingston BP, Roetert EP: Shoulder range of motion in elite tennis players. Effect of age and years of tournament play. *Am J Sports Med* 24:279-285, 1996.
    Notes that measurements of shoulder internal rotation based upon the vertebrae to which the thumb reaches is not reliable.

14. Wolf EM, Agrawal V: Transdeltoid palpation (the rent test) in the diagnosis of rotator cuff tears. *J Shoulder Elbow Surg* 10:470-473, 2001.
    Transdeltoid palpation had sensitivity of 95.7%, specificity of 96.8%, and accuracy of 96.3% for the diagnosis of full-thickness rotator cuff tear.

15. Neer CS 2nd: Impingement lesions. *Clin Orthop* 173:70-77, 1983.
    Describes the Neer test for rotator cuff pathology.

16. Hawkins RJ, Kennedy JC: Impingement syndrome in athletes. *Am J Sports Med* 8:151-158, 1980.
    Describes the Hawkins test for rotator cuff pathology.

17. Kelly BT, Kadrmas WR, Speer KP: Empty can versus full can exercise for rotator cuff rehabilitation: an electromyographic analysis. *Orthop Trans* 21:147-148, 1997.
    Discusses the thumb down or empty can test and the thumb up or full can test for rotator cuff pathology.

18. Savoie FH 3rd, Field LD, Atchinson S: Anterior superior instability with rotator cuff tearing: SLAC lesion. *Orthop Clin North Am* 32:457-461, 2001.
    Discusses the Whipple test for anterior supraspinatus pathology.

19. Burkhart SS, Tehrany AM: Arthroscopic subscapularis tendon repair: technique and preliminary results. *Arthroscopy* 18:454-463, 2002
    Discusses the Napoleon test for subscapularis dysfunction.

20. Bennett WF: Specificity of the Speed's test: arthroscopic technique for evaluating the biceps tendon at the level of the bicipital groove. *Arthroscopy* 14:789-796, 1998.
    Reports Speed's test to be 90% sensitive and 13.8% specific. The test was positive with a variety of shoulder pathologies other than bicipital tendinosis.

21. O'Brien SJ, Pagnani MJ, Fealy S et al: The active compression test: a new and effective test for diagnosing labral tears and acromioclavicular joint abnormality. *Am J Sports Med* 26:610-613, 1998.

Reports the O'Brien active compression test for SLAP lesions and acromioclavicular joint abnormalities.

22. Kim SH, Ha KI, Ahn JH et al: Biceps load test II: A clinical test for SLAP lesions of the shoulder. *Arthroscopy* 17:160-164, 2001.
The biceps load test II is described and is reported as 89.7% sensitive and 96.9% specific.

23. Andrews JR, Dugas JR: Diagnosis and treatment of shoulder injuries in the throwing athlete: the role of thermal-assisted capsular shrinkage. *Instr Course Lect* 50:17-21, 2001.
Describes the Lachman test for glenohumeral instability.

24. Cofield RH, Irving JF: Evaluation and classification of shoulder instability. With special reference to examination under anesthesia. *Clin Orthop* 223:32-43, 1987.
Excellent discussion of the examination under anesthesia.

25. Payne LZ, Altchek DW: The surgical treatment of anterior shoulder instability. *Clin Sports Med* 14:863-883, 1995.

Physical examination of the unstable shoulder and grading systems are presented. Open stabilization technique is discussed.

26. Jobe FW, Kvitne RS, Giangarra CE: Shoulder pain in the overhand or throwing athlete. The relationship of anterior instability and rotator cuff impingement. *Orthop Rev* 18:1268, 1989.
The Jobe anterior apprehension and posterior relocation tests are described.

27. Pollock RG, Bigliani LU: Glenohumeral instability: evaluation and treatment. *J Am Acad Orthop Surg* 1:24-32, 1993.
The posterior stress test for posterior instability is discussed.

28. Neer CS 2nd: Four-segment classification of proximal humeral fractures: purpose and reliable use. *J Shoulder Elbow Surg* 11:389-400, 2002.
Discusses the Velpeau axillary view for patients unable or unwilling to abduct the shoulder.

# CHAPTER 41

# Tendinopathy of the Rotator Cuff and Proximal Biceps

Jeffrey E. Budoff

MD, Assistant Professor, Hand and Upper Extremity Institute, Department of Orthopaedic Surgery, Baylor College of Medicine; Houston Veterans Affairs Medical Center, Houston, TX

## Rotator Cuff Injuries

- The anatomy and function of the rotator cuff were discussed in Chapter 40. The rotator cuff is the most common source of shoulder pain and disability. Most rotator cuff injuries occur without a history of trauma and result from overuse.

### Etiology

#### Classic Teaching (Primary Extrinsic Coracoacromial Arch Impingement)

- Congenital variations in acromial morphology exist. Some acromions are flatter, whereas others have inferior subacromial spurs or hooks on them. With repetitive arm elevation, these subacromial spurs mechanically abrade or cut into the rotator cuff, progressively leading to tendon injury.
  - In his classic 1972 article, Neer[1] implicated the anterior acromion and its "spurs" in the etiology of rotator cuff injuries. Subacromial abrasion caused rotator cuff inflammation, which progressed to partial-thickness tears and later full-thickness tears.[1]
  - In 1986, Bigliani, Morrison, and April[2] characterized acromial morphology as type I (flat), type II curved (parallel to the humeral head), or type III hooked (converging on the humeral head). They found that full-thickness rotator cuff tears were associated with type III acromions and anterior undersurface spurs.[2]
  - The classic theory of the etiology of rotator cuff pathology has been challenged.

## Primary Intrinsic Degenerative Tendinopathy (Tendinosis)

- The rotator cuff fails from tensile, not compressive, overload. Pathoetiology and mechanism are identical to tendon pathology in many other areas of the body (i.e., tennis elbow, patellar tendinosis, Achilles tendinosis). Evidence strongly suggests that most rotator cuff symptoms are caused by primary intrinsic degeneration, not extrinsic subacromial compression.[3–5]
- Histologic studies of symptomatic rotator cuff disease have repeatedly noted an absence of acute inflammatory cells. These studies have consistently noted the changes of degenerative tendinopathy, for which the pathologic name is *angiofibroblastic hyperplasia*.
  - The term *impingement syndrome* has been used to describe symptoms related to the rotator cuff in the absence of a full-thickness tear. Commonly used synonyms include *bursitis* and *tendinitis*. However, use of the term *tendinosis* is now recommended in lieu of the histologically inaccurate term *tendinitis*, because it more accurately describes the true pathology.[3]
- Clinical and cadaveric studies have noted that more than 90% of partial-thickness rotator cuff tears occur on the articular side, away from the acromion.[3,4]
  - Degeneration begins on the articular sides of the supraspinatus and infraspinatus tendon insertions rather than the bursal sides probably because of their poor blood supply.[3]

- Acromial spurs form with age and are degenerative.
  - The type III acromion is rare (2%–4%) in young, asymptomatic athletes. A higher incidence of type III acromions is seen in older populations.[6]
- Cadaveric studies have demonstrated that rotator cuff pathology predates that of the acromion.[3,5]
- Spur reformation has been noted following subacromial decompression.[7]
- A study using mineral apposition analysis and quantitative cytochemical techniques demonstrated active bone formation at the acromial insertion of the coracoacromial (CA) ligament, supporting the concept that spur formation is a secondary phenomenon. Thus the spur is actually an enthesophyte (bone growth) at the CA ligament's acromial insertion, probably in response to dynamic loading.[8]
- Nonoperative management has been reported to successfully treat most full-thickness rotator cuff tears. Because therapy cannot modify pathologic osseous prominences, another etiology is implied.[9]

## Pathomechanics

- Tissue damage occurs when the stresses placed on the rotator cuff exceed its stress tolerance, which is related to its strength. The rotator cuff muscles are small and weak and therefore are vulnerable to overuse. Overuse injuries occur when the rate of tissue damage over time exceeds the body's rate of repair. As a natural part of the aging process, the deltoid retains its strength longer than the smaller rotator cuff. When rotator cuff injury, degeneration, fatigue, or weakness occurs, the rotator cuff is unable to effectively oppose (via concavity-compression) the superior shear stresses imparted by the larger and stronger deltoid muscle. This situation leads to dynamic superior instability of the humeral head with arm elevation. This inappropriate superior migration of the humeral head causes *secondary* impingement of the rotator cuff against the CA arch, leading to further injury, in a self-perpetuating cycle. Therefore, subacromial impingement is a secondary and not a primary process.[3]
- The CA ligament and undersurface of the acromion function as secondary, static stabilizers of the humeral head against anterosuperior migration. With rotator cuff dysfunction, the CA ligament may experience increased stress and undergo degenerative changes, forming a traction spur at its insertion into the anteromedial corner of the acromion. These acromial changes are the result of rotator cuff injury; they are not the cause.[3,5,8] This traction spur often is mistaken for an abnormal acromial hook, or type III acromion.[3,8]
  - As rotator cuff dysfunction increases with age, the CA arch may function as a fulcrum for the superiorly migrated humeral head, allowing continued glenohumeral elevation.[10]

- *Relationship to instability:* In patients with anterior glenohumeral instability resulting from ligamentous insufficiency, the dynamic stabilizers, including the supraspinatus, infraspinatus, and biceps, compensate with increased activity.[11] This overuse may predispose patients to injury.

## Diagnosis

- The history and physical examination of rotator cuff disorders are discussed in Chapter 40. Concomitant loss of passive motion, instability, and scapulothoracic dysfunction should be noted.

## Radiography

- Subtle superior migration of the humeral head can be detected by the presence of a "break" in the arch formed by the medial cortex of the humerus and the lateral cortex of the scapula (Figure 41–1).[12]
- Marked elevation of the humeral head with narrowing of the acromiohumeral distance to less than 5 mm is highly suggestive of a large rotator cuff tear.[12]
- Sclerosis, osteophytes, and subchondral cysts of the greater tuberosity are associated with rotator cuff tears.[13]

## Magnetic Resonance Imaging

- According to Frost, Andersen, and Lundorf,[14] supraspinatus pathology as seen on magnetic resonance imaging (MRI) is related to age, not to symptoms. According to Shuman,[15] conventional MRI has not performed well in distinguishing partial-thickness rotator cuff tears from small full-thickness rotator cuff tears or normal tendon. According to Torstensen and Hollinshead,[16] MRI is not an effective or accurate tool for assessing shoulder pathology when the clinical picture is unclear.
- From 33% to 80% of partial-thickness rotator cuff tears can be missed on MRI.[16–19]

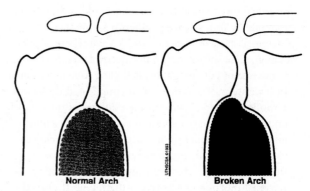

**Figure 41–1:**

**Model of an anteroposterior radiograph. Normal rotator cuff function presents with a smooth unbroken scapulohumeral arch. Rotator cuff dysfunction leads to superior migration of the humeral head with a broken scapulohumeral arch. (From Burkhart SS: Reconciling the paradox of rotator cuff repair versus debridement: a unified biomechanical rationale for the treatment of rotator cuff tears.** *Arthroscopy* **10:4-19, 1994.)**

- MRI is 68% to 92% accurate, 78% to 96% sensitive, and 49% to 94% specific for assessing full-thickness rotator cuff tears. MR arthrography may be more accurate.[15,16,18,19]
- Studies by Needell et al.,[20] Tempelhof, Rupp, and Seil,[22] and Sher et al[21] demonstrated that between the ages of 40 and 60 years, 24% to 27% of asymptomatic volunteers had partial-thickness rotator cuff tears. Above age 60 years, 27% to 28% of asymptomatic volunteers had full-thickness rotator cuff tears, and another 26% to 27% had partial-thickness rotator cuff tears. Above age 80 years, 51% of asymptomatic volunteers had full-thickness rotator cuff tears.
  - *Pearl:* Because conservative management of full-thickness tears is identical to that for partial-thickness tears, diagnosing the thickness of the tear may be initially irrelevant. Initial treatment in most cases should not be based on the presence or absence of a full-thickness tear because most full-thickness rotator cuff tears are asymptomatic.[12]
- Decisions regarding operative treatment are best made based on the patient's symptoms, wishes, and response to nonoperative management and not the presence or absence of a hole in the cuff.

## Nonoperative Management

- Rotator cuff and scapulothoracic stabilizer strengthening reportedly was successful in treating 50% to 82% *full*-thickness rotator cuff tears.[9,23–26]
- Nonoperative management may be considered if the patient can actively elevate the arm above the horizontal. This ability implies the tear is functional and does not involve the rotator cuff cable (described in Chapter 40.
  - No significant relationship exists between the length of preoperative symptoms and the final outcome following repair of nonacute rotator cuff tears. Therefore, no evidence indicates that a "penalty" exists for attempting nonoperative management of nonacute rotator cuff tears.[9]
- At least 3 months of nonoperative management is recommended in most cases before undertaking operative management.
- Because rotator cuff pathology results from degeneration and weakness, not from inflammation, nonsteroidal antiinflammatory drugs, corticosteroid injections, and modalities should be used only as adjuncts to increase patient comfort and promote effective strengthening given that they have no proven long-term efficacy or curative potential.
  - The efficacy of steroid injections has been questioned. A randomized prospective trial found no difference in symptoms between patients (with medial tennis elbow; a disorder with identical histopathology) injected with steroid and lidocaine and those injected with only

saline at 3 and 12 months.[27] In addition, a meta-analysis performed by the Cochrane Database found that although subacromial steroid injections had a small benefit over placebo in some trials, no benefit of subacromial steroid injections over oral nonsteroidal antiinflammatory drugs was observed.[28] Repetitive injections are inappropriate because they may cause cellular death, further tissue weakness, and actually slow the healing process.[27]
- Any rest should be relative, with activity allowed within the limits of pain to prevent further deconditioning.
- Physical therapists may educate the patient and facilitate this program, but patients must assume responsibility for their own daily exercise program. Once the motivated patient can properly perform the exercises, he or she can perform therapy exclusively at home.
- Acute large traumatic tears
  - Although the patient usually retains nearly full passive motion, the arm cannot be actively elevated above the horizontal, even following a lidocaine injection. The other elements in the differential diagnosis are fracture and dislocation, which are excluded by radiography, and suprascapular and axillary neuropathies, which are uncommon. Conservative management is ineffective in this setting. Early repairs performed within 3 weeks of injury have yielded better results, with greater postoperative motion and function, than repairs performed later.[29] Therefore, the diagnosis should be confirmed by MRI and operative management strongly considered.

## Treatment Specifics

- The mainstay of nonoperative management is strengthening of the rotator cuff, deltoid, and scapulothoracic stabilizers. Strengthening the rotator cuff may help decrease symptoms for the following reasons:
  - A stronger rotator cuff can better oppose superior translation of the humeral head and avoid subsequent secondary impingement.
  - Muscles are the "shock absorbers" of the musculoskeletal system and protect their tendons from excessive stress. Therefore, muscle strengthening increases the stress tolerance of the myotendinous unit.
  - Strengthening may enhance tendon healing via increased tissue turnover.
- Scapular strengthening may help decrease symptoms by restoring normal scapular motion, which allows the acromion to clear the rotator cuff during arm elevation. Scapulothoracic weakness causes decreased acromial clearance and increased rotator cuff compression, exacerbating symptoms.[30]
- Rotator cuff and deltoid strengthening exercises include
  - Internal rotation, external rotation, forward flexion, abduction, and extension, and a diagonal proprioceptive

neuromuscular facilitation pattern similar to the motion used to draw a sword (Figures 41–2 and 41–3). In cases of significant weakness, closed chain exercises may be substituted, which create less stress in the rotator cuff.

- Scapulothoracic strengthening exercises include
  - The seated row, pull-downs, the "push-up plus," the "bench press plus," and the "press-up plus." These exercises should be carried out to a "four-count" to avoid substituting biceps and triceps function for scapulothoracic retraction and protraction, respectively (Figures 41–4 through 41–8)
  - The middle and lower trapezius may be strengthened by prone dumbbell flies performed with the shoulder abducted 90 and 135 degrees, respectively. A four-count is not necessary for these exercises (Figure 41–9).
  - An elastic resistance can be used in lieu of a weight.
  - Exercises optimally should be performed until the muscles fatigue, which is when mechanics become abnormal, rather than completing a specified number of sets and repetitions. For deconditioned patients, a rough goal is one set of 10 to 12 repetitions for each exercise, performed once or twice a day, to start. A well-conditioned athlete can begin with a more advanced program.
  - Exercise should not cause pain. If pain occurs during or after exercises, then (1) the resistance should be decreased, (2) the number of repetitions should be decreased, or (3) the patient should restrict the exercise motion to within the pain-free arc.
- The posterior joint capsule and pectoralis minor should be stretched (Figures 41–10 and 41–11). A tight posterior capsule may negatively affect glenohumeral biomechanics, whereas pectoralis minor tightness may exacerbate scapular protraction.[30,31]

## Surgical Management

- *Pearl:* Instability should be ruled out using examination under anesthesia and/or diagnostic arthroscopy. Failure to address underlying glenohumeral instability will compromise the surgical result.

### Subacromial Decompression (Acromioplasty)

- Subacromial decompression (SAD; acromioplasty) is the most common shoulder procedure performed today. This procedure is designed to alleviate rotator cuff problems caused by subacromial spurs, per the classic theory of extrinsic CA impingement.
- According to the theory of intrinsic degenerative tendinosis, SAD may provide pain relief by removing the CA ligament and acromial undersurface, the sources of secondary impingement, thereby removing pressure from a sensitive tendon.

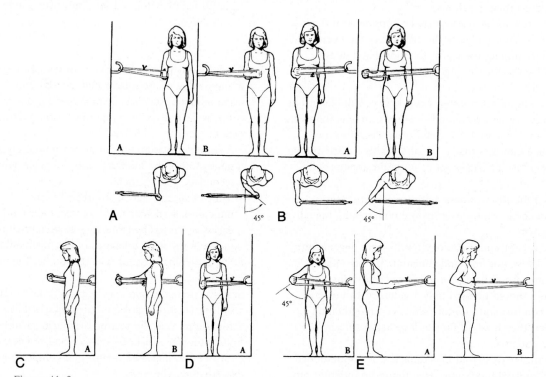

Figure 41–2:
**A,** Internal rotation. **B,** External rotation. **C,** Forward flexion. **D,** Abduction. **E,** Extension. (From Wirth MA, Basamania C, Rockwood CA Jr: Nonoperative management of full-thickness tears of the rotator cuff. *Orthop Clin North Am* 28:59-67, 1997.)

Figure 41–3:
**Diagonal proprioceptive neuromuscular facilitation.**

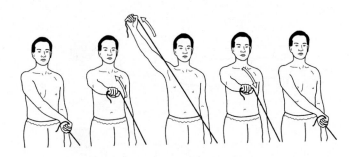

Figure 41–4:
**Rows.**

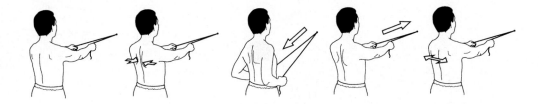

- Other plausible explanations include denervation of the CA arch[32] or the institution of relative rest and meaningful postoperative rehabilitation.[33]
- SAD alone does not directly address the primary degenerative tendinosis and, as noted by Weber[34] and Hyvonen, Lohi, and Jalovaara,[35] does not prevent tear progression from rotator cuff tendinosis/partial-thickness tears to full-thickness tears.
- If pathologic reactive subacromial exostoses are seen in combination with a bursal-sided partial-thickness tear, the offending exostosis should be removed. This procedure does not require a formal SAD, because the acromial body itself rarely is abnormal.[3,36]
- Two common arthroscopic techniques can be used to "check" each other:
  1. Burr lateral/scope posterior: A burr is buried into the anterolateral corner of the acromion to the desired depth, and the anterior border of the acromion is resected at this depth to its medial border. The depth of resection decreases as the burr is brought posteriorly.

  2. Cutting block technique (burr posterior/scope lateral): The posterior acromion is used to guide resection of the anterior acromion to create a flat undersurface.

## Results

- Short-term results of arthroscopic SAD (ASAD) are favorable overall, with between 46% and 100% success at a mean 17- to 48-month follow-up.[3] Stephens et al.[37] reported 81% surgical success for ASAD at average follow-up of 8 years 5 months. Of these patients, 34% underwent concomitant rotator cuff debridement.
- Meta-analysis by Checroun, Dennis, and Zuckerman[38] revealed 83.3% surgical success for 698 open subacromial decompressions at 6 to 62 months and 81.4% surgical success for 1237 arthroscopic SADs at 6 to 41 months. At 25-month follow-up, Spangehl et al.[39] found no significant difference between open and ASAD for strength and patient satisfaction, although patients who had open SAD had less pain and better function.

Figure 41–5:
**Pull-downs.**

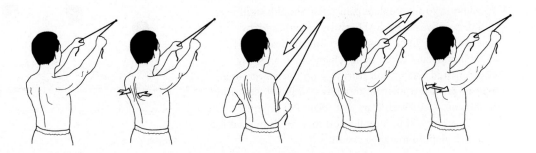

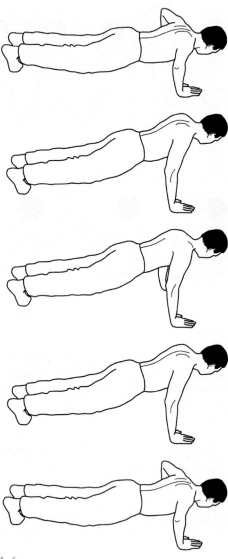

Figure 41–6:
**Push-up plus.**

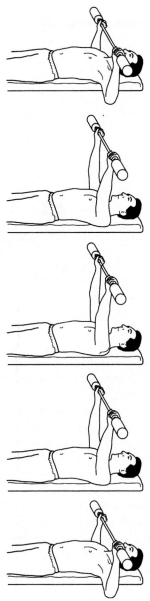

Figure 41–7:
**Bench press plus.**

- Hyvonen, Lohi, and Jalovaara[35] reported 72% good or excellent results for open SAD for impingement syndrome at mean follow-up of 9 years (range 6–15 years). Stuart reported 73% good to excellent results at minimum 3-year follow-up.[3]
- Fukuda[40] reported 93.9% satisfactory results at 4.5-year follow-up of partial-thickness rotator cuff tears treated with open SAD followed by rotator cuff debridement and repair.
- In addition to incomplete pain relief, shoulder stiffness, and deltoid weakness, SAD can be complicated by anterosuperior instability of the humeral head. The instability occurs when biomechanically marginally compensated rotator cuff tears rely on the subacromial arch to provide a fulcrum to allow continued elevation.[10] It also can occur with tears that recur and progress despite surgery. This complication may result in total loss of active glenohumeral elevation.[41–43]

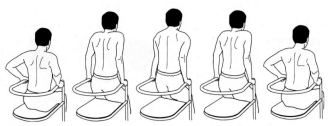

Figure 41–8:
**Press-up plus.**

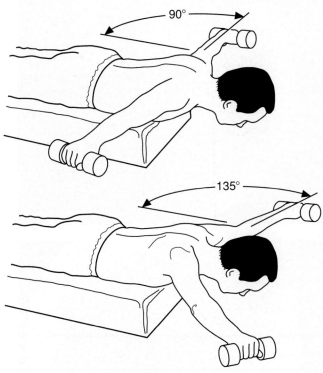

Figure 41–9:
**Prone flies.**

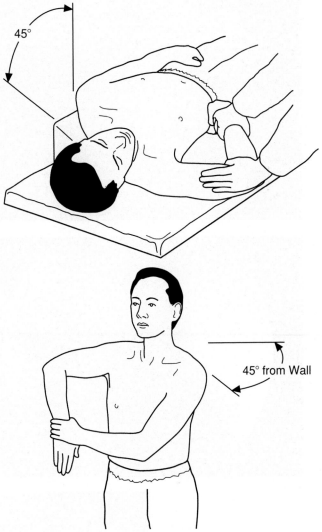

Figure 41–10:
**Posterior glenohumeral capsule stretch.**

## Arthroscopic Rotator Cuff Debridement

- Arthroscopic rotator cuff debridement (ARCD) is an alternative, or complementary procedure to subacromial decompression. ARCD addresses the primary pathology directly without additional iatrogenic injury to the shoulder. Postoperative pain and morbidity are less than experienced with ASAD.

### Technique (Figure 41–12)

- ARCD is best performed with the patient in the lateral decubitus position because of the traction applied. ARCD is extremely difficult to perform effectively with the patient in the beach chair position.
- Instability should be ruled out by examination with the patient under anesthesia and/or by diagnostic arthroscopy. Failure to address underlying glenohumeral instability will compromise the surgical result.
- An angled, motorized shaver is used to debride the insertions of the rotator cuff tendons. The area of tendinosis corresponds to the crescent area described by Burkhart,[10,12] just lateral to the rotator cuff's cable. The cable itself is essentially never degenerative.
  - *Pearl:* The deepest layer of soft tissue surrounding any synovial articulation is the joint capsule. Therefore, when the arthroscope is introduced into a relatively

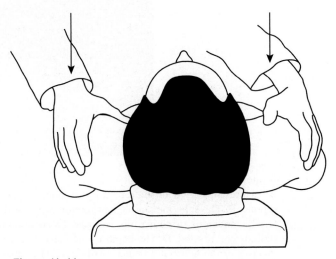

Figure 41–11:
**Pectoralis minor stretch.**

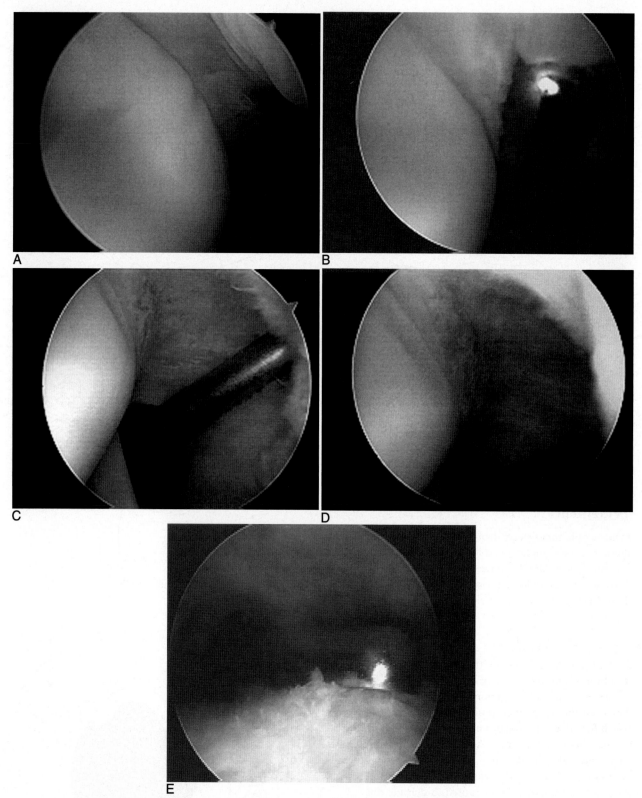

Figure 41–12:

**A,** Arthroscopic view of the superior glenohumeral joint. The pathology is hidden behind the superior joint capsule. **B,** The superior capsule and rotator cuff insertion are challenged with an aggressive motorized shaver. **C,** The tendinotic tissue is easily removed. Normal tendon, including the cable of Burkhart seen on the far right, is not affected. **D,** The depth of the defect can be estimated from the size of the newly created bare spot superior to the humeral articular cartilage. **E,** The subacromial space is free from underhanging pathologic osseous prominences. Debridement of the bursal surface of the rotator cuff usually removes significantly less pathologic tissue compared to debridement of the articular surface.

normal glenohumeral joint and the lens is directed superiorly, the surgeon is viewing the superior joint capsule, *not* the rotator cuff. To assess the rotator cuff, you need to debride the superior capsule and challenge the rotator cuff insertion with a motorized shaver.

- Normal tendon is composed of white, shiny fibers of parallel orientation. A motorized shaver used in a windshield wiper fashion will not injure normal tendon. However, the more friable tendinosis tissue will be quickly and easily debrided. Debridement is continued until normal tendon is reached, at which point continued debridement becomes ineffective.
- The CA ligament is not released. Pathologic subacromial osteophytes can be debrided if necessary, but the procedure is uncommon. A traditional SAD is not performed.

## Results

- Budoff, Nirschl, and Guidi[3] reported 89% good to excellent results at average 53-month follow-up, 93% if workers' compensation cases were excluded. Long-term results at minimum 5-year follow-up were 81% good to excellent, 86% if workers' compensation cases were excluded.[3]
- Snyder et al.[44] reported 93% success, with the addition of SAD making no difference.
- Andrews, Broussard, and Carson[45] reported 85% success in treating young athletes.
- Altchek and Carson[46] reported 80% success in throwing athletes, 10% of whom also underwent ASAD. They believed that untreated instability was responsible for the failures.[46]

## Rotator Cuff Repair

- Open repairs involve deltoid takedown and reattachment, necessitating more conservative postoperative therapy and predisposing to the devastating complication of deltoid detachment.
- Mini-open repairs split the deltoid without takedown, are versatile, and prevent the potentially devastating complication of deltoid detachment.
- Arthroscopic repairs have benefited from improved techniques, equipment, and experience. Even large tears can be routinely repaired arthroscopically.
  - From 84% to 95% satisfactory results at 2.5- to 4-year follow-up have been reported, rates equal to open repair. Less postoperative pain and stiffness have been noted. Postoperative rehabilitation may be less aggressive than following open repair.[47-49]
- Common rotator cuff tear patterns[50]:
  - Longitudinal: These longitudinal splits can simply be repaired side to side.
  - Crescent-shaped: Minimally retracted. The tendon is simply repaired back to the greater tuberosity (Figure 41–13).

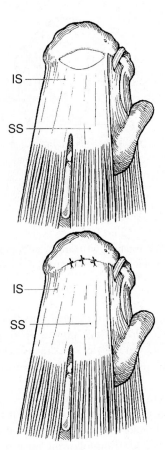

Figure 41–13:
**Crescent-shaped rotator cuff fear. *IS,* infraspinatus; *SS,* supraspinatus. (From Lo IK, Burkhart SS: Current concepts in arthroscopic rotator cuff repair. *Am J Sports Med* 31:308-324, 2003.)**

- U-shaped: These often extend medially. The longitudinal component should first be repaired in a side-to-side fashion from medial to lateral (margin convergence) to create a crescent-shaped tear, which reduces strain at the cuff edge. The tear then can be repaired back to the greater tuberosity with minimal tension. Attempts to bring the medial margin laterally to the tuberosity will fail (Figure 41–14).
- L-shaped: This tear is similar to the U-shaped tear, except that one of the cuff's leaves (usually the posterior leaf) is torn from the greater tuberosity and the adjacent tendon. This leaf is more mobile than the other and is repaired side to side along the longitudinal split then back to the greater tuberosity. It may occasionally be easiest to first repair its free corner back to the greater tuberosity and then sew its free longitudinal edge back to the adjacent rotator cuff tendon (Figure 41–15).
- Massive: These tears often are chronic and immobile, requiring surgical release(s) to accomplish a minimal

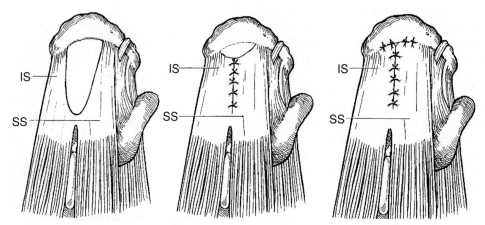

Figure 41–14:

**U-shaped rotator cuff tear.** *IS,* infraspinatus; *SS,* supraspinatus; (From Lo IK, Burkhart SS: Current concepts in arthroscopic rotator cuff repair. *Am J Sports Med* 31:308-324, 2003.)

tension repair. Poorly mobilized tears that are repaired under tension have a high propensity to fail.

- Reported results of full-thickness rotator cuff repairs performed with or without SAD demonstrate similar results.
  - From 80% to 94% surgical success has been reported for open repair with SAD at 2- to 13.4-year follow-up.[51–53]
  - Goldberg, Lippitt, and Matsen[54] reported good results and improved function following open repair performed without acromioplasty at average 4-year follow-up.
  - Gartsman and O'Connor[55] performed a prospective, randomized study of 92 patients with full-thickness tears of the supraspinatus tendon and a type II acromion undergoing arthroscopic repair. At

minimum 1-year follow-up, they noted no significant difference in outcomes whether or not an acromioplasty was performed.

## Mini-Open Rotator Cuff Repair

- I routinely perform arthroscopy before mini-open repair to avoid missing additional pathology, and to be able to debride the undersurface of the rotator cuff.
1. A longitudinal incision in Langer lines is performed over the lateral acromion, centered at its anterolateral corner (Figure 41–16). The skin is mobilized from the superficial deltoid fascia and retracted with a Gelpi retractor.
2. The anterolateral raphe of the deltoid is split (Figure 41–17). The proximal anterolateral raphe often runs

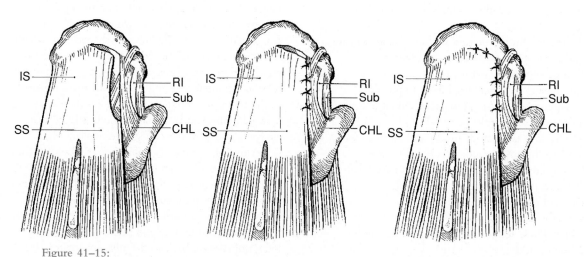

Figure 41–15:

**L-shaped rotator cuff tear.** *CHL,* coraco-humeral ligament; *IS,* infraspinatus; *RI,* rotator interval; *SS,* supraspinatus; *Sub,* subscapularis. (Reprinted from: Lo IK, Burkhart SS: Current concepts in arthroscopic rotator cuff repair. *Am J Sports Med* 31:308-324, 2003 with permission.)

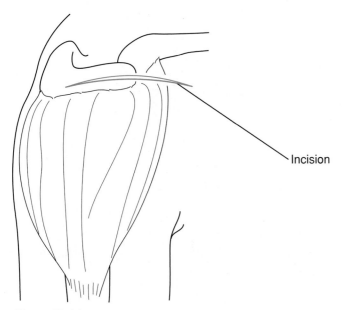

Figure 41–16:
**Mini-open rotator cuff repair: sabre incision.**

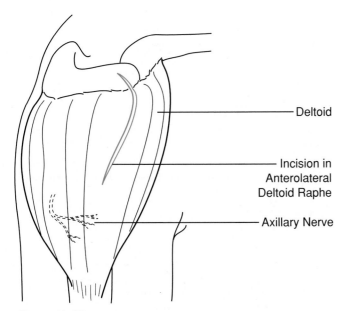

Figure 41–17:
**Mini-open rotator cuff repair: deltoid split.**

along the anterior margin of the acromion. Extension of the raphe along this margin can compromise the anterior deltoid origin. To avoid this situation, once the anterolateral corner of the acromion is reached, the incision is angled toward the center of the acromion, in a direction 45 degrees from the anterior and lateral acromial border. To maximize exposure, electrocautery should be used to incise the deltoid's deep fascial origin at the acromion.

3. To avoid injuring the axillary nerve, classic teaching is to not split the deltoid raphe distally more than 5 cm from the acromion. Although the classic teaching is correct, a more accurate technique is to realize that the nerve courses distal to the distal margin of the subacromial bursa. The pouch-like distal extent of the subacromial bursa can be palpated and the deltoid split just short of this level. A Gelpi retractor is used to maintain the deltoid split.

4. The bursa is resected. This procedure exposes the rotator cuff and may partially denervate the subacromial space, potentially relieving pain.[32] To identify the bursa, remember that the bursa does not move with humeral rotation but the rotator cuff does (Figure 41–18).

5. The tear pattern is recognized and repaired appropriately. Margin convergence (side-to-side repair of the tendon, starting medially and progressing laterally) is used as needed, especially in U-shaped tears (Figure 41–19). Massive tears may require release of the rotator interval (between the supraspinatus and subscapularis), including release of the supraspinatus from the coracohumeral ligament, which tethers it to the base of the coracoid process. Occasionally, a release between the contracted supraspinatus and infraspinatus is also necessary.

6. The tendon should be repaired to bone. A rongeur is used to remove degenerative tendinosis and sclerotic cortex just lateral to the articular cartilage margin. However, the entire cortical thickness does not need to be removed, nor does cancellous bone need to be exposed or a trough created. Doing so may only weaken the suture anchor fixation.

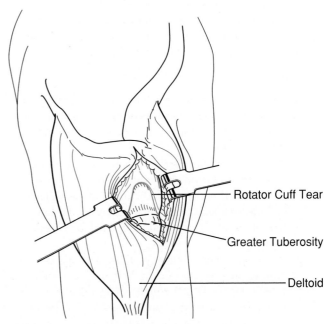

Figure 41–18:
**Mini-open rotator cuff repair: exposure.**

Margin Convergence Stitches

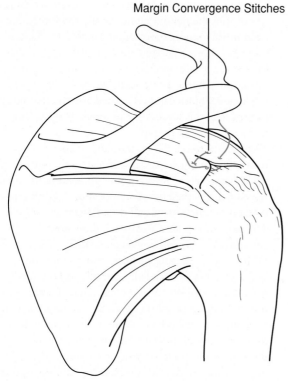

Figure 41–19:

**Mini-open rotator cuff repair: margin convergence.**

7. Suture anchors and/or sutures through drill holes can be used to coapt the tendon to bone. Suture anchors are placed at a 45-degree "dead man's angle" just lateral to the decorticated bone. I prefer a modified Mason-Allen stitch with no. 2 Fiberwire suture (Arthrex; Naples, FL) (Figure 41–20).

• Postoperatively, early passive and gentle active assisted motion is performed. Active motion is delayed for 4 to 6 weeks and strengthening for 10 to 12 weeks.

## Arthroscopic Rotator Cuff Repair

• This particular technique is my preference, but there are many variations, and other surgeons have other excellent techniques. I have no financial interest in any of the products mentioned.

1. The posterior and anterior portals are made more superiorly to provide better angles for suture passage. The anterior portal should be made in the superior and medial extent of the rotator interval, not low on the subscapularis (as would be optimal for a Bankart repair).

2. A complete bursectomy is performed, taking care to remove the posterior wall of the bursa (the "veil of tears") (Figure 41–21). I prefer using a shaver on forward to prepare the "landing pad" on the greater tuberosity instead of a burr. Sclerotic bone is removed, but a full decortication is not performed.

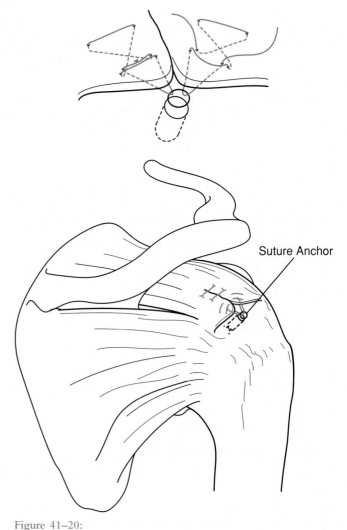

Suture Anchor

Figure 41–20:

**Mini-open rotator cuff repair: tendon-bone fixation with modified Mason-Allen stitches.**

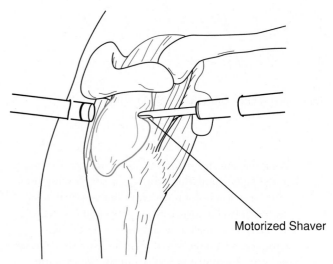

Motorized Shaver

Figure 41–21:

**Arthroscopic rotator cuff repair: subacromial bursectomy.**

3. The lateral portal is used for visualization. It is localized with a spinal needle approximately 3 to 4 cm lateral to the lateral border of the acromion, at the anteroposterior center of the rotator cuff tear (Figure 41–22). Before transferring the arthroscope to the lateral portal, any soft tissue around the localizing needle is debrided, otherwise it will obstruct your view once the arthroscope is moved.

   ○ The anterolateral portal is used to place suture anchors into the greater tuberosity. It is localized with a spinal needle close to the lateral border of the acromion (for a better angle for anchor placement) in line with an axis bisecting the acromioclavicular (AC) joint. Metal anchors can be screwed through needle holes in the skin without the need to create a formal portal.

   ○ Additional portals can be created as necessary to facilitate the procedure, analogous to extending an open incision. The "safe zone" for portal placement is within 5 cm of the acromial edge in a 180-degree arc lateral to the coracoid, anteriorly and posteriorly.

4. There are four types of tears, in addition to massive tears: longitudinal, U-shaped, L-shaped, and crescent-shaped. Longitudinal tears are repaired side to side and are the easiest to start with. U-shaped tears are repaired by margin convergence (side to side) and then anchored to bone. Following margin convergence, the anterior and posterior leafs of the rotator cuff should lie against the tuberosity without tension. One suture anchor, with two loaded sutures, often is sufficient to anchor both leaves of a U-tear with a "single-row" repair. Crescent tears are repaired by multiple suture anchors, usually proceeding from anterior to posterior. L-shaped supraspinatus tears are repaired by pulling the avulsed corner laterally with a locking grasper and repairing this corner to a suture anchor in the tuberosity. Two anchors (four sutures) often are required to coapt the entire tear to bone. Side-to-side stitches are then placed to repair the longitudinal component of the tear. Alternatively, the side-to-side stitches may be placed before the suture anchor.

5. It is crucial for margin convergence stitch placement to have an unobstructed view of the anterior and posterior cannulas; debride more bursa until this occurs. In my experience, I have found it easiest to pass sutures with the 45-degree Arthrex lasso. After passing the lasso through the posterior cannula, its tip is rotated inferiorly and pushed through the rotator cuff's posterior leaf. It is important to capture enough tissue (5–10 mm) but not so much that the tendon bunches up excessively when the knot is tied. The lasso then is passed through the anterior leaf of the rotator cuff. It is helpful to use a grasper passed through the anterior cannula, or the anterior cannula itself, to provide "back-pressure" to facilitate penetration of the anterior leaf.

   ○ The lasso's suture loop is grasped and pulled out of the anterior cannula, where it is loaded with a free fiber wire (Arthrex) suture (Figures 41–23 and 41–24). The lasso is pulled back out of the posterior cannula, bringing one end of the Fiberwire stitch out with it (Figure 41–25). It is important to pull the metal shaft of the lasso and its suture loop back simultaneously as one unit. If the suture loop is simply pulled through the lasso's shaft, the fiber wire can be damaged against its sharp tip.

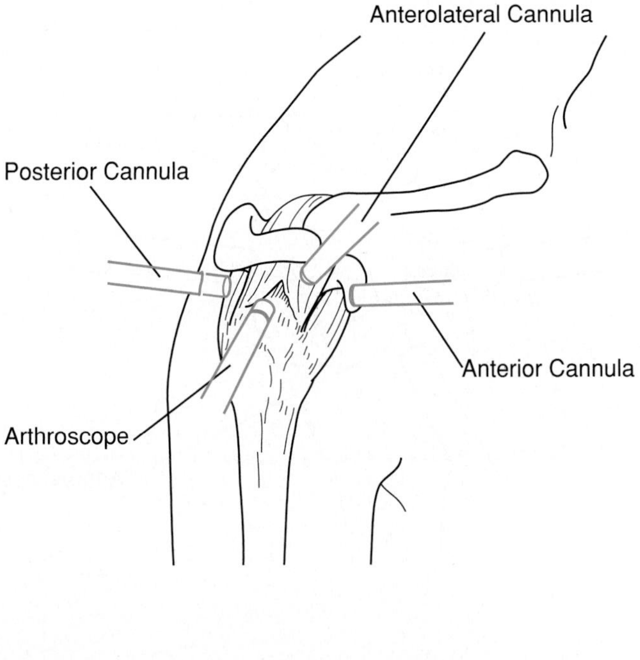

Figure 41–22:
**Arthroscopic rotator cuff repair: portal placement.**

Anterolateral Cannula

Posterior Cannula

Anterior Cannula

Arthroscope

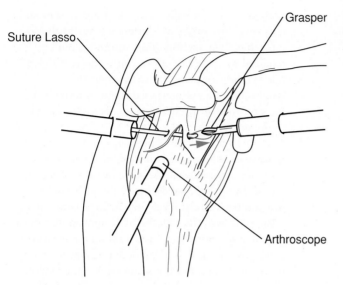

Figure 41–23:
Arthroscopic rotator cuff repair: margin convergence stitch placement.

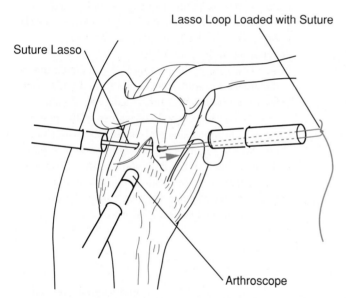

Figure 41–24:
Arthroscopic rotator cuff repair: margin convergence stitch placement.

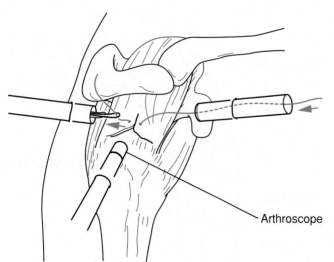

Figure 41–25:
Arthroscopic rotator cuff repair: margin convergence stitch placement.

○ The first end of the fiber wire suture retrieved through the posterior portal is tagged with a hemostat and will be the "post strand" during arthroscopic knot tying. This method ensures that the knot opposes the two rotator cuff leafs to each other and does not become interposed in the repair between them. The grasper is deployed through the posterior cannula, and the other end of the fiber wire suture is grasped close to its exit from the anterior cannula and pulled out of the posterior cannula. An arthroscopic knot is tied through the posterior cannula, as the posterior tendon leaf usually is more mobile than the anterior leaf. I prefer the SMC (Seoul Medical Center) sliding knot, backed up with three half-hitches, but many others work just as well.

6. The suture anchor is placed through the anterolateral portal at a 45-degree "dead man's angle" just lateral to the decorticated "landing pad (Figure 41–26). The laser markings on the anchor's inserter correspond to its eyelet and should be oriented medial to lateral to best oppose the tendon to the tuberosity.

○ Passing the anchor sutures (Figure 41–27): The arthroscope is in the lateral portal. To pass an anchor suture through the posterior leaf of the rotator cuff, first take the medial free end of the suture through the opposite (anterior) portal.

○ *Pearl:* Take care that the anchor is not unloaded during this step: Visualize the anchor's eyelet. If the suture doesn't move as its free end is shuttled between portals, then the correct end is being pulled. If the suture moves through the eyelet as it is being pulled, then the wrong end is being shuttled, which will result in anchor unloading if the process is continued.

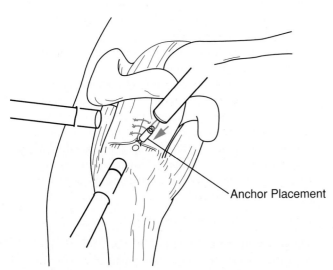

Figure 41–26:
**Arthroscopic rotator cuff repair: suture anchor placement.**

○ I prefer to use the 90-degree Arthrex lasso for this step. The lasso passes through the posterior cannula and penetrates the posterior leaf 5 to 10 mm medial to its free margin. A grasper is inserted through the anterior portal to retrieve the lasso's suture loop. The preplaced (medial) end of the anchor's suture is extracorporeally placed inside the lasso's loop outside of the anterior cannula. The lasso, its suture loop, and the anchor suture's medial free end are pulled back through the posterior portal. A hemostat is placed on the medial end of the anchor suture, which has just been shuttled through the posterior leaf; this will be the "post" strand during arthroscopic knot tying. The other (lateral) free end of the anchor suture is retrieved through the posterior portal and an arthroscopic knot tied. This process is repeated for the anterior leaf, with the medial free end of the remaining anchor suture preplaced out of the opposite (posterior) cannula.

7. I place and tie knots as I go to prevent tangles. To best oppose the tendon to the bone (or to other tissue), the suture end that is passed through the tendon should be your post. Otherwise the knot can become interposed between the tissues that you are trying to oppose.

• Postoperative rehabilitation is slightly less aggressive than following mini-open rotator cuff repairs. Passive and gentle active assisted motion is started after 1 to 2 weeks and is limited to 90 degrees of elevation for 3 to 4 weeks. Active motion and return to activities are similar to that following mini-open repair.

## Bicipital Tendinosis

• In abduction-external rotation, the biceps tendon runs almost perpendicular to the glenoid surface. In this position, it can function as a secondary dynamic stabilizer, increasing compression of the humeral head into the glenoid.[56]

• The biceps tendon assists in preventing superior migration of the humeral head, especially in patients with rotator cuff dysfunction. Symptoms related to the biceps tendon are strongly correlated with rotator cuff disease, possibly because a dysfunctional rotator cuff increases the use of the biceps in this role.[56] Anterior instability leads to even greater biceps activity, especially during the throwing motion.[57]

• Bicipital tendinosis is most commonly (95%) secondary to other pathologic conditions about the shoulder. Most cases are secondary to rotator cuff tendinosis, although bicipital tendinosis also is associated with glenohumeral instablity.[58] Failure to address symptomatic bicipital tendinosis may lead to recalcitrant pain following treatment of these other conditions.

• Primary bicipital tendinosis, which accounts for only approximately 5% of cases, most often occurs in younger patients

Grasper Retrieving Lasso Loop

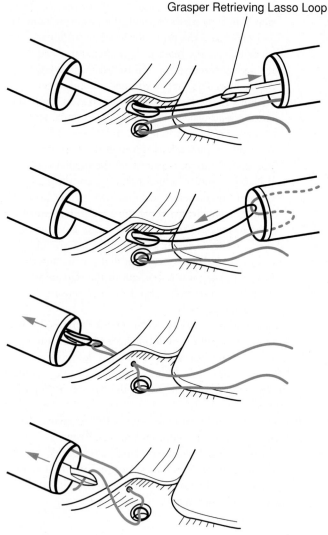

Figure 41–27:

**Passing the anchor suture through the rotator cuff tendon.**

following acute trauma.[58] However, rotator cuff dysfunction must be excluded before this diagnosis is made.[56]

## Diagnosis

- Bicipital tendinosis is suspected based on its clinical presentation. It causes anterior shoulder pain, often overlapping with symptoms caused by the rotator cuff. Pain of biceps origin often radiates down to the biceps muscle belly.
- Instability of the biceps tendon may present in a young overhead athlete with a painful snapping or clicking, especially in overhead positions, going from internal to external rotation.[56]
- Tenderness is noted in the bicipital groove. Unlike rotator cuff tenderness, this moves laterally with external humeral rotation and medially with internal humeral rotation. The speed test is discussed in Chapter 40.

- Diagnostic injections may be difficult to interpret, because the bicep's sheath communicates with the glenohumeral joint. Consequently, biceps sheath injections may relieve symptoms caused by intraarticular pathology and vice versa.
- If biceps sheath pathology is suspected, MRI can be used to identify biceps tendon instability, tenosynovitis, or other extraarticular tendon pathology. Contrary to common belief, most cases of biceps tendon subluxation do not intermittently reduce with arm motion. Instead, this subluxation appears to be fixed. Biceps tendon instability may be difficult to assess preoperatively.[56]
- The intraarticular portion of the biceps tendon is best assessed at the time of arthroscopy.
- During arthroscopy, the biceps tendon itself should look shiny and white without significant fraying. As noted by Bennett,[59] the tendon in the proximal bicipital groove can be examined by flexing the patient's elbow and using a probe to pull it into the joint.

## Treatment

- Nonoperative management should be directed toward the rotator cuff.[56] If nonoperative management fails, surgical treatment for the rotator cuff and biceps tendon can be considered.
- Intraarticular tendinosis most commonly affects the base of the biceps near its origin from the superior labrum. Tendinosis in this area can be debrided similarly to the rotator cuff. Normal biceps tendon will not be injured by a motorized shaver.
- Following debridement, if more than 25% to 50% of the tendon is involved, a tenotomy or tenodesis can be considered.[56,60] The superiority of one technique over the other is not completely resolved. However, in higher-demand patients younger than 50 to 60 years, a tenodesis is generally favored. In lower-demand patients, an arthroscopic tenotomy may be just as satisfactory.[61] Good or excellent results have been reported in up to 92% of patients following tenodesis.[58]
- Symptomatic subluxation or dislocation of the biceps is another indication for tenodesis or tenotomy.
- Isolated rupture of the long head of the biceps can be treated nonoperatively. Residual pain or weakness of elbow flexion is uncommon. Supination strength has been noted to decrease 10% to 21% in patients treated nonoperatively and in 8% in patients tenodesed. Although surgical tenodesis may improve cosmesis and possibly supination strength, patients treated nonoperatively may return to work earlier.[56]

## Technique for Open Biceps Tenodesis

- Preoperatively mark the point of the patient's maximal tenderness, which may locate the proximal end of the biceps stump. In my experience, arthroscopy is routinely performed to evaluate and treat any rotator cuff pathology.

1. If the long biceps tendon is torn, its intraarticular proximal stump is debrided. If it is incompletely torn and a tenodesis is indicated, then, before releasing the biceps tendon, it is marked with cautery just as it enters its groove to guide later tensioning.

2. Once arthroscopy is discontinued, the adducted arm is externally rotated. A longitudinal incision is made over the bicipital groove on the anterior aspect of the shoulder (Figure 41–28). Dissection is carried down via a muscle-splitting approach to the biceps sheath, which is opened and the tendon identified. The incision may have to be extended distally in more chronic situations.

3. Longitudinally incise and elevate the periosteum on either side of the tenodesis site. Use a curette to roughen the bone. Flex the elbow 90 degrees and advance the tendon proximally until it is appropriately tensioned. If the tendon was marked prior to arthroscopic tenotomy, it is tensioned by bringing the cautery mark to the level of the proximal bicipital groove.

4. Place two suture anchors. Weave one end of each suture through the tendon in Bunnell fashion to grasp it firmly. When tying your knot, this end will be your "loop" strand. The other free end goes through the tendon only once so that it slides easily. This sliding end is your "post" strand. This will allow the well-grasped tendon to

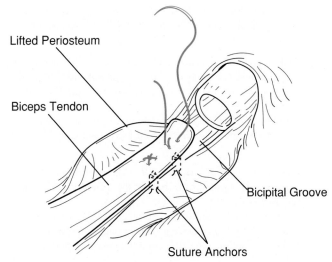

Figure 41–29:
**Open biceps tenodesis: tendon-bone fixation.**

slide down to the bone when the knot is tied. Place all sutures first, then tie the knots (Figure 41–29).

5. Oversew the tendon into the raised periosteal flaps or other local tissue.

- Postoperatively, keep the elbow flexed 90 degrees for 2 to 3 weeks, then allow active extension and passive flexion. Gradually regain extension. Active flexion is allowed at 4 weeks. Full range of motion should be accomplished by 6 weeks. Light strengthening is allowed at 2 months. Full activity and lifting are allowed at 3 to 4 months.

## References

1. Neer CS II: Anterior acromioplasty for the chronic impingement syndrome in the shoulder: a preliminary report. *J Bone Joint Surg Am* 54:41-50, 1972.
   Neer's classic article about extrinsic coracoacromial impingement and its treatment by subacromial decompression.

2. Bigliani LU, Morrison DS, April EW: The morphology of the acromion and its relationship to rotator cuff tears. *Orthop Trans* 10:228, 1986.
   The authors classified acromions into types I, II, and III. Type III acromions were associated with full-thickness rotator cuff tears.

3. Budoff JE, Nirschl RP, Guidi EJ: Debridement of partial-thickness tears of the rotator cuff without acromioplasty: long-term follow-up and review of the literature. *J Bone Joint Surg* 80A: 733-748, 1998.
   Eighty-seven percent good or excellent results are reported for 79 shoulders at a mean of 53 months following arthroscopic rotator cuff debridement.

4. Sano H, Ishii H, Trudel G, Uhthoff HK: Histologic evidence of degeneration at the insertion of 3 rotator cuff tendons: a comparative study with human cadaveric shoulders. *J Shoulder Elbow Surg* 8:574-579, 1999.

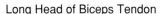

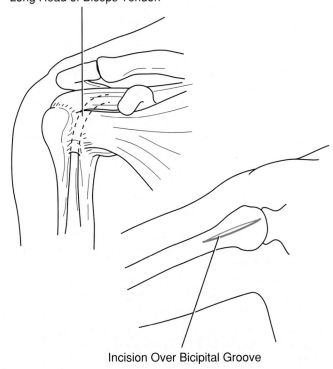

Figure 41–28:
**Open biceps tenodesis: incision.**

The authors found that rotator cuff insertional degeneration was more prominent on the articular side compared with the bursal side.

5. Ozaki J, Fujimoto S, Nakagawa Y et al: Tears of the rotator cuff of the shoulder associated with pathological changes in the acromion. A study in cadavera. *J Bone Joint Surg* 70A:1224-1230, 1988.
   The authors examined cadaveric shoulders and noted that acromial changes are secondary to primary rotator cuff changes.

6. Speer KP, Osbahr DC, Montella BJ et al: Acromial morphotype in the young asymptomatic athletic shoulder. *J Shoulder Elbow Surg* 10:434-437, 2001.
   The type III acromion occurs in only 2% to 4% of young athletes. A higher incidence is seen in older populations, suggesting that the type III acromion is reactive, not congenital.

7. Anderson K, Bowen MK: Spur reformation after arthroscopic acromioplasty. *Arthroscopy* 15:788-791, 1999.
   The authors describe reformation of the subacromial spur following arthroscopic subacromial decompression.

8. Chambler AF, Pitsillides AA, Emery RJ: Acromial spur formation in patients with rotator cuff tears. *J Shoulder Elbow Surg* 12:314-321, 2003.
   The acromial "spur," located at the insertion of the CA ligament, demonstrates active bone formation, implying that spur formation is a secondary phenomenon.

9. Wirth MA, Basamania C, Rockwood CA Jr: Nonoperative management of full-thickness tears of the rotator cuff. *Orthop Clin North Am* 28:59-67, 1997.
   Sixty-two percent good or excellent results are reported for treatment of full-thickness rotator cuff tears with nonoperative management at minimum 2-year follow-up.

10. Burkhart SS: Arthroscopic debridement and decompression for selected rotator cuff tears. Clinical results, pathomechanics, and patient selection based on biomechanical parameters. *Orthop Clin North Am* 24:111-123, 1993.
    The author discusses the biomechanics of the rotator cuff cable, force couples, and the fact that not all "successful" rotator cuff repairs have fully healed tendons.

11. Itoi E, Newman SR, Kuechle DK et al: Dynamic anterior stabilizers of the shoulder with the arm in abduction. *J Bone Joint Surg* 76B:834-836, 1994.
    The authors discuss the active and passive stabilizers of the shoulder.

12. Burkhart SS: Reconciling the paradox of rotator cuff repair versus debridement: a unified biomechanical rationale for the treatment of rotator cuff tears. *Arthroscopy* 10:4-19, 1994.
    Functional and nonfunctional rotator cuff tears are discussed with reference to the force couples of the shoulder.

13. Pearsall AW IV, Bonsell S, Heitman RJ et al: Radiographic findings associated with symptomatic rotator cuff tears. *J Shoulder Elbow Surg* 12:122-127, 2003.
    Sclerosis, osteophytes, and subchondral cysts of the greater tuberosity are associated with rotator cuff tears.

14. Frost P, Andersen JH, Lundorf E: Is supraspinatus pathology as defined by magnetic resonance imaging associated with clinical signs of shoulder impingement? *J Shoulder Elbow Surg* 8:565-568, 1999.
    Supraspinatus pathology as seen on MRI is related to age rather than rotator cuff symptoms.

15. Shuman WP: Gadolinium MR arthrography of the rotator cuff. *Semin Musculoskelet Radiol* 2:377-384, 1998.
    The author notes that MRI has not performed well in distinguishing normal tendon from partial-thickness or small full-thickness rotator cuff tears. MR angiography has performed better.

16. Torstensen ET, Hollinshead RM: Comparison of magnetic resonance imaging and arthroscopy in the evaluation of shoulder pathology. *J Shoulder Elbow Surg* 8:42-45, 1999.
    MRI is not an effective or accurate tool for assessing shoulder pathology when the clinical picture is not clear.

17. Struhl S: Anterior internal impingement. *Arthroscopy* 18:2-7, 2002.
    Eight of 10 arthroscopically proven partial-thickness rotator cuff tears were not seen on MRI.

18. Wnorowski DC, Levinsohn EM, Chamberlain BC, McAndrew DL: Magnetic resonance imaging assessment of the rotator cuff: is it really accurate? *Arthroscopy* 13:710-719, 1997.
    MRI was reported to be up to 78% sensitive, 83% specific, and 82% accurate for detecting full-thickness rotator cuff tears.

19. Balich SM, Sheley RC, Brown TR et al: MR imaging of the rotator cuff tendon: interobserver agreement and analysis of interpretive errors. *Radiology* 204:191-194, 1997.
    MRI was reported to be 84% sensitive, 94% specific, and 92% accurate for detecting full-thickness rotator cuff tears.

20. Needell SD, Zlatkin MB, Sher JS et al: MR imaging of the rotator cuff: peritendinous and bone abnormalities in an asymptomatic population. *AJR Am J Roentgenol* 166:863-867, 1996.
    MRI demonstrated a high prevalence of partial-thickness and full-thickness rotator cuff tears in asymptomatic shoulders.

21. Sher JS, Uribe JW, Posada A et al: Abnormal findings on magnetic resonance images of asymptomatic shoulders. *J Bone Joint Surg* 77A:10-15, 1995.
    MRI examination revealed that 28% of asymptomatic volunteers older than 60 years had full-thickness rotator cuff tears, and 26% had partial-thickness tears.

22. Tempelhof S, Rupp S, Seil R: Age-related prevalence of rotator cuff tears in asymptomatic shoulders. *J Shoulder Elbow Surg* 8:296-299, 1999.
    The authors report full-thickness rotator cuff tears in asymptomatic volunteers and conclude that these tears can be regarded as "normal" degenerative attrition.

23. Bokor DJ, Hawkins RJ, Huckell GH et al: Results of nonoperative management of full-thickness tears of the rotator cuff. *Clin Orthop Relat Res* 294:103-110, 1993.
    Seventy-four percent success is reported for treatment of full-thickness rotator cuff tears with nonoperative management at

mean 7.6 year follow-up. The program consisted of non-steroidal anti-inflammatory medications, stretching, strengthening and occasional steroid injections.

24. Goldberg BA, Nowinski RJ, Matsen FA: Outcome of nonoperative management of full-thickness rotator cuff tears. *Clin Orthop Relat Res* 382:99-107, 2001.
Reports 59% of patients had a significant improvement in symptoms at mean 2.5 year follow-up of non-operative management of full-thickness rotator cuff tears. The program was based on patient education and a home program of strengthening and stretching.

25. Hawkins HR, Dunlop R: Nonoperative treatment of rotator cuff tears. *Clin Orthop Relat Res* 321:178-188, 1995.
Reports 58% of patients were satisfied at mean 3.8 follow-up of non-operative management of full-thickness rotator cuff tears. The program was based on rotator cuff strengthening exercises.

26. Itoi E, Tabata S: Conservative treatment of rotator cuff tears. *Clin Orthop Relat Res* 275:165-173, 1992.
Eight-two percent good or excellent results are reported for treatment of full-thickness rotator cuff tears with nonoperative management at mean 3.4 year follow-up. The program consisted of rest, anti-inflammatory medications, local injection of analgesia with or without streoid, and motion and strengthening exercises.

27. Wolf BR, Altchek DW: Elbow problems in elite tennis players. *Tech Shoulder Elbow Surg* 4:55-68, 2003.
The authors question the efficacy of steroid injections and note that repetitive injections can cause cellular death, further tissue weakness, and slow the healing process.

28. Buchbinder R, Green S, Youd JM: Corticosteroid injections for shoulder pain. *Cochrane Database Syst Rev* CD004016, 2003.
No benefit of subacromial steroid injection compared with oral nonsteroidal antiinflammatory drugs was demonstrated; however a small benefit of subacromial steroid injection compared with placebo was found in some studies.

29. Bassett RW, Cofield RH: Acute tears of the rotator cuff. The timing of surgical repair. *Clin Orthop Relat Res* 175:18-24, 1983.
For large traumatic rotator cuff tears, early repairs performed within 3 weeks of injury yielded better results than repairs performed later.

30. Kibler WB: The role of the scapula in athletic shoulder function. *Am J Sports Med* 26:325-337, 1998.
The author discusses the relationship between scapulothoracic and glenohumeral pathology and the physical examination and management of scapulothoracic dysfunction.

31. Burkhart SS, Morgan CD, Kibler WB: The disabled throwing shoulder: spectrum of pathology part III: The SICK scapula, scapular dyskinesis, the kinetic chain, and rehabilitation. *Arthroscopy* 19:641-661, 2003.
Tightness of the posteroinferior glenohumeral capsule may predispose to glenohumeral pathology, especially SLAP lesions.

32. Soifer TB, Levy HJ, Soifer FM et al: Neurohistology of the subacromial space. *Arthroscopy* 12:182-186, 1996.

A rich supply of neural elements was identified within the subacromial bursa.

33. Ryu RK: Arthroscopic subacromial decompression: a clinical review. *Arthroscopy* 8:141-147, 1992.
Improvement following ASAD in patients with articular-sided partial-thickness rotator cuff tears may result from postoperative rest rather than the surgery.

34. Weber SC: Arthroscopic debridement and acromioplasty versus mini-open repair in the treatment of significant partial-thickness rotator cuff tears. *Arthroscopy* 15:126-131, 1999.
The author noted that acromioplasty alone does not prevent rotator cuff tear progression.

35. Hyvonen P, Lohi S, Jalovaara P: Open acromioplasty does not prevent the progression of an impingement syndrome to a tear. Nine-year follow-up of 96 cases. *J Bone Joint Surg* 80B:813-816, 1998.
The authors report 72% good or excellent results at a mean of 9 years following open SAD, with the development of rotator cuff tears following SAD.

36. Ogata S, Uhthoff HK: Acromial enthesopathy and rotator cuff tear. A radiologic and histologic postmortem investigation of the coracoacromial arch. *Clin Orthop Relat Res* 254:39-48, 1990.
This cadaveric study notes that rotator cuff tears likely are not initiated by impingement; rather, they develop as an intrinsic degenerative tendinopathy.

37. Stephens SR, Warren RF, Payne LZ et al: Arthroscopic acromioplasty: a 6- to 10-year follow-up. *Arthroscopy* 14:382-388, 1998.
The authors report 81% success at average 8.4-year follow-up. Thirty-three percent could not return to throwing, and those who did experienced pain. Fifty percent could not serve a tennis ball.

38. Checroun AJ, Dennis MG, Zuckerman JD: Open versus arthroscopic decompression for subacromial impingement. A comprehensive review of the literature from the last 25 years. *Bull Hosp Joint Dis* 57:145-151, 1998.
Using meta-analysis, the authors report 83.3% surgical success for 698 open SAD at 6 to 62 months and 81.4% surgical success for 1237 ASAD at 6 to 41 months.

39. Spangehl MJ, Hawkins RH, McCormack RG, Loomer RL. Arthroscopic versus open acromioplasty: a prospective, randomized, blinded study. *J Shoulder Elbow Surg* 11:101-107, 2002.
The authors report no significant difference between open and arthroscopic subacromial decompression at 25-month follow-up.

40. Fukuda H: Partial-thickness rotator cuff tears: a modern view on Codman's classic. *J Shoulder Elbow Surg* 9:163-168, 2000.
Open SAD followed by rotator cuff debridement and repair was performed for partial-thickness rotator cuff tears, leading to 93.9% satisfactory results at 4.5 years.

41. Lee SB, Itoi E, O'Driscoll SW, An KN: Contact geometry at the undersurface of the acromion with and without a rotator cuff tear. *Arthroscopy* 17:365-372, 2001.
Factors other than acromial shape play a significant role in the pathogenesis of rotator cuff tears.

42. Wiley A: Superior humeral dislocation. *Clin Orthop Relat Res* 263:135-141, 1991.
Four cases of anterosuperior humeral instability are reported following CA ligament division and SAD.

43. Watson M: Major ruptures of the rotator cuff: the results of surgical repair in 89 patients. *J Bone Joint Surg* 67B:618-624, 1985.
The authors, having reviewed large rotator cuff repairs, note that CA ligament excision leads to a poor result by allowing superior humeral migration, which may stretch the repair.

44. Snyder SJ, Pachelli AF, Del Pizzo W et al: Partial thickness rotator cuff tears: results of arthroscopic treatment. *Arthroscopy* 7:1-7, 1991.
The authors report 93% good or excellent results for arthroscopic debridement of partial-thickness rotator cuff tears. Results were similar whether or not an SAD was performed.

45. Andrews JR, Broussard TS, Carson WG: Arthroscopy of the shoulder in the management of partial tears of the rotator cuff: a preliminary report. *Arthroscopy* 1:117-122, 1985.
Arthroscopic rotator cuff debridement was performed on 36 young competitive athletes, 64% of whom were baseball pitchers. Eighty-five percent had good or excellent results.

46. Altchek DW, Carson EW: Arthroscopic acromioplasty: current status. *Orthop Clin North Am* 28:157-168, 1997.
The authors discuss the rationale for primary rotator cuff dysfunction and weakness leading to superior migration of the humeral head and secondary CA arch impingement. The authors report good results in 80% following arthroscopic rotator cuff debridement.

47. Burkhart SS, Danaceau SM, Pearce CE Jr: Arthroscopic rotator cuff repair: analysis of results by tear size and by repair technique-margin convergence versus direct tendon-to-bone repair. *Arthroscopy* 17:905-912, 2001.
The authors report 95% good or excellent results at mean 3.5-year follow-up.

48. Gartsman GM, Khan M, Hammerman SM: Arthroscopic repair of full-thickness tears of the rotator cuff. *J Bone Joint Surg* 80A:832-840, 1998.
The authors report 84% good or excellent results at mean 30-month follow-up.

49. Wilson F, Hinov V, Adams G: Arthroscopic repair of full-thickness tears of the rotator cuff: 2- to 14-year follow-up. *Arthroscopy* 18:136-144, 2002.
The authors report 91% good or excellent results using suture anchors.

50. Lo IK, Burkhart SS: Current concepts in arthroscopic rotator cuff repair. *Am J Sports Med* 31:308-324, 2003.
The authors review rotator cuff tear patterns and strategies for arthroscopic repair.

51. Cofield RH, Parvizi J, Hoffmeyer PJ et al: Surgical repair of chronic rotator cuff tears. A prospective long-term study. *J Bone Joint Surg Am* 83A:71-77, 2001.
The authors report 80% satisfactory results following open repair at 13.4-year follow-up.

52. Liu SH, Baker CL: Arthroscopically assisted rotator cuff repair: correlation of functional results with integrity of the cuff. *Arthroscopy* 10:54-60, 1994.
The authors report 86% good or excellent results following mini-open rotator cuff repair.

53. Romeo AA, Hang DW, Bach BR Jr, Shott S: Repair of full thickness rotator cuff tears. Gender, age, and other factors affecting outcome. *Clin Orthop Relat Res* 367:243-255, 1999.
The authors report 94% of patients were satisfied following open repair.

54. Goldberg BA, Lippitt SB, Matsen FA III: Improvement in comfort and function after cuff repair without acromioplasty. *Clin Orthop Relat Res* 390:142-150, 2001.
The authors report good results for rotator cuff repairs without acromioplasty at 4 years.

55. Gartsman GM, O'Connor DP: Arthroscopic rotator cuff repair with and without arthroscopic subacromial decompression: a prospective, randomized study of one-year outcomes. *J Shoulder Elbow Surg* 13:424-426, 2004.
No significant difference in outcomes was noted whether or not an acromioplasty was performed with a full-thickness rotator cuff repair.

56. Sethi N, Wright R, Yamaguchi K: Disorders of the long head of the biceps tendon. *J Shoulder Elbow Surg* 8:644-654, 1999.
The authors provide a good review of the topic.

57. Itoi E, Hsu HS, An KN: Biomechanical investigation of the glenohumeral joint. *J Shoulder Elbow Surg* 5:407-424, 1996.
The authors provide a good review of the topic. They note that anterior instability leads to increased biceps activity, especially during the throwing motion.

58. Post M, Benca P: Primary tendinitis of the long head of the biceps. *Clin Orthop Relat Res* 246:117-125, 1989.
The authors note that 95% of bicipital tendonitis is secondary to other glenohumeral disorders and report 92% good or excellent results following tenodesis.

59. Bennett WF: Specificity of the Speed's test: arthroscopic technique for evaluating the biceps tendon at the level of the bicipital groove. *Arthroscopy* 14:789-796, 1998.
The author discusses arthroscopic assessment of the long biceps tendon.

60. Lo IK, Burkhart SS: Arthroscopic biceps tenodesis: indications and technique. *Oper Tech Sports Med* 10:105-112, 2002.
Indications, techniques and results of arthroscopic biceps tenodesis are discussed.

61. Osbahr DC, Diamond AB, Speer KP: The cosmetic appearance of the biceps muscle after long-head tenotomy versus tenodesis. *Arthroscopy* 18:483-487, 2002.
The authors found no difference in cosmetics, pain, or spasm between tenodesis and tenotomy in most patients (average age 58 years).

# CHAPTER 42

# Glenohumeral Instability, Adhesive Capsulitis, and Superior Labral Anteroposterior Lesions

Jeffrey E. Budoff

MD, Assistant Professor, Hand and Upper Extremity Institute, Department of Orthopaedic Surgery, Baylor College of Medicine; Houston Veterans Affairs Medical Center, Houston, TX

## Glenohumeral Instability

- The anatomy and function of the glenohumeral ligaments were discussed in Chapter 40. Glenohumeral instability now is understood to comprise a spectrum from frank dislocation to subtle degrees of recurrent subluxation.

### Etiology

- The existence of an "essential lesion" remains controversial.
  - A Bankart lesion (avulsion of the anteroinferior labrum and attached ligaments from the glenoid rim) alone leads to only a small increase in translation, not to glenohumeral dislocation (Figure 42–1).[1]
  - Dislocation may require plastic deformation of the capsuloligamentous stabilizers in addition to a Bankart lesion. The amount of plastic deformation may vary with the patient's body habitus. "Ligamentously loose" individuals may stretch more before failure, whereas "tight-jointed" individuals may avulse their labrum with lesser degrees of permanent ligament stretch. Subsequent episodes of instability can lead to further plastic deformation/elongation.[2]
  - Pathologic glenohumeral subluxation may occur in the absence of labral detachment.
  - If surgical treatment is elected, increased capsular volume should be addressed.[2]

### Direction of Instability

- Glenohumeral instability may occur in the anterior direction, posterior direction, or both (multidirectional instability). In addition, ligamentously lax individuals may have a significant degree of inferior hyperlaxity imposed upon their primary instability. This loose ligamentous habitus may be considered a biologic predisposition upon which repetitive or macrotrauma is superimposed.[2]
- Patients with glenohumeral instability present a spectrum from traumatic instability associated with a capsuloligamentous avulsion (Bankart lesion) to a more atraumatic condition associated with generalized ligamentous laxity, a positive sulcus sign, a patulous capsule, and no Bankart lesion.[2] Multidirectional instability is associated with increased capsular volume and inferior glenohumeral hyperlaxity.[2]

### Diagnosis

- Glenohumeral instability is a clinical diagnosis. Its history and physical examination is discussed in Chapter 40. Radiographs should be assessed to determine the presence of an avulsion (Bankart) fracture, Hill-Sachs lesion, posttraumatic arthritis, or a nonconcentric reduction.
- Examination of the anesthetized patient and arthroscopic findings may help confirm the diagnosis in subtle cases.

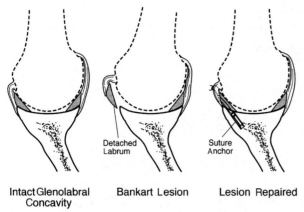

Detached Labrum

Suture Anchor

Intact Glenolabral Concavity | Bankart Lesion | Lesion Repaired

**Figure 42–1:**
**Bankart lesion involves detachment of the labrum from the glenoid. It is optimally repaired with appropriately placed suture anchors. (Modified from Lippitt S, Matsen F:** *Clin Orthop* **291:20-28, 1993.)**

Arthroscopic findings indicative of instability include Hill-Sachs lesions, Bankart lesions, and anteroinferior labral or chondral injury. According to McFarland et al, a positive drive-through sign, in which the arthroscope is easily placed from a posterior portal between the humeral head and the glenoid into the anterior joint is 92% sensitive but is only 38% specific for instability, as it may be associated with physiologic shoulder laxity.[3]

## Nonoperative Management

### Closed Reduction of Anterior Glenohumeral Dislocations

- Relatively contraindicated in the presence of a humeral head, neck, or shaft fracture. If attempted, great care should be taken to avoid fracture displacement.
- Closed reduction should be performed as gently and as early after the dislocation as possible. If closed reduction is not possible without great force, open reduction should be considered.
- Can be facilitated with an intraarticular injection of lidocaine into the vacant glenoid fossa, posterior to the humeral head in lieu of or in addition to intravenous sedation and muscle relaxation.[4]
  - Postreduction radiographs, including an axillary view, are always taken to confirm concentric reduction. Prereduction and postreduction neurovascular checks are routine.
  - *Author's preferred technique:* Scapular manipulation: This technique focuses on repositioning the glenoid and bringing it to the humeral head, instead of bringing the humeral head to the glenoid. The technique is simple, quick, relatively painless, minimally traumatic, and safe. It can be performed with the patient prone or seated.
    - *Scapular manipulation technique:* The patient is placed prone, with the affected arm off the side of the

gurney. From 5 to 10 lb traction can be applied to the arm, or an assistant can provide traction (Figure 42–2).
  - Alternatively, the patient can be seated, with the lateral side of the unaffected shoulder placed firmly against the raised head of the stretcher or the wall. This position prevents the discomfort of assuming the prone position. The assistant provides firm but gentle forward traction by grasping the wrist of the affected side and slowly flexing it 90 degrees, with countertraction provided by placing the palm of his/her other arm against the midclavicle, with his/her elbow extended (Figure 42–3).[5,6]
  - The scapula is manipulated by rotating its inferior angle medially. The other hand stabilizes the superior scapula, pushing it slightly inferolaterally (see Figure 42–2). The physician can stand on the injured or the uninjured side. Standing on the uninjured side may be easier, because the physician's fingertips can more easily grasp the lateral margin of the scapula and pull its inferior angle toward the midline rather than pushing it from the injured side. The glenohumeral joint often reduces with a palpable pop, but reduction may be subtle.
- Reported 86% to 96% success. No complications have been reported, probably because the reduction can be accomplished with minimal exertion.[5,6]

## Traction-Countertraction Technique

- Excessive force should not be used, especially during humeral rotation, as fracture, brachial plexus, and vascular injuries have been reported. This technique also is effective for posterior dislocations.

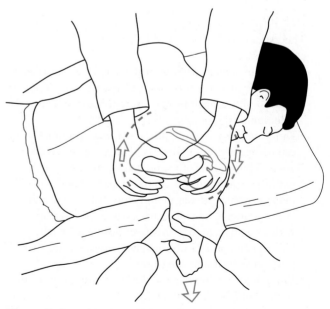

**Figure 42–2:**
**Prone scapular manipulation.**

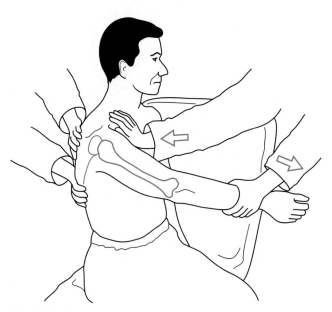

Figure 42–3:
**Seated scapular manipulation.**

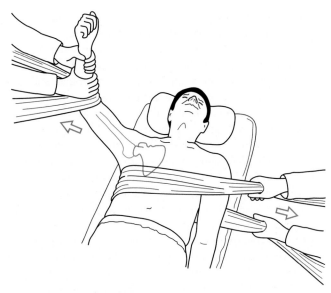

Figure 42–4:
**Traction/countertraction technique of closed glenohumeral reduction.**

- The patient is placed in the supine position. The physician wraps a sheet around his/her waist and the forearm of the injured arm just distal to the elbow, which is flexed 90 degrees (elbow flexion relaxes the biceps and neurovascular structures). The assistant wraps a sheet around his/her waist and the patient's thorax for countertraction. The affected arm is gently abducted and flexed. The surgeon and assistant apply gentle traction-countertraction by leaning back. Gentle but firm traction is gradually increased and maintained. The surgeon *gently* externally rotates the arm, applies slightly more traction, and then gently internally rotates the arm. Lateral pressure can be applied on the proximal humerus from the axilla (Figure 42–4).

## Subacute Management

- Although immobilization has not been shown to decrease recurrence rates, the recommendation is 3 weeks following dislocations in young active patients and 1 week in older individuals more predisposed to developing shoulder stiffness.[7,8] Restriction of activity and sports for 6 weeks or more has been shown to decrease the recurrence rate.[9]
- Magnetic resonance imaging (MRI) studies have shown that following anterior dislocation, immobilization with the shoulder in external rotation more closely approximates the Bankart lesion to the glenoid neck than does the conventional position of internal rotation. Conversely, following posterior dislocation, internal rotation better coapts the posterior labrum to the glenoid rim.[10,11]
- Rehabilitation should include posterior capsular stretching and rotator cuff and scapulothoracic strengthening (detailed in Chapter 41). Burkhead and

Rockwood[12] reported 80% good or excellent results in patients with an atraumatic onset of instability associated with ligament laxity, with only 16% good or excellent results in cases of acute unidirectional instability with Bankart lesions.[7] Savoie and Field[13] reported 90% satisfactory results with 6 months of rehabilitation for patients with multidirectional instability.

## Results

- Redislocation rates vary by age and activity, with younger, more active patients having higher rates of recurrent instability. The results reported in the literature vary, noting a 17% to 94% recurrence rate following initial dislocation in patients younger than 20 to 22 years, 37% to 61% for patients between 21 and 30 years, and 9% to 35% in patients older than 30 to 40 years. Recurrent instability is uncommon following initial dislocation in patients older than 40 years.[7–9,14]
- In older patients, future disability may be more related to traumatic rotator cuff tearing than to recurrent dislocation. Rotator cuff repair alone may be adequate to stabilize the joint in elderly patients, even in the presence of an unrepaired Bankart lesion.[15]
- Hovelius et al.[16] noted a 20% rate of posttraumatic arthritis at 10 years (11% mild and 9% moderate to severe). The risk of damage to capsule, labrum, and cartilage is believed to increase with subsequent dislocations.

## Surgical Stabilization

- Surgical stabilization should include repair of any Bankart lesion, repair of any significant rotator interval tear, and treatment of pathologically increased capsular volume as needed. This may be done by open or arthroscopic technique. Although open stabilizations traditionally have provided more security, improved arthroscopic techniques, equipment, and experience may allow the surgeon to attain excellent results even in high-demand contact athletes with a lower degree of morbidity and stiffness. The capsule can be shifted, capsular volume decreased, and rotator interval repairs performed.

- Rotator interval tears may be responsible for increased inferior or posterior laxity and should be suspected in cases of a sulcus sign that does not reduce with external rotation. Its closure is especially important in patients with posterior or multidirectional instability. In the absence of significant inferior hyperlaxity, rotator interval tightening may limit external rotation.

- Open stabilization may be preferred in young or high-demand patients, contact athletes, or patients with decreased tissue quality (as may occur following multiple dislocations), or for revision of a failed arthroscopic stabilization. It also may be favored in patients with a loose ligamentous habitus. Such patients have less tendency to lose motion and a higher tendency toward recurrent instability. Capsular volume can be significantly decreased by "shifting" the capsular leafs in a superior/inferior direction.

- Although treatment of an initial dislocation traditionally has been nonoperative, arthroscopic treatment of first time dislocations in young, active patients has been advocated by some because of the poor results of nonoperative management in this patient group. Studies comparing nonoperative management to arthroscopic stabilization showed decreased recurrence rates from 47% to 75% to 11% to 16% at follow-up of 24 to 36 months, with improved quality of life and less labral, capsular, and cartilage damage. Compared to nonoperative management, arthroscopic stabilization demonstrated improved overall results and function, with no significant difference in range of motion.[17,18]

- Arthroscopic stabilization is contraindicated in cases of large bony deficits (>20%–25% loss) of the anterior glenoid, large Hill-Sachs lesions (>25%–35% of the arc), or Hill-Sachs lesions that engage the anterior glenoid rim in abduction-external rotation, poor-quality, attenuated capsulolabral tissue, and avulsion of the capsulolabral tissue from the humerus ("HAGL" lesion).[19]

  - *Author's preferred technique:* The particular techniques included in this chapter are my preference, but "there is more than one way to skin a cat," and other surgeons have other excellent techniques. I have no financial interest in any of the products mentioned. Note that, in the absence of contraindications, I prefer arthroscopic stabilization.

    ○ *Open anterior stabilization:* I believe that arthroscopy should be performed first, in order to assess and treat any coexisting pathologies.
    ○ I have found open stabilization technically easier to perform with the patient supine, as opposed to the

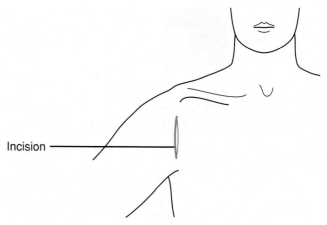

Figure 42–5:
**Open stabilization: incision.**

"beach chair" position. I place two folded towels under the scapula to stabilize it.

1. Make a longitudinal incision in the anterior axillary skin fold, starting at the level of the coracoid and extending inferiorly 4 to 5 cm (Figure 42–5). Mobilize the skin.

2. Identify the deltopectoral interval and retract the cephalic vein laterally (Figure 42–6). Release the superior 1 to 2 cm of the pectoralis major tendon. Release the inferior 20% of the coracoacromial (CA) ligament to ease rehabilitation but do not fully transect it. The CA ligament is in the same layer as the conjoined tendon layer. Incise the lateral 30% of the conjoined tendon just below its origin from the coracoid to ease exposure (Figure 42–7).

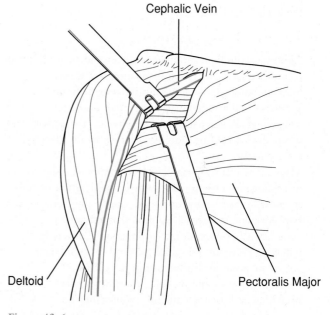

Figure 42–6:
**Open stabilization: deltopectoral approach.**

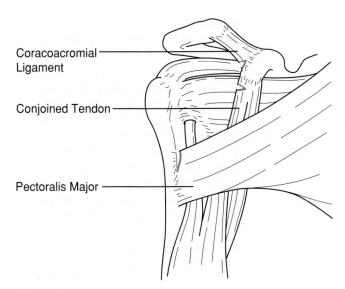

Coracoacromial Ligament

Conjoined Tendon

Pectoralis Major

Figure 42–7:
**Open stabilization: releases.**

3. Externally rotate and adduct the shoulder to tension the subscapularis and move the axillary nerve medially. Palpate the axillary nerve as it crosses anterior to the inferior border of the subscapularis. Ligate the anterior humeral circumflex vessels (the "three sisters").

4. The two options for subscapularis takedown are (1) releasing the subscapularis off of its origin or (2) splitting it. I prefer the former option if more exposure is needed to perform a humeral shift or a rotator cuff interval repair. However, the subscapularis split also works well and is preferred in overhead athletes. The subscapularis split allows adequate exposure for a Bankart repair or a glenoid-sided shift but not a humeral shift.
   - A. *Subscapularis takedown* (Figure 42–8): Use a Bovie to take the subscapularis off its insertion on the lesser tuberosity by cutting vertically at

the medial edge of the bicipital groove from the top of the subscapularis (the rotator cuff interval) to its inferior edge (identified by the anterior humeral circumflex vessels). The subscapularis tendon is approximately 7 to 8 mm thick. After cutting to this depth, angle the Bovie and dissect in the coronal plane medially. Alternate using the Bovie to cut and the corner of a ½-inch key elevator to scrape and elevate. Identify and dissect the plane between the joint capsule and the subscapularis. It is easier to find the plane inferiorly and then work superiorly. Free up the superolateral and inferolateral corners of the subscapularis to facilitate dissection. Place two no. 2 Ethibond (Ethicon; Sommerville, NJ) tag stitches on the subscapularis to generate tension. The subscapularis is tendinous laterally and muscular medially. The joint capsule is white, smooth, and shiny. Reduce the humeral head with shoulder flexion to increase visualization. If there is no Bankart lesion (as determined at arthroscopy), the subscapularis need only be taken off the capsule to a level 1 cm lateral to the glenoid. If there is a Bankart lesion, dissection should be continued medial to the glenoid. It is important for subscapularis function to free its tendon 360 degrees around. Place a Richardson retractor under the subscapularis for a humeral shift, and three-pronged "pitchfork" retractor on the equator of the glenoid neck for a Bankart repair.
   - B. *Subscapularis split* (Figure 42–9): When the shoulder is externally rotated, the subscapular nerves enter the muscle more than 2 cm medial to the glenoid rim. Therefore, splitting this tendon over the glenohumeral joint will not denervate it. Split it at the level of the glenoid's equator. Start medially in the muscle with a needle-tipped Bovie. Then use a small key

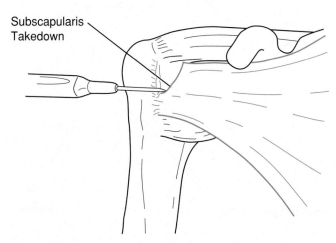

Subscapularis Takedown

Figure 42–8:
**Open stabilization: subscapularis takedown.**

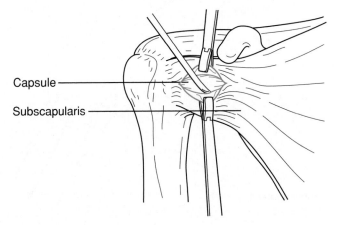

Capsule

Subscapularis

Figure 42–9:
**Open stabilization: subscapularis split.**

elevator to dissect down to the capsule. Place a Kocher clamp on each leaf of the subscapularis muscle to provide tension. Use a key elevator and then your finger to dissect between the subscapularis muscle and the capsule. Use a scalpel to sharply dissect between the subscapularis tendon and the capsule laterally, followed by a key elevator. Take the time to obtain a generous exposure now because it will be difficult to gain more separation between these two layers once the capsule is cut and tension is lost. The two layers should be separated to a level 1 cm lateral to the glenoid margin to provide enough exposure to place a humeral head retractor in the glenohumeral joint. Place a deep Gelpi retractor between the leaves of the subscapularis, and a three-pronged pitchfork retractor on the equator of the glenoid neck.

5. Taking down the subscapularis allows visualization of any rotator interval tear. The subscapularis split will not allow you to see this, which is a disadvantage of this approach. Pull distally on the arm to make any rotator interval tear obvious, and fix this superior capsular tear *before* you incise the joint capsule. Have the arm abducted 45 degrees and externally rotated 45 to 60 degrees as you close this interval. Abduct and externally rotate it only 30 degrees for patients with multidirectional instability. Use a running no. 2 Arthrex (Naples, FL) Fiberwire suture from medial to lateral (Figure 42–10). Be careful to not incorporate the biceps tendon into the repair (it is located under the superior capsular leaf).

6A. *Humeral shift:* This procedure is technically easier than the glenoid-sided shift because the operation takes place in the shallow end of the field. The capsule is taken vertically off its humeral insertion. Avoid injuring the biceps tendon superiorly. An elevator, knife, or Bovie may be needed to mobilize the capsular flaps. Below the 6 o'clock position (6:00), the capsule's insertion veers medially and superiorly. Flex, adduct, and externally rotate the humerus to bring the inferior capsule into view. Keep the elevator on bone as you dissect inferiorly and posterosuperiorly to prevent injury to the axillary nerve. Do not plunge posteroinferiorly into the neurovascular structures. Stay sutures in the capsule help to tension it. Place a finger in the inferior pouch. Release the inferior capsule from the humerus until tensioning it obliterates the pouch and forces your finger out.

Split the capsule transversely along the glenoid's equator, with the arm in adduction-external rotation to protect the axillary nerve. Start laterally and work medially. Have an assistant help hold the capsule up while you cut to prevent injury to the underlying articular cartilage (Figure 42–11).

Gently abrade the anterior humeral neck with a curette for 1 cm lateral to the articular margin. Place suture anchors just lateral to the articular margin at 2:00, 3:00, and 5:00. The articular margin runs from inferomedially to superolaterally (Figure 42–12).

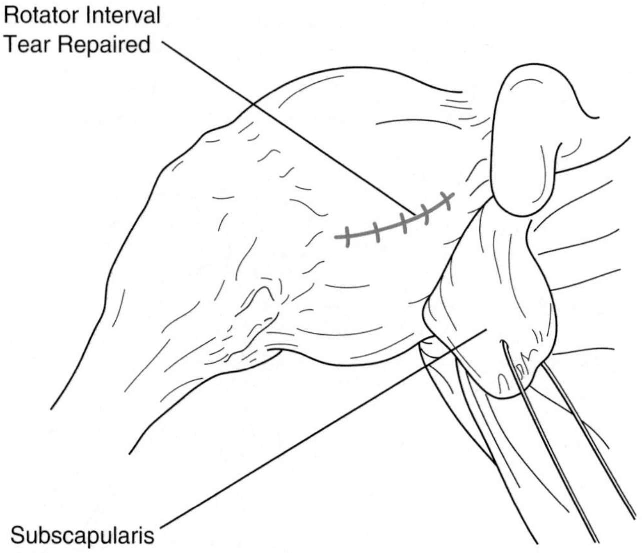

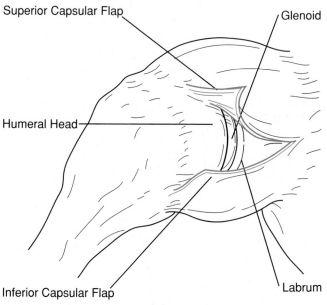

**Figure 42–10:**
Open stabilization: rotator interval repair.

**Figure 42–11:**
Open stabilization: capsular incisions for humeral-sided capsular shift.

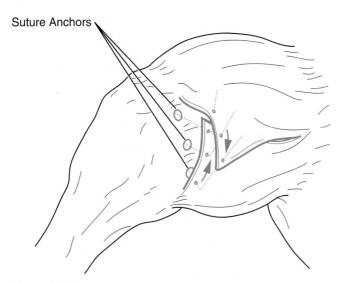

Figure 42–12:
**Open stabilization: anchor placement for humeral-sided capsular shift.**

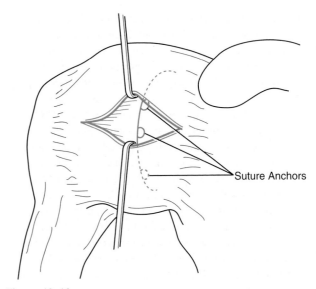

Figure 42–13:
**Open stabilization: transverse capsular incision for glenoid-sided capsular shift.**

Pull up on the superolateral corner of the inferior capsular leaf until the capsular pouch is obliterated. Place the inferior sutures, then the middle sutures, then the superior sutures. When these sutures are tensioned, a finger placed in the axillary pouch should be extruded. Tie the sutures from inferior to superior with the humerus held in 45 degrees abduction and 45 degrees external rotation. Use more abduction-external rotation for throwers and less for those with ligamentous hyperlaxity. Flex the humerus 10 degrees and push its head posteriorly to ensure it is reduced as the stitches are tied. Shift the superior leaf inferiorly and place and tie its sutures from superior to inferior. Do not cut the sutures off the anchors because they will be used to reattach the subscapularis. Oversew the superior and inferior capsular flap to each other. If additional tightening is required, the two flaps can be imbricated using vest-over-pants stitches.

6B. *Bankart repair:* Split the capsule transversely along the glenoid's equator, with the arm in adduction-external rotation to protect the axillary nerve. Start laterally and work medially. Have an assistant help hold the capsule up while you cut to prevent injury to the underlying articular cartilage (Figure 42–13).

- *Pearl:* The glenohumeral capsule has two medial insertions: (1) a synovial insertion onto the labrum and (2) a fibrous insertion onto the glenoid neck. If a glenoid shift with or without a Bankart repair is to be performed, take the synovial insertion coronally off of the labrum for approximately 1 cm superiorly and inferiorly to its equator. Place a tag suture in the capsule at the level of its synovial insertion onto the

labrum. Your repair stitches should be at this same mediolateral level to avoid medializing (and overtightening) the anterior capsule. The capsule's fibrous insertion onto the glenoid neck is left intact.

After carefully placing a narrow double-pronged humeral head retractor in the joint (this requires lateral traction and rotation), gently retract the labrum and abrade the anterior glenoid neck with a curette for 1 cm medial to the articular margin. Place suture anchors in the glenoid at 2:00, 3:00, and 5:00 (Figure 42–14). Place them at the bone–cartilage junction, erring slightly onto the cartilage to ensure the labrum is placed laterally enough to restore normal concavity. At least 50% of the anchor's hole should be in the articular cartilage. Aim the drill medially and toward the center of the glenoid to get good fixation within bone. Hooking the drill guide over the glenoid lip usually positions the drill appropriately.

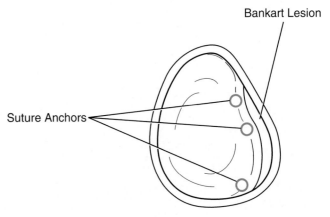

Figure 42–14:
**Bankart repair: suture anchor placement.**

- *Pearl:* Visualization and placement of the labral and inferior capsular stitches is significantly easier if the surgeon moves *out* of the axilla, *superior* to the shoulder. Take a few seconds to switch positions with your assistant until this step is finished, and then move back into the axilla to place the superior capsular stitches.

Tie the labrum back down onto the glenoid rim anatomically but do not cut the suture ends. You will use these same sutures to tie the medial capsule down to the labrum. Do not make the knot between the labrum and the capsule so bulky that the capsule does not approximate to the labrum.

The inferior capsule may be shifted superiorly (Figure 42–15). Use a traction stitch to tension the inferior capsular leaf in a superior direction; advancement of 1 cm is usually enough. To avoid medialization of the capsule, the anchor's stitches are placed at the medial-lateral level of the capsule's synovial attachment to the labrum. Place the inferior sutures, then the middle sutures, then the superior sutures. The stitches are placed and tied with the arm in 30 to 40 degrees abduction, neutral rotation. A small bump of folded towels can be placed under distal humerus to provide slight flexion, keeping the humeral head reduced. The superior capsule is shifted inferiorly as needed; the same anchor sutures are placed from superior to inferior, and then tied. Note that the narrow two-pronged humeral head retractor is removed after the superior capsular stitches are placed but before they are tied. Wider retractors, such as the Fakuda, may need to be removed after the inferior capsular stitches are placed but before they are tied. Oversew the superior and inferior flap to each other. If additional tightening is required, these two flaps can be imbricated using vest-over-pants stitches.

6C. *Glenoid shift:* If a glenoid shift is desired in the absence of a Bankart lesion (usually through a

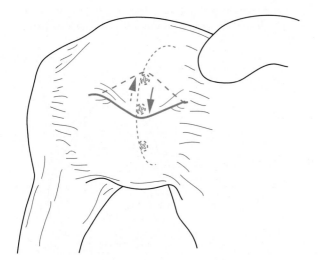

Figure 42–15:

**Open stabilization: glenoid-sided capsular shift.**

subscapularis split), then no suture anchors are needed. The synovial capsular insertion is released as for a Bankart repair, and the capsular leaves are mobilized and shifted superiorly and inferiorly as needed. The capsule is tied down to the intact labrum with no. 2 Fiberwire sutures. Oversew the superior and inferior flap to each other. If additional tightening is required, the two flaps can be imbricated using vest-over-pants stitches.

7. Check motion. Approximately 90 degrees abduction with 60 degrees external rotation should be possible before the capsule is fully tensioned. Under gentle stress, the anterior instability should be eliminated and the sulcus sign reduced. The amount of external rotation that can be obtained postoperatively without stressing the repair is determined.

8. Repair the subscapularis back with suture anchors; for the humeral shift the same anchors that secured the capsule may be used. For glenoid-sided procedures, three anchors can be placed along the subscapularis' normal insertion. Alternatively, the subscapularis can be initially taken down, leaving a 1-cm lateral cuff of tendon for a soft tissue repair. The deltopectoral interval and skin are routinely closed.

## Postoperative

- The protocol varies depending on the patient and the procedure, but early active and active assisted motion can be started, especially in cases performed through a subscapularis split. In cases of subscapularis takedown, active assisted and passive motion can be started early, with active motion allowed after 2 to 3 weeks. Rotator cuff and scapulothoracic strengthening (except internal rotation in cases of subscapularis takedown) can be started early. Motion is gradually advanced so that full motion is obtained by 10 to 12 weeks. The increases in motion often must be individualized. External rotation is limited to the constraints determined intraoperatively for 4 to 6 weeks. Contact sports and throwing can be allowed at 6 months.
- *Author's preferred technique:* Arthroscopic anterior stabilization
  ○ The patient is placed in the lateral decubitus position, and an examination with the patient under anesthesia is used to confirm anterior instability.
  1. Make the anterior portal as inferior and as lateral as possible, to give yourself a better angle for glenoid suture anchor placement. Perform diagnostic arthroscopy and debride the rotator cuff insertion to remove any tendinosis.
  2. Create an anterosuperior portal 1 cm anterior to the anterolateral corner of the acromion. Place a cannula through this portal, anterior to the biceps.

3. If an anterior labral periosteal sleeve avulsion (ALPSA) lesion exists (indicating the Bankart healed medially along the glenoid neck), it is mobilized with a shaver or elevator. This is an important step and should not be rushed. The labral tissue is freed until red subscapularis muscle is seen under the freed labrum. The glenoid neck is abraded with a 4-mm oblong burr for 1 to 2 cm medial to its edge. I prefer not to enlarge the Bankart lesion.

4. Three drill holes are made for the Mitek (Norwood, MA) Bioknotless anchors, at 2:00, 3:00, and 5:00 (Figure 42–16). This technique allows the arthroscope to be maintained posteriorly, facilitating orientation. To prevent having the 5:00 hole too close to the anterior rim, leading to a thin anterior wall that predisposes to anchor "breakout," the 5:00 hole is centered 3 mm onto the glenoid cartilage. The 3:00 and 2:00 holes are centered 2 mm onto the glenoid cartilage. Placing the holes onto the articular cartilage ensures restoration of the glenoid concavity, recreates the labral "bumper," and allows tensioning of the capsulolabral tissue as the anchors are impacted. Aim the drill 45 degrees into the glenoid; you may have to lever up slightly on the humeral head to obtain the appropriate angle. Note that bioabsorbable devices cannot tolerate the amount of leverage that metal devices can, so the levering must be done gently. The process is easier if your anterior portal was placed more laterally. Press the hypothenar eminence of the hand that is holding

the drill guide firmly against the patient's shoulder to keep the drill from migrating. After each hole is drilled, mark it well by cauterizing the remaining cartilage anterior to the hole and using a biter to clean out the hole so it can be easily found.

5. Capsular imbrication is performed by (1) capturing capsule inferior to the anchor it is tied to and (2) folding the lateral capsule to the glenoid anchors (Figure 42–17). For example, for the 5:00 anchor hole, the capsule is captured at 5:30 to 6:00 in order to advance it superiorly. The labrum is captured at 5:00, as it need not be routinely advanced. In my hands, the easiest devices for performing this are the Arthrex 90-degree lasso and the Arthrex corkscrew lasso, using a right-sided corkscrew for right shoulders and a left-sided corkscrew for left shoulders. Although effective, the

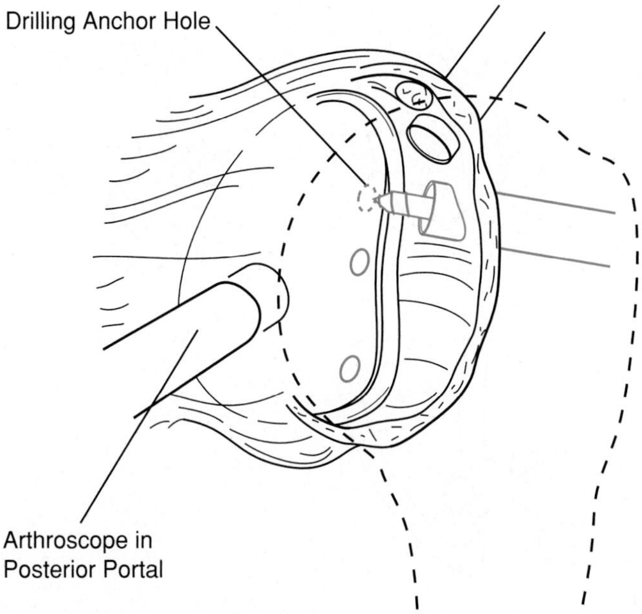

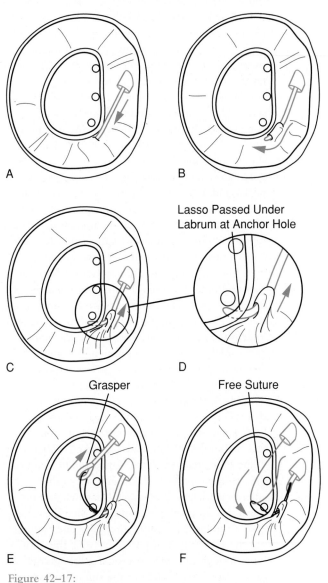

**Drilling Anchor Hole**

**Arthroscope in Posterior Portal**

**Figure 42–16:**
**Arthroscopic stabilization: anchor hole placement.**

A    B

Lasso Passed Under Labrum at Anchor Hole

C    D

Grasper    Free Suture

E    F

**Figure 42–17:**
**Arthroscopic stabilization: capsular shift via suture placement.**

90-degree lasso will not allow you to capture capsule as far inferior to the anchor as will the corkscrew. The lasso passes through the capsule from inside-out at 5:30 to 6:00, approximately 1 cm lateral to the labrum and 1 cm inferior to the anchor hole (Figure 42–17, *A*). It then reenters the joint through the capsule to capture a "tuck" of capsular tissue, which is folded against the labrum (Figure 42–17, *B*). It is easiest to "pop" the lasso through the capsule at a perpendicular angle. The lasso then is slid underneath the labrum, between it and the glenoid, at 5:00 (Figure 42–17, *C* and *D*). The correct amount of capsule to plicate should be individualized.

The lasso's suture loop is deployed and brought out of the anterosuperior cannula (Figure 42–17, *E*). A no. 1 Prolene (Ethicon; Sommerville, NJ) shuttle stitch is placed through the lasso, which then is pulled back (Figure 42–17, *F*). This step brings one end of the Prolene shuttle stitch through the previously captured capsulolabral tissue and out the anteroinferior cannula. Care is taken to pull the lasso's metal and suture components at the same time. Pulling back on the suture loop without withdrawing its metal component will shear the Prolene suture against the lasso's sharp tip, damaging it. The Prolene shuttle loop now has one end out of the anterior portal and one end out of the anterosuperior portal, and it goes through the capsulolabral tissue.

If a greater amount of anteroinferior instability is present, necessitating a greater amount of capsular shifting, an inferior capsular split (i.e., the "Tauro tuck") can be used.[20] A narrow biter is used to cut through the anteroinferior labrum and capsule at 5:00 for 5 to 10 mm. This step allows a superior capsulolabral shift of twice the amount of the length of the cut. The axillary nerve is safe as long as the biter stays within 1 cm of the labrum. A tag stitch can be placed through the capsule and taken out through a separate superior stab wound to apply superior traction to the capsule.

6. The Mitek Bioknotless anchor has two prongs that will be used to secure the anchor's suture loop. There is a green Ethibond anchor loop attached to the anchor, with a longer 2-0 Vicryl utility loop attached to this. Using the free end of the Prolene shuttle stitch coming out of the anterior portal, tie one simple half-hitch around this utility loop and gently pull on the other free end of the Prolene shuttle stitch (the one coming out the anterosuperior portal) to bring the utility loop through the anterior cannula, through the capsulolabral tissue, and out the anterosuperior cannula (Figure 42–18, *A*). Continue to pull on

the utility loop to pass the anchor loop through the capsulolabrous tissue (Figure 42–18, *B*). Pass the prongs of the anchor around the inferior anchor loop (Figure 42–18, *C*). Gently place the anchor into the predrilled hole at the appropriate orientation at which it was drilled and gently mallet it into the hole (Figure 42–18, *D*). The capsulolabral tissue will be brought up onto the anterior glenoid rim as the anchor is malleted in (Figure 42–18, *E*). Some control of the amount of tensioning is available, but be careful not to mallet the anchor in too far or the anchor's suture loop may cut through the labrum like a wire through cheese, leaving you in a difficult situation. Of course, the anchor must be malleted in far enough so that it is buried beneath the subchondral bone. Traction may be reduced to 5 lb, the shoulder gently internally rotated, and a posteriorly directed force placed on the humeral head as the anchors are being placed. The utility loop can be pulled to ensure the anchor is secure within the glenoid,

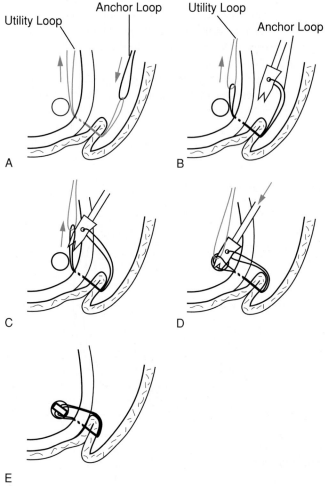

Figure 42–18:
**Arthroscopic stabilization: Mitek Bioknotless anchor placement.**

and then one end of the utility loop is grasped and pulled to remove it from the joint.

7. The 3:00 and 1:00 anchors are similarly placed. Again, these anchors should be placed 2 mm onto the glenoid surface. In my hands, a 45-degree Arthrex lasso is the easiest device to use to capture the capsulolabral tissue at this level. The capsule is captured inferior to the anchor for advancement, and the labrum is captured at the level of the anchor. Less capsular plication should be performed for the superior anchors to prevent loss of external rotation. In general, the middle glenohumeral ligament (MGHL) should be superiorly advanced to the 2:00 anchor.

8. *Rotator interval repair* should be performed for patients with significant inferior (or posterior) hyperlaxity, especially those with a sulcus sign that does not reduce with external rotation.

Pull the anterior cannula back just outside of the joint capsule. Use a 45-degree lasso through the anterior cannula to penetrate the MGHL, then bring the lasso's suture loop out of the anterosuperior portal (Figure 42–19). Shuttle a no. 2 Fiberwire stitch back through the MGHL and out the anterior portal (Figure 42–20). Move the extraarticular anterior cannula superiorly, and use an Arthrex 22-degree bird beak grasper, or similar retrieving device, to penetrate the SGHL or tissue in the superior rotator interval. Grasp the superior end of the Fiberwire stitch and bring it back out through the same anterior cannula (Figure 42–21). Tie an extraarticular knot to close down this

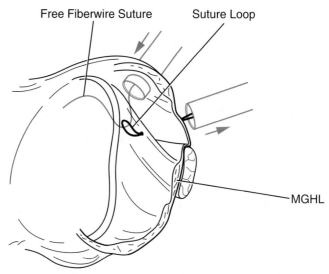

Figure 42–20:
Arthroscopic rotator interval closure: Suture retrieval. *MGHL,* Middle glenohumeral ligament.

interval (Figure 42–22). One to two stitches can be placed in the lateral interval, but the medial interval should be left open to prevent loss of external rotation, unless significant tightening is required.

## Capsular Plication

- In the presence of instability without a Bankart lesion, the capsule and labrum are captured as in arthroscopic anterior stabilization, step 5. The appropriate Lasso device penetrates the capsule from inside-out, then outside-in, then captures the labrum by coming between the labrum

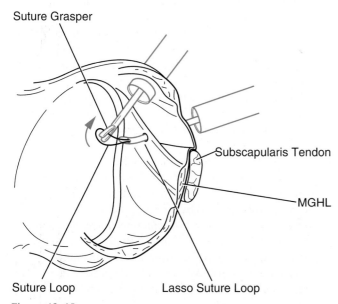

Figure 42–19:
Arthroscopic rotator interval closure: Middle glenohumeral ligament (MGHL) penetration.

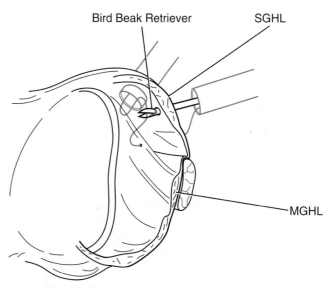

Figure 42–21:
Arthroscopic rotator interval closure: Superior glenohumeral ligament *(SGHL)* penetration. *MGHL,* Middle glenohumeral ligament.

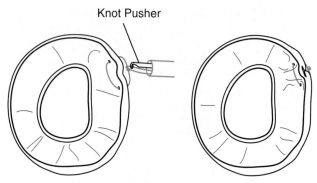

Figure 42–22:

**Arthroscopic rotator interval closure: Knot tying.**

and the glenoid. The capsule is captured inferior to the labrum to shift it superiorly. However, instead of placing anchors, the suture loop is pulled out through the anterosuperior cannula, and a no. 2 Fiberwire stitch is shuttled back through the capsulolabral tissue. This stitch is tied to secure the folded capsule against the intact labrum. Three to four stitches can be placed as needed (Figure 42–23). The traction should be decreased to 5 lb, the shoulder internally rotated, and a posterior force placed on the humeral head as these knots are tied.

## Postoperative

- Initially keep the arm "between the nose and toes." Active and passive motion can be performed below the horizontal. External rotation at the side should be limited to 0 to 30 degrees to protect the repair, depending on the patient's propensity for stiffness. Deltoid, rotator cuff, and scapulothoracic strengthening can be started early.

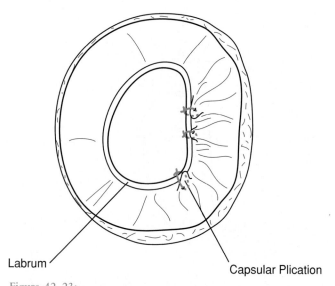

Labrum

Capsular Plication

Figure 42–23:

**Arthroscopic capsular plication for stabilization in patients without a Bankart lesion.**

At 3 weeks, motion can be increased gradually to obtain full elevation and 50% of external rotation by 6 weeks. A sling is used for 6 weeks when the patient is not performing therapeutic exercises. Abduction-external rotation is avoided for 2 months. Plyometrics may be started to regain full elevation and abduction-external rotation at 10 to 12 weeks. Light throwing can commence at 4 months and overhead and contact athletics at 6 months.

## Results

- Many still consider open stabilization the "gold standard," with reported recurrence rates of 4% to 17% (average 7%).[21–23]
- Much of the criticism leveled at arthroscopic techniques arose from literature reporting results of techniques still "early on the learning curve," such as absorbable tacks and the transglenoid technique. Although these techniques reported good initial success, results appear to deteriorate with time and increased activity of the patient, leading to a high rate of recurrent instability at long-term follow-up.
- Speer et al.[24] showed 79% good results at mean 42-month follow-up using a bioabsorbable tack for Bankart repair. Manta et al.[25] showed a recurrent instability rate of 60% at minimum 5-year follow-up after transglenoid stabilization.
- Series of arthroscopic suture anchor repairs have reported recurrence rates equal to the rates of open techniques, with less postoperative morbidity, less loss of motion (especially abduction-external rotation), and improved function, especially in overhead-throwing athletics.[20,26,27]
- In cases of traumatic anterior instability, arthroscopic suture anchor techniques have reported 92% to 97% good to excellent results at 2- to 5-year follow-up, with 91% returning to the same or a higher level of athletic activity. These results are equivalent to the rates of open repair, even in contact athletes.[19,27–30] Abrams et al.[28] reported that 100% of 662 patients regained a minimum of 170 degrees flexion and abduction; at 90 degrees abduction, external rotation averaged 110 degrees. In a prospective comparison study, Kim, Ha, and Kim[26] noted 86.6% good or excellent results for open stabilizations, compared to 91.5% for arthroscopic stabilization at average 39-month follow-up. Residual instability was 10% in the open group and 10.2% in the arthroscopic group. There was no significant difference in loss of external rotation or return to prior activity.[26]
- In cases of bidirectional or multidirectional instability, 88% to 94% success has been reported at 2- to 5-year follow-up, with good return of motion including abduction-external rotation, and 85% of patients returning to athletics.[31–33] This result is similar to that of open capsular shift, which has 59% to 94% good or excellent results at 4.5 to 8.3 years, with 76% returning to athletics and 57% still active in athletics.[34–36]

- Thermal capsulorraphy/electrothermal shrinkage has been shown to reduce capsular laxity but alters its viscoelastic properties, placing it at risk for recurrent stretching. Reports of early failures and complications, such as axillary nerve injury, severe refractory stiffness, and capsular necrosis, have led many to advocate arthroscopic suture plication techniques instead.[27,28] Risk factors for early failure include previous surgery and recurrent dislocations.[27]
- From 61% to 96% good or excellent results have been reported for thermal capsulorraphy at 25- to 46-month follow-up.[13,28,37] However, studies with longer follow-up tended to have higher recurrence rates. At average 46-month follow-up, Abrams et al.[28] found 45% unsatisfactory results with treatment of multidirectional instability, 32% unsatisfactory results with treatment of recurrent anterior subluxation, and 25% unsatisfactory results with treatment of anterior dislocations. Young athletic females with multidirectional instability had 50% unsatisfactory results.
- In conclusion, thermal capsulorraphy probably should be used only as an adjunct to more traditional arthroscopic stabilizations, if at all.

# Adhesive Capsulitis ("Frozen Shoulder")

## Etiology

- The etiology of this disorder is unclear. However, it is an inflammatory disease characterized by acute synovitis. Its origin may be idiopathic or secondary to diabetes mellitus, surgery, or trauma. It has been associated with hyperthyroidism, hypothyroidism, collagen vascular diseases, and crystal arthropathy. It often coexists with rotator cuff pathology, which is not inflammatory.[38]
- Idiopathic and diabetic adhesive capsulitis result mainly from capsular fibrosis, thickening, and contracture, although extraarticular and subacromial adhesions also may exist. Posttraumatic and postsurgical frozen shoulder may have significant extraarticular adhesions in the subacromial, subdeltoid, and subcoracoid spaces in addition to capsular contracture.[39] Tethering of the long head of the biceps in its groove may exacerbate motion loss for adhesive capsulitis of all causes.

## Natural History

- Three phases[38]:
  1. The initial freezing phase lasts 3 to 9 months. It presents with painful shoulder stiffness in all planes. During this phase, aggressive attempts at manipulation or surgery may increase the inflammatory response and be counterproductive.
  2. The frozen phase may last 4 to 12 months or more.
  3. The thawing phase lasts 12 to 42 months, during which motion gradually improves. However, complete recovery may not occur. Without treatment, most cases should resolve within 2 to 3 years, with a mean of 30 months before comfort and motion return. However, a significant percentage (7%–42%) may continue to experience chronic motion restriction. Even in cases that may be self-limited, the long duration of morbidity has major implications for patient function and satisfaction.

## Diagnosis

- The diagnosis of adhesive capsulitis is clinical and is suspected with decreased passive range of motion. Standard radiographs can rule out posttraumatic deformity and arthritis, which are the other elements in the differential diagnosis.
- Because painful motion can lead to stiffness, secondary stiffness may mask underlying pathology, such as instability, rotator cuff pathology, or even tumors.[38]
- In idiopathic, diabetic, and posttraumatic cases, motion restriction will be global.
- In postsurgical cases, motion restriction may be limited to certain planes.[38]

## Nonoperative Management

- The mainstay of nonoperative management is therapeutic stretching, which should not cause undue pain. Overaggressive manipulation is ineffective and may be counterproductive. Although intraarticular steroid injections may be a helpful adjuvant, injections alone will not lead to long-term recovery.[38]
- If strengthening exercises are performed because of concomitant rotator cuff tendinosis, they should be pain-free in order to avoid increasing inflammation.

## Operative Management

- Indicated for failure after 3 to 6 months of nonoperative management.[38]
- Gentle manipulation under anesthesia, often followed by arthroscopic debridement or capsular release, has been shown to be effective. Only gentle, "two-finger" force should be used. Forceful manipulation can be complicated by glenohumeral dislocation, humeral fracture, rotator cuff tear, or complete plexus palsy and is not recommended.[38] If manipulation succeeds, the intervention can be stopped or arthroscopic treatment performed as an adjunct.
- If manipulation fails to restore motion, a capsular release should be performed.[38]
- Compared to open release, arthroscopic capsular release has the advantage of not requiring subscapularis takedown and repair, allowing aggressive postoperative therapy.[38] The tight portions of the capsule are released from the labrum with an arthroscopic biter. By staying

adjacent to the labrum and performing extraarticular dissection with the biter in the inferior joint, axillary nerve injury can be reliably avoided. In cases of global loss of motion, the entire 360 degrees of capsule can be incised adjacent to the labrum, in addition to release of the rotator interval. Following arthroscopic capsular release, manipulation is performed to free up unaddressed extraarticular adhesions.[39]

- Open excision of extraarticular adhesions can be performed in the subacromial space, subcoracoid space, and/or subdeltoid space in cases of posttraumatic or postoperative stiffness. This procedure does not require modification of postoperative rehabilitation.[39]

- *Author's preferred technique:* Arthroscopic capsular release

  1. Use a shaver or blunt dissection to free the subscapularis from the MGHL deep to it, and from the coracohumeral ligament superficial to it.

  2. Use a meniscal biter/basket forceps to open the rotator interval, from the glenoid to the humeral head, from the subscapularis to the biceps tendon.

  3. Use a biter to cut the capsule just lateral to the labrum for 360 degrees around the joint (Figure 42–24). Do not injure the labrum or the biceps tendon. The subscapularis tendon does not have to be cut. Start with the biter in the anterior portal. Cut through the capsule inferiorly. The axillary nerve is located approximately 2 cm lateral to the labrum and is safe if the biter is kept within 1 cm of the labrum. For extra safety, the closed biter can be used to dissect extraarticularly just outside of the capsule, to create a space between the capsule and the extraarticular structures. In my experience, cutting the capsule

mechanically may cause less postoperative pain than burning through the capsule with electrocautery, although this has not been proven. Internal rotation relaxes the anterior capsule and may provide more room to work anteriorly. External rotation relaxes the posterior capsule and may provide more room to work posteriorly. The capsule should be cut until rotator cuff muscle is visible through the gap.

  4. An accessory posterior-inferior portal may facilitate cutting the inferior capsule. A spinal needle is placed 2–4 cm inferior and 2–4 cm lateral to the posterior portal and directed to enter the joint. A switching stick or sharp trocar can be inserted along the same path to puncture the capsule and the biter placed through this opening to cut the inferior capsule. A cannula is not routinely necessary.

  5. To cut the superior-posterior capsule, the portals should be reversed with the arthroscope viewing from the anterior portal. If visualization of the posterior-inferior capsule is required, the scope can be placed through an anterosuperior portal, 1 cm anterior to the anterolateral corner of the acromion.

  6. After the capsule has been cut, a motorized shaver should be used to shave the cut edges of the capsule, which widens the gap, and hopefully prevents recurrent contracture. Any inflamed adhesive capsulitis synovitis should then be removed. If this synovectomy is performed earlier, the resultant bleeding can impede visualization.

  7. The subacromial space should be inspected and all adhesions excised.

  8. Methylprednisolone can be injected into the glenohumeral joint, subacromial space and/or intravenously as desired.

  9. In cases of post-fracture or postoperative stiffness, an open release of the shoulder as described by Goldberg, Scarlat, and Harryman[39] may be considered to clear adhesions from the subdeltoid, subacromial, and subcoracoid locations.

## Postoperative

- Begin full active and passive range of motion on postoperative day 1 to 3. A methylprednisolone (Medrol) dose pack can be prescribed for immediate postoperative use.

## Results

- Manipulation alone has reported satisfactory results in 94% to 97% at a mean 11- to 58-month follow-up, although in one series 8% required a second manipulation to obtain a successful result. Most patients continued to improve with time.[40,41]

- Manipulation combined with arthroscopy has reported 75% satisfactory results at minimum 1-year follow-up, with normal or near-normal motion and minimal pain.[42]

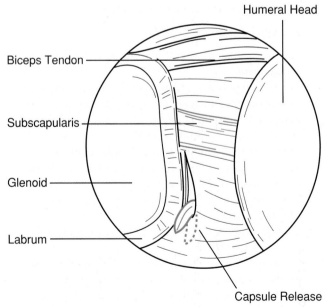

**Humeral Head**

**Biceps Tendon**

**Subscapularis**

**Glenoid**

**Labrum**

**Capsule Release**

Figure 42–24:

**Arthroscopic capsular release.**

- Arthroscopic release has been reported to be safe and effective with improved motion and pain relief in 83% at 22-month follow-up. Arthroscopic release may be less traumatic than manipulation. Instability following capsular release is rare, even in patients who developed stiffness following procedures initially performed to treat instability.[39,43]
- Arthroscopic capsular release combined with open extraarticular release as needed has reported 90% surgical success.[39]
- Diabetic frozen shoulder may be more refractory to nonoperative and surgical treatment than the idiopathic variety, although this observation is not universally accepted.
- Patients with frozen shoulder because of prior surgery had significantly more pain, less function, and less satisfaction than those with idiopathic or postfracture causes.[44]
- The prognosis is better for patients who have experienced stiffness for less than 6 months.[38]

# Superior Labral Anteroposterior (SLAP) Lesions

- Originally described and classified by Snyder et al, this entity refers to injury of the superior labrum about the biceps root. Type 1 refers to labral fraying, type 2 is detachment of the superior labrum from the glenoid, type 3 is a bucket handle tear of the superior labrum without detachment, and type 4 is a bucket handle tear (like type 3) but with extension into the biceps root (Figure 42–25).[45]

## Etiology

- The exact mechanism of injury is still debated. Although superior labral anteroposterior (SLAP) lesions originally were thought to be avulsion injuries of the biceps tendon that occurred during the deceleration phase of throwing, Burkhart, Morgan, and Kibler[46] showed that SLAP lesions most commonly are caused by "peel back" of the biceps root and attached labrum from the superior glenoid during abduction-external rotation. This process may occur during the acceleration phase of the throwing motion.
- A tight posterior-inferior capsule may predispose to SLAP lesions in throwers by causing inappropriate posterosuperior migration of the humeral head as the shoulder moves into full external rotation during the late cocking phase of throwing. This process may overload the posterosuperior labrum as the peel-back mechanism produces maximum torsional force in abduction-external rotation. Posterior capsular stretching appears to help prevent this injury in throwing athletes.[47]

## Diagnosis

- Preoperative diagnosis is difficult. Often, the definitive diagnosis can be made only at the time of arthroscopy.[47]

- Symptoms may include pain or the "dead arm" syndrome in throwers (loss of velocity and control because of pain and unease). A prodrome of posterior shoulder soreness and tightness may occur in combination with decreased internal rotation of the abducted shoulder.[48]
- Although SLAP lesions may coexist with glenohumeral instability, type 2 SLAP lesions alone may lead to increased anterior translation, or pseudo-laxity, of the glenohumeral joint in the absence of capsulolabral pathology.[47]
- Speed and O'Brien tests may be positive in the presence of anterior SLAP lesions.[46]
- The posterior relocation test may be positive with posterior or combined anterior-posterior SLAP lesions.[46]
- Clinical tests have not proved consistently accurate in the diagnosis of SLAP lesions.
- MRI is reported to be only 42% to 65% sensitive and 74% to 92% specific in detecting SLAP lesions.[49,50] MR arthrography is reported to be 84% to 92% sensitive, 69% to 91% specific, and 74% to 90% accurate.[51,52]

## Treatment

- Type 1 lesions probably are incidental, asymptomatic findings. They can be debrided along with treatment of the symptomatic pathology.[53]
- Type 2 lesions should be surgically reattached to the glenoid. A suture anchor placed just posterior to the biceps root is most effective at resisting torsional peel-back forces. True instability resulting from capsulolabral pathology should be addressed simultaneously, but often the anteroinferior "pseudo-instability" and positive "drive-through" sign is eliminated following SLAP repair, making formal stabilization unnecessary. Good to excellent results have been reported in 71% to 82.3%, with 52% to 87% of patients returning to their preinjury level of sporting activity.[46,47,54,55] Suture anchor repairs seem to have better results, with 87% of patients returning to their previous level of sport compared to 52% following bioabsorbable tack repair.[47,55]
    - *Pearl:* SLAP lesions occur most commonly in the dominant shoulder of young throwing athletes. In other settings, be aware of normal anatomic variants, whose "repair" is not indicated and may lead to complications, especially stiffness.
- Type 3 lesions can be treated by surgical resection of the torn labrum, analogous to treatment of bucket handle meniscal tears.[45]
- Type 4 lesions are treated similar to type 3 lesions. In addition, the biceps tendon should be debrided and tenotomized or tenodesed if greater than 30% to 50% is involved.[45]
- In throwing athletes, posterior capsular stretching should be continued postoperatively throughout their athletic career.[47]
- *Author's preferred technique:* SLAP repair
    1. Debride the superior glenoid rim with burr or a shaver on forward. A full decortication is not necessary or desirable.

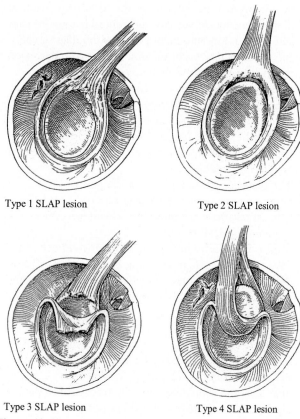

Type 1 SLAP lesion

Type 2 SLAP lesion

Type 3 SLAP lesion

Type 4 SLAP lesion

**Figure 42–25:**
Superior labral anteroposterior *(SLAP)* lesions. (From Snyder SJ, Karzel RP, Del Pizzo W et al: *Arthroscopy* 6:274-279, 1990.)

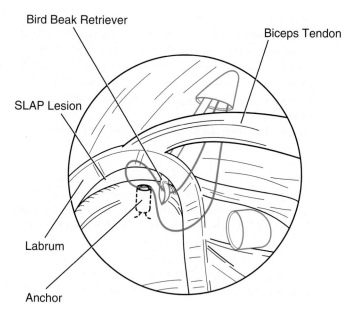

**Figure 42–26:**
Bird beak retriever passed under labrum, retrieving the medial end of the anchor suture. *SLAP,* Superior labral anteroposterior.

2. Create an anterosuperior portal 1 cm lateral to the anterolateral corner of the acromion; this is in a more lateral location than the portal created for the Bankart repair, in order to obtain a better angle to drill the anchor hole. The portal is localized with a spinal needle, the capsule is penetrated in the rotator interval with a switching stick or sharp obturator, and a cannula is placed. If an anterior anchor is desired, it should be drilled through this cannula. The most biomechanically important stitch is the one placed just posterior to the biceps root. Other anchors are used as needed. The suture anchors are placed and their sutures tied, one at a time.

3. To drill a posterior anchor, the "portal of Wilmington" is optimal. This portal is localized by a spinal needle entering 1 cm inferior and 1 cm anterior to the posterolateral corner of the acromion. Angle the needle toward the coracoid. It may help to adduct the arm in traction so that this portal goes through the rotator cuff muscle instead of its tendon. Because this portal is used for anchor placement only, no cannula is needed.

4. Anchor holes should be drilled at a 45-degree angle into the superior glenoid. Anchors should be placed on the superior aspect of the glenoid; they do not have to come onto the glenoid cartilage (note that this is different than for Bankart repairs). Take care that the eyelet of the anchor (often identified by a laser mark on the anchor) is oriented medial-lateral, to allow the labrum to be easily opposed to the glenoid.

5. Once the anchor is placed, a 45-degree Arthrex bird beak or similar retriever is passed under the labrum to retrieve the medial free end of the anchor's suture (Figure 42–26). This is then brought out of the anterosuperior portal (Figure 42–27). When tied with

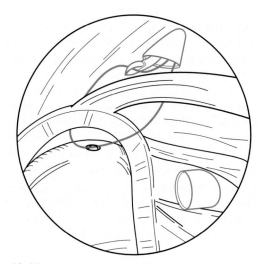

**Figure 42–27:**
Bird beak grasper retrieving anchor suture out anterosuperior portal.

Knot Pusher

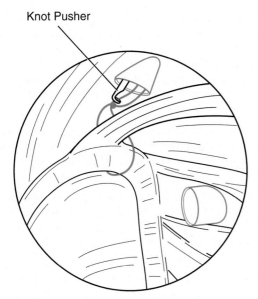

**Figure 42–28:**
**Arthroscopic knot tying.**

an arthroscopic knot, this forms a simple loop around the labrum, securing it to the glenoid (Figures 42–28 and 42–29).

For posterior anchors placed through other portals, both suture ends are first shuttled into the anterosuperior portal before passing the medial end under the labrum and tying the knot.

6. If the patient has posteroinferior capsular tightness resistant to preoperative stretching, this quadrant should be released with a biter, using a similar technique to that described for the arthroscopic capsular release.

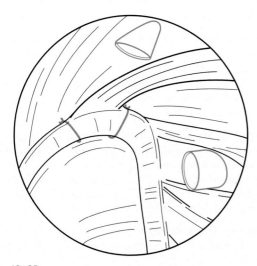

**Figure 42–29:**
**Completed repair.**

## Postoperative

- Prevent stiffness by allowing early active and passive motion. However, abduction-external rotation greater than 90 degrees/90 degrees should be avoided for 6 weeks, as should resisted biceps loading. The posteroinferior capsule should be stretched as demonstrated in Chapter 41 for the duration of the patient's athletic career. Light throwing can begin at 4 months, and overhead and contact sports can resume at 6 to 7 months.

## References

1. Speer KP, Deng X, Borrero S et al: Biomechanical evaluation of a simulated Bankart lesion. *J Bone Joint Surg Am* 76:1819-1826, 1994.
   A simulated Bankart lesion resulted in only small increases in anterior glenohumeral translation, with a maximum of only 3.4 mm.

2. Bigliani LU, Kurzweil PR, Schwartzbach CC et al: Inferior capsular shift procedure for anterior-inferior shoulder instability in athletes. *Am J Sports Med* 22:578-584, 1994.
   Reports 84% good or excellent results following a capsular shift for anterior-inferior glenohumeral instability. Discusses the pathoanatomy and surgical technique.

3. McFarland EG, Neira CA, Gutierrez MI et al: Clinical significance of the arthroscopic drive-through sign in shoulder surgery. *Arthroscopy* 17:38-43, 2001.
   Reports that a positive drive-through sign is not specific for shoulder instability but may be associated with shoulder laxity.

4. Matthews DE, Roberts T: Intraarticular lidocaine versus intravenous analgesic for reduction of acute anterior shoulder dislocations. A prospective randomized study. *Am J Sports Med* 23:54-58, 1995.
   Compared to intravenous sedation, intraarticular lidocaine injections showed no significant difference in difficulty of reduction or subjective pain.

5. McNamara RM: Reduction of anterior shoulder dislocations by scapular manipulation. *Ann Emerg Med* 22:1140-1144, 1993.
   Good description of the technique.

6. Kothari RU, Dronen SC: Prospective evaluation of the scapular manipulation technique in reducing anterior shoulder dislocations. *Ann Emerg Med* 21:1349-1352, 1992.
   Good description of the technique.

7. Pollock RG, Bigliani LU: Glenohumeral instability: evaluation and treatment. *J Am Acad Orthop Surg* 1:24-32, 1993.
   Recommends full-time immobilization for at least 3 weeks following primary traumatic dislocation in patients younger than 30 years but only 1 week in older patients.

8. Arciero RA, St Pierre P: Acute shoulder dislocation. Indications and techniques for operative management. *Clin Sports Med* 14:937-953, 1995.
   Discusses recurrence rates following primary anterior glenohumeral dislocation and notes that immobilization has little effect on recurrence, especially in young patients.

9. Simonet WT, Cofield RH: Prognosis in anterior shoulder dislocation. *Am J Sports Med* 12:19-24, 1984.
Discusses rates of redislocation for patients of various ages following primary anterior dislocation. Restricting patients from resuming sports for 6 weeks helped.

10. Itoi E, Sashi R, Minagawa H et al: Position of immobilization after dislocation of the glenohumeral joint. A study with use of magnetic resonance imaging. *J Bone Joint Surg Am* 83A: 661-667, 2001.
Immobilization of the arm in external rotation better approximates the Bankart lesion to the glenoid neck than does the conventional position of internal rotation.

11. Edwards BT, Lassiter TE Jr, Easterbrook J: Immobilization of anterior and posterior glenohumeral dislocation. *J Bone Joint Surg Am* 84A:873-874, 2002; author reply 84A:874, 2002.
Following posterior dislocation, internal rotation better reduced the posterior labral tear to the glenoid rim.

12. Burkhead WZ, Jr., Rockwood CA, Jr.: Treatment of instability of the shoulder with an exercise program. J Bone Joint Surg Am 74:890–896, 1992.

13. Savoie FH 3rd, Field LD: Thermal versus suture treatment of symptomatic capsular laxity. *Clin Sports Med* 19:63-75, vi, 2000.
Nonoperative management of patients with capsular laxity, emphasizing rotator cuff and scapulothoracic strengthening, had 90% satisfactory results.

14. Hovelius L: Anterior dislocation of the shoulder in teen-agers and young adults. Five-year prognosis. *J Bone Joint Surg Am* 69:393-399, 1987.
Discusses recurrence rates following primary anterior dislocation according to age.

15. Itoi E, Tabata S: Rotator cuff tears in anterior dislocation of the shoulder. *Int Orthop* 16:240-244, 1992.
Following traumatic anterior dislocation, rotator cuff repair is sufficient to stabilize the shoulder in elderly patients, even when the Bankart lesion is not repaired.

16. Hovelius L, Augustini BG, Fredin H et al: Primary anterior dislocation of the shoulder in young patients. A ten-year prospective study. *J Bone Joint Surg Am* 78:1677-1684, 1996.
Reports long-term rates of recurrence and posttraumatic arthritis following initial glenohumeral dislocation.

17. Bottoni CR, Wilckens JH, DeBerardino TM, et al: A prospective, randomized evaluation of arthroscopic stabilization versus nonoperative treatment in patients with acute, traumatic, first-time shoulder dislocations. *Am J Sports Med* 30:576-580, 2002.
Arthroscopic stabilization of traumatic, first-time anterior shoulder dislocations is an effective and safe treatment that significantly reduces the recurrence rate.

18. Kirkley A, Griffin S, Richards C et al: Prospective randomized clinical trial comparing the effectiveness of immediate arthroscopic stabilization versus immobilization and rehabilitation in first traumatic anterior dislocations of the shoulder. *Arthroscopy* 15:507-514, 1999.
A significant reduction in redislocation and improvement in quality of life is afforded by early arthroscopic stabilization in patients younger than 30 years.

19. Burkhart SS, De Beer JF: Traumatic glenohumeral bone defects and their relationship to failure of arthroscopic Bankart repairs: significance of the inverted-pear glenoid and the humeral engaging Hill-Sachs lesion. *Arthroscopy* 16:677-694, 2000.
Even in contact athletes, arthroscopic and open Bankart repairs have equal results in the absence of engaging Hill-Sachs lesions or significant anterior glenoid defects.

20. Tauro JC: Arthroscopic inferior capsular split and advancement for anterior and inferior shoulder instability: technique and results at 2- to 5-year follow-up. *Arthroscopy* 16:451-456, 2000.
The inferior capsular split technique is described.

21. Nelson BJ, Arciero RA: Arthroscopic management of glenohumeral instability. *Am J Sports Med* 28:602-614, 2000.
Reviews the literature regarding open and arthroscopic stabilizations, including first-time dislocators.

22. Payne LZ, Altchek DW: The surgical treatment of anterior shoulder instability. *Clin Sports Med* 14:863-883, 1995.
A grading system for the physical examination of glenohumeral instability is presented.

23. Magnusson L, Kartus J, Ejerhed L et al: Revisiting the open Bankart experience: a four- to nine-year follow-up. *Am J Sports Med* 30:778-782, 2002.
Reports the unexpectedly high recurrent instability rate of 17%.

24. Speer KP, Warren RF, Pagnani M, Warner JJ: An arthroscopic technique for anterior stabilization of the shoulder with a bioabsorbable tack. *J Bone Joint Surg Am* 78:1801-1807, 1996.
Reported 79% good results using a bioabsorbable tack for Bankart repair.

25. Manta JP, Organ S, Nirschl RP, Pettrone FA: Arthroscopic transglenoid suture capsulolabral repair. Five-year followup. *Am J Sports Med* 25:614-618, 1997.
Reported a recurrent instability rate of 60% at minimum 5-year follow-up of transglenoid stabilization.

26. Kim SH, Ha KI, Kim SH: Bankart repair in traumatic anterior shoulder instability: open versus arthroscopic technique. *Arthroscopy* 18:755-763, 2002.
Showed similar results between arthroscopic and open Bankart repair.

27. Stein DA, Jazrawi L, Bartolozzi AR: Arthroscopic stabilization of anterior shoulder instability: a review of the literature. *Arthroscopy* 18:912-924, 2002.
Compared to open stabilization, arthroscopic stabilization leads to better cosmesis, decreased perioperative morbidity, and less loss of external rotation.

28. Abrams JS, Savoie FH III, Tauro JC, Bradley JP: Recent advances in the evaluation and treatment of shoulder instability: anterior, posterior, and multidirectional. *Arthroscopy* 18(suppl 2):1-13, 2002.
The authors recommend that thermal devices be used solely to augment arthroscopic suture stabilizations, not as a primary means of shoulder stabilization.

29. Weiss KS, Savoie FH 3rd: Recent advances in arthroscopic repair of traumatic anterior glenohumeral instability. *Clin Orthop Relat Res* 400:117-122, 2002.

Reports 93% stable shoulders following arthroscopic repair of traumatic anterior glenohumeral instability in a high-demand patient population.

30. Gartsman GM, Roddey TS, Hammerman SM: Arthroscopic treatment of anterior-inferior glenohumeral instability. Two to five-year follow-up. *J Bone Joint Surg Am* 82A:991-1003, 2000.
    Reports 92% good or excellent results following arthroscopic treatment of anterior-inferior glenohumeral instability.

31. Gartsman GM, Roddey TS, Hammerman SM: Arthroscopic treatment of bidirectional glenohumeral instability: two- to five-year follow-up. *J Shoulder Elbow Surg* 10:28-36, 2001.
    Reports 91% good or excellent results following arthroscopic treatment of bidirectional glenohumeral instability.

32. Gartsman GM, Roddey TS, Hammerman SM: Arthroscopic treatment of multidirectional glenohumeral instability: 2- to 5-year follow-up. *Arthroscopy* 17:236-243, 2001.
    Reports 94% good or excellent results following arthroscopic treatment of multidirectional glenohumeral instability.

33. Treacy SH, Savoie FH 3rd, Field LD: Arthroscopic treatment of multidirectional instability. *J Shoulder Elbow Surg* 8:345-350, 1999.
    Reports 88% good or excellent results following arthroscopic treatment of multidirectional glenohumeral instability at mean 60-month follow-up.

34. Pollock RG, Owens JM, Flatow EL, Bigliani LU: Operative results of the inferior capsular shift procedure for multidirectional instability of the shoulder. *J Bone Joint Surg Am* 82A:919-928, 2000.
    Reports 94% good or excellent results following open treatment of multidirectional glenohumeral instability at mean 61-month follow-up.

35. Bak K, Spring BJ, Henderson JP: Inferior capsular shift procedure in athletes with multidirectional instability based on isolated capsular and ligamentous redundancy. *Am J Sports Med* 28:466-471, 2000.
    Reports 92% good or excellent results following open treatment of multidirectional glenohumeral instability at mean 54-month follow-up.

36. Hamada K, Fukuda H, Nakajima T, Yamada N: The inferior capsular shift operation for instability of the shoulder. Long-term results in 34 shoulders. *J Bone Joint Surg Br* 81:218-225, 1999.
    Reports 59% good or excellent (85% satisfactory) results following open treatment of inferior or multidirectional glenohumeral instability at 8.3 years.

37. Lyons TR, Griffith PL, Savoie FH 3rd, Field LD: Laser-assisted capsulorrhaphy for multidirectional instability of the shoulder. *Arthroscopy* 17:25-30, 2001.
    Reports that 96% shoulders were stable and asymptomatic at minimum 2-year follow-up after laser-assisted capsulorrhaphy for multidirectional instability.

38. Harryman DT 2nd: Shoulders: frozen and stiff. *Instr Course Lect* 42:247-257, 1993.
    Discusses the clinical presentation and three phases of adhesive capsulitis.

39. Goldberg BA, Scarlat MM, Harryman DT 2nd: Management of the stiff shoulder. *J Orthop Sci* 4:462-471, 1999.
    Discusses the pathoetiology and treatment of the stiff shoulder and notes that the disease is not necessarily self-limited.

40. Reichmister JP, Friedman SL: Long-term functional results after manipulation of the frozen shoulder. *Md Med J* 48:7-11, 1999.
    Reports that 97% of patients had relief of pain and near-complete recovery of motion following shoulder manipulation, although 8% required a second manipulation.

41. Dodenhoff RM, Levy O, Wilson A, Copeland SA: Manipulation under anesthesia for primary frozen shoulder: effect on early recovery and return to activity. *J Shoulder Elbow Surg* 9:23-26, 2000.
    Reports that 59% had no or only mild disability at mean 11 month follow-up after manipulation under anesthesia for primary frozen shoulder.

42. Andersen NH, Sojbjerg JO, Johannsen HV, Sneppen O: Frozen shoulder: arthroscopy and manipulation under general anesthesia and early passive motion. *J Shoulder Elbow Surg* 7:218-222, 1998.
    Reports 75% satisfactory results with normal or near-normal motion and minimal pain at minimum 1-year follow-up of manipulation combined with arthroscopy.

43. Pearsall AW, Osbahr DC, Speer KP: An arthroscopic technique for treating patients with frozen shoulder. *Arthroscopy* 15:2-11, 1999.
    Reported that all patients showed substantial gains in range of motion and diminished shoulder pain following arthroscopic capsular release.

44. Holloway GB, Schenk T, Williams GR et al: Arthroscopic capsular release for the treatment of refractory postoperative or post-fracture shoulder stiffness. *J Bone Joint Surg Am* 83A:1682-1687, 2001.
    Patients with postoperative frozen shoulder had significantly more pain, less function, and less satisfaction than those with idiopathic or postfracture causes.

45. Snyder SJ, Karzel RP, Del Pizzo W et al: SLAP lesions of the shoulder. *Arthroscopy* 6:274-279, 1990.
    The four types of SLAP lesions, and their treatment, are described.

46. Burkhart SS, Morgan CD, Kibler WB: Shoulder injuries in overhead athletes. The "dead arm" revisited. *Clin Sports Med* 19:125-158, 2000.
    Excellent discussion on the pathoetiology, symptoms, diagnosis, and treatment of SLAP lesions.

47. Burkhart SS, Parten PM: Dead arm syndrome: torsional SLAP lesions versus internal impingement. *Tech Shoulder Elbow Surg* 2:74-84, 2001.
    SLAP lesions are predisposed to by a tight posteroinferior capsule, result from a "peel-back" mechanism during external rotation, lead to the "dead arm" syndrome, and produce "pseudo-laxity." Definitive diagnosis often only can be made arthroscopically.

48. Burkhart SS, Morgan CD, Ben Kibler W: The disabled throwing shoulder: spectrum of pathology part III: the SICK scapula,

scapular dyskinesis, the kinetic chain, and rehabilitation. *Arthroscopy* 19:641-661, 2003.

Symptoms of SLAP lesions may include pain or the "dead arm" syndrome in throwers (loss of velocity and control because of pain and unease).

49. Stetson WB, Templin K: The crank test, the O'Brien test, and routine magnetic resonance imaging scans in the diagnosis of labral tears. *Am J Sports Med* 30:806-809, 2002.

Reports MRI was 92% specific but only 42% sensitive for detecting SLAP lesions. Clinical testing was not accurate in predicting SLAP lesions.

50. Tuite MJ, Cirillo RL, De Smet AA, Orwin JF: Superior labrum anterior-posterior (SLAP) tears: evaluation of three MR signs on T2-weighted images. *Radiology* 215:841-845, 2000.

MRI had 65% sensitivity and 74% to 84% specificity in detecting type 2, 3, or 4 SLAP lesions.

51. Bencardino JT, Beltran J, Rosenberg ZS et al: Superior labrum anterior-posterior lesions: diagnosis with MR arthrography of the shoulder. *Radiology* 214:267-271, 2000.

MR arthrography had 89% sensitivity, 91% specificity, and 90% accuracy in detecting SLAP lesions.

52. Jee WH, McCauley TR, Katz LD et al: Superior labral anterior posterior (SLAP) lesions of the glenoid labrum: reliability and accuracy of MR arthrography for diagnosis. *Radiology* 218:127-132, 2001.

MR arthrography had 84% to 92% sensitivity, 69% to 84% specificity, and 74% to 86% accuracy in detecting SLAP lesions.

53. Budoff JE, Nirschl RP, Ilahi OA, Rodin DM: Internal impingement in the etiology of rotator cuff tendinosis revisited. *Arthroscopy* 19:810-814, 2003.

The "kissing lesions" of undersurface rotator cuff tears and posterosuperior labral damage may be explained by mechanisms other than "internal impingement."

54. Segmuller HE, Hayes MG, Saies AD: Arthroscopic repair of glenolabral injuries with an absorbable fixation device. *J Shoulder Elbow Surg* 6:383-392, 1997.

Reports 82.3% good or excellent results, with 53% of patients returning to their preinjury level of sporting activities following SLAP repair with a bioabsorbable tack.

55. O'Brien SJ, Allen AA, Coleman SH, Drakos MC: The trans-rotator cuff approach to SLAP lesions: technical aspects for repair and a clinical follow-up of 31 patients at a minimum of 2 years. *Arthroscopy* 18:372-377, 2002.

Reports 71% good or excellent results at an average of 3.7 years following SLAP repair with a bioabsorbable tack.

# CHAPTER 43

# Fractures About the Shoulder

David P. Barei*, Lisa A. Taitsman†, and Sean E. Nork‡

*MD, FRCSC, Assistant Professor, Department of Orthopaedics and Sports Medicine, University of Washington, Harborview Medical Center, Seattle, WA
†MD, MPH, Assistant Professor, Department of Orthopaedics and Sports Medicine, University of Washington; Attending Surgeon, Department of Orthopaedics, Harborview Medical Center, Seattle, WA
‡MD, Associate Professor, Department of Orthopaedics and Sports Medicine, University of Washington, Harborview Medical Center, Seattle, WA

## Fractures of the Proximal Humerus

### Introduction

- Fractures of the proximal humerus are commonly encountered and represent approximately 5% of all fractures.[1]
- Fractures that occur in the elderly usually result from a low-energy fall. Younger patients with these injuries more likely are involved in high-energy trauma and present with significant associated injuries.[2]

### Anatomy

- Four main osseous structures are surgically relevant when managing fractures of the proximal humerus: the humeral head, greater tuberosity, lesser tuberosity, and humeral shaft.
- When viewed in the frontal plane, the humeral neck-shaft angle is approximately 130 to 150 degrees. When viewed in the sagittal plane, the humeral head appears retroverted relative to the humeral shaft approximately 20 to 40 degrees. Although there is significant variation among patients, individuals tend to be symmetrical bilaterally.
- The subscapularis, supraspinatus, infraspinatus, and teres minor compose the rotator cuff muscles. The latter three insert into the greater tuberosity, whereas the subscapularis inserts into the lesser tuberosity. The tuberosities are anatomically separated by the bicipital groove, which contains the tendinous portion of the long head of the biceps muscle. The attachments of the rotator cuff play a role in determining fracture displacement.
- Humeral head vascularity mainly comes from the anterior branch of the anterior humeral circumflex artery. This branch ascends within the bicipital groove and terminates as the arcuate artery, which penetrates the cortex of the proximal humerus. Lesser contributions arise from the posterior humeral circumflex artery as it terminates into numerous penetrating branches along the posterior aspect of the proximal humerus. Additional vascularity is provided by the attachment of the rotator cuff tendons into their respective tuberosities.
- After an acute fracture, the remaining soft tissue attachments to the humeral head, particularly those from the capsule and medial periosteal vessels, play a predominant role in preserving vascularity to the head.[3,4]

### Physical Examination

- The initial physical examination should identify associated injuries and, in conjunction with a full history, begin to ascertain the patient's functional status. The functional evaluation of the patient often has a significant influence on management decisions and patient expectations.

- A focused examination of the involved shoulder region and ipsilateral upper extremity begins with the identification of deformity, areas of tenderness, swelling, and the presence of open wounds. Open injuries are exceptionally uncommon around the proximal humerus because of the surrounding muscle bulk. They usually occur in patients involved in high-energy trauma. Less commonly, cachectic elderly patients present with open injuries after lesser degrees of trauma.
- The clinical diagnosis of associated nerve injuries in fractures of the proximal humerus is exceptionally inaccurate and significantly underestimates their presence. Electromyographic studies have identified nerve lesions in approximately 82% of displaced proximal humerus fractures. A lesser incidence (59%) was identified in undisplaced fractures. The axillary nerve, followed by the suprascapular nerve, are most commonly injured.[5]
- The difficulty in clinical diagnosis, particularly of the axillary and suprascapular nerves, is not surprising given the associated pain and swelling in the region being tested.
- Major arterial injury is a rare, but devastating, complication of these fractures.[6] Age greater than 50 years and the presence of a brachial plexus injury are associated factors. Almost 90% of these cases involve the third part of the axillary artery. Diminished distal pulses, altered skin temperature, and altered digital sensation are indications for prompt further investigation.

## Radiographic Examination

- The standard trauma series radiographs obtained for suspected fractures about the glenohumeral joint include the anteroposterior (AP) and lateral images, both obtained in the plane of the scapula. In addition, the axillary view is essential to the diagnosis of an associated glenohumeral dislocation. Obtaining an axillary lateral view may be difficult because of the pain involved in appropriately positioning the upper extremity. An alternative technique is the Velpeau axillary lateral view.[7] While wearing a sling or Velpeau bandage, the patient leans backward 30 to 45 degrees over the x-ray table. The x-ray tube is placed above the shoulder, and the beam is projected vertically down through the shoulder onto the underlying cassette (see Figure 40–28).
- A study demonstrated the effect of arm position on the accuracy of the axillary projection in determining fracture angulation in simulated fractures of the proximal humerus.[8] Increased apparent angulation is encountered with decreasing amounts of abduction, with 30 degrees abduction creating the most apparent angulation. This same increased apparent angulation effect occurs with increasing shoulder extension, whereas shoulder flexion decreases the apparent angulation. Because of pain, a technically sound axillary lateral projection (90 degrees abduction, neutral flexion/extension, neutral rotation) is

rarely obtained in the emergency room setting. Although still useful for diagnosis of glenohumeral dislocations, accurate assessment of fracture angulation on nonstandardized axillary projections is questionable.[8]
- The vast majority of clinical decision making is based upon information obtained from the plain radiographs.
- Computerized tomography (CT) allows improved definition of fracture fragments and their relative relationships.[9,10] Articular injuries of the humeral head, such as head-splitting fractures and impaction injuries, are easily identified and quantified. CT scanning is not routinely used but is beneficial in situations of fracture-dislocations or when associated humeral head injuries are suspected.
- Magnetic resonance imaging or ultrasound imaging is rarely indicated in fractures of the proximal humerus.

## Classification

### Neer

- The Neer classification was introduced in 1970 and remains the most commonly used classification system for the diagnosis and treatment of proximal humerus fractures (Figure 43–1).[11,12]
- The key to the Neer classification system is the identification that the proximal humerus reproducibly fractures into two, three, or four major segments. These segments are the humeral head, greater tuberosity, lesser tuberosity, and humeral shaft.
- Displaced fractures are classified as two-part, three-part, or four-part fractures. They can be further classified into fracture-dislocations, depending on the presence of an associated dislocation. To be considered displaced, however, at least 1 cm or at least 45 degrees of angulation must be present between one anatomic segment compared to the others on biplanar radiographs. Fractures with less than this displacement are termed *minimally displaced fractures*.
- Articular injuries of the humeral head, such as head-splitting or impaction injuries, are grouped as fracture-dislocations because the resultant head deformity often has significant impact on glenohumeral stability.
- Increasing vascular isolation of the humeral head segment occurs as the number of displaced fracture fragments or "parts" occurs.

### AO/ASIF

- The AO/ASIF (Arbeitsgemeinschaft für Osteosynthesefragen/Association for the Study of Internal Fixation) is a comprehensive alphanumeric classification system that, like the Neer system, emphasizes the remaining vascular supply to the humeral head segment (Figure 43–2).[13,14]
- Types A, B, and C are the three main categories. The system groups the injuries according to increasing

Figure 43–1:
Original Neer four-segment classification system for proximal humeral fractures and fracture-dislocations. (From Neer CS: *J Bone Joint Surg Am* 52A:1077–1089, 1970.)

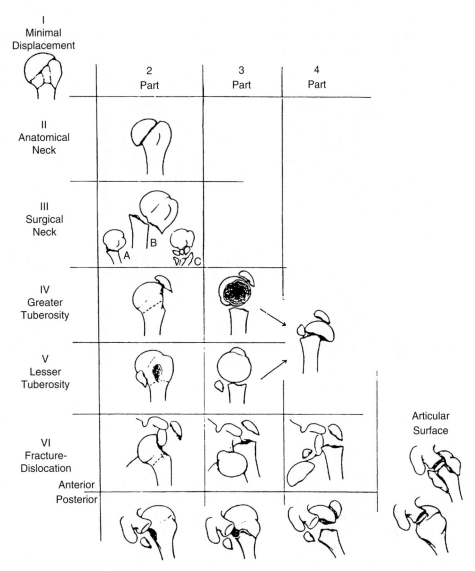

severity and likelihood of avascular necrosis of the humeral head. All three types are extensively subdivided to include the vast majority of fracture patterns. With this system, type C injuries are associated with the highest risk of osteonecrosis.

- Although more commonly used for periarticular fractures throughout the appendicular skeleton, the AO/ASIF classification is less commonly used to guide treatment decisions. However, the system will be increasingly referred to in the proximal humeral fracture literature.

## Limitations

- Like many other classification systems, the Neer and AO/ASIF systems demonstrate poor intraobserver and interobserver variability.[15–17]
- Other shortcomings include the inability to classify all fracture types.[2] Furthermore, despite being heavily based on the predictability of osteonecrosis of the humeral

head, variable avascular necrosis rates have been noted within groups.

- This finding suggests that the vascular viability of the humeral head is more complex than simply the number of fragments present. Factors such as the orientation of the humeral head in multifragmentary fractures may have a significant effect on the presence or absence of soft tissue attachments remaining to the humeral head.[3,18]
- The Neer classification provides guidelines, not rules, for fracture management. Whereas 5 mm of displacement may be well tolerated in a two-part fracture at the surgical neck of the humerus in an older individual, this degree of displacement in a young, active patient with a superiorly displaced greater tuberosity fracture may be an indication for surgical management.[19]

## Emergency Room Management

- After obtaining a thorough history and performing a physical examination, the shoulder trauma series of

Groups:

Humerus Proximal Segment, Extraarticular Unifocal (11-A)

Humerus, Proximal Segment, Extraarticular, Bifocal (11-B)

Humerus, Proximal Segment, Articular Fractures (11-C)

1. Avulsion of Tuberosity (11-A1)

1. With Metaphyseal Impaction (11-B1)

1. Articular Fracture with Slight Displacement Impacted Valgus Fracture (11-C1)

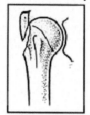

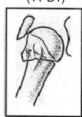

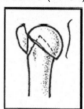

2. Impacted Metaphysis (11-A2)

2. Without Metaphyseal Impaction (11-B2)

2. Articular Fracture Impacted with Marked Displacement (11-C2)

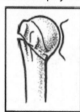

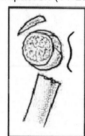

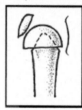

3. Non-Impacted Metaphysis Fracture (11-A3)

3. With Glenohumeral Dislocation (11-B3)

3. Articular Fracture with Glenohumeral Dislocation (11C3)

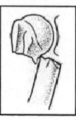

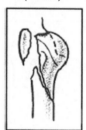

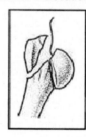

A

B

C

Figure 43–2:
AO/ASIF classification of proximal humerus fractures. (Courtesy Orthopaedic Trauma Association.)

radiographs should be obtained and reviewed. Most fractures without dislocations can be initially placed in a sling or a collar-and-cuff immobilizer (Box 43–1).

- Patients with an anterior glenohumeral dislocation with an associated greater tuberosity fracture or those with a posterior dislocation with lesser tuberosity fracture may benefit from an attempt at closed reduction under satisfactory sedation.
- Patients with glenohumeral dislocations and associated surgical neck fractures likely will not be reduced by closed means. Attempts at closed reduction in patients

with this injury complex may displace the fracture and are best performed in the operating room under general anesthesia to allow maximal muscle relaxation. Failure of gentle attempts at closed reduction then allows rapid conversion to open methods.

## Treatment

- Though commonly used in the therapeutic decision-making process, the final management decision should not be based solely on the presence of the number of fracture fragments as dictated by the classification schemes described. The decision must be individualized according to age, associated injuries, functional demands of the patient, and fracture characteristics.

## Minimally Displaced Fractures

- The vast majority of proximal humerus fractures (80%–85%) reported are minimally displaced,[20] according to the criteria described by Neer,[11] and can be managed nonoperatively.
- As pain subsides, patients are instructed on a supervised physical therapy program to restore glenohumeral motion. Range of motion exercises are started once the clinical stability of the fracture is assessed. Impacted fractures typically are stable at first presentation and are immediately started on pendulum and passive range of motion exercises. Active assisted motion is instituted as union and comfort progress.
- Unimpacted and unstable proximal humeral fractures are treated with a 1- to 2-week period of shoulder immobilization. After this period, physical examination should demonstrate that gentle passive rotation of the humeral shaft is accompanied by palpable, synchronous humeral head motion. This finding ensures that gentle passive motion can be started, because the majority of motion now is occurring at the glenohumeral joint and not at the fracture site. Range of motion may be slowly progressed as tolerated.
- Even in unstable fractures, a supervised physical therapy program should be instituted within 2 weeks of injury. Koval et al.[21] reviewed 104 patients with minimally displaced proximal humerus fractures managed with a standardized protocol. At a minimum 1-year follow-up, 77% of their patients obtained a good or excellent result. Ninety percent of patients had minimal or no residual pain with functional recovery greater than 90%. Final recovery of forward elevation, external rotation, and internal rotation approached 90% of the contralateral uninjured extremity.

## Displaced Fractures

- The best treatment for proximal humerus fractures remains controversial and elusive.
- Published literature is inadequate to make evidence-based recommendations for treatment of these complex injuries.[22] What seems apparent is that open methods of treatment for displaced fractures appear to result in

superior pain relief with improved return of a functional arc of motion compared to patients managed nonoperatively.

- Because of these deficiencies in the literature, treatment should be individualized until high-quality studies can better guide treatment decisions.
- An important first step in managing these injuries is in differentiating "physiologically active" patients from "physiologically inactive" or "low-demand" individuals. It is important to note that this definition should not be based simply on the patient's age, as an increasing number of older individuals remain independent, active, and functional members of the community.

### Displaced Fractures in Physiologically Active Patients

- The goal of surgical treatment of proximal humerus fractures is to:
  1. Restore anatomic alignment of the neck and shaft in the coronal, sagittal, and transverse planes.
  2. Anatomically reduce and secure the greater and lesser tuberosities, if involved.
  3. Maintain reduction with sufficient stability to allow early range of motion without the need for postoperative immobilization.
- The most common operative techniques include open reduction and internal fixation (ORIF), intramedullary nailing, closed reduction, and percutaneous pin fixation.
- Studies that compare these operative techniques in a randomly assigned method among similar fracture groups are lacking. Studies have failed to demonstrate any significant advantages in patient outcomes with one technique compared to others. Understanding the relative advantages, disadvantages, and rationale for use of these techniques allows the surgeon to manage the spectrum of fracture types that occur in disparate patient populations.

#### Surgical Procedures

- Open Reduction and Internal Fixation
  - ORIF allows direct visualization and stabilization of critical fracture fragments, namely, the humeral head, humeral shaft, and the greater and lesser tuberosities. The major concern with open techniques is the potential for further devitalization of fracture fragments, leading to delayed union, nonunion, and avascular necrosis.
  - The selection of stabilizing implants is variable and has ranged from conventional screw/plate devices, cerclage wires, blade plates, suture fixation, and newer locking screw/plate devices (Figure 43–3).
  - The choice of implant should be tailored to the specific fracture pattern, bone quality, and anticipated time to union, with the goal of achieving rigid fracture fixation that allows unrestricted range of motion. For example, standard screw/plate devices typically demonstrate poor

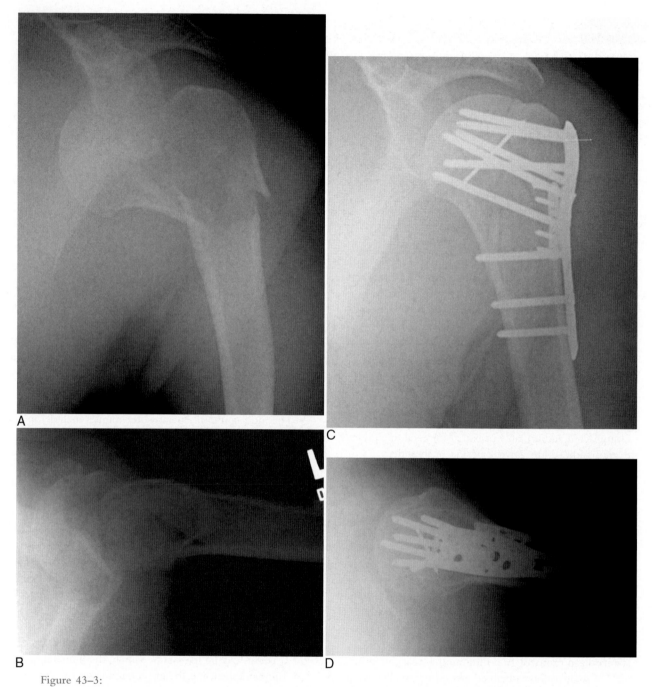

Figure 43–3:

**A, B,** Anteroposterior and axillary lateral images show a three-part fracture-dislocation of the proximal humerus in a 28-year-old man involved in a motorcycle collision. Associated injuries included an open unstable pelvic ring disruption and a moderate closed head injury. **C, D,** Postoperative anteroposterior and lateral radiographs show satisfactory reduction and fixation with a screw/plate construct using a deltopectoral approach.

fixation ability in osteoporotic bone. Alternatives such as locking screw/plate implants or blade plate fixation are better choices. Similarly, comminuted tuberosity fragments often are better secured with suture techniques rather than screws.
• Patients usually are given a general anesthetic and positioned in the beach chair or supine position.

• The vast majority of multifragmentary proximal humeral fractures are approached using the deltopectoral interval via an anterior skin incision. The incision begins at the region of the coracoid process and proceeds distally toward the deltoid insertion. The cephalic vein marks the deltopectoral interval and is mobilized, allowing it to be retracted, usually with the deltoid. Once this interval is traversed, the fracture should be immediately encountered. The tendon of the long head of biceps is valuable in identifying the greater and lesser tuberosity fragments. Further soft tissue dissection is limited to the cortical margins of the fracture edges.

- Initial reduction of the head/neck relationship subsequently makes "space" available for reduction of the greater and lesser tuberosities. This is particularly important when treating proximal humeral fractures with valgus angulation of the head/neck region.
- Temporary fixation is performed with small Kirschner (K) wires and should be placed out of the way of the anticipated definitive implants.
- Plates are placed along the lateral aspect of the proximal humerus and are distal to the tip of the greater tuberosity to prevent impingement during shoulder flexion and abduction. Conventional screws directed into the humeral head should be placed as subchondral and central as possible because bone quality typically is best in this region.[23]
- Tuberosity fixation can be achieved with screws, provided the bone quality is excellent and the fragment is of sufficient size, which frequently is not the case. In these situations, suturing the tendinous portion of the rotator cuff insertion to the adjacent bone or plate provides satisfactory stability of the tuberosities.
- At the conclusion of the procedure, the adequacy of reduction and the position of the implants are assessed radiographically. The shoulder is placed through a range of motion, and fracture stability is assured.
- Using proper soft tissue handling, satisfactory results have been demonstrated.[4,24–27]
- Intramedullary Nailing
  - Locked intramedullary devices specifically designed for fractures of the proximal humerus have been developed and are commercially available. Several multiplanar screws can be placed through the nail and into the humeral head, creating control of the proximal segment (Figure 43–4).
  - Standard humeral nail systems are not designed for these fractures because of the relatively low proximal interlocking location.
  - Potential benefits of intramedullary nailing of proximal humeral fractures include the ability to independently capture greater and lesser tuberosity fragments with the proximal interlocking screws, a minimally invasive insertion technique, load-sharing ability of the implant, and management of fractures with associated humeral shaft extension.
  - Patients are placed supine on a radiolucent table, and a small incision is made distally from the lateral border of the acromion. The deltoid muscle is split in line with its fibers, and the rotator cuff is incised in line with its fibers and retracted. Avoid excessive distal dissection of the deltoid muscle, which may injure the anterior branch of the axillary nerve.
  - Fractures typically are reduced with closed manipulative or percutaneous techniques, and the nail is inserted medial to the greater tuberosity. At the conclusion of the procedure, careful attention is paid to proper closure of the rotator cuff tendon with nonabsorbable suture.
  - Despite satisfactory early results demonstrated in two-, three-, and four-part fractures, care must be taken when considering this technique for highly comminuted fractures of the proximal humerus.[28–30] The main indication for use of locked intramedullary nailing of proximal humerus fractures is for treatment of combined surgical neck and shaft fractures.
  - Rehabilitation After Open Reduction and Internal Fixation or Intramedullary Nailing
    - Patients are started immediately on pendulum and gravity assisted range of motion exercises. Motion restrictions do not need to be imposed, provided stable and secure fixation is obtained in the operating room. Active assisted and pulley exercises are instituted gradually, and the importance of physical therapy is reinforced.
    - At 6 weeks, active range of motion is introduced gradually. At this point, radiographs are obtained and fracture union should be progressing.
    - At 12 weeks, radiographs are repeated. Fracture union should be complete to the point that stretching and strengthening exercises can be initiated. Strengthening and rehabilitation of the rotator cuff are performed prior to strengthening the major shoulder motors (deltoid, pectoralis, latissimus).
- Percutaneous Pinning
  - Because this technique is performed using closed manipulation, the most significant theoretical benefit is maximal preservation of soft tissue attachments to the proximal humeral fragments (Figure 43–5).
  - The patient is placed supine on a radiolucent table. Image intensification (anteroposterior and axillary lateral) is necessary during both closed reduction and pinning of these fractures.
  - Several multiplanar 2.5-mm Schanz pins are placed from the lateral cortex of the humerus to the subchondral bone of the humeral head in a divergent pattern to maximize fixation. Additional pins are placed to secure the greater and lesser tuberosity fragments if required.
  - This technique has been most frequently described in two-part fractures, although three-part fractures, four-part fractures, and fracture dislocations can be managed successfully.[31,32]
  - Understanding the location of the axillary and musculocutaneous nerves, cephalic vein, and posterior humeral circumflex artery is critical for safe use of this technique.[33]

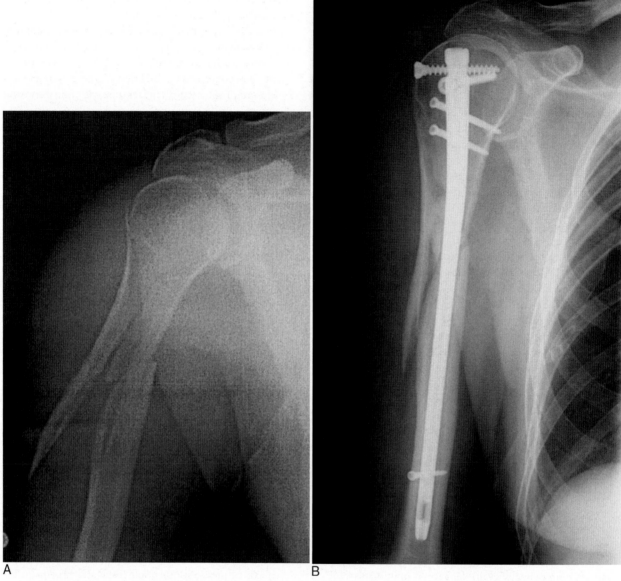

A

B

Figure 43–4:
Comminuted surgical neck fracture with extension into the diaphysis of the humerus. **A,** Preoperative anteroposterior radiograph. **B,** Postoperative anteroposterior radiograph shows satisfactory reduction and fixation
using an intramedullary implant. This nail is specifically designed for fractures of the proximal humerus and
allows for placement of several multiplanar proximal interlocking screws into the humeral head.

- Rehabilitation
  - Contrary to the basic concept of rigid fixation that
    allows early range of motion, percutaneous pin
    fixation typically results in the transfixation of some
    amount of the surrounding soft tissue envelope that
    hampers early, unrestricted range of motion. It is
    important to recognize how this technique differs
    from modern fracture fixation ideas. Despite this
    difference, patients appear to ultimately achieve
    satisfactory shoulder range of motion.[31]
  - Patients are started on pendulum and passive range of
    motion exercises of the shoulder within the confines
    of tolerable pain levels. Often this is approximately 30
    to 40 degrees forward elevation, 20 degrees
    abduction, and external rotation to neutral (0
    degrees). It is important to understand that restriction
    of abduction is secondary to the greater tuberosity
    pins abutting the lateral aspect of the acromion.
    Therefore, aggressive abduction should not be
    attempted until these pins are removed.
  - At 3 weeks, lesser tuberosity pins are removed in the
    clinic, and patients are allowed to increase their range
    of motion as comfort allows. Of the three main pin
    clusters (lesser tuberosity, greater tuberosity, humeral

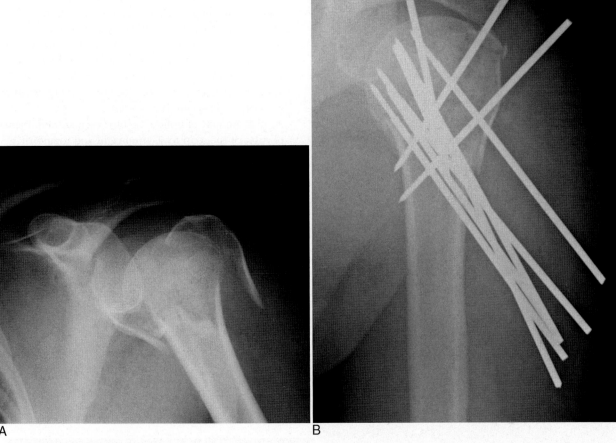

A

B

Figure 43–5:

A healthy 40-year-old woman fell while she was hiking. Her proximal humerus fracture was managed with closed manipulative techniques and percutaneous pinning. **A,** Anteroposterior injury radiograph shows a displaced four-part fracture of the proximal humerus. The articular segment is in extreme valgus, with impaction into the proximal humeral metaphysis. Note that the humeral head segment does not appear to be laterally translated. This finding suggests that the medial soft tissue hinge remains intact, improving the chances of humeral head viability. Both tuberosities are well visualized and are widely displaced. **B,** Postoperative anteroposterior radiograph shows satisfactory reduction of the humeral neck-shaft angle and humeral head retroversion. Reduction of the greater and lesser tuberosity fragments is performed once the humeral head is elevated from its impacted position.

shaft), the lesser tuberosity pin cluster seems to bother patients the most.

○ At 6 weeks, the greater tuberosity pins are removed. Commonly, this procedure improves patient comfort, allowing increased forward elevation, abduction, and external rotation.

○ Depending on radiographic union, typically at 8 to 12 weeks, the remainder of the pins can be removed and patients started on a stretching and strengthening program as described for ORIF and intramedullary nailing.

## Displaced Fractures in the Physiologically Elderly

• Critical to the successful management of displaced proximal humerus fractures in this population is accurate assessment of the patient's functionality and bone quality. The best treatment remains controversial.

• Three studies have demonstrated satisfactory results with nonoperative management of translated two-part surgical neck fractures and three-part valgus impacted fractures in the physiologically elderly population.[34,35]

- Indications for nonoperative management include two-part fractures with translation of less than approximately two thirds the diameter of the proximal humeral metaphysis and valgus-impacted three-part injuries without significant angulation. We prefer to manage widely displaced two-part fractures and unstable three- and four-part fractures operatively, provided the patient has reasonable cognitive and functional capabilities.

- Reasonable options for obtaining satisfactory fracture stability in osteoporotic bone include locking screw/plate implants, blade plate implants, or tension band fixation with supplemental intramedullary Ender nails. In functional patients with significant osteoporosis, we preferentially manage two- and three-part fractures with locking screw/plate devices, because these devices appear to demonstrate improved fracture stability in osteoporotic bone (see Figure 43–3, C and D).[36,37] The procedure is performed via the deltopectoral approach with the reduction and fixation strategies outlined in the section on open reduction and internal fixation. If stable fixation cannot be achieved, then hemiarthroplasty should be performed.

- Displaced three-part fracture-dislocations and four-part fractures are managed with hemiarthroplasty.

*Hemiarthroplasty*

- The goals of hemiarthroplasty are (1) stable replacement of the humeral head, (2) restoration of proximal humeral length and retroversion, (3) secure and stable fixation of the tuberosities, (4) repair of the rotator cuff, and (5) institution of early motion (Figure 43–6).

- A deltopectoral approach is performed. The humeral head is removed, and the cancellous bone is used for supplemental bone graft around the tuberosities. The bicipital groove and transepicondylar axis of the distal humerus are intraoperative landmarks that can be used to determine the appropriate retroversion of the prosthesis. The height of the prosthesis often is difficult to accurately assess in the fracture situation but is critical to obtaining a satisfactory outcome (Box 43–2).

- A small amount of bone cement is used at the proximal portion of the stem to secure height and rotational control of the prosthesis. The tuberosities are anatomically repaired to the humeral shaft and to the prosthesis using heavy nonabsorbable suture. Cerclage wire is used less often because of its comparatively poor handling characteristics and potential for crowding the subacromial space.

- In a prospective, multicenter study, Boileau et al.[39] demonstrated that the functional results after hemiarthroplasty for three- and four-part proximal humerus fractures appeared to be directly correlated with satisfactory reduction and union of the greater tuberosity. Complications associated with the greater tuberosity, such as malposition and migration, led to unsatisfactory results. To decrease these complications, attention should be directed at obtaining appropriate prosthesis height and retroversion as well as anatomic and secure fixation of the greater tuberosity.

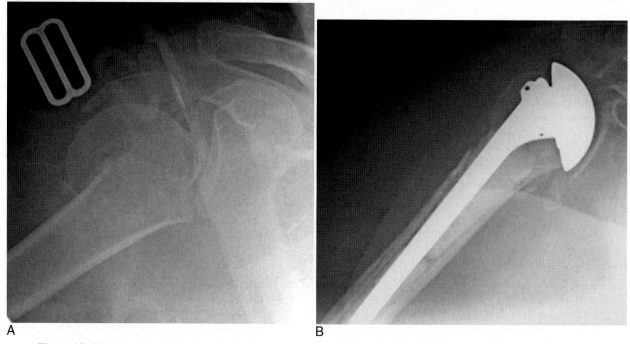

A                                                                      B

Figure 43–6:
**A,** 70-year-old man sustained a comminuted four-part fracture of the proximal humerus after he was involved in a motorcycle collision. **B,** The postoperative anteroposterior radiograph shows satisfactory position of a cemented hemiarthroplasty.

| Box 43–2 | Clinical Pearl |
| --- | --- |

- The humeral head should translate approximately 50% of the glenoid surface, yet allow stable, anatomic repair of the tuberosities.[38]
- Inferior traction should translate the humeral head approximately 50% of the glenoid surface.
- With gentle traction and the arm held in neutral rotation, match the height of the humeral head prosthesis with the native glenoid. Specifically, the superior aspect of the humeral head should match the superior aspect of the glenoid.
- With slight abduction, the superior aspect of the greater tuberosity should be approximately 5 to 8 mm inferior to the superior aspect of the prosthetic humeral head.

- Several studies showed hemiarthroplasty is a satisfactory method for achieving a relatively painless shoulder, but patients should be informed of the expected restrictions in forward elevation, strength, and functional activity.[12,26,39,40] Most patients will obtain between 90 and 120 degrees of forward elevation, 25 degrees of external rotation, and internal rotation to the first lumbar vertebrae.

## Complications

- The most common complications after fractures of the proximal humerus are nonunion, malunion, stiffness, and avascular necrosis.
- Most nonunions occur at the surgical neck and can be managed successfully with plate fixation and bone grafting. Fixed-angled devices, such as blade plates, give improved fixation in the often osteopenic humeral head.[41,42]
- Avascular necrosis with associated collapse frequently is responsible for poor outcomes in displaced four-part fractures.[4,24,25] Prosthetic replacement may be indicated when nonsurgical methods fail to provide satisfactory pain relief, although delayed hemiarthroplasty results are inconsistent because of less reliable pain relief than anticipated.[24–26]
- Posttraumatic shoulder stiffness remains a difficult therapeutic problem. Physical therapy is the mainstay of treatment. Operative procedures include open or arthroscopic mobilization of the glenohumeral articulation, subacromial space, and scapulothoracic region. Surgical success is greatly dependent upon aggressive and consistent postoperative physical therapy.

## Fractures of the Clavicle

### Introduction

- Clavicle fractures represent 2% to 5% of all fractures and 25% to 40% of all shoulder girdle fractures.[43]
- Can be secondary to low- or high-energy injury.[43] Can occur as an isolated fracture or in the polytraumatized patient.

- Commonly result from a fall on the shoulder and less often from a fall on the outstretched arm.[44]
- Most clavicle fractures are managed nonoperatively. The majority occur in the middle third and heal without complications.[43]
- Nonunion rates of 0.1% to 5% are reported, with significantly higher nonunion rates (>10% in some series) in operatively treated patients.[45] Poor technique and suboptimal fixation devices likely played an important role in these nonunion cases.
- Increasing evidence indicates that not all clavicle fractures result in satisfactory outcomes.[46–48] High-energy injuries with comminution and substantial shortening (2–3 cm) appear to have lower functional results secondary to the inevitable malunion that occurs with nonoperative treatment. This finding has prompted recommendations for surgical management of some of these high-energy injuries.

### Anatomy

- The clavicle is an **S**-shaped bone that varies in thickness when viewed from its superior and anterior aspects. It presents a subcutaneous anterosuperior border along its entire length.
- It articulates with the sternum (sternoclavicular joint) and the acromion (acromioclavicular joint) at its proximal and distal extents, respectively. Biomechanically, the clavicle serves as a strut between the shoulder and the chest wall, allowing the shoulder to function at a distance from the center of the body. Clavicle fractures with significant shortening allow the shoulder to displace anteriorly and centrally, potentially compromising normal glenohumeral and scapulothoracic function.
- The stability of the sternoclavicular joint is secondary to its stout ligamentous connections, particularly the posterior contributions. The acromioclavicular joint is secured via numerous ligamentous attachments distally:
  - The superiorly located acromioclavicular ligament surrounds the joint capsule and provides minor support.
  - The coracoclavicular ligaments maintain the relationship of the clavicle to the coracoid. This relationship indirectly maintains the stability of the acromioclavicular joint. The coracoclavicular ligaments are composed of two major contributions: the conoid ligament (medial, and the stronger of the two) and the trapezoid ligament (lateral).
- The major muscle attachments include the deltoid, trapezius, pectoralis major, and sternocleidomastoid. Fracture displacement is related to muscle attachments. Midshaft fractures typically result in superior displacement of the medial portion secondary to pull of the sternocleidomastoid and trapezius. Similarly, the weight of the arm displaces the distal segment inferiorly.
- The subclavian artery and vein and the brachial plexus are important structures that lie immediately below the

clavicle. They can be injured at the time of fracture, during surgical fixation, or in a delayed fashion secondary to excessive callus formation. The supraclavicular nerves cross the anterior aspect of the clavicle and innervate the skin of the anterior, superior portion of the chest wall. They can be injured during surgical exposure of the clavicle.

## Physical Examination

- Examine the skin. Most of these fractures result from direct injury to the shoulder, so abrasions are common[44] whereas open fractures are rare.
- Neurovascular evaluation must be comprehensive and well documented.
- Pneumothorax must be considered in patients with isolated fractures and more commonly in polytraumatized patients. It is reported in up to 3% of patients with clavicle fractures.[49]

## Radiographic Examination

- Most clavicle fractures can be identified on an AP chest x-ray film. Shoulder films are useful for assessing fractures of the distal clavicle and associated shoulder/scapular injuries.
- In addition to an AP view, a 20- to 45-degree cephalad tilt view of the fractured clavicle is obtained to better assess the anteroposterior relationship of the main clavicle fragments.
- A posteroanterior view with 15 degrees caudal tilt has been described as beneficial in assessing the clavicle shaft for length/shortening.[50]
- The 45-degree anterior and posterior oblique views (off the coronal plane) can assist in demonstrating displacement of distal one-third clavicle fractures.[51]
- Weighted views can be useful in evaluating distal clavicle fractures if concern about fracture stability and potential displacement exists. This radiograph is taken as a standard AP view with a weight (often 10 lb) strapped to the patient's affected extremity. Comparison is made to a similar unweighted view. True displacement may be potentially altered, however, because several shoulder girdle muscles may be recruited to support the weight.
- The "serendipity view" of the sternoclavicular joints is taken with 40 to 45 degrees cephalad tilt. This view should be centered on the manubrium and should include both sternoclavicular joints for comparison.
- CT scan can be useful in evaluating very medial fractures or sternoclavicular dislocations.

## Classification

- Most fractures are characterized descriptively by location, comminution, and displacement.
- Allman[52] classified clavicle fractures into three groups (Figure 43–7):

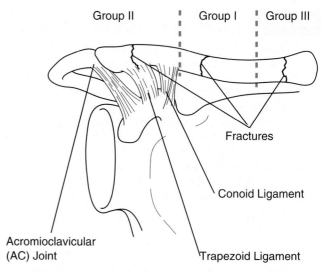

Figure 43–7:

**Allman classification groups clavicle fractures according to their anatomic location: middle (Group I), distal (Group II), or proximal (Group III).**

- Group I: middle third diaphyseal fractures. Most common location (approximately 80%).[43,53] Fracture is medial to coracoclavicular ligament insertions.
- Group II: lateral (distal) third fractures. Less common (approximately 12%–15%).[53]
- Group III: medial third fractures. Least common (approximately 5%–8%).[53] They often result from a direct blow and usually are minimally displaced because of the stout costoclavicular ligaments.
- Neer[51] subclassified distal clavicle fractures (Figure 43–8) as follows:
  - Type I distal fracture, coracoclavicular ligaments intact, minimal displacement (stable)
  - Type II: distal fracture with conoid (and possibly part of trapezoid) ligament disrupted from shaft, usually significant displacement (unstable)
- Additional classification has been added[49]:
  - Type III: distal fracture involving the acromioclavicular joint
  - Type IV: physeal separation

## Treatment

- The vast majority of clavicle fractures can be managed nonoperatively.
- Performing a closed manipulation is of limited use because reduction is difficult to achieve and maintain.
- Nonoperative treatment focuses on patient comfort and early functional rehabilitation of the shoulder. Initially, the injured arm is placed in a sling for comfort, and the patient is encouraged to remove the sling for hygiene, personal care, and elbow range of motion.
- Pendulum exercises are started immediately, with passive and active assisted exercises beginning once the acute pain has improved.

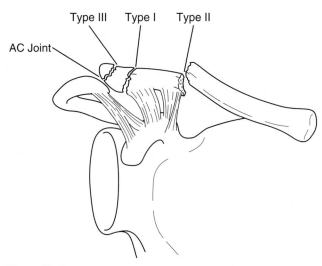

**Figure 43–8:**
Group 2 distal clavicle fractures are subdivided according to their relationship with the coracoclavicular ligaments. Type I distal clavicle fractures are nondisplaced and do not have disruption of these ligaments. Type II fractures are just medial to the coracoclavicular ligaments and often are unstable, with a higher risk of nonunion. Type III fractures are distal to the coracoclavicular ligaments and involve the articular surface of the distal clavicle at the acromioclavicular (AC) joint.

- Follow-up should begin within the first 1 to 2 weeks after injury to reinforce the benefits of early motion and to reassure the patient who may be anxious about pain and motion at the fracture site. It is reasonable at this time to discuss the residual cosmetic effect that may persist after union.
- By the 6- to 8-week mark, the fracture should demonstrate clinical union and substantially less pain with palpation. Motion should be approaching full range. At this time, patients may be concerned about the mass (healing callus) that develops at the site of the fracture and should be reassured that this is a common occurrence that will regress as the fracture remodels. Strengthening activities are instituted in a progressive fashion and are guided by pain. A return to contact sports should be avoided for a minimum of 3 months to allow for solid union and muscle rehabilitation to a competitive level.
- Figure-of-eight splints applied in an effort to minimize excessive shortening were recommended in the past; however, functional and cosmetic results are similar to simple sling management.[54]

## Indications for Operative Management

- The majority of clavicle fractures can be successfully managed with nonoperative means, but several relative indications for surgical management exist. The indications continue to evolve.

## Open Fractures

- Open fractures are rare and usually result from high-energy trauma.
- In addition to a thorough surgical debridement and irrigation, fracture stabilization often is beneficial, particularly in allowing soft tissue recovery.

## Skin at Risk

- Displaced clavicle fractures can place skin at risk for necrosis with delayed presentation of an open wound. Significant superior-anterior displacement can result in tenting of the skin with ischemic changes. Blanched skin that is no longer mobile over the fracture site can result from a fragment of bone that penetrated the dermis or a severely displaced fragment. In these unusual situations, the fracture is operatively reduced and stabilized to prevent skin necrosis and to allow soft tissue recovery.

## Scapulothoracic Dissociation

- *Pearl:* Because of normal muscle forces, the majority of clavicle fractures demonstrate shortening of the clavicle through the fracture. Patients that demonstrate distraction of a clavicle fracture should raise suspicion for traction-type mechanisms and suggest a scapulothoracic dissociation (Figure 43–9).
- This rare injury often is accompanied by devastating neurovascular injury, with the clinical picture often

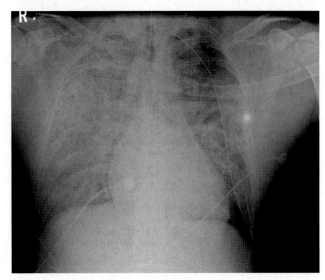

**Figure 43–9:**
Anteroposterior chest radiograph of a 38-year-old man who was severely injured after he was struck by a car while riding his bicycle. Note the distracted appearance of the clavicle fracture, associated rib fractures, and lateral displacement of the scapula relative to the chest wall. In addition to this scapulothoracic dissociation, the patient had a significant brachial plexus injury and an open wound along the lateral base of the neck.

demonstrating some degree of paralysis of the upper extremity (secondary to brachial plexus injury) and/or a dysvascular limb. Despite limited literature support, we advocate fracture fixation, especially in cases of significant displacement and/or associated vascular disruption requiring surgical repair.

## Floating Shoulder

- Clavicle fractures with ipsilateral scapular neck fractures create a glenohumeral articulation that is no longer in continuity with the axial skeleton. This combination injury is commonly referred to as a *floating shoulder.*
- Stabilization of the clavicular component has been advocated in the past to allow improved shoulder

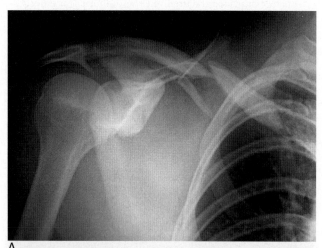

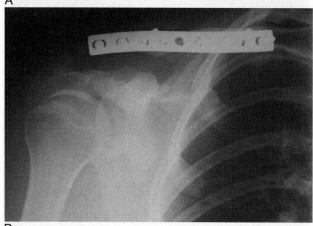

Figure 43–10:
**A,** A 29-year-old man sustained a closed clavicle fracture with associated displaced glenoid neck fracture after a fall from a significant height. Theoretical complications of this injury complex include a foreshortened extremity with muscular weakness and the potential for chronic brachial plexopathy from the weight of the arm. **B,** Although currently controversial, the patient's clavicle was reduced and stabilized with anteroinferior plating using a 3.5-mm DC (dynamic compression) plate to prevent the possible theoretical complications.

function (Figure 43–10). Contemporary clinical and biomechanical literature questions this concept, suggesting that satisfactory results can be obtained with nonoperative treatment.[55–57] At present, management of this injury complex should be individualized and dependent on the displacement of the clavicle and scapular neck fractures.[55]

- When nonoperative treatment is selected, routine x-ray films obtained during the first few weeks are important to ensure that unacceptable displacement does not occur.

## Neurovascular Injury

- Repair of the clavicle should be considered with concomitant vascular injury requiring repair to protect against further bony injury. Likewise, if a brachial plexus repair is performed, clavicle fixation may be prudent to avoid disruption by bony fragments.

## Distal Clavicle Fractures

- A controversial and relative indication.[58–60]
- Significantly displaced distal fractures (type II) have a higher rate of nonunion and functional problems and may benefit from operative fixation.[61,62]
- Careful consideration is needed because fixation of these fractures can be particularly challenging.

## Special Situations

- A relative indication for fixation of clavicle fractures are patients with neuromuscular conditions, such as Parkinson's disease, where immobilization is difficult.[63]
- Polytrauma, bilateral fractures, and elite athlete status of the patient have been described as relative indications for operative treatment.[49]

## Surgical Procedures

### Open Reduction Internal Fixation

- Open reduction and plate osteosynthesis is our preferred technique for operative management.
- Patients are placed in the supine or beach chair position on a radiolucent table. A small towel bump is placed between the scapulae, allowing the involved shoulder to be relatively extended.
- The surgical incision parallels the clavicle and is placed just inferior to the prominent anterosuperior border. Care is taken to preserve supraclavicular nerve branches.
- Contoured 2.7-mm dynamic compression plates or 3.5-mm limited contact dynamic compression plates are used, with supplemental lag screws when possible. Reconstruction plates also can be used. Adequate plate length is critical, as many prior studies of nonunion following ORIF attribute failure to technical errors such as inadequate plate length (Figure 43–11).
- Plates can be applied superiorly or anteroinferiorly. Mechanical studies suggest that superior plate placement

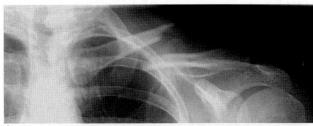

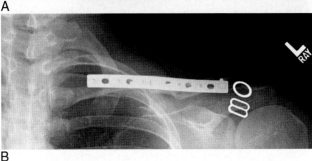

**Figure 43–11:**
A 22-year-old woman was involved in a low-speed motor vehicle collision. **A,** Anteroposterior clavicle radiograph shows an isolated left clavicle fracture sustained by the patient. Ten months postinjury, the fracture had failed to unite, leading to complaints of persisting pain, shoulder weakness, and inability to lift objects above her head. Autogenous bone grafting and stabilization with an anteroinferior 2.7-mm DC (dynamic compression) plate was performed. **B,** Four months later, the anteroposterior radiograph shows union. Clinically, all of the patient's preoperative symptoms resolved.

offers increased fracture stability,[64] but clinical studies of anteroinferior placement demonstrate comparable union rates, with substantially less complications related to implant prominence.[65] For these reasons, we prefer anteroinferior plate placement.

### External Fixation

- Described in the literature as effective for management of acute fractures and nonunions but is used infrequently.[66,67]
- Patient comfort is the biggest drawback of this technique.

### *Intramedullary Implants*

- K-wires, threaded Steinman pins, intramedullary screws, rush rods, elastic nails, and other devices all have been described for successful fixation of clavicle fractures.[45,68–71]
- Despite successful reports, K-wire stabilization is associated with implant migration[72] and is not used at our institution for management of these fractures. Implants have been found within numerous organ systems, including the lung, heart, and spinal canal. Smooth wires, rather than threaded pins, appear to be particularly problematic.

### *Rehabilitation*

- Patients are started on immediate pendulum exercises with their sling still in place. Gravity assisted and passive

range of motion are subsequently started. The sling should be worn for the majority of the day, except during physical therapy. Until early fracture union occurs, the weight of the arm presents a significant displacing force after fixation, so the arm needs to be supported with the sling.
- Progressive strengthening exercises usually can begin at approximately 8 weeks, depending on radiographic stability and union.

## Complications

### Malunion

- Symptomatic malunions of the clavicle can lead to patient dissatisfaction.[46,47,73,74] McKee, Wild, and Schemitsch[47] reviewed 15 patients who underwent corrective osteotomy for clavicular malunion. Preoperative symptoms included weakness, pain, neurologic/thoracic outlet symptoms, and appearance concerns ("droopy" shoulder, with other symptoms). Fourteen of the 15 patients subsequently achieved union and significant symptom improvement.
- Shortening of 2 cm or more is the most consistent risk factor for symptomatic malunion.[46,47]

### Nonunion

- More common in operatively treated fractures, especially in older studies. Overall, nonunion rates of less than 1% to greater than 10% have been reported.
- Most common in distal third fractures, but functional results appear to be satisfactory.[58]
- Operative management includes stabilization and the addition of bone graft (see Figure 43–11). Satisfactory results have been reported with both plate fixation and intramedullary devices.[65,67,75–77]
- Midshaft fractures with more than 2 cm of shortening and lateral third fractures appear to be at higher risk for nonunion.[46,48]

## Fractures of the Scapula and Glenoid

### Introduction

- Scapula and glenoid fractures occur uncommonly.
- Frequently result from high-energy trauma.
- Scapular body fractures typically occur after a direct blow to the thorax or shoulder girdle after vehicular accidents or a fall from significant height. Associated skeletal and soft tissue injuries occur commonly.
- Intraarticular glenoid fractures occur in 20% to 30% of scapula fractures and are associated with similar violent trauma and associated injuries. The exception is the glenoid rim fracture, which may occur in association with an anterior glenohumeral dislocation.

- The vast majority of scapular body fractures are treated nonoperatively.
- Surgical indications for scapular (glenoid) neck fractures are unclear.
- Intraarticular glenoid fractures may require operative treatment, depending on the displacement and the amount of articular surface involvement.

## Anatomy

- The scapula is encased in muscle and is minimally constrained by osseous attachments to the axial skeleton.
- This generous muscular coverage of the majority of the scapula imparts rapid healing but makes surgical access difficult, except to the palpable subcutaneous portions such as the scapular spine, acromion process, and medial scapular border.
- The osseus anatomy is complex, with significant variability in cortical thickness from the central body to the borders and processes.[78]
- The portions of the scapula useful for screw purchase include the glenoid neck, acromion process, coracoid process, scapular spine, and medial and lateral borders.
- The glenoid articular surface is small and relatively flat, making the glenohumeral joint poorly constrained.
- Shoulder joint stability results primarily from the dynamic muscular forces acting across the glenohumeral articulation.
- Important articulations include the glenohumeral joint, acromioclavicular joint, and scapulothoracic articulation.
- Thorough understanding of the location of the primary muscular attachments, nerve supply, and vascular supply of the anterior and posterior scapula is necessary for a complete assessment and treatment plan.
  - For posterior approaches to the shoulder, the interval between the teres minor and the infraspinatus allows safe access to the shoulder joint.
  - The axillary nerve is located between the teres minor and the teres major.
  - The circumflex scapular artery crosses the lateral border of the scapula near the glenoid neck and requires identification in posterior approaches that expose the lateral border.
  - The deltopectoral interval is used for anterior access to the shoulder for anterior glenoid fractures.
- The muscular and ligamentous attachments to the coracoid process include the coracoclavicular ligaments, coracoacromial ligament, pectoralis minor, coracobrachialis, and short head of the biceps brachii. The displacement patterns of glenoid articular fractures involving the anterosuperior portion of the joint are determined by the relative integrity of these attachments.

## Physical Examination

- Associated shoulder girdle injuries, such as those to the clavicle, acromioclavicular joint, and proximal humerus, occur commonly and should be identified.

- Although open fractures of the scapula and glenoid are rare, a careful assessment of the skin integrity should be performed.
- An accurate upper extremity neurologic examination should include assessment of the entire brachial plexus because associated nerve injuries are common.
- Special attention should be directed to assessment of the axillary, suprascapular, and musculocutaneous nerves.[79]
- To adequately assess the vascular supply of the upper extremity, the presence and quality of pulses and the ankle-brachial index should be documented.

## Radiographic Examination

- Radiographic studies include AP and lateral shoulder views in the plane of the scapula (true AP and lateral), a true AP of the entire scapula (frequently lacking on a true AP shoulder view), and an axillary lateral shoulder view. The glenoid articular surface is best visualized on the scapular (true) AP and the axillary lateral. Glenohumeral subluxations and dislocations are most evident on the axillary lateral view.[80,81]
- Comparison views of the contralateral shoulder frequently are helpful in determining angulatory and translational deformities of glenoid neck and fossa injuries.
- In most glenoid articular fractures, radiographic evaluation with CT is important in fracture pattern comprehension, preoperative planning, and determination of the surgical approach. Three-dimensional reconstructions may enhance planning of some difficult patterns.
- The role of CT scans in scapular body fractures is poorly defined and limited because surgical indications are unusual.
- Angiographic studies are warranted in patients with altered upper extremity blood flow, as predicted by physical examination and ankle-brachial indices. Further evaluation of the brachial plexus may be indicated in patients demonstrating associated extensive neurologic upper extremity impairment.

## Classification

- Classification of scapula fractures is primarily descriptive and based on the anatomic location of the primary injury pattern. Key anatomic locations for classification purposes include the acromion, scapular spine, glenoid neck, glenoid articular surface, and scapular body.[81–83]
- Glenoid articular fractures have been further classified according the anatomic location of the primary fracture lines as follows (Figure 43–12): fractures of the glenoid rim (type I), inferior lateral partial articular injuries (type II), superior partial articular injuries (type III), transverse fractures extending to the medial scapular border (type IV), combined patterns involving the entire fossa (type V), and severely comminuted fractures (type VI).[84–86]

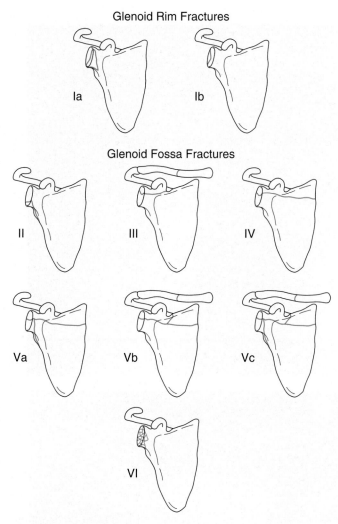

**Figure 43–12:**
**Modified Ideberg classification system of glenoid fractures.**

## Emergency Room Management

- Most scapular and glenoid articular injuries can be initially managed with a sling for comfort. Open scapula fractures are surgical emergencies and require early debridement and irrigation. Fixation may be required, depending on the particular skeletal and soft tissue injury. Associated vascular injuries require a coordinated approach with an appropriate vascular consultant.

## Treatment

- The vast majority of scapular body fractures heal rapidly with nonoperative management. Following an initial sling for comfort, early and unrestricted active and passive shoulder range of motion exercises can be instituted.
- Scapular neck and glenoid articular fractures that are treated nonoperatively are initially managed with a sling for comfort.[81,82] Early passive range of motion exercises

can be initiated based upon patient comfort. Resistive exercises should be restricted for 6 weeks in patients with neck fractures and 12 weeks in those with articular fractures.

- Indications for fixation of acromial fractures are poorly described. Significant displacement and associated shoulder girdle injuries are relative indications. The approach is directed by the fracture configuration. Fractures of the lateral acromial process usually can be approached posteriorly along the posterior border, carefully elevating the deltoid origin. Fixation frequently is difficult because of the complex anatomy and limited scapular bone stock.
- Surgical indications for fractures confined to the scapular body are unusual. Even open scapular bodies do not necessarily require fixation after an appropriate and timely debridement and irrigation.
- Surgical indications for glenoid neck fractures are not well described. Significant displacement, translation, and angulation of the entire glenohumeral joint relative to the scapular body may affect shoulder joint motion and the mechanical advantage of the rotator cuff and shoulder girdle muscles, producing a surgical indication.[87] The exact displacement, translation, and angulation that produce functional abnormalities are unknown, so treatment must be individualized (Figure 43–13). Associated clavicle fractures create the so-called *floating shoulder injury* and have been identified as a strong indication for fixation of the glenoid neck and/or clavicle fracture. Clinical and biomechanical studies have questioned this condition as a surgical indication.
- Surgical indications for operative fixation of glenoid fractures include displacement of 3 to 5 mm and/or humeral head subluxation (Figure 43–14). The amount (percentage) of articular surface involved and the fracture location also influence the treatment decision.[86,88–97]
- Anterior rim fractures may represent labral avulsion fractures in patients with an associated dislocation. Treatment decisions parallel glenohumeral instability without an anterior rim fracture.

### Surgical Management

#### Exposures

##### Anterior

- For anterior glenoid rim or articular fractures, the deltopectoral approach is used. These fracture patterns are unusual and represent the exception.

##### Posterior

- The majority of glenoid articular fractures and all scapular neck fractures are approached posteriorly.[84,86,97–99]
- Positioning can be either lateral or prone.
- The lateral position allows simultaneous access to the coracoid for manipulation of fractures involving the

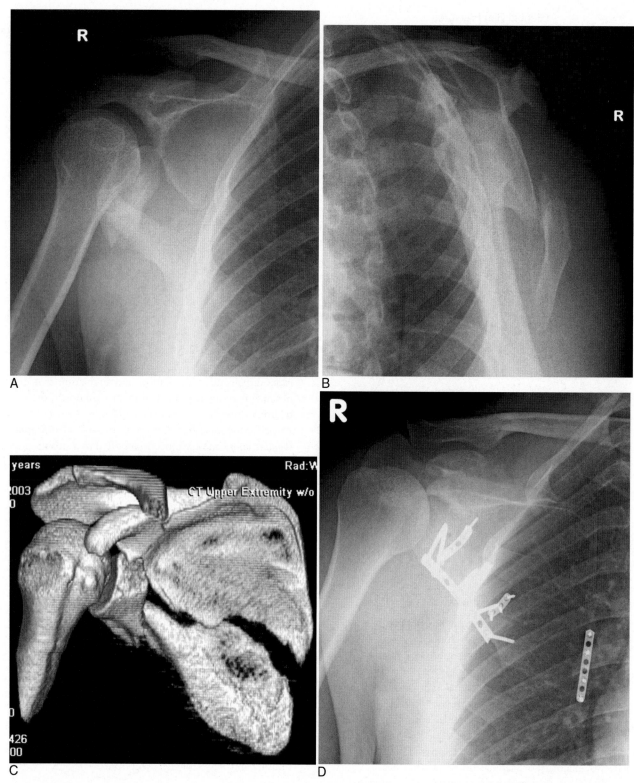

Figure 43–13:

**A, B,** Injury anteroposterior and scapular Y radiographs of the right shoulder of a 38-year-old man after he slipped and fell down a flight of stairs. Note the marked inferior displacement of the glenoid fossa. **C,** Three-dimensional CT reconstruction was obtained to improve the comprehension of the fracture pattern. The anterior view of the right scapula is shown.
**D, E, F:** Using a posterior surgical exposure, multiple minifragment scapular body plates and a single one-third tubular antiglide plate placed along the inferior glenoid neck were used for fixation. Anteroposterior, axillary, and scapular Y radiographs show satisfactory union 4 months later. An excellent functional result was obtained.

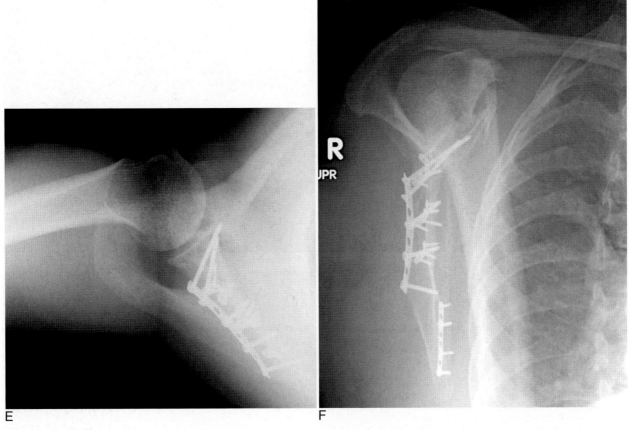

E                    F

Figure 43–13: cont'd

entire articular surface. However, intraoperative fluoroscopic imaging is limited.

- Prone positioning allows intraoperative fluoroscopic images but limits manipulation of anterior fracture fragments.
- For combined glenoid articular and scapular body fractures, one approach consists of a modification of a posterior approach to the shoulder combined with aspects of the posterior (Judet) approach to the scapula.[86,97]

## Technique

- An incision is made along the spine of the scapula extending from the lateral acromion to the medial scapular border. The incision curves distally and parallels the medial scapular border along the scapular length. A full-thickness flap of the skin and subcutaneous tissues is developed, exposing the overlying fascia of the deltoid and the shoulder external rotators.
- The deltoid muscle belly, with its investing fascia, is reflected off the underlying infraspinatus muscle and the scapular spine. With the deltoid retracted laterally, the interval between the teres minor and the infraspinatus is

identified and developed, exposing the lateral border of the scapula and the posterior joint capsule. Care is taken to identify the circumflex scapular artery at the lateral scapular border and to avoid dissection inferior to the teres minor (axillary nerve) (Box 43–3).

- Exposure of the scapular spine and medial scapular border is important in fractures with extensions to these locations. In fractures not involving the medial or lateral scapular borders (types II and III), further exposure in these locations for reduction and plate applications is not necessary. The shoulder joint can then be exposed. The interval between the infraspinatus and the teres minor can be extended laterally to uncover the posterior joint capsule. Typically, the posterior exit of an intraarticular fracture component produces a capsular disruption that can be used to view the articular surface and the subsequent reduction. The capsular and labral attachments to the posterior glenoid rim should be left intact. However, a vertical capsular incision can be extended to improve the exposure. For fractures of the scapular neck, lateral exposure to the joint capsule is unnecessary.
- The suprascapular nerve and vessels at the spinoglenoid notch should be protected throughout.

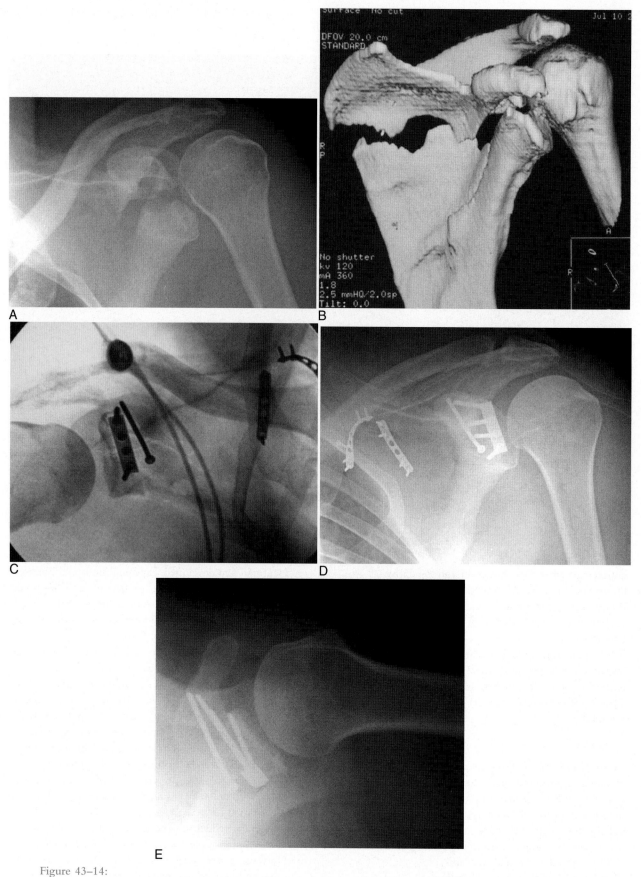

Figure 43–14:

**A, B,** Injury anteroposterior plain radiograph and three-dimensional CT reconstruction show a type IV glenoid fossa fracture in a 42-year-old man involved in a motorcycle collision. Marked articular congruity of the glenoid articular surface is seen. **C,** Intraoperative anteroposterior fluorograph shows satisfactory reduction and stabilization via a posterior exposure. **D, E,** Anteroposterior and axillary radiographs show satisfactory union.

> **Box 43–3   Pitfall**
>
> • Occasionally, a large fat stripe is present between the two heads of the infraspinatus. Mistakenly assuming that this interval is the infraspinatus–teres minor interval may result in denervation of the inferior head of the infraspinatus.

## Fixation Strategies

• The choice of implant for fixation is governed by the cortical thickness, complex scapular geometry, and limited space for plate application.

• Scapular neck fractures can be stabilized with a plate placed along the lateral aspect of the lateral border of the scapula.

• Glenoid articular fractures require a more comprehensive surgical approach.

• Smaller (2.0, 2.4, or 2.7 mm) plates combine adequate stiffness, flexibility, and contouring characteristics for the medial scapular border and scapular spine. Plates spanning the thinner, frequently unicortical scapular body usually are 2.0 mm; the maximum screw length in this location usually is 6 to 8 mm. One-quarter tubular, one-third tubular, or 2.7-mm reconstruction plates can be easily contoured to stabilize the glenoid neck.

• The most important location for fixation of type Va, Vc, and VI fractures usually is at the lateral scapular border, extending to inferior articular margin. One-quarter tubular and one-third tubular plates can be placed on the lateral aspect of the lateral border (see Figure 43–13, *D* and *E)*. This step allows fixation through the plate and into the coracoid process, supporting both the inferior articular fracture and the caudal scapular body component. It should be understood that the coracoid process base actually is lateral and cephalad in location relative to the lateral border.

• The medial border fracture (in type IV, V, and VI patterns) usually is stabilized prior to the articular reduction in glenoid articular fractures. Although fixation of the medial border of the scapula is not needed for stability, scapular body reduction facilitates articular reduction.

## Rehabilitation

• Postoperatively, immediate, unrestricted passive range of motion exercises are encouraged. Active shoulder exercises are delayed for 6 weeks to allow for healing of the repaired deltoid origin.

• Resistive exercises are instituted beginning at 12 weeks.

• Radiographic evaluation includes scapular anteroposterior and axillary lateral views postoperatively and at 6, 12, and 24 weeks.

## Complications

• Infections are unusual given the generous vascular supply to the scapula.

• Healing complications after scapular body fractures are rare. Union is predictable and rapid because of the abundant vascular supply.

• Glenoid neck fractures heal predictably, but the impact of significant angular or translational deformities is unknown. Glenohumeral stiffness after a glenoid neck or articular fracture occurs commonly but can be managed with early, aggressive physical therapy.

• Traumatic peripheral nerve injuries occur relatively frequently, and their management usually is expectant.

• Iatrogenic intraoperative nerve injuries, especially to the axillary and suprascapular nerves, usually can be prevented by understanding the surgical anatomy and safe planes of dissection and implant placement.

## References

1. Horak J, Nilsson BE: Epidemiology of fracture of the upper end of the humerus. *Clin Orthop* 112:250-253, 1975.

2. Court-Brown CM, Garg A, McQueen MM: The epidemiology of proximal humeral fractures. *Acta Orthop Scand* 72:365-371, 2001.

3. Jakob RP, Miniaci A, Anson PS et al: Four-part valgus impacted fractures of the proximal humerus. *J Bone Joint Surg Br* 73: 295-298, 1991.
   The valgus four-part fracture of the proximal humerus is identified. The rate of avascular necrosis was lower than that of other displaced four-part fractures.

4. Wijgman AJ, Roolker W, Patt TW et al: Open reduction and internal fixation of three and four-part fractures of the proximal part of the humerus. *J Bone Joint Surg Am* 84A:1919-1925, 2002.
   ORIF yields good functional results in most patients and should be considered even for patients with fracture-dislocation patterns that are associated with a high risk for avascular necrosis.

5. Visser CP, Coene LN, Brand R, Tavy DL: Nerve lesions in proximal humeral fractures. *J Shoulder Elbow Surg* 10:421-427, 2001.
   The nerves most frequently injured were the axillary nerve (58%) and the suprascapular nerve (48%). These injuries occurred more frequently in displaced fractures than in nondisplaced fractures.

6. McLaughlin JA, Light R, Lustrin I: Axillary artery injury as a complication of proximal humerus fractures. *J Shoulder Elbow Surg* 7:292-294, 1998.

7. Bloom MH, Obata WG: Diagnosis of posterior dislocation of the shoulder with use of Velpeau axillary and angle-up roentgenographic views. *J Bone Joint Surg Am* 49:943-949, 1967.

8. Simon JA, Puopolo SM, Capla EL et al: Accuracy of the axillary projection to determine fracture angulation of the proximal humerus. *Orthopedics* 27:205-207, 2004.
   The axillary view is not accurate for measuring proximal humerus angulation at the arm positions commonly encountered in the trauma setting.

9. Jurik AG, Albrechtsen J: The use of computed tomography with two- and three-dimensional reconstructions in the diagnosis of three- and four-part fractures of the proximal humerus. *Clin Radiol* 49:800-804, 1994.

10. Castagno AA, Shuman WP, Kilcoyne RF et al: Complex fractures of the proximal humerus: role of CT in treatment. *Radiology* 165:759-762, 1987.

11. Neer CS 2nd: Displaced proximal humeral fractures. I. Classification and evaluation. *J Bone Joint Surg Am* 52:1077-1089, 1970.

12. Neer CS 2nd: Displaced proximal humeral fractures. II. Treatment of three-part and four-part displacement. *J Bone Joint Surg Am* 52:1090-1103, 1970.

13. Orthopaedic Trauma Association Committee for Coding and Classification: Fracture and dislocation compendium. *J Orthop Trauma* 10(suppl 1):31-34, 1996.

14. Muller ME, Nazarian S, Koch P, Schatzker J: *The comprehensive classification of fractures of long bones.* Berlin, 1990, Springer-Verlag.

15. Siebenrock KA, Gerber C: The reproducibility of classification of fractures of the proximal end of the humerus. *J Bone Joint Surg Am* 75:1751-1755, 1993.
    Neither the Neer nor the AO/ASIF fracture classification is sufficiently reproducible to allow meaningful comparison of similarly classified fractures in different studies.

16. Sidor ML, Zuckerman JD, Lyon T et al: The Neer classification system for proximal humeral fractures. An assessment of inter-observer reliability and intraobserver reproducibility. *J Bone Joint Surg Am* 75:1745-1750, 1993.
    The authors identified suboptimal interobserver reliability and intraobserver reproducibility with the Neer classification system for fractures of the proximal humerus.

17. Bernstein J, Adler LM, Blank JE et al: Evaluation of the Neer system of classification of proximal humeral fractures with computerized tomographic scans and plain radiographs. *J Bone Joint Surg Am* 78:1371-1375, 1996.
    The classification of proximal humerus fractures remains difficult because of the lack of uniform agreement about which fragments are fractured. Intraobserver reliability was marginally improved with CT scanning, but interobserver reproducibility was not.

18. Tamai K, Hamada J, Ohno W, Saotome K: Surgical anatomy of multipart fractures of the proximal humerus. *J Shoulder Elbow Surg* 11:421-427, 2002.
    This study identifies and confirms the inaccuracies of the current classification schemes in proximal humerus fractures.

19. Green A, Izzi J Jr: Isolated fractures of the greater tuberosity of the proximal humerus. *J Shoulder Elbow Surg* 12:641-649, 2003.
    Review of isolated greater tuberosity fractures of the proximal humerus.

20. Cuomo F, Goss TP: Shoulder trauma: bone. In Kasser JR, editor: *Orthopaedic knowledge update 5*, ed 5. Rosemont, 1996, American Academy of Orthopaedic Surgeons.

21. Koval KJ, Gallagher MA, Marsicano JG et al: Functional outcome after minimally displaced fractures of the proximal part of the humerus. *J Bone Joint Surg Am* 79:203-207, 1997.
    Reports 77% good or excellent results for minimally displaced proximal humerus fractures, with an improved prognosis for those who started supervised physical therapy in less than 14 days.

22. Misra A, Kapur R, Maffulli N: Complex proximal humeral fractures in adults—a systematic review of management. *Injury* 32:363-372, 2001.
    Nonoperative treatment of three- and four-part proximal humerus fractures leads to more pain and poorer motion than ORIF or arthroplasty.

23. Liew AS, Johnson JA, Patterson SD et al: Effect of screw placement on fixation in the humeral head. *J Shoulder Elbow Surg* 9:423-426, 2000.
    Optimal screw purchase is achieved by placing screws in the center of the humeral head abutting the subchondral bone. The anterosuperior position provided the least fixation.

24. Hessmann M, Baumgaertel F, Gehling H et al: Plate fixation of proximal humeral fractures with indirect reduction: surgical technique and results utilizing three shoulder scores. *Injury* 30:453-462, 1999.
    Indirect reduction and plate fixation is an adequate procedure for treating unstable and displaced two- to four-part fractures of the proximal humerus, enabling early functional rehabilitation.

25. Hintermann B, Trouillier HH, Schafer D: Rigid internal fixation of fractures of the proximal humerus in older patients. *J Bone Joint Surg Br* 82:1107-1112, 2000.
    Rigid fixation of displaced fractures of the proximal humerus with a blade plate in the elderly patient provides sufficient primary stability to allow early functional treatment.

26. Becker R, Pap G, Machner A, Neumann WH: Strength and motion after hemiarthroplasty in displaced four-fragment fracture of the proximal humerus: 27 patients followed for 1-6 years. *Acta Orthop Scand* 73:44-49, 2002.
    Impaired function seems to be caused by stiffness rather than weakness. A better outcome was observed following early rather than late hemiarthroplasty.

27. Esser RD: Treatment of three- and four-part fractures of the proximal humerus with a modified cloverleaf plate. *J Orthop Trauma* 8:15-22, 1994.
    This study supports ORIF of multifragmentary proximal humerus fractures.

28. Agel J, Jones CB, Sanzone AG et al: Treatment of proximal humeral fractures with Polarus nail fixation. *J Shoulder Elbow Surg* 13:191-195, 2004.
    The authors identify some of the limitations of intramedullary nail fixation of proximal humerus fractures, particularly those with comminution extending to the nail starting point.

29. Adedapo AO, Ikpeme JO: The results of internal fixation of three- and four-part proximal humeral fractures with the Polarus nail. *Injury* 32:115-121, 2001.
    Reports good results following closed intramedullary nailing using a Polarus nail for displaced three- and four-part proximal humerus fractures, except for 13%, all of whom had four-part fractures, who continued to have significant pain.

30. Rajasekhar C, Ray PS, Bhamra MS: Fixation of proximal humeral fractures with the Polarus nail. *J Shoulder Elbow Surg* 10:7-10, 2001.

31. Jaberg H, Warner JJ, Jakob RP: Percutaneous stabilization of unstable fractures of the humerus. *J Bone Joint Surg Am* 74: 508-515, 1992.
Results of percutaneous pinning were comparable or superior to those obtained in previously described operative methods for treatment of these fractures.

32. Williams GR Jr, Wong KL: Two-part and three-part fractures: open reduction and internal fixation versus closed reduction and percutaneous pinning. *Orthop Clin North Am* 31:1-21, 2000.

33. Rowles DJ, McGrory JE: Percutaneous pinning of the proximal part of the humerus. An anatomic study. *J Bone Joint Surg Am* 83A:1695-1699, 2001.
In this cadaveric model, the authors describe the proximity of neurovascular structures to the pin location in percutaneous techniques for fracture stabilization of the proximal humerus.

34. Court-Brown CM, Garg A, McQueen MM: The translated two-part fracture of the proximal humerus. Epidemiology and outcome in the older patient. *J Bone Joint Surg Br* 83:799-804, 2001.
Patients with two-part translated fractures of the surgical neck tended to be independent and relatively fit, even though their mean age was 72 years. Outcome was determined by the age of each patient and the degree of translation on the initial anteroposterior radiograph.

35. Court-Brown CM, Cattermole H, McQueen MM: Impacted valgus fractures (B1.1) of the proximal humerus. The results of non-operative treatment. *J Bone Joint Surg Br* 84:504-508, 2002.
This study reported 80.6% of patients with an impacted valgus fracture treated nonsurgically had a good or excellent result, the quality of which depended on the age of the patient and the degree of displacement. Operative fixation of these fractures is not necessary.

36. Fankhauser F, Gruber G, Schippinger G et al: Minimal-invasive treatment of distal femoral fractures with the LISS (Less Invasive Stabilization System): a prospective study of 30 fractures with a follow-up of 20 months. *Acta Orthop Scand* 75:56-60, 2004.

37. Wenzl ME, Porte T, Fuchs S et al: Delayed and non-union of the humeral diaphysis: compression plate or internal plate fixator? *Injury* 35:55-60, 2004.

38. Compito CA, Self EB, Bigliani LU: Arthroplasty and acute shoulder trauma. Reasons for success and failure. *Clin Orthop* 307:27-36, 1994.

39. Boileau P, Krishnan SG, Tinsi L et al: Tuberosity malposition and migration: reasons for poor outcomes after hemiarthroplasty for displaced fractures of the proximal humerus. *J Shoulder Elbow Surg* 11:401-412, 2002.
Satisfactory tuberosity position and union correlated with the success or failure of hemiarthroplasty for treatment of displaced fractures of the proximal humerus.

40. Prakash U, McGurty DW, Dent JA: Hemiarthroplasty for severe fractures of the proximal humerus. *J Shoulder Elbow Surg* 11:428-430, 2002.
Fracture severity and timing of the operation did not appear to have a bearing on the outcome. Technical problems at surgery, greater tuberosity displacement, late rotator cuff rupture, and poorly motivated patients were the main reasons for failure.

41. Ring D, McKee MD, Perey BH, Jupiter JB: The use of a blade plate and autogenous cancellous bone graft in the treatment of ununited fractures of the proximal humerus. *J Shoulder Elbow Surg* 10:501-507, 2001.
Blade plates and autograft were used to repair ununited fractures of the proximal humerus. A 92% rate of healing and 80% good or excellent results with few complications were reported.

42. Galatz LM, Iannotti JP: Management of surgical neck nonunions. *Orthop Clin North Am* 31:51-61, 2000.

43. Postacchini F, Gumina S, De Santis P, Albo F: Epidemiology of clavicle fractures. *J Shoulder Elbow Surg* 11:452-456, 2002.
Clavicle fractures represented 2.6% of all fractures and 44% of those in the shoulder girdle. Fractures of the middle third were most common (81%), whereas fractures of the medial third were the least common (2%).

44. Stanley D, Trowbridge EA, Norris SH: The mechanism of clavicular fracture. A clinical and biomechanical analysis. *J Bone Joint Surg Br* 70:461-464, 1988.
Study reported that 94% of patients fractured their clavicle from a direct blow on the shoulder; only 6% had fallen on an outstretched hand.

45. Grassi FA, Tajana MS, D'Angelo F: Management of midclavicular fractures: comparison between nonoperative treatment and open intramedullary fixation in 80 patients. *J Trauma* 50:1096-1100, 2001.

46. Hill JM, McGuire MH, Crosby LA: Closed treatment of displaced middle-third fractures of the clavicle gives poor results. *J Bone Joint Surg Br* 79:537-539, 1997.
Unsatisfactory results were reported by 16 of 52 patients with displaced, midshaft clavicle fractures. Shortening of 2 cm or more was highly correlated with nonunion and unsatisfactory results.

47. McKee MD, Wild LM, Schemitsch EH: Midshaft malunions of the clavicle. *J Bone Joint Surg Am* 85A:790-797, 2003.
Corrective osteotomy was performed for 15 patients with clavicle midshaft malunion; 14 of 15 healed. Satisfaction and function improved significantly in all patients.

48. Wick M, Muller EJ, Kollig E, Murh G: Midshaft fractures of the clavicle with a shortening of more than 2 cm are predispose to nonunion. *Arch Orthop Trauma Surg* 121:207-211, 2001.
Midshaft clavicle fractures with shortening greater than 2 cm are predisposed to nonunion. ORIF should be undertaken in symptomatic patients if no signs of healing are observed after 6 weeks.

49. Ring D, Jupiter JB, Miller ME, Ada JR: Fractures of the clavicle. In Browner BD, Jupiter JB, Levine AM, Trafton PG, editors: *Skeletal trauma,* vol 2. Philadelphia, 1998, WB Saunders.

50. Sharr JR, Mohammed KD: Optimizing the radiographic technique in clavicular fractures. *J Shoulder Elbow Surg* 12:170-172, 2003.

The authors describe the advantage of obtaining a posteroanterior 15-degree caudal view in assessing clavicle fractures and evaluating shortening.

51. Neer CS 2nd: Fractures of the distal third of the clavicle. *Clin Orthop* 58:43-50, 1968.
Distal clavicle fractures are reviewed. A classification with division into two types as related to stability is described.

52. Allman FL Jr: Fractures and ligamentous injuries of the clavicle and its articulation. *J Bone Joint Surg Am* 49:774-784, 1967.
A review of clavicle fractures, acromioclavicular and sternoclavicular sprains. Classifications are defined. Evaluation protocols and treatment options are described.

53. Rowe CR: An atlas of anatomy and treatment of midclavicular fractures. *Clin Orthop* 58:29-42, 1968.

54. Andersen K, Jensen PO, Lauritzen J: Treatment of clavicular fractures. Figure-of-eight bandage versus a simple sling. *Acta Orthop Scand* 58:71-74, 1987.
Treatment with a simple sling caused less discomfort and perhaps fewer complications than a figure-of-eight bandage, with identical functional and cosmetic results.

55. Egol KA, Conner PM, Karunakar MA et al: The floating shoulder: clinical and functional results. *J Bone Joint Surg Am* 83:1188-1194, 2001.
Good results may be seen both with and without operative treatment for patients with a displaced fracture of the glenoid neck and an ipsilateral clavicular fracture or acromioclavicular separation.

56. Edwards SG, Whittle AP, Wood GW 2nd: Nonoperative treatment of ipsilateral fractures of the scapula and clavicle. *J Bone Joint Surg Am* 82:774-780, 2000.
Twenty patients with a floating shoulder were treated nonoperatively. Nineteen fractures united; one clavicular nonunion resulted. The majority of patients had excellent shoulder motion and functioning scores.

57. van Noort A, te Slaa RL, Marti R, van der Werken C: The floating shoulder. A multicentre study. *J Bone Joint Surg Br* 83:795-798, 2001.
Ipsilateral clavicle and scapula fractures are not inherently unstable. In the absence of caudal dislocation of the glenoid, nonoperative treatment leads to good outcomes.

58. Anderson K: Evaluation and treatment of distal clavicle fractures. *Clin Sports Med* 22:319-326, 2003.
A review article evaluating the controversies involving the management of distal clavicle fractures.

59. Nordqvist A, Petersson C, Redlund-Johnell I: The natural course of lateral clavicle fracture. 15 (11-21) year follow-up of 110 cases. *Acta Orthop Scand* 64:87-91, 1993.
Most distal clavicle fractures do not require surgical intervention.

60. Robinson CM, Cairns DA: Primary nonoperative treatment of displaced lateral fractures of the clavicle. *J Bone Joint Surg Am* 86A:778-782, 2004.
Nonoperative treatment of most displaced lateral clavicle fractures results in good functional outcomes.

61. Webber MC, Haines JF: The treatment of lateral clavicle fractures. *Injury* 31:175-179, 2000.
The authors describe their technique of using a Dacron arterial graft as a sling around the clavicle and coracoid process to treat distal clavicle fractures. All fractures healed.

62. Yamaguchi H, Arakawa H, Kobayashi M: Results of the Bosworth method for unstable fractures of the distal clavicle. *Int Orthop* 22:366-368, 1998.
Eleven Neer type II distal clavicle fractures were treated by open reduction internal fixation with a Bosworth-type screw. All fractures healed within 10 weeks.

63. Zenni EJ Jr, Krieg JK, Rosen MJ: Open reduction and internal fixation of clavicular fractures. *J Bone Joint Surg Am* 63:147-151, 1981.

64. Iannotti MR, Crosby LA, Stafford P et al: Effects of plate location and selection on the stability of midshaft clavicle osteotomies: a biomechanical study. *J Shoulder Elbow Surg* 11:457-462, 2002.
Clavicles plated superiorly exhibit significantly greater stability than those plated anteriorly. Limited contact dynamic compression (LCDC) plates provide greater stability than reconstruction and dynamic compression (DC) plates.

65. Kloen P, Sorkin AT, Rubel IF, Helfet DL: Anteroinferior plating of midshaft clavicular nonunions. *J Orthop Trauma* 16:425-430, 2002.
The authors describe their technique for open reduction internal fixation of clavicular nonunion with anteroinferior placement of a 3.5-mm reconstruction plate.

66. Schuind F, Pay-Pay E, Andrianne Y et al: External fixation of the clavicle for fracture or non-union in adults. *J Bone Joint Surg Am* 70:692-695, 1988.
Fifteen patients with clavicle fractures and five patients with nonunions were treated with external fixation. All fractures united with shoulder function and minimal complications.

67. Nowak J, Rahme H, Holgersson M et al: A prospective comparison between external fixation and plates for treatment of midshaft nonunions of the clavicle. *Ann Chir Gynaecol* 90:280-285, 2001.

68. Chu CM, Wang SJ, Lin LC: Fixation of mid-third clavicular fractures with Knowles pins: 78 patients followed for 2-7 years. *Acta Orthop Scand* 73:134-139, 2002.

69. Jubel A, Andermahr J, Schiffer G et al: Elastic stable intramedullary nailing of midclavicular fractures with a titanium nail. *Clin Orthop* 408:279-285, 2003.
The authors describe a technique for fixation of displaced midshaft clavicle fractures with flexible titanium nails, leading to healing in 57 of 58 fractures.

70. Neviaser RJ, Neviaser JS, Neviaser TJ: A simple technique for internal fixation of the clavicle. A long term evaluation. *Clin Orthop* 109:103-107, 1975.

71. Ngarmukos C, Parkpian V, Patradul A: Fixation of fractures of the midshaft of the clavicle with Kirschner wires. Results in 108 patients. *J Bone Joint Surg Br* 80:106-108, 1998.

72. Leppilahti J, Jalovaara P: Migration of Kirschner wires following fixation of the clavicle: a report of 2 cases. *Acta Orthop Scand* 70:517-519, 1999.

73. Chan KY, Jupiter JB, Leffert RD, Marti R: Clavicle malunion. *J Shoulder Elbow Surg* 8:287-290, 1999.
The functional status of four patients was improved after corrective osteotomy of a clavicle malunion, realignment, and plate fixation.

74. Kitsis CK, Marino AJ, Krikler SJ, Birch R: Late complications following clavicular fractures and their operative management. *Injury* 34:69-74, 2003.
Seventeen patients were treated surgically following clavicle fracture. Overall, patients had improvement, but some residual symptoms remained.

75. Boehme D, Curtis RJ Jr, DeHaan JT et al: Non-union of fractures of the mid-shaft of the clavicle. Treatment with a modified Hagie intramedullary pin and autogenous bone-grafting. *J Bone Joint Surg Am* 73:1219-1226, 1991.
Twenty of the 21 patients with a clavicle nonunion healed when treated with open reduction internal fixation with a modified Hagie intramedullary pin and bone grafting.

76. Enneking TJ, Hartlief MT, Fontijne WP: Rushpin fixation for midshaft clavicular nonunions: good results in 13/14 cases. *Acta Orthop Scand* 70:514-516, 1999.

77. Manske DJ, Szabo RM: The operative treatment of mid-shaft clavicular non-unions. *J Bone Joint Surg Am* 67:1367-1371, 1985.

78. Ebraheim NA, Xu R, Haman SP et al: Quantitative anatomy of the scapula. *Am J Orthop* 29:287-292, 2000.
The relative thickness of the bone of the glenoid, coracoid, scapular spine, and body was measured and quantified.

79. Boerger TO, Limb D: Suprascapular nerve injury at the spino-glenoid notch after glenoid neck fracture. *J Shoulder Elbow Surg* 9:236-237, 2000.

80. Ebraheim NA, Mekhail AO, Haman SP: Axillary view of the glenoid articular surface. *J Shoulder Elbow Surg* 9:115-119, 2000.
The true scapular lateral view should demonstrate a continuous line of the coracoid and glenoid articular surfaces.

81. Ada JR, Miller ME: Scapular fractures. Analysis of 113 cases. *Clin Orthop* 269:174-180, 1991.
Displaced scapular spine and neck fractures were associated with functional limitations, and operative fixation should be considered.

82. Ideberg R, Grevsten S, Larsson S: Epidemiology of scapular fractures. Incidence and classification of 338 fractures. *Acta Orthop Scand* 66:395-397, 1995.
A 10-year review of scapular and glenoid articular fractures was studied to determine the etiology and incidence. A classification system is proposed.

83. Nordqvist A, Petersson C: Fracture of the body, neck, or spine of the scapula. A long-term follow-up study. *Clin Orthop* 283:139-144, 1992.

Fourteen years after nonoperative treatment for scapula fractures, the majority of patients had satisfactory outcomes, but half with residual deformity had slight or moderate shoulder disability.

84. Goss TP: Fractures of the glenoid cavity. *J Bone Joint Surg Am* 74:299-305, 1992.
An extensive review of intraarticular glenoid fractures and their management. The classification system is further elucidated.

85. Goss TP: The scapula: coracoid, acromial, and avulsion fractures. *Am J Orthop* 25:106-115, 1996.

86. Mayo KA, Benirschke SK, Mast JW: Displaced fractures of the glenoid fossa. Results of open reduction and internal fixation. *Clin Orthop* 347:122-130, 1998.
Good outcomes were obtained following ORIF of displaced glenoid fossa fractures.

87. Goss TP: Double disruptions of the superior shoulder suspensory complex. *J Orthop Trauma* 7:99-106, 1993.
The superior shoulder suspensory complex is described. Surgical reconstruction and stabilization of injuries to this complex is recommended.

88. Bauer G, Fleischmann W, Dussler E: Displaced scapular fractures: indication and long-term results of open reduction and internal fixation. *Arch Orthop Trauma Surg* 114:215-219, 1995.

89. Adam FF: Surgical treatment of displaced fractures of the glenoid cavity. *Int Orthop* 26:150-153, 2002.

90. Aulicino PL, Reinert C, Kornberg M, Williamson S: Displaced intra-articular glenoid fractures treated by open reduction and internal fixation. *J Trauma* 26:1137-1141, 1986.

91. Cameron SE: Arthroscopic reduction and internal fixation of an anterior glenoid fracture. *Arthroscopy* 14:743-746, 1998.
Case report of fixation of an anterior glenoid rim fracture associated with anterior shoulder instability.

92. Carro LP, Nunez MP, Llata JI: Arthroscopic-assisted reduction and percutaneous external fixation of a displaced intra-articular glenoid fracture. *Arthroscopy* 15:211-214, 1999.
The authors describe the principles of arthroscopically assisted fixation of glenoid rim fractures.

93. Hardegger FH, Simpson LA, Weber BG: The operative treatment of scapular fractures. *J Bone Joint Surg Br* 66:725-731, 1984.
The indications for fixation include displaced intraarticular fractures, fractures of the glenoid rim associated with glenohumeral subluxation, and unstable fractures of the scapular neck.

94. Kavanagh BF, Bradway JK, Cofield RH: Open reduction and internal fixation of displaced intra-articular fractures of the glenoid fossa. *J Bone Joint Surg Am* 75:479-484, 1993.
Ten displaced intraarticular glenoid fractures were treated with ORIF. No patients developed arthritic changes, and good outcomes were obtained.

95. Kligman M, Roffman M: Glenoid fracture: conservative treatment versus surgical treatment. *J South Orthop Assoc* 7:1-5, 1998.
Based on a limited experience, the authors recommend nonoperative treatment for most displaced intraarticular fractures of the glenoid.

96. Leung KS, Lam TP, Poon KM: Operative treatment of displaced intra-articular glenoid fractures. *Injury* 24:324-328, 1993.
At an average of almost 2.5 years after operative fixation of displaced glenoid articular fractures, good results were obtained in 14 patients.

97. Schandelmaier P, Blauth M, Schneider C, Krettek C: Fractures of the glenoid treated by operation. A 5- to 23-year follow-up of 22 cases. *J Bone Joint Surg Br* 84:173-177, 2002.
Good results were obtained in patients that did not have a deep infection or an associated brachial plexus palsy. The surgical approach and reduction of displaced glenoid fractures are described in detail.

98. Kligman M, Roffman M: Posterior approach for glenoid fracture. *J Trauma* 42:733-735, 1997.
A posterior surgical approach and reduction maneuvers are described.

99. Ebraheim NA, Mekhail AO, Padanilum TG, Yeasting RA: Anatomic considerations for a modified posterior approach to the scapula. *Clin Orthop* 334:136-143, 1997.
The suprascapular nerve is located an average of 1.4 cm from the glenoid rim. The circumflex scapular artery is an average of 2.8 cm from the inferior glenoid margin.

# CHAPTER 44

# Shoulder Arthritis

Phani K. Dantuluri

MD, Clinical Instructor, Department of Orthopaedic Surgery, Thomas Jefferson University,
Jefferson Medical College, Philadelphia, PA

## Introduction

- Normal shoulder function depends on the humeral head and glenoid smoothly articulating via congruent, well-lubricated joint surfaces. When these surfaces are damaged, this normally congruent relationship deteriorates, leading to pain, stiffness, and loss of function.
- Glenohumeral arthritis of the shoulder is a relatively common condition, although it occurs less frequently than arthritis of the hip and knee.
- In addition to rotator cuff disease, it is one of the most common causes of shoulder pain and functional loss in elderly patients.
- Incidence of osteoarthritis of the shoulder seems to increase with age, with patients typically presenting in the sixth and seventh decades of life.
- Treatment of symptomatic arthritis of the shoulder is nonoperative in the majority of patients. Surgical intervention may become necessary in advanced cases with significant degenerative change and loss of range of motion leading to functional loss.
- The degree of degenerative change, patient age, and functional demands of the patient help determine the most appropriate treatment plan. With the improvement of biomaterials and the modularity of prosthetic replacement, glenohumeral arthroplasty is becoming an increasingly viable option in properly indicated patients.

## Clinical Etiologies of Glenohumeral Arthritis

- A number of different etiologies can lead to arthritic changes of the shoulder joint.

### Primary Degenerative Arthritis

- Primary degenerative arthritis or osteoarthritis typically presents with increased posterior wear of the glenoid cartilage and subchondral bone. Significant central wearing of the humeral head cartilage with a rim of residual cartilage and peripheral osteophytes is seen. Osteophytes are common inferiorly and posteriorly along the glenoid and the anterior, inferior, and posterior aspects of the humeral head, leading to a flattened appearance. Subchondral sclerosis and degenerative cystic changes may be present in the humeral head or glenoid (Figure 44–1). In addition to significant posterior glenoid wear, there often is posterior humeral subluxation and tightness of the anterior capsular structures. Often there is an enlarged inferior capsule with laxity of posterior structures. Loose bodies are often seen in the glenohumeral joint, but rotator cuff pathology is rare.

### Secondary Degenerative Arthritis

- Arthritic changes result from posttraumatic alterations, recurrent instability, prior surgery, or other conditions leading to secondary degenerative changes. Fracture

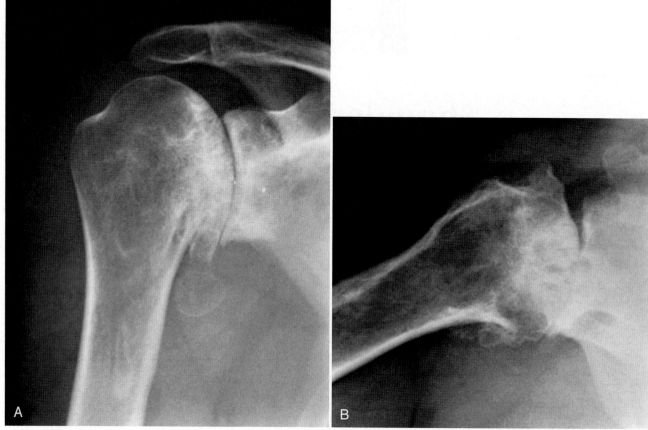

Figure 44–1:
Osteoarthritis of the shoulder. **A,** Stereotypical radiographic, pathoanatomic appearance. The humeral head is somewhat enlarged and flattened. Peripheral osteophytes are particularly prominent inferiorly. There is flattening of the humeral head with subchondral sclerosis, best seen centrally and central-superiorly. Interosseous cysts may be present and are best seen on the axillary projection. **B,** In the axillary view, asymmetric glenoid wear with slightly greater wear of the posterior aspect of the glenoid is seen. This radiographic appearance of the glenoid is typical of that of a biconcave glenoid that, unless otherwise contraindicated, is best treated by implanting a glenoid component. (From Matsen FA, Rockwood CA, Wirth MA, Lippitt SB: Glenohumeral arthritis and its management. In Rockwood CA, Matsen FA, editors: *The shoulder,* ed 2. Philadelphia, 1998, WB Saunders.)

leading to malunion can result in altered joint congruity precipitating significant cartilage erosion (Figure 44–2). Prosthetic arthroplasty in malunion cases show that satisfactory long-term pain relief and function can result in 75% of cases, but with a relatively high complication rate. Dislocation can lead to instability, which also disrupts normal glenohumeral motion, leading to wear. Radiographic patterns in secondary degenerative arthritis are generally similar to primary degenerative arthritis with subchondral sclerosis, osteophytes, and joint space narrowing.

## Inflammatory Arthritis

- Most commonly rheumatoid arthritis. Rheumatoid arthritis typically presents with even cartilage destruction across joint surfaces (Figure 44–3). Glenoid erosion typically is medial and central as opposed to the posterior

erosion seen in osteoarthritis.[1] Significant marginal erosions can be present along the humeral head. Osteopenia is present, and there usually is significant involvement of the soft tissues, including the rotator cuff. Significant soft tissue swelling, weakness, and contractures often are present. Ipsilateral upper extremity rheumatoid involvement of the sternoclavicular and acromioclavicular joints, hand, wrist, and elbow can lead to significant loss of function. Other inflammatory and crystalline arthropathies, such as pigmented villonodular synovitis, gout, and pseudogout, can present similarly.

## Rotator Cuff Tear Arthropathy

- Degenerative changes are the result of a chronic large rotator cuff defect that allows superior migration of the humerus, leading to arthritic change superiorly and erosion of the coracoacromial arch. Glenoid wear

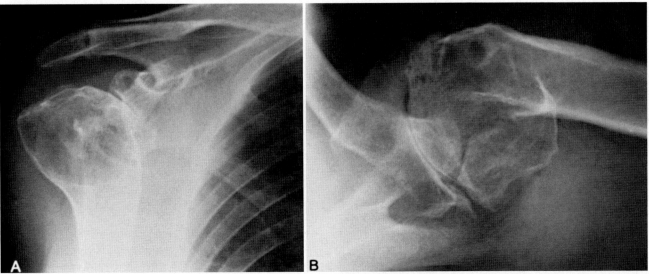

Figure 44–2:
Posttraumatic arthritis with loss of glenohumeral cartilage developed after malunion of a comminuted proximal humeral fracture. **A,** Anthroposterior view, **B,** Axillary view showing apex anterior malunion of the head-neck junction. (From Matsen FA, Rockwood CA, Wirth MA, Lippitt SB: Glenohumeral arthritis and its management. In Rockwood CA, Matsen FA, editors: *The shoulder,* ed 2. Philadelphia, 1998, WB Saunders.)

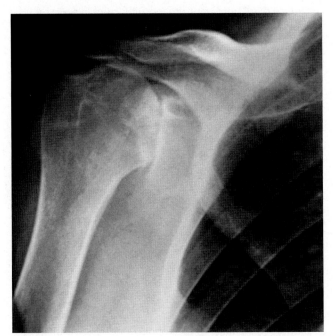

Figure 44–3:
Rheumatoid arthritis of the shoulder. Radiograph shows a slight amount of osteopenia, cartilage loss, mild subchondral bone loss, and superior translation of the humeral head. In this patient, as in many patients with rheumatoid arthritis of the shoulder, the rotator cuff, although not frankly torn, has become attenuated and functionally compromised. (From Matsen FA, Rockwood CA, Wirth MA, Lippitt SB: Glenohumeral arthritis and its management. In Rockwood CA, Matsen FA, editors: *The shoulder,* ed 2. Philadelphia, 1998, WB Saunders.)

typically is superior as well. The resulting superior instability resulting from cuff deficiency makes glenoid replacement a poor option, because lack of glenohumeral stability leads to eccentric loading forces on the glenoid component and early loosening. Radiographic changes are notable for the "femoralization" of the proximal humerus and the "acetabularization" of the coracoacromial arch as the incompetent rotator cuff allows the superior migration of the proximal humerus and this new pathologic articulation (Figure 44–4).[2]

## Capsulorrhaphy Arthropathy

- Capsulorrhaphy arthropathy is a secondary degenerative process caused by prior surgery performed for recurrent instability. It typically is seen in shoulders that underwent prior anterior surgical procedures to tighten the anterior capsule for recurrent dislocations. If overtightening is done, posterior subluxation and posterior wear of the glenohumeral joint can occur. Similarly, excessive posterior capsular tightening can lead to anterior translation, wear, and subsequent degenerative changes. It may also be seen secondary to surgical structural alteration of the glenohumeral joint or to surgical implants left in the joint, such as screws or staples. It is a common cause of glenohumeral arthritis in the younger demographic group.

## Avascular Necrosis

- Avascular necrosis of the humeral head can lead to collapse and irregularity of the humeral head. This irregular humeral head causes wear of the glenoid and

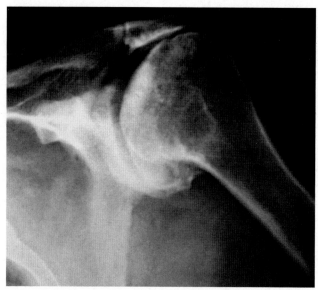

Figure 44–4:

Rotator cuff tear arthropathy. Radiograph depicts cartilage loss, mild but definite bone loss of the humeral head and glenoid, severe superior translation of the humeral head against the acromion with rotator cuff tearing, and some erosion of the abutting acromion. The patient had significant multitissue involvement of the cartilage, bone, capsule, and rotator cuff. (From Matsen FA, Rockwood CA, Wirth MA, Lippitt SB: Glenohumeral arthritis and its management. In Rockwood CA, Matsen FA, editors: *The shoulder,* ed 2. Philadelphia, 1998, WB Saunders.)

leads to secondary degenerative changes. Causes of avascular necrosis are numerous. Steroids, vascular causes, dysbaric conditions, alcoholism, transplantation, Gaucher's disease, radiation, lipid metabolism disorders, cytotoxic drugs, sickle cell disease, and idiopathic etiologies all have been implicated as causal factors.[2] Pathologic changes can be detected in the early stages by magnetic resonance imaging (MRI), but radiographic changes occur later in the process. Relative osteopenia or osteosclerosis and eventual subchondral fracture leading to the classic crescent sign can be seen (Figure 44–5). End-stage changes occur on both sides of the joint and involve the humeral head and the glenoid.

## Additional Causes of Glenohumeral Arthritis

- Septic arthropathy is an uncommon cause of glenohumeral arthritis but should be suspected in patients who are immunosuppressed and who show systemic signs of infection. Destructive changes are secondary to the infectious process, with collagenases and proteases believed to contribute to cartilage destruction. Aspiration, an elevated white blood cell count, and an elevated erythrocyte sedimentation rate all can help confirm the

diagnosis. Neuropathic arthropathy often is associated with syringomyelia, diabetes, or other causes of joint denervation and often can be confused for septic arthritis because of extensive destruction of the glenohumeral joint (Figure 44–6). Neoplasia can be another cause of destructive changes of the glenohumeral joint and may present with night pain or nonmechanical pain. Furthermore, the pain may be unresponsive to rest. Additional imaging studies and biopsy may be necessary to confirm the diagnosis.

## Clinical Presentation

### History

- The history is critically important in making the proper diagnosis when dealing with patients having shoulder pathology. Obtaining the chief complaint, age, extremity dominance, occupation, activities, trauma history, and functional demands are critical in determining the etiology, presentation, and treatment plan in patients with glenohumeral arthritis. Symptoms can vary, depending on the extent of articular involvement, but typically patients present with pain, stiffness, and loss of function that are refractory to rest, nonsteroidal antiinflammatory drugs, and exercise. Important prognostic factors include the presence of systemic disease and the etiology of the degenerative changes.

### Physical Examination

- Careful examination of the deltoid and rotator cuff should be performed because these areas are important factors in surgical decision making.
- A complete neurovascular examination including isometric testing is essential.
- Examination of the ipsilateral wrist, elbow, and hand to evaluate the impact of surgical intervention is beneficial.
- Careful examination of overall body function is crucial. The findings may affect surgical timing because patients may also present with significant lower body involvement. Lower extremity involvement may influence the timing of shoulder surgery because upper extremity weight bearing cannot be considered until 4 to 6 months after arthroplasty.

### Findings on Physical Examination

- Limited joint range of motion. Loss of external rotation and forward flexion is typical of advanced stages. In patients with capsulorrhaphy arthropathy, this loss of external rotation can be severe, and symptoms of instability can still be present.
- Pain can be elicited, depending on the location of arthritic change, by placing the arm in a provocative position.
- Patients who have loose bodies or osteophytes may experience locking or popping during range of motion.
- Crepitus may be felt through passive range of motion of the shoulder.

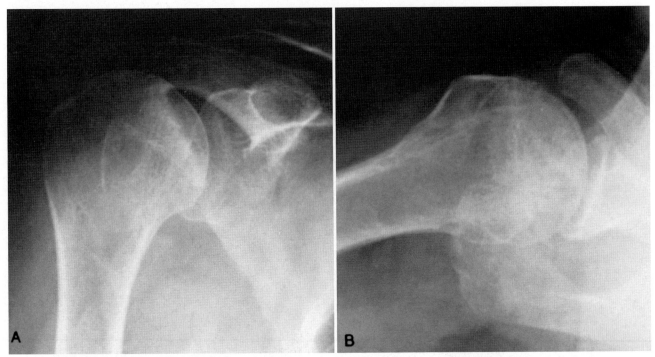

Figure 44–5:
Osteonecrosis of the proximal humerus. There is an osteochondral fracture with minimal distortion of the artic-
ular surface of the humerus, best seen in the anteroposterior view (**A**). In the axillary view (**B**), a crescent sign
in the anterocentral part of the humeral head is seen. (From Matsen FA, Rockwood CA, Wirth MA, Lippitt
SB: Glenohumeral arthritis and its management. In Rockwood CA, Matsen FA, editors: *The shoulder*, ed 2.
Philadelphia, 1998, WB Saunders.)

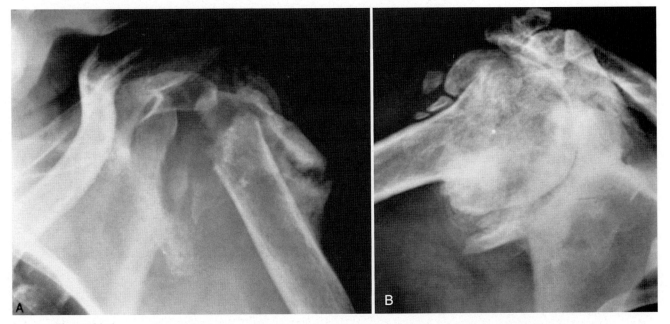

Figure 44–6:
Neuropathic arthritis. Occasionally, neuropathic arthritis can be confused with the more common forms of
glenohumeral arthritis. **A,** Fragmentation of the proximal humerus with bone debris scattered throughout the
joint region. **B,** Bone fragmentation is seen, but this predominantly sclerotic response is associated with neuropathic arthritis. The underlying condition in both of these patients was syringomyelia of the cervical portion of
the spinal cord. (From Matsen FA, Rockwood CA, Wirth MA, Lippitt SB: Glenohumeral arthritis and its management. In Rockwood CA, Matsen FA, editors: *The shoulder*, ed 2. Philadelphia, 1998, WB Saunders.)

- Muscle wasting can be seen around the glenohumeral joint, depending on the severity and duration of involvement.

## Diagnostic Imaging

- Careful assessment of the shoulder via various imaging studies can provide a better understanding of the extent of disease and guide treatment. Many imaging studies are available. Each has its advantages and disadvantages and provides different information.
- As in all surgical interventions, careful preoperative planning can allow a successful result and help prevent

unexpected surprises. Imaging studies can aid in this preoperative planning.

## Radiographic Evaluation

- Radiography is always the starting point for diagnostic evaluation of the glenohumeral joint. Tremendous amounts of information can be determined from careful examination of plain films. Understanding the three-dimensional orientation of the glenohumeral joint is necessary to understand the radiographs and to acquire the appropriate views. Standard views include a scapular anteroposterior (AP) view and a true axillary view (Figure 44–7). These views can allow the examiner to evaluate

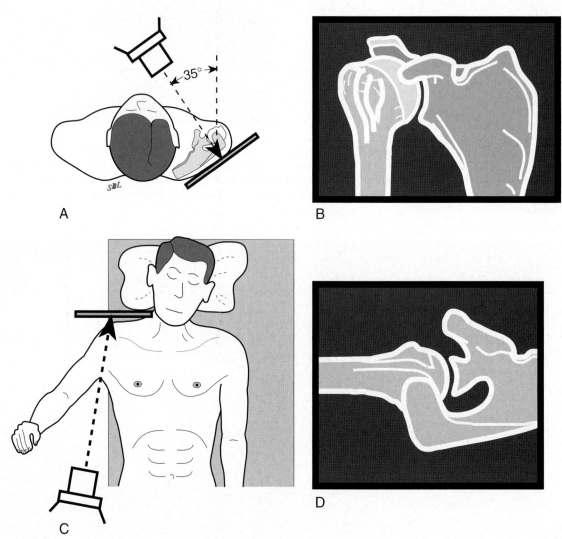

Figure 44–7:

**Radiographic series for a stiff shoulder. A,** The anteroposterior view in the plane of the scapula is obtained by orienting the beam perpendicular to the plane of the scapula and centering it on the coracoid tip while the film is parallel to the plane of the scapula. **B,** The resultant radiograph should clearly reveal the radiographic joint space between the humeral head and the glenoid. **C,** The axillary view is obtained by centering the beam between the coracoid tip and the posterior angle of the acromion. **D,** The resultant radiograph should project the glenoid midway between the coracoid and the acromion, providing a clear view of the joint space. (From Matsen FA, Rockwood CA, Wirth MA, Lippitt SB: Glenohumeral arthritis and its management. In Rockwood CA, Matsen FA, editors: *The shoulder,* ed 2. Philadelphia, 1998, WB Saunders.)

bony architecture, relative cartilage thickness, humeral head position in relation to the glenoid, degree of osteopenia or osteosclerosis, presence and location of osteophytes, and extent of deformity present. Furthermore, internal and external rotation views of the humerus can aid in preoperative arthroplasty planning by allowing a truer understanding of the anatomy of the proximal humerus. Superior displacement of the humeral head on the scapular AP view can be suggestive of rotator cuff deficiency. An AP radiograph taken with the arm in 45 degrees abduction can help demonstrate central humeral head cartilage loss, which may not be apparent on the standard scapular AP view. The glenoid can be well visualized on the axillary view, allowing careful evaluation of posterior erosion, subluxation of the humeral head, and available bone stock for glenoid resurfacing.

## Computed Tomography

- Glenoid morphology and version can be better visualized with the three-dimensional information available through computed tomography (CT). Three-dimensional reconstructions also can provide an excellent idea of bony architecture and help determine reconstructive options. Both shoulders should be included in the scan in order to allow comparison. Preoperative CT scans can help prevent shoulder arthroplasty malposition and subsequent failure because of unrecognized posterior glenoid wear. A CT scan is recommended prior to shoulder arthroplasty if there is significantly decreased external rotation or a history of prior surgery, or if the plain radiographs are suggestive of posterior subluxation of the humeral head or significant posterior glenoid erosion (Figure 44–8).[2] Furthermore, a CT arthrogram can provide additional information on the pathologic joint changes present.

## Magnetic Resonance Imaging

- MRI provides excellent visualization of the soft tissues surrounding the glenohumeral joint, allowing careful evaluation of the rotator cuff and surrounding musculature. MRI also can provide information on labral and capsular pathology, and MRI arthrography may be superior to CT arthrography in assessing labral pathology. Furthermore, in patients in whom osteonecrosis is suspected, early changes may be visualized on MRI before any radiographic changes are apparent. Although MRI can provide excellent visualization of the soft tissues, CT scans may allow better evaluation of the bony architecture and aid in preoperative planning of cases where shoulder arthroplasty is considered.

## Management

### Nonoperative Management

- Treatment of early glenohumeral arthritis should always be nonoperative before surgical intervention is considered.

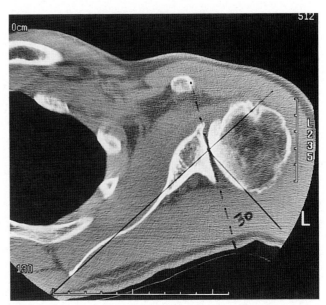

Figure 44–8:
Computed tomography scan of the shoulder reveals the posterior subluxation of the humeral head along with posterior glenoid erosion of 30 degrees. This radiographic appearance of the glenoid is typical of that of a biconcave glenoid that, unless otherwise contraindicated, is best treated by implanting a glenoid component. (From Rockwood CA, Jensen KL: X-ray evaluation of shoulder problems. In Rockwood CA, Matsen FA, editors: *The shoulder,* ed 2. Philadelphia, 1998, WB Saunders.)

### Physical Therapy and Range of Motion Exercises

- A proper physical therapy and rehabilitation protocol can be greatly beneficial in improving range of motion and strength. Passive and active ranges of motion exercises are important in increasing the flexibility and pliability of the soft tissues around the shoulder in order to improve function. Furthermore, scapulothoracic strengthening may improve the biomechanics of the shoulder joint complex. Strengthening the muscles around the shoulder girdle, including the rotator cuff and deltoid, can lead to significant functional gains and allow improvements in the activities of daily living while decreasing concomitant pain from possible coexisting rotator cuff pathology.

### Nonsteroidal Antiinflammatory Drugs

- Nonsteroidal medications can be effective because of their analgesic and antiinflammatory effects. Care must be taken to take a safe, effective NSAID based on one's general medical condition and comorbidities.

### Pain Medications

- Pain medications should be used judiciously and only on a short-term basis if necessary because of the great potential for abuse.

## Steroid Injections

- Steroid injections have been beneficial in relieving symptoms of the arthritic glenohumeral joint, particularly in patients with an inflammatory component to their arthritis. However, care should be taken when administering steroid injections to diabetic or immunocompromised patients. Repeat steroid injections may cause additional damage to the soft tissues within and around the glenohumeral joint.

# General Surgical Indications

- Surgery should be considered only after nonoperative management has failed. Patients must be made fully aware of the risks, complications, limitations, and expectations of the proposed surgical procedure. Patient selection is one the most important determinants to achieving a successful surgical outcome. The patient's age, comorbidities, and functional demands also dictate surgical options. Surgical options include synovectomy, arthroscopic debridement, capsular release, resection arthroplasty, interpositional arthroplasty, arthrodesis, corrective osteotomies, and prosthetic arthroplasty.

## Synovectomy

- Synovectomy is most often indicated in patients with inflammatory arthropathies, including rheumatoid arthritis, with intact articular surfaces. Patients with severe synovitis and significant soft tissue swelling that is unresponsive to nonoperative treatment may be candidates for synovectomy. Synovectomy can be performed either arthroscopically or via an open approach, but in both cases great care must be taken to avoid iatrogenic nerve injury because abundant inflamed synovium and soft tissues can alter the normal anatomy.

## Arthroscopic Debridement

- Arthritis of the glenohumeral joint may include a degenerative labrum, loose bodies, articular defects, and osteophytes. Arthroscopic debridement may be a reasonable treatment in patients after nonoperative methods have been unsuccessful and when prosthetic arthroplasty is not desired.[3] However, this procedure is best indicated when severe arthritic change has not occurred, as little benefit is seen in patients with advanced disease. Long-term studies are needed to clearly evaluate this treatment option. Capsular release often is performed as part of the procedure, and should also be considered in patients with early capsulorrhaphy arthropathy. It can be performed either open or arthroscopically.

## Resection Arthroplasty

- Resection arthroplasty is indicated primarily as a salvage procedure. It can be useful in septic arthropathy with significant involvement of the humeral head and glenoid. It also is used in the setting of an infected prosthetic arthroplasty or component failure. Typically postoperative instability is seen initially, but stiffness usually develops over time. Weakness often is present because of the lack of bony stability and mechanical advantage. Pain relief can be variable.

## Arthrodesis

- Indications for arthrodesis have become rare. It can be used in patients with strenuous physical demands, such as heavy manual laborers who are not candidates for prosthetic arthroplasty. It also is a treatment option for patients with multiple failed surgeries. Other indications include patients with septic arthritis, loss of deltoid and rotator cuff function, and refractory instability.

## Interpositional Arthroplasty

- Interpositional arthroplasty has relatively few indications but can be an option in younger patients with severe rheumatoid arthritis. Interposition has been performed in a variety of ways using local capsular tissue, fascia lata autograft, Achilles tendon allograft, and lateral meniscal allograft. Results are less favorable than prosthetic arthroplasty and can be highly variable. However, the combination of biologic resurfacing of the glenoid and hemiarthroplasty of the shoulder is a viable option in younger patients.

## Corrective Osteotomies

- Opening wedge osteotomies of the glenoid have been used in patients with fixed posterior subluxation of the humeral head and posterior glenoid wear, but the technique is reserved for selected cases. Varus/valgus and derotational osteotomies of the humerus can rarely be considered in posttraumatic deformity, but indications are limited and corrective osteotomy should be performed before significant arthritic changes occur.

## Prosthetic Arthroplasty

- Main indications for prosthetic arthroplasty of the glenohumeral joint are pain, severe loss of function, and end-stage arthritic change of the joint refractory to conservative measures. The different causes leading to end-stage disease influence surgical management and present unique considerations that must be addressed. Common contraindications to prosthetic arthroplasty include the presence of infection, deltoid and rotator cuff insufficiency, neuropathic arthropathy, and intractable instability. Relative contraindications may include patients who are younger, patients with inadequate bone stock for glenoid replacement, and patients with rotator cuff defects that cannot be repaired.

# Unique Disease Considerations in Prosthetic Arthroplasty

## Osteoarthritis

- Prosthetic replacement has led to consistently good results in most reports.[4-6] Prospective long-term studies of total shoulder arthroplasty have shown good survivorships at 10 to 15 years and have shown that total shoulder arthroplasty has yielded better results than hemiarthroplasty alone.[7] Hemiarthroplasty can be considered without glenoid resurfacing if the articular surface of the glenoid is preserved, but the glenoid often will need to be resurfaced at a later date if glenoid wear continues. Hemiarthroplasty also is preferred in cases of avascular necrosis or proximal humeral fracture, or in revisions with poor glenoid bone stock. Hemiarthroplasty in combination with an interpositional allograft, such as the lateral meniscal allograft, may be a reasonable option in younger patients. Hemiarthroplasty is contraindicated in cases where posterior humeral subluxation and subsequent posterior wear have resulted in formation of a biconcave glenoid.[5] Long-term posterior subluxation of the humeral head may lead to posterior capsular laxity, which may require plication in some cases. Rotator cuff pathology is relatively uncommon in osteoarthritis patients compared to rheumatoid patients.

## Rheumatoid Arthritis

- Rotator cuff pathology and more soft tissue involvement is common in patients with rheumatoid arthritis. Functional improvement after arthroplasty may be less predictable. Most reports show better outcomes with total shoulder arthroplasty, provided good soft tissues and viable rotator cuff function are present.[1] Careful examination of an AP radiograph demonstrating the lack of superior humeral head migration may indicate a balanced rotator cuff force couple, suggesting that a glenoid component may be placed. However, as glenoid erosion is central and more osteopenia is present, inadequate bone stock may preclude glenoid fixation, and a hemiarthroplasty may be indicated. A deficient or irreparable rotator cuff is another indication for a hemiarthroplasty.

## Rotator Cuff Arthropathy

- In rotator cuff arthropathy where the rotator cuff is not functional, glenoid resurfacing is generally not indicated because the lack of a functioning rotator cuff leads to

eccentric loading on the glenoid component and early component loosening. Hemiarthroplasty often is the treatment of choice with a prosthetic head roughly the same size as the native humeral head. Use of a humeral head prosthesis that is too large may overstuff the joint and lead to pain, decreased range of motion, and early failure. Preserving the integrity of the coracoacromial arch is crucial in these patients to prevent anterosuperior instability, as patients who previously underwent subacromial decompression with coracoacromial ligament compromise have demonstrated significant anterosuperior instability with subsequent loss of active elevation. Some surgeons have considered further retroverting the humeral head in cases involving loss of integrity of the coracoacromial arch. New directions in dealing with patients with rotator cuff arthropathy are on the horizon. A newly developed reverse ball and socket prosthesis, which effectively reverses the ball and socket in the shoulder joint (Figure 44–9), uses the deltoid to achieve active elevation. This prosthesis has just received US Food

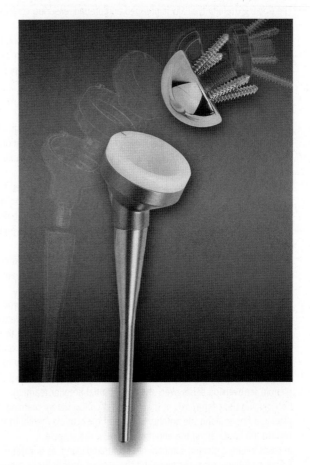

Figure 44–9:
This newly developed prosthesis reverses the ball and socket locations, allowing for stability of the implant without relying on the rotator cuff. This prosthesis may be a treatment option for patients with rotator cuff arthropathy.

and Drug Administration approval, and further studies are needed before widespread use is considered.

## Capsulorrhaphy Arthropathy

- Several factors are relevant in these patients, including the younger age demographic, soft tissue contractures, and potential bony deficiencies. A long-term study reviewing the results of arthroplasty in this patient group demonstrated that arthroplasty provides pain relief and improved motion but is associated with higher rates of revision surgery and unsatisfactory results because of component failure, instability, and pain caused by arthritic change of the glenoid.[8]

## Proximal Humeral Malunions

- A study evaluating patients who had undergone arthroplasty after they developed posttraumatic arthritic change secondary to malunion demonstrated satisfactory pain relief and function in 75% of cases, but with a high rate of complications.[9] Patients who were treated operatively at the time of initial injury and patients who had tuberosity osteotomy at the time of arthroplasty were at risk for a poor result.

## Prosthetic Arthroplasty

(Box 44–1, and Figures 44–10 through 44–24).

---

**Box 44–1    Surgical Pearls for Prosthetic Arthroplasty**

- I prefer to place the patient in a modified beach chair position with the head of table flexed approximately 20 to 30 degrees and a small folded towel placed under the scapula.
- The upper extremity typically is prepped and draped, ensuring complete access to the entire shoulder girdle region and allowing full passive range of motion of the shoulder.
- A number of surgical approaches have been described, but the long anterior deltopectoral approach is the most commonly used.
- When exposing the glenohumeral joint, the superior portion of the pectoralis major tendon insertion can be released to improve exposure. Superiorly, a portion of the coracoacromial ligament can be released, but the structural integrity of the ligament should be maintained because it may become important in preventing anterosuperior instability.
- Measuring preoperative external rotation allows determination of whether effective lengthening of the subscapularis is necessary to increase postoperative external rotation.
- A 360-degree release of all adhesions around the subscapularis should be performed after release from the humerus to provide more external rotation and prevent postoperative scarring and loss of range of motion.
- Great care must be taken when removing the humeral head articular surface to ensure the humeral cut is at the correct angle and to avoid injuring the posterior rotator cuff.
- The correct starting point for humeral reaming must be determined to avoid humeral component malposition. Varus malalignment of the humeral prosthesis may lead to overstuffing of the joint, which can result in pain, loss of motion, and early failure.
- Pay close attention to determining the correct amount of version before broaching the humeral canal.
- Leave the humeral broach in place when exposing the glenoid to prevent iatrogenic injury or fracture to the proximal humerus from vigorous retraction.
- Be aware of posterior glenoid wear and determine if preferential anterior reaming can correct this deformity or if posterior bone grafting is necessary. Typically, approximately 1 cm of preferential anterior reaming can be performed to correct the glenoid version to neutral, but this step depends on the amount of glenoid bone stock available.
- Posterior bone grafting should rarely be performed because this procedure can be technically demanding and is associated with higher complication rates. Many advocate accepting almost 15 degrees retroversion of the glenoid after anterior reaming rather than performing posterior bone grafting. If the retroversion of the glenoid appears to be greater than 15 degrees after reaming, posterior bone grafting may be necessary. Some commonly used bone graft choices include bone grafts fashioned from the resected humeral head or grafts taken from the iliac crest. My preference is tricortical iliac crest bone grafts with screw fixation. Some have advocated using less retroversion of the humeral component to address this problem, but my preference is to correct the retroversion of the glenoid with bone grafting if greater than 15 degrees glenoid retroversion exists even after preferential anterior reaming.
- Determining the central axis of the glenoid is critical before reaming the glenoid to avoid component malposition. This can be accomplished by placing a finger along the anterior surface of the scapula medial to the glenoid and then reaming the glenoid with the tip of the reamer aimed toward the finger along the anterior surface of the scapula.
- In cases where a glenoid component is contraindicated, as in rotator cuff arthropathy or rheumatoid arthritis with an irreparable rotator cuff tear, I do not routinely ream the glenoid if the glenoid surface is not too irregular and relatively congruent. If the surface is too irregular, I do a very gentle ream to provide a smooth congruent surface for the humeral head to articulate with.
- Do not overstuff the joint with components that are too large, as doing so can lead to pain, decreased motion, and early component loosening.
- Above all, realize that total shoulder arthroplasty is an operation where proper balancing of the soft tissues is critically important, as the components are not as constrained as in total hip and total knee arthroplasties.

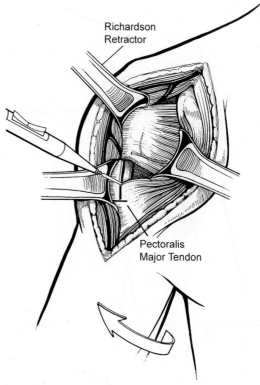

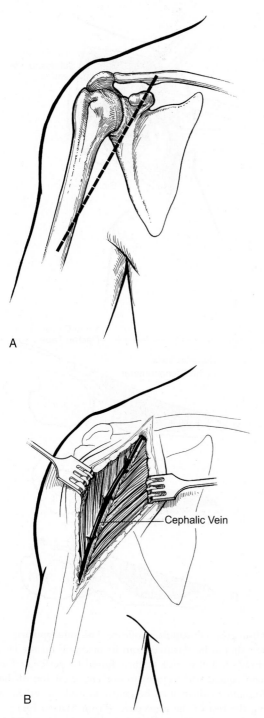

**Figure 44–11:**
Subscapularis exposure. The deltoid and pectoralis major tendons are retracted, and the upper portion of the pectoralis major tendon can be released to aid exposure. Care should be taken not to injure the underlying long head of the biceps tendon if it is to be preserved. (From Matsen FA, Rockwood CA, Wirth MA, Lippitt SB: Glenohumeral arthritis and its management. In Rockwood CA, Matsen FA, editors: *The shoulder,* ed 2. Philadelphia, 1998, WB Saunders.)

## Complications of Arthroplasty

- Two series have examined the long-term outcome and results of shoulder arthroplasty and noted the complications associated with glenohumeral arthroplasty.[10]
- Common complications include glenoid component wear and loosening, glenohumeral instability, intraoperative humeral fractures, neurologic injury, rotator cuff tears, infection, humeral component subsidence or loosening, and deltoid dysfunction.

## Rehabilitation after Prosthetic Arthroplasty

- Intraoperative range of motion should be recorded after implant fixation and subscapularis repair to help guide postoperative protocols.

**Figure 44–10:**
Deltopectoral incision. **A,** Placement of the surgical incision from the clavicle across the top of the coracoid down to the anterior aspect of the arm. **B,** The cephalic vein should be preserved. Although most surgeons prefer to take it medially to prevent iatrogenic trauma to the vein during the procedure, taking it either medially or laterally is acceptable. (From Matsen FA, Rockwood CA, Wirth MA, Lippitt SB: Glenohumeral arthritis and its management. In Rockwood CA, Matsen FA, editors: *The shoulder,* ed 2. Philadelphia, 1998, WB Saunders.)

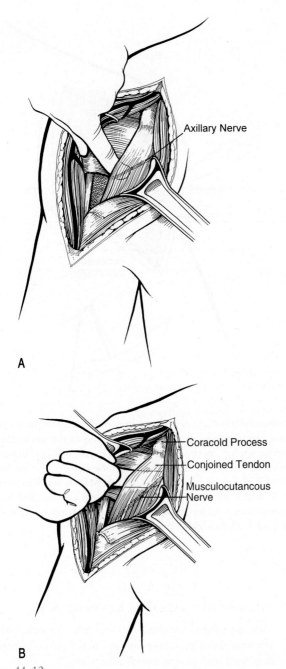

**A**

**B**

**Figure 44–12:**

**A,** Identification and protection of axillary and **B,** musculocutaneous nerves. (From Matsen FA, Rockwood CA, Wirth MA, Lippitt SB: Glenohumeral arthritis and its management. In Rockwood CA, Matsen FA, editors: *The shoulder,* ed 2. Philadelphia, 1998, WB Saunders.)

- Typically, pendulum and passive range of motion exercises are started on postoperative day 1. Limits on range of motion depend on intraoperative measurements and the quality of soft tissue repairs. External rotation limits are noted in the operating room.
- Two weeks postoperatively, additional assisted range of motion exercises and isometric strengthening can be added.

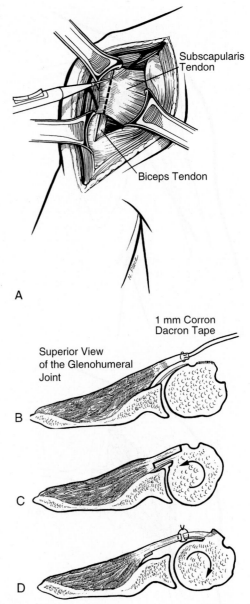

**A**

**B**

**C**

**D**

**Figure 44–13:**

A 360-degree subscapularis release. The subscapularis tendon should be released from its insertion on the lesser tuberosity. A 360-degree release should be performed and the end tagged with sutures to prevent retraction of the tendon and to allow it to be gently moved out of the way during the rest of the procedure. (From Matsen FA, Rockwood CA, Wirth MA, Lippitt SB: Glenohumeral arthritis and its management. In Rockwood CA, Matsen FA, editors: *The shoulder,* ed 2. Philadelphia, 1998, WB Saunders.)

- Six weeks postoperatively, assisted motion in all planes is started, and light resistive exercises can be added in all planes.
- Twelve weeks postoperatively, more resistance and stretching are added. Final outcomes typically are seen 6 to 8 months after surgery.

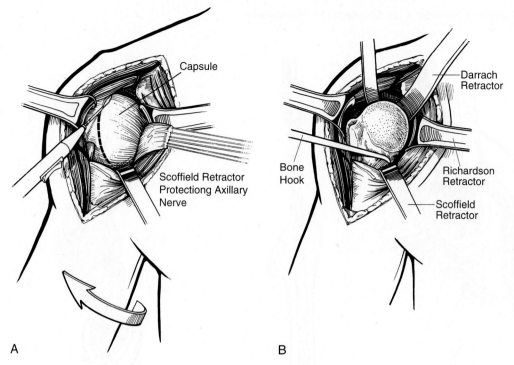

Figure 44–14:

Humeral head exposure. **A,** The capsule should be released from the neck of the humerus from top to bottom. Failure to release the capsule all the way inferiorly leads to difficulty in displacing the head of the humerus up and out of the glenoid fossa. **B,** With Darrach retractors in the shoulder as a skid, a bone hook can be used to gently lift the head of the humerus out of the glenoid fossa while the arm is externally rotated and extended off the edge of the table. (From Matsen FA, Rockwood CA, Wirth MA, Lippitt SB: Glenohumeral arthritis and its management. In Rockwood CA, Matsen FA, editors: *The shoulder,* ed 2. Philadelphia, 1998, WB Saunders.)

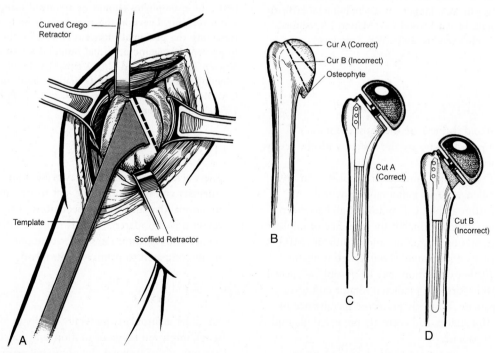

Figure 44–15:

Humeral head resection. **A,** The template should be used to determine the proper angle of humeral head resection. **B–D,** Failure to use the template when removing the head may lead to insufficient bony support for the neck of the prosthesis. (From Matsen FA, Rockwood CA, Wirth MA, Lippitt SB: Glenohumeral arthritis and its management. In Rockwood CA, Matsen FA, editors: *The shoulder,* ed 2. Philadelphia, 1998, WB Saunders.)

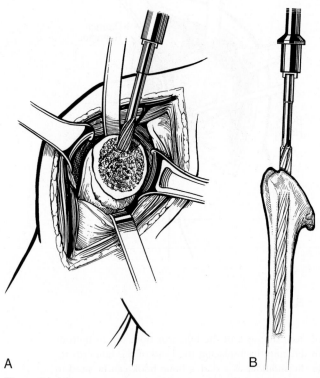

A    B

**Figure 44–16:**
Proximal humeral preparation. **A,** Place the intramedullary reamers as far laterally and superiorly as possible into the proximal humerus to allow proper component positioning. **B,** Progressive reamers are used until the reamer begins to obtain purchase in the cortical bone. (From Matsen FA, Rockwood CA, Wirth MA, Lippitt SB: Glenohumeral arthritis and its management. In Rockwood CA, Matsen FA, editors: *The shoulder,* ed 2. Philadelphia, 1998, WB Saunders.)

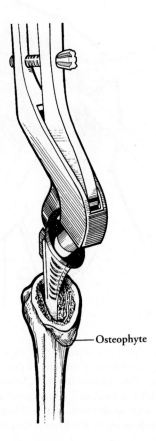

—Osteophyte

**Figure 44–17:**
Proximal humeral broaching and osteophyte removal. After insertion of the driver extractor tool into the trial broach body, the osteophytes should be removed using an osteome and a rongeur. Leave in the trial broach body while retracting the proximal humerus to expose the glenoid to prevent iatrogenic proximal humeral fracture. (From Matsen FA, Rockwood CA, Wirth MA, Lippitt SB: Glenohumeral arthritis and its management. In Rockwood CA, Matsen FA, editors: *The shoulder,* ed 2. Philadelphia, 1998, WB Saunders.)

## Failed Shoulder Arthroplasty

- Shoulder pain and stiffness are the most common complaints of patients who are dissatisfied with the results of shoulder arthroplasty.[11]
- Evaluation of the painful shoulder arthroplasty can be a diagnostic challenge. Serial radiographs, physical examination, arthrography, CT, and MRI all have been used to provide information, but the presence of implants can make interpreting diagnostic studies difficult. MRI studies in patients with painful shoulder arthroplasties showed that further evaluation may be possible, as special technique MRIs correctly predicted rotator cuff tears in 10 of 11 patients, correctly predicted the absence of tears in 8 of 10 patients, and correctly predicted glenoid wear in 8 of 9 patients.[12]
- Diagnostic arthroscopy can be considered in patients in whom no cause is found with less invasive investigations.
- Revision shoulder arthroplasty can be considered in selected patients with failed shoulder arthroplasty. An

assessment must be made of available bone stock, the integrity and function of the soft tissues, and the functional demands and expectations of the patient before revision is considered. Patients must be advised of the higher complication rates and worse outcomes that can result compared to primary arthroplasty.

## Conclusions

- Shoulder arthroplasty generally results in excellent pain relief, improved range of motion, and functional gains in patients with advanced glenohumeral arthritis.
- Nonoperative modalities, including rest, physical therapy, activity modification, medications, and careful use of steroid injections, should be considered before surgical intervention is contemplated.

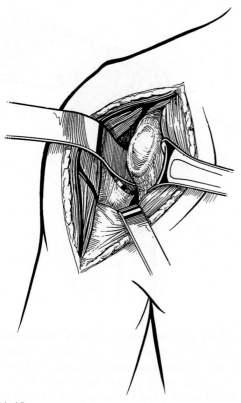

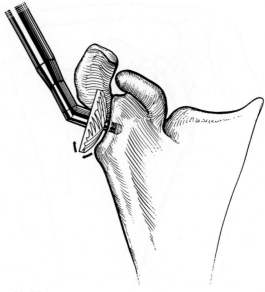

Figure 44–20:

Glenoid preparation. The hub of the glenoid reamer can be placed into the central hole. Reaming of the glenoid should be performed until the glenoid fossa is perfectly smooth and matches the back surface of the glenoid component. (From Matsen FA, Rockwood CA, Wirth MA, Lippitt SB: Glenohumeral arthritis and its management. In Rockwood CA, Matsen FA, editors: *The shoulder,* ed 2. Philadelphia, 1998, WB Saunders.)

Figure 44–18:

Glenoid exposure. When resurfacing the glenoid fossa and placing a glenoid component, various types of humeral head retractors can be gently used to expose the glenoid fossa. (From Matsen FA, Rockwood CA, Wirth MA, Lippitt SB: Glenohumeral arthritis and its management. In Rockwood CA, Matsen FA, editors: *The shoulder,* ed 2. Philadelphia, 1998, WB Saunders.)

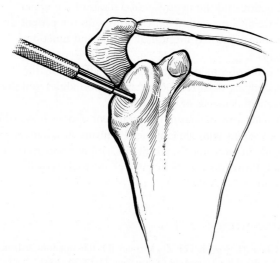

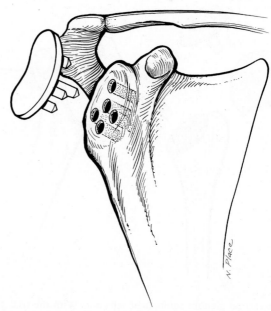

Figure 44–19:

Location of the glenoid center. After the center of the glenoid fossa is located, a central hole is placed in the glenoid fossa using a punch or an air burr. (From Matsen FA, Rockwood CA, Wirth MA, Lippitt SB: Glenohumeral arthritis and its management. In Rockwood CA, Matsen FA, editors: *The shoulder,* ed 2. Philadelphia, 1998, WB Saunders.)

Figures 44–21:

Glenoid component placement. A trial pegged glenoid component is placed into position. (From Matsen FA, Rockwood CA, Wirth MA, Lippitt SB: Glenohumeral arthritis and its management. In Rockwood CA, Matsen FA, editors: *The shoulder,* ed 2. Philadelphia, 1998, WB Saunders.)

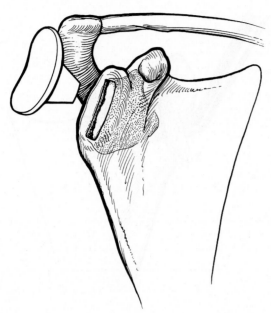

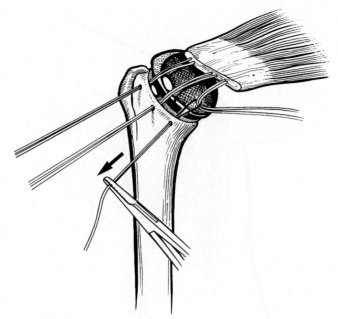

Figures 44–22:
Glenoid component placement. If a keeled glenoid component is being placed, an air burr is used to create a slot in the glenoid fossa. After the glenoid fossa has been reamed, a trial keeled component is placed into position. (From Matsen FA, Rockwood CA, Wirth MA, Lippitt SB: Glenohumeral arthritis and its management. In Rockwood CA, Matsen FA, editors: *The shoulder*, ed 2. Philadelphia, 1998, WB Saunders.)

Figure 44–24:
Subscapularis reattachment. After the final humeral and glenoid components are in place, the subscapularis tendon is reattached to the humerus using sutures through drill holes. (From Matsen FA, Rockwood CA, Wirth MA, Lippitt SB: Glenohumeral arthritis and its management. In Rockwood CA, Matsen FA, editors: *The shoulder*, ed 2. Philadelphia, 1998, WB Saunders.)

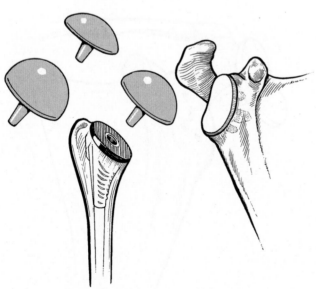

Figure 44–23:
Humeral and glenoid component selection. With the trial glenoid component and humeral broach body in place, the appropriate-size humeral head that will balance the soft tissues is selected. (From Matsen FA, Rockwood CA, Wirth MA, Lippitt SB: Glenohumeral arthritis and its management. In Rockwood CA, Matsen FA, editors: *The shoulder*, ed 2. Philadelphia, 1998, WB Saunders.)

- Careful preoperative planning is crucial prior to any surgical procedure. Evaluation of rotator cuff and deltoid function and the neurovascular status of the upper extremity are critical. Discussions with the patient must include expected surgical outcomes and functional gains.
- Results of shoulder arthroplasty are affected by the underlying disease, concomitant comorbidities, and the age and demands of the patient.
- A wide armamentarium of treatment options is available for patients with glenohumeral arthritis. As advances are made in biomaterials, prosthetics, and our understanding of arthritic disease, the science of arthroplasty will continue to evolve.

## References

1. Chen AL, Joseph TN, Zuckerman JD: Rheumatoid arthritis of the shoulder. *J Am Acad Orthop Surg* 11:12-24, 2003.
   Thorough review article on the manifestations of rheumatoid arthritis in the shoulder.

2. Rockwood CA, Matsen FA: *The shoulder*, ed 2. Philadelphia, 1998, WB Saunders.
   Comprehensive and thoughtful chapter on glenohumeral arthroplasty is presented in this superb resource.

3. Weinstein DM, Bucchieri JS, Pollock RG et al: Arthroscopic debridement of the shoulder for osteoarthritis. *Arthroscopy* 16:471-476, 2000.
   Reported good to excellent in 80% of 25 patients following arthroscopic debridement for early glenohumeral arthritis at mean 34-month follow-up.

4. Norris TR, Iannotti JP: Functional outcome after shoulder arthroplasty for primary osteoarthritis: a multicenter study. *J Shoulder Elbow Surg* 11:130-135, 2002.
   Reported greater than 90% of 176 shoulders with primary osteoarthritis had excellent pain relief, satisfaction, and functional gains following both hemiarthroplasty and total shoulder arthroplasty.

5. Iannotti JP, Norris TR: Influence of preoperative factors on outcome of shoulder arthroplasty for glenohumeral osteoarthritis. *J Bone Joint Surg* 85A:251-258, 2003.
   Patients with less than 10 degrees of preoperative passive external rotation had significantly less postoperative external rotation, a repairable rotator cuff tear was not a contraindication to glenoid replacement, patients with glenoid erosion should have a glenoid component placed, and humeral head subluxation preoperatively was associated with a poor result regardless of whether hemiarthroplasty or total shoulder arthroplasty was performed.

6. Godeneche A, Boileau P, Favard L et al: Prosthetic replacement in the treatment of osteoarthritis of the shoulder: early results of 268 cases. *J Shoulder Elbow Surg* 11:11-18, 2002.
   At mean 30-month follow-up, good or excellent results were seen in 77% of patients. Mean active forward elevation was 145 degrees.

7. Edwards TB, Kadakia NR, Boulahia A et al: A comparison of hemiarthroplasty and total shoulder arthroplasty in the treatment of primary glenohumeral osteoarthritis: results of a multicenter study. *J Shoulder Elbow Surg* 12:207-213, 2003.
   Largest series comparing hemiarthroplasty and total shoulder arthroplasty (TSA) in patients with primary osteoarthritis, with a mean follow-up of 43.3 months. TSA provided better scores for pain, mobility, and activity.

8. Sperling JW, Antuna SA, Sanchez-Sotelo J et al: Shoulder arthroplasty for arthritis after instability surgery. *J Bone Joint Surg* 84A:1775-1781, 2002.
   Shoulder arthroplasty for arthritis following instability surgery in a relatively young patient group provided improved motion and significant pain relief but was associated with high rates of revision surgery and unsatisfactory results.

9. Antuna SA, Sperling JW, Sanchez-Sotelo J, Cofield RH: Shoulder arthroplasty for proximal humeral malunions: long-term results. *J Shoulder Elbow Surg* 11:122-129, 2002.
   Proximal humeral malunions treated with shoulder arthroplasty had satisfactory pain relief and good function in 75% at a mean of 50 months, but with a high rate of complications.

10. Hasan SS, Leith JM, Campbell B et al: Characteristics of unsatisfactory shoulder arthroplasties. *J Shoulder Elbow Surg* 11:431-441, 2002.
    Shoulder pain and stiffness were the most common complaints, but instability, rotator cuff tears, and glenoid erosions in shoulders with a hemiarthroplasty and glenoid polyethylene wear and loosening in patients with total shoulder arthroplasty were commonly seen.

11. Boileau P, Avidor C, Krishnan SG et al: Cemented polyethylene versus uncemented metal-backed glenoid components in total shoulder arthroplasty: a prospective, double-blind, randomized study. *J Shoulder Elbow Surg* 11:351-359, 2002.
    Periprosthetic radiolucent lines were seen more frequently with cemented polyethylene components but did not correlate with functional results. Loosening occurred in 20% of metal-backed glenoids and correlated with poor results. The authors subsequently abandoned metal-backed glenoid implantation.

12. Sperling JW, Potter HG, Craig EV et al: Magnetic resonance imaging of painful shoulder arthroplasty. *J Shoulder Elbow Surg* 11:315-321, 2002.
    New developments in MRI techniques were used in patients with painful shoulder arthroplasty. MRI correctly predicted rotator cuff tears in 10 of 11 patients, correctly predicted the absence of tears in 8 of 10 patients, and correctly predicted glenoid wear in 8 of 9 patients.

# Index

Page numbers followed by "f" denotes figures; "b" denotes boxes; and "t" denotes tables.